Fishman's

MANUAL of
PULMONARY
DISEASES and
DISORDERS

W9-CUI-947

Fishman's
MANUAL of PULMONARY DISEASES and DISORDERS

Third Edition

Alfred P. Fishman
Jack A. Elias
Jay A. Fishman
Michael A. Grippi
Larry R. Kaiser
Robert M. Senior

McGRAW-HILL
Medical Publishing Division

New York Chicago San Francisco Lisbon London Madrid Mexico City Milan New Delhi San Juan Seoul Singapore Sydney Toronto

McGraw-Hill

A Division of The McGraw·Hill Companies

Notice

Medicine is an ever-changing science. As new research and clinical experience broaden our knowledge, changes in treatment and drug therapy are required. The editors and the publisher of this work have checked with sources believed to be reliable in their efforts to provide information that is complete and generally in accord with the standards accepted at the time of publication. However, in view of the possibility of human error or changes in medical sciences, neither the editors nor the publisher nor any other party who has been involved in the preparation or publication of this work warrants that the information contained herein is in every respect accurate or complete, and they disclaim all responsibility for any errors or omissions or for the results obtained from use of the information contained in this work. Readers are encouraged to confirm the information contained herein with other sources. For example and in particular, readers are advised to check the product information sheet included in the package of each drug they plan to administer to be certain that the information contained in this work is accurate and that changes have not been made in the recommended dose or in the contraindications for administration. This recommendation is of particular importance in connection with new or infrequently used drugs.

Contents

v

Contributors

Lisa M. Bellini, M.D. Vice Chair for Education, Department of Medicine, Hospital of the University of Pennsylvania, Philadelphia, Pennsylvania, Chapters 2, 12–14, 21–23, 72–74, 76, 78

Murali Chakinala, M.D. Pulmonary and Critical Care Unit, Department of Internal Medicine, Washington University School of Medicine, St. Louis, Missouri, Chapter 41

Jack A. Elias, M.D. Professor and Chief, Pulmonary and Critical Care Medicine, Department of Internal Medicine, Yale University School of Medicine, New Haven, Connecticut, Chapters 9, 10, 24, 34–36

Alan M. Fein, M.D. Critical Care Medicine, North Shore University Hospital, Manhasset, New York, Chapter 54

Alfred P. Fishman, M.D. Senior Associate Dean for Program Development, William Maul Measey Professor Emeritus of Medicine, University of Pennsylvania School of Medicine, Philadelphia, Pennsylvania, Chapters 1, 6, 8, 39, 40

Jay A. Fishman, M.D. Associate Professor of Medicine, Harvard Medical School, Director, Transplant Infectious Disease Program, Boston, Massachusetts, Chapters 58–67

Michael A. Grippi, M.D. Chief of Medicine, Veterans Administration Hospital, Philadelphia, Pennsylvania, Chapters 2, 5, 11–14, 21–23, 68–71, 74, 75, 77–79

Bruce E. Johnson, M.D. Dana-Farber Cancer Center, Lowe Center for Thoracic Oncology, Boston, Massachusetts, Chapter 57

Larry R. Kaiser, M.D. The John Rhea Barton Professor and Chairman, Department of Surgery, University of Pennsylvania School of Medicine, Philadelphia, Pennsylvania, Chapters 47, 51–57

Steven M. Keller, M.D. Chief, Division of Thoracic Surgery, Director, David B. Kriser Lung Cancer Center, Department of Surgery, New York, New York, Chapter 56

C. Glen Mayhall, M.D. Division of Infectious Diseases, Department of Internal Medicine, University of Texas Med Branch at Galveston, Galveston, Texas, Chapter 61

Wallace T. Miller, Jr., M.D. Department of Radiology, Thomas Jefferson University Hospital, Philadelphia, Pennsylvania, Chapter 3

Reynold A. Panettieri, Jr., M.D. Associate Professor, Pulmonary Allergy and Critical Care Division, University of Pennsylvania Medical Center, Philadelphia, Pennsylvania, Chapters 6, 8

Joe B. Putnam, Jr., M.D. Associate Professor of Surgery, Thoracic and Cardiovascular Surgery, University of Texas, M.D. Anderson Cancer Center, Houston, Texas, Chapter 47

Daniel B. Rosenbluth, M.D. Pulmonary and Critical Care Division, Washington University School of Medicine, St. Louis, Missouri, Chapters 37, 38, 42–46

William A. Rutala, Ph.D. M.P.H. Professor of Medicine, Division of Infectious Diseases, University of North Carolina at Chapel Hill, Chapel Hill, North Carolina, Chapter 61

Daniel P. Schuster, M.D. Associate Professor of Medicine and Radiology, Pulmonary and Critical Care Division, Department of Internal Medicine, Washington University School of Medicine, St. Louis, Missouri, Chapter 41

Richard J. Schwab, M.D. Assistant Professor of Medicine, Pulmonary, Allergy and Critical Care Division, University of Pennsylvania Medical Center, Philadelphia, Pennsylvania, Chapter 50

Robert M. Senior, M.D. Dorothy R. and Hubert C. Moog Professor of Pulmonary Diseases in Medicine, Division of Pulmonary & Critical Care Medicine, Washington University Medical Center, Barnes-Jewish Hospital, St. Louis, Missouri, Chapters 7, 48, 49

Daniel H. Sterman, M.D. Pulmonary Allergy and Critical Care Division, University of Pennsylvania Medical Center, Philadelphia, Pennsylvania, Chapter 4

Lynn T. Tanoue, M.D. Associate Professor of Medicine, Pulmonary and Critical Care Medicine, Yale University School of Medicine, New Haven, Connecticut, Chapters 15–20, 25–33

John C. Wain, Jr., M.D. Thoracic Surgery Unit, Massachussets General Hospital, Boston, Massachusetts, Chapter 53

David J. Weber, M.D., M.P.H. Associate Professor of Medicine, Division of Infectious Diseases, University of North Carolina at Chapel Hill, Chapel Hill, North Carolina, Chapter 61

Preface

By definition, a manual is "a book partly held in the hand, especially one giving information or instructions."* This book satisfies this definition. Moreover, this small volume also qualifies as a compendium; that is, "a brief summary of a larger work or a field of knowledge."* The larger work is *Fishman's Pulmonary Diseases and Disorders,* which in reality is the third edition of *Pulmonary Diseases and Disorders,* which began life in 1980 with Alfred P. Fishman, M.D., as the sole editor.

This Manual is more of a distillate than a condensate. It is intended to provide the physician in the office, clinic, or hospital with a handy, up-to-date manual of pulmonary medicine. Preparation of the individual chapters entailed fractional distillation to preserve the essential and practical features of the big book, while leaving behind much of the mechanisms of disease, anatomy, and pathology that are detailed and depicted in the larger work. But, as a guide to scientific underpinnings, illustrative materials, and extensive bibliographies that constitute the basis of the Manual, each chapter of the compendium makes reference to relevant pages in the big book.

Most chapters in this Manual were not prepared by their original authors in the third edition of *Fishman's Pulmonary Diseases and Disorders.* The authors in the big book are given credit at the beginning of each chapter of the Manual. The editors of this book are grateful both to the authors of the original chapters in the larger work as well as to those who adapted them for the purposes of the Manual. Their considerable time and effort spent in preparing their individual contributions are appreciated.

Webster's New Collegiate Dictionary. Springfield, Massachusetts, G. & C. Merriam Co., 1981.

Fishman's

MANUAL of PULMONARY DISEASES and DISORDERS

Part One | SYMPTOMS AND SIGNS OF RESPIRATORY DISEASE

1 | Approach to the Patient*

Alfred P. Fishman

INTRODUCTION

The most common respiratory complaint for which a person seeks medical help is either shortness of breath or cough. Less common are hemoptysis, thoracic pain, cyanosis, and an abnormal breathing pattern. As in the case of any medical evaluation, the paramount diagnostic mainstays are the history and physical examination. Chest radiography is generally reserved for patients who have clinical manifestations of chest disease or are from families or populations known to be particularly vulnerable to chest disease. More sophisticated diagnostic measures and interventions are described in subsequent chapters.

HISTORY

There still is no substitute for a comprehensive, penetrating medical history. The personal history should include a detailed inventory of cigarette smoking. When did it begin? When did it stop? How many cigarettes per day (expressed in number of pack-years)? The workplace is often a site where toxic air is breathed. An almost forgotten exposure to asbestos 20 years ago may explain an enigmatic pulmonary or pleural disease. A newly installed home humidifier or an air-conditioning system that incorporates stagnant pools of water can point the way to resolving a mysterious illness. A brief residence in an area where either cryptococcosis (southwestern United States) or histoplasmosis (southern and midwestern United States) is endemic may help to clarify the nature of an illness that mimics tuberculosis. A recent visit to a Latin American country may bring into focus a more remote possibility (e.g., South American blastomycosis).

Personal habits of the patient, such as intravenous drug abuse or unorthodox sexual practices, may also help to uncover the cause of an unusual pulmonary disorder. Recent treatment of a neoplastic disorder with immunosuppressive agents can raise suspicion of toxicity caused by the therapeutic agent or pulmonary infection by organisms that are usually noninvasive.

---

*Edited from Chap. 28, "Approach to the Patient with Respiratory Symptoms," by Fishman AP, and from Chap. 110, "The Solitary Pulmonary Nodule: A Systematic Approach," by Fein AM, Feinsilver SH, Ares CA. In: *Fishman's Pulmonary Diseases and Disorders,* 3d ed., edited by Fishman AP, Elias JA, Fishman JA, Grippi MA, Kaiser LR, Senior RM. New York, McGraw-Hill, 1998, pp 361–393; 1727–1737. For fuller discussion of topics dealt with in this chapter, the reader is referred to the original text, as noted above.

Certain pharmacologic agents have the propensity for inflicting lung damage. Among these are bleomycin, nitrofurantoin, and methotrexate. Beta blockers, administered as part of a cardiac regimen, can evoke undesirable bronchoconstriction. Even a common agent like aspirin may, on rare occasions, cause a severe pulmonary disorder (e.g., pulmonary edema).

The family history is an essential ingredient of the medical inventory. This history can be particularly helpful in uncovering heritable diseases of the lungs (e.g., cystic fibrosis, α_1-antitrypsin deficiency, alveolar microlithiasis, and hereditary telangiectasia). It may also disclose susceptibility, as for asthma.

PHYSICAL EXAMINATION

General Aspects

Important clues are often available before examination of the chest. Neglected pyorrheal teeth raise the prospect of a necrotizing aspiration pneumonia. A lacerated tongue suggests that a convulsive episode may have led to aspiration. Subtle changes in consciousness or coordination may signal that metastasis has occurred to the brain from a primary carcinoma of the lung. In the patient with chronic obstructive pulmonary disease (COPD), a clouded sensorium or a disturbed personality can signify acute CO_2 retention.

Evidence to support the diagnosis of pulmonary sarcoidosis is sought in the eyes and skin. Petechiae in the skin may reflect a systemic vasculitis that also affects the vessels of the lungs. The presence of a gallop rhythm alerts the examiner to a cardiac, rather than a pulmonary, origin of an asthmatic attack. The skin lesions of von Recklinghausen's disease may signify that a solitary pulmonary nodule in the paraspinal region may be a neurofibroma.

A variety of endocrine syndromes can accompany a carcinoma of the lung. Also, a number of clinical disorders can be associated with clubbing of the digits (Table 1-1).

TABLE 1-1 Clinical Disorders Commonly Associated with Clubbing of Digits

Pulmonary and thoracic
  Primary lung cancer
  Metastatic lung cancer
  Bronchiectasis
  Cystic fibrosis
  Lung abscess
  Pulmonary fibrosis
  Pulmonary arteriovenous malformations
  Empyema
  Mesothelioma
  Neurogenic diaphragmatic tumors
Cardiac
  Congenital
  Subacute bacterial endocarditis
Gastrointestinal and hepatic
  Hepatic cirrhosis
  Chronic ulcerative colitis
  Regional enteritis (Crohn's disease)
Miscellaneous
  Hemiplegia

A minute skin abscess can turn out to be the source of multiple lung abscesses. Distinctive scars over the antecubital veins of a drug addict can help to clarify the etiology of old lesions in the lungs as well as fresh abscesses. Erythema nodosum and erythema multiforme occasionally complicate sarcoidosis, tuberculosis, histoplasmosis, and coccidioidomycosis; sometimes they are part of a drug reaction.

A puffy face, neck, and eyelids coupled with dilated veins of the neck, shoulder, thorax, and upper arm (i.e., superior vena cava syndrome) occasionally constitute the first clinical evidence of extrinsic obstruction of the superior vena cava by a neoplasm of the lung. The detection of Horner's syndrome—unilateral ptosis, miosis, and anhidrosis—in a patient with carcinoma of the lung suggests a pulmonary sulcus tumor with involvement of the ipsilateral sympathetic pathway within the thorax.

Inspection

Observation of the chest from the foot of the bed can be informative: a visible lag of one side of the thorax localizes a pleural effusion, pulmonary infection, or paralyzed diaphragm. The position of the trachea with respect to the midline can be a useful clue to atelectasis of one lobe or to obstruction of a major bronchus. Inspection of the chest and abdomen during sleep may reveal the paradoxical inward movement of the abdomen that is characteristic of obstructive sleep apnea. Thoracoabdominal discoordination in the supine position raises the possibility of diaphragmatic paresis or paralysis.

Palpation

Palpation can provide helpful diagnostic clues. For example, the position of the trachea determined by palpation in the suprasternal notch can be helpful in detecting a lateral shift of the upper mediastinum. Displacement of the apical impulse and cardiac dullness can be useful as indices in detecting shift of the lower mediastinum. Tenderness over a rib may reflect a fracture, a metastasis, or an underlying pleuritis. Enlargement of the right ventricle can be more readily detected by palpation in the subxiphoid region than by other surface examination. Hoover's sign can be useful in disclosing a unilateral lag in motion of one side of the chest due to pleuritis or a pleural effusion.

Percussion

The response to percussion is impaired whenever something other than air-filled lung lies directly beneath the chest wall. Common causes are consolidation or atelectasis of the lung, fluid in the pleural space, pleural thickening, and a large mass at the surface of the lung. Distinction should be made between dullness and flatness: dullness is characteristic of pneumonic consolidation or atelectasis, whereas flatness is characteristic of a large pleural effusion or a high diaphragm. Widespread hyperresonance can often be elicited in emphysema and circumscribed hyperresonance over a pneumothorax or large bulla. As a rule, a decrease in breath sounds, as over a large bulla, is more characteristic than an increase in resonance.

Auscultation

A global decrease in the intensity of breath sounds over the thorax or hemithorax can be due to a variety of abnormalities: impaired movement of air (e.g., in emphysema), paralysis of a diaphragm, complete obstruction of a bronchus, and impaired transmission of sounds to the chest wall (e.g., in pleural effusion, pleural thickening, pneumothorax). A bulla gives rise to a more circumscribed diminution in breath sounds. In a patient with COPD, regional variations in breath sounds correspond to the distribution of ventilation.

An abnormal increase in intensity of breath sounds is accompanied by a change in their character (the sounds become either harsh or bronchial). The abnormal sounds are heard over consolidated, atelectatic, or compressed lung as long as the airway to the affected portion of the lung remains patent.

Transmission of Lung Sounds

Changes in voice sounds are often easier to appreciate than changes in breath sounds. Large pleural effusions, pneumothorax, and bronchial occlusion produce distant or inaudible breath sounds. Transmission of voice sounds is enhanced by consolidation, infarction, atelectasis, or compression of lung tissue. Accompanying the increased transmission is a change in the character of the voice sounds that causes them to be higher-pitched and less muffled than normal (bronchophony). When bronchophony is extreme, spoken words assume a nasal or bleating quality (egophony) and the sound "ee" is heard through the stethoscope as "ay." Egophony is most common when consolidated lung and pleural fluid coexist; sometimes it is heard over an uncomplicated lobar pneumonia or pulmonary infarction. Transmission of whispered voice sounds with abnormal clarity (whispered pectoriloquy) has the same significance as bronchophony.

A pleural friction rub is a coarse, grating, or leathery sound that is usually heard late in inspiration and early in expiration, most often low in the axilla or over the lung base posteriorly. It sounds close to the ear and usually is not altered by coughing.

Adventitious Lung Sounds

Lung sounds are categorized as continuous (wheezes, rhonchi, or stridor) or discontinuous (crackles). Crackles (or rales) are further identified as fine or coarse.

Wheezes originate in airways narrowed by spasm, thickening of the mucosa, or luminal obstruction. Although wheezes are more apt to occur during forced expiration, which further narrows airways, they generally occur during both inspiration and expiration in asthma. Wheezes presumably originate through a combination of limitation to airflow and vibrations in the walls of the airways.

Stridor is predominantly inspiratory and best heard over the neck. The common causes of stridor are a foreign body in the upper intrathoracic airway or esophagus and an acquired lesion of the airway (e.g., carcinoma in adults and a congenital lesion in children).

Early Inspiratory Crackles

Early inspiratory crackles are probably due to a rapid succession of explosive openings of small airways that closed prematurely during the previous expiration. Crackles that clear after a cough or two probably reflect secretions in the airways; those that linger, as in COPD, are presumably the consequences of a decrease in elastic recoil (emphysema) or increase in airway secretions (bronchitis).

Late Inspiratory Crackles

The late inspiratory crackles that occur at the lung bases in the elderly or bedridden can be made to disappear with a few deep breaths. Late inspiratory crackles also occur in interstitial lung disease (e.g., fibrosing alveolitis, asbestosis, pulmonary edema) and in pneumonia. With the patient upright, they are best heard at the lung base.

Wheezing

Wheezes, rhonchi, and stridor are musical adventitious sounds. Wheezes originate in airways narrowed by bronchospasm, thickened mucosa, or luminal obstruction. Wheezes are most apt to occur during expiration, but—as in asthma—may occur during both inspiration and expiration. Wheezes are presumably due to limitation to airflow coupled with vibrations in the walls of the airways.

Wheezing is the most characteristic physical sign of asthma, even though it is not specific for asthma. It is caused by high-velocity, turbulent flow through narrowed airways. Inspiratory and expiratory wheezes, which are best heard over the upper airways, should prompt a search for causes of upper airway obstruction, including dysfunction of the vocal cords, vocal cord paralysis, tumors of the upper airways, and thyroid enlargement encroaching on the airways. Recognition of vocal cord dysfunction often requires fiberoptic laryngoscopy during an acute episode.

Stridor occurs predominantly during inspiration. In adults, the most common cause is a foreign body in the upper intrathoracic airway or esophagus. Not uncommonly, stridor may be due to a carcinoma of the airways. Stridor is best heard over the neck.

BRONCHOSCOPY

Flexible fiberoptic bronchoscopy and video bronchoscopy feature prominently in the armamentarium of the pulmonologist. In contrast, rigid, larger-bore bronchoscopy is a surgical procedure that provides better visualization and control. It is useful for aspiration of secretions and for the introduction of accessories, such as biopsy forceps, bronchial brushes, or ultrasound probes. The rigid bronchoscope has proved useful in such interventions as cryotherapy, brachytherapy, laser therapy, and stenting.

Bronchoscopy may be diagnostic or therapeutic. For the various applications, choice of a proper bronchoscope is essential. The diagnostic applications include assessment of the structure, functions, and integrity of the airways; identification of the source of hemoptysis; performance of bronchial and parenchymal biopsies; sampling of constituents of the airways and alveoli; and transbronchial needle aspiration and biopsy. The therapeutic applications include removal of foreign bodies, control of hemoptysis, aspiration of secretions, relief of bronchial obstruction, closure of bronchial fistulae, and application of accessories and therapies such as thermal lasers, brachytherapy, electrocautery, cryotherapy, photodynamic therapy, placement of stents, and airway dilation.

DYSPNEA

Clinical Presentations

Dyspnea is the medical term for breathlessness or shortness of breath.

TABLE 1-2 Causes of Acute and Chronic Dyspnea[a]

Acute
  Pulmonary edema
  Asthma
  Injury to chest wall and intrathoracic structures
  Spontaneous pneumothorax
  Pulmonary embolism
  Pneumonia
  Adult respiratory distress syndrome
  Pleural effusion
  Pulmonary hemorrhage
Chronic, progressive
  Chronic obstructive pulmonary disease
  Left ventricular failure
  Diffuse interstitial fibrosis
  Asthma
  Pleural effusions
  Pulmonary thromboembolic disease
  Pulmonary vascular disease
  Psychogenic dyspnea
  Anemia, severe
  Postintubation tracheal stenosis
  Hypersensitivity disorders

[a]Asthma and acute left ventricular failure represent chronic causes with paroxysmal exacerbations.

Acute Dyspnea

The causes of acute dyspnea in children differ from those in adults. In children, upper airway infection (epiglottitis, laryngitis, or acute laryngo-tracheobronchitis) is a common cause. In adults, the causes of acute dyspnea are much more varied (Table 1-2). Among the most common are an episode of acute left ventricular failure, a thromboembolic event, pneumonia, and spontaneous pneumothorax. Less common but not unusual is massive collapse of one lung due to inability to clear the airways of thick, tenacious secretions (e.g., chronic bronchitis or asthma) or the first attack of asthma.

Chronic (and Progressive) Dyspnea

Chronic dyspnea is almost invariably progressive. As a rule, this type of dyspnea begins with breathlessness on exertion, which in time progresses to dyspnea at rest. The most common cause of recurrent bouts of dyspnea is asthma. As a rule, in these patients breathlessness is accompanied by cough and wheezing. One special type of asthma, especially in middle-aged or elderly persons, is cardiac asthma, which is a manifestation of paroxysmal nocturnal dyspnea due to acute left ventricular failure and resultant pulmonary edema. Another, much less frequent cause of paroxysmal nocturnal dyspnea is acute left ventricular failure and the ensuing pulmonary edema. Another, much less frequent cause of paroxysmal wheezing and breathlessness is bronchopulmonary aspergillosis.

Attempts to understand the physiologic bases of dyspnea have evolved along four separate lines: ventilatory performance, mechanics of breathing, chemoreception, and exercise testing.

TABLE 1-3 Modified Borg Category Scale

Rating	Intensity of sensation
0	Nothing at all
0.5	Very, very slight (just noticeable)
1	Very slight
2	Slight
3	Moderate
4	Somewhat severe
5	Severe
6	
7	Very severe
8	
9	Very, very severe (almost maximal)
10	Maximal

Scaling

A variety of scaling methods have been devised in the attempt to quantify dyspnea during exercise and various experimental conditions. Some, such as the Borg Category Scale (Table 1-3), use numbers and descriptive terms to depict a change in the intensity of the stimulus ("threshold stimulus detection methods"). Others rely on visual analog scales, which are straight lines, usually 10 cm long, that extend from "not breathless" at one end to "extremely breathless" at the other. The Shortness of Breath Scale issued by the American Thoracic Society has been used for years in one form or another, particularly in epidemiologic studies. No single scale is applicable to all subjects or patients.

Dyspnea in Chronic Pulmonary Disease

Two common types of pulmonary disease in which dyspnea features prominently are chronic obstructive airway disease and restrictive lung disease.

Chronic Obstructive Pulmonary Disease (COPD)

COPD refers to a spectrum of airway diseases in which obstruction to airflow is the common denominator. Cigarette smoking is the leading cause of COPD. The outer limits of the spectrum are marked by chronic bronchitis at one end and emphysema at the other. Most patients with COPD fall into categories between those limits (i.e., they manifest mixtures of chronic bronchitis and emphysema that vary in degree). Patients with COPD suffer from disturbances in the mechanics of breathing, abnormal lung volumes, and derangements in gas exchange. The minute ventilation, which may be only slightly increased at rest, constitutes an abnormally large fraction of the maximum breathing capacity (i.e., the "breathing reserve" is low).

In COPD, abnormalities in the mechanics of breathing dominate the scene: resistance to airflow is high; the thorax assumes a hyperinflated position, placing the inspiratory muscles at a mechanical disadvantage; the work of breathing is greatly increased. The O_2 cost of breathing is correspondingly high. Derangements in dead-space ventilation and in alveolar-capillary gas exchange add to the afferent stimuli. As a result of the disturbances in mechanics and gas exchange, swings in pleural pressure (a measure of force applied to the lungs) are large, and a considerable muscular effort is expended in breathing. Some patients with COPD settle for a lower ventilation than do others; the result is CO_2 retention. One teleologic explanation is that the lower ventilation in the CO_2 retainer causes less dyspnea.

Asthma

Asthma constitutes a different entity, not only in its clinical expressions but also because it is usually episodic, is unrelated to smoking, is often related to allergic manifestations, and generally affects younger people. The mechanisms described above for COPD apply as well to asthma. However, these mechanisms do not account for the sensation of "tightness in the chest" or the inordinate sense of labored breathing that accompanies the breathlessness.

Cystic Fibrosis

Cystic fibrosis is another distinct entity because of its genetic basis, clinical and radiographic presentations, nature of the airway obstruction (i.e., by inspissated mucus), and proclivity to superinfection.

Restrictive Lung Disease

Restrictive lung diseases can be due to different causes, but usually they have in common a reduction in lung volumes and diffusing capacity (Table 1-4). One major category of restrictive lung disease is diffuse interstitial disease. This, in turn, has many different causes and may be either acute or chronic in onset (Table 1-5). Characteristically, in widespread interstitial disease, diffusing capacity is low and accompanied by a considerable decrease in total lung capacity and vital capacity in association with lesser decrements in functional residual capacity and residual volume. Similar findings occur in severe kyphoscoliosis or encasement of the lung by pleural thickening. Neuromuscular disease that affects the inspiratory muscles sufficiently to diminish maximum inspiratory pressures may decrease only the vital and total lung capacities, leaving the functional residual capacity and residual volume unaffected.

Patients with widespread pulmonary fibrosis breathe faster and maintain a higher minute ventilation than do normal subjects, both at rest and during exercise. The work and O_2 cost of ventilating the stiff lungs are increased. The maximum breathing capacity is well preserved. In these patients, dyspnea is attributable to the considerable effort by the respiratory muscles in ventilating the stiff lungs and in sustaining the high ventilatory rate. During exercise, dyspnea may become intolerable.

TABLE 1-4 Common Causes of Restrictive Lung Disease

Cause	Example
Interstitium	
Interstitial fibrosis and/or infiltration	Asbestosis
Pulmonary edema	Left ventricular failure
Pleura	
Pleural disease	Fibrothorax
Thoracic cage and abdomen	
Neuromuscular disease	Poliomyelitis
Skeletal abnormalities	Severe kyphoscoliosis
Marked obesity	Grossly overweight
Pulmonary vascular disease	
Pulmonary hypertensive disorders	Primary pulmonary hypertension

TABLE 1-5 Common Types of Diffuse Interstitial Disease

Etiology	Example	Common features
Acute		
Infection	Miliary tuberculosis, histoplasmosis	Exposure to organism
	Pneumocystis carinii, cytomegalic inclusion Virus, fungus	Immunosuppression
Radiation therapy	After mastectomy	Shortly after treatment
Pulmonary edema	Narcotic overdose, nitrogen dioxide (silo-filler's disease), uremia	Distinctive history
Inhalation	Byssinosis	Monday-morning asthma and fever
Aspiration	After loss of consciousness	History and alcoholism or epilepsy
Immunologic	Goodpasture's syndrome	Renal and pulmonary involvement
Carcinoma of lung	Alveolar cell carcinoma	
Idiopathic	Idiopathic pulmonary fibrosis	
Chronic		
Inhalation	Pneumoconioses	History of exposure
Radiation therapy	After mastectomy	Gradual evolution after treatment
Lymphangitic spread	Carcinoma of breast, lung, stomach, pancreas	Evidence of primary carcinoma
Medications	Hexamethonium, hydralazine, bleomycin, busulfan, nitrofurantoin	History, suggestive chest radiograph
Systemic disorders	Sarcoidosis, collagen disorders, histiocytosis X, amyloidosis, tuberous sclerosis	Multiorgan involvement, biopsy

Dyspnea in Chronic Cardiac Disease

The mechanisms responsible for dyspnea in cardiac disease vary with the extent to which the lungs are stiffened.

Without Stiff Lungs

Dyspnea occurs in many forms of heart disease that are not associated with congestion of the lungs; pulmonic stenosis is an excellent example. The likely mechanism is an inadequate cardiac output. In cyanotic heart disease, both dyspnea and fatigue appear during exertion when the arterial oxyhemoglobin saturation has fallen appreciably below the resting level.

With Stiff Lungs

Cardiac dyspnea is associated with expanded blood and water content of the lungs. It is a common occurrence in left ventricular failure and mitral stenosis, both of which are accompanied by increases in pulmonary venous and capillary pressures. In chronic left ventricular failure, pulmonary fibrosis, consequent to long-standing interstitial edema, contributes to the stiff lungs. Edema of the tracheobronchial mucosa increases airway resistance.

In patients with pulmonary congestion and edema, tachypnea is a regular feature at rest and increases during exercise. Although tachypnea is consistent, its degree is generally modest and probably not entirely responsible for the dyspnea. Fatigue is a common concomitant of low cardiac output.

Orthopnea and Other Positional Forms of Breathlessness

Orthopnea signifies dyspnea in the recumbent but not in the upright or semi-vertical position; it is usually relieved by two or three pillows under the head and back. Oppositely, *platypnea* signifies dyspnea induced by assuming the upright position and relieved by assuming the recumbent position. Orthopnea is a hallmark of pulmonary congestion that stiffens the lungs (i.e., decreases their compliance).

Some patients with chronic lung disease or asthma are intolerant of recumbency. In these people, the discomfort is attributed to the greater difficulty of performing vigorous movements of the chest bellows in the recumbent position.

Paroxysmal Nocturnal Dyspnea

In an episode of paroxysmal nocturnal dyspnea, the patient is aroused from sleep gasping for air and must sit up or stand to catch his or her breath; sweating may be profuse. Sometimes the patient throws a window open wide in an attempt to relieve the oppressive sensation of suffocation. Both inspiratory and expiratory wheezes, often simulating typical asthma, are heard. In some instances, overt, acute pulmonary edema occurs, accompanied by many crackles at end-inspiration; this rarely terminates fatally. Occasionally, the attacks recur several times a night, forcing the patient to sleep upright in a chair.

The episode represents precipitous failure of the left ventricle caused by the factors that produce orthopnea (see above), abetted by acute pulmonary hypervolemia caused by a surge in systemic venous return.

Cardiac Asthma

The asthmatic wheezes often heard in patients with pulmonary congestion have given rise to the term *cardiac asthma*. The wheezes are a manifestation of tracheobronchial edema and often are accompanied by overt signs of pulmonary edema.

Dyspnea in Anemia

Shortness of breath during exercise or excitement is a common complaint in severe anemia (e.g., hemoglobin concentration less than 6 to 7 g/dL). It is more common in acute than in chronic anemia. Although the pathogenesis of the dyspnea is not clear, inadequate O_2 delivery to the respiratory muscles has been proposed.

Miscellaneous Disorders

Breathlessness is not uncommon in patients with musculoskeletal disorders. The usual explanation is the heightened motor drive that is needed to activate the weakened respiratory muscles. In the intensive care unit, inadequate ventilator settings for flow and tidal volume may fail to satisfy the intrinsic ventilatory drive of the patient, generating the sensation of breathlessness.

ABNORMAL BREATHING PATTERNS

An important clue to the nature of a clinical problem in pulmonary disease is sometimes provided by bedside observation of a patient's respiratory pattern. The pertinent features are the rate, regularity, depth, and apparent effort being expended in breathing. A normal person at rest breathes about 12 to 15 times per minute, with a tidal volume of 400 to 800 mL. As a result, minute ventilation is normally greater than 5 L/min. The pattern is quite regular except for an occasional slow, deep breath, and the respiratory movements appear effortless. In the patient with lobar pneumonia, both the rate and depth of breathing increase, along with the increase in body temperature.

Severe skeletal deformity as well as massive obesity can limit chest excursions to cause alveolar hypoventilation. Neuromuscular weakness, as in myasthenia gravis or Guillain-Barré syndrome, can do the same, not only by diminishing ventilatory excursions as a result of generalized weakness of the respiratory muscles but also by overloading of unaffected muscles (e.g., residual effects of poliomyelitis). Unilateral involvement of one pleural space by pneumothorax, effusion, or fibrothorax limits excursions on the affected side. Massive chest trauma can cause flail chest.

In COPD, a slow respiratory rate and large tidal volumes are characteristic. This pattern presumably serves to minimize the work of breathing in these patients. Pursed-lip breathing, a self-induced type of positive-pressure breathing, is often part of the picture. In contrast, persons with restrictive lung disease adopt a breathing pattern that is characterized by small tidal volumes and a rapid respiration rate, often with little apparent effort. It is seen in patients with a decrease in distensibility of the lung or chest wall or with reduction of the vital capacity from any other cause. During exercise, minute ventilation increases inordinately with respect to the level of O_2 uptake and frequency increases more than tidal volume.

Fatigue of the diaphragm and intercostal muscles, sufficient to disturb their coordinated contractions, can give rise to paradoxical breathing, heralding the onset of respiratory failure.

Cheyne-Stokes Respiration

Cheyne-Stokes breathing is characterized by alternating periods of hypoventilation and hyperventilation. In its typical form, an apneic phase lasting for 15 to 60 s is followed by a phase during which tidal volume increases with each breath to a peak level and then decreases in a progressive fashion to the apneic phase. At the onset of apnea, CO_2 tension P_{CO_2} in brachial or femoral arterial blood is at its lowest, while the arterial oxyhemoglobin saturation is at its highest.

In patients with congestive heart failure, the respiratory oscillations are attributable to slowing of the circulation so that the blood gases reaching the respiratory centers in the brain are 180 degrees out of phase with those in pulmonary capillary blood.

Fluctuations in mental state and electroencephalographic patterns and evidence of nervous system dysfunction may occur during Cheyne-Stokes breathing because of swings in cerebral blood flow. In neurologic disorders, Cheyne-Stokes breathing can be due to supramedullary dysfunction, particularly in patients who have destructive lesions in the tegmentum of the pons. Less common than in heart failure or neurologic disorders is the occurrence of Cheyne-Stokes respiration in normal infants, in healthy elderly persons, and in normal persons at high altitude. It is also seen occasionally after the administration of respiratory depressants (e.g., morphine) and often accompanies an increase in intracranial pressure, uremia, or coma.

Kussmaul Breathing

This pattern of breathing at rest resembles that seen in normals during exercise: deep regular breaths are accomplished with little apparent effort. It usually occurs in severe metabolic acidosis (e.g., diabetic, alcoholic).

Other Abnormal Breathing Patterns

Gasping respirations are characteristic of severe cerebral hypoxia. The pattern is commonly seen in shock or in other conditions associated with severe reductions in cardiac output.

Hyperventilation is commonly seen in anxious patients without structural disease of the lungs. In some of these patients, striking, deep sighs dominate the ventilatory pattern.

COUGH

A cough is an explosive expiration that protects the lungs against aspiration and promotes the movement of secretions and other airway constituents upward toward the mouth. It is a reflex act that usually but not invariably arises from stimulation of the bronchial mucosa somewhere between the larynx and the second-order bronchi. The stimuli that can elicit a cough are diverse: inhaled particles, mucus that has been elaborated by the lining of the airways, inflammatory exudate in airways or parenchyma, a new growth or foreign body in an airway, and pressure on the external wall of the bronchus.

The site and significance of a cough can sometimes be localized from telltale signs and symptoms (Table 1-6). Interpretation of the significance of a cough depends on the clinical company that it keeps. A cough that is productive of purulent sputum is generally a reliable indication of infection in the tracheobronchial tree or lungs. When this symptom is associated with an acute illness, the characteristics of the sputum can be of considerable diagnostic help. Purulent sputum with a foul odor usually indicates an anaerobic infection, commonly due to streptococci or *Bacteroides* in a lung abscess. A persistent cough that is productive of purulent sputum occurs in chronic bronchitis, bronchiectasis, and a variety of other suppurative disorders.

Workup for Chronic Cough

Five general causes of chronic cough are kept in mind in the course of a diagnostic workup: infection, inflammation of the lungs and/or airways, tumor, foreign body, and cardiovascular deficits.

Diagnostic workup begins with a thorough history and physical examination, including the nasopharynx, oropharynx, and sinuses (Table 1-7). If the cough is productive, sputum is examined microscopically and collected for culture. A white blood cell count may help to pinpoint infection versus allergy. A chest radiograph, posteroanterior (PA) and lateral, rounds out the general appraisal.

Special tests are chosen in accord with the clinical impression. Spirometry may disclose obstructive or restrictive lung disease. If obstructive disease

TABLE 1-6 Some Causes and Characteristics of Cough

Cause	Characteristics
Acute infections of lungs	
Tracheobronchitis	Cough associated with sore thorat, running nose and eyes
Lobar pneumonia	Cough often preceded by symptoms of upper respiratory infection; cough dry, painful at first; later becomes productive
Bronchopneumonia	Cough dry or productive, usually begins as acute bronchitis
Mycoplasmal and viral pneumonia	Paroxysmal cough, productive of mucoid or blood-stained sputum associated with flu-like syndrome
Exacerbation of chronic bronchitis	Cough productive of mucoid sputum; becomes purulent
Chronic infections of lungs	
Bronchitis	Cough productive of sputum on most days for more than 3 consecutive months and for more than 2 years
	Sputum mucoid until acute exacerbation, when it becomes mucopurulent
Bronchiectasis	Cough copious, foul, purulent, often since childhood; forms layers upon standing
Tuberculosis or fungus	Persistent cough for weeks to months, often with blood-tinged sputum
Parenchymal inflammatory processes	
Interstitial fibrosis and infiltrations	Cough nonproductive, persistent; depends on origin
Smoking	Cough usually associated with injected pharynx; persistent, most marked in morning, usually only slightly productive unless succeeded by chronic bronchitis
Tumors	
Bronchogenic carcinoma	Cough nonproductive to productive for weeks to months; recurrent small hemoptysis common
Alveolar cell carcinoma	Cough similar to that with bronchogenic carcinoma except in occasional instances, when large quantities of watery, mucoid sputum are produced
Benign tumors in airways	Cough nonproductive; occasionally hemoptysis
Mediastinal tumors	Cough, often with breathlessness, caused by compression of trachea and bronchi
Aortic aneurysm	Brassy cough
Foreign body	
Immediate, while still in upper airway	Cough associated with progressive evidence of asphyxiation
Later, when lodged in lower airway	Nonproductive cough, persistent, associated with localizing wheeze
Cardiovascular	
Left ventricular failure	Cough intensifies while supine, along with aggravation of dyspnea
Pulmonary infarction	Cough associated with hemoptysis, usually with pleural effusion

TABLE 1-7 Persistent Cough: Sequence of Diagnostic Tests

General	1. History and physical examination
	2. Chest radiograph, posteroanterior and lateral
	3. Sputum examination, Gram's stain and culture, cytology
	4. Differential leukocyte count
Special	1. Lung spirometry
	2. Provocative bronchoconstriction test
	3. Sinus radiography
	4. Bronchoscopy
	5. Esophageal reflux tests: motility; pH

is suspected but spirometry is normal, a provocative bronchoconstrictor test, as with methacholine, may disclose bronchial hyperactivity. Sinus radiographs may reveal a chronic sinusitis responsible for a postnasal drip. More invasive measures are called for in a persistent, troubling cough: bronchoscopy for lesions of the larynx and tracheobronchial tree and esophageal studies to exclude gastroesophageal reflux.

Posttussive Syncope

An abrupt and inordinate increase in intrathoracic pressure, greater than that reached during a cough, can precipitate an episode of posttussive syncope. Men are predominantly affected. The increase in intrathoracic pressure elicits systemic vasodilation accompanied by a drop in systemic blood pressure and cerebral blood flow. Syncope usually develops within a few seconds of a paroxysm of coughing and ends soon after coughing stops.

Treatment of Chronic Cough

Treatment centers around removing the cause, such as smoking, or relieving the underlying condition, such as sinusitis. Attempts are made to render an ineffective cough productive, as by posttussive agents (e.g., glyceryl guaiacolate).

HEMOPTYSIS

The coughing up of blood is termed *hemoptysis*. The material that is produced varies from blood-tinged sputum to virtually pure blood. Although any portion of the respiratory tract can be the source, bleeding more often comes from a main bronchus or the lungs than from the nose or throat.

Massive or life-threatening hemoptysis is usually defined as the expectoration of blood at a rate of 300 to 600 mL/24 h. Unfortunately, such estimates rely on quantification by a frightened patient. For practical purposes, an expectorated volume of 150 mL or more is generally defined as life-threatening. Asphyxia is the usual cause of death in massive hemoptysis.

Among the more common causes of massive hemoptysis are infections, such as tuberculosis, lung abscess, necrotizing pneumonia, mycetoma, bronchiectasis, and cystic fibrosis (Table 1-8). However, brisk hemoptysis can also occur in mitral stenosis and alveolar-capillary syndromes, such as Goodpasture's syndrome.

The appearance of the bloody material helps to distinguish between hemoptysis and hematemesis: blood that originates in the airways is usually

TABLE 1-8 Some Common Causes of Hemoptysis

Infections	**Trauma**
Bronchitis	Foreign body
Tuberculosis	Blood dyscrasia
Fungal infection (mycetoma)	Goodpasture's syndrome
Pneumonia	**Systemic disorders**
Lung abscess	Goodpasture's syndrome
Bronchiectasis	Wegener's granulomatosis
Necrotizing pneumonia	**Miscellaneous**
Neoplasms	Vicarious menstruation
Bronchogenic carcinoma	Aspirated foreign body
Bronchial adenoma	Extruded calcified lesion
Cardiovascular disorders	Blood dyscrasias
Pulmonary infarction	Arteriovenous malformation
Mitral stenosis	Coagulopathy

bright red, is mixed with frothy sputum, has an alkaline pH, and contains alveolar macrophages that are laden with hemosiderin; in contrast, blood from the stomach is usually dark, has an acid pH, contains food particles, and occurs in patients with a long history of gastric complaints.

The patient can be exceedingly helpful in localizing the intrapulmonary site of bleeding. Occasionally, the detection of rales or rhonchi over one side or area of the lung directs the search. Sputum is collected and examined: venous blood comes from the pulmonary arterial tree; bright-red blood stems either from a bronchial vein (as in mitral stenosis) or from a bronchial artery (as in bronchiectasis). Expectorated blood clots indicate that blood has been sitting in the lung for a while.

The list of causes of hemoptysis is long and diverse (Table 1-8). The clinical setting is usually helpful in identifying the cause. Hemoptysis before middle age usually brings to mind mitral stenosis, tuberculosis, pneumonia, or bronchiectasis; after 40 to 45 years of age, bronchogenic carcinoma and tuberculosis head the list. In patients who are left with a pulmonary cavity after a pulmonary disease (such as tuberculosis) has healed, especially in regions of the country where pulmonary fungal diseases are prevalent, a bout of hemoptysis may occasionally be the first sign of a mycetoma. In patients who have a predisposing cause, such as chronic heart failure, pulmonary embolism must be considered.

Clinical Manifestations

The most common clue to the etiology of hemoptysis is a history of underlying chest disease. Age and personal habits can also point the way: carcinoma of the lung is rare before the age of 40 years; a history of heavy smoking often precedes carcinoma of the lung. Cystic fibrosis and bronchiectasis affect young populations.

Physical examination is usually complicated by manifestations of apprehension on the part of the patient. Examination of the oropharynx and nasopharynx can eliminate possible supraglottic sources of bleeding. Auscultation and percussion may help to localize a site of pulmonary bleeding, but interpretation can be complicated by signs of aspirated blood.

The chest radiograph is usually the most defining diagnostic aid to etiology. Not only localized pulmonary lesions, such as a mycetoma or neoplasm, but also diffuse pulmonary lesions, such as Goodpasture's syndrome, and cardiac lesions, such as mitral stenosis, may become evident. However, aspiration of blood to the opposite lung often complicates attempts at radiographic localization.

Bronchoscopy is an essential tool for localizing and diagnosing the source of bleeding. The type of bronchoscopy depends on the degree of hemoptysis: a large volume and/or rapid flow, as in massive hemoptysis, calls for rigid bronchoscopy, whereas lesser volumes and flows can be handled by the smaller lumens of the fiberoptic bronchoscope. Bronchoscopic evaluation is urgent when bleeding is massive; less threatening hemoptysis can be investigated more leisurely, but within 24 h.

Special tests may help to identify specific etiologies. For example, computed tomography (CT) is useful for diagnosing bronchiectasis noninvasively. Similarly, angiography can clinch the diagnosis of pulmonary embolism. Both tests may disclose pulmonary arteriovenous malformations.

Specific Entities

Neoplasm

Hemoptysis is so common in bronchogenic carcinoma that it should be regarded as the likeliest possibility in patients between 40 and 60 years of age. The likelihood is greatly increased if there is a long history of cigarette smoking. Most often the bleeding is a consequence of ulceration caused by the expanding tumor; sometimes it is due to a pneumonic process of an abscess in the lung behind the obstruction. Hemoptysis rarely complicates metastatic tumors of the lungs, since few (primarily renal and colon carcinomas) intrude on the airways until preterminal stages.

Not only malignant but also benign tumors of the lung cause bleeding. The classic example is bronchial carcinoid, which often causes bleeding that is generally difficult to arrest.

Infections

Hemoptysis can accompany a severe infection anywhere from the top to the bottom of the respiratory tract. It is uncommon in the usual viral or bacterial pneumonia. Conversely, it is not uncommon in the pneumonia that complicates bronchogenic carcinoma or in that caused by staphylococci, influenza virus, or *Klebsiella.*

The organism determines the appearance and composition of the material that is expectorated with the blood. In pneumococcal lobar pneumonia, the sputum at the onset is characteristically rusty-looking, but sometimes it is faintly or grossly bloody. In staphylococcal pneumonia, the blood is mixed with pus. In *Klebsiella* pneumonia, the bloody sputum often resembles currant jelly. Brisk bleeding is common in lung abscess; the blood is mixed with copious amounts of foul-smelling pus. In lung gangrene, blood is associated with necrotic lung tissue.

In bronchiectasis, bleeding is common. Because bleeding usually originates in a bronchial artery, it is often brisk. Although rarely life-threatening, it tends to recur; and almost invariably each episode stops spontaneously.

Fungal infections of the lungs can cause hemoptysis. As in tuberculosis, hemoptysis is generally a consequence of a continuing necrotizing and ulcerating inflammatory process or of bronchiectasis. The most common fungal disease associated with hemoptysis is a "fungus ball" (mycetoma) that resides either in a healed tuberculous or bronchiectatic area or in a cystic residue of sarcoidosis. *Aspergillus* is the usual fungal agent. The most common source of hemoptysis used to be an active tuberculous cavity. But now tuberculous pneumonia is more common.

The right-middle-lobe syndrome is frequently associated with hemoptysis. It is due to a partial or complete obstruction of the right-middle-lobe bronchus, resulting in atelectasis and/or pneumonitis of the lobe. The obstruction is more often caused by scarring and/or inflammation than by physical compression of the lumen by an enlarged lymph node. The cause is usually infectious, and the infection can be tuberculosis.

Amebiasis in parts of the world where amebiasis is endemic can cause hemoptysis. Hemoptysis results from perforation into the airways of a lung abscess that is continuous with hepatic abscess. The sputum resembles anchovy paste.

Cardiovascular Disorders

Pulmonary congestion and alveolar edema sometimes produce blood-tinged sputum.

Pulmonary embolism and, less often, pulmonary thrombosis produce hemoptysis only when associated with infarction. The hemoptysis of pulmonary infarction is usually associated with pleuritic pain and often with a small pleural effusion because of the peripheral location of the infarct.

Tight mitral stenosis is sometimes first manifest by a bout of brisk, bright-red hemoptysis that is difficult to control. The source of the bleeding is the submucosal bronchial veins, which proliferate considerably in this disorder. Massive hemoptysis due to mitral stenosis is a medical emergency and an indication for surgical intervention to relieve the obstruction at the mitral valve.

Alveolar Hemorrhage Syndromes

An increasing number of alveolar hemorrhage syndromes have been characterized by an increasing number of serologic tests. These disorders may present insidiously or abruptly, the latter quickly culminating in respiratory failure. They affect the lungs alone or as part of a systemic disease, often with renal involvement. Prompt diagnosis and treatment may be lifesaving, but diagnosis is often complicated (e.g., the specificity of circulating anti–glomerular basement membrane (GBM) antibodies for the diagnosis of Goodpasture's syndrome, uncertain serologic tests, and reluctance to perform lung biopsy in critically ill patients). The diverse diseases and conditions include Goodpasture's syndrome, Wegener's granulomatosis, systemic lupus erythematosus, idiopathic pulmonary hemosiderosis, bone marrow transplantation, and lymphangiomatosis.

Massive Hemoptysis

Stabilization of the patient is prerequisite for definitive therapy. This involves placement of intravenous lines for the administration of fluids to sustain blood pressure, maintenance of oxygenation, avoidance of cough suppressants, and correction of any coagulopathy. For particular sites of bleeding, such as the bronchial veins in mitral stenosis, the intravenous administration of Pitressin may be helpful.

Definitive therapy is directed at ensuring patent airways, protecting the uninvolved lung, and arresting the bleeding. Endotracheal intubation is generally involved; the choice of tube is considered above. Considerable technical skill is required for proper placement and to avoid injury to the airways.

Uncontrollable bleeding raises the question of surgery once the patient has been stabilized. This option then applies if the patient's lung function is adequate and if the lesion is local, such as carcinoid, a foreign body, bronchiectasis, or arteriovenous malformation. Bleeding from an aspergilloma may be difficult to arrest medically. In such patients, amphotericin B instilled within the cavity may prove successful in delaying or avoiding surgery.

Embolization of the feeder vessels may be an option to arrest life-threatening bleeding in certain diseases in which the source can be identified by angiography. These diseases include a lung cancer, tuberculosis, lung abscess, bronchiectasis, aspergilloma, or an arteriovenous malformation. Effective embolization requires great technical skill and runs the risk of inadvertent embolization of extrapulmonary sites, such as the spinal cord, and infarction of a bronchus.

Trauma

Hemoptysis follows a variety of chest injuries: puncture of a lung by a fractured rib, contusion of a lung by severe blunt trauma to the chest, and necrosis of the lining of the tracheobronchial tree by inhaled fumes or smoke. Blunt trauma from the steering wheel during an automobile collision sometimes lacerates or fractures the tracheobronchial tree. Stab or gunshot wounds often tear the lungs or airways.

Treatment

Management of the patient with hemoptysis depends on the urgency and cause. Massive hemoptysis calls for clearing of the airways to prevent asphyxia, protection of the uninvolved lung, and arrest or elimination of the cause. Nonmassive hemoptysis, because of less urgency, can be directed at controlling the underlying disease (e.g., an infectious process, a coagulopathy, or a neoplasm).

Bronchoscopy can be helpful for both diagnosis and treatment. The type of bronchoscope depends on the clinical situation. For nonmassive hemoptysis, fiberoptic bronchoscopy may suffice to slow bleeding, to provide access to a bleeding source in the airways, for topical treatment (e.g., epinephrine, 1:20,000), for application of fibrin precursors, or for tamponade (e.g., via a Fogerty balloon catheter).

However, rigid bronchoscopy is the method of choice for large-scale bleeding. The large bore of the instrument enables it to deal more efficiently with large volumes of blood secretions and clots and for lavage with cold scaling; it also provides safer access to the bleeding site for photocoagulation and for more efficient packing of the airway than does the fiberoptic bronchoscope. Moreover, a ventilating bronchoscope may prove useful in ensuring adequate ventilation. Finally, a single-bore tube may be useful diagnostically.

Nonmassive Hemoptysis

Treatment of nonmassive hemoptysis varies according to the underlying disease. Pulmonary infections generally respond to antibiotics. Bleeding from a neoplasm can be managed by radiation, surgery, laser therapy, or chemotherapy, the choice depending on the feasibility of surgical resection and the clinical state and lung function of the patient. Bleeding from bronchial veins in mitral stenosis may only be arrested by valve repair or replacement.

Medical treatment is generally the only recourse in alveolar hemorrhage syndromes, such as Goodpasture's syndrome, lupus erythematosus, and necrotizing vasculitis. In addition to high-dose corticosteroids and cytotoxic agents, plasmapheresis is often used.

CYANOSIS

Cyanosis refers to a bluish discoloration of the skin that is caused by a high level of reduced hemoglobin in the subcutaneous minute vessels of the skin. For cyanosis to become discernible, the concentration of reduced hemoglobin in the subdermal capillaries must reach 5 g/dL. The discoloration is most evident in the lobes of the ears, the cutaneous surfaces of the lips, and the nail beds. In patients with dark skin, the mucous membranes and the retinae are important sites to examine for cyanosis. Unless flow through the skin is slowed, as in heart failure, cyanosis implies arterial hypoxemia. Cyanosis does not appear in CO poisoning or in severe anemia in which arterial O_2 content is extremely low. The presence of abnormal pigments in blood, such as methemoglobin or bilirubin, complicates the detection of cyanosis.

Causes of Cyanosis

Pulmonary Disease

Cyanosis in pulmonary disease varies with the mechanism. In chronic bronchitis and emphysema, the cause is usually a derangement in ventilation-perfusion relationships. In interstitial fibrosis, a low diffusing capacity may cause arterial hypoxemia and cyanosis during exercise. In right-to-left shunts, venous admixture to arterial blood is responsible.

Methemoglobinemia is an occasional cause of cyanosis. Methemoglobinemic blood is chocolate-brown, and spectrophotometric examination of blood reveals the characteristic pigment. Arterial blood examination discloses a normal P_{O_2}.

The cause of methemoglobinemia may be hereditary (i.e., due to the presence of hemoglobin M or a deficiency in methemoglobin reductase) or, more often, acquired (e.g., by exposure to chemical agents such as aniline dyes, chlorates, nitrates, and nitrites); or it may derive from use of drugs such as acetanilide, nitroglycerin, phenacetin, and primaquine. Nitrates are a common cause of methemoglobinemia, in which the ferrous iron is oxidized to ferric iron, rendering the hemoglobin molecule incapable of binding O_2 or CO_2. Clinical manifestations of methemoglobinemia vary with the blood levels. Concentrations of methemoglobin between 10 and 25 percent usually cause asymptomatic cyanosis. When these levels are exceeded, dizziness, fatigue, and headache appear.

Peripheral Cyanosis

The most common cause of peripheral cyanosis is a low cardiac output associated with peripheral vasoconstriction. The cyanosis is due to the abnormally large extraction of O_2 as blood flows through peripheral capillaries. In Raynaud's disease, peripheral vasoconstriction per se produces cyanosis of the nail beds.

Venous Admixture

Cyanosis may be due to shunting of venous blood into the systemic circulation by way of anatomic communications between blood vessels or in the heart or, as in chronic obstructive pulmonary disease, due to ventilation-perfusion inhomogeneities.

CLUBBING AND HYPERTROPHIC OSTEOARTHROPATHY

Clubbing of the fingers designates the selective bulbous enlargement of the distal segments of the digits due to an increase in soft tissue. Most often it is painless.

Clubbing is generally acquired, but it may be hereditary. Acquired clubbing is seen in a wide variety of disorders, both extrathoracic and thoracic (see Table 1-1). As a rule, clubbing is bilaterally symmetrical, affecting hands and feet; on occasion, local factors, such as injury of a finger or of the median nerve, may cause clubbing that is confined to a single finger. On rare occasions, clubbing may be confined to the digits of one hand (e.g., in an ipsilateral pulmonary sulcus tumor that has invaded the brachial plexus or following hemiplegia). In patent ductus arteriosus associated with reversal of shunt through the ductus, clubbing affects only the toes.

The pathogenesis of clubbing is unknown, but a common denominator appears to be vasodilation of vessels in the fingertip, including formation of arteriovenous connections.

Hypertrophic Osteoarthropathy

Occasionally, clubbing of the digits is accompanied by hypertrophic osteoarthropathy, a separate entity both clinically and radiographically. Clinically, hypertrophic osteoarthropathy is manifest by pain and swelling of the soft tissues over the distal ends of the long and tubular bones. Radiographically, the distinctive feature of hypertrophic osteoarthropathy is the formation of new bone beneath the periosteum of the distal diaphyses of the long bones of the extremities. The most common disorder associated with hypertrophic osteoarthropathy is carcinoma of the lung. In contrast to clubbing of the digits, which is rarely painful, hypertrophic osteoarthritis associated with carcinoma of the lung often causes severe rheumatic symptoms.

PAIN

Thoracic Pain

Cardiac pain is the most common type of thoracic pain. However, cardiac pain is generally distinguishable from other types of chest pain because of its vise-like nature; its characteristic radiation to the left arm, shoulder, or neck; and its lack of relation to breathing. Pain may also be referred to the thorax as a result of gastroesophageal reflux. Within the thorax, pain may arise from the pleura, lungs, or chest wall.

Pleuritic Pain

The most characteristic pain associated with the respiratory apparatus is pleural pain. It originates in the parietal pleura and endothoracic fascia; the visceral pleura is insensitive to pain. It is predominantly an inspiratory pain reflecting the stretching of inflamed parietal pleura during movement of the thorax; coughing or laughing is exceedingly distressing, and the patient often clutches his or her chest to minimize its excursion. Irritation of the diaphragmatic pleura by an inflammatory process either below or above the diaphragm often causes ipsilateral shoulder pain; sometimes the pain is referred to the abdomen.

Pulmonary Pain

A second distinctive type of respiratory chest pain accompanies a tracheitis or tracheobronchitis. The pain is searing and is most pronounced after cough. Invariably this central chest pain is associated with evidence of upper respiratory infection.

An uncommon type of respiratory pain is due to pulmonary hypertension. It is usually absent at rest and appears during exertion. The pain is substernal and is invariably associated with dyspnea; it subsides promptly when exercise stops. It is often mistaken for angina until the presence of pulmonary hypertension is uncovered.

Chest Wall Pain

In addition to pleuritic and tracheobronchial sources of chest pain, musculoskeletal pain originating in the muscles of the chest is a common disorder. A fractured rib is usually identified as the source of pain by history of injury, fall, or trauma accompanied by point tenderness and crepitus of the affected area. Chest radiography usually demonstrates the lesion.

The pain of a pulmonary sulcus tumor arises along the distribution of the eighth cervical and the first and second thoracic nerves. In Horner's syndrome, there is local destruction of bone by the tumor and atrophy of hand muscles. The chest radiograph is distinctive in showing a small, sharply defined shadow at one apex. Destruction of one or more of the upper three ribs posteriorly and of their adjacent transverse processes may also be observed.

Cardiac Pain

In addition to the pain of myocardial ischemia, another type of cardiac pain is that of pericarditis. Pericardial pain is often aggravated by deep breathing and is almost invariably accompanied by a telltale rub that is synchronous with the heartbeat. Another type of cardiac pain is the postcommissurotomy (postpericardiotomy) syndrome, which is characterized by chest pain that develops within a few days to weeks after cardiac surgery or pericardiotomy. The pain is usually sudden in onset and substernal, with radiation to the left side of the neck; often it is aggravated by deep breathing. Low-grade fever and a high sedimentation rate are regular concomitants.

Miscellaneous Sources of Chest Pain

Other structures in the mediastinum can be the source of chest pain. Noteworthy are the types of pain arising from the esophagus (peptic esophagitis) and dissection of the aorta. Their patterns and intensity serve to distinguish them from respiratory pain.

Arthritis of the cervical spine is a common cause of thoracic pain. Usually the cause is quite clear because of the characteristic distribution of the pain. Cervical spondylosis occasionally causes severe pain in the chest and arms, but it is more apt to mimic myocardial infarction than respiratory pain. A metastatic tumor to the thoracic spine often causes bilateral symmetrical pain, whereas unilateral pain, along with distribution of an intercostal nerve, is characteristic of herpes zoster before the appearance of a skin eruption.

Anxiety can produce or intensify the chest pain. Usually, pain related to anxiety is accompanied by dyspnea and hyperventilation. Manifestations of vasomotor instability—such as excessive palmar sweating, flushing, and tachycardia—may accompany the complaint of chest pain. The pain rarely conforms to a characteristic or consistent pattern. Anxiety also interferes with the quantification of pain originating in a somatic lesion and with its management.

FEVER

In the patient with lung disease, fever usually but not invariably signifies infection. When the lung disease is chronic, as in bronchitis and emphysema, a bout of acute bronchitis usually elicits only a modest fever, even though the sputum turns purulent. In contrast, an acute pneumonia or lung abscess may be associated with high fever.

Often overlooked at its outset is miliary tuberculosis, which occasionally escapes detection on the initial chest radiograph. Favoring this diagnosis is a history of recent contact with active tuberculosis, general malaise, easy fatigability, and anorexia during the previous few weeks.

Neoplasms are also associated with fever. In certain neoplasms, such as carcinoma of the bronchus, the fever is generally a secondary effect attributable to infection distal to obstruction; necrosis within the tumor is a less common cause. In others, such as hypernephroma, fever and chills are striking even though evidence of infection is absent. A mesothelioma of the pleura is often associated with fever; removal of the tumor is generally followed by defervescence. In patients with neoplasms who have no evidence of infection, necrosis within the tumor presumably leads to the elaboration of pyogenic substances within and around the tumor.

Extrinsic allergic alveolitis is sometimes followed by fever as well as by pulmonary disability after exposure to the offending antigen. Usually, the diagnosis poses no problem once the nature of the illness is suspected.

In contrast to the pulmonary disorders in which fever is a characteristic feature, pulmonary sarcoidosis is uncommonly associated with fever unless widespread extrapulmonary impairment or erythema nodosum coexists. Nor is pneumoconiosis associated with fever unless it is complicated by necrosis in the midst of conglomerate fibrosis or by superimposed tuberculosis. Among the other extensive disorders of the lungs that cause no fever (and few systemic complaints) are idiopathic pulmonary fibrosis, lymphangitic carcinomatosis, multiple pulmonary metastases, alveolar proteinosis, idiopathic pulmonary hemosiderosis, and alveolar microlithiasis.

RADIOLOGIC EVALUATION

The radiologic evaluation of the patient presenting with respiratory symptoms is dealt with in considerable detail elsewhere in this book. In recent years, the conventional chest radiograph has been supplemented by a succession of imaging techniques, such as computed tomography (CT), magnetic resonance imaging (MRI), and positron emission tomography (PET). Although these powerful tools are generally used as complementary techniques, they often assume primary roles (e.g., examination of the mediastinum for lymphadenopathy or invasion of the chest wall in a patient with carcinoma of the lung).

TESTS IN THE EVALUATION OF PULMONARY DISORDERS

Elsewhere in this book, pulmonary function testing is discussed in some detail. Often a combination of pulmonary function tests is needed to characterize a patient's abnormalities. Table 1-9 summarizes some practical initial approaches to pulmonary disorders.

TABLE 1-9 Practical Initial Approaches to Assessing Pulmonary Disorders[a]

Clinical state	First-order tests	Comments
Obstructive diseases of airways *Expiration*		
Asthma	FEV_1; before and after bronchodilator	Detect bronchospasm
	Arterial blood-gas levels	Increasing P_{CO_2} requires assisted ventilation
Chronic bronchitis	FEV_1; before and after bronchodilator	Degree of obstruction-reversibility
	Arterial blood-gas levels	Magnitude of ventilation-perfusion abnormalities
Emphysema	FEV_1	Degree of obstruction-reversibility
	Arterial blood-gas levels	Extent of ventilation-perfusion abnormalities
	Elastic recoil pressure	Abnormally low if emphysema predominates over bronchitis
Inspiration	FEV_1	Normal
	Maximal inspiratory and expiratory flow curves	Characteristic configurations of curves
Restrictive lung disease		
Diffuse interstitial inflammation, infiltration, fibrosis, thickened pleura	Chest radiograph	Characteristic patterns
	Lung volumes	Concentric reduction
	Arterial P_{O_2} at rest and exercise	Arterial hypoxemia during exercise
	Diffusing capacity	Conformity
Alveolar hypoventilation		
Secondary to obstructive disease of airways ("net")	Same as for obstructive diseases of airways	Seriously abnormal lungs
	Arterial blood-gas levels	Hypoxemia, hypercapnia, respiratory acidosis
Primary mechanism lungs, respiratory centers, chest bellows, coordinating mechanisms	FEV_1; spirometry	Normal
	Arterial blood-gas levels	Hypoxemia, hypercapnia, respiratory
	Response to assisted ventilation	Normalization of blood-gas levels
	Maximum inspiratory & expiratory pressures	Access muscle weakness
Obliterative pulmonary vascular disease	Chest radiograph	Characteristic
	Electrocardiogram	Right ventricular hypertrophy
	Spirometry; FEV_1	Normal
	Right-sided heart catheterization	Pulmonary hypertension
Complications or sources of ambiguity		
Respiratory failure	Arterial blood-gas levels; identify cause	Guide to therapy
Pulmonary congestion edema	Chest radiograph	Enlarged heart; vascular and interstitial
	Vital capacity	Response to diuretics and cardiotonic agents
Cyanosis		
Polycythemia vera	Spirometry; FEV_1; arterial blood-gas levels	All near normal
Anatomic right-to-left shunt	Arterial blood-gas levels	Severe hypoxemia without hypercapnia
Abnormal pigment	Arterial blood-gas levels; spectroscopy	Normal; identify pigments

[a]Emphasizing simplicity as well as specificity in substantiating clinical diagnosis.

PULMONARY NODULES

Solitary pulmonary nodules are usually asymptomatic and are discovered on the chest radiograph. (See Chap. 3.) Distinction is made between a nodule, which is 3 cm or less in diameter, and a mass, which is larger and usually less well defined. This distinction has both diagnostic and prognostic implications, because a mass is more apt to be neoplastic than is a nodule.

Solitary Pulmonary Nodule

The frequency with which solitary nodules prove to be malignant depends on the population under study. In parts of the country that are endemic for histoplasmosis and coccidioidomycosis, the frequency of malignant nodules in the general population is low—10 to 15 percent. In surgical series that include a large number of heavy smokers, the incidence of malignant lesions will be much higher—30 to 50 percent. With these reservations in mind, Table 1-10 provides some idea of the incidence of various etiologies of solitary pulmonary nodules based on published reports.

Because the incidence of malignancy in solitary nodules is high and because a malignant solitary nodule should be removed promptly if there is no evidence of local or distant spread, evaluation of a solitary nodule is pursued

---

TABLE 1-10 Causes of Multiple Pulmonary Nodules

Malignant nodules
  Metastatic malignancy
  Alveolar cell carcinoma of the lung, multicentric lymphomas
  Multiple primary neoplasms (bronchogenic carcinomas, adenomas)
  Plasmacytomas
  Lymphomatoid granulomas
Benign nodules
  Neoplasms
   Hamartomas
   Juvenile papillomatosis
   Chondromas
   Benign metastasizing leiomyomas
  Other benign lesions
   Infectious granulomas (tuberculosis, atypical mycobacterial infection,
   histoplasmosis, coccidioidomycosis)
   Pyogenic abscesses
   Noninfectious granulomas (sarcoid, Wegener's, rheumatoid nodules,
   paraffinomas, lymphomatoid granulomatosis)
   Vasculitis
   Parasitic (paragonimiasis, hydatid cysts, dirofilariasis)
   Pneumoconioses
   Bronchial lesions (cystic bronchiectasis, mucoid impaction syndrome,
   allergic bronchopulmonary aspergillosis)
   Rheumatoid nodules
   Multiple mycetomas
   Multiple amyloidomas
   Arteriovenous malformations
   Sjögren's disease (pseudolymphomas)
Combinations (neoplastic and inflammatory)

SOURCE: Modified after Table 124-2 of Lillington GA."Systematic Diagnostic Approach to Pulmonary Nodules." In: Fishman AP, *Pulmonary Diseases and Disorders,* 2d ed. New York, McGraw-Hill, 1988, p 1951.

aggressively. Several criteria favor benignity: (1) the absence of risk factors, e.g., the patient is a nonsmoker; (2) the patient is <35 years old; (3) the absence of current or prior primary extrapulmonary tumor; (4) a nodule that is small, circumscribed, and has not grown radiographically for 2 or more years; and (5) a distinctive pattern of calcification (see below). Of these five criteria, the last two carry the most weight. Although it is reasonable to use these criteria to determine the aggressiveness with which histologic proof of the nature of the lesion is sought, final proof of benignity often rests on histologic diagnosis.

Chest Radiography

Chest radiography is pivotal to the diagnosis and management of pulmonary nodules (see Chap. 3). Benign solitary nodules are usually small, with distinct margins. Cavitation is uncommon. Calcification, if present, can be helpful in establishing the benign nature of the nodule. Calcification is common in benign nodules, especially in healed infectious granulomas, and rare in malignant nodules. For example, central, laminated, diffuse, and popcorn patterns occur almost exclusively in benign lesions.

The standard chest radiograph may fail to disclose calcification in a nodule. Chest radiographs enable measurement of the diameter of the nodule, assessment of the nature of its edge (fuzzy edges and protrusions are usually malignant), and detection of calcification. CT has largely replaced conventional chest tomography as a follow-up in the search for calcification. CT is not only more effective in uncovering calcification and delineating the edge of the nodule but may also disclose other nodules that were indiscernible on the conventional chest radiograph. It also enables examination of the mediastinum and hilar areas for adenopathy and, if adenopathy is present, for staging.

Growth Rate and Doubling Times

The time that it takes for the nodule to double its volume radiographically (doubling time) is much less for a benign than for a malignant lesion—e.g., of the order of 20 to 400 days for a malignant lesion versus >400 days for a benign lesion. (A benign lesion usually does not grow at all; in contrast, an acute infectious nodule may have a doubling time of 2 to 3 weeks or less.)

Primary Carcinoma of the Lung as a Solitary Nodule

About 40 percent of solitary nodules are malignant. Of these, about three-quarters (30 percent) are bronchogenic carcinomas. Adenocarcinomas and squamous cell carcinomas are the more common and occur with about the same frequency; the incidence of large-cell carcinomas is somewhat less. Small-cell carcinomas and carcinoids rarely present as solitary nodules.

The guiding principle in dealing with a solitary nodule is that it must be promptly removed unless it can be proved to be benign. The criteria useful as a guide to benignity have been noted above. However, if doubt remains, histologic proof is required. Bronchoscopy is often a preliminary if the nodule is located centrally, less for histology than searching for airway lesions or extrinsic compression by cancerous nodes. Transthoracic needle aspiration is much more rewarding; it provides histologic diagnosis in 80 to 95 percent of malignant nodules. Thoracoscopy and thoracotomy are the most reliable but are also more invasive. Mediastinoscopy is generally reserved for those patients.

Solitary Metastatic Nodule

About 5 to 10 percent of solitary pulmonary nodules are metastatic. Histologic evidence is often required to settle whether a lesion is primary in the lungs or arises elsewhere. However, this histologic distinction is not always easy to make. Adenocarcinomas are particularly troublesome in this regard. In patients who are known to have extrapulmonary primary neoplasms, the likelihood that a solitary nodule is a metastasis to the lungs increases greatly; 25 to 50 percent of solitary nodules in these patients are metastatic. Surgical resection is commonly done for a solitary metastatic nodule, but the influence of this intervention on the course of the disease is unclear.

Benign Solitary Nodule

About 50 percent of all solitary nodules are infectious granulomas. The major interest in these lesions is to prove that they are not neoplastic. Often this can be done by taking into account the history of exposure (e.g., coccidioidomycosis); by skin testing (e.g., tuberculosis); and by serial chest radiographs (e.g., at monthly intervals to determine rate and pattern of growth or resolution). Histologic evidence is obtained by bronchoscopy, needle biopsy, thoracoscopic biopsy, or thoracotomy. Of these procedures, bronchoscopy is least likely to establish that a lesion is benign; needle biopsy is apt to provide proof of benignity in only about 50 percent of patients. Thoracoscopy and thoracotomy are much more rewarding.

Multiple Pulmonary Nodules

A wide variety of etiologies can cause multiple pulmonary nodules (see Table 1-10). However, widespread metastatic carcinoma is the most common cause. Cavitation is common. Usually, metastatic nodules are peripheral or subpleural in location. Both lungs are usually involved and the lesions are more often at the bases. As a rule, the primary extrapulmonary site is known or materializes in the course of workup or serial observations. However, in some instances, despite intensive search, an extrapulmonary site cannot be identified.

In metastatic lesions, the nodules usually grow rapidly and new nodules generally appear in the course of serial radiographs. CT scanning can reveal multiple nodules that are not evident on the chest radiograph. However, CT can be a mixed blessing. Indeed, it has the potential for creating ambiguity by uncovering not only malignant lesions but also artifacts and residua of old inflammatory processes that may be indistinguishable from neoplastic nodules. Histologic evidence obtained by biopsy is prerequisite for treatment of malignant lesions.

Approach to Management

The probability that a solitary pulmonary nodule is malignant is the most important guide to therapy: the lower the probability of cancer, the more reasonable the "wait and see" approach. On the other hand, when probability is high—as in the older patient with a lesion that radiographically shows fuzzy or spiculated margins, a history of smoking, and rapid growth—early histologic diagnosis is critical.

BIBLIOGRAPHY

Caskey CI, Templeton PA, Zerhouni EA: Current evaluation of the solitary pulmonary nodule. *Radiol Clin North Am* 28:511–521, 1990.

Jaakkola MS, Jaakkola JJK, Ernst P, Becklake MP: Respiratory symptoms should not be overlooked. *Am Rev Respir Dis* 147:359–366, 1993.

Johnston H, Reisz G: Changing spectrum of hemoptysis. *Arch Intern Med* 149:1666–1668, 1989.

Kamin SS (ed): Lung sounds. *Semin Respir Med* 6:157–242, 1985.

Lemanske RF, Busse WW: Asthma. *JAMA* 278:1855–1873,1997.

Lillington GA: Investigating solitary pulmonary nodules. *Intern Med* 21:11–17, 2000.

Mahler DA, Horowitz MB: Clinical evaluation of exertional dyspnea. *Clin Chest Med* 15:259–269, 1994.

Miller DL, Allen MS, Deschamps C, et al: Video-assisted thoracic surgical procedure: Management of a solitary pulmonary nodule. *Mayo Clin Proc* 67:462–464, 1992.

Ost D, Fein A: Evaluation and management of the solitary pulmonary nodule. *Am J Respir Crit Care Med* 162:782–787, 2000.

Patrick H, Patrick FG: Chronic cough. *Med Clin North Am* 79:361–372, 1995.

Sharma OP: Symptoms and signs in pulmonary medicine: Old observations and new interpretations. *Dis Mon* 41:577–638, 1995.

Viggiano RW, Swenson SJ, Rosenow EC III: Evaluation and management of solitary and multiple pulmonary nodules. *Clin Chest Med* 13:83–95, 1992.

DIAGNOSTIC PROCEDURES

2 | Pulmonary Function and Cardiopulmonary Exercise Testing*

Michael A. Grippi and Lisa M. Bellini

INTRODUCTION

Pulmonary function testing and assessment of integrated cardiovascular and pulmonary performance during exercise constitute important diagnostic techniques commonly used to assess a wide variety of disorders affecting the lungs and cardiovascular system. Standardized test approaches have been developed that enable comparisons of results obtained sequentially in the same laboratory as well as those derived from different laboratories.

MECHANICAL PROPERTIES OF THE RESPIRATORY SYSTEM

The total volume of gas in the lungs is conventionally subdivided into compartments (*volumes*) and combinations of two or more volumes (*capacities*). For many of these subdivisions, the end-expiratory volume—the volume of gas remaining in the lungs at the end of normal expiration—is the point of reference. Lung volumes and capacities are depicted schematically in Fig. 2-1.

The elastic properties of the respiratory system are altered by diseases that affect the lung parenchyma or, less commonly, the chest wall. *Static lung compliance* (Cst,L) is a measure of lung distensibility and is determined over the linear portion of the pressure-volume curve of the lung. Cst,L decreases with age and is higher in males than in females. In diseases characterized by increased elastic recoil pressure (e.g., interstitial fibrosis), static lung compliance decreases, as do *functional residual capacity* (FRC) and *total lung capacity* (TLC). In contrast, in emphysema, lung elastic recoil pressure is reduced, while lung compliance, TLC, and FRC are increased. Disorders of the chest wall (e.g., obesity, kyphoscoliosis, and fibrothorax) limit chest wall excursion and lung expansion and reduce FRC. In addition, they produce decreases in static compliance of the lung and chest wall and maximal recoil pressure.

*Edited from Chap. 36, "Pulmonary Function Testing," by Grippi MA, Metzger LF, Sacks AV, Fishman AP, and Chap. 37, "Principles and Applications of Cardiopulmonary Exercise Testing," by Weber KT. In: *Fishman's Pulmonary Diseases and Disorders,* 3d ed., edited by Fishman AP, Elias JA, Fishman JA, Grippi MA, Kaiser LR, Senior RM. New York, McGraw-Hill, 1998, pp 533–588. For fuller discussion of topics dealt with in this chapter, the reader is referred to the original text, as noted above.

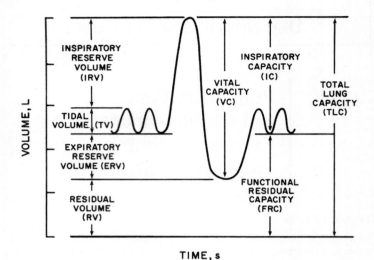

FIG. 2-1 The subdivisions of lung volume as recorded by a spirometer. The record is generated on paper calibrated for volume in the vertical direction and time in the horizontal. The term *capacity* is applied to a subdivision composed of two or more *volumes.*

Ventilatory performance also depends on respiratory muscle strength. The maximal pressure generated by an isometric contraction varies directly with the resting muscle length. When TLC is less than 70 percent of predicted, *maximal expiratory pressure* (PE_{max}) is low. When RV exceeds 40 percent of predicted, *maximal inspiratory pressure* (PI_{max}) is low. Maximal inspiratory and expiratory pressures can be measured using an aneroid vacuum and pressure gauge.

Additional information can be gained from tests done during airflow—i.e., under "dynamic" conditions. These tests are included under the designation *spirometry,* discussed below.

Forced Vital Capacity

Expiratory and inspiratory measurements of the *forced vital capacity* (FVC) are standard in pulmonary function laboratories. Unless otherwise specified, FVC refers to the forced *expiratory* maneuver. The FVC maneuver entails a full inspiration to total lung capacity followed by a rapid, forceful, maximal expiration to *residual volume* (RV). The FVC is normally equal to the slow *vital capacity* (VC), which represents a more relaxed expiration to RV. In obstructive disease of the airways, the FVC is less than the VC. The FVC is displayed in one of two ways: expired volume plotted against time or airflow plotted against lung volume—i.e., an expiratory "flow-volume curve."

Values determined from the volume-time plot of the forced vital capacity include (1) the *volume expired in the first second,* expressed either as an absolute volume (FEV_1) or as a percentage of the forced vital capacity (FEV_1/FVC%); (2) the *volume expired in the first 3 s,* expressed either as an absolute volume (FEV_3) or as a percentage of the forced vital capacity

(FEV$_3$/FVC%); and (3) the *forced midexpiratory flow rate* (FEF$_{25-75\%}$). The FEF$_{25-75\%}$ is determined by locating the points on the volume-time curve corresponding to 25 and 75 percent of the FVC and then calculating the slope of a straight line passing through those two points. The slope of this line represents the average airflow over the midportion of the FVC.

Although the slow vital capacity (VC) may be normal or only modestly reduced in obstructive airway disease, the volume-time relationship of the FVC maneuver is usually distinctly abnormal. The slope of the curve is flattened at any given lung volume, reflecting reduced airflow. In addition, the duration of the forced expiratory maneuver is prolonged. Normally, expiration is complete within 5 s; in obstructive airway disease, expiratory airflow may continue for 10 to 12 s. These changes in expiratory airflow reduce the FEV$_1$ and FEV$_3$, FEV$_1$/FVC%, FEV$_3$/FVC%, and FEF$_{25-75\%}$.

Restrictive lung disorders reduce the slow vital capacity. However, the *configuration* of the volume-time relationship may not be abnormal. Although the FEV$_1$ and FEV$_3$ are reduced because of the reduced vital capacity, the FEV$_1$/FVC% and FEV$_3$/FVC% remain normal or even exceed normal values. Often, because of the reduced vital capacity, the FEF$_{25-75\%}$ is also less than predicted.

Measurement of the *forced inspiratory vital capacity* (FIVC) involves full expiration to residual volume, followed by a rapid maximal inspiratory effort. The rate of airflow over the middle half of the forced inspiratory vital capacity (FIF$_{25-75\%}$) is determined using a procedure similar to that described previously for the FEF$_{25-75\%}$. In normal subjects, the FIF$_{25-75\%}$ is greater than the FEF$_{25-75\%}$. When airway resistance is high, a disproportionate fall in FIF$_{25-75\%}$ relative to FEF$_{25-75\%}$ suggests an extrathoracic site of airway obstruction.

Flow-Volume Curve

A *flow-volume curve* shows the relationship between lung volume and maximal airflow as lung volume changes during a forced expiration. While breathing into a spirometer, the subject makes several tidal breaths and then a maximal inspiratory effort to TLC followed by a maximal expiration to RV. Subsequently, another maximal inspiratory effort to TLC is made. Volume is displayed on the horizontal axis and airflow on the vertical axis.

Maximal Voluntary Ventilation

The *maximal voluntary ventilation* (MVV) depends on the movement of air into and out of the lungs during continued maximal effort throughout a preset interval. The MVV is a simple, informative test that provides an overall assessment of effort, coordination, and the elastic and flow-resistive properties of the respiratory system. In performing the test, the patient is urged to breathe as hard and as fast as possible. The total volume that is expired during a 12-s interval, expressed in liters per minute (BTPS), is the maximal voluntary ventilation. The difference between the MVV and the resting minute ventilation is the *breathing reserve*.

Airway Resistance

Total respiratory resistance is the resistance to airflow and chest expansion offered by the airways, chest wall, and lung tissue. The only clinically useful measurement of resistance is airway resistance (Raw), defined as the ratio of driving pressure to airflow along the airways (i.e., the mouth, nasopharynx, larynx, and central and peripheral airways). Raw varies inversely with lung volume, increasing curvilinearly as lung volume and, consequently, airway diameters are reduced. In contrast, the inverse of Raw, *airway conductance,* is linearly related to lung volume. Interpretation of a given value for Raw or airway conductance requires that the lung volume at which the measurement is made be taken into account. *Specific conductance* (SGaw) is calculated by dividing airway conductance by the lung volume.

AIRWAY REACTIVITY

Bronchoprovocation tests quantify bronchoconstriction following exposure to particular inhaled agents (methacholine, histamine, or carbacholine), specific antigens, inhalation of cold or dry air, isocapnic hyperventilation, or exercise. The principal indication for bronchoprovocation testing is a history suggestive of bronchospasm induced by an environmental or occupational agent in the setting of normal pulmonary function tests, including determination of airflow before and after administering a bronchodilator.

Methacholine evokes constriction of both the central and peripheral airways. The delivered dose of methacholine corresponding to the point at which the FEV_1 is 80 percent of the control FEV_1 is designated as the *provocation dose,* or PD_{20} FEV_1. If specific conductance (SGaw) is used as the index of bronchial reactivity, the dose that produces a 35 percent drop in the baseline SGaw is regarded as the "provocation dose" and is designated as PD_{35} SGaw.

Persons without a history of asthma who develop cough, wheezing, or dyspnea after exercise may have *exercise-induced asthma* (EIA). Measurement of FEV_1 and peak expiratory flow just before and immediately after exercise and at 2- to 5-min intervals for 30 min make up the test for EIA. A decrease in FEV_1 of 10 percent or more below the preexercise value constitutes a positive test.

Bronchoprovocation testing with a specific antigen is unpredictable and potentially hazardous. Too much of the antigen may be given, and a late response, far more severe than the initial one, often develops about 6 h after the challenge. However, testing may be warranted to uncover a particular agent in the environment that causes bronchoconstriction, to establish the diagnosis of occupational asthma, or to prove that bronchoconstriction is caused by a particular antigen after routine skin tests have failed to support the clinical suspicion.

In patients who manifest appreciable airway obstruction by conventional testing (e.g., $FEV_1/FVC\% < 70$), life-threatening airway narrowing during a bronchoprovocation test may occur. In such patients, a bronchodilator study is more appropriate.

SMALL AIRWAY FUNCTION

Normally, the peripheral airways contribute little to total airway resistance; hence, the small airways can undergo considerable damage before the usual tests of lung function become abnormal. With obstruction of peripheral airways, their contribution to overall resistance increases and the narrowing may be evident as an isolated reduction in the $FEF_{25-75\%}$. The basis for this finding is that $FEF_{25-75\%}$ measures airflow during the effort-independent part of the FVC, when the small airways contribute substantially to the limitation of airflow. Small airways obstruction also results in abnormal distribution of ventilation to peripheral lung units, as assessed by tests of frequency dependence of dynamic compliance and closing volume. The helium-oxygen flow-volume curve is also used to assess small airways function.

Dynamic compliance—the change in lung volume during airflow produced by a given change in transpulmonary pressure—is normally independent of breathing frequency. However, under conditions of nonuniformity of ventilation throughout the lung, increases in breathing frequency are associated with a fall in dynamic compliance. In normal subjects, Cdyn,L/Cst,L remains above 0.8, even at frequencies greater than 60 breaths per minute. However, in the presence of obstructive disease of the small airways, Cdyn,L/Cst,L falls progressively to values below 0.8 as breathing frequency increases. The interpretation of frequency dependence of compliance with regard to small airway disease is valid only if the static compliance and overall airway resistance are normal.

Measurement of *closing volume*—the lung volume at which small airways close during expiration—entails measurement of expired volume and N_2 concentration in the expirate after a maximal breath of 100 percent O_2. The initial expirate contains virtually no N_2, since it derives from the O_2-containing dead space. The second phase represents a mixture of gases from the dead space and the alveoli, while the third phase represents a mixture of gases from alveoli located at the apices, midlung fields, and bases. The final phase, characterized by an upward shift in N_2 concentration, is attributable to closure of alveoli in the dependent parts of the lungs at low lung volumes and preferential emptying of alveoli in the middle and upper lung regions. The volume from the onset of the final phase of the tracing to the completion of the full expiratory maneuver is termed the *closing volume* (CV), generally expressed as a percentage of the VC. The *closing capacity* (CC), expressed as a percentage of TLC, is calculated by adding RV to CV and dividing the sum by TLC. In healthy young adults, normal CV averages about 10 percent of VC. Narrowing or obstruction of peripheral airways causes CV to enlarge. CV also increases progressively with aging, so that by the age of 50, CV may reach 25 percent of VC. Cigarette smokers consistently demonstrate an increase in CV.

In normal subjects, at lung volumes greater than 10 percent of VC, the primary site of resistance to airflow is in the larger airways, where flow is turbulent and, therefore, density-dependent. At these lung volumes, the flow attained with breathing a less dense helium-oxygen mixture is higher than that attained with breathing air. At lung volumes less than 10 percent of the VC, the primary site of resistance is in the smaller airways, where flow is laminar and, therefore, not density-dependent. In this circumstance, the helium-oxygen mixture has no effect on flow. In disease of the small airways, the primary site of resistance shifts at large volumes from the larger to the smaller airways. As a result, the flow-enhancing effect of the less dense gas disappears at volumes well above 10 percent of the VC.

Comparison of the helium-oxygen and room air flow-volume curves is made at 50 percent of VC (the $\Delta\dot{V}_{max}$, 50 percent) and at the volume at which the flows become identical [*volume of isoflow* (Viso $\dot{V}$)]. As noted previously, the volume of isoflow is normally less than 10 percent of VC; when it is increased, it indicates small airway obstruction.

Despite their intellectual appeal, the practical value of helium-oxygen flow-volume curves in detecting small airway disease is debatable.

GAS EXCHANGE FUNCTIONS

The gas exchange function of the lung is assessed by measurement of the *diffusing capacity* for carbon monoxide ($D_{L_{CO}}$), known in Europe as the transfer factor. $D_{L_{CO}}$ can be determined by steady-state, rebreathing, and single-breath methods.

A reduction in the lung volume alone can reduce the $D_{L_{CO}}$, as may ventilation/perfusion inequalities and anemia. The blood of a heavy smoker sometimes contains as much as 10 percent COHb. Such levels of COHb are accompanied by appreciable concentrations of dissolved CO in the plasma. The resulting back pressure of CO reduces the $D_{L_{CO}}$. Conversely, polycythemia, intrapulmonary hemorrhage, and high altitude increase $D_{L_{CO}}$ (Pa_{O_2} falls with increasing altitude and the reduction in Pa_{O_2} allows CO to diffuse more rapidly into the blood).

CONTROL OF BREATHING

The rate, depth, and pattern of breathing reflect a complex interplay of neurohumoral and chemical regulatory mechanisms that drive the respiratory apparatus. Evaluation of control of breathing is based on assessment of the ventilatory response to controlled hypercapnia or hypoxia.

Ventilatory Response to Hypercapnia

The ventilatory response to changes in Pa_{CO_2} is linear over a broad range. Blunting of the ventilatory response is seen in endurance athletes, with aging, and in certain racial groups (e.g., the Enges of New Guinea). Low concentrations of bicarbonate in serum and in the brain enhance the response; high concentrations of bicarbonate have the opposite effect. Aminophylline, salicylates, thyroxine, and progesterone increase responsiveness, whereas narcotics, barbiturates, and other central nervous system (CNS) depressants decrease it. Finally, the ventilatory response to CO_2 is sometimes reduced in certain neurologic diseases (e.g., encephalitis and brainstem disease), metabolic disorders (e.g., myxedema), obesity-hypoventilation syndrome, and chronic obstructive pulmonary disease.

Ventilatory Response to Hypoxia

The response to hypoxemia is curvilinear; the magnitude depends on the Pa_{CO_2}, increasing as the concentration of CO_2 in arterial blood increases. Tests for assessing the ventilatory response to hypoxia are also based on steady-state and non–steady-state methods. A high ventilatory response to CO_2 may be associated with a high sensitivity to hypoxia. In addition, at higher levels of arterial P_{CO_2}, the ventilatory response to hypoxia increases. Native residents at high altitude and persons with cyanotic congenital heart disease manifest a diminished sensitivity to acute hypoxia. In cardiac patients, hypoxic insensitivity is reversed after successful surgery. The normal aging process is also associated with a depressed response, as are a variety of other clinical disorders, including myxedema and hypothyroidism, autonomic nervous system dysfunction, carotid endarterectomy, chronic narcotic addiction, and the chronic use of methadone.

APPROACH TO INTERPRETING PULMONARY FUNCTION TESTS

As a rule, results of pulmonary function tests are interpreted with respect to predicted values for normal subjects. For most pulmonary function tests, normal values fall in a broad range that is assumed to follow a normal (Gaussian) distribution. Traditionally, but without sound statistical basis, most laboratories have arbitrarily set upper and lower limits of normal as well as gradations of abnormality, using percentage of predicted normal mean values.

Two alternative methods for expressing results have been proposed. One, the *95 percentile method,* defines the lower limit of normal as the value above which lie values for 95 percent of the normal population. The other method uses *95 percent confidence intervals.* This method defines the limits of normal as the predicted value plus or minus the 95 percent confidence interval. The degree of abnormality for a particular test is expressed in terms of the *number* of 95 percent confidence intervals above or below the predicted normal; this number is calculated as the predicted normal value minus the measured value, divided by the confidence interval.

Classification of Abnormal Patterns

The following categories of test pattern abnormalities are practical for clinical use: (1) *obstructive* (due to airway narrowing and reduced airflow), (2) *restrictive* (due to diseases of the lung, chest wall, pleural space, or neuromuscular respiratory apparatus that reduce the vital capacity and lung volumes), (3) *combined obstructive-restrictive* (due to pathologic processes that reduce lung volumes, vital capacity, and airflow and that also include an element of airway narrowing), and (4) *abnormal gas transfer* (in which an abnormality in the alveolar-capillary membrane impairs oxygen uptake from alveolar gas to pulmonary capillary blood). Overlap among categories is not uncommon.

Analysis of test results begins with assessment of respiratory muscle strength; peak inspiratory and expiratory pressures provide an index of patient effort. In addition, a poor response calls attention to the possibility of neuromuscular or respiratory disease. Next, $FEV_1/FVC\%$, FVC, and FEV_1 are examined in turn. This panel of studies constitutes "screening spirometry" and may suffice to exclude significant disease. If the results are abnormal, additional insight may be gained from examination of the lung volumes. Finally, the $D_{L_{CO}}$ is determined and interpreted with regard to any abnormalities that may have been uncovered by the tests.

Assessing Respiratory Muscle Strength and Effort

Respiratory muscle strength is expressed in terms of peak inspiratory (PI_{max}) and peak expiratory (PE_{max}) pressures. Suboptimal effort, fatigue, weakness of the respiratory muscles, deformity of the chest wall, or intrinsic diseases of the lungs or chest wall may reduce the measurements. Although the first three factors noted characteristically reduce both peak inspiratory and expiratory pressures, disease of the lungs or chest wall often reduces, selectively, one or the other. Thus, diseases that reduce lung volumes (e.g., widespread interstitial fibrosis) and shorten the length of the expiratory muscles at the end-inspiratory position generally reduce maximal expiratory pressure. Conversely, diseases that increase lung volume, such as obstructive airway disease, increase inspiratory muscle length at end-expiration and generally reduce maximal inspiratory pressure. Consistently low values on spirometry despite maximal patient effort, coupled with reduced maximal pressures, may signal neuromuscular disease.

Obstructive Pattern

Included in this group of disorders are chronic obstructive diseases of the airways (chronic bronchitis and emphysema), cystic fibrosis, asthma, small

TABLE 2-1 Categorization of Obstruction: Measurement of FEV$_1$/FVC%

| | % Predicted Method | | 95% Confidence Interval (CI) Method | |
| | | | Predicted Minus Measured FEV$_1$/FVC% | |
Category	Absolute FEV$_1$/FVC%	No. CIs below mean	Male	Female
Normal	>69	<1	<8.3	<9.1
Mild obstruction	61–69	≥1–<2	8.3–16.5	9.1–18.1
Moderate obstruction	45–60	≥2–<4	16.6–33.1	18.2–36.3
Severe obstruction	<45	≥4	≥33.2	≥36.4

SOURCE: From Kanner and Morris: *Clinical Pulmonary Function Testing: A Manual of Uniform Laboratory Procedures.* Salt Lake City, Intermountain Thoracic Society, 1975.

airway disease, and upper airway obstruction. Except for diseases confined to the small airways, the hallmark of the obstructive pattern is a reduction in the FEV$_1$/FVC%. This measurement is also useful in quantifying the magnitude of the disorder (Table 2-1). In addition, the FEV$_1$ is consistently reduced and usually accompanied by a reduction in FVC. As a rule, the slow vital capacity is also low. A greater reduction in the forced vital capacity than in the slow vital capacity indicates air trapping. Changes in lung volume commonly accompany the abnormal findings on spirometry. Frequently, but not invariably, lung volumes are elevated. The increase in TLC or RV is useful in quantifying the degree of "hyperinflation" (Table 2-2).

The response to inhaled bronchodilators (Table 2-3) is helpful in distinguishing between chronic obstructive pulmonary disease (COPD) and asthma. Inhalation of a bronchodilator significantly improves expiratory airflow in asthma but not in chronic bronchitis or emphysema. One indication of responsiveness to a bronchodilator is a decrease in lung volumes.

TABLE 2-2 Categorization of Hyperinflation: Measurement of TLC and RV

| | % Predicted Method | | 95% Confidence Interval (CI) Method | |
| | | | Measured Minus Predicted TLC, L | |
Category	TLC or RV, % Predicted	No. CIs above mean TLC	Male	Female
Normal[a]	≤120	<1.0	<1.61	<1.08
Mild hyperinflation	121–<134	≥1.0–<1.5	1.61–2.41	1.08–1.61
Moderate hyperinflation	135–<149	≥1.5–<2.0	2.42–3.21	1.62–2.15
Severe hyperinflation	≥150	≥2	≥3.22	≥2.16

[a]The classification of normal is based additionally on a difference between predicted and measured RV of <0.76 L for males and <0.78 L for females. Differences in RV exceeding these values when differences in TLC are normal are suggestive of hyperinflation.
SOURCE: From Kanner and Morris: *Clinical Pulmonary Function Testing: A Manual of Uniform Laboratory Procedures.* Salt Lake City, Intermountain Thoracic Society, 1975.

TABLE 2-3 Categorization of Bronchodilator Response: Measurement of Vital Capacity and Expiratory Flow Rates before and after Bronchodilator Administration

Category	Measurement[a]		
	FVC	FEV_1	$FEF_{25-75\%}$
Not responsive	<1.05	<1.05	<1.10
Not clearly responsive	1.05–1.14	1.05–1.11	1.10–1.44
Responsive	1.15–1.24	1.12–1.24	1.45–1.99
Markedly responsive	≥1.25	≥1.25	≥2.00

[a]Each value represents the ratio of the measurement made after administration of a bronchodilator to that made before.
SOURCE: From Kanner and Morris: *Clinical Pulmonary Function Testing: A Manual of Uniform Laboratory Procedures.* Salt Lake City, Intermountain Thoracic Society, 1975.

Although chronic bronchitis and emphysema usually coexist, they occasionally exist in virtually pure forms. Measurement of $D_{L_{CO}}$ can help make the distinction. Emphysema, characterized by a loss of alveolar units and a decrease in alveolar surface area, is associated with a low $D_{L_{CO}}$, whereas the $D_{L_{CO}}$ in chronic bronchitis is usually normal or near normal.

In obstructive disease of the small airways (less than 2 mm in diameter), expiratory flow is usually normal except at low lung volumes; i.e., the FEV_3 and $FEF_{25-75\%}$ are reduced. Other tests of small airway function—including the helium-oxygen flow-volume loop, nitrogen washout test, and frequency dependence of dynamic compliance—are also usually abnormal. Lung volumes and $D_{L_{CO}}$ are normal. Bronchodilators are virtually without effect. The practical value of tests of small airway function is problematic. Enthusiasm for testing for small airway disease has waned, since it is still unclear whether small airway disease is a reversible phase in the evolution of clinically significant obstructive airway disease that affects larger bronchi.

Upper Airway Obstruction

The designation *upper airway obstruction* (UAO) is an umbrella for anatomic or functional narrowing of the large upper airways—the larynx, extra- and intrathoracic trachea, and lobar bronchi. Although upper airway obstruction of any cause (see Chap. 11) may reduce expiratory or inspiratory airflow, an alteration in the contour of the flow-volume loop has proved to be the most reliable abnormality in conventional pulmonary function testing. Three major functional categories of UAO are recognized: (1) fixed obstruction, (2) variable extrathoracic obstruction, and (3) variable intrathoracic obstruction.

A *fixed obstruction,* such as tracheal narrowing by scar tissue at the site of a previous tracheotomy, is one in which the geometry and cross-sectional area of the lesion do not change during the respiratory cycle. Characteristically, both inspiratory and expiratory flows are affected about equally (Fig. 2-2*A*).

A *variable obstruction* is one in which the configuration of the obstructive lesion changes with the phases of respiration. Depending on its location in the tracheobronchial tree (extra- or intrathoracic), this type of lesion usually affects predominantly either inspiration or expiration. The inspiratory arm of the flow-volume loop is primarily affected by a *variable extrathoracic* obstruction, leaving the expiratory limb relatively unaffected (Fig. 2-2*B*).

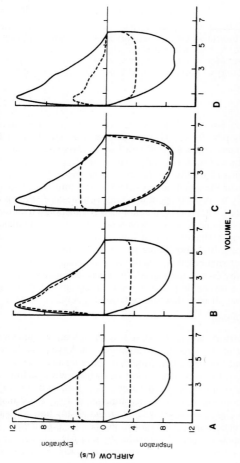

FIG. 2-2 Schematic flow-volume loops in four pathologic conditions (each depicted by broken line in figure). *A.* In a fixed upper airway obstruction, both inspiratory and expiratory limbs are truncated. *B.* In a variable extrathoracic obstruction, the inspiratory limb is flattened while the expiratory limb is not altered. *C.* In a variable intrathoracic obstruction, the expiratory limb is flattened while the inspiratory portion is unchanged. *D.* In chronic obstructive airway disease, although expiratory airflow is reduced, the tapering in airflow during expiration is generally maintained so that the configuration of the loop is different from that in variable intrathoracic obstruction.

During forced expiration, tracheal pressure exceeds atmospheric, so that the degree of obstruction decreases; conversely, during forced inspiration, intratracheal pressure becomes less than atmospheric and the trachea tends to collapse. The expiratory arm of the flow-volume loop is primarily affected by a *variable intrathoracic* obstruction (Fig. 2-2C). In this case, during forced expiration, as pleural pressure reaches and then exceeds intratracheal pressure downstream from the lesion (i.e., toward the mouth), the obstruction tends to increase; conversely, during a forced inspiration, as intratracheal pressure exceeds pleural pressure, the intrathoracic obstruction decreases.

Not infrequently, variable intrathoracic lesions coexist with obstructive airway disease. Although both UAO and obstructive airway disease (reversible and irreversible) decrease maximal expiratory flow, the shapes of the flow-volume cures are frequently quite distinctive (Fig. 2-2C and D). In obstructive airway disease, despite a decrease in airflow, the expiratory limb of the loop generally retains its normal configuration (Fig. 2-2D)—i.e., an early peak in flow, followed by gradual tapering. In contrast, in UAO (fixed and variable intrathoracic), the expiratory limb is flat and flow is decreased throughout most of expiration (Fig. 2-2C).

In addition to changes in the shape of the flow-volume loop, clues from routine pulmonary function tests may signal the possibility of UAO: (1) $FEF_{50\%}/FIF_{50\%}$ of at least 1, where $FEF_{50\%}$ and $FIF_{50\%}$ are the forced expiratory flow at 50 percent of FVC and the forced inspiratory flow at 50 percent of FIVC, respectively; (2) $FEV_1/PEFR$ greater than 10 ml/L/min, where PEFR is the peak expiratory flow; (3) $FIF_{50\%}$ less than 100 L/min; and (4) $FEV_1/FEV_{0.5}$ of at least 1.5.

Restrictive Pattern

The restrictive pattern characteristically occurs in several groups of disorders: (1) a primary disorder of the lung parenchyma in which functional tissue is lost through disease (e.g., an alveolar filling process, such as pneumonia, tumor, atelectasis, or fibrosis); (2) surgical removal of lung tissue (e.g., lobectomy); (3) constrictive disease of the pleura and chest wall (e.g., extensive pleural fibrosis, large pleural effusion or pleural mass, kyphoscoliosis, obesity); and (4) neuromuscular diseases, notably those in which the generation of respiratory force is reduced (e.g., disorders of the spinal cord, peripheral nerves, neuromuscular junction, and muscle).

The hallmark of the restrictive pattern is a reduction in the vital capacity, accompanied by a proportional drop in the FEV_1. As a result, $FEV_1/FVC\%$ remains normal. Indeed, not uncommonly, because of an increase in elastic recoil pressure caused by many of the disease processes that evoke a restrictive pattern, $FEV_1/FVC\%$ is greater than normal. Characteristically, lung volumes are reduced. However, different compartments are primarily affected in the four categories enumerated above. TLC generally is reduced in all. However, while FRC is usually preserved in disorders characterized by decreased respiratory force (e.g., the neuromuscular disorders), it is reduced in the others. In the neuromuscular disorders, expiratory reserve volume is decreased because of loss of expiratory force, so that RV is often increased. In the other types of restrictive disorders, RV is usually reduced. Both the VC and lung volumes have been used to categorize the degree of restriction (Table 2-4). Whether or not the $D_{L_{CO}}$ is reduced in the restrictive disorders depends on the underlying disease process. Primary parenchymal disorders and removal

TABLE 2-4 Quantitation of Restriction: Measurement of VC and TLC

| | % Predicted Method | | | | 95% Confidence Interval (CI) Method | | | |
| | | | No. CIs below mean | | Male | | Female | |
Category	VC, % Predicted	TLC, % Predicted	VC	TLC	VC	TLC	VC	TLC
Normal	≥81	≥81	<1	<1	<1.12	<1.61	<0.68	<1.08
Mild restriction	66–80	66–80	≥1–1.75	≥1–1.5	1.12–1.95	1.61–2.41	0.68–1.18	1.08–1.61
Moderate restriction	51–65	51–65	≥1.75–2.5	≥1.5–2	1.96–2.79	2.42–3.21	1.19–1.69	1.62–2.15
Severe restriction	≤50	≤50	≥2.5	≥2	≥2.80	≥3.22	≥1.70	≥2.16

SOURCE: From Kanner and Morris: *Clinical Pulmonary Function Testing: A Manual of Uniform Laboratory Procedures.* Salt Lake City, Intermountain Thoracic Society, 1975.

of lung tissue decrease the diffusing surface area and reduce $D_{L_{CO}}$. Diseases of the pleura and chest wall that limit thoracic excursion during the inspiratory vital capacity maneuver, which is part of the technique for determining $D_{L_{CO}}$, also reduce this measurement.

Mixed Obstructive-Restrictive Pattern

A mixed test pattern is characterized by a low $FEV_1/FVC\%$ (indicating obstructive airway disease) and small lung volumes (indicating coexisting restrictive disease). Sarcoidosis and interstitial fibrosis, when severe, generally result in this pattern because parenchymal disease causes restriction and narrowing of the airways by adjacent fibrosis, evoking airway obstruction. Another example is the patient with lobar pneumonia or large pleural effusion who also has underlying chronic bronchitis or emphysema.

Isolated Decrease in the Efficiency of Gas Transfer

An isolated reduction in the $D_{L_{CO}}$ suggests one of two possible abnormalities: (1) interstitial lung disease that is so mild as not to affect measurements of airflow or lung volume or (2) widespread occlusive disease of the pulmonary microcirculation (e.g., due to an inflammatory process or multiple small emboli). In occlusive vascular disorders, tests of airflow and lung volume are usually normal. Although other disorders can also decrease $D_{L_{CO}}$, almost invariably they also reduce airflow, lung volumes, or both. Quantification of the degree to which the $D_{L_{CO}}$ is reduced by any of these processes is indicated in Table 2-5.

CARDIOPULMONARY EXERCISE TESTING

Exercise testing represents a useful approach in the clinical evaluation of a wide variety of respiratory and cardiovascular disorders.

Physiologic Principles

In an average-sized person, resting oxygen consumption ($\dot{V}_{O_2}$) is approximately 250 mL/min or 3.5 mL/min/kg body weight (one *metabolic equivalent* or *MET*) and is associated with a $\dot{V}_E$ of 8 to 10 L/min and a cardiac output of 4 to 6 L/min. O_2 extraction is about 75 percent of arterial O_2 content.

TABLE 2-5 Categorization of Reduction in Efficacy of Gas Transfer: Measurement of $D_{L_{CO}}$

Category	% Predicted method	95% Confidence Interval (CI) Method		
		No. CIs below mean	Predicted Minus Measured $D_{L_{CO}}$, mL/min/mmHg	
			Male	Female
Normal	81–140	<1	<8.2	<6.1
Mild reduction	61–80	≥1–1.75	8.2–14.3	6.1–10.6
Moderate reduction	41–60	≥1.75–2.5	14.4–20.4	10.7–15.2
Severe reduction	≤41	≥2.5	≥20.5	≥15.3

SOURCE: From Kanner and Morris: *Clinical Pulmonary Function Testing: A Manual of Uniform Laboratory Procedures.* Salt Lake City, Intermountain Thoracic Society, 1975.

$\dot{V}_E$ may rise 8 to 10 times above baseline during strenuous work. Unlike cardiac output, ventilation normally poses no limitation to performance of aerobic work. Enhanced O_2 extraction and circulatory autoregulation further ensure O_2 availability during physical activity. Physiologic limits to the elevation in cardiac output and O_2 extraction determine the aerobic capacity of untrained subjects. Beyond these physiologic limits, any additional increment in work is not accompanied by an elevation in $\dot{V}_{O_2}$; this plateau in $\dot{V}_{O_2}$ is the *maximal oxygen uptake* ($\dot{V}_{O_2max}$). In athletes, a greater cardiac reserve and enhanced capacity for oxidative metabolism by trained skeletal muscle provide for greater aerobic capacity.

Resting carbon dioxide production ($\dot{V}_{CO_2}$) averages 190 mL/min. The resting $\dot{V}_{CO_2}/\dot{V}_{O_2}$ ratio, or *respiratory gas exchange ratio* (R), is typically between 0.75 and 0.85. The absolute value of R depends on the proportion of dietary carbohydrates and fats. $\dot{V}_{O_2}$ and $\dot{V}_{CO_2}$ rise in proportion to one another during physical activity as long as an adequate amount of O_2 is available to sustain oxidative metabolism.

With strenuous levels of muscular work, $\dot{V}_{O_2}$ rises to a level where the heart is unable to provide adequate O_2 delivery. Working skeletal muscle enhances its use of less efficient anaerobic metabolism, resulting in lactate production. This nonmetabolic source of CO_2 is derived from rapid buffering of lactate by bicarbonate; the CO_2 generated stimulates respiration. The accompanying increase in $\dot{V}_E$ maintains eucapnia and raises the respiratory gas exchange ratio above that associated with aerobic metabolism. Anaerobic metabolism during a progressive exercise test is heralded by this disproportionate rise in $\dot{V}_E$ and $\dot{V}_{CO_2}$ relative to $\dot{V}_{O_2}$. The corresponding level of $\dot{V}_{O_2}$ at which anaerobic metabolism occurs is termed the *anaerobic threshold* (AT). Anaerobiosis normally occurs when 60 percent of more of a person's aerobic capacity ($\dot{V}_{O_2max}$) has been attained.

Exercise Testing Methods

Re-creating muscular work by using a treadmill or bicycle ergometer in a monitored setting permits evaluation of the nature and severity of respiratory or cardiac symptoms and the potential contributions of abnormal heart or lung function.

$\dot{V}_{O_2max}$ is defined as $\dot{V}_{O_2}$ that remains invariant (less than 1 mL/min/kg for 30 s or more) despite an increment in workload. $\dot{V}_{O_2max}$ follows the AT, which can be determined during progressive exercise as a disproportionate rise in $\dot{V}_{CO_2}$, $\dot{V}_E$, or R relative to $\dot{V}_{O_2}$ or in end-tidal O_2 relative to end-tidal CO_2.

The normal ventilatory response to incremental treadmill exercise consists of an increase in $\dot{V}_E$ achieved through an increase in respiratory rate and tidal volume. Normally, ventilatory "reserve," as reflected in the maximal voluntary ventilation (MVV), is only partly utilized during light, moderate, or maximal exercise. The ratio of $\dot{V}_E$ at maximal exercise to MVV reflects use of this ventilatory reserve. $\dot{V}_E$ during exercise in normal subjects and patients with predominant cardiovascular disease rarely exceeds 50 percent of MVV.

Invasive hemodynamic monitoring may be useful in defining the nature and severity of an underlying cardiopulmonary disorder. A triple-lumen pulmonary artery flotation catheter can be safely used for hemodynamic monitoring during upright exercise. The hemodynamic response to incremental treadmill exercise in normal subjects is characterized by a progressive rise in cardiac output, accomplished with minimal elevations in left- and right-ventricular filling pressures. The rise in cardiac output occurs because of an increment in stroke volume and an elevation in heart rate. Systemic O_2 extraction rises progressively with incremental exercise and exceeds 70 percent at maximal workloads. A rise in mixed venous lactate concentration occurs when O_2 extraction exceeds 60 percent and when the subject is working at greater than 60 percent of $\dot{V}_{O_2max}$.

Systolic and mean arterial pressures rise during upright exercise. Because of skeletal muscle vasodilatation, arterial diastolic pressure remains essentially constant. Systemic vascular resistance falls by 50 percent to approximately 600 dynes $\cdot$ s $\cdot$ cm^{-5}. Normally, pulmonary artery systolic, mean, and diastolic pressures rise only minimally and only with higher work loads. Pulmonary vascular resistance, like systemic vascular resistance, falls by 50 percent, to about 60 dynes $\cdot$ s $\cdot$ cm^{-5}.

Clinical Applications

Cardiopulmonary exercise testing is used commonly to diagnose and assess respiratory and cardiovascular disease, assess preoperative risk, and uncover the cause of puzzling dyspnea.

Exercise Testing in Lung Disease

In a normal subject performing maximal exercise, $\dot{V}_E$ rarely exceeds 50 percent of MVV. Given this large ventilatory reserve, exercise is not normally limited by ventilation. With lung disease, ventilatory reserve is reduced.

Exercise intolerance commonly accompanies chronic obstructive pulmonary disease (COPD), with dyspnea limiting physical activity to modest levels of work. Patients with COPD have a higher $\dot{V}_E$ for any given work load largely due to increased dead space ventilation. Given their reduction in MVV and greater exercise $\dot{V}_E$, these patients often exercise with a $\dot{V}_E$/MVV ratio that exceeds 75 percent. Use of such a large portion of the ventilatory reserve cannot be sustained, accounting for breathlessness and termination of exercise. This generally occurs in patients with moderate to severe COPD before they have reached their AT, implying a ventilatory rather than cardiac limitation to exercise. The workload at which patients terminate exercise represents peak $\dot{V}_{O_2}$.

In severe emphysema, $D_{L_{CO}}$ is reduced, in keeping with alveolar capillary destruction. In such patients, exercise-induced hypoxemia often occurs. This is in contrast to patients with chronic bronchitis, in whom O_2 saturation may actually increase due to improved ventilation in areas with low ventilation/perfusion ratios. Patients with a $D_{L_{CO}}$ less than 55 percent of predicted are most likely to experience hypoxemia with exercise.

Patients with interstitial lung disease experience limiting dyspnea on exertion. This may be secondary to reduced ventilatory reserve or development of arterial O_2 desaturation. These patients tend to breathe at a higher respiratory rate and lower tidal volume than do normal subjects for any given $\dot{V}_{O_2}$. Because of a reduced MVV, exercise capacity is limited by nearly full utilization of the reduced ventilatory reserve. As in patients with airway disease, the $D_{L_{CO}}$ is a good predictor of arterial O_2 desaturation during exercise. The degree of arterial O_2 desaturation during exercise correlates with the reduction in $D_{L_{CO}}$.

Pulmonary hypertension frequently accompanies intrinsic pulmonary vascular disease or arteriolar vasoconstriction associated with hypoxemia due to intrinsic lung disease. Right ventricular pressure overload may lead to impaired left ventricular filling. Accordingly, exercise cardiac output is compromised and aerobic capacity declines.

Exercise Testing in Cardiovascular Disease

In chronic cardiac failure, $\dot{V}_{O_2max}$ attained during incremental treadmill exercise is primarily a function of maximal cardiac output. Impaired aerobic capacity is gauged according to the exercise AT and $\dot{V}_{O_2max}$ and assigned a functional class. These parameters are, in turn, used to predict maximal exercise cardiac index (or cardiac reserve).

For each functional class of chronic cardiac failure, the heart rate–$\dot{V}_{O_2}$ response to upright incremental exercise is represented by a common slope. The average slope is 3.6 beats per minute for every increment of 1 mL/min/kg in $\dot{V}_{O_2}$. Some patients with chronic cardiac failure deviate from this heart rate–$\dot{V}_{O_2}$ relation by having an inappropriate sinus tachycardia at rest or throughout exercise. In the presence of a reduced ejection fraction and ventricular dilation, an inappropriately rapid heart rate further compromises exercise cardiac output and reduces aerobic capacity.

As in normal persons, lactate production appears in chronic cardiac failure when systemic O_2 extraction exceeds 60 percent. Mixed venous lactate concentration during exercise rises above resting values when 60 percent or more of $\dot{V}_{O_2max}$ is attained.

Dyspnea corresponds with the lactate threshold and a disproportionate rise in $\dot{V}_E$ relative to $\dot{V}_{O_2}$. Patients can be encouraged to exercise to exhaustion, attaining $\dot{V}_{O_2max}$ in the presence of dyspnea. $\dot{V}_E$ rises appropriately during incremental exercise in patients with chronic cardiac failure. The response in $\dot{V}_E$ most closely corresponds to $\dot{V}_{CO_2}$ throughout exercise (aerobic and anaerobic work) and is sufficient to sustain alveolar ventilation, thereby preventing hypoxemia and hypercapnia. Maximum $\dot{V}_E$ attained with exercise is less than 50 percent of MVV. Thus, these patients do not exhaust their ventilatory reserve in responding to exercise.

TABLE 2-6 Ventilatory versus Cardiovascular Causes of Exertional Dyspnea

Ventilatory failure
1. Exercise maximum $\dot{V}_E$ utilizes >70% of MVV.
2. Exercise-associated arterial hypoxemia.
3. Failure to cross AT and to achieve $\dot{V}_{O_2max}$.

Cardiac/circulatory failure
1. Cross AT and can achieve $\dot{V}_{O_2max}$.
2. Maximum exercise $\dot{V}_E$ does not exceed 50% of MVV.
3. Does not develop arterial hypoxemia with exercise.

KEY: AT, anaerobic threshold; MVV, maximal voluntary ventilation.

Preoperative Risk Assessment

Preoperative incremental exercise testing has proved useful in assessing postoperative morbidity and mortality in the elderly and patients with underlying heart or lung disease who are scheduled for major intrathoracic or intraabdominal surgery. The premise underlying this approach is based on a recognition that during and after surgery, there may be a need to call on cardiac and ventilatory reserves—namely, the ability to increase cardiac output and maintain O_2 delivery, and to increase $\dot{V}_E$ and prevent hypoxemia.

Assessment of Dyspnea

An objective and reliable estimate of dyspnea on exertion and its severity can be gauged from exercise testing. Dyspnea occurs when $\dot{V}_E$ is excessive relative to $\dot{V}_{O_2}$ and when $\dot{V}_E$ is driven by chemical stimuli or altered lung mechanics. Dyspnea with exercise can appear when $\dot{V}_E$ occupies an excessive proportion of MVV. More than 70 percent of the MVV cannot be sustained by normal subjects for greater than several minutes. Hence, the ventilatory response to exercise that is associated with dyspnea in heart or lung disease follows a similar pattern of short-lived, near-maximal ventilation.

Patients with mild, moderate, or severe cardiac or circulatory failure rarely use more than 50 percent of their ventilatory reserve at maximal exercise, and they do not experience arterial O_2 desaturation during exercise. Unless there is a major reduction in MVV (or in FEV_1 to less than 3 L), patients will not have a ventilatory limitation to exercise. They are able to cross their AT and, if encouraged, may reach their point of exhaustion attaining $\dot{V}_{O_2max}$. These endpoints are not attained in patients with lung disease or those with coexistent heart and lung disease in whom the respiratory system is the primary limitation to exercise. Table 2-6 summarizes the salient exercise test features used to differentiate ventilatory from cardiovascular causes of exertional dyspnea.

BIBLIOGRAPHY

ATS Statement: Single breath carbon monoxide diffusing capacity (transfer factor): Recommendations for a standard technique—1995 update. *Am J Respir Crit Care Med* 152:2185–2198, 1995.

ATS Statement: Standardization of spirometry—1994 update. *Am J Respir Crit Care Med* 152:1107–1136, 1995.

Britton J, Pavord I, Richards K, et al: Factors influencing the occurrence of airway hyperreactivity in the general population: The importance of atopy and airway calibre. *Eur Respir J* 7:881–887, 1994.

Glindmeyer HW, Lefante JJ, McColloster C, et al: Blue-collar normative spirometric values for Caucasian and African-American men and women aged 18 to 65. *Am J Respir Crit Care Med* 151:412–422, 1995.

Johnson, BD, Beck KC, Zeballos RJ, Weisman IM: Advances in pulmonary laboratory testing, *Chest* 116:1377–1387, 1999.

Neas LM, Schwartz J: The determinants of pulmonary diffusing capacity in a national sample of U.S. adults. *Am J Respir Crit Care Med* 153:656–664, 1996.

O'Connor GT, Sparrow D, Weiss ST: A prospective longitudinal study of methacholine airway responsiveness as a predictor of pulmonary-function decline: The Normative Aging Study. *Am J Respir Crit Care Med* 152:87–92, 1995.

Paoletti P, Carrozzi L, Viegi G, et al: Distribution of bronchial responsiveness in a general population: Effect of sex, age, smoking, and level of pulmonary function. *Am J Respir Crit Care Med* 151:1770–1777, 1995.

Wasserman K (ed): *Exercise Gas Exchange in Heart Disease*. Armonk, NY, Futura, 1996.

3 | Evaluation of Pulmonary Diseases by Imaging*

Wallace T. Miller, Jr.

Imaging of the lung is an important component of the overall evaluation of pulmonary diseases. Although the chest radiograph remains the primary diagnostic imaging test, computed tomography (CT) and magnetic resonance imaging (MRI) have shown increasing indications in thoracic imaging. Ultrasound (US) is limited to applications in the thorax and, except for rare circumstances, is used only in the detection and evaluation of pleural effusions.

PRINCIPLES OF IMAGING TECHNIQUES

Transmission Radiographs

Since x-rays are generated at a point source, the x-ray beam diverges as it passes toward the detector. Thus the image produced by the x-ray detector is magnified relative to the object it represents. The standard posteroanterior (PA) and lateral chest radiograph is performed at a fixed x-ray source-to-film distance of 72 in. This fixed distance ensures constant magnification from film to film and allows accurate comparison of the size of objects, such as the heart and pulmonary masses, from one exam to the next. The PA position, with the anterior chest closest to the film cassette, is chosen to minimize magnification of the heart. For the same reason, a left lateral chest radiograph, with the left side closest to the film cassette, is chosen as well.

Portable chest radiographs are usually taken in the anteroposterior (AP) projection, which results in greater magnification of the heart and other anterior structures as compared with the PA projection. In addition, there is no fixed distance between the x-ray source and detector; therefore there is variable magnification of the x-ray image. Consequently, care must be taken in evaluating changes in the size of the heart, masses, or other objects detected by portable radiographs. Apparent changes in size may be a result of the variable magnification rather than a change in the size of the object.

The absorption and scatter of x-rays by an object is dictated by a variety of complex physical principles; however, the dominant determinant of x-ray absorption is the physical density of the object. Thus air, with a low density, absorbs few x-rays. Bone, with a relatively high density, absorbs a larger fraction of x-rays; and soft tissues, with an intermediate density, absorb an intermediate fraction of the incident x-rays. The net result of this is that lung appears black, bone appears white, and soft tissues are seen as intermediate gray areas on standard chest radiographs. Soft copy images on a digital monitor usually preserve the same convention.

---

*Edited from Chap. 32, "Radiographic Evaluation of the Chest" by Miller WT. In: *Fishman's Pulmonary Diseases and Disorders,* 3d ed, edited by Fishman AP, Elias JA, Fishman JA, Grippi MA, Kaiser LR, Senior RM. New York, McGraw-Hill, 1998, pp 433–486. For fuller discussion of the topics dealt with in this chapter, the reader is referred to the original text, as noted above.

Computed Tomography

Computed tomography (CT) is a form of x-ray imaging in which the x-ray transmission data are mathematically reconstructed to produce axial tomographic images of an object, usually a human body. Within the ring of a CT scanner is both an x-ray source and a row of detectors spaced 18 degrees apart from one another. These rotate synchronously and the detectors count the fraction of x-rays transmitted through the object. The number of x-rays transmitted along each path of the x-ray beam is dependent on the ability of the sum of objects along that path to absorb x-rays. A computer built into the CT scanner mathematically calculates the ability of each point in the x-ray path to absorb x-rays, a feature known as the x-ray attenuation coefficient. Each CT image is essentially a map of the x-ray attenuation coefficients for that slice of tissue. Since each organ has slightly different x-ray attenuation, this map provides a tomographic image of the internal organs of the body.

Owing to limitations in the ability of a monitor to display shades of gray, the entire range of x-ray attenuation coefficients cannot be displayed in a single CT image. This limitation is overcome by viewing the data in several modes. The most common viewing modes are termed *lung windows, soft tissue windows,* and *bone windows;* their parameters are set in a fashion which optimizes conspicuity of the lung, soft tissues, and bones, respectively.

CT remains the only cross-sectional imaging technique that adequately evaluates the lung parenchyma and is as good or nearly as good as MRI at evaluating the mediastinum, pleura, and chest wall. Thus CT remains the primary cross-sectional imaging technique for evaluation of the thorax.

Magnetic Resonance Imaging

Magnetic resonance imaging (MRI) is a form of imaging based on the resonance of hydrogen atoms in a magnetic field. The nucleus of the hydrogen atom is composed of a single proton that has a spin producing a small magnetic field. When placed in a large magnetic field, these protons will align with the external magnetic field. If these protons are then stimulated with a radiofrequency pulse of energy, they will first absorb and then emit radiofrequency pulses of electromagnetic energy. The absorption and emission of these electromagnetic waves is affected by the local environment of the protons. The local magnetic field of the liver is different from that of the kidney, which is different from the local magnetic fields of other tissues. These differences are mapped by the MR computer, creating images of the internal structures of the body.

MRI evaluation of the thorax is somewhat limited in its capabilities because of limited resolution of the lungs. Consequently, most of the indications for thoracic MRI are related to mediastinal and chest wall abnormalities. In this arena, however, MRI has distinct advantages over CT because of its greater inherent tissue contrast and because of its ability to image directly in planes other than the axial projection.

Ultrasound

Ultrasound (US) scanners create images by sending high-frequency sound waves through tissue and then listening for returning echoes. The time between transmission of the signal and reception of the echo is a function of the depth of the structure producing the reflected sound wave. This time interval and directional data are used to map the tissues according to their ability to reflect sound waves. Unfortunately, evaluation of the thorax is limited by the poor sound transmission of air in the lung, which results in nearly 100 percent reflection of the signal at the pleural surface. Consequently, the only significant indication for thoracic ultrasound is in the evaluation of pleural effusions. In this situation, ultrasound can determine the location and extent of pleural effusions as well as evaluate the extent and severity of loculations. Ultrasound can also be used to guide thoracentesis.

Ultrasound has proved valuable in diseases of the pulmonary circulation for estimating levels of pulmonary arterial blood pressure and for assessing the performance and anatomic features of the right ventricle. In patients with pulmonary hypertension, ultrasound enables consecutive determinations of pulmonary arterial pressure, the presence of cor pulmonale, tricuspid insufficiency, and the behavior of the interventricular septum.

Nuclear Medicine Imaging

In nuclear medicine imaging, a radiation-emitting compound, called a radiopharmaceutical, with either a short biologic or short physical half-life, is administered to the patient. These compounds contain two components. One is specifically designed to aggregate in a target organ such as the kidney, bone, brain, or lung. This component is linked to a radiation-emitting compound. The result is emission of radiation dependent on anatomic location and physiologic principles. These emissions can be detected by a special device known as a gamma camera, which can be used to create images of the radiations.

Most radiopharmaceuticals emit gamma rays, a form of high-energy photon. Some, however, emit beta rays, which are electrons and as such are more damaging to tissues. Recently, positron emitters, used for positron emission tomography (PET), have been developed. Gamma and beta emitters are the product of fission of high-molecular-weight atoms. These types of products can be created at a distant laboratory and delivered to hospitals for use in nuclear medicine imaging. Their main limitation is the difficult radiochemistry necessary to create clinically safe radiopharmaceuticals and limited shelf life. Positron emitters have a very short half-life and must be created in a cyclotron. Only large, research-oriented hospitals have access to such equipment and consequently to PET scanning. The advantage to PET scanning is, however, that common biologic compounds such as glucose can be radiolabeled and used to track common biologic processes.

The most important nuclear medicine examination for imaging the lung is the ventilation/perfusion ($\dot{V}/\dot{Q}$) scan: ventilation of the lung is imaged by administering either a radioactive gas or radioactive aerosol during inspiration; perfusion of the lung is imaged by the intravenous administration of the radiopharmaceutical technetium-99m macroaggregated albumin (99mTc MAA) designed to be trapped in the pulmonary arterial capillary bed. This technology is used most often to evaluate patients suspected to have pulmonary emboli. However, it is also relative to blood flow or ventilation to different regions of the lung.

TERMINOLOGY

Consolidation	Alveolar filling.
Infiltrate	A term sometimes used as a synonym for *pneumonia.* Also, used to mean any parenchymal opacity, alveolar or

interstitial in character; i.e. nonspecifically to indicate pneumonia, atelectasis, pulmonary infarct, vasculitis or other entity.

Atelectasis The loss of volume of pulmonary parenchyma. Usually but not invariably associated with consolidation of the alveoli.

Pneumonia Infection of the pulmonary parenchyma.

Pneumonitis Sometimes used to signify inflammation of the pulmonary parenchyma due to pneumonia or other inflammatory processes.

Opacity A nonspecific term indicating increased whiteness on the chest radiograph. This can be due to pneumonia, atelectasis, pleural effusion, carcinoma, chest wall lesions, or other entities.

PRINCIPLES OF IMAGE INTERPRETATION

The chest radiograph continues to be the primary technique for imaging the thorax. Despite its simplicity, it is often the only imaging modality required to make a diagnosis.

The first task in evaluating the chest radiograph is to determine whether it falls within the range of normal variation or whether an abnormality is present. There is a wide range of normal appearance of the chest radiograph, which can only be confidently understood though repeated observations of normal.

Once a radiographic abnormality is detected, the next task is to determine from which general space— the lung, the pleura, mediastinum, or chest wall— the abnormality originates.

The cardinal tenet of chest radiology is that structures are identifiable because they are surrounded by air. The heart, mediastinal, diaphragmatic, and vascular silhouettes are seen because of the adjacent air in the lung; the same is true of pneumonias, pulmonary masses, pleural effusions, and many other abnormalities.

To evaluate an abnormality of the pulmonary parenchyma, it is useful to begin by categorizing the abnormality according to whether it is interstitial or alveolar in character.

The radiographic clue suggesting interstitial disease is an excessive number of lines or dots on the chest radiograph. These must be distinguished from normal pulmonary vessels, which radiate from the pulmonary hila and become progressively smaller as they extend peripherally. The appearance of the vessels varies considerably. However, in the normal individual, the vessels are not detectable in the most peripheral 1 to 2 cm. Any lines in this outer zone or the presence of extra lines more centrally usually indicates an interstitial process. In general, interstitial diseases alter the opacity of the radiograph only minimally.

The radiographic hallmark of alveolar diseases is the presence of markedly increased opacity of the lung parenchyma. This usually takes the form of a fluffy, cloud- or cotton-like opacity. Other characteristic features of alveolar diseases are air bronchograms and the silhouette sign.

Air bronchograms occur when alveoli become opacified with fluid causing relative differences in opacity between the air in the bronchi and fluid in the alveoli. Air bronchograms are seen most commonly in pneumonia but can also be seen in other alveolar processes, including atelectasis, pulmonary edema, alveolar cell carcinoma, and so on.

The *silhouette sign* is one of the most important concepts in chest radiology and is essentially a corollary to the cardinal tenet above. If the surrounding air within the alveoli makes it possible to detect normal structures, then the absence of a normally observed structure implies the presence of fluid in the alveoli of the lung adjacent to the normal structure. For example, a pneumonia in the lingula fills the alveoli adjacent to the heart with fluid, causing the left cardiac border to disappear. Similarly, the right cardiac silhouette is obscured by alveolar disease in the adjacent right middle lobe, and the diaphragmatic silhouette can be obscured by alveolar disease in the right or left lower lobe. Moreover, the absence of the branching white lines of the pulmonary vasculature also implies an alveolar process—an observation that can be helpful in detecting focal infiltrates in the lung behind the heart.

The *hilar overlay sign* is the obverse of the silhouette sign. It denotes a mass or infiltrate that overlaps the hilum but through which the hilum is still visible. It indicates that the lesion is either in front of or behind the hilum. If it were in the hilum, the hilar shadows would be obscured because of the principles of the silhouette sign.

The terms *interstitial* and *alveolar* are in some respects poor choices for describing abnormalities on the chest radiograph, because some pathologically alveolar diseases will produce a pattern on the radiograph which may appear "interstitial"—and vice versa. The utility of the radiographic designation *interstitial* or *alveolar* lies in helping the reader to generate a differential diagnosis. The histologic character of an abnormality cannot be determined by chest radiograph; nevertheless, the majority of diseases that produce an interstitial radiographic pattern are in fact interstitial abnormalities pathologically, and the majority of diseases that produce an alveolar radiographic pattern are histologically alveolar abnormalities.

DIFFUSE INTERSTITIAL DISEASES

Once the abnormality is identified as interstitial or alveolar, it must be decided whether it is focal or diffuse. The designation *diffuse* implies a relatively uniform involvement of both lungs. Accordingly, an abnormality that involves one lung uniformly but spares the other lung is still a "focal" process. In contrast to diffuse disease, which reflects either a global pulmonary process or systemic disease, focal disease is generally local—e.g., inflammatory or neoplastic.

In considering diffuse interstitial diseases, the first factor to consider is whether the process is acute or chronic. The clinical history will often help in making this distinction. Old chest radiographs can also be helpful in distinguishing acute from chronic processes.

Interstitial Edema

Acute interstitial diseases predominantly fit into two groups: interstitial edema and interstitial pneumonia. The most common *diffuse* interstitial disease is interstitial pulmonary edema due to congestive heart failure. The characteristic findings include pulmonary vascular engorgement, increased interstitial markings, Kerley B lines, and cephalization of the pulmonary vasculature (see below). Kerley B lines are fine horizontal lines seen in the peripheralmost portion of the lung adjacent to the chest wall. These lines are due to engorgement of fine pulmonary septa. Although congestive heart failure (CHF) is the most common cause of Kerley B lines, they sometimes occur in other interstitial diseases. Moreover, Kerley B lines should not be considered pathognomonic of CHF. In addition, they are not always present in CHF. Therefore Kerley B lines are neither sensitive nor specific for CHF.

Cephalization or vascular redistribution is a radiographic manifestation of pulmonary venous hypertension. It is diagnosed when the diameter of the upper lobe pulmonary vessels is equal to or greater than that of the corresponding lower lobe pulmonary vessels. Most often it is a sign of CHF. In the supine patient, vascular redistribution to the upper lobes is a normal finding because of the effects of gravity, which direct pulmonary blood flow to the bases of the lungs in the upright position and no longer distribute blood flow preferentially to the lung bases, as in the supine position.

The most common cause of pulmonary venous hypertension is left ventricular failure. Failure of the left ventricle to maintain adequate cardiac output results in increased left ventricular end-diastolic pressure. This elevated pressure is propagated backward into the left atrium and further to the pulmonary veins, resulting in pulmonary venous hypertension.

In addition to CHF, other conditions—mitral stenosis, mitral regurgitation, and pulmonary venoocclusive disease—may cause pulmonary venous hypertension. Cardiomegaly and pleural effusions may accompany cephalization, but CHF may be present without either of these findings. Because it is so common, CHF should be considered in virtually all cases of interstitial lung disease. A trial of diuretics followed by a repeat chest radiograph often helps to distinguish CHF from other causes of interstitial lung disease.

Interstitial Pneumonia

Pneumonias are rarely interstitial. Organisms that may produce interstitial pneumonias include *Pneumocystis carinii, Mycoplasma pneumoniae,* and many viral species. These are often referred to as primary atypical pneumonias because of their clinical presentation, with low-grade fevers ($< 101°F$) and nonproductive cough. In urban centers, the most common cause of interstitial pneumonia is *P. carinii.*

Although mycoplasmal pneumonia is commonly regarded as a type of interstitial pneumonia, its radiologic appearance in two-thirds of patients is alveolar. The term *viral* pneumonia covers a wide variety of organisms. Children are more likely to have increased interstitial markings in viral pneumonias than are adults. This is particularly true of bronchiolitis caused by respiratory syncytial virus (RSV). In adults, the only virus commonly associated with interstitial pneumonia is caused by cytomegalovirus.

Chronic interstitial disease has multiple causes. Some of the more common areas are listed in Table 3-1. Clinical history is the most important factor in determining the etiology of the various interstitial diseases; however, certain radiographic and CT features may help in narrowing the differential, including (1) the pattern of interstitial disease—nodular, reticular, linear or cystic; (2) the distribution of findings—upper lung zone predominant, lower lung zone predominant, or diffuse; or (3) the presence of associated findings such as bone or soft tissue abnormalities in collagen vascular disorders and eosinophilic granuloma or the presence of pleural plaques in asbestosis. The specifics of the evaluation of interstitial lung diseases are beyond the scope of this chapter.

TABLE 3-1 Interstitial Lung Diseases

A. Acute
   1. Interstitial edema due to congestive heart failure[a]
   2. Interstitial pneumonias
      a. *Pneumocystis carinii*[a]
      b. *Mycoplasma*
      c. Viruses
      d. *Chlamydia,* congenital infections
      e. Miliary tuberculosis
      f. Miliary fungal infections
         i. *Cryptococcus*
         ii. Coccidioidomycosis
         iii. Histoplasmosis
B. Chronic
   1. Idiopathic pulmonary fibrosis[a]
   2. Collagen vascular diseases[a]
      a. Scleroderma
      b. Rheumatoid arthritis
      c. Mixed connective tissue disorder
      d. Dermatomyositis
      e. Systemic lupus erythematosis
   3. Pneumoconiosis
      a. Asbestosis
      b. Silicosis
      c. Coal workers pneumoconiosis
      d. Berylliosis
      e. Other
   4. Sarcoidosis[a]
   5. Chronic hypersensitivity pneumonitis
      a. Farmer's lung
      b. Mushroom worker's lung
      c. Pigeon breeder's lung
      d. Air conditioner lung
      e. Humidifier lung
      f. Other
   6. Metastasis
      a. Nodular
      b. Lymphangitic
   7. Diffuse bronchiectasis
      a. Cystic fibrosis
      b. Allergic bronchopulmonary aspergillosis
      c. Immotile cilia syndrome
      d. Immunodeficiency states
   8. Lymphangiomyomatosis
   9. Tuberous sclerosis
   10. Eosinophilic granuloma of the lung (histiocytosis X)
   11. Bronchiolitis obliterans organizing pneumonia

[a]The most common causes of interstitial lung disease

DIFFUSE ALVEOLAR DISEASES

By definition, an alveolar disease is one that involves filling of the alveolus by fluid of one type or another. Basically, three types of fluid can fill an alveolus: "blood, pus, or water"—i.e., alveolar hemorrhage, pneumonia, or edema. Some of the various causes of diffuse alveolar disease are presented in Table 3-2.

TABLE 3-2 Diffuse Alveolar Diseases

A. Diffuse alveolar hemorrhage
    1. Pulmonary-renal syndromes
        a. Goodpasture's disease
        b. Wegener's granulomatosis
        c. Systemic lupus erythematosus
        d. Other
    2. Primary pulmonary hemosiderosis
    3. Anticoagulation
    4. Leukemia, lymphoma
    5. Bone marrow transplantation
B. Pneumonia
    1. Aspiration
    2. Viral
    3. *Pneumocystis carinii*
    4. Bacterial
C. Pulmonary edema
    1. Cardiogenic (hydrostatic edema)[a]
    2. Noncardiogenic (increased permeability edema)
        a. Adult respiratory distress syndrome (ARDS)[a]
        b. Acute hypersensitivity pneumonitis
            i. Intravenous or ingested allergens
                (1) Blood products
                (2) Medications
                (3) Other
            ii. Inhaled allergens
                (1) Farmer's lung
                (2) Mushroom worker's lung
                (3) Pigeon breeder's lung
                (4) Air conditioner lung
                (5) Humidifier lung
                (6) Other
        c. Inhaled pulmonary toxins
            i. Smoke
            ii. N_2O (silo filler's lung)
            iii. SO_2 (industrial accidents)
        d. Narcotics
        e. Neurogenic edema
        f. Near drowning
        g. Fat emboli syndrome
        h. Amniotic fluid embolus
        i. Hyoproteinemia
            i. Cirrhosis
            ii. Nephrotic syndrome
D. Other
    1. Alveolar cell carcinoma
    2. Pulmonary alveolar proteinosis

[a]Common causes.

Although some of these entities present subtle distinctions in radiographic pattern, in most instances the radiographic appearances are similar or identical. Consequently, clinical history is often the discriminator for a specific diagnosis.

Pulmonary Edema

Pulmonary edema, especially cardiogenic pulmonary edema and adult respiratory distress syndrome (ARDS), are by large measure the most common causes of diffuse alveolar diseases and should be considered in virtually every case. As noted above, cardiogenic pulmonary edema is often associated with an enlarged heart. Characteristically, the edema is greater in the perihilar or central region of the lung—i.e., in the so-called butterfly or batwing pattern of pulmonary edema. Since most instances of cardiogenic pulmonary edema improve in response to diuretic therapy, serial radiographs following diuresis will usually show radiographic improvement.

ARDS may also cause an alveolar density throughout the lung, but the heart is generally normal in size unless the patient has preexisting heart disease. As a rule, respiratory distress requiring ventilator support is clinically evident before the radiograph indicates pulmonary edema. Therefore, in general, the radiographic diagnosis of ARDS should not be made in a patient who is not intubated. Unlike cardiogenic pulmonary edema, ARDS characteristically remains unchanged radiographically for days and often weeks. The radiographic pattern will often persist despite clinical improvement. Therefore the radiograph should not be employed as a measure of response to therapy.

Other noncardiogenic causes of pulmonary edema are listed in Table 3-2. These are uncommon.

Diffuse Pneumonia

Pneumonias usually result in focal alveolar opacities. On rare occasion, however, they may produce diffuse lung disease. Most often, the pneumonia is due to aspiration, typically in debilitated or obtunded hospital patients. In outpatients, the most common diffuse type of pneumonia is caused by viruses, which may ultimately result in ARDS. Diffuse alveolar opacities may also be due to *P. carinii*. Although aspiration, viruses, and *P. carinii* are the most common causes of diffuse pneumonia, nearly any etiology of pneumonia can on occasion manifest diffuse alveolar opacities on chest radiographs.

Diffuse Alveolar Hemorrhage

Alveolar hemorrhage is a rare cause of diffuse alveolar opacity. Often, but not invariably, the patients present with hemoptysis. The most common etiologies of diffuse alveolar hemorrhage are the "pulmonary-renal syndromes," especially Goodpasture's disease, Wegener's granulomatosis, and systemic lupus erythematosus. Occasionally vasculitides other than Wegener's granulomatosis, such as Churg-Strauss vasculitis or pauci-immune vasculitis, may cause diffuse hemorrhage. Patients with diffuse diseases of bone marrow such as leukemia or lymphoma are also apt to develop alveolar hemorrhage. Finally, diffuse hemorrhage may be a life-threatening complication of bone marrow transplantation.

Other Causes of Diffuse Alveolar Disease

Rarely, diffuse alveolar disease may be due to processes other than edema, pneumonia, or alveolar hemorrhage. For example, diffuse bronchoalveolar carcinoma and pulmonary alveolar proteinosis can cause diffuse alveolar disease. Bronchoalveolar carcinoma is an unusual form of bronchogenic carcinoma that grows preferentially within the alveolar spaces. It may appear as a rounded nodule, a focal alveolar opacity mimicking pneumonia, or a diffuse alveolar opacity. Pulmonary alveolar proteinosis is a rare disorder in which thick, tenacious alveolar secretions fill the alveoli and produce diffuse alveolar opacities on the chest radiograph. CT shows so-called crazy paving, characterized by a combination of ground-glass opacities and interlobular septal thickening.

Radiologic distinction between pulmonary edema and other forms of diffuse alveolar disease, such as alveolar hemorrhage, is rarely possible. As a rule, clinical history is the primary discriminator.

FOCAL LUNG DISEASE

Pneumonia and Atelectasis

The vast majority of focal lung diseases are alveolar. Of the focal alveolar diseases, pneumonia and atelectasis account for greater than 95 percent of cases.

In general, the more fluffy an opacity, the more likely it is to point to a pneumonia. The more dense and dependent an opacity, the more likely it is to be atelectasis. Although there are radiographic clues to distinguish pneumonia from atelectasis, these entities may appear identically. Therefore, the final and most powerful discriminator is not the chest radiograph but the clinical history.

A good rule of thumb is that a focal infiltrate is a pneumonia unless the patient has a known cause of atelectasis. In general, outpatients rarely have conditions that cause atelectasis; therefore most focal infiltrates in outpatients are caused by pneumonia. Hospitalized patients, however, frequently have conditions causing atelectasis. Therefore most focal infiltrates in inpatients are caused by atelectasis. Table 3-3 lists some of the more common causes of atelectasis.

Atelectasis can be subdivided into several general categories. The two most important are "obstructive" and "passive" atelectasis. Obstructive atelectasis occurs when a lobar bronchus is occluded, so that air distal to the obstruction is gradually absorbed by the pulmonary blood flow. The resulting loss of volume of the lobe is, by definition, atelectasis. Obstructive atelectasis produces characteristic opacities in the lung in accord with the location of the interlobar fissures. The locations of the lobes and interlobar fissures on the PA and lateral chest radiographs are depicted in Fig. 3-1. All three fissures are seen in profile on the lateral view. In contrast, on the PA view, the two major fissures pass obliquely from superoposterior to anteroinferior and consequently are not identified as lines. As a result, obstructive atelectasis is often more easily identified on the lateral view. The volume of the thorax is relatively fixed because of the rigidity of bony thorax; therefore as one lobe decreases in volume, the other lobes expand to fill the thorax. Thus, the atelectatic lobe is displaced as the other lobes expand. The lower lobes are displaced posteriorly and inferiorly by the upper and middle lobes. Similar responses occur in the other lobes. Since all the lobes are attached at the hilum, they will all collapse centrally toward it. Diagrams of the characteristic patterns of collapse are illustrated in Fig. 3-2.

Passive atelectasis reflects the natural tendency of the lung to collapse because of the elastic recoil of the pulmonary parenchyma. If this elastic recoil is unopposed by the elastic recoil of the chest wall, atelectasis results. Gravity favors collapse of the more dependent parts of the lung—i.e., the posterior

---

TABLE 3-3 Causes of Atelectasis

A. Obstructive atelectasis
    1. Malignancy
       a. Bronchogenic carcinoma[a]
       b. Metastasis
       c. Carcinoid
       d. Mucoepidermoid carcinoma
       e. Adenoid cystic carcinoma
       f. Other
    2. Mucous plug
       a. Bland plug[a]
       b. Allergic bronchopulmonary aspergillosis (ABPA)
    3. Foreign body
    4. Granulomatous disease
       a. Sarcoidosis
       b. Histoplasmosis
       c. Tuberculosis
       d. Other
B. Passive atelectasis
    1. Causes of chest or abdominal pain
       a. Thoracic and abdominal surgery[a]
       b. Chest trauma[a]
       c. Pulmonary embolus
       d. Viral pleuritis
       e. Inflammatory disease below the diaphragm[a]
          i. Peritonitis
          ii. Subphrenic abscess
          iii. Pancreatitis
          iv. Cholecystitis
          v. Other
    2. Diseases that expand the pleural space
       a. Pleural effusion[a]
       b. Pneumothorax
       c. Other
    3. Neuromuscular disorders
       a. Myasthenia gravis
       b. Muscular dystrophy
       c. CNS depression
       d. Phrenic nerve paralysis
       e. Other
    4. Ascites and other space-occupying lesions below the diaphragm
    5. Diseases that encase the lung
       a. Pleural fibrosis
       b. Mesothelioma
       c. Pleural metastasis
C. Cicatricial atelectasis
    1. Right middle lobe syndrome[a]
    2. Chronic infection
       a. Tuberculosis
       b. Nontuberculous mycobacterial infection
       c. Other
    3. Other

---

[a]Common causes.

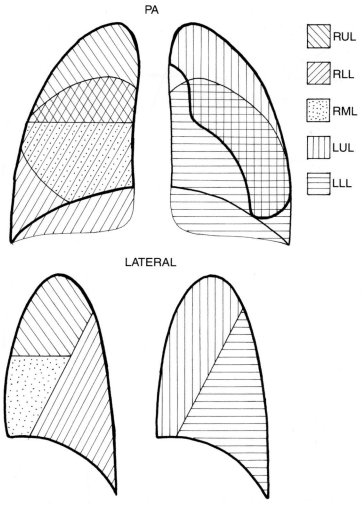

FIG. 3-1   Lobar anatomy. Posteroanterior (PA) and lateral chest radiographs. RUL, right upper lobe; RLL, right lower lobe; RML, right middle lobe; LUL, left upper lobe; LLL, left lower lobe.

and inferior aspects. Therefore passive atelectasis is usually manifest as opacity of the lower and posterior lung zones.

Cicatricial atelectasis is due to parenchymal or pleural scarring. It is usually manifested as linear bands that represents areas of scarring, sometimes accompanied by shifting of the fissures.

Most often, bacterial pneumonias appear as unilobar areas of alveolar filling. Except for aspiration pneumonia, multilobar pneumonias are rare. Unfortunately,

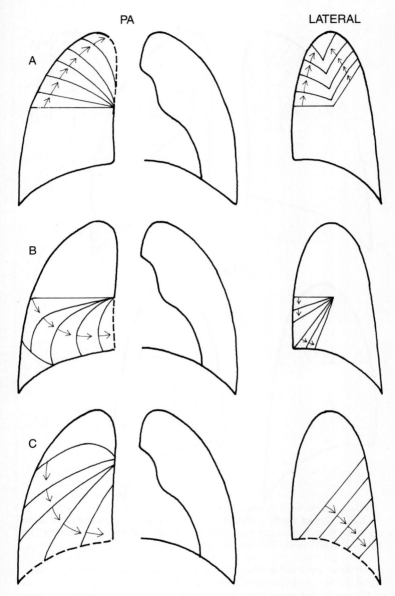

PA   LATERAL

FIG. 3-2   Schematics of lobar atelectasis. (*A*) Right-upper-lobe atelectasis. (*B*) Right-middle-lobe atelectasis. (*C*) Right-lower-lobe atelectasis.

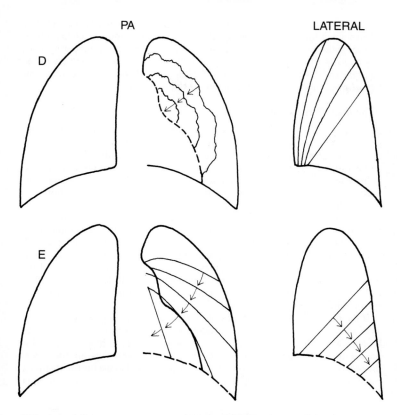

FIG. 3-2   (*continued*) (*D*) Left-upper-lobe atelectasis.(*E*) Left-lower-lobe atelectasis. Dashed lines indicate absence of border seen in normals on the chest radiographs.

there are few reliable radiographic features that distinguish one bacterial pneumonia from another; acute viral pneumonias may also appear as focal alveolar infiltrates identical to those of bacterial pneumonias. Therefore differentiation of most pneumonias depends on analysis of sputum and sputum cultures.

Unlike that of acute infections, the radiographic appearance of some chronic infections may suggest specific or limited differential diagnoses. The most important of these is reactivation or postprimary tuberculosis. Reactivation tuberculosis characteristically occurs as apical lung disease with appearances that range from coarse fibrotic bands and nodules, the "fibronodular appearance," to alveolar consolidation with associated multiple areas of cavitation, the "fibroproductive appearance." Recognition of either of these patterns should lead to careful clinical investigation for active tuberculosis.

Several other infections may mimic the appearance of tuberculosis. These include nontuberculous mycobacteria, especially *Mycobacterium avium* complex and *Mycobacterium kansasii*, and some endemic fungi such as *Cryptococcus, Histoplasma,* and *Coccidioidomyces* species.

Chronic aspergillosis may be recognized radiographically by its tendency to produce a mobile mass, or mycetoma, within a pulmonary cavity. Other chronic pulmonary infections—most notably actinomycosis, mucormycosis, tuberculosis, and nocardiosis—may manifest themselves by invasion of the adjacent chest wall tissues. CT or MR images will demonstrate such soft tissue invasion and suggest the nature of the infection.

Pulmonary Masses and Nodules

Pulmonary opacities that are round or oval with rather well-defined borders are more aptly called *masses* or *nodules. Mass* also implies a somewhat different appearance than *nodule:* a nodule is smaller, usually less than 3 cm, and is usually better defined. Tables 3-4 to 3-6 categorize pulmonary masses, pulmonary nodules, and multiple pulmonary nodules. The lists are quite similar. The differences stem from the listing of the different presentations according to frequency of radiographic appearance.

Most solitary masses represent primary carcinomas of the lung. But if the mass is at all indistinct, it may represent a circumscribed pneumonia. Most individuals with a new, rounded opacity should be given an empiric course of antibiotics and the chest radiograph repeated in 2 to 3 weeks. If it improves or completely resolves, the opacity was a pneumonia. However, if the opacity should diminish in size, the lesion should be followed radiographically until complete clearance; on occasion, a carcinoma will hide within a surrounding inflammatory infiltrate.

If the mass does not change in size, a tissue diagnosis is usually necessary. This can be achieved by either endobronchial, transthoracic, or surgical biopsy. Some clinicians perform a CT of the chest prior to biopsy to look for mediastinal adenopathy and provide a possible fourth option for tissue diagnosis—i.e., mediastinoscopic biopsy. The CT is also useful for staging a carcinoma by detecting lung, hepatic, or adrenal metastases, by delimiting

---

TABLE 3-4 Etiologies of Pulmonary Masses According to Frequency

A. Neoplasm
  1. Bronchogenic carcinoma[a]
  2. Metastasis
  3. Lymphoma
  4. Other pulmonary neoplasms
B. Lung abscess[a]
C. Round pneumonia
  1. Acute bacterial[a]
  2. Chronic pneumonias
    a. Blastomycosis
    b. Actinomycosis
    c. Nocardiosis
    d. Cryptococcosis
D. Rounded atelectasis
E. Vasculitis
  1. Wegener's granulomatosis
  2. Churg-Strauss vasculitis
  3. Pauci-immune vasculitis
  4. Other
F. Pulmonary hematoma

[a]Common causes.

TABLE 3-5 Etiologies of Solitary Pulmonary Nodules According to Frequency

A. Neoplasm
   1. Bronchogenic carcinoma[a]
   2. Metastasis[a]
   3. Bronchial adenoma
   4. Lymphoma
   5. Hamartoma
   6. Other pulmonary neoplasms
B. Granuloma[a]
   1. Histoplasmoma
   2. Tuberculoma
   3. Coccidioidoma
   4. Cryptococcoma
   5. Other
C. Pulmonary hematoma
D. Vasculitis
   1. Wegener's granulomatosis
   2. Churg-Strauss vasculitis
   3. Pauci-immune vasculitis
   4. Other
E. Pulmonary arteriovenous malformation (AVM)

[a]Common causes.

macroscopic adenopathy, and by suggesting chest wall and mediastinal invasion.

Radiographically, pulmonary masses may be produced by lung abscesses, unusual primary pulmonary malignancies, unusual chronic pneumonias, and a variety of other conditions. The nature of such lesions usually depends on the clinical history and often on biopsy for diagnosis and exclusion of malignancy. One important exception is rounded atelectasis. This form of atelectasis secondary to visceral pleural fibrosis has CT features that are often sufficiently characteristic for diagnosis. Rounded atelectasis produces a

TABLE 3-6 Etiologies of Multiple Pulmonary Nodules According to Frequency

A. Neoplasm
   1. Metastasis[a]
   2. Multiple bronchogenic carcinomas
   3. Lymphoma
B. Granulomas
   1. Histoplasmoma[a]
   2. Tuberculoma
   3. Coccidioidoma
   4. Cryptococcoma
   5 Other
C. Septic emboli[a]
D. Vasculitis
E. Rheumatoid nodules
F. Arteriovenous malformation (Osler-Weber-Rendu syndrome)
G. Sarcoidosis
H. Papillomatosis

[a]Common causes.

dome-shaped, mass-like opacity that directly abuts an area of diffuse pleural thickening. A series of radiating vessels may be seen extending from the mass into the adjacent lung. These represent the normal pulmonary vessels crowded together as a result of the atelectasis.

A small, well-defined nodule is often more likely to represent a granuloma than a malignancy. In this setting, it is exceedingly important to attempt to obtain previous chest radiographs of the patient. Often, previous radiographs demonstrate that the nodule has remained without change for several years, indicating that the lesion is benign, most often a granuloma. If no previous radiographs are available, some physicians prefer to postpone biopsy of a small, well-defined nodule, opting to follow the nodule radiographically over increasing intervals (e.g., serial radiographs of 1, 3, and 6 months). An unchanging nodule suggests a benign process, usually a granuloma.

The radiographic appearance of most pulmonary nodules is nonspecific, so that clinical and radiographic follow-up or tissue biopsy is necessary to exclude malignancy. One notable exception is pulmonary arteriovenous malformation (AVM). The nodule produced by a pulmonary AVM is, in fact, a markedly dilated segment of vein at the junction of a pulmonary arteriovenous connection. Careful scrutiny of the chest radiographs, CT, or MRI will demonstrate the small artery feeding the AVM and a large serpentine vein draining the AVM. This appearance is usually sufficiently distinctive to obviate further evaluation. If necessary, specifically designed CT or MRI examinations or pulmonary angiography will diagnose an AVM conclusively.

Interest is high in imaging techniques to avoid biopsy. Demonstration of calcification or fat by chest radiograph, CT, or MRI indicates a benign lesion that does not require biopsy. Thus, central calcification, diffuse calcification, or concentric rings of calcification in a smooth, round, or oval nodule less than 3 cm in diameter is diagnostic of a benign nodule and nearly always indicates a granuloma. Demonstration of popcorn-like calcification or of fat is also evidence of a benign lesion and indicates a pulmonary hamartoma. Although these features may be evident on the chest radiograph, CT or MRI is often necessary to uncover more subtle areas of calcification or fat. It is important to remember that the CT scan must be performed without intravenous contrast to avoid confusion between contrast enhancement and calcification.

Attempts are under way to increase the specificity of contrast-enhanced CT for the diagnosis of benign conditions. One recent approach entails sequential CT images through the center of a nodule during intravenous infusion of contrast material and calculation of the peak enhancement of the nodule. Enhancement less than 20 Hounsfield units (HU) is reported to have 100 percent specificity for benign conditions.[1] But, this test has yet to attain wide acceptance in the medical community.

Positron emission tomography (PET) is another imaging technique that shows promise of separating benign from malignant conditions.[2] Fludeoxyglucose F 18 is injected intravenously and images are made of the nodule, adenopathy, or other abnormal condition. If the lesion does not have high radiation activity, it is interpreted as having a low metabolic rate and likely to be benign. Unfortunately, PET scanning requires a cyclotron to manufacture the radioactive label and is therefore available only at large, research-oriented medical centers.

Other Causes of Focal Lung Disease

Among the other causes of focal pulmonary infiltrates are pulmonary infarction, contusion, vasculitis, eosinophilic pneumonia, and bronchiolitis obliterans organizing pneumonia (BOOP). Although these are often indistinguishable from pneumonias, they may have some suggestive features. Pulmonary infarction characteristically appears as a wedge-shaped opacity with its base on the pleural surface of the lung. As it resolves, this opacity shrinks toward the pleural surface, producing a small hill-shaped opacity called "Hampton's hump." Vasculitides, such as Wegener's granulomatosis and Churg-Strauss vasculitis, and BOOP often produce multiple pulmonary opacities that shift position on serial radiographs. Chronic eosinophilic pneumonia characteristically causes opacities in the upper lung zone that preferentially involve lung parenchyma immediately beneath the pleura. Blunt trauma to the chest can cause an opacity representing pulmonary contusion or laceration.

OBSTRUCTIVE LUNG DISEASES

In the vast majority of obstructive lung diseases, imaging will play no significant role in diagnosis, which is usually made by a combination of clinical evaluation and pulmonary function testing. However, in rare instances, imaging, especially CT, may play an important role in detecting structural abnormalities responsible for the airways obstruction. For example, extrinsic compression of the trachea by a mass (such as a thyroid goiter, lymphoma, esophageal carcinoma, and lung carcinoma) or by aberrant vascular structures (such as double aortic arch, right aortic arch with an aberrant left subclavian and pulmonary sling) may be demonstrated by CT and MRI. Such entities appear as masses arising from their organ of origin on the cross-sectional evaluation. Intrinsic tracheal masses—such as squamous, adenoid cystic, and mucoepidermoid carcinomas—may also be demonstrated by CT or MRI as focal masses arising from the tracheal wall. Diffuse disorders of the tracheal wall—including tracheomalacia, amyloidosis, relapsing polychondritis, and tracheopathia osteochondroplastica—may produce distinctive CT abnormalities, usually some combination of airway narrowing, airway wall thickening, and wall calcification.

Although bronchiectasis is not a cause of obstructive lung disease, it can produce airways obstruction by enhancing interference with bronchial clearance mechanisms. Ring-shaped opacities or groups of parallel lines called "tram tracks" on the chest radiograph may strongly suggest the diagnosis of bronchiectasis. However, chest radiographs often show only nonspecific, irregular opacities in the region of the bronchiectasis.

Thin-section (high-resolution) CT scanning has replaced bronchography as the primary radiographic technique for the diagnosis of bronchiectasis. The characteristic CT findings are the tram-track and "signet ring" signs. The tram-track sign signifies that instead of tapering as they proceed distal, the airways are dilated and run parallel, indicating cylindrical bronchiectasis. If the diameter of the airway is greater than 1.5 times that of the adjacent artery, there is also evidence of bronchiectasis. The signet ring sign is formed by a ring of air containing bronchus capped by the round opacity of the adjacent artery, which, together resemble a signet ring.

Saccular bronchiectasis may appear as cystic spaces in the central portions of the lung. Normal bronchi in the outer third of the lung are too small to be seen by current CT technology. Visible airways in this zone of the lung indicates dilatation of the small airways, or bronchioloectasis. If these small airways become filled with mucus, they produce small, Y-shaped opacities that are additional evidence of bronchioloectasis.

Chest radiographs of patients with asthma are usually normal. Occasionally nonspecific increases in interstitial markings may be present. Often, on the lateral radiograph, the anterior-to-posterior (AP) diameter of the thorax may be increased and the diaphragm flattened. These radiographic findings are more frequently seen in patients with emphysema than in those with asthma or chronic bronchitis. CT is more sensitive for the diagnosis of emphysema and may distinguish between the morphologic subtypes of emphysema: centrilobular, panlobular, and paraseptal emphysema. CT scoring techniques have been developed that correlate with the distribution and extent of emphysema at histologic evaluation. These are currently being investigated as selection criteria for surgical lung volume reduction.

CT images obtained at different lung volumes can disclose "air trapping." Most CT images are obtained at end-inspiration. As they are obtained at lower and lower inspiratory volumes and at greater expiration, the attenuation (whiteness) of the lung increases as the ratio of air to tissue in the lungs decreases. If egress of air is impeded, a focal region of lung will remain less attenuated (black) and stand out among the relatively high-attenuated (whiter) lung. This phenomenon of air trapping is a manifestation of small airways disease. Although small degrees of air trapping may be seen in clinically asymptomatic individuals and may be assumed to be within the range of normal variation, greater degrees of air trapping may indicate small airways disease. Disorders that have been shown to cause air trapping include asthma, bronchiectasis, bronchiolitis obliterans, panbronchiolitis, and some diseases that cause endobronchial granulomas, such as sarcoidosis.

PULMONARY VASCULAR DISORDERS

Pulmonary Embolism

The standard approach to the diagnosis of pulmonary embolism (PE) begins with the chest radiograph. Although the chest radiograph cannot definitively diagnose PE because most of the radiographic findings are nonspecific, the chest radiograph is useful in two ways: (1) it excludes causes of dyspnea and chest pain, such as pneumothorax and pneumonia, and (2) ventilation/perfusion ($\dot{V}/\dot{Q}$) scans are interpreted with respect to certain radiographic findings.

Common findings on the chest radiograph in patients with pulmonary embolism include pleural effusions and atelectasis; however, the chest radiograph may be normal. Much more specific is Westermark's sign, which is a decrease in the size of pulmonary vessels in a region of the lung; this is a highly specific sign of pulmonary oligemia due to embolism.

Pulmonary infarction is suggestive but not diagnostic of pulmonary embolism. It appears as a wedge-shaped lesion of alveolar opacification with one side abutting on the pleura. When present, the appearance of pulmonary infarction is suggestive but not diagnostic of pulmonary embolism. Pulmonary infarction is an uncommon manifestation of pulmonary embolism because of the dual blood supply of the lung parenchyma by both pulmonary and bronchial arteries. This dual blood supply usually suffices to prevent pulmonary infarction except when the bronchial circulation is compromised, as in congestive heart failure.

In pulmonary embolism, ventilation/perfusion scans demonstrate areas of ventilation without perfusion—i.e., a mismatched defect. Areas in which both perfusion and corresponding ventilation defects are present are most often due to parenchymal lung disease or pleural effusions.

Evaluation of pulmonary embolism with spiral CT scans is in the early stages of clinical development. Several reports have demonstrated high sensitivity and specificity of spiral CT for detection of pulmonary embolism, especially emboli proximal to the pulmonary segmental arteries.[3–5] Enhanced CT demonstrates intraluminal masses indicative of emboli. Although promising, the use of CT is not yet universally accepted.

The "gold standard" for the diagnosis of pulmonary embolism is pulmonary angiography. Its shortcoming is that it is an invasive test requiring placement of an arterial catheter in the right or left pulmonary artery for injection of contrast material. The strength of this technique is its ability to demonstrate perfusion defects the lung or intraluminal filling defects.

Pulmonary Hypertension

Pulmonary hypertension can be secondary to a variety of disorders, including chronic heart failure, chronic pulmonary disease, and more unusual disorders such as chronic pulmonary embolism. It can also be of unknown etiology, the so-called primary pulmonary hypertensions. Pulmonary hypertension is manifest radiographically by enlargement of the central pulmonary arteries in association with decreased caliber of the peripheral pulmonary vessels—i.e., "pruning." The cause of secondary pulmonary hypertension may be inferred from other radiographic findings, such as the presence of cardiomegaly, interstitial lung disease, or pulmonary hyperinflation. In severe pulmonary hypertension, cor pulmonale occurs with enlargement of the right ventricle.

On CT and MR images, the diameter of the main pulmonary artery should be equal to or smaller than the diameter of the adjacent ascending aorta in normal individuals. Enlargement of the main pulmonary artery to an area greater than that of the ascending aorta is evidence of pulmonary hypertension.

PLEURAL DISEASES

Pleural Effusion

Some of the most common causes of pleural effusion are listed in Table 3-7.

The appearances of pleural effusions on chest radiographs may vary considerably, depending on the position of the patient when the image is obtained and the character of the effusion itself: transudate, exudate, chylous, or other.

The most common manifestation on the erect radiograph of pleural effusion is a curvilinear density that obscures the costophrenic angle—i.e., a meniscus (Fig. 3-3A). Because the posterior costophrenic angle is the most dependent aspect of the pleural space, the lateral view, which displays the posterior costophrenic angle, is more capable of disclosing small pleural effusions than the PA view.

Sometimes, a pleural effusion fails to obscure the costophrenic angle. In this situation, the effusion is manifest as a density that displaces the pleura away from the ribs. However, this appearance is not specific for pleural effusion and may be seen with pleural thickening without effusion.

TABLE 3-7 Etiologies of Pleural Effusions

A. Malignancy
    1. Metastasis
    2. Mesothelioma
    3. Lymphoma
B. Infection
    1. Parapneumonic
    2. Tuberculous pleuritis
    3. Viral pleuritis
    4. Fungal pleuritis
       a. Cryptococcosis
       b. Coccidioidomycosis
       c. Blastomycosis
       d. Other
    5. Mediastinitis
C. Trauma
D. Congestive heart failure
E. Pulmonary embolism
F. Diseases below the diaphragm
    1. Ascites
    2. Inflammatory diseases
       a. Cholecystitis
       b. Pancreatitis
       c. Peritonitis
       d. Pyelonephritis
       e. Subphrenic abscess
       f. Other
G. Collagen vascular disease
    1. Systemic lupus erythematosus (SLE)
    2. Rheumatoid arthritis (RA)
    3. Mixed connective tissue disorder (MCTD)
H. Drugs
    1. SLE-causing medications
       a. Procainamide
       b. Hydralazine
       c. Other
    2. Bromocriptine
    3. Methysergide
    4. Nitrofurantoin
I. Postoperative

Occasionally, pleural effusions collect between the lung and the diaphragm, causing a "subpulmonic effusion." This is manifest on the left side by an increase in the distance between the bottom of the lung and the top of the stomach bubble. Other evidence of subpulmonic effusion is a lateral shift of the apex of the hemidiaphragm displaced from the normal position of the apex, which is from one-half to the medial one-third of the distance between the spine and the lateral chest wall.

On supine films, pleural effusions do not obscure the lateral costophrenic angle because the fluid moves to the posterior position, the most dependent aspect of the pleural space. Consequently, pleural effusions usually appear as a hazy opacity overlying the hemithorax. A uniform opacity is characteristic of pleural and chest wall processes, in contrast with diseases involving the lung parenchyma. The latter have a variegated appearance because they are

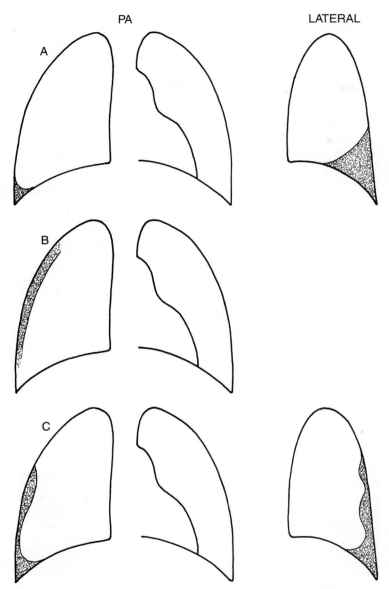

FIG. 3-3 Schematics of the appearances of pleural effusion. (*A*) Meniscus on PA and lateral chest radiographs. (*B*) Meniscus en face (anteroposterior view). (*C*) Loculated effusion.

composed of a mixture of air and soft tissue, in which some alveoli remain aerated while others are filled with fluid. Chest wall masses and pleural effusions are usually composed only of water or soft tissue, so that the density is uniform. Thus, on a supine film, a unilateral pleural effusion will appear as increased opacity over one hemithorax.

The more upright the patient, the more the pleural fluid will collect at the base of the pleural space. In this case, the pleural effusion will appear as a gradient of increasing opacity from the superior to the inferior aspect of the hemithorax.

Regardless of the position of the patient, pleural effusions form a meniscus because of the surface tension of the fluid. When the patient is erect, the meniscus appears as a curvilinear, triangular opacity in the costophrenic angles. When the patient is supine, the pleural fluid tracks along the posterior lateral pleural space, decreasing in amount anteriorly. On an PA or AP chest radiograph, the fluid appears as an opacity which displaces the lung from the internal border of the ribs—the "meniscus en face" (Fig. 3-3B).

Up to this juncture, it has been assumed that the pleural fluid is unrestricted in the pleural space. This is usually true of transudative effusions, whereas exudative or bloody effusions are prone to producing pleural adhesions. These pleural adhesions restrict the flow of pleural fluid causing loculations.

A loculated pleural effusion remains in the same position regardless of change in the patient's position. Effusions usually collect in the inferior and posterior aspects of the pleural space, and thus these are the locations where they most commonly loculate. Decubitus films are often useful in determining whether an effusion is loculated or free by determining if changes in body position shift the location of fluid.

Often a loculated effusion appears as an opacity adjacent to the chest wall; the opacity has a smooth margin with the lung and forms obtuse angles with the chest wall (Fig. 3-3C). This appearance is not distinctive for loculated effusion since it may occur in other pleural lesions, especially benign pleural masses.

CT, US, and MRI are superior to the chest radiograph for the detection of pleural effusions.

Pleural Thickening

Pleural thickening may be secondary to pleural fibrosis or pleural malignancy, such as metastasis or mesothelioma. Some causes of pleural thickening are listed in Table 3-8. On the chest radiograph, pleural thickening usually appears as a wavy opacity separating the lung from the chest wall. The more lumpy or nodular the appearance, the more likely it is to be malignant. Distinguishing pleural thickening from loculated pleural effusions may be impossible on chest radiographs; however, if the thickness of the pleural opacity exceeds 2 cm, there is nearly always some pleural fluid present. CT, MRI, and US examinations can distinguish loculated pleural fluid from pleural thickening.

Pneumothorax

Unless it is suspected, pneumothorax may be among the most problematic diagnoses to make on the chest radiograph. Characteristically, a pneumothorax appears as a thin white line that parallels the chest wall. This line is the visceral pleura, which is seen because there is air on both sides of it: air in

---

TABLE 3-8 Etiologies of Pleural Thickening

A. Malignancy
   1. Metastasis
   2. Mesothelioma
   3. Lymphoma

B. Fibrosis
   1. Asbestos-related
      a. Pleural plaques
      b. Prior benign asbestos effusion
   2. Prior hemothorax
   3. Prior exudative effusion
      a. Empyema
      b. Collagen vascular diseases
         i. Rheumatoid arthritis (RA)
         ii. Systemic lupus erythematosus (SLE)
         iii. Mixed connective tissue disorder (MCTD)
      c. Tuberculous and fungal effusions
   4. Drugs
      a. Bromocriptine
      b. Methysergide
      c. Ergot alkaloids
      d. Other

---

the lung and air in the pleural space. This is the most reliable sign of pneumothorax but is difficult to detect because pleura is so thin.

Pneumothorax is also manifest by the absence of pulmonary parenchymal markings in the region of pneumothorax. Although this finding can be helpful, it is not reliable as the sole diagnostic criterion, since there are no parenchymal lines in the peripheral 1 to 2 cm of the normal lung.

If the pleural space is free of adhesions, air will shift in the pleural space, rising to its uppermost portion. Therefore it is important to know the position of the patient when the chest radiograph is taken. On the erect chest radiograph, the pneumothorax collects in the apex. In the supine position, the air rises to the anterior chest, where a pneumothorax can also be seen as a thin white line at the lung base, paralleling the diaphragm, heart border, or lateral chest wall. If the patient is able to sit or stand, a decubitus view of the chest should be taken in order to image the most nondependent portion of the pleural space in profile and maximizing the detection of pneumothoraces.

CT examinations are more sensitive for the detection of tiny pneumothoraces than are chest radiographs. Therefore, CT exams can be utilized to detect radiographically occult pneumothoraces.

MEDIASTINAL DISORDERS

Chest radiographs are relatively insensitive for the diagnosis of mediastinal disorders because of the lack of contrast between the various mediastinal structures. Thus, with a few exceptions, the chest radiographic detection of mediastinal disorders is confined to mediastinal masses that distort the mediastinal contour.

Mediastinal masses are traditionally categorized as anterior, middle, and posterior, according to their position on the lateral radiograph (Fig. 3-4). The

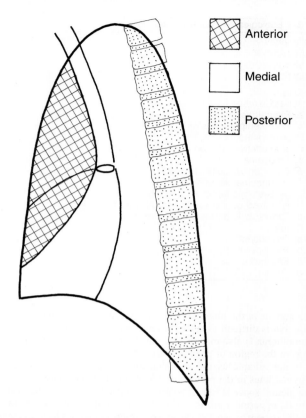

Anterior

Medial

Posterior

FIG. 3-4 Schematics showing classification of mediastinal masses using the lateral chest radiograph.

major organs in the anterior mediastinum are the thymus and thyroid glands;
the most common tumors are lymphomas, thymomas, tumors of the thyroid,
and teratomas arising from embryologic rests. The middle mediastinum contains the great vessels, esophagus, trachea, heart, and pericardium; the most
common middle mediastinal tumors are aortic aneurysms and dissection, lymphadenopathy, bronchopulmonary foregut cysts derived from the trachea or
esophagus, hiatal hernias, and pericardial cysts. The posterior mediastinum
contains the thoracic spine, spinal cord, and thoracic nerves; the most common masses of the posterior mediastinum are neurogenic tumors, spinal
osteomyelitis, and bone malignancies. Table 3-9 provides a more complete
listing of mediastinal masses.

   CT and MRI examinations have much greater tissue contrast resolution
than do chest radiographs, thus enabling more precise localization and diagnosis of mediastinal masses. Anterior mediastinal masses except for thyroid tumors are also indistinguishable. However, masses of the middle and
posterior mediastinum are often easily distinguished by their CT or MRI

TABLE 3-9 Mediastinal Masses

A. Anterior
   1. Thymic tumors
      a. Lymphoma
      b. Thymoma
      c. Thymolipoma
      d. Thymic cyst
      e. Thymic carcinoid
   2. Germ cell tumors
      a. Teratoma and teratocarcinoma
      b. Seminoma
      c. Choriocarcinoma
      d. Other
   3. Thyroid tumors
      a. Goiter
      b. Carcinoma
      c. Other
B. Middle
   1. Vascular masses
      a. Aortic aneurysm/pseudoaneurysm
      b. Aortic dissection
      c. Vascular anomalies
         i. Double aortic arch
         ii. Right aortic arch with an aberrant left subclavian artery
         iii. Pulmonary sling
         iv. Other
   2. Lymphadenopathy
      a. Metastatic tumor
      b. Sarcoidosis
      c. Lymphoma
      d. Chronic lymphocytic leukemia
      e. Other
   3. Bronchopulmonary cysts
      a. Bronchogenic cyst
      b. Esophageal duplication cyst
      c. Neuroenteric cyst
   4. Esophageal masses
      a. Hiatal hernia
      b. Achalasia
      c. Carcinoma
      d. Leiomyoma and other tumors of the esophageal wall
   5. Pericardial masses
      a. Pericardial cyst
      b. Pericardial neoplasms
         i. Hemangioma
         ii. Lymphangioma
         iii. Other
   6. Cardiac masses
      a. Myocardial aneurysm
      b. Cardiac malignancy
         i. Rhabdomyosarcoma
         ii. Other
C. Posterior
   1. Neurogenic tumors
      a. Schwannoma
      b. Neurofibroma
      c. Other

(*continued*)

TABLE 3-9 (*continued*)

2. Masses of the thoracic spine
   a. Spinal osteomyelitis
      i. Bacterial
      ii. Fungal
      iii. Tuberculous
   b. Primary malignancy
      i. Multiple myeloma
      ii. Ewing's sarcoma
      iii. Other
   c. Metastasis
   d. Extramedullary hematopoiesis

characteristics. CT and MRI are also more sensitive for mediastinal disorders than are chest radiographs. In particular, CT and MRI exhibit greater sensitivity for adenopathy.

CHEST WALL ABNORMALITIES

Abnormalities of the bones are well evaluated by chest radiographs because the bones have a distinct radiation attentuation. These abnormalities include fractures, primary and metastatic bone tumors, and some metabolic bone disorders. CT and MRI provide greater detail of chest wall abnormalities than does the chest radiograph. This is particularly true of the soft tissue structures of the chest wall.

CONCLUSIONS

The chest radiograph continues to play an important role in the diagnosis of abnormalities of the lungs and thorax. In situations where greater sensitivity is necessary or where radiographic findings are inconclusive or confusing, CT is the cross-sectional imaging modality of choice for imaging the thorax. Ultrasound, MRI, and nuclear medicine examinations often provide additional information in certain clinical situations.

REFERENCES

1. Swenson SJ, Brown, LR, Cloby TV, Weaver AL: Pulmonary nodules: CT evaluation of enhancement with iodinated contrast material. *Radiology* 194:393–398, 1995.
2. Patz EF, Lowe VJ, Hoffman JM, et al: Focal pulmonary abnormalities: Evaluation with F-18 fluorodeoxyglucose PET scanning. *Radiology* 188:487–490, 1993.
3. Goodman LR, Curtin JJ, Mewissen MW, et al: Detection of pulmonary embolism in patients with unresolved clinical and scintigraphic diagnosis: Helical CT vs angiography. *AJR* 164:1369–1374, 1995.
4. Remy-Jardin MJ, Remy J, Deshildre F, et al: Diagnosis of acute pulmonary emboism with spiral CT: Comparison with pulmonary angiography and scintigraphy. *Radiology* 200:699–706, 1996.
5. Teigen CL Maus TP, Sheedy PF II, et al: Pulmonary embolism: Diagnosis with contrast-enhanced electron beam CT and comparison with pulmonary angiography. *Radiology* 194:313–319, 1995.
6. Maki DD, Gefter WB, Alavi A: Recent advances in pulmonary imaging. *Chest* 115:1388–1402, 1999.

4 | Bronchoscopy, Transthoracic Needle Aspiration, and Related Procedures*

Daniel H. Sterman

Gustav Killian reported his experience with the first bronchoscopy in 1898. Technologic advances during the next century facilitated development of bronchoscopy as a pivotal diagnostic and therapeutic tool in pulmonary medicine. Although a number of bronchoesophagologists contributed to refinement of the technique based upon use of a rigid instrument, the advent of flexible fiberoptic bronchoscopy, pioneered by Ikeda in 1967, opened new horizons to clinicians.

More recently, transthoracic needle aspiration and biopsy added to the pulmonologist's diagnostic armamentarium. These techniques are particularly useful for evaluating localized or peripheral lung lesions. Transthoracic needle aspiration permits acquisition of material for cytologic and microbiologic analysis, while transthoracic needle biopsy provides tissue for histologic study.

This chapter comprises an overview of bronchoscopy, transthoracic needle aspiration and biopsy, and related techniques. Contradictions to bronchoscopy appear in Table 4-1. Following a general discussion of bronchoscopy and

---

TABLE 4-1 Contraindications to Bronchoscopy

Cardiovascular
  Recent myocardial infarction
  Unstable angina
  Unstable cardiac arrhythmias
  Severe hypertension
  Severe carotid or cerebrovascular disease
Pulmonary
  Severe hypoxemia despite maximal oxygen supplementation
  Hypoventilation with hypercapnia
  Severe bronchospasm or unstable asthma
Neurologic
  Active seizures
  Increased intracranial pressure
  Severe agitation
Other medical conditions
  Bleeding diathesis
  Platelet dysfunction or thrombocytopenia
  Severe anemia
  Cirrhosis with portal hypertension
  Uremia

---

*Edited from Chap. 38, "Bronchoscopy, Transthoracic Needle Aspiration, and Related Procedures," by Unger M, Sterman DH. In: *Fishman's Pulmonary Diseases and Disorders*, 3d ed., edited by Fishman, AP, Elias JA, Fishman JA, Grippi MA, Kaiser LR, Senior RM. New York, McGraw-Hill, 1998, pp. 589–606. For fuller discussion of the topics dealt with in this chapter, the reader is referred to the original text, as noted above.

associated general instrumentation, indications for the technique and patient preparation are considered. Specific applications of diagnostic and therapeutic bronchoscopy are discussed. Subsequently, safety factors related to bronchoscopy and complications of the technique are reviewed. Finally, transthoracic needle aspiration and biopsy are described.

TYPES OF BRONCHOSCOPY AND GENERAL INSTRUMENTATION

Rigid Bronchoscopy

The initial bronchoscope, developed by Killian in Europe and further perfected by Jackson in the United States, was a rigid metal tube that permitted either spontaneous or mechanical ventilation. Over the decades, rigid bronchoscopes of various lengths and sizes, which are adaptable for diverse applications in children and adults, have become available. With the development of fiberoptic and advanced electronic technology, the flexible bronchoscope has, to a large extent, replaced the rigid bronchoscope for diagnostic and some therapeutic indications.

Both rigid and flexible modern systems are equipped with optic capabilities for airway observation. Various diagnostic and therapeutic accessories can be inserted through the rigid bronchoscope while the patient remains ventilated.

In recent years, development of small cameras based on charged couple device (CCD) technology has facilitated transmission of bronchoscopic images to television monitors, enhancing the education of trainees and permitting improved documentation of bronchoscopic findings.

Flexible Fiberoptic and Videobronchoscopy

Although the optical resolution of early fiberoptic bronchoscopes was inferior to that of rigid devices, their flexibility, ease of manipulation, and simplicity of use, which permit rapid examination under topical anesthesia, have made flexible bronchoscopy the primary endoscopic procedure in pulmonary diseases.

The flexible bronchoscope varies from ultrathin, allowing for neonatal endoscopy, to larger, adult-size therapeutic devices. The diameter of the working channel permits aspiration of secretions or introduction of accessories required for diagnostic or therapeutic purposes. With flexible bronchoscopy, the patient's ventilation is assured by airflow between the external wall of the device and the tracheobronchial tree. Thus, the appropriate selection of bronchoscope size is crucial.

Recent technologic advances have permitted the replacement of fiberoptic systems by a miniaturized CCD camera at the tip of the scope that provides electronic transmission of images to a television monitor.

Diagnostic Bronchoscopy Accessories

The working channel of the fiberoptic or videobronchoscope, although of relatively small diameter, allows the insertion of various diagnostic and therapeutic accessories. Specially constructed accessories of larger caliber have been developed for use with the rigid bronchoscope.

Biopsy Forceps

Simple visualization of lesions is usually not sufficient to determine a precise diagnosis and to guide management. Pathologic confirmation through biopsy is frequently required. A variety of instruments have been developed that permit retrieval of biopsy specimens.

The cutting cups of biopsy forceps may be round or elliptic and may have smooth or jagged edges. The use of nonserrated edges, however, seems to reduce tissue trauma and the concomitant risk of bleeding. The biopsy procedure is simple and generally associated with only minimal complications in the case of a visible lesion. Even peripheral lesions, which are not visible through the bronchoscope, may be biopsied. With diffuse parenchymal or interstitial lung disease, specimens may be obtained without fluoroscopic guidance. With smaller lesions, however, the diagnostic yield of biopsies increases when fluoroscopy is utilized.

Bronchial Brushes

Lesions not accessible to direct biopsy with a forceps can be approached with a bronchial brush. This device consists of a rigid central wire surrounded by brushes of various sizes and shapes. To-and-fro movement of the brush against the adjacent tissue enables collection of specimens for cytologic or microbiologic analysis.

In some clinical circumstances, there is a need to obtain from the lower respiratory tract an uncontaminated specimen for microbiologic studies. A brush protected by an additional sheath and tip may be passed through the working channel of the bronchoscope.

Needles for Aspiration and Biopsy

Transbronchoscopic needle biopsy via rigid bronchoscopy was first reported by Schieppati, but the technique was subsequently adapted by Wang, utilizing a flexible needle with a fiberoptic bronchoscope. Initially, several models of needles were designed to obtain cytologic material; subsequently, histologic specimens from submucosal lesions and peribronchial mediastinal and hilar lymph nodes were obtained with larger-bore needles. These methods are useful in obtaining diagnostic material from areas that cannot be sampled with simple bronchoscopy forceps or brushes. The main indication for use of this type of cytology needle is staging of lung carcinoma. The procedure is particularly useful for patients who are marginal or poor surgical candidates; in these patients, more invasive approaches, such as mediastinoscopy or mediastinotomy, may be obviated.

The diagnostic yield depends on two factors: optimization of the bend of the tip of the bronchoscope and proper performance of bronchial wall puncture by the needle through the intercartilaginous space.

Dedicated Catheters and Balloons

Bronchoscopically guided double-lumen catheters allow for collection of uncontaminated specimens via bronchoalveolar lavage for study of lung diseases. These are wedged in the selected bronchus, the balloon inflated for isolation of the bronchus, and fluid instilled and then reaspirated through the central lumen of the catheter. Other low-pressure balloon catheters contribute to estimation of airway diameter prior to stent insertion. In addition, inflation of a balloon at the tip of the bronchoscope permits enlargement of the lumen and eventual passage of the bronchoscope beyond an area of stenosis, allowing exploration of peripheral airways.

Ultrasound Probes

Recent technologic advances, including miniaturization of various instruments, have allowed for the integration of ultrasound equipment into the body of the bronchoscope and development of separate ultrasound probes that can be introduced through the working channel. The integrated ultrasound bronchoscope may provide either linear-array images, with sectional visualization of the bronchial wall and peribronchial structures, or circumferential pictures. To avoid any interposition of air between the probe and the bronchus, specially designed fluid-filled balloons secure intimate contact with the airway wall, which allows better resolution of the peribronchial structures. With further refinements, these devices should provide guidance for more precise biopsies, *in vivo* diagnosis of infiltrative diseases of the bronchi, and more reliable delineation of clear surgical margins in lung cancer surgery.

PATIENT PREPARATION AND MONITORING DURING BRONCHOSCOPY

Most fiberoptic bronchoscopies are performed under conscious sedation with the short-acting agents fentanyl, codeine, midazolam, hydroxyzine, and diazepam. Patients undergoing bronchoscopy are often premedicated with anticholinergic drugs (e.g., atropine or glycopyrrolate) to reduce the risk of vasovagal reactions (bradycardia) and minimize airway secretions. Local anesthesia of the upper airway, larynx, and tracheobronchial tree is achieved with topical, inhaled and/or bronchoscopically instilled lidocaine.

Although rigid bronchoscopy was performed initially with topical anesthesia, the recent trend has been to perform the procedure under intravenous general anesthesia (propofol) with patients breathing spontaneously or ventilated with a jet ventilator. With appropriate technique and monitoring, good oxygenation and adequate ventilation can be assured.

Success of bronchoscopy, whether diagnostic or therapeutic, depends in large part on proper preparation of the patient, including relief of anxiety, muscle relaxation, cough suppression, and adequate anesthesia. Time spent in achieving these goals will be well worthwhile in reducing the risks of complications and increasing the ease of performance of the procedure. During and shortly after the procedure, appropriate monitoring of hemodynamic parameters, oxygenation, and ventilation contributes to the safety of bronchoscopy.

In the case of diffuse lung disease, use of fluoroscopy has not been demonstrated to improve the yield of transbronchial biopsies. Fluoroscopy is useful, however, in providing information regarding the proximity of the forceps to the pleura and in more rapidly diagnosing complications (e.g., pneumothorax). The role of fluoroscopy is essential in cases of focal peripheral lesions when attempts are made to obtain tissue by transbronchial (forceps or needle) biopsy. Also, the risk of biopsy-induced pneumothorax is reduced with use of fluoroscopy.

Insertion of brachytherapy catheters and their precise localization must be accomplished with fluoroscopic guidance. Similarly, placement of various types of stents is facilitated by fluoroscopic control (see below).

APPLICATIONS OF DIAGNOSTIC BRONCHOSCOPY

Bronchoscopy is the means for visual examination of the tracheobronchial tree and plays an essential role in the diagnosis of pulmonary malignancies. The instrument permits the acquisition of tissue biopsy specimens, selective mucosal brushings, and bronchoalveolar washings. In addition, a transbronchoscopic approach permits selective sampling of mediastinal structures, as described below.

Assessment of Airway Anatomy and Function

Thorough bronchoscopic evaluation begins with examination of the upper airways. It is of paramount importance to distinguish among normal anatomy, anatomic variations without clinical significance, and frankly pathologic conditions. For example, abnormal bronchial branching could be a normal variant or the source of frequent infections due to impaired drainage. Expertise is required for bronchoscopic examination after thoracic surgery, especially following bronchoplastic procedures or lung transplantation.

Flexible bronchoscopy with spontaneous respiration is superior to rigid bronchoscopy under general anesthesia for the assessment of airway integrity, with special attention to dynamic changes in airway caliber. Prolapse of the membranous portion of the trachea and main bronchi secondary to destruction of elastic connective tissue may account for greater than expected expiratory airflow obstruction. On the other hand, the finding of localized, posttraumatic chondromalacia may respond to surgical correction or bronchoscopic stent placement.

Bronchoscopic examination also permits evaluation and localization of congenital or postsurgical pathologic changes in bronchial integrity, such as tracheoesophageal or bronchopleural fistulas. Bronchoscopic observation and early diagnosis of bronchial rupture after chest trauma also greatly influence further therapy and prognosis. The same is true for the evaluation of anastomoses in bronchoplastic surgery or lung transplantation.

Critically ill patients who require prolonged intubation or tracheotomy have a higher incidence of delayed tracheal injuries (malacia, stricture, granulation tissue) that are best documented by bronchoscopy. Such complications can have significant bearing on clinical outcome.

Evaluation of Tracheobronchial Mucosa

Careful examination of the mucosal surface during diagnostic bronchoscopy is crucial. Rapid development of granulation tissue is frequently associated with reaction to a foreign body. Inflammatory mucosal reactions should raise the possibility of mycobacterial infection, other granulomatous diseases such as sarcoidosis, and some viral infections such as herpes simplex.

The distinction between normal, pale-pink mucosa and hypervascular areas in the tracheobronchial tree may provide important diagnostic clues. Most commonly, changes in mucosal coloration are associated with an inflammatory reaction due to bronchitis. These findings are, however, very distinct from those involving small hemangiomas or vascular ectasias due to compression by enlarged lymph nodes. Similarly, enlarged mucosal lymphatics may be visible in the setting of lymphatic interruption due to surgery, radiation therapy, fibrosis, or malignancy. In addition, distinct purplish mucosal discoloration can be observed in Kaposi's sarcoma.

Bronchial mucosal ulcerations are characteristic of Wegener's granulomatosis or malignancy. Loss of the usual mucosal luster and presence of a roughened surface may alert the expert bronchoscopist to an early infiltrative or neoplastic process. Prior mucosal trauma may induce the delayed formation of mucosal and submucosal fibrosis, resulting in airway retraction or distortion.

Various photosensitizer agents have been applied for bronchoscopic evaluation of the tracheobronchial mucosa. Photosensitizers, such as hematoporphyrin derivative (HPD) and delta-aminolevulinic acid (ALA), are retained more selectively by neoplastic tissues and are beneficial in the diagnosis of early-stage central lung cancers. When stimulated by blue light (440 nm), tissues containing these photosensitizers (i.e., tumors but not normal tissues) emit weak fluorescence in the red spectrum (630 nm). Use of photosensitizers, however, is cumbersome and associated with skin photosensitivity. Recent technologic developments permit the observation and analysis of tracheobronchial mucosal surfaces without photosensitizing agents, using the characteristic of tissue autofluorescence. When stimulated with light of a particular wavelength, all normal tissues emit specific fluorescence. Changes in the structural integrity of the same tissues due to pathologic processes modify or suppress the autofluorescence. The fluorescent emissions are too low in intensity to be seen by the human eye, but they can be imaged in real time with the use of a sophisticated camera, computer-controlled image analysis, and lung-imaging fluorescent endoscopy (LIFE system) attached to a fiberoptic bronchoscope.

Biopsies from areas of abnormal fluorescence increase the rate of detection of dysplasia or carcinoma in situ lesions in the tracheobronchial tree. Currently under development are bronchoscopic spectrophotometric techniques for study of metabolic functions in vivo and the performance of "optical biopsies," which provide information noninvasively on specific tissue components—e.g., changes in intracellular concentrations of NADPH or other cellular constituents.

Evaluation of Hemoptysis

One of the most frequent indications for bronchoscopy is hemoptysis. Bronchoscopic evaluation can be of help in determining the precise location and source of bleeding. Studies have shown that bronchoscopy is more effective in localizing the site of bleeding if performed early (91 percent yield) than if performed late (50 percent yield). In the case of a normal chest radiograph and hemoptysis, it is common to find traces of bleeding but not the site of origin. In these circumstances, examination with an ultrathin flexible instrument may be beneficial in identifying the source of bleeding in a peripheral airway. In some instances, bronchoscopy becomes useful not only as a diagnostic method but also as a therapeutic procedure (see below).

Evaluation of Peribronchial Structures

The trachea and bronchi are surrounded by mediastinal and parenchymal structures. Developmental or pathologic changes in these organs may be noted during bronchoscopic evaluation. An enlarged goiter or thymus can compress upper airways, resulting in airflow obstruction. Lymphadenopathy may produce structural changes, such as carinal widening or bronchial compression. Calcification of peribronchial lymph nodes may result in erosion of the bronchial wall and formation of a broncholith. These lesions are potential sources of airway obstruction, infection, and hemoptysis.

Development of the techniques of transbronchoscopic needle aspiration and biopsy has permitted sampling of the peribronchial lymph nodes with less risk, lower cost, and fewer complications than mediastinoscopy. The transbronchial approach also facilitates, to a certain extent, more accurate staging of bronchogenic carcinoma in that aortopulmonary, retrocarinal, and hilar lymph nodes can be routinely sampled for involvement. Bronchoscopy with transbronchial needle aspiration and biopsy can be performed on an outpatient basis, through fiberoptic instruments, using real-time fluoroscopic or computed tomographic (CT) guidance.

New developments in bronchoscopic ultrasonography should further assist in the precise localization of lesions and guidance of diagnostic biopsies and needle aspirations.

Performance of Bronchial and Parenchymal Biopsies

Improvements in bronchoscopic instrumentation since the days of Chevalier Jackson have permitted performance of endobronchial biopsies as well as biopsy of peripheral lung lesions. Transbronchial biopsies for diffuse parenchymal diseases such as sarcoidosis are usually of low risk and do not necessitate fluoroscopic guidance. In cases of small, peripheral, localized lesions, fluoroscopy is nevertheless mandatory to assure proper positioning of the brush, biopsy forceps, or needle. The diagnosis of various infectious diseases can be established with a variety of transbronchoscopic sampling techniques. The role of bronchoscopic lung biopsy is established in immunocompromised hosts, in whom documentation of the precise pathogen is crucial for appropriate therapy. Simple, cost-effective transbronchoscopic tissue sampling can obviate much more complicated, expensive, and higher-risk thoracic surgical procedures.

Sampling of Airway and Alveolar Constituents

Bronchoscopy provides easy and relatively safe access to material in the tracheobronchial tree and distal alveolar spaces. Aspirated secretions can be sent for microscopy and for cultures to determine the offending organism in cases of suspected infection. Cytologic analysis of bronchoscopically obtained materials can diagnose malignancy. The most commonly employed bronchoscopic techniques for sampling the airways and alveolar spaces include "bronchial washing," bronchial brushing (see above), and bronchoalveolar lavage.

Bronchoalveolar Lavage

Bronchoalveolar lavage (BAL) is a useful bronchoscopic technique that is safe, even in critically ill patients, wherein lung biopsy or brushings may not be recommended because of the risk of bleeding. BAL involves the instillation of sterile normal saline solution into distal airspaces through a "wedged" bronchoscope and then aspirated through the instrument's suction channel. The fluid collected in this manner can be grossly analyzed for detection of alveolar hemorrhage or subjected to microbiologic testing, cytologic analysis, cell count and differential, polymerase chain reaction, electron microscopy, flow cytometry, and evaluated for immunologic parameters or tissue markers.

The role of BAL is well documented in the diagnosis of some diffuse parenchymal diseases such as eosinophilic pneumonia, eosinophilic granuloma, and pulmonary alveolar proteinosis. It remains investigational in the evaluation of many other diseases—e.g., sarcoidosis, hypersensitivity pneumonitis, and idiopathic pulmonary fibrosis.

Application of Quantitative Microbiologic Techniques

Two bronchoscopic methods that are useful in the diagnosis of pulmonary infections are quantitative BAL and protected-specimen brushing (PSB).

They are, perhaps, most useful in the setting of suspected ventilator-associated pneumonia (VAP), wherein a patient who is endotracheally intubated and receiving mechanical ventilation has signs of infection and an abnormal chest radiograph. Intubated patients experience colonization of their upper and lower airways with nosocomial organisms. Because of an abnormal mucociliary clearance mechanism, these patients are at greater risk for developing pulmonary infections. In addition, mechanically ventilated, intubated patients are often treated empirically with broad-spectrum antibiotics and therefore are at greater risk for infection with resistant organisms and unusual lower respiratory tract pathogens. Quantitative BAL and PSB aid tremendously in the distinction between benign distal airway bacterial colonization and clinically significant infection that warrants antibiotic therapy.

Protected Brush Catheter Specimen

PSB utilizes a double-catheter system in which an outer cannula and distal, biodegradable plug protect the bronchoscopic brush within the inner cannula from contamination with secretions in the upper airway and suction channel of the bronchoscope. When the bronchoscope is positioned proximal to the segmental orifice of interest, the PSB inner cannula is advanced into a subsegment and the protective distal plug ejected. The brush is then advanced peripherally, rotated gently, and retracted into the inner cannula. The inner cannula is subsequently retracted into the outer cannula and the bronchoscope removed from the airway. The distal portion of the catheter is cleaned with 70% alcohol and the brush clipped into saline solution under sterile conditions. The PSB is then submitted for quantitative bacterial culture within 15 min of the performance of the procedure. The threshold for diagnosis of VAP with PSB is 10^3 colony-forming units (CFU) per milliliter, which corresponds to an initial concentration of 10^5 to 10^6 organisms in the original respiratory sample. In studies from various centers, PSB sampling has been shown to have a predictive value for the presence or absence of pneumonia of 72 to 100 percent.

Quantitative Bronchoalveolar Lavage

Quantitative BAL entails the performance of a standardized BAL, with infusion of at least 120 mL of saline for adequate sampling of a pulmonary subsegment. Quantitative culture of the aspirated material is performed to determine the number of CFU recovered. For quantitative BAL, a threshold of 10^4 CFU per milliliter is used for the diagnosis of pneumonia, reflecting a concentration of 10^5 to 10^6 bacteria per milliliter in the original specimen. Several groups have reported sensitivity and specificity rates for the detection of pneumonia by quantitative BAL culture in the range of 70 to 100 percent.

Although PSB is more commonly used in bronchoscopic clinical investigations, quantitative BAL may be superior to PSB in the diagnosis of VAP, since BAL samples a much larger proportion of lung parenchyma and is estimated to recover 5 to 10 times as many organisms as PSB. Protected BAL, which requires the use of a balloon-tipped catheter with a distal ejectable plug inserted through the suction channel of the bronchoscope, has a greater specificity than standard BAL; its sensitivity is at least as good as that of PSB. Combining the techniques of PSB and quantitative BAL may significantly improve the sensitivity of diagnosing nosocomial pneumonia.

APPLICATIONS OF THERAPEUTIC BRONCHOSCOPY

Removal of Foreign Bodies

The earliest therapeutic use of the rigid bronchoscope was for extraction of aspirated foreign bodies via various types of grasping forceps, retrieval baskets, and magnetic devices. The rigid bronchoscope remains the tool of choice for the removal of foreign bodies, especially in children, as it has a larger access channel, permitting insertion of retrieval tools, and the ability to provide and control the patient's ventilation. After removal of the foreign body, patients should be observed for hemoptysis or subglottic edema.

Control of Hemoptysis

In cases of hemoptysis, bronchoscopy may be of value not only for diagnosis but for emergency management of endobronchial bleeding. Because of difficulties with visualization, instruments with large and maximally effective suction channels should be used. Rigid bronchoscopy is generally preferred with massive bleeding, when the need to remove large clots is anticipated.

When continuous suctioning of blood fails to clear the airways, other means can be used. An iced saline solution can be instilled along with vasoactive drugs, such as epinephrine, to induce spasm of the bleeding vessels. The bronchoscope itself can also be used to stem the bleeding by tamponade of the bleeding site or to occlude the lumen of the bronchus from which the bleeding originates. The same effect, perhaps with better local control, can be achieved with bronchoscopic balloon catheters. Another effective method for control of visible sources of bleeding, particularly from endobronchial neoplasms, is neodymium-YAG laser photocoagulation (see below).

Aspiration of Secretions

Removal of retained secretions is a leading indication for therapeutic bronchoscopy. Bronchoscopic aspiration of secretions may be indicated in patients presenting with weakness of respiratory muscles (e.g., due to underlying neuromuscular disease or the postoperative state) or disorders leading to recurrent aspiration of food or excessive upper airway secretions. In critically ill or mechanically ventilated patients, removal of secretions and mucous plugs causing segmental or lobar atelectasis can usually be rapidly achieved with the flexible bronchoscope. Underlying pulmonary diseases, such as bronchiectasis, may aggravate the retention of airway secretions.

Two specific disorders are worth highlighting in the context of therapeutic bronchoscopy: pulmonary alveolar proteinosis (PAP) and allergic bronchopulmonary aspergillosis (ABPA). In PAP, BAL for clearance of alveolar material can be both diagnostic and therapeutic. In ABPA, lavage with saline solution may be insufficient to remove tenacious impactions (described as "plastic bronchitis"). In these circumstances, use of bronchoscopic forceps may prove helpful.

Treatment of Endobronchial Obstruction

Thermal Lasers

Debulking of endobronchial lesions, particularly benign and malignant tumors, can be accomplished with biopsy forceps or with the flange of the rigid bronchoscope. These techniques carry the risk of significant bleeding, which can be obviated via use of coagulative technologies such as thermal lasers.

The first laser used in treating lesions of the tracheobronchial tree was the CO_2 laser. Because of its far-infrared (wavelength 10,600 nm) beam, this laser can be transmitted only via special mirrors and a rigid bronchoscope. The CO_2 laser provides tissue vaporization and cutting with minimal depth of penetration of target tissues.

The neodymium-YAG laser is in the near-infrared spectrum (wavelength 1064 nm). The laser can penetrate deeply, leading to coagulation of blood vessels and other viable tissues. With a contact technique using specially designed sapphire tips, the YAG laser can be used bronchoscopically for coagulation of bleeding sources and tumors prior to mechanical debulking. Success rates and complications directly related to laser therapy are not different when the procedure is performed under general anesthesia through the rigid bronchoscope or under topical anesthesia through a flexible bronchoscope.

Photodynamic Therapy

The concept of photodynamic therapy (PDT) is based on three independent factors: use of a photosensitizer, light of a specific wavelength capable of activating the photosensitizer, and oxygen. Each of these factors is nontoxic when administered individually. In combination, however, these agents can destroy tissue, particularly neoplasms. When, in the presence of oxygen, the tissue is exposed to stimulating energy from light at a specific wavelength, a photochemical reaction occurs, resulting in the release of oxygen free radicals. Oxygen free radicals are very toxic and destroy the tissue in which they are produced.

"Nonthermal" lasers of very low power in the red spectrum (wavelength of about 630 nm), when delivered with the flexible bronchoscope, are capable of stimulating photosensitivity and are effective in the treatment of early endobronchial lung cancer. PDT is also approved by the U.S. Food and Drug Administration (FDA) for palliative debulking of unresectable endobronchial tumors.

Patients selected for PDT are pretreated with an intravenous injection of a photosensitizing compound (e.g., a hematoporphyrin derivative), which is preferentially localized and retained in neoplastic tissue. About 48 h after injection, the patient undergoes bronchoscopy. The tumor, as well as surrounding normal tissue, is exposed to the red light generated by the nonthermal laser. Within 24 to 48 h after treatment, the malignant bronchial tumor becomes necrotic. Generally, "cleanup" bronchoscopy is then required to remove the necrotic eschar.

Recent well-controlled studies from Japan have confirmed excellent results when this therapy is used in radiographically occult carcinoma of the central airways. The complete response rate during a 5-year follow-up period was 95.2 percent.

Among the more appealing photosensitizers for future clinical use is delta aminolevulinic acid (ALA), which can be given orally or topically. ALA has a shorter tissue half-life, decreasing the risk of prolonged photosensitivity.

Brachytherapy

Attempts to deliver a maximal therapeutic dose of radiation with minimal effects on unaffected surrounding tissues have fostered development of the technique of brachytherapy, in which radiation is introduced as close as possible to the target.

Endobronchial irradiation for bronchial carcinoma first used implantable radioactive sources. Many isotopes have been tried in pulmonary medicine, such as cobalt 60 and cesium 137. At present, most treatments are performed with iridium 192 (^{192}Ir).

The bronchial lesion is measured during a diagnostic bronchoscopy; then, under fluoroscopic guidance and direct bronchoscopic control, a special catheter is placed in proximity of the treated area. After appropriate calculation of the precise dose to be delivered, radioactive ^{192}Ir is introduced through the catheter. The radiation can be delivered either by high-dose-rate equipment or by a medium- or low-dose radioactive isotope, inserted manually. The high dose rate (more than 12 Gy/h) delivered by a remote-control introducer requires an average of at least three bronchoscopic procedures, while the medium (2 to 12 Gy/h) and lower dose (0.4 to 2 Gy/h) rates can be completed in one session.

The effectiveness of brachytherapy in symptom palliation is most pronounced when the procedure is performed shortly after removal of most of the endobronchial tumor by photoradiation therapy with the neodymium-YAG laser.

Electrocautery and Cryotherapy

Other techniques of tissue destruction can be applied through the bronchoscope. Electrocautery, proven effective in surgery and gastrointestinal endoscopy, also involves tissue destruction by coagulation and vaporization. Specially designed bronchoscopes have been developed to prevent potential electrical injury to both the patient and the endoscopist. Also, creating an electric spark in an oxygen-enriched environment may result in combustion and severe burns. This technique has been demonstrated by several investigators to be equally effective and less expensive than laser therapy.

Bronchoscopic cryotherapy involves insertion of specially designed probes containing liquid nitrous oxide or nitrogen (approximate temperature 20°C), resulting in the rapid creation of an "ice ball" at the tip of the probe. The target tissue is then rewarmed, resulting in thawing. Inappropriate manipulations, excessively rapid thawing, or premature detachment of the probe may result in bleeding or tissue fracture. Cryotherapy is inappropriate for patients requiring rapid reopening of airways, since the beneficial effects of this method are delayed and are achieved only after subsequent removal of the sloughed necrotic tissue. Cryotherapy is also not very effective in paucicellular or paucivascular lesions—e.g., fibrotic strictures and lipomas.

Airway Dilation

Rigid Scope Dilation   If obstruction is limited only to the proximal airways, correction of a short stenotic segment can result in significant clinical and physiologic improvement. Immediate but often transitory improvement can be achieved via rigid bronchoscopic dilation, as with tracheal webs. Once an acceptable bronchial lumen diameter is achieved, insertion of endobronchial prostheses can be considered.

Stent Placement   Since the beginning of interventional bronchoscopy, various endobronchial prostheses (airway stents) have been evaluated, but often with disappointing long-term results. Initially the stents were rigid devices made of rubber, metal, plastic, or composite materials. More recently, however, implantation of airway stents made of silicone or special metal alloys such as nitonol (a nickel-titanium alloy with shape memory) has been associated with improved long-term results. Airway stent insertion should be guided by three basic safety principles: satisfactory stent placement, maintenance of adequate ventilation and oxygenation, and skilled handling of potential complications. The role of the prosthesis is prevention of airway collapse and maintenance of airway integrity and an acceptable airflow. The ideal indication for prosthetic placement is a short segment of stenosis (in two or three cartilaginous rings) in the left mainstem bronchus or the trachea, preferably due to tracheobronchomalacia or extrinsic compression.

The most popular tracheobronchial stents were developed in France by Dumon and colleagues. These silicone prostheses are of various lengths and diameters and have external studs, which maintain better endobronchial stability. Placement of the stents requires special training in advanced rigid bronchoscopy. The advantage of the Dumon stents is their ease of removal. The most frequently reported complications are stent migration and occlusive overgrowth of tumor or granulation tissue at the end of the prosthesis.

Another recently developed endoprosthesis is the so-called dynamic stent, which was designed specifically for management of lower tracheal and main carinal stenosis. The stent is constructed from silicone and metal "scaffolding," mimicking the cartilaginous rings of the trachea; it has a soft posterior for better mobilization of secretions with coughing. As with the Dumon stent, the dynamic stent must be introduced with the help of a special introducer. During introduction of the dynamic stent through the stenotic area and before the stent's full deployment, the patient's ventilation can be severely compromised. There is much less risk of migration with this type of stent. As in the case of any synthetic prosthesis, however, there is a risk of the plugging of the lumen by secretions or necrotic debris.

Self-expanding stents were developed initially for vascular and biliary applications; only later were they modified for endobronchial use. The primary advantage of self-expanding stents is that they can be introduced with fiberoptic bronchoscopy. However, these prostheses carry a higher risk of granulation tissue formation at their distal and proximal aspects, potentially resulting in airway obstruction. Improved models have been introduced that have a polyethylene or polyurethane membrane covering the metallic mesh in an attempt to prevent tissue overgrowth. The major risk with older, high-pressure, self-expanding metal stents is perforation of the tracheobronchial tree. Because of their relatively rigid structure and overgrowth of tissue, removal of metallic stents is difficult and often requires rigid bronchoscopy.

Balloon Dilatation

For fibrotic bronchial stenosis, another bronchoscopic approach of dilatation has been developed, borrowing from the technique and equipment used in angioplasty procedures. After the nature, length, and initial diameter of bronchial stenosis have been determined, a high-pressure angioplasty balloon catheter is introduced through the working channel of the bronchoscope or over a guidewire under fluoroscopy. The diameter of the inflated balloon should match the optimal dilatation of the stenotic segment. The major risks of this technique are rupture of a bronchial wall, bleeding, and postprocedure airway edema. The advantage of the technique is that it obviates permanent introduction of foreign bodies into the tracheobronchial tree, which, by their presence, create a potential source of irritation, infection, or stasis of secretions.

Closure of Bronchial Fistulas

Fiberoptic bronchoscopy can be a useful intervention in identifying and treating bronchopleural and bronchoesophageal fistulas. Many different techniques have been employed, including introduction of irritating substances to stimulate formation of reactive granulation tissue as well as proclotting agents such as Gelfoam, autologous blood patch, cryoprecipitate, and thrombin injection to create occlusive fibrin clot. Small bronchopleural fistulas following thoracic surgery are associated with a higher rate of success of bronchoscopic sealing. It is much more difficult to achieve good obliteration of the fistula in the presence of infection or malignancy.

Therapeutic Bronchoscopic Accessories

Foreign-Body Retrieval Forceps and Baskets

Aspiration of foreign bodies is much more common in children than in adults. Ideally, a specialized bronchoscopic unit should be equipped with a large array of devices for foreign-body extraction. In particular, rigid bronchoscopy should be available. Unfortunately, however, removal of foreign bodies may need to be done on an emergency basis, in places where there is no ready access to specialized instrumentation.

Basic biopsy forceps may be of some value in foreign-body removal, particularly forceps with jagged edges. These devices may be helpful in the retrieval of hard objects with an irregular surface. Smooth objects or organic materials (e.g., nuts, food particles) require use of expandable baskets, balloon catheters, suction devices, or grasping forceps. Special dexterity is required of the bronchoscopist to guide the retrieval forceps or basket at the proper angle, so as to avoid any additional perforation or injury to the tracheobronchial tree or upper airway during the withdrawal.

Contact and Noncontact Laser Fibers

Laser beams, which can be transmitted via fiberoptic technique, are useful for deep coagulation and vaporization of tissue. The crucial aspects in this technique are the constant visualization of the aiming beam, maintenance of the tip of the laser guide free of debris, and observation of changes occurring in the targeted tissue during the procedure. Coagulation of the tumor vasculature results in reduction in tumor volume and progressive enlargement of the airway lumen. Specially designed sapphire contact tips require lower laser power, but provide improved control of tissue effects, and are useful as cutting or debulking tools. The disadvantage of the technique is that precise observation of tissue reaction is obscured.

In response to specific needs of PDT, special light guides have been developed. Patients with small, superficial, well-circumscribed tumors benefit from a microlens quartz fiber that delivers nonthermal laser light in a uniform fashion at the tip. Fibers with radial light distribution patterns over a specified length at the tip, which are capable of affecting the lumen of the bronchus circumferentially, are preferred for treating more extensive tumors. The same fibers can also be used for interstitial insertion into large tumors.

The precise time of treatment and the total energy to be delivered to the tissues are calculated according to protocols.

Balloon Catheters

High-pressure angioplasty catheters with various balloon lengths and diameters have been used for airway dilation. None of the widely used balloon catheters, such as Fogarty embolectomy balloon catheters, were developed specifically for bronchoscopic use. These catheters have proved to be very helpful in removing accumulated secretions, blood clots, debris, and foreign bodies. Given the potential risk of bronchial rupture, the general recommendation is to avoid exceeding a balloon pressure above 6 atm.

In the double-lumen catheter, the balloon is inflated for anchoring the catheter in place, and the central lumen is used for insertion of the radioactive source. Similarly, balloon-tipped catheters are very useful in selective obstruction of a bronchial lumen, for tamponading bronchial bleeding, or for temporary interruption of a bronchopleural communication. Selective delivery catheters have been used for endobronchial administration of antineoplastic drugs, antibiotics, radiolabeled monoclonal antibodies, and photosensitizers.

Prostheses Introducers

Dedicated tracheobronchial stents, however, are inserted using specially constructed introductory devices. The Dumon stent must first be folded, then compressed and introduced into a tube, which is then inserted through a rigid bronchoscope. Once the distal tip of this tube has reached beyond the estimated area of stenosis, the stent is pushed out from the proximal end with a special device. Proper positioning of the stent is achieved with a grasping forceps.

Similarly, the "dynamic" stent is inserted over a specially designed dual-function grasping forceps and integrated "pusher" device. Once the device holding the compressed, Y-shaped stent passes through the upper airways, the grasping forceps, which approximates the two small limbs of the Y, is opened. The integrated pusher anchors the stent at the level of the carina, while the introducer is withdrawn. The two Silastic arms remain in the left and right main-stem bronchi, and the main, "dynamic" part of the stent extends into the trachea.

SAFETY FACTORS IN BRONCHOSCOPY

Bronchoscopy is a specialized procedure that requires extensive training. Familiarity with both the physiology and anatomy of the airways is essential. Any diagnostic or therapeutic manipulation should be considered in relation to the underlying condition of the patient, localization of the area of investigation, and other surrounding structures in the thorax. It is critical to have nursing or respiratory therapy assistance during the procedure for patient monitoring (oxygen saturation, blood pressure, heart rhythm, etc.) and checking and maintaining the adequacy of ancillary equipment (suction, oxygenation, accessories such as forceps, balloons, catheters, laser light guides). Risks are decreased if, for example, special attention is paid to the control of accessories during their manipulation beyond the tip of the bronchoscope. Premature deployment of the needle biopsy device or inappropriate bending of the bronchoscope while an instrument is inside the flexible portion can result in

TABLE 4-2 Safety Measures to Avoid Bronchoscopic Complications

Attention to proper indications
Attention to contraindications
Experienced team and appropriate facilities
Appropriate instrumentation
Appropriate pre-, peri-, and postbronchoscopic monitoring
Proper preparation for emergencies

perforation of the bronchoscope. Activation of the laser with a broken light guide inside the bronchoscope or inadequate protrusion of the tip of the fiber beyond the bronchoscope may result in airway fires or severe burns to the patient. Attention to details and proper maintenance of the equipment, including accessories, enhance safety for the patient and staff and improve diagnostic yields and therapeutic results (Table 4-2).

COMPLICATIONS OF BRONCHOSCOPY

Anesthesia and Related Blood Gas Abnormalities

A significant proportion of the life-threatening complications of diagnostic bronchoscopy are associated with sedation and topical anesthesia. Risk is significantly increased in the elderly and those with underlying medical problems, including cardiovascular disease, chronic pulmonary disease, renal and hepatic dysfunction, seizures, and altered mental status. Doses of sedatives and topical anesthetics must be adjusted for underlying organ dysfunction. Conscious sedation techniques using short-acting benzodiazepines (e.g., midazolam) seem to have reduced the incidence of potentially dangerous hypotension and respiratory depression.

Inadequate topical anesthesia potentiates coughing, gagging, and patient discomfort and increases the risk of injury during bronchoscopy. However, topical anesthetics such as lidocaine, the most frequently used agent, are absorbed systemically through the respiratory mucosa, increasing the risk of arrhythmias and seizures. These complications are more likely to occur in patients with underlying cardiac dysfunction, hepatic dysfunction, and oropharyngeal candidiasis. Another, less frequent complication of lidocaine use is methemoglobinemia and tissue hypoxia.

Introduction of the bronchoscope under general anesthesia or under conscious sedation with topical anesthesia frequently results in a decrease in oxygenation and in hypoventilation, with a significant increase in Pa_{CO_2}. In patients with underlying chronic lung disease, severe hypoxemia may occur, triggering life-threatening cardiac arrhythmias, unless corrected by supplemental oxygen. After rigid and flexible bronchoscopy, patients with predisposing factors should be monitored carefully for laryngospasm or bronchospasm.

All patients undergoing bronchoscopic procedures should be monitored continuously (ECG, blood pressure, O_2 saturation, and, if indicated, expiratory CO_2 concentration). Use of supplemental oxygen during the procedure should be routine. Bronchoscopy should probably not be performed in patients who are unable to maintain a Pa_{O_2} of 65 mmHg while an $F_{I_{O_2}}$ of 1.0 and full ventilatory support are administered.

Significant oxygen desaturation may occur during BAL. The degree of desaturation is directly related to the duration of the procedure and the volume of lavage fluid used. Return to the prebronchoscopy level of O_2 saturation may be prolonged after removal of the bronchoscope, and supplemental O_2 should be continued throughout the procedure and during the postbronchoscopy observation period.

Fever and Infection

In patients with underlying valvular cardiac disease and those predisposed to endocarditis, the American Heart Association recommends use of prophylactic antibiotics before rigid bronchoscopy but not before flexible bronchoscopy. Appearance of transient fever after bronchoscopy is not unusual and generally does not require any therapy. However, persistent fever in the setting of progressive radiographic infiltrates necessitates antibiotic therapy. The incidence of postbronchoscopy fever is increased in the elderly and in those with underlying chronic obstructive pulmonary disease (COPD) or malignant endobronchial obstruction. The incidence of postbronchoscopic infections is higher in immunocompromised hosts.

Airway Obstruction and Perforation

The advent of interventional bronchoscopy has resulted in complications not ordinarily seen with diagnostic bronchoscopy. Inappropriate use of lasers has resulted in endobronchial burns and bronchial perforations associated with catastrophic bleeding, pneumomediastinum, or pneumothorax.

Following photodynamic therapy, formation of a necrotic eschar, airway edema, or rapid, potentially complete airway obstruction should be anticipated and treated with "cleanup" bronchoscopy.

As noted previously, insertion of airway stents is associated with many potential complications, including incomplete stent deployment or stent migration, resulting in life-threatening airway obstruction.

Pneumothorax

Most of the serious complications directly due to diagnostic bronchoscopy have been reported in association with performance of transbronchial biopsies. Pneumothorax following transbronchial biopsy occurs in about 4 percent of cases, even when the procedure is done under fluoroscopic guidance.

The incidence of pneumothorax is increased greatly (three or four times) in immunocompromised hosts, mechanically ventilated patients, and in the presence of bullous lung disease. For these reasons, a postbronchoscopic expiratory chest radiograph is performed routinely. In the case of a significant pneumothorax, a chest tube should be inserted immediately to avoid tension pneumothorax.

Hemorrhage

One of the most frequently reported complications related to bronchoscopy is hemorrhage. The risks of hemorrhage during bronchoscopy are increased in uremia and bleeding disorders. For these reasons, a blood urea nitrogen (BUN) level above 30 mg/dL or a creatinine level above 3 mg/dL should be considered relative a contraindication to bronchoscopy. Bronchoscopy should not be performed if the platelet count is below 50,000/mm^3, and transbronchial biopsy or aggressive interventional procedures (laser therapy, bronchoplasty, or stent placement) are probably safe only with platelet counts above 75,000/mm^3.

Manipulation of the bronchoscope, mechanical trauma, vigorous suctioning, endobronchial brushing, and biopsy may result in significant bleeding in 1 to 4 percent of patients without underlying risks for hemorrhage. Hemorrhage can also occur with inadvertent perforation of pulmonary vessels during transbronchial needle aspiration or biopsy.

Overall, when bronchoscopy is performed by an experienced endoscopist, backed up by a well-trained team and appropriate facilities, mortality and morbidity are very low.

TRANSTHORACIC NEEDLE ASPIRATION AND BIOPSY

Transthoracic needle aspiration (TTNA) is a useful technique for the diagnosis of a variety of benign and malignant thoracic lesions, using fluoroscopic, CT, or ultrasound guidance. In the past, many pulmonologists performed TTNA as the initial diagnostic procedure for intrapulmonary lesions, especially those in the lung periphery. With the development of video-assisted thoracic surgical techniques, patients can more easily undergo complete excision of pulmonary nodules. Transthoracic needle biopsy (TTNB) provides core biopsy material from pulmonary nodules for histologic examination. The ability to analyze histology is critical in establishing a definitive diagnosis for certain disease states (e.g., sarcoidosis) in which cytologic aspiration is inadequate in documenting the characteristic noncaseating granulomas. TTNB also provides improved diagnostic accuracy in lymphomas. TTNB plays a minor role in the diagnosis of suspected bronchogenic carcinomas, since most can be diagnosed accurately with cytologic analysis alone, and since subtyping of non–small cell carcinomas has little bearing on prognosis, therapeutic approach, or tumor response to therapy. Histologic specimens may improve the yield in the diagnosis of pulmonary hamartomas, characterized by the presence of cartilage or adipose tissue.

Indications and Contraindications

In 1989, the American Thoracic Society published guidelines for percutaneous needle aspiration biopsy. The major indications include evaluation of solitary lung nodules and masses, mediastinal and hilar lesions, metastatic disease to the lung from a known extrathoracic malignancy, chest wall invasion by lung carcinoma, and pulmonary consolidation or infiltrates that are likely to be of infectious origin. The most common indication for TTNA is evaluation of a solitary pulmonary nodule that arouses suspicions of bronchogenic carcinoma.

TTNA can affect therapeutic decisions by establishing a definitive benign diagnosis, such as pulmonary hamartoma, by differentiating small cell and non–small cell carcinoma of the lung and distinguishing between primary and metastatic lung tumors. The latter distinction is often difficult, particularly in the case of adenocarcinomas. Diagnosis of benign disease, small cell lung cancer, metastatic cancer, or synchronous primaries may obviate thoracotomy. One must also distinguish clinical circumstances in which transthoracic needle biopsy is more appropriate than transthoracic needle aspiration. A cytology sample may be inadequate for diagnosing certain pulmonary lesions, such as lymphoma and sarcoidosis. When these disorders are suspected, transthoracic needle biopsy is more appropriate.

Absolute contraindications to TTNA include an uncooperative patient or one with an intractable cough, as patients must suspend respirations while the needle crosses the pleura. In addition, TTNA is absolutely contraindicated in patients with a suspected pulmonary hydatid cyst because of the risk of capsule rupture and systemic dissemination. Relative contraindications include bullous emphysema, pulmonary arterial hypertension, and coagulation or platelet disorders. Patients with bullous emphysema are at increased risk of developing symptomatic pneumothoraces after TTNA, although most induced pneumothoraces are small and can be treated conservatively. Those with pulmonary hypertension and coagulation disorders who undergo TTNA have a higher chance of developing pulmonary hemorrhage and significant hemoptysis.

Technique

Choice of Needle

In the early 1960s, TTNA was performed with large-bore cutting needles; significant hemmorhagic complications were reported. More recently, thin-needle aspiration has become standard; it uses devices ranging in size from 18 to 22 gauge. Coaxial needle systems have been introduced for the purpose of obtaining multiple samples from a single pleural penetration. These systems are also useful for procuring specimens for histologic evaluation.

Radiographic Guidance

Most transthoracic needle procedures are performed with fluoroscopic guidance, typically using a C-arm or biplane device capable of rotation of over 180 degrees in a single plane. C-arm fluoroscopy allows for real-time imaging of pulmonary lesions during needle insertion and specimen retrieval. CT has been used to guide TTNA of pulmonary lesions, most commonly lesions that are too small to be seen fluoroscopically or those that are centrally located and adjacent to major vascular structures. Core biopsy for obtaining histologic specimens is commonly done with CT guidance. An automated biopsy system with a diagnostic sensitivity of 81 percent and a pneumothorax rate of 9 percent has been described.

Ultrasound guidance of TTNA offers the advantage of real-time lesion imaging, easy portability, and absence of exposure to ionizing radiation for both the clinician and the patient. Ultrasound is used most commonly for peripheral lung lesions that extend to the pleural edge or for anterior mediastinal masses. The sensitivity of ultrasound-guided TTNB of pulmonary and mediastinal lesions larger than 3 cm is over 95 percent, with a pneumothorax rate less than 2 percent.

Needle Insertion

The procedure is best performed with the patient lying on a table that is fluoroscopy-compatible; positioning should be either supine or prone, depending on the location of the lesion. A lateral approach can be considered if the target lesion is large and apposed to the lateral pleural surface.

The lesion is localized by fluoroscopic guidance, and the overlying skin is marked and anesthetized with 1% lidocaine. Conscious sedation may be indicated for patients who are particularly anxious or agitated. Throughout the procedure, the patient's pulse, blood pressure, heart rate, cardiac rhythm, and oxyhemoglobin saturation should be monitored closely.

The aspiration needle is inserted perpendicularly through the anesthetized region into the lesion, as seen under fluoroscopy. Rotation of a C-arm fluoroscopy unit for visualization of the lesion in another plane aids in proper positioning of the needle. Under fluoroscopy, the needle may be seen to displace the lesion or, if properly positioned, the needle will move in concert with the lesion during quiet breathing. If the needle is seen to move independently of the lesion during respiration, it is positioned unsatisfactorily. Several samples should be obtained so as to increase the diagnostic yield. With a necrotic mass, aspiration should also be performed in peripheral locations of the lesion in order to obtain viable cells and to decrease the risk of false-negative results.

Noncoaxial transthoracic needles require an initial aspiration and immediate examination of a touch preparation to determine the adequacy of the specimen. If the aspirated material is insufficient, a second puncture must be made, increasing the likelihood of pneumothorax or intraparenchymal hemorrhage. Coaxial TTNA systems allow for multiple aspirations with a single pleural puncture and therefore have a lower rate of pneumothorax without reduced diagnostic accuracy.

The technique of TTNB is similar to that of TTNA and is performed primarily with a coaxial needle system. These systems typically consist of a 19-gauge, beveled-tip outer needle with a cutting edge and a 21-gauge inner needle that acts as a trocar, facilitating passage of the instrument toward the lesion. The inner needle may be used as a standard TTNA device to obtain multiple aspirates from the target lesion with a single puncture of the pleural surface. The distal lumen of the outer needle is used to core out and store the biopsy specimen. Occasionally, in patients who have a large amount of subcutaneous adipose tissue or muscle, insertion of a 14-gauge catheter proximal to the pleura as a guide for the TTNB needle is helpful in preventing alterations in the angle of the TTNB toward the lesion.

Because of the need for complete withdrawal before a core biopsy is obtained, obtaining a second sample necessitates a second pleural puncture, increasing the risk of pneumothorax. In addition, by virtue of its larger diameter, the hollow outer needle carries a greater overall risk of complications than does the thinner cytology needle. TTNB has a higher pneumothorax rate per pleural puncture than does TTNA; TTNB is also associated with a greater chance of significant pulmonary hemorrhage.

TTNB is most useful for pulmonary lesions extending to the pleural surface, which are easily visualized fluoroscopically and are less likely to require multiple passes to obtain diagnostic material. In expert hands, the pneumothorax rate for TTNB may be as low as 21 percent, with negligible rates of pulmonary hemorrhage and air embolism.

Specimen Processing

Specimens obtained with TTNA or TTNB can be placed into a glutaraldehyde solution for delayed analysis; however, evaluation is much more successful if a cytopathologist is present at the time of the procedure. Cytopathologists can immediately process the aspirated material with a modified Diff-Quik stain (Baxter Scientific Products) for on-site light microscopic examination. Cell blocks can also be created from multiple tissue fragments fixed in 95% ethanol.

Cytologic evaluation alone can often distinguish between non-small cell and small cell carcinoma of the lung, and primary and metastatic pulmonary tumors. Electron microscopy may be utilized to aid in identification of poorly differentiated tumors or to determine the primary malignancy of origin of a metastatic pulmonary lesion. Immunohistochemical analysis of aspirated cells can help differentiate epithelial from mesenchymal tumors and can identify a specific tumor of origin through analysis of cell surface markers (e.g., estrogen or progesterone receptors in metastatic breast carcinoma).

TTNA is commonly conducted as an outpatient procedure. It is standard to perform a chest radiograph 1 to 2 h after the procedure to rule out pneumothorax. Most clinically significant pneumothoraces necessitating medical intervention have been shown to occur within the first hour. A patient with small, asymptomatic pneumothorax may be discharged home after an additional 1 to 2 h of observation if a repeat radiograph documents no interval enlargement of the pneumothorax.

Results

TTNA and TTNB have excellent success rates in the diagnosis of primary or metastatic pulmonary malignancies; for TTNA, the sensitivity is 85 to 95 percent. Major causes of false-negative results in malignant disease are inadequate sampling of the lesion and aspiration in an area of necrosis or postobstructive pneumonia. In addition, small, central malignant lesions may be difficult to diagnose accurately with TTNA. Aspiration of vascular tumors—such as angiosarcoma, carcinoid, or metastatic renal cell carcinoma—may yield a bloody aspirate with few if any malignant cells. TTNA rarely leads to misclassification of primary pulmonary neoplasms, with a reported rate of misdiagnosis of small cell carcinoma of 0 to 1.1 percent. False-positive results are extremely rare (under 0.5 percent) and are typically reported in the setting of inflammatory processes such as tuberculosis, radiation fibrosis, organizing pneumonia, and pulmonary infarction.

Specific diagnosis of a benign lesion with TTNA is more problematic, with published sensitivities ranging widely, from 11.7 to 68 percent. A TTNA that is negative for malignancy does not rule out the presence of neoplastic disease, especially if the aspirate was unsatisfactory. The degree of suspicion of malignancy in a particular clinical situation becomes extremely important in dictating the next step following a negative TTNA. For a smoker with a high risk of bronchogenic carcinoma, the proper course may lead to videothoracoscopic biopsy of the lesion; whereas in a young, otherwise healthy nonsmoker, close observation with serial chest radiographs may be the preferred option.

Complications

As mentioned previously, the most common complication of both TTNA and TTNB is pneumothorax; incidence rates reported in the literature vary from 8 to 61 percent. A small percentage of the pneumothoraces are clinically significant; only about 8 percent require thoracostomy tube drainage. Most symptomatic pneumothoraces can be managed successfully with insertion of a pneumothorax catheter connected to a Heimlich valve. Tension pneumothoraces are true medical emergencies, typically occurring within minutes of the procedure; they should be treated with immediate decompression. Preexisting lung disease—in particular, bullous emphysema—is the most significant predisposing factor to development of pneumothorax after TTNA or TTNB. Other risk factors are deep lesions, increased number of passes, more than one pleural surface crossed, and increased patient age.

Uncommon complications of TTNA and TTNB include hemorrhage and hemoptysis, although these are typically minor. Cases of fatal hemorrhage with clot-induced tracheobronchial obstruction and subsequent asphyxia after use of large-bore (18-gauge) cutting needles have been reported.

Air embolism is a rare complication caused by creation of a communication between atmospheric air and a pulmonary vein. To minimize this risk, the needle should never be left open to air while in the chest, and the patient should be discouraged from deep breathing, straining, or coughing during the procedure. The procedure should be halted and the needle withdrawn if the patient is actively coughing. If an air embolism is suspected, 100% oxygen should be administered through a nonrebreather face mask and the patient placed in the left lateral decubitus position, with the head down; this position optimizes capture of air in the right atrium. The patient should be transferred immediately to a hyperbaric chamber.

BIBLIOGRAPHY

Cavaliere S, Foccoli P, Farina PL: Nd:YAG laser bronchoscopy: A five-year experience with 1396 applications in 1000 patients. *Chest* 94:15–21, 1988.

Dumon JF, Cavaliere S, Diaz-Jimenez JP, et al: Seven-year experience with the Dumon prosthesis. *J Bronchol* 3:6–10, 1996.

Edell ES, Cortese DA: Photodynamic therapy in management of early superficial squamous cell carcinoma as an alternative to surgical resection. *Chest* 102:1319–1322, 1992.

Falguera M, Nogues A, Ruiz-Gonzalez A, et al: Transthoracic needle aspiration in the study of pulmonary infections in patients with HIV. *Chest* 106:697–702, 1994.

Guidelines for percutaneous needle aspiration biopsy. *Am Rev Respir Dis* 140:255–256, 1989.

Jackson C, Jackson CL: Bronchoscopy, in *Bronchoesophagology.* Philadelphia, Saunders, 1950 pp 50–67.

Killian G: Ueber directe Bronchoscopie. *Munich Med Wochenschr* 27:844–847, 1898.

Lam S, MacAulay C, LeRiche JC, et al: Detection of dysplasia and carcinoma in situ by lung imaging fluorescence endoscope (LIFE) device. *J Thorac Cardiovasc Surg* 105:1035–1040, 1993.

McManigle JE, Fletcher GL, Tenholder MF: Bronchoscopy in the management of bronchopleural fistula. *Chest* 97:1235–1238, 1990.

Meduri GU: Diagnosis and differential diagnosis of ventilator-associated pneumonia. *Clin Chest Med* 16:61–93, 1995.

Prakash UBS, Offord KP, Stubbs SE: Bronchoscopy in North America: The ACCP survey. *Chest* 100:1668–1675, 1991.

Saumench J, Escarabill J, Padro L, et al: Value of fiberoptic bronchoscopy and angiography for diagnosis of the bleeding site in hemoptysis. *Ann Thorac Surg* 48:272–274, 1989.

Shure D: Transbronchial biopsy and needle aspiration. *Chest* 95:1130–1138, 1989.

Unger M: Nd:YAG laser therapy for malignant and benign endobronchial obstructions. *Clin Chest Med* 6:277–290, 1985.

Wang KP: Staging of bronchogenic carcinoma by bronchoscopy. *Chest* 106: 588–593, 1994.

Westcott JL: Direct percutaneous needle aspiration of localized pulmonary lesions: Results in 422 patients. *Radiology* 137:31–35, 1980.

Zavala DC, Schoell JE: Ultrathin needle aspiration of the lung in infections and malignant disease. *Am Rev Respir Dis* 123:125–131, 1981.

5 | Impairment and Disability Evaluation*

Michael A. Grippi

INTRODUCTION

The physician's role in the evaluation of impairment or disability complements others' assessment of the patient's education, alternative job potential, and regional work opportunities. Indeed, the physician plays a *supporting* rather than a *deciding* role in determining whether financial benefits are to be awarded on the basis of a work-related injury. *Impairment* is a medical condition resulting from a functional abnormality. Impairment exists if an environmental sensitivity precludes a worker from performing a specific job, if a nontreatable lethal disease is present, or if the worker constitutes a public health hazard (e.g., untreated tuberculosis). *Disability* is the composite effect that an impairment has on an individual's life and, by definition, includes many nonmedical factors. While a physician evaluates impairment, a nonmedical adjudicator determines disability.

CLINICAL EVALUATION

A chronologically complete medical and occupational history includes delineation of workplace exposures that may account for loss of lung function. Symptoms should be quantified. The American Thoracic Society (ATS), adapting a scale from the British Medical Research Council, grades shortness of breath as mild, moderate, severe, or very severe based on the level of everyday activity that causes dyspnea. A dyspnea scale is useful in evaluating symptoms disproportionate to the results of pulmonary function testing. A complete physical examination should be performed in order to confirm the presence of respiratory disease and to detect disease in other organs that affect respiratory symptoms or function. However, the physical examination plays only a supportive role in impairment and disability evaluation.

Frequently, the chest x-ray initiates an impairment or disability evaluation, particularly in the setting of a suspected pneumoconiosis. The National Institute of Occupational Safety and Health (NIOSH) designates qualified physicians as experts ("B readers") in application of the International Labor Organization (ILO) classification for assessment of radiographic severity of pneumoconioses. The ILO classification is based on a set of standard films. However, the severity of pulmonary function abnormalities and radiographic readings among patients with pneumoconioses correlate poorly, particularly in patients with obstructive lung disease. In general, radiographic findings are not reliable measures of impairment or disability.

---

*Edited from Chap. 41, "Impairment and Disability Evaluation," by Epstein PE. In: *Fishman's Pulmonary Diseases and Disorders,* 3d ed., edited by Fishman AP, Elias JA, Grippi MA, Kaiser LR, Senior RM. New York, McGraw-Hill, 1998, pp 631–644. For fuller discussion of the topics dealt with in this chapter, the reader is referred to the original text, as noted above.

Pulmonary function testing constitutes an important element in the evaluation of impairment and disability. The ATS has published standards for pulmonary function test equipment and test performance. The older practice of judging FVC or FEV_1 as abnormal if less than 80 percent of predicted does not appear to be justified, since there is no statistical support for such an approach (see Chap. 2); alternatively, the lowest 5 percent of a reference population may be defined as abnormal. However, certain entitlement programs for the evaluation of impairment mandate specific test results as cutoff points between normal and abnormal, based on sex, height, and age.

Cardiopulmonary exercise testing (see Chap. 2) is frequently performed to determine the highest level of exertion achievable, as denoted by the patient's maximal oxygen utilization ($\dot{V}_{O_2max}$). By noting when limiting symptoms develop during progressive exercise, it may be possible to match exercise capacity with the job requirements. Measured $\dot{V}_{O_2max}$ may be compared to normal predicted values and reflects whether the individual can perform a normal amount of exertion. The level of exertion at which lactate begins to accumulate in the blood (the *anaerobic threshold*) is also an important indicator of work capacity. Measurement of $\dot{V}_{O_2}$ at the anaerobic threshold helps in evaluating the level of exertion that can be sustained for long periods, since anaerobic exertion clearly cannot be sustained indefinitely. However, neither the ATS nor the American Medical Association recommends exercise testing if pulmonary function tests are normal or if severe impairment is evident according to other criteria. In addition, exercise studies should not be performed when coexisting conditions (e.g., cardiac arrhythmias or unstable angina) make maximal exertion dangerous. Exercise testing is rarely indicated when no disparity exists between symptoms and pulmonary function test abnormalities.

GUIDELINES FOR ASSESSING IMPAIRMENT AND DISABILITY

Three sets of guidelines for impairment and disability evaluation—including those of the American Medical Association, the American Thoracic Society, and the Social Security Administration—are briefly summarized below.

American Medical Association Guidelines

According to the American Medical Association (AMA) *Guides to the Evaluation of Permanent Impairment,* the underlying disease should be stable and maximally treated. Spirometry and diffusing capacity measurements should be made and results expressed as "percent predicted," using published standards. If spirometry and diffusing capacity results appear to underestimate the true severity of the disease, cardiopulmonary exercise testing may be performed.

Four functional categories are recognized, ranging from class I (normal) to class IV (severely impaired) (Table 5-1). The most abnormal test result determines the class of impairment. The AMA *Guides* also identify impairment associated with specific disorders, including asthma, sleep apnea, pneumoconiosis, hypersensitivity pneumonitis, and lung cancer.

Impairment due to asthma is based on the optimally treated patient's pulmonary function abnormalities measured on three separate occasions, at least 1 week apart.

Obstructive or central sleep apnea is considered a severely impairing illness in the untreated patient because of the secondary effects of the illness

TABLE 5-1 Classes of Respiratory Impairment According to AMA *"Guides to the Evaluation of Permanent Impairment"*

	Class 1 (0%, no impairment of the whole person)	Class 2 (10–25%, mild impairment of the whole person)	Class 3 (26–50%, moderate impairment of the whole person)	Class 4 (51–100%, severe impairment of the whole person)
FVC, FEV_1, $FEV_1FVC\%$, D_{LCO}	FVC≥80% predicted, *and* FEV_1≥80% predicted, *and* FEV_1/FVC%≥ 70, and D_{LCO} ≥70% predicted or	FVC between 60 and 79% predicted, *or* FEV_1 between 60 and 79% predicted, *or* D_{LCO} between 60 and 69% predicted or	FVC between 51 and 59% predicted, *or* FEV_1 between 41 and 59% predicted, *or* D_{LCO} between 41 and 59% predicted or	FVC≤50% predicted, or FEV_1≤40% predicted, *or* D_{LCO} ≤40% predicted or
$\dot{V}_{O_2max}$	>25 mL/(kg·min) *or* >7.1 METs	Between 20 and 25 mL/(kg·min); *or* 5.7–7.1 METs	Between 15 and 20 mL/(kg·min); *or* 4.3–5.7 METs	<15 mL/(kg·min); *or* <1.05 L/min; *or* <4.3 METs

SOURCE: Reproduced with permission from *Guides to the Evaluation of Permanent Impairment.* American Medical Association, Chicago, 1994.

on job performance. In those treated, polysomnography results are used to determine the severity of persistent impairment.

Patients with pneumoconioses must be assessed functionally and for risk of further damage from remaining in the current job. Some experience disease progression even without further dust exposure. If continued exposure might occur, susceptible individuals should be removed from the workplace. In evaluating an individual for impairment or disability, future employment should be restricted to jobs that eliminate any further fibrogenic dust exposure. Hypersensitivity pneumonitis usually relapses upon exposure to the offending agent, and repeated exposures may lead to pulmonary fibrosis. Impairment rating in hypersensitivity pneumonitis is based on test results noted in Table 5-1; however, subjects may be considered impaired for specific jobs entailing exposure to the causative agent even if pulmonary function is normal.

All patients with lung cancer are considered severely impaired at diagnosis. If reevaluation at 1 year following treatment reveals recurrence of the cancer, the designation of severe impairment is continued. If there is no recurrence, assessment is made on the basis of tests noted in Table 5-1.

American Thoracic Society Guidelines

According to American Thoracic Society (ATS) criteria (Table 5-2), most individuals can be assessed by using spirometry and diffusing capacity measurements. *Mild impairment* is not expected to diminish the ability to perform most jobs. *Moderate impairment* correlates with diminished ability to perform many jobs. *Severe impairment* suggests that the individual cannot perform most jobs and probably cannot even travel to the workplace. Arterial blood gas analysis is not generally recommended, since most patients with exercise-induced hypoxia already have demonstrated impairment on the basis of less invasive tests, such as spirometry or D_{LCO} measurements. When

TABLE 5-2 Factors to Be Considered in Rating Impairment Due to Asthma

Score	Reversibility of FEV$_1$ or Degree of Airway Hyperresponsiveness			
	Postbronchodilator FEV$_1$, % Predicted	% FEV$_1$ Change	PC$_{20}$, mg/mL or Equivalent	Minimum Medication Needed
0	>Lower limit of normal	<10	>8	No medication
1	Between 70 and lower limit of normal	10–19	Between 8 and 0.5	Occasional bronchodilator (not daily) and/or occasional cromolyn (not daily)
2	60–69	20–29	Between 0.5 and 0.125	Daily bronchodilator and/or daily cromolyn and/or daily low-dose inhaled corticosteroid (<800 mg beclomethasone or equivalent)
3	50–59	>30	<0.125	Bronchodilator on demand and daily, high-dose inhaled corticosteroid (>800 μg beclomethasone or equivalent), or occasional course (1–3 times annually) systemic corticosteroid
4	<50	—	—	Bronchodilator on demand and daily high-dose, inhaled corticosteroid (>1000 mg beclomethasone or equivalent) and daily systemic corticosteroid

SOURCE: American Thoracic Society. Modified with permission.

performed, arterial blood gas analysis requires confirmation with a repeat study over an interval of at least 4 weeks in clinically stable patients. Hypoxemia, either at rest or with exercise, is not considered evidence of severe impairment unless accompanied by cor pulmonale. Cor pulmonale alone is proof of severe impairment, regardless of spirometric results.

The ATS guidelines distinguish asthma from chronic obstructive and restrictive lung diseases. If the FEV$_1$/FVC% is below normal, an inhaled beta-adrenergic agonist is administered and spirometry repeated. An increase of 12 percent or more in the FEV$_1$ is indicative of asthma, while an increase of less than 12 percent is further evaluated by corticosteroid administration and repeat spirometry after 1 to 2 weeks. If spirometric results following corticosteroid administration show an increase in the FEV_1 of 20 percent or more, the diagnosis of asthma is confirmed. If initial spirometry performed on a patient with asthma-like symptoms shows an $FEV_1/FVC\%$ above the lower limit of normal, methacholine or histamine challenge testing should be performed using standardized methods. Airway hyperresponsiveness is confirmed by a fall in FEV_1 of 20 percent or greater when the concentration of the provocative agent administered by the tidal breathing method is ≤8 mg/mL (see Chap. 2). Impairment or disability due to asthma may be temporary or permanent. If treatment objectives have not been fully achieved at the time of evaluation, only a rating for temporary impairment can be assigned. Reevaluation is performed for assessment of permanent impairment when the treatment objectives are achieved or after 6 months, whichever comes first.

Social Security Administration Guidelines

The legal definition of disability under the program of the Social Security Administration (SSA) is an inability to engage in any substantial gainful activity over a period that has lasted (or can be expected to last) for at least 12 months or that is expected to result in death. Medical information may be provided by the claimant's own physician or an authorized consultant. In addition to the usual medical history, the consultant must provide a statement about what the claimant can still do despite his or her impairment. SSA provides a listing of impairments considered severe enough to preclude gainful employment.

Evaluation of respiratory impairment under SSA guidelines includes a chest radiograph and spirometry. If airways obstruction is noted, bronchodilator responsiveness is assessed; if interstitial lung disease or cor pulmonale is suspected, diffusing capacity measurement or arterial blood gas analysis may also be performed. Although cardiopulmonary exercise testing is generally discouraged, it may be performed if chronic pulmonary disease has been documented and other studies fail to satisfy the criteria for disability consideration.

Under SSA guidelines, asthma is considered severe if, despite adherence to a prescribed therapeutic regimen, acute exacerbations requiring intensive treatment in a hospital emergency department or its equivalent occur six times yearly or if hospitalization for longer than 24 h is required. Each hospitalization is counted as the equivalent of two asthma attacks.

WORKERS' COMPENSATION PROGRAM

Workers compensation programs protect employees injured on the job. When disputes arise regarding causation of injury, the issue is adjudicated before a referee appointed by the workers' compensation board. A medical expert who has examined the injured worker provides testimony; the employer may have the worker reevaluated by an independent medical examiner. The referee may accept or reject the disability claim.

The first federal program for workers' compensation—the Federal Coal Mine Health and Safety Act of 1969—provides for benefits as a result of coal worker's pneumoconiosis. The program is based on length of service in the coal industry and assessment of chest radiograph findings using the ILO International Classification of Pneumoconioses. Once having qualified for the diagnosis of pneumoconiosis, the miner is considered "totally disabled" if the disease prevents him from working in the immediate area of his residence using skills and abilities comparable to those he used in the coal mine. Medical criteria for total disability are arbitrarily stated in the act. No age requirement for the spirometric findings is listed. Since FEV_1 normally decreases with age, qualification for black lung benefits becomes easier as the miner grows older. Even if the miner fails to qualify through spirometric testing, he can still be judged totally disabled on the basis of a medical opinion furnished by one or more physicians designated by the government.

Outside the United States, workers' compensation claims are usually processed by national agencies that generally obtain medical consultation from recognized experts or boards of experts. Lists or schedules of specific diseases accepted as employment-related are used to determine when compensation is allowed. Disabled individuals who do not qualify for benefits under workers' compensation schedules are often covered by secondary sources of health and disability insurance that provide similar levels of support.

AMERICANS WITH DISABILITIES ACT

The Americans with Disabilities Act (ADA) of 1990 prevents exclusion of employees from jobs because of handicaps that have little or nothing to do with ability to perform the specific job being offered. According to ADA regulations, initial evaluation for a job must be performed on the basis of nonmedical criteria. The employer is specifically prohibited from asking any questions regarding health or physical impairment and may not perform medical examinations until an actual offer of employment has been made. Following the job offer, the employer is allowed to perform a "fitness for duty" examination prior to the start of work. Any withdrawals of job offers following examinations must be supported by convincing medical evidence that the individual cannot perform the job or that the prospective employee would pose a substantial danger to himself or coworkers in the performance of a particular job. It is not sufficient to conclude that a worker with a particular disease, in general, cannot perform a job; rather, the specific worker being considered must be assessed with regard to his or her ability to perform the specific job being offered. Furthermore, as long as the worker can perform most of the essential tasks of the job, the employer is obligated to make reasonable accommodations to the employee's handicap.

The physician's obligation under the provisions of the ADA is to evaluate the physical condition of the job applicant in terms of his or her ability to perform specific tasks. The decision to hire does not belong to the physician: it is solely the responsibility of the company requesting the evaluation. The physician must maintain confidentiality regarding all other aspects of the applicant's health. Medical files are kept separate from other employment files, and only health professionals may have access to this information. The physician must supply enough information for the personnel office to judge fitness to perform a particular job, but he or she must not disclose other health-related information.

BIBLIOGRAPHY

American Medical Association: *Guides to the Evaluation of Permanent Impairment* 4th ed. Chicago, American Medical Association, 1993.

American Thoracic Society: Guidelines for evaluation of impairment/disability in patients with asthma. *Am Rev Respir Dis* 147:1056–1061, 1993.

Cotes JE, Reed JW, Elliott C: Breathing and exercise requirements of the work place, in Whipp BJ, Wasserman K (eds): *Exercise, Pulmonary Physiology and Pathophysiology*. New York, Marcel Dekker, 1991.

Dewitte JD, Chan-Yeung M, Malo JL: Medicolegal and compensation aspects of occupational asthma. *Eur Respir J* 7:969–980, 1994.

Mahowald MW, Schenck CH: Medical-legal aspects of sleep medicine. *Neurol Clin* 17:215–234, 1999.

National Institute of Health: Guidelines for the diagnosis and management of asthma. Expert panel report. National Asthma Education Program. Pub no 91-3042A. Bethesda, MD: National Heart, Lung and Blood Institute. 1991.

Social Security Administration: *Disability Evaluation under Social Security*. SSA pub no 64-039. Washington, DC: US Government Printing Office, 1995.

Sood A, Beckett WS: Determination of disability for patients with advanced lung disease. *Clin Chest Med* 18:471–482, 1997.

Sue DY: Exercise testing in the evaluation of impairment and disability. *Clin Chest Med* 15:369–387, 1994.

Part Two | **OBSTRUCTIVE LUNG DISEASES**

CHRONIC OBSTRUCTIVE PULMONARY DISEASE DISORDERS

6 | Chronic Obstructive Pulmonary Disease: Overview*

Reynold A. Panettieri, Jr., and Alfred P. Fishman

DEFINITIONS

During the past half-century, definitions of chronic obstructive diseases have been refined because of fresh clinical observations, new diagnostic tools, and sophisticated epidemiologic studies.

Although the term *chronic obstructive pulmonary disease* (COPD) may be used to describe a variety of pulmonary disorders, including asthma, chronic bronchitis, emphysema, cystic fibrosis, and bronchiectasis, COPD usually refers to chronic bronchitis and emphysema. Unlike asthma, COPD implies, in part, irreversible airways obstruction. There also exists considerable overlap in the clinical manifestations of these diseases, such that many of the features of asthma, emphysema, and/or chronic bronchitis may coexist in an individual with airways obstruction. Two syndromes with particular significance are described below.

Emphysema

This entity continues to be defined in anatomic terms—i.e., abnormal permanent enlargement of the gas-exchanging units of the lungs (acini) in association with destruction of alveolar walls, without obvious fibrosis. The predominant physiologic consequence of these anatomic abnormalities is a decrease in the elastic recoil of the lungs—which, in turn, causes outward displacement of the chest wall and flattening of the diaphragm, hyperinflation of the lungs, and increased resistance to airflow due to circumferential traction on the small airways by the overdistended lungs. The hyperinflation places the respiratory muscles at mechanical disadvantage, increasing the work and the oxygen cost of breathing. Although imbalances in ventilation perfusion are observed less frequently than in chronic (clinically significant) bronchitis, derangements sufficient to cause arterial hypoxemia are common.

*Edited from Chap. 42, "Chronic Obstructive Lung Disease," by Fishman AP. In: *Fishman's Pulmonary Diseases and Disorders,* 3d ed., edited by Fishman AP, Elias JA, Fishman JA, Grippi MA, Kaiser LR, Senior RM. New York, McGraw-Hill, 1998, pp 645–658. For fuller discussion of topics dealt with in this chapter, the reader is referred to the original text, as noted above.

Chronic Bronchitis

The American Thoracic Society has defined chronic bronchitis as the persistence of cough and excessive secretion of mucus on most days over a 3-month period for at least 2 consecutive years. The cough is due to hypersecretion of mucus and need not be associated with airflow limitation. The majority of patients with chronic bronchitis do not have airflow limitation. Such limitation is usually demonstrated by a decrease in FEV_1 and even earlier by flow-volume loops, obtained during a forced expiration. Patients with airflow limitation, i.e., with "chronic obstructive bronchitis," make up most of the patients with COPD.

Chronic Obstructive Pulmonary Disease (COPD)

This term recognizes that chronic bronchitis and emphysema generally coexist but that generally it is not possible to quantify the relative contributions of each to the clinical syndrome. The most recent definition, described by the American Thoracic Society, defines "chronic obstructive pulmonary disease (COPD) as a disease state characterized by the presence of airflow obstruction due to chronic bronchitis or emphysema; the airflow obstruction is generally progressive, may be accompanied by airway hyperreactivity, and may be partially reversible." Diagnostic features of this inclusive nonspecific entity are chronic productive cough, breathlessness on exertion, physiologic evidence of airflow limitation (e.g., reduced FEV_1), and poor reversibility (e.g., poor response to bronchodilators). General functional hallmarks by which predominant bronchitis or emphysema can be distinguished are shown in Table 6-1.

TABLE 6-1 Functional Hallmarks: Predominant Bronchitis versus Predominant Emphysema

	Predominant bronchitis	Predominant emphysema
FEV_1/FVC	Reduced	Reduced
FRC	Mildly increased	Markedly increased
TLC	Normal or slightly increased	Considerably increased
RV	Moderately increased	Markedly increased
Lung compliance	Normal or low	Normal or low
Recoil pressure	Normal or high	Low
MVV	Moderately decreased	Markedly decreased
Airway resistance	Increased	Normal or slightly increased
$D_{L_{CO}}$	Normal or low	Low
Arterial P_{O_2}	Moderately to severely reduced	Slightly to moderately reduced
Arterial hypercapnia	Chronic	Only during acute respiratory infection
Hematocrit	Generally high, may reach 70%	Normal or slightly high, rarely above 55%
Pulmonary artery pressure	Generally increased	Normal or slightly increased

KEY: TLC, total lung capacity; RV, residual volume; $D_{L_{CO}}$, diffusing capacity of carbon monoxide.

Bronchiectasis

Bronchiectasis is characterized by dilation of airways rather than by narrowing and does not contribute to obstruction to airflow. In cystic fibrosis, bronchiectasis is a consistent concomitant. Characteristically, proximal airways are dilated and distal airways obstructed by mucopurulent exudate and by narrowed, obliterated terminal airways.

Small Airways Disease

The designation *small airways disease* began with observations made at autopsy. It refers to obstruction of small airways (<2 mm in diameter), i.e., a combination of small bronchi and bronchioles, by inflammation and mucous plugs. This term has been carried over to in vivo measurements of small airway function, such as closing volume, particularly in cigarette smokers.

Bronchiolitis Obliterans (and BOOP)

The term *bronchiolitis obliterans* was coined in 1901 to designate an acute respiratory illness of unknown cause due to lesions in the terminal branches of the bronchial tree. By the 1970s, it was appreciated that bronchiolitis obliterans could be caused by plugging of the terminal bronchioles either from within by organizing exudate; by constriction, inflammation, and fibrosis within bronchiolar walls; or by concomitant involvement of terminal bronchioles and adjacent alveoli. During the 1970s and 1980s, the list of causes of bronchiolitis obliterans expanded greatly to include connective tissue disorders, toxic inhalants, cigarette smoking, immunologic disorders, and infections in immunocompromised hosts.

In 1985, bronchiolitis obliterans organizing pneumonia (BOOP) was described. Its hallmarks are the presence of plugs of granulation tissue in the small airways, often with extension of the granulation tissue into alveolar ducts and alveoli. As in the case of bronchiolitis obliterans, a pulmonary and heterogeneous list of etiologic agents has been described for BOOP.

PATHOLOGY AND PATHOGENESIS

Although defined as a clinical disorder, chronic bronchitis is manifest by chronic excessive secretion of mucus that is associated with airway obstruction and mucus plugging. Pathologically, there is enlargement of bronchial mucus glands with an increase in the number of mucus-secreting cells (hyperplasia). As determined by histologic examination of the airways, an increased ratio of the thickness of bronchial mucous glands to that of the bronchial wall (Reid index) has been associated with chronic bronchitis. This index, however, may not be specific for chronic bronchitis, since a variety of other obstructive airway diseases also induce alterations in this ratio.

Emphysema is characterized by a permanent, abnormal increase in the size of airspaces distal to the terminal bronchiole (acinus). Emphysema is also classified according to the site where the terminal bronchiole is affected. Centrilobular emphysema, which occurs most commonly as a result of or in association with cigarette smoking, affects the proximal segment of the respiratory bronchiole. Panacinar emphysema, which occurs in the elderly and in patients with alpha$_1$-antiprotease deficiency, uniformly affects the entire respiratory bronchiole. Such classifications are not unique to specific disorders, since panacinar and centrilobular emphysema may coexist in the same lung. Further, the degree of functional impairment from emphysema, not the type, determines the clinical significance of the disease.

In the United States, the majority of patients with emphysema and chronic bronchitis smoke cigarettes or were former smokers. Only a minority of smokers (approximately 15 percent) develop COPD. Two possible hypotheses have been developed to explain the relationship between smoking and the pathogenesis of emphysema. First, bronchial hyperresponsiveness predisposes smokers to the development of chronic irreversible airflow limitation. The findings of airway hyperresponsiveness to histamine, increased IgE levels, and eosinophil counts in smokers support this hypothesis. However, the specificity of these findings remains to be determined, since nonspecific airway responsiveness has been characterized in other obstructive lung diseases unassociated with emphysema.

A second hypothesis emphasizes an imbalance between protease and antiprotease activity in the lung, resulting in a relative increase in elastase activity. The unchecked intrapulmonary elastase activity then destroys alveolar walls, resulting in emphysema. Since tobacco smoke has potent antioxidant activity that inactivates endogenous antiproteases, this theory is compatible with the notion that cigarette smoking may induce emphysema. Further, the recognition that patients with alpha$_1$-antiprotease deficiency, a hereditary disease characterized by a lack of alpha$_1$-antitrypsin activity in homozygotic individuals, also develop emphysema supports this hypothesis. Unfortunately, the precise mechanisms that induce emphysema remain unknown.

As in emphysema, the exact mechanisms that induce the pathologic findings of chronic bronchitis are unknown; however, cigarette smoking appears to be causally related. In addition, acute or chronic exposure to dusts, fumes, air pollution, and respiratory viruses has been associated with the onset of chronic bronchitis in susceptible individuals.

Tobacco Smoking and COPD

Overwhelming evidence links tobacco smoking with the development of emphysema and/or chronic bronchitis. Smoking-related diseases account for approximately 434,000 deaths per year with approximately 47 percent due to cardiovascular disease, 33 percent due to cancer, and 20 percent due to respiratory disease. The incidence of smoking-related disease also appears to be dose-dependent, since those patients who smoke more cigarettes per day appear to have proportionally more cardiovascular and respiratory disease than those who smoke less.

The benefits of smoking cessation are well established. Studies have demonstrated that smoking cessation has been associated with dramatic reductions in respiratory symptoms within a month of cessation. At 1 year after cessation, former smokers reduce their risk of ischemic heart disease by 50 percent and, after 15 years of abstinence, risk from all smoking-related mortality approaches that of individuals who never smoked (Table 6-2).

PATHOPHYSIOLOGY

Pulmonary Mechanics

Chronic airflow limitation, which is a hallmark of emphysema and chronic bronchitis, may occur through several mechanisms. First, the airway lumen may be partially occluded by excessive and tenacious secretions, as described

TABLE 6-2 Life Expectancy as a Function of Smoking History

	Life Expectancy (Years)		
	Age 35	Age 45	Age 65
Nonsmoker	78.5	79.0	82.0
Current cigarette smoker (1–2 packs/day)	71.7	72.5	77.6
Previous cigarette smoker	77.1	77.5	80.9
Years lost by smoking (1–2 packs/day)	6.8	6.5	4.4
Years regained by stopping smoking at age indicated	5.4	5.0	3.3

SOURCE: Adapted from Sachs DPL: Advances in smoking cessation treatment, in Simmons (ed): *Current Pulmonology*. Chicago, Year Book, 1991, pp 139–198.

in patients with chronic bronchitis. Second, airway smooth muscle contraction and/or bronchial wall edema and inflammation also induce airway obstruction by decreasing airway luminal diameter, which may be reversible, as recognized in patients with asthma. Last, destruction of lung parenchyma, as described in patients with emphysema, may alter the tethering forces exerted on the airway lumen. In emphysema, moderate-sized airways, which are those not surrounded by cartilage, become "floppy" and limit airflow, especially during forced expiratory maneuvers. Importantly, all three mechanisms may occur concomitantly; therefore, therapeutic efforts should be directed at reversing airway smooth muscle contraction, decreasing airway inflammation, and augmenting sputum expectoration. Unfortunately, the loss of radial traction of the airways and decrease in the elastic recoil of the lung, as seen in emphysema, is irreversible.

Despite a variety of mechanisms that can induce airway obstruction, chronic airway obstruction alters pulmonary mechanics in a predictable manner. Expiratory flow rates and volumes are diminished throughout the expiratory cycle. Since airflow limitation prolongs expiration time and prevents complete emptying of affected alveoli, lung volumes also increase. These increases in lung volume alter the length-tension relationship of the diaphragm, which then places respiratory muscles at a mechanical disadvantage.

Gas Exchange

In patients with COPD, ventilation/perfusion mismatch occurs commonly and induces hypoxemia with or without CO_2 retention. The alveolar-arterial difference for P_{O_2} is usually increased, with a large proportion of ventilation preferentially directed to areas of the lung with high ventilation/perfusion ratios (increased dead space ventilation).

Control of Ventilation

Although patients with severe airflow limitation (less than 0.8 L) are more likely to retain CO_2, there is considerable individual variation. Some patients with COPD, particularly those with severe chronic bronchitis, develop CO_2 retention, while others with comparable airflow limitation do not.

Studies suggest that patients with COPD may experience an increased work of breathing due in part to increased airway resistance and altered respiratory muscle mechanics. In addition, these patients may have a blunted ventilatory response to inhaled CO_2 as compared with normal subjects. Despite the concept that patients with COPD may retain CO_2 in order to compensate for an increased work of breathing, the exact mechanism that induces CO_2 retention in these patients is likely to be multifactorial and remains unknown.

CLINICAL MANIFESTATIONS

History

Dyspnea or an upper respiratory tract illness usually brings the patient with COPD to the physician. A careful history reveals a chronic cough, most often on awakening in the morning, and moderate shortness of breath with exertion that has been insidious in onset. These symptoms usually occur in the sixth or seventh decade of life and are associated with a history of cigarette smoking. Similar symptoms that occur in the fourth or fifth decade of life should prompt the physician to consider alternative diagnoses such as asthma, chronic bronchitis, alpha$_1$-antitrypsin deficiency, or congenital lung disease. Although cough is a frequent symptom, it is rarely debilitating. Hemoptysis, weight loss, and/or a severe cough may occur in patients with chronic bronchitis or emphysema; however, these symptoms should raise the suspicion of lung cancer or tuberculosis.

Other symptoms that may occur late in the course of the disease are associated with complications from COPD. The presence of leg swelling suggests that there is significant right-sided congestive heart failure or pulmonary hypertension. Morning headache, lethargy, and confusion are common symptoms of CO_2 retention or hypercapnia. Although exertional dyspnea often occurs in patients with moderate to severe COPD, exertional dyspnea may also be a manifestation of ischemic heart disease, especially in those patients with a significant smoking history.

The "pink puffer" (type A) and the "blue bloater" (type B) syndromes are historical descriptions of two subsets of patients with COPD. *Blue bloater* referred to patients with moderate or severe COPD who presented predominantly with obesity, copious sputum production, hypercapnia, leg swelling, and right-sided congestive heart disease. *Pink puffer* referred to patients with moderate or severe COPD who presented with scant sputum production, cachexia, and normal arterial P_{O_2}. It was originally thought that pink puffers were primarily patients with emphysema and blue bloaters were primarily patients with chronic bronchitis. Pathologic studies confirmed that both groups of patients have emphysema. Although this classification of COPD patients demonstrates the spectrum of the disease, few patients fall exclusively into one or the other subset. Therefore, describing patients with COPD as blue bloaters or pink puffers is no longer valuable in understanding the basic mechanisms responsible for these patterns.

Physical Examination

On auscultation, examination of the chest often reveals a lack of breath sounds, an occasional wheeze, or a prolonged expiratory phase. If airways obstruction is moderately severe, increased lung volumes are manifest by an increased anteroposterior diameter of the chest, diaphragm movement is ᵈd, and breath sounds are diminished. A palpable liver edge without evidence of hepatomegaly is the result of increased lung volumes that displace the diaphragm downward. Hypertrophy of accessory muscles of respiration (sternocleidomastoid and trapezius) also suggests severe chronic airflow limitation. Cyanosis is uncommon in patients with stable COPD; however, during acute exacerbations, cyanosis indicates significant arterial oxygen desaturation. Hepatomegaly and neck vein distention, which are signs of pulmonary hypertension and right-sided congestive heart failure, are seen infrequently in patients with emphysema.

Chest Radiology

The chest radiograph of a patient with emphysema characteristically shows hyperinflation, manifest by radiolucent lung fields, a flattened diaphragm, and a slender cardiac silhouette. In chronic bronchitis, the pulmonary vasculature can be prominent and suggests pulmonary hypertension, but this finding may also occur with severe emphysema. Although the chest radiograph is useful in confirming a diagnosis of COPD, the specificity of the findings is not limited to emphysema, since patients with acute exacerbations of asthma, cystic fibrosis, bronchiectasis, or chronic bronchitis may have identical chest radiographs. Further, findings on the chest radiograph may not correlate with the severity of COPD as determined by pulmonary function testing.

Pulmonary Function Testing

Pulmonary function testing in patients with COPD is valuable in assessing the severity of the disease, confirming the diagnosis, evaluating the presence of reversibility, and determining the prognosis. Spirometry reveals decreases in both the forced expiratory volume in 1 s (FEV_1) and the forced vital capacity (FVC). The FEV_1/FVC ratio is also decreased and is diagnostic of obstructive airways disease. Unfortunately, these findings are not unique to emphysema, since any disease characterized by airways obstruction will manifest decreases in the FEV_1 and FVC. Although most patients with COPD have no increase in their FEV_1 with bronchodilator treatment, approximately 20 percent of COPD patients are bronchodilator-responsive, as defined as an increase in the FEV_1 by 20 percent after beta-agonist treatment. Lung volumes, as determined by body plethysmography, are increased in emphysema and asthma but may be normal in chronic bronchitis. Increases in total lung volume are a consequence of airflow limitation and air trapping that also induce increases in the functional residual volume and residual volume. Lung volumes measured by body plethysmography may differ from those measured by helium dilution techniques in COPD patients. Slow emptying of high ventilation/perfusion ($\dot{V}/\dot{Q}$) units may not equilibrate with the inspired helium; thus the measured lung volumes using this technique may report artificially low volumes. In emphysema, the single-breath diffusing capacity ($D_{L_{CO}}$), which correlates well with severity of illness, is decreased and results from alveolar-capillary membrane destruction. Interestingly, the $D_{L_{CO}}$ is preserved in patients with chronic bronchitis or asthma and is a valuable test in characterizing COPD patients with emphysema from those with asthma or chronic bronchitis.

Arterial blood gases are relatively insensitive measures of COPD severity. In early stages of emphysema, increases in the arterial-alveolar oxygen differences occur frequently. In later stages of the disease, the presence of hypoxemia at rest and/or hypercapnia (increased Pa_{CO_2}) may occur. Reactive

TABLE 6-3 Differential Diagnosis of Obstructive Airways Disease

Asthma
Chronic bronchitis
Emphysema
Bronchiectasis
Cystic fibrosis
Congenital bullous lung disease

erythrocytosis, which is manifest by increases in hematocrit, results from chronic hypoxemia and chronically elevated carboxyhemoglobin levels from tobacco smoking.

DIAGNOSIS

The diagnosis of COPD requires identification of the clinical manifestations and pulmonary function tests that confirm obstructive airway disease (Table 6-3). Emphysema, chronic bronchitis, and asthma in their early stages are often indistinguishable.

NATURAL HISTORY AND PROGNOSIS

Prognosis correlates in part with measurements of the FEV_1. In young smokers (<35 years old) who have mild obstructive airways disease (80 percent predicted >FEV_1 >60 percent predicted), the FEV_1 will return to normal with smoking cessation. In older patients, smoking cessation will slow but not eliminate further decrements in the FEV_1. Poor prognosis in COPD is associated with cor pulmonale and hypercapnia. In patients presenting with values of FEV_1 less than 0.75 L, the mortality rate at 1 year is 30 percent and at 10 years is 95 percent.

Respiratory failure is the most common cause of death in these patients. Recent studies suggest that some patients with severe airway obstruction may survive significantly longer than current median survival rates. In these studies, aggressive management of acute exacerbations of COPD appeared to improve overall survival rates.

MANAGEMENT

Pharmacologic Therapy

Bronchodilators

As a single agent, inhaled ipratropium bromide is at least equal to and, in many studies, a better bronchodilator than methylxanthines or inhaled beta agonists. Ipratropium bromide, which blocks muscarinic receptors on airway smooth muscle, decreases vagal tone, inhibits smooth muscle contraction, and decreases secretion of mucus. In a few studies, the addition of anticholinergics to beta-agonist therapy appeared to have an additive effect. As first-line therapy, inhaled quaternary anticholinergic agents (ipratropium) offer greater bronchodilator effect and fewer side effects than do other available bronchodilating agents in the majority of COPD patients. In addition, the bronchodilator potency of the anticholinergic agents is not attenuated by continued administration, whereas patients treated with beta agonists for prolonged periods may experience blunted bronchodilator responses to beta agonists. Further, beta agonists may also induce pulmonary vasodilation, which worsens $\dot{V}/\dot{Q}$ matching and occasionally

TABLE 6-4 Theophylline Dosing [a,b] in Adults with Acute Bronchospasm

Dosing	Intravenous aminophylline
Loading dose[c]	
History of theophylline use	
None	6 mg/kg over 20 min
Oral theophylline use	0–3 mg/kg over 20 min
Maintenance dose[c]	
Patient category	
Nonsmoker	0.5 mg/kg/h
Smoker	0.3 mg/kg/h
Critically ill	0.5 mg/kg/h
Congestive heart failure	0.2 mg/kg/h
Severe pneumonia	0.2 mg/kg/h

[a]Dosing expressed in aminophylline equivalents (theophylline dose = 0.8 × aminophylline dose).
[b]Theophylline levels should be measured 12 to 24 h after loading and more frequently if symptoms or signs of theophylline toxicity are evident.
[c]If possible, serum theophylline levels should be obtained prior to administration. The initial target serum concentration for theophylline is 10 μg/mL.

results in a decrease in the arterial P_{O_2}. Inhaled beta-agonist dosing is reviewed in Chap. 8. Ipratropium is delivered by metered-dose inhaler (18 μg per puff), two puffs four times daily to a maximum of four puffs four times daily. Recent evidence also suggests that salmeterol, a long-acting bronchodilator, improves COPD management.

Theophylline

Despite the use of methylxanthines in the treatment of COPD for over 100 years, the mechanism by which this agent improves dyspnea or decreases airway obstruction remains unknown. Theophylline is a weak bronchodilator in comparison to beta agonists or ipratropium. Given the narrow therapeutic window, the use of theophylline should be tailored to the individual patient, and "optimal" bronchodilator effects may occur in the low therapeutic range (5 to 15 mg/L) (Table 6-4). Theophylline clearance may be affected by a variety of other medications; therefore dosing regimens should be individualized and serum levels checked regularly (Table 6-5).

TABLE 6-5 Physiologic Factors and Drug Interactions Altering Theophylline Metabolism

Increases serum levels	Decreases serum levels
Advanced age	Carbamazepine
Obesity	Dilantin
Erythromycin	Rifampin
Cimetidine	Cigarette smoking
Oral contraceptives	Phenobarbital
Propranolol	
Allopurinol	
Hepatic disease/congestion	
Congestive heart disease	
Quinolones (ciprofloxacin, etc.)	

In COPD patients, the therapeutic benefit of theophylline may be a consequence of its nonbronchodilator actions. Apart from increasing cAMP levels by inhibiting phosphodiesterase activity, methylxanthines have been reported to increase the contractility of "fatigued" diaphragms and to increase mucociliary action in normal airways. Moreover, methylxanthines also increase hypoxic drive to ventilation in hypercapnic COPD patients and increase right and left ventricular ejection fractions through vasodilation and direct myocardial stimulation.

Steroids

Although the benefit of steroids is well established in the management of asthma, the efficacy of steroids in the management of COPD is less well established. Therapy with corticosteroids has been reported to provide both subjective and objective benefits in some patients with COPD. Unfortunately, there are few clinical predictors that identify which patients will respond. Despite the notion that COPD patients with reversible airways disease may respond to steroids, some COPD patients who are not bronchodilator responsive improve with steroid therapy. Thus, a therapeutic trial of corticosteroids seems justified in any patient with COPD. The patient undergoes pretreatment pulmonary function testing and then receives a 2-week course of methylprednisolone or prednisone at a dose of 20 to 40 mg/day. Repeat pulmonary function testing is then performed, and if there is objective improvement, the dose of steroids is slowly tapered to a maintenance level; otherwise, steroid therapy is discontinued. Current evidence suggests that some patients with COPD may benefit from inhaled or alternate-day steroid therapy.

Mucolytics

Adjunctive use of mucolytic-expectorants appears to improve the quality of life, decreases cough, and decreases the duration of acute exacerbations of dyspnea in some COPD patients with excessive production of mucus. Although 1 to 8 weeks of iodinated glycerol therapy at a dose of 60 mg four times daily has been reported to reduce symptoms in these patients, other mucolytic agents such as acetylcysteine (inhaled or oral), glyceryl guaiacolate (guaifenesin), and ambuxol have not been shown to be consistently effective. If conventional therapy fails to improve symptoms of cough or chest tightness, an 8-week trial of oral iodinated glycerol may determine whether a patient will respond to mucolytic therapy.

Antibiotics and Vaccines

Antibiotics (trimethoprim-sulfamethoxazole, amoxicillin, or doxycycline) used in patients with acute exacerbations of COPD decrease the duration of the COPD exacerbation and results in more rapid improvement of peak expiratory flow rates when compared with controls. There is, however, no evidence to support the prophylactic use of antibiotics in COPD patients. Current data support the use of antibiotics for 7 to 10 days in the management of acute exacerbations of COPD.

Although pneumococcus is one of the two most commonly cultured pathogens in the sputum of patients with COPD exacerbations, most exacerbations are not due to bacterial infections. There is no evidence to support the hypothesis that pneumococcal bacteremia or sepsis is more common or more severe in COPD patients. Although the cost-benefit ratio of pneumo-coccal vaccine is low, this therapy should be regarded as potentially useful but not yet of proven efficacy.

Supplemental Oxygen

When administered for a minimum of at least 12 h per day, supplemental O_2 is the *only drug* that has reduced mortality in the management of COPD. The current indications for home O_2 therapy include (1) resting Pa_{O_2} <55 mmHg or an arterial oxygen saturation <90%, (2) Pa_{O_2} 55 to 59 mmHg with evidence of cor pulmonale or polycythemia, or (3) significant exercise- or sleep-induced hypoxemia/arterial oxygen desaturation that reverses with supplemental O_2 therapy. Supplemental O_2 should be titrated to maintain the Pa_{O_2} between 65 to 80 mmHg.

Pulmonary Rehabilitation

Exercise limitation in patients with COPD may be due to a variety of patho-physiologic mechanisms including abnormal pulmonary mechanics, impaired gas exchange, abnormal perceptions of dyspnea, impaired cardiac perform-ance, and poor nutritional status. Pulmonary rehabilitation programs have been reported to decrease the need for hospitalization, improve quality of life, decrease respiratory symptoms (dyspnea), and improve endurance time or exercise tolerance in patients with severe COPD. Unfortunately, because ex-ercise is ventilation-limited, classic training effects do not occur and im-provements may be task-specific.

Lung Volume Reduction Surgery

End-stage emphysema leads to incapacity largely because of dyspnea on mild exertion, which imposes severe restrictions on daily activity and the quality of life. The rationale for lung volume reduction surgery is that excision of wedges of emphysematous lung tissue will decrease lung volume, with sev-eral desirable consequences: (1) improvement in elastic recoil of the thorax and patency of the intrathoracic airways, (2) improvement in the mechanical function of the muscles of respiration by diminishing the expansion of the thoracic cage and repositioning the diaphragm, and (3) relief of compression of normal lung caused by localized areas of emphysema.

Experience to date indicates that the procedure helps certain patients with emphysema. However, the features of such a group have not yet been de-fined and are being investigated as part of the National Emphysema Treatment Trial (NETT). Currently, the surgical outlook seems to be better for the individual with heterogeneous distribution of emphysema than for the individual with more homogeneous distribution. Computed tomogra-phy (CT) and newer imaging techniques hold promise of improving the preoperative assessment of the extent and distribution of destroyed lung. The reported mortality from the surgical procedure is of the order of 5 to 10 percent, the most common complication being persistent air leak. Less frequent complications include pneumonia, sepsis, myocardial infarction, and stroke.

Although, as noted above, some patients have experienced benefit from the procedure, long-term data are sparse, inclusion-exclusion criteria have been variable, morbidity has been considerable, complications frequent, and mortality high. Because of the uncontrolled nature of the experience to date with lung volume reduction surgery and the widespread interest in its use, the National Institutes of Health are conducting the NETT, in which 18 centers are evaluating the efficacy and safety of the surgical approaches, establishing suitable inclusion-exclusion criteria, comparing the efficacy and effectiveness of medical versus surgical management, and identifying optimal surgical approaches.

Lung Transplantation

Both unilateral and bilateral lung replacement can be performed in patients with COPD. Some centers use unilateral procedures for patients over the age of 50 and bilateral procedures for those under the age of 50. The criteria for lung transplantation may vary slightly among institutions; however, COPD patients who fail medical therapy are considered for transplant if they have severe obstructive disease that substantially limits daily activities. In addition, the patient must be ambulatory with rehabilitative potential, have adequate cardiac function without significant coronary heart disease, and have adequate nutritional and psychosocial profiles. Patients are excluded if there is significant nonpulmonary disease, coronary artery disease, or if patients continue to smoke.

Investigational Therapy

Respiratory Muscle Training/Strengthening

Repetitive inspiration against resistive loads improves respiratory muscle strength and endurance in COPD patients. Although there is some improvement in exercise tolerance after resistive load conditioning, there is generally no improvement in spirometry, maximal voluntary ventilation, or maximal sustainable ventilation.

Continuous Positive Airway Pressure (CPAP)

CPAP ventilation during acute exacerbations, during sleep, and/or during exercise may be beneficial in some COPD patients. CPAP ventilation appears to decrease dyspnea and the work of breathing in COPD patients weaning from mechanical ventilation and improves exercise tolerance during exercise testing. The use of CPAP in weaning COPD patients from mechanical ventilation remains investigational.

Antielastase Therapy

Since emphysema may be induced by an imbalance between neutrophil elastases and serum antiproteases, therapy directed toward increasing serum antiproteases or decreasing neutrophil elastases may prove beneficial in the management of patients with emphysema. In patients with alpha$_1$-antitrypsin deficiency, plasma alpha$_1$-antitrypsin may be given intravenously once weekly (60 mg/kg) or once monthly (250 mg/mL) to maintain serum levels above 11 μM. These doses increase lung alpha$_1$-antitrypsin levels and restore lung antineutrophil elastase defense mechanisms into the normal range. Although alpha$_1$-antitrypsin replacement therapy is efficacious in restoring serum levels of antiprotease activity, its clinical efficacy remains unproven in regard to reducing the decline in lung function or improving survival in patients with alpha$_1$-antitrypsin deficiency.

BIBLIOGRAPHY

Barnes PJ: Chronic obstructive pulmonary disease. *N Engl J Med* 343:269–280, 2000.

Barnes PJ: Novel approaches and targets for treatment of chronic obstructive pulmonary disease. *Am J Respir Crit Care Med* 160:S72–S79, 1999.

Barnes PJ: Mechanisms in COPD: differences from asthma. *Chest* 117:10S–14S, 2000.

Campbell EJ, Senior RM: Emphysema, in Fishman AP (ed): *Update: Pulmonary Diseases and Disorders*. New York, McGraw-Hill, 1992, pp 37–51.

Chapman KR: Therapeutic algorithm for chronic obstructive pulmonary disease. *Am J Med* 91(suppl 4A):17S–23S, 1991.

7 | Chronic Obstructive Pulmonary Disease: Epidemiology, Pathophysiology, Pathogenesis, Clinical Course, Management, and Rehabilitation*

Robert M. Senior

The American Thoracic Society defines chronic obstructive pulmonary disease (COPD) as "a disease state characterized by the presence of airflow obstruction due to chronic bronchitis or emphysema; the airflow obstruction is generally progressive, may be accompanied by airflow hyperreactivity, and may be viewed as partially reversible." This definition excludes asthma. In some patients, the distinction between asthma and COPD can be difficult.

EPIDEMIOLOGY

COPD occurs worldwide. It is a major health problem where cigarette smoking is common and the average lifespan extends into the sixth decade or beyond. Nonsmokers in occupations associated with high levels of particulates in the inspired air and women in undeveloped countries chronically exposed to indoor open fires for cooking and heating are groups prone to develop COPD without smoking cigarettes. With the current marketing of tobacco products to developing countries, an increased prevalence of COPD can be expected throughout the world in the future.

The incidence of COPD in the United States has been rising sharply in recent decades. It is estimated that 4 to 6 percent of adult white males and 1 to 3 percent of adult white females have COPD. The death rate from COPD in the United States has also been rising in recent decades and contrasts with the falling death rates from heart and cerebrovascular diseases. COPD is now the fourth most common cause of death in the United States. The highest mortality exists among white men, and the lowest rate is among Hispanic women. African Americans have intermediate death rates. Although the

*Edited from Chap. 43, "Chronic Obstructive Pulmonary Disease: Epidemiology, Pathophysiology, and Pathogenesis," by Senior RM, Shapiro SD; Chap. 44, "Chronic Obstructive Pulmonary Disease: Clinical Course and Management," by George RB, San Pedro GS; Chap. 45, "Cigarette Smoking and Disease," by Rennard SI, Daughton DM; and Chap. 46, "Rehabilitation in Chronic Obstructive Pulmonary Disease and Other Respiratory Disorders," by Ries AL. In: *Fishman's Pulmonary Diseases and Disorders,* 3d ed., edited by Fishman AP, Elias JA, Fishman JA, Grippi MA, Kaiser LR, Senior RM. New York, McGraw-Hill, 1998, pp 659–682, 683–696, 697–708, and 709–720. For fuller discussion of topics dealt with in this chapter, the reader is referred to the original text, as noted above.

percentage of smokers in the adult population in the United States has dropped over the past 30 years, especially among men, COPD will continue to be common in the foreseeable future, since there are 48 million smokers in the United States and 3000 people, mostly teenagers, take up the habit daily.

RISK FACTORS

Smoking

Smoking is the overwhelming risk factor for COPD. Nearly all patients with symptomatic COPD are smokers or former smokers. Accelerated deterioration of ventilatory function is common among smokers, but its magnitude is usually small and only 10 to 20 percent of long-time smokers develop symptomatic COPD. The basis for heightened susceptibility in this group is unknown, but genetic factors are almost certainly key. The relationship between amount of smoking and risk of COPD is unpredictable on an individual basis. However, on average, in men who smoke one pack per day, the reduction in FEV_1 per year is 9 mL more than the decline in nonsmokers; in women, the excess rate of decline is 6 mL. In the Lung Health Study, middle-aged smokers who already had a significant decrease in FEV_1 cut their rate of loss of FEV_1 to normal by stopping smoking. Young adult smokers commonly show mild disturbances of lung function even while their FEV_1 is still normal, but these abnormalities do not predict later development of clinical COPD.

Other Adverse Health Effects of Smoking

The risk of developing lung cancer is about 20-fold greater in smokers than in nonsmokers, and smoking is the major risk factor associated with lung cancer. The risk of lung cancer increases with the amount smoked and the duration of smoking. The risk of lung cancer among passive smokers also seems to be increased, suggesting that low-dose exposure to cigarette smoke is a risk.

Cigarette smoking is also a major risk factor for the development of cardiovascular disease. Cigarette smoking may contribute to the development of chronic cardiovascular diseases by a variety of mechanisms, including direct endothelial injury, tachycardia, hyperlipidemia with increased levels of low-density-lipoprotein (LDL) cholesterol, increase in circulating neutrophils, and increased blood coagulability. Cigarette smoking is the major risk factor for thromboangiitis obliterans and accelerates the development of microvascular disease in persons with diabetes mellitus; a smoking history is almost uniformly present in individuals with abdominal aortic aneurysm.

Cigarette smoking has also been implicated in acute cardiac events in a variety of ways: myocardial ischemia can result from an increase in myocardial oxygen requirements; increased concentrations of carbon monoxide in blood, which impair oxygen delivery; increased blood viscosity, which predisposes to a hypercoagulable state; and increased circulating catecholamines, which can evoke coronary vasospasm and arrhythmias.

Cigarette smoking has also been implicated in a variety of nonmalignant lung diseases, including eosinophilic granuloma and spontaneous pneumothorax, and with many nonrespiratory diseases (e.g., peptic ulcer disease). These associations are typically based on epidemiologic studies.

Occupational Exposure

Studies from around the world implicate occupations producing exposures to dusts, gases, and fumes as risk factors for COPD. Dusts appear to be most significant. The presence of chronic bronchitis does not correlate with airflow obstruction. The risk generally relates to the intensity of exposure, but there is considerable individual variability, indicating the importance of host factors in determining susceptibility.

Airway Hyperresponsiveness

Airway hyperresponsiveness is common in COPD; however, whether this precedes or follows the development of COPD has been difficult to sort out. In some individuals COPD seems to develop out of an asthmatic predisposition that may include childhood respiratory problems and allergic features such as an elevated serum IgE and eosinophilia (the so-called Dutch hypothesis for the cause of COPD), while in other individuals airway hyperresponsiveness seems to be a consequence of COPD.

PATHOPHYSIOLOGY

Airflow Obstruction

Reductions in FEV_1 and $FEV_1/FVC\%$, indicative of airflow obstruction, are the characteristic physiologic abnormalities of COPD. The reduced FEV_1 seldom shows increases >15 percent with a bronchodilator. Maximal inspiratory flow may be relatively well preserved. In the early stages of COPD, reduced maximal expiratory airflow is evident only at lung volumes at or below functional residual capacity, appearing as a "scooped out" lower part of the descending limb of the flow-volume curve. The arterial P_{O_2} (Pa_{O_2}) usually remains normal at rest until the FEV_1 is decreased to about 50 percent of the predicted level and may be near normal even when the FEV_1 is as low as 25 percent of predicted. Elevation of arterial P_{CO_2} (Pa_{CO_2}) is not expected in COPD until the FEV_1 is <25 percent of predicted. Cor pulmonale and right ventricular failure occur only in persons who have chronic hypoxemia (Pa_{O_2} <55 mmHg).

Nonuniform Ventilation and Ventilation/Perfusion Mismatching

Nonuniform ventilation and ventilation/perfusion ($\dot{V}/\dot{Q}$) mismatching are characteristic of COPD and reflect the heterogeneous nature of the disease process in the airways and lung parenchyma. In type A ("pink puffer") COPD, there is a substantial amount of ventilation distributed to high-$\dot{V}/\dot{Q}$ regions. In a second pattern, called type B ("blue bloater") COPD, there is a substantial amount of pulmonary blood flow perfusing low-$\dot{V}/\dot{Q}$ regions. This classification has limitations, because persons with the clinical features of type A or type B do not necessarily have the expected $\dot{V}/\dot{Q}$ pattern, and most people with COPD are not easily classified as either type A or type B. $\dot{V}/\dot{Q}$ mismatching accounts for essentially all of the reduction in Pa_{O_2} in COPD.

Hyperinflation

Increased residual volume and an increased ratio of residual volume to total lung capacity are characteristic of COPD. The total lung capacity is also often increased. Hyperinflation of the thorax helps compensate for airway obstruction by helping to dilate airways, but hyperinflation makes the thorax less efficient as a bellows and increases the work of breathing.

Dyspnea

Most people with COPD seek medical care because of dyspnea. Dyspnea is seldom a complaint until the FEV_1 is <60 percent of predicted. An increased sense of effort relating to the pressures needed from the respiratory muscles relative to their maximum pressure-generating capacity is thought to be one factor in producing dyspnea. Signals of "length-tension inappropriateness" from the respiratory muscles due to hyperinflation constitute another factor. Impulses from airways undergoing abnormal dynamic compression during exhalation may also be involved. Hypercapnia and hypoxemia play only a small role except in acute situations. Oxygen administration may decrease dyspnea by reducing ventilation during exertion.

Pathologic Correlations

Airways ≤ 2 mm in diameter are the principal sites of increased airway resistance in COPD. Therefore COPD is called a "small-airway disease." Although the obstruction to airflow in COPD is in the small airways, the relative importance of emphysema causing functional closure of small airways versus intrinsic abnormalities of the structure of small airways varies between individuals; even in the same patient, there is not a single pathologic feature that accounts for the obstruction. Emphysema and small-airway pathology are both present in most persons with COPD.

Cigarette smoking often results in mucous gland enlargement and goblet cell hyperplasia in large airways. These changes are proportional to the cough and mucus production that define chronic bronchitis, but they do not cause airflow obstruction.

The small airways of smokers typically show goblet cell metaplasia, infiltrating mononuclear inflammatory cells, and replacement of surfactant-secreting Clara cells with mucus-secreting cells. Smooth-muscle hypertrophy may be present. Together, these abnormalities may cause luminal narrowing. Reduced surfactant may predispose to airway narrowing or collapse. Fibrosis in the wall may cause airway narrowing in some patients. Because small airway patency is maintained by the surrounding lung parenchyma, providing radial traction on bronchioles at points where alveolar septa attach, loss of bronchiolar attachments as a result of extracellular matrix destruction may cause airway distortion and narrowing. Macrophage accumulation in respiratory bronchioles is typical in cigarette smokers. Proteolytic enzymes and oxidants from these cells may contribute to the destruction of elastic fibers and other matrix in respiratory bronchioles.

Emphysema is defined "as a condition of the lung characterized by abnormal, permanent enlargement of airspaces distal to the terminal bronchiole, accompanied by destruction of their walls, and without obvious fibrosis." *Centriacinar emphysema,* the type most frequently associated with cigarette smoking, is characterized by enlarged airspaces found (initially) in association with respiratory bronchioles. It is most prominent in the upper lobes and superior segments of lower lobes. *Panacinar emphysema* refers to abnormally large airspaces evenly distributed within and across acinar units. Panacinar emphysema is usually observed in patients with alpha$_1$-antitrypsin (α_1-AT) deficiency; it has a predilection for the lower lobes. In most smokers with advanced COPD, both pathologic patterns of emphysema are present. As currently defined, emphysema is diagnosed by direct inspection of lung tissue; however, computed tomography (CT) of the chest is increasingly being accepted as a sensitive, reliable means of locating and quantifying emphysema.

Pathogenesis of Emphysema in Smokers

The proteinase-antiproteinase hypothesis is the prevailing concept of the pathogenesis of emphysema. According to this hypothesis, there is a steady or episodic release of proteolytic enzymes into the lung parenchyma. Normally, plasma proteinase inhibitors, especially α_1-AT, and inhibitors made in the lungs permeate lung tissue and prevent proteolytic enzymes, especially elastases, from digesting lung structural proteins, especially elastin. Emphysema results when there is an imbalance between proteinases and antiproteinases in favor of proteinases. Inflammatory cells are regarded as the main sources of the proteinases, but structural cells of the lungs may also produce matrix-degrading enzymes. Destruction and aberrant repair of alveolar collagen also occur, and reports of these processes have led to the "inflammatory repair hypothesis" of the pathogenesis of emphysema. Recently, apoptosis of alveolar cells has been introduced as another basic mechanism involved in emphysema. Oxidants in cigarette smoke or produced by leukocytes recruited to the lungs by smoking are also involved in emphysema. Oxidants can inactivate α_1-AT. They may also increase the susceptibility of elastin and other matrix molecules to proteinases, and may impair the function of cells that synthesize extracellular matrix. In brief, the biology of emphysema associated with smoking is complex, involving inflammatory cell recruitment, proteinase-antiproteinase balance, and oxidant-antioxidant balance, and responses of lung cells to proteinases and oxidants from inflammatory cells and to constituents of tobacco smoke. The relative importance of these factors is likely to vary on a genetic basis among different individuals.

Emphysema Associated with Alpha₁-Antitrypsin Deficiency

Emphysema associated with alpha₁-antitrypsin (α_1-AT) deficiency is the most compelling example of the role of elastase activity in the pathogenesis of emphysema and of a genetic predisposition to emphysema. At a normal concentration of 150 to 350 mg/dL, α_1-AT has the highest concentration of all of the plasma protease inhibitors. It is a glycoprotein synthesized primarily by the liver. It inhibits many serine proteinases but inactivates neutrophil elastase so much faster than other serine proteinases that inhibition of neutrophil elastase is likely to be its primary function .

α_1-AT is transmitted in a codominant fashion, meaning that the gene product from each parent is expressed in the offspring. More than 75 different α_1-AT alleles are known, most of which result in single amino acid changes that do not alter the levels of the protein or its function. The normal phenotype, Pi M, exists in more than 90 percent of the population, with the MS and MZ phenotypes being the next most common. These latter phenotypes are associated with about half of normal serum levels. Levels of >35 percent of normal are thought to be enough to avoid increased risk of emphysema, but some evidence indicates that people who are Pi MZ (who typically have about 60 percent of normal levels) account for more than the expected number among patients with COPD and are predisposed to accelerated decline of lung function.

TABLE 7-1 Alpha$_1$-Antitrypsin Deficiency: Indications for Screening

Premature onset of COPD, with moderate or severe impairment by age 50
Predominance of basilar emphysema
Unremitting asthma, especially in a person under age 50 (screening is indicated even in the presence of atopy)
Chronic bronchitis with airflow obstruction in a never-smoker
Bronchiectasis without other identifiable cause
Family history of alpha$_1$-antitrypsin deficiency or COPD before age 50
Cirrhosis without apparent risk factors

Source: Adapted from the American Thoracic Society.

A severe deficiency of α_1-AT can be detected by serum protein electrophoresis, but quantification of serum α_1-AT concentration is done routinely by immunoassay. The deficiency should be suspected with characteristics listed in Table 7-1. Isoelectric focusing is done for determination of α_1-AT phenotype. Several α_1-AT phenotypes are associated with <15 percent of normal serum concentration, but the Pi Z phenotype is by far the most common, accounting for more than 95 percent. Typically, Pi Z individuals have about 15 percent of the normal serum concentration of α_1-AT. The prevalence of the Pi Z phenotype in the United States is about 1 in 3000 people. The Z allele is rare in Asians and African Americans. The Z form of the α_1-AT protein inactivates neutrophil elastase more slowly than the M, so that persons with the Pi Z phenotype have both a deficiency of α_1-AT protein and a form of α_1-AT that is less effective than normal. The low levels of the Z protein in the plasma are due to an alteration in the structure of the α_1-AT molecules that prevents efficient secretion from the liver. Retention of α_1-AT in the liver can lead to cirrhosis and hepatoma. Most people with the Pi Z phenotype eventually become symptomatic with COPD, but there is considerable variation. Smoking has a marked effect on the age at which shortness of breath appears. On average, the Pi Z smoker has symptoms by age 40, about 15 years earlier than a Pi Z nonsmoker.

CLINICAL COURSE

In the early stages of COPD, dyspnea is restricted to exertion or not even apparent. The only symptoms may be cough and sputum production. However, as the disease develops, progressively lower levels of routine activity result in dyspnea; finally, dyspnea occurs at rest, so that activities of daily living, such as bathing and dressing, become burdensome. During the late stages of COPD, appetite is often decreased and weight loss occurs. Weight loss is thought to be due to several factors, including decreased caloric intake and increased energy expended on breathing. As lung function declines, the alveolar-arterial gradient for oxygen increases, primarily because of an increase in $\dot{V}/\dot{Q}$ imbalance. Psychological effects of advanced COPD may be observed, including anxiety and depression. A number of factors are associated with clinical course and survival (Table 7-2).

Hypercapnia, hypoxemia, cor pulmonale, and weight loss are late features of COPD. Their presence correlates with significant disability and reduced longevity. The onset of respiratory disability occurs late in the course of COPD, after the FEV$_1$ has decreased to about 30 percent of predicted. Associated findings—e.g., resting tachycardia—are due to hypoxemia,

TABLE 7-2 Factors Associated with Clinical Course and Survival in Patients with COPD

Cigarette smoking	Hypercapnia
Passive smoking exposure	Pulmonary artery pressure
Age	Resting heart rate
Rate of decline of FEV_1	Weight loss
Type of lung disease (reversibility)	

pulmonary hypertension, and right heart failure. Acute exacerbations of symptoms are common in the more advanced stages of COPD. Although these are usually treated as infections, the etiology of most of these episodes is not certain. Severe exacerbations may culminate in the need for hospitalization; sometimes mechanical ventilation is necessary.

MANAGEMENT

Smoking Cessation

Smoking cessation will decrease the rate of decline in lung function. Therefore smoking cessation is an essential component of the management of all smokers with COPD. Nicotine, a potent euphoriant, is the active psychopharmaceutical drug in the leaves of the tobacco plant. It may improve task performance and, measurably, attention time in nonhabituated subjects; it can also alleviate anxiety and depression and induce a sense of well-being as well as a state of arousal. Unfortunately, it is also addicting, so that smoking cessation represents dealing with nicotine addiction. Most people who become addicted to nicotine do so before adulthood. In the United States, the peak incidence for developing a regular nicotine habit occurs in adolescence. Persons who do not acquire a nicotine habit before the age of 20 years are very unlikely to do so later.

Pragmatic Approaches to Smoking Cessation

There is no single "best" approach for smoking cessation. While nicotine replacement therapy may help one smoker quit, the identical regimen may be of absolutely no benefit to another. In the past, 95 percent of successful quitters stopped smoking on their own. Approximately 25 percent stop without developing tobacco withdrawal symptoms. Many who quit by themselves develop withdrawal symptoms, but the discomfort does not overwhelm their desire to quit. There are two critical ingredients required for successful abstinence, a *reason for quitting* and the *ability to quit.*

Most smokers know reasons for quitting smoking, such as serious health risks, expense, and social unacceptibility, but these seldom are enough to drive smokers to quit. Many patients at risk will make a genuine effort to quit when they have an immediate reason for quitting, such as a recent myocardial infarction or recurrent pneumonia.

Two categories of smokers experience considerable difficulty in quitting despite powerful reasons, such as disabling emphysema or cardiac disease. The first comprises those with significant psychiatric disorders. The incidence of smoking among such individuals is notoriously high. The second group includes heavily nicotine-dependent individuals. An evaluation of the smoker's habit is useful. This can be done quickly with the Fagerström test, a brief questionnaire for nicotine dependence (Table 7-3). Individuals with

TABLE 7-3 The Fagerström Tolerance Questionnaire

1. How soon after you wake do you smoke your first cigarette?	___	1 = within 30 min 0 = after 30 min
2. Do you find it difficult to refrain from smoking in places where it is forbidden; e.g., in church, at the library, in cinemas, etc.?	___	1 = yes 0 = no
3. Which cigarette would you most hate to give up?	___	1 = the first one in the morning 0 = any other
4. How many cigarettes a day do you smoke?	___	2 = 26 or more 1 = 16 to 25 0 = 15 or fewer
5. Do you smoke more frequently during the early morning than the rest of the day?	___	1 = yes 0 = no
6. Do you smoke if you are so ill that you are in bed most of the day?	___	1 = yes 0 = no
7. What is the nicotine level of your usual brand of cigarettes?	___	2 = more than 1.0 mg 1 = 0.61 to 1.0 mg 0 = 0.6 mg or fewer
8. Do you inhale?	___	2 = always 1 = sometimes 0 = never
TOTAL SCORE ___		

SOURCE: Used with permission of Karl-Olov Fagerström.

high scores are likely to benefit from nicotine replacement therapy while those with low scores should be encouraged to quit on their own.

Smoking Intervention Models

In one popular model, the smoking cessation process consists of five stages: *precontemplation, contemplation, preparation, action,* and *maintenance.* A model recommended by the US Public Health Service for smoking cessation, popularly referred to as the "5 As," emphasizes the role of medical professionals to *ask* patients about their smoking status, to *advise* smokers to stop, to *assess* whether patients are willing to make a quit attempt at this time, to *assist* them in their stop-smoking efforts, and to *arrange* for follow-up visits to support the patients' efforts. The approach utilizes brief intervention techniques and emphasizes the role of physicians as facilitators in the quitting process.

Preparing Smokers for Quitting

Several obstacles challenge smokers during their first 3 months of quitting. By anticipating the problems smokers will likely encounter, clinicians can help guide patients through the pitfalls that await them. The process begins with the setting of a quit day, when the smoker will make an all-out effort to stop smoking.

Pharmacologic Measures to Assist Quitting

A wide spectrum of behavioral techniques have been used to treat cigarette addiction. Most of these have had poor overall success rates. As a result, a variety of pharmacologic agents are currently in use or under review. The principal agents among these are the antidepressant bupropion, the antihypertensive clonidine, and various forms of nicotine replacement. Bupropion relieves or suppresses nicotine withdrawal symptoms in individuals irrespective of whether they are depressed. It may be used with nicotine replacement therapy.

Nicotine Replacement Therapies

Several forms of nicotine replacement have been devised. Current forms include gum, transdermal patches, nasal sprays, and inhalers. All of the approved forms increase long-term smoking cessation rates, and the higher the nicotine dose delivered, the greater the success in smoking cessation. None of these forms at recommended dosages increase the risk of myocardial infarction, stroke, or peripheral vascular disease.

Nicotine polacrilex (nicotine gum) Nicotine polacrilex was the first nicotine replacement therapy to gain FDA approval. Available in 2- and 4-mg doses, the nicotine is bound to a buffered resin. Mouth pH and rate of chewing influence nicotine absorption. Ad lib use of 2 mg of nicotine polacrilex is associated with blood nicotine levels less than 40 percent of those associated with customary smoking, so that many patients using nicotine gum still experience discomforting symptoms of tobacco withdrawal. Because gum can provide a rapid increases in blood nicotine, it, unlike the patch, may be most effective as an adjunct to the patch to curb sudden cravings for a cigarette. In this regard it resembles nicotine nasal sprays and the nicotine inhaler, which also produce rapid increments in nicotine levels.

Transdermal nicotine Transdermal nicotine systems reduce tobacco withdrawal symptoms and enhance smoking cessation rates. Abstinence rates associated with use of the nicotine patch are generally double those of placebo controls. Unlike gum, transdermal nicotine systems have consistently improved quit rates in the primary care setting. Plasma nicotine concentrations obtained with patches that deliver 21 mg per day provide about 40 to 50 percent of the nicotine levels achieved by customary smoking. The recommended use period for patches varies according to manufacturers' recommendations, but 6 to 12 weeks with termination or gradual taper is standard. The 1-year rates of abstinence are 10 to 20 percent. Side effects other than minor skin irritation are uncommon.

Perhaps because the replacement of nicotine is only partial, most smokers who use patches still experience some tobacco withdrawal symptoms during the first few days of quitting and are tempted to smoke *and* to wear patches. As noted, for such individuals, supplementation with rapid-delivery nicotine systems such as gum, nasal spray, or inhaler may combat the cravings for a cigarette. Patients who continue to smoke and use patches are unlikely to achieve abstinence, so the simultaneous wearing of nicotine patches while smoking is continued should be strongly discouraged.

Tobacco Withdrawal Period

The symptoms of smoking cessation include restlessness, anxiety, difficulty concentrating, irritability, frustration, depression, and an almost relentless craving for cigarettes. These symptoms generally peak during the first 72 h and then gradually subside over 3 to 4 weeks. To help smokers cope with these early withdrawal symptoms, the following are recommended in addition to nicotine replacement therapy: (1) Be active. Increased activity may curtail some of the drive to smoke. (2) Avoid caffeine. Caffeine is a stimulant that, theoretically, may exacerbate withdrawal symptoms. (3) Use deep-breathing exercises. The simplest breathing exercise requires nothing more than extended breath-holding, followed by slow exhalation through pursed lips. (4) Avoid high-risk situations for smoking during the first 3 weeks of quitting. (5) Use plenty of gum or chewable candies. (6) Know that strong urges to smoke will go away, without smoking. Craving waves usually occur less frequently after 2 to 3 weeks but can sometimes catch smokers off guard because of their unexpected intensity.

Depression

At some time during the first 3 months of abstinence, some smokers experience depression. For many, the depression is mild and transient. For very few, quitting smoking may produce clinical depression that requires antidepressant therapy, counseling, or a return to smoking.

Weight Gain

One of the most disheartening components of quitting smoking is weight gain during the first 6 to 8 weeks of cigarette abstinence, followed by a gradual increase in weight to roughly 10 lb at 6 months. Average weight gain at 10 years after cessation is about 10 lb for men and 12 lb for women.

Desire for an Occasional Cigarette

The desire for an occasional cigarette may extend beyond the first year of abstinence. Strong urges to smoke periodically recur during times of extreme stress or while drinking alcohol with friends who smoke. Smoking one cigarette is a reliable predictor of relapse. Ex-smokers should see themselves as "smokeaholics" who will not be able to stop at just one cigarette.

Bronchodilators

Several classes of bronchodilator agents are used routinely in the management of COPD, including beta-adrenergic agonists, anticholinergic agents, and methylxanthines. Other agents such as D2 dopamine receptor agonists may be forthcoming in the near future. Whether use of an inhaled bronchodilator will slow the rate of decline is unclear but seems doubtful. Regular use of ipratropium in the Lung Health Study did not affect the long-term decline in FEV_1.

Beta-Adrenergic Agonists

Beta-Adrenergic agonists are the mainstay rescue treatment of COPD. Onset of action is usually more rapid with these agents than with inhaled ipratropium bromide, but their duration of action is usually shorter. Salmeterol is an exception, showing a long duration of action. Because of their high incidence of side effects by the oral route, oral formulations are generally not used unless patients are unable to use the inhaled forms. The various inhaled agents provide similar bronchodilation in equivalent doses. Choice of agent depends on such factors as patient preference, physician experience, availability, and cost. The drugs are best taken on an "as needed" basis; hence, they may be used as primary therapy in patients who have dyspnea only intermittently.

They may be added to regular doses of ipratropium when patients have daily symptoms. Excessive use of beta agonists may result in tachyphylaxis. The side effects include tachycardia, dysrhythmias, exacerbation of myocardial ischemia, and hypo- or hypertension, tremor, agitation, and insomnia, and hypokalemia in patients receiving large doses.

Anticholinergic Agents

Atropine sulfate has long been available in aerosolized and oral forms; however, its use has been limited by excessive side effects. Quaternary ammonium atropine derivatives have less mucosal absorption and fewer side effects. Currently, ipratropium bromide is the only such agent available in the United States, but the longer-acting tiotropium may become available soon. Ipratropium bromide is available in a metered-dose inhaler and as a solution for nebulization. The drug has a relatively slow onset of action (60 to 90 min); however, it has a longer duration of bronchodilation (6 to 8 h) than do most beta-adrenergic agonists. The incidence of side effects is low, and side effects are generally not seen even when the recommended dose of two puffs four times daily is doubled or tripled. No tachyphylaxis has been reported, even when ipratropium bromide was used for as long as 5 years. Extended use of the agent does not appear to influence the long-term decline in FEV_1. Given its effectiveness, prolonged duration of effect, low incidence of side effects, and freedom from tachyphylaxis, ipratropium bromide has become the first-line agent for patients with symptomatic COPD.

In some studies, ipratropium bromide has been reported to produce greater bronchodilation than do conventional doses of beta agonists. However, other investigations show that maximal doses of beta agonists produce the same degree of bronchodilation.

Theophylline

The exact mechanism of action of theophylline remains unclear. The drug relaxes bronchial smooth muscle (although only to relatively mild degrees) and increases diaphragmatic contractility and endurance. It also improves cardiac output, reduces pulmonary vascular resistance, and improves perfusion to ischemic myocardium. It has a narrow therapeutic window, with minimal improvement in lung function at serum levels less than 10 μg/mL; significant toxic effects are observed at levels greater than 20 μg/mL. Theophylline's unique multisystem effects, additive actions with other bronchodilators, and availability in sustained-release oral formulations provide a role for the agent in maintenance regimens for patients with COPD. Nevertheless, the potential for serious side effects (nausea, vomiting, insomnia, agitation, seizures, cardiac dysrhythmias) requires that serum levels be monitored, especially in the elderly and in patients with hepatic dysfunction and congestive heart failure. A number of drugs commonly prescribed for patients with COPD (e.g., macrolide and quinolone antibiotics, H_2 blockers, propranolol) may prolong theophylline's half-life, resulting in toxic blood levels.

Corticosteroids

Based on the common pathologic finding of airway inflammation in COPD, use of systemic corticosteroids would seem rational; however, benefits have been difficult to establish except for acute exacerbations, in which they accelerate recovery of lung function. Only a small percentage of COPD patients will show significant improvement in spirometry and symptomatology with a trial of prednisone during periods of stability.

Recent studies of chronic administration of inhaled corticosteroids point to improvement in health status and reduction in acute exacerbations without adverse effects. There is not, however, a slowing of the rate of decline of FEV_1. Thus, chronic usage of inhaled corticosteroids, unlike systemic corticosteroids, may have a role in the regimen of COPD patients having moderate or more advanced disease and appear to be safe.

Cough Control

Chronic cough is the defining symptom in chronic bronchitis; however, cough may be a sign of associated diseases, such as cancer and acute respiratory infection. Nonnarcotic antitussives and expectorants may be tried to control the cough. Patients with ineffective, exhausting coughs can be trained to cough more effectively. Mucolytics are of doubtful benefit.

Immunizations

Administration of influenza and pneumococcal vaccinations is advised.

Pulmonary Rehabilitation

As the FEV_1 falls, the capacity to carry out essential activities of daily living commonly becomes restricted. This limitation develops against a background of an already compromised quality of life due to shortness of breath and psychosocial disability. A vicious cycle can ensue in which the patient performs less exercise and becomes more disabled from deconditioning and more depressed. Pulmonary rehabilitation is aimed at interrupting the cycle and improving the patient's overall health status (see below).

Oxygen Therapy

The value of long-term supplemental oxygen therapy for hypoxemic patients with severe COPD has been demonstrated in major controlled trials. In the National Heart, Lung, and Blood Institute's Nocturnal Oxygen Therapy Trial among patients with COPD and hypoxemia, mortality was approximately one-half as great in patients receiving continuous oxygen (actually for an average of 19 h/day) than in those who received it for only 12 h/day. In addition, morbidity in the continuous group was less than that in the other group. These findings, along with those reported in a study from the British Medical Research Council, serve as the basis for current recommendations regarding supplemental oxygen use in patients with COPD.

Indications

Indications for long-term supplemental oxygen include a resting Pa_{O_2} of 55 mmHg or less or arterial oxygen saturation (Sa_{O_2}) of 88% or less. The criteria are slightly less stringent (resting Pa_{O_2} of 56 to 59 mmHg or Sa_{O_2} of 89%) if there is electrocardiographic evidence of cor pulmonale, secondary polycythemia, or edema from right-sided heart failure. Evaluation for nocturnal oxygen use should also be considered, since patients with COPD may have episodic desaturation during sleep without daytime hypoxemia. Likewise, patients who are normoxemic at rest may become hypoxemic during exercise; exercise capacity and endurance may be improved with oxygen supplementation.

Administration of Supplemental Oxygen

Home oxygen can be supplied with an oxygen concentrator, a cylinder of compressed oxygen, or a source of liquid oxygen. The most cost-effective and reliable method is the oxygen concentrator, since it requires only an electrical source and periodic maintenance; backup sources of oxygen, such as a cylinder or liquid oxygen, should be available for extenuating circumstances (e.g., electrical power failure). Liquid oxygen and compressed oxygen cylinders permit patient mobility.

Oxygen is usually delivered by nasal cannula at continuous flows of 0.5 to 4 L/min. Oxygen-conserving devices use reservoirs that allow delivery at lower flow rates. The goal of oxygen therapy is to achieve a Pa_{O_2} of 60–70 mmHg; higher levels of oxygenation will accomplish little clinically. The patient should be reevaluated with arterial blood gases after 1, 6, and 12 months. Follow-up arterial blood gases are important, since about 20 percent of patients initially eligible for supplemental oxygen no longer need it after aggressive bronchodilator therapy.

Transtracheal oxygen delivery via a small-bore catheter offers several advantages over use of nasal cannula, including a 50 percent reduction in supplemental oxygen requirement, decreased dyspnea, improved exercise tolerance, decreased rate of hospitalization, and protection against hypoxemia during obstructive sleep disturbances. Because the device can easily be covered by clothing, acceptance of oxygen therapy is improved with some patients. The main disadvantages are that insertion is an invasive procedure; mucous balls can form in the airway, causing respiratory distress; and the catheter requires some maintenance.

Acute Exacerbations

Acute decompensation of COPD is characterized by varying combinations of increased dyspnea, cough, and production of purulent sputum. Many such episodes can be managed on an outpatient basis. The decision to hospitalize a patient with an acute exacerbation is usually based on the physician's subjective interpretation of clinical symptoms, including severity of dyspnea, short-term response to therapeutic efforts, and the presence of other conditions—e.g., bronchitis, pneumonia, or other comorbidities. Not rarely, patients discharged after emergency department management will relapse and require hospitalization. The American Thoracic Society has devised guidelines for hospitalization (Table 7-4) and intensive care unit (ICU) admission (Table 7-5) for patients with an acute exacerbation of COPD. Similar guidelines have been devised by the recent Global Initiative for Chronic Obstructive Lung Disease (GOLD). Mortality among patients who require hospitalization is substantial. Factors associated with increased mortality include advanced age, a markedly widened alveolar-arterial oxygen gradient, and presence of atrial fibrillation or ventricular dysrhythmias. Typical therapy of acute exacerbations consists of intensive administration of inhaled bronchodilators, intravenous corticosteroids, and antibiotics.

Bronchodilators

Pharmacologic therapy centers on the use of beta agonists administered by either a metered-dose inhaler (MDI) or nebulizer. Studies confirm the equal efficacy of the two techniques. The safety and efficacy of continuous nebulization of beta agonists have not been established in COPD. The relatively slow onset of action of ipratropium bromide has relegated this drug to

TABLE 7-4 Indications for Hospitalization of Patients with COPD

I. Acute exacerbation (increased dyspnea, cough, or sputum production)
   plus one or more of the following:
      Inadequate response to outpatient management
      In a patient previously mobile, inability to ambulate due to dyspnea
      Inability to eat or sleep due to dyspnea
      Inadequate home care resources
      Serious comorbid condition
      Prolonged progressive symptoms before emergency visit
      Altered mentation
      Worsening hypoxemia
      New or worsening hypercapnia
II. New or worsening cor pulmonale unresponsive to outpatient management
III. Planned invasive surgical or diagnostic procedure requiring analgesics
   or sedatives that may worsen pulmonary function
IV. Comorbid condition—e.g., severe steroid myopathy or acute vertebral
   compression fractures—that has worsened pulmonary function

SOURCE: Adapted from Celli et al., 1995.

a minor role in the acute setting; however, its apparent additive effects with beta agonists should be considered.

Theophylline has been used in the management of acute exacerbations of COPD, but its efficacy in this setting is uncertain. If it is used, levels of the agent should be monitored so that overdosage is avoided. Serum levels of 8 to 12 μg/mL are appropriate for most patients, although some patients may tolerate higher levels (up to 18 to 20 μg/mL).

Corticosteroids

Corticosteroids are used routinely for the hospitalized patient and are often prescribed for outpatients who have severe COPD but do not meet the criteria for hospitalization. In a large, controlled, prospective study of Veterans Administration (VA) patients given intravenous methylprednisolone for 72 h, followed by prednisone, the hospital stay was shorter and the FEV_1 recovered more rapidly in those given corticosteroids. However, mortality was not affected. Hyperglycemia was the only complication of the therapy. Two weeks of corticosteroids appeared to yield maximum benefit.

Antibiotics

Even though bacterial infection is seldom proved, a meta-analysis of the randomized trials of antibiotics for exacerbations of COPD confirmed a small but statistically and clinically significant improvement in symptoms and airflow with antibiotic therapy. *Streptococcus pneumoniae* and *Haemophilus influenzae* are the most common pathogenic bacteria isolated in the sputum

TABLE 7-5 Indications for ICU Admission of Patients with Acute Exacerbation of COPD

Severe dyspnea that responds inadequately to initial emergency therapy
Confusion or lethargy
Respiratory muscle fatigue (especially paradoxical diaphragmatic motion)
Persistent or worsening hypoxemia despite supplemental oxygen or severe/worsening respiratory acidosis (pH <7.30)
Need for noninvasive or invasive assisted mechanical ventilation

SOURCE: Adapted from Celli et al., 1995.

of patients experiencing an acute exacerbation, but the same bacteria can be isolated from stable patients. Any of many antibiotics may be administered— for example, trimethoprim-sulfamethoxazole, amoxicillin, doxycycline, azithromycin, or levofloxacin.

Oxygen and Hydration

Supplemental oxygen will be administered to hospitalized patients with an exacerbation, since deterioration usually leads to increased $\dot{V}/\dot{Q}$ inequalities and worsening hypoxemia. For outpatients who use oxygen, flows may be increased. Sputum may be tenacious and copious, so adequate hydration should be provided: 2 to 3 L of fluid daily should be supplied by mouth or parenterally unless cardiac or renal insufficiency is of concern.

Ventilatory Support

Noninvasive positive-pressure ventilation (NPPV) is beneficial in selected hospitalized patients. It may accelerate improvement in alveolar gas exchange, prevent the need for invasive mechanical ventilation, and lower in-hospital mortality.

SURGERY FOR COPD

Although removal of localized large bullae (bullectomy) has long been recognized as potentially beneficial in a carefully selected group of patients with emphysema, lung transplantation and volume reduction surgery have become available for patients with far advanced COPD and emphysema.

Lung Transplantation

Selection criteria for lung transplantation in COPD include an FEV_1 of ≤25 percent predicted; age <60 years; life expectancy without transplantation of 2 years or less; progressive deterioration of clinical status; emotional stability; adequate nutrition; and a history of compliance with medical regimens, including abstinence from cigarette smoking. Coronary artery disease and renal or hepatic dysfunction should be absent. With increasing transplantation experience, some of these restrictions (e.g., age limit) are becoming less rigid. Actuarial survival rates for 1, 3, and 5 years are in the range 80, 70, and 50 percent. Cost of the procedure and lack of an adequate supply of donor lungs are problematic, but a high incidence of progressive bronchiolititis obliterans is a devastating and common complication, occurring in nearly half of the patients within 5 years after surgery.

Lung Volume Reduction Surgery

Studies thus far appear to confirm a symptomatic, physiologic, and even longevity benefit in carefully selected individuals who undergo lung volume reduction surgery for advanced emphysema. However, the status of this procedure is under scrutiny in a muticenter trial sponsored by the National Heart, Lung and Blood Institute.

PULMONARY REHABILITATION

Pulmonary rehabilitation is appropriate for any patient with stable lung disease who is disabled by respiratory symptoms. Even patients with advanced disease may benefit if they are selected appropriately and realistic goals are set.

Historically, pulmonary rehabilitation strategies have been used primarily for patients with COPD. However, pulmonary rehabilitation has also been applied successfully to patients with other chronic lung conditions, including interstitial diseases, cystic fibrosis, bronchiectasis, and thoracic cage abnormalities. It has been used successfully in the evaluation and preparation of patients for surgery, such as lung transplantation and lung volume reduction surgery, maximizing recovery after surgery, recovery from acute lung injury, and exacerbations of chronic lung disease requiring mechanical ventilation or acute hospital care.

Definition

A definition of pulmonary rehabilitation proposed by a National Institutes of Health (NIH) Workshop on Pulmonary Rehabilitation Research emphasizes the importance of multidimensional services, an interdisciplinary team, involvement of patients and families, and individual goals for patient independence and function in the community. The definition is as follows: "Pulmonary rehabilitation is a multidimensional continuum of services directed to persons with pulmonary disease and their families, usually by an interdisciplinary team of specialists, with the goal of achieving and maintaining the individual's maximum level of independence and functioning in the community."

Successful pulmonary rehabilitation programs have been established in both outpatient and inpatient settings and with different formats. A key to success is a dedicated, enthusiastic staff that is familiar with respiratory problems and relates well to pulmonary patients.

Patient Selection

Any patient with symptomatic chronic lung disease is a candidate for pulmonary rehabilitation. The ideal patient for pulmonary rehabilitation is one with functional limitation from moderate to severe lung disease who is stable on standard therapy, not distracted or limited by other serious or unstable medical conditions, willing and able to learn about his or her disease, and motivated to devote the time and effort necessary to benefit from a comprehensive care program (Table 7-6). Criteria based on arbitrary lung function parameters or age alone should not be used in selecting patients, as pulmonary function is not a good predictor of symptoms, function, or improvement after rehabilitation. Patients should be evaluated and stabilized on standard medical therapy before beginning a program.

Patient Evaluation

Interview

The screening interview serves to evaluate the patient's medical status, identify psychosocial problems and needs, and set realistic goals. Family members

---

TABLE 7-6 Patient Selection Criteria for Pulmonary Rehabilitation

Symptomatic chronic lung disease
Stable on standard therapy
Functional limitation from disease
Relationship with primary care provider
Motivated to be actively involved in and take responsibility for own health care
No other interfering or unstable medical conditions
No arbitrary lung function or age criteria

and significant others should be included in the interview. Communication with the primary care physician is also important to establish the vital link for the rehabilitation staff in clarifying medical questions and in facilitating recommendations during and after treatment.

Medical Evaluation and Diagnostic Testing

A review of the medical history is necessary to identify the patient's lung disease and to assess its severity. Other medical problems that might preclude or delay participation may be identified. Available laboratory data should be reviewed.

Planning an appropriate rehabilitation program requires accurate, current information. The need for testing depends upon the individual patient and program goals as well as the facilities and expertise available. Spirometry and lung volumes are the most useful pulmonary function measurements. Exercise testing helps to assess the patient's exercise tolerance and to evaluate changes in arterial blood gases (e.g., development of hypoxemia or hypercapnia) with exercise. This may also uncover coexisting diseases (e.g., heart disease). The exercise test is also used to establish a safe and appropriate prescription for subsequent training. Maximal exercise of patients with chronic lung disease is limited largely by their breathing reserve. Simple pulmonary function tests such as spirometry can be used to estimate a patient's capacity for sustained breathing (maximal ventilation) during exercise, but an individual patient's maximum work capacity can be estimated only from exercise testing. Exercise tolerance depends also on the patient's perception and tolerance of the subjective symptom of breathlessness.

Exercise evaluation for rehabilitation is most easily performed with the type of activity planned for training (e.g., treadmill for a walking training program). Variables measured or monitored during testing should include workload, heart rate, electrocardiogram, arterial oxygenation, and symptoms (e.g., breathlessness). Other measures, such as ventilation or expired gas analysis to calculate oxygen uptake and related variables, may be obtained depending on the interest and expertise of the program staff and laboratory. Measurement of arterial blood gases at rest and during exercise is important because of the frequent but unpredictable occurrence of exercise-induced hypoxemia, but arterial blood-gas sampling during exercise makes testing more complex. The noninvasive estimate of arterial oxygen saturation by pulse oximetry is useful for continuous monitoring, but it has limited accuracy (95 percent confidence limits, ± 4 to 5 percent).

Psychosocial Assessment

Successful rehabilitation requires attention to psychological, emotional, and social issues. Commonly, patients with chronic lung diseases become depressed, frightened, anxious, and more dependent on others. Progressive dyspnea is a frightening symptom and may lead to a vicious "fear-dyspnea" cycle: with progressive disease, less exertion results in more dyspnea, which produces more fear and anxiety, which, in turn, lead to more dyspnea so that ultimately the patient avoids any physical activity associated with these unpleasant symptoms.

The initial evaluation should include an assessment of the patient's psychological state and attention should be directed to "psychosocial clues" that may be apparent during the screening interview (e.g., the level of family and social support and the patient's living arrangement, activities of daily living, hobbies, and employment potential). Family members and significant others may provide valuable insight.

Setting Goals

Specific, realistic goals should be set that are compatible with the patient's disease, needs, and expectations. Family members and significant others should be included in this process so that everyone understands what can and cannot be achieved.

Program Content

Comprehensive pulmonary rehabilitation programs typically include several key components: education, instruction in respiratory and chest physiotherapy, psychosocial support, and exercise training.

Education Successful pulmonary rehabilitation depends upon an understanding of lung disease. Education is an integral component; even patients with severe disease can gain a better understanding of their disease and learn specific means to deal with problems. Despite the importance of education, increased patient knowledge alone seldom leads to improved health status.

Physiotherapy techniques and breathing retraining techniques Each patient's needs for respiratory care should be assessed and instruction provided in the proper use of these techniques, which may include chest physiotherapy to control secretions; breathing retraining techniques to relieve and control dyspnea and improve ventilatory function; and proper use and care of respiratory equipment, including nebulizers, MDIs, and supplemental oxygen.

Pulmonary rehabilitation typically includes instruction in breathing techniques, such as diaphragmatic and pursed-lips breathing to prevent dynamic airway compression, improve respiratory synchrony of the abdominal and thoracic musculature, and improve gas exchange. The primary effect of the diaphragmatic breathing technique in which the patient coordinates abdominal wall expansion with inspiration and slows expiration through pursed lips is to slow the respiratory rate and increase the tidal volume. Pursed-lips breathing is commonly taught to pulmonary patients, particularly those with COPD, to slow the expiratory phase and maintain positive airway pressure in order to "stent the airways open." It is a maneuver assumed naturally by many patients.

Bronchial hygiene Rehabilitation programs provide teaching of a variety of chest physiotherapy techniques for secretion control (e.g., coughing, postural drainage, and chest vibration and percussion). These methods are important for patients who experience excess mucus production during exacerbations of their lung disease as well as for those who chronically produce sputum.

Oxygen When chronic oxygen therapy is required, the available delivery methods should be reviewed with the patient to help select the best system for his or her needs. Long-term continuous oxygen therapy has been clearly shown to improve survival and reduce mortality and morbidity in hypoxemic patients with COPD. Maintaining patients on supplemental oxygen presents several challenges. Handling equipment is particularly difficult for physically disabled and frail patients. Therefore it is important to assess each person's oxygen needs and to provide instruction on appropriate techniques.

Exercise Considerable evidence demonstrates favorable responses to exercise training in patients with chronic lung diseases. Benefits are physiologic and psychological. Patients may increase their maximum capacity and endurance for physical activity even though objective measures of lung function do not usually change. Patients may also benefit from learning to perform physical tasks more efficiently. Exercise training provides an ideal opportunity for patients to learn their capacity for physical work and to use and practice methods for controlling dyspnea.

The exercise program should be tailored to the individual's physical abilities, interests, resources, and environment. Techniques should be simple and inexpensive. Patients tend to do best with activities and exercises for which they are trained. Walking programs are particularly useful. They have the added benefit of encouraging patients to expand social horizons. In inclement weather, many can walk indoors (e.g., at shopping malls). Other types of exercise (e.g., cycling, swimming) are also effective. Since many persons with chronic lung disease have limited exercise tolerance, emphasis during training should be on increasing endurance. Changes in endurance with rehabilitation are often greater than changes in maximal exercise tolerance.

Patients who are not hypoxemic at rest may develop changes in arterial oxygenation that cannot be predicted reliably from resting measurements of pulmonary function or gas exchange. In patients with mild COPD, the Pa_{O_2} typically does not change with exercise; it may even improve. However, in patients with moderate to severe COPD, Pa_{O_2} may increase, decrease, or remain the same. Patients with interstitial lung disease commonly develop worsening oxygenation with exercise. Thus, it is important to evaluate a patient's oxygenation both at rest and during exercise. With the availability of ambulatory oxygen delivery systems, hypoxemia is not a contraindication to safe exercise training.

In patients with chronic lung diseases, the best method of choosing an appropriate training prescription is not clearly defined. Exercise tolerance in pulmonary patients is typically limited by maximal achievable ventilation and breathlessness. Such patients frequently do not reach their limits of cardiac or peripheral muscle performance.

Much controversy exists regarding the appropriate training intensity target for patients with chronic lung disease. Use of a target heart rate has been advocated by some, although it is recognized that such a target may not be reliable for patients with more severe disease. Many patients can be trained at a high percentage of their maximal activity level, with work levels approaching or even exceeding the maximal level reached on the initial exercise test. Even patients with advanced disease can be trained successfully at or near maximal exercise levels.

Some pulmonary rehabilitation programs define exercise targets and progression during training more by symptom tolerance than by heart rate, work level, or other physiologic measurements. Ratings of perceived symptoms (e.g., breathlessness) help teach patients to exercise to "target" levels of breathing discomfort. A typical approach is to begin training at a level that the patient can sustain with reasonable comfort for several minutes and then to increase the time or exercise level according to symptom tolerance. Patients are encouraged to exercise daily and to increase exercise duration up to 15 to 30 min of continuous activity. This graduated program helps patients to achieve a goal of improved tolerance for tasks of daily living.

Although exercise programs for pulmonary patients typically emphasize lower extremity training (i.e.,walking), inclusion of other forms of exercise may be valuable. Many patients with chronic lung disease report disabling dyspnea with daily activities involving the upper extremities (e.g., lifting, grooming) at work levels that are much lower than activities involving the lower extremities. Upper extremity exercise is accompanied by a higher ventilatory demand for a given level of work than is lower extremity exercise. Because there is specificity of training for muscle, upper extremity exercises may help pulmonary patients cope better with common daily activities.

Techniques of isocapnic hyperventilation, inspiratory resistive loading, and inspiratory threshold loading improve function of the respiratory muscles in both normals and patients. In patients with COPD, the patient group most extensively studied, improvement in general exercise performance from ventilatory muscle training alone has not been demonstrated consistently, so respiratory muscle training as a routine component of pulmonary rehabilitation has not been clearly established.

Psychosocial Support

Depression is common in patients with chronic pulmonary disorders, as are anxiety (especially anxiety over dyspnea), denial, anger, and isolation. Patients become sedentary and dependent upon others. Excessive concern over other physical problems and psychosomatic complaints arises. Sexual dysfunction and fear are common and represent often unspoken consequences of chronic lung disease. Psychosocial support is provided best by a warm and enthusiastic staff. Family members and significant others should be included in activities so that they can understand the disease and help the patient cope. Support groups are also effective. Patients with severe psychological disorders may benefit from individual counseling and therapy. Psychotropic drugs should generally be reserved for patients with more severe psychological dysfunction. Progressive muscle relaxation, a technique in which patients are taught to sequentially tense and then relax different muscle groups, may help to relieve dyspnea and anxiety.

Pulmonary Rehabilitation in Conjunction with Surgery for COPD

In recent years, surgical options for patients with severe, disabling lung disease have been used more frequently. Pulmonary rehabilitation is a valuable adjunct in preparing these patients for surgery and in the postsurgery recovery phase.

Lung Transplantation

Patients with advanced lung disease who are candidates for lung transplantation are usually evaluated by the transplant team and then referred for pulmonary rehabilitation after their transplant candidacy is approved. Rehabilitation staff plans a program that can be maintained throughout a waiting period, which may last months to years. The overall goals of pulmonary rehabilitation in the pretransplant setting are to maintain function, monitor disease progression, prevent complications, provide education about the underlying lung disease and lung transplantation, and offer psychosocial support for patients and families in coping with the stresses of waiting for a potentially lifesaving procedure. The exercise training program may be similar to that for other chronic lung disease patients except that patients with primary pulmonary vascular diseases do not typically participate in exercise or other physical activities because of the increased risk of sudden death. Although patients may have some initial improvement in exercise tolerance or endurance, the primary goal is to maintain mobility and exercise capacity.

Education in the pretransplant period aims to teach patients about their underlying lung disease, the transplant procedure itself, and expectations following transplantation.

The psychosocial stresses of waiting for transplantation are considerable. Many patients feel as though their lives are "on hold." Some may have moved away from family and their usual social support network to live close to the transplant center. Providing support for patients and family members during this time, whether through formal group support sessions or informal contact with supportive staff and other patients, helps patients to cope with these problems.

After lung transplantation, patients must learn to cope with a new level of function, new expectations, and a new set of problems. Rehabilitation for patients in this phase can facilitate physical reconditioning, help implement self-care and assessment techniques, and assist the psychosocial adaptations to a new lifestyle.

Goals of exercise training after transplantation are improved physical work tolerance and assessment of symptoms and oxygenation as early warning signs of complications, including rejection and infection. Educational goals are focused on self-care and assessment and the importance of compliance with a new medical regimen. Psychosocial support can assist with adaptation to a new set of stresses related to additional demands and expectations that patients have of themselves and their significant others. Patients who are used to being sick, disabled, and cared for by others may now be expected to be well and independent, to return to work, and to support other people.

Lung Volume Reduction Surgery

Pulmonary rehabilitation has become an important modality in evaluating patients and preparing them for volume reduction lung surgery for sever emphysema. In addition, rehabilitation has been employed in the postoperative recovery phase. Enrolling patients in rehabilitation prior to surgery has several advantages: (1) optimizing functional status, (2) improving physical and psychological symptoms, (3) helping patients to learn more about their disease, and (4) improving skills for coping with their disease. Rehabilitation following volume reduction surgery helps patients to adapt to new levels of function and to reassess symptoms and needs for supplemental oxygen.

Results of Pulmonary Rehabilitation

Several randomized clinical trials demonstrate important and significant benefits of pulmonary rehabilitation (Table 7-7).

Hospitalizations and Medical Resources

Pulmonary rehabilitation is effective in reducing hospital utilization. Given the high cost of hospitalization for acute care for these often sick patients, the potential savings from a reduction in inpatient days alone is significant.

TABLE 7-7 Results of Pulmonary Rehabilitation

Decreases in:
  Medical resource utilization (e.g., hospitalizations, emergency room visits)
  Respiratory symptoms (e.g., breathlessness)
  Psychological symptoms (e.g., depression, fear)
Increases in:
  Quality of life
  Physical activity
  Exercise tolerance (endurance or maximal level of activities of daily living)
  Knowledge
  Independence

Quality of Life

After rehabilitation, improvements occur in respiratory and psychological symptoms, exercise tolerance, and social activity. These changes are measured by quality-of-life instruments that incorporate aspects of physical, emotional, and psychological function into one or a small number of measures. Three of the popular instruments are the Chronic Respiratory Questionnaire (CRQ), the St. George's Respiratory Questionnaire (SGRQ), and the Quality of Well-Being Scale (QWB). The CRQ utilizes a questionnaire that focuses on four measured dimensions of quality of life—dyspnea, fatigue, emotional function, and mastery. The SGRQ is a self-administered questionnaire that permits calculation of a composite score based on three component scores: symptoms, activity, and impacts on daily life. The QWB is a comprehensive measure of health-related quality of life shown to have validity as an outcome measure for evaluating interventions that affect general health status. Although these instruments have generally shown quality-of-life improvements following rehabilitation, this is not always the case. Sometimes, quality of life is not affected despite marked improvements in exercise tolerance and breathlessness following rehabilitation.

Exercise Tolerance

Exercise plays an important and well-established role in pulmonary rehabilitation, producing both physiologic and psychological benefits. Many studies are in agreement that pulmonary rehabilitation results in improvement in exercise endurance or maximal exercise tolerance. Generally, these studies find highly significant improvements in exercise endurance and maximal exercise tolerance after rehabilitation that can persist for long periods.

Pulmonary Function and Symptoms

Pulmonary rehabilitation does not result in any consistent changes in lung function in chronic lung disease if the patient is on a good medical regimen prior to beginning the program. Nevertheless, many patients report improvement in respiratory symptoms, particularly breathlessness. Improvement in psychological symptoms has also been demonstrated consistently after rehabilitation.

Knowledge

Pulmonary rehabilitation emphasizes educating patients, family members, and significant others to be actively involved in the patient's care, improving their understanding of disease, and learning practical ways of coping with disabling symptoms. Even patients with severe disease can learn to understand their disease better.

Survival

Whether the survival of patients with chronic lung disease is improved by pulmonary rehabilitation is uncertain. In studies showing a benefit from rehabilitation, the difference appears to be small compared to controls.

BIBLIOGRAPHY

Epidemiology, Pathophysiology, Pathogenesis

Barnes PJ: Chronic obstructive pulmonary disease. *N Engl J Med* 343:269–280, 2000.

Eriksson S: A 30-year perspective on α_1-antitrypsin deficiency. *Chest* 110:237S–242S, 1996.

42d Annual Thomas L. Petty Lung Conference: Mechanisms of COPD. *Chest* 117:219S–323S, 2000.

Sandford AJ, Chagani T, Weir TD, et al: Susceptibility genes for rapid recline of lung function in the lung health study. *Am J Respir Crit Care Med* 163:469–473, 2001.

Clinical Course and Management

Anthonisen NR, Connett JE, Kiley JP, et al: Effects of smoking intervention and the use of an inhaled anticholinergic bronchodilator on the rate of decline of FEV_1: The Lung Health Study. *JAMA* 272:1497–1505, 1994.

Burge PS, Calverley PM, Jones PW, et al: Randomised, double blind, placebo controlled study of fluticasone propionate in patients with moderate to severe chronic obstructive pulmonary disease: The ISOLDE trial. *Br Med J* 320:1297–1303, 2000.

Celli BR, Snider GL, Heffner J, et al: Standards for the diagnosis and care of patients with chronic obstructive pulmonary disease. *Am J Respir Crit Care Med* 152:S77–S120, 1995.

Ferguson GT: Recommendations for the management of COPD. *Chest* 117:23S–28S, 2000.

Gierada DS, Yusen RD, Villanueva IA, et al: Patient selection for lung volume reduction surgery: An objective model based on prior clinical decisions and quantitative CT analysis. *Chest* 117:991–998, 2000.

Meyers BF, Lynch J, Trulock EP, et al. Lung transplantation: A decade of experience. *Ann Surg* 230(3):362–370, 1999.

Niewoehner DE, Collins D, Erbland ML: Relation of FEV_1 to clinical outcomes during exacerbations of chronic obstructive pulmonary disease. *Am J Respir Crit Care Med* 161:1201–1205, 2000.

O'Donohue WJ Jr: Home oxygen therapy. *Clin Chest Med* 18:535–545, 1997.

Pauwels RA, Buist AS, Calverley PMA, et al: Global strategy for the diagnosis, management, and prevention of chronic obstructive pulmonary disease. NHLBIWHO Global Initiative for Chronic Obstructive Lung Disease (GOLD) Workshop Summary. *Am J Respir Crit Care Med* 163:1256–1276, 2001.

Plant PK, Owen JL, Elliott MW: Early use of non-invasive ventilation for acute exacerbations of chronic obstructive pulmonary disease on general respiratory wards: A multicentre randomised controlled trial. *Lancet* 355:1931–1935, 2000.

Snow V, Lascher S, Mottur-Pilson C, et al: The evidence base for management of acute exacerbations of COPD. Clinical Practice Guideline, Part 1. *Chest* 119:1185–1189, 2001.

Smoking

Aubry MC, Wright JL, Myers JL: The pathology of smoking-related lung diseases. *Clin Chest Med* 11:35, 2000.

Kumra V, Markoff BA: Who's smoking now? The epidemiology of tobacco use in the United States and abroad. *Clin Chest Med* 21(1):1–9, 2000.

Lillington GA, Leonard CT, Sachs DP: Smoking cessation. Techniques and benefits. *Clin Chest Med* 21:199–208, 2000.

Sethi JM, Rochester CL: Smoking and chronic obstructive pulmonary disease. *Clin Chest Med* 21:67–86, 2000.

The Tobacco Use and Dependence Clinical Practice Guideline Panel, Staff, and Consortium Representatives. A clinical practice guideline for treating tobacco use and dependence: A US Public Health Service Report. JAMA 283:3244–3254, 2000.

Rehabilitation

Anonymous: Pulmonary rehabilitation: Joint ACCP/AACVPR evidence-based guidelines. ACCP/AACVPR Pulmonary Rehabilitation Guidelines Panel. American College of Chest Physicians. American Association of Cardiovascular and Pulmonary Rehabilitation. *Chest* 112:1363–1396, 1997.

Bowen JB, Votto JJ, Thrall RS, et al: Functional status and survival following pulmonary rehabilitation. *Chest* 118:697–703, 2000.

Celli BR: Pulmonary rehabilitation for patients with advanced lung disease. *Clin Chest Med* 18(3):521–534, 1997.

Mahler DA: Pulmonary rehabilitation. *Chest* 113:263S–268S, 1998.

Troosters T, Gosselink R, Decramer M: Short- and long-term effects of outpatient rehabilitation in patients with chronic obstructive pulmonary disease: A randomized trial. *Am J Med* 109:207–212, 2000.

8 | Asthma

Reynold A. Panettieri, Jr., and Alfred P. Fishman

DEFINITION AND ETIOLOGY

Asthma is a chronic disease characterized in part by reversible obstruction to airflow within the lungs. In contrast to emphysema or chronic bronchitis, patients with asthma may have essentially normal lung function between episodes. Although the etiology of asthma remains unknown, airway hyperreactivity in response to inhalational challenge using methacholine or aerosolized allergen is a hallmark of this disease. In some patients, narrowing of the airways may be part of an allergic reaction triggering the release of biologically active mediators. In other patients, specific stimuli trigger episodes and suggest an etiologic relationship (exercise, airway cooling, or stress). In the majority of patients, the cause of the airway hyperreactivity is unknown. Specific causes that have been proposed include imbalances within the nervous system, deficiency of beta receptors, excess contraction of airway smooth muscle, imbalances in mediator production, and immune regulatory defects.

Epidemiology

Asthma is a prevalent disease now affecting approximately 4 to 8 percent of the U.S. population. The prevalence of asthma has increased by 25 percent over the last decade independent of demographic factors. In addition, the mortality of asthma has increased by 31 percent during the past decade, with a disproportionate rise in mortality in young African Americans, particularly from urban areas.

Pathology

The pathology of asthma includes narrowing of the airway lumen and thickening of the airway wall. Mucus and sloughed epithelial cells are seen within the airway lumen and an infiltrate of inflammatory cells, especially eosinophils, is seen within the airway wall. Edema within the airway wall is also a prominent finding. Recent studies of biopsies in asthmatics have shown increased numbers of T lymphocytes (CD4+ cells), mast cells, macrophages, and eosinophils than in normals.

*Edited from Chap. 47, "The Biology of Asthma," by Busse WW, Parry DE. In: *Fishman's Pulmonary Diseases and Disorders,* 3d ed., edited by Fishman AP, Elias JA, Fishman JA, Grippi MA, Kaiser LR, Senior RM. New York, McGraw-Hill, 1998, pp 721–734. For fuller discussion of topics dealt with in this chapter, the reader is referred to the original text, as noted above.

ABNORMAL PHYSIOLOGY

Increased resistance to airflow is the sine qua non of the asthmatic attack. In large part, the increase in airway resistance is due to contraction of airway smooth muscle cells, but other mechanisms contribute to the obstruction to airflow, notably thickening of the airways by edema and cellular infiltration as well as intraluminal collections of mucus, secretions, and cellular debris. Small changes in airway diameter have dramatic effects on airway resistance.

An increase in resistance to airflow causes a series of physiologic alterations, including abnormalities of lung mechanics and gas exchange. Spirometry reveals an obstructive pattern manifest by a decrease in FVC and FEV_1 and a decrease in the FEV_1/FVC ratio. The functional residual capacity (FRC) is increased and the lungs appear hyperinflated on the chest radiograph. The work of breathing is increased and the efficiency of the respiratory pump is decreased because of altered compliance and a pressure-volume relationship that places the respiratory muscles at a suboptimal length-tension relationship. Thus, as airflow is restricted, the work of breathing is increased.

Regional inhomogeneity in the distribution of inspired air leads to ventilation/perfusion ($\dot{V}/\dot{Q}$) mismatch and impaired gas exchange. Areas of low $\dot{V}/\dot{Q}$ contribute to the development of hypoxemia in patients with acute attacks of asthma. In stable asthmatics, the Pa_{O_2} is normal. Dead-space ventilation is increased but adequate elimination of CO_2 is maintained in mild to moderate asthma by a compensatory increase in minute ventilation. In severe asthma, the combined effects of augmented CO_2 production, impaired CO_2 elimination, and respiratory muscle fatigue lead to the development of hypercapnea and respiratory acidosis, eventuating in respiratory failure if therapy is unsuccessful.

CLINICAL MANIFESTATIONS

History

A detailed history is an essential part of formulating a diagnosis of asthma in a patient with unexplained dyspnea. Patients with asthma typically have a history of intermittent episodes of shortness of breath, wheezing, and chest tightness. In some patients, cough, unaccompanied by wheezing or breathlessness, may be the sole manifestation.

A history should attempt to determine whether any enviromental factors or other exposures appear temporally or causally linked to the exacerbation of symptoms. For example, some patients will report exercise- or cold-induced symptoms, suggesting the diagnosis of exercise-induced asthma. Other patients may report symptoms that are related to prior upper respiratory tract infections or exposure to specific irritants. Exacerbation of symptoms early in the week followed by improvement over the weekend suggests an occupationally induced cause for the asthma. A detailed history concerning pet exposures, travel history, how symptoms change seasonally, type of home heating and air conditioning, and effects of vacations may suggest other specific trigger factors that may be avoided by the patient.

If the patient already carries the diagnosis of asthma, the history should also focus on number of emergency room visits, pattern of exacerbations, admissions to the hospital, admissions to the intensive care unit, or prior need for intubation. These factors, along with a history of prior steroid requirements to control asthma, may help identify those patients who are at increased risk for severe or fatal asthma.

Physical Examination

The physical examination of the asthmatic during an acute attack frequently reveals an uncomfortable and anxious patient obviously short of breath. Use of accessory muscles and nasal flaring suggests particularly severe obstruction. The chest is resonant to percussion, and the diaphragms may be low, with reduced movement. Auscultation frequently reveals polyphonic wheezes radiating throughout the chest during expiration. Although such wheezing is usually described as diffuse in that it may be heard in many locations over the chest wall, acoustic analysis usually reveals only two or three discrete wheezes in a given patient. The finding of only a single localized wheeze favors a tracheal or endobronchial obstruction, as may be seen with tumor or a foreign body. The expiratory phase is prolonged up to four or five times the inspiratory phase; thus inspiration is brief and forceful. Auscultation of the heart should be normal other than for tachycardia and distant heart sounds. The heart examination is important because an S_3 suggests an alternative diagnosis [congestive heart failure (CHF)/cardiac asthma] for the patient's dyspnea and wheezing. Pulsus paradoxus may result from wide swings in intrapleural pressure. Cyanosis may be seen in severely ill patients; clubbing or edema should not be present. The presence of nasal polyps suggests triad asthma as a possible etiology (aspirin sensitivity, asthma, and nasal polyps). In those patients with hysterical vocal cord dysfunction presenting as asthma, direct laryngoscopy examination may show inappropriate apposition of the vocal cords during expiration.

Usual Diagnostic Tests

It is important to remember that asthma is a clinical diagnosis suggested by the onset of wheezing, breathlessness, and cough in patients exposed to certain trigger factors. The "gold standard" for the diagnosis of asthma is the reversibility of symptoms either spontaneously or in response to therapy. Not all signs and symptoms or laboratory abnormalities need be present at one time in a particular patient.

Pulmonary Function Testing

Since the symptoms and signs of asthma often do not correlate with the severity of the bronchoconstriction, objective measures of lung function are essential for the diagnosis and assessment of patients with asthma. Simple spirometry, which provides a measure of the forced expiratory volume in 1 s (FEV_1) and the forced vital capacity (FVC) are the most useful ways to diagnose increased resistance to airflow. Even when a patient is asymptomatic, the FEV_1 and the FVC are usually low in cases of asthma. The reduction in peak expiratory flow rate (PEFR), which correlates well with a reduction in the FEV_1, may also be used to objectively assess airflow obstruction. Patients can measure their PEFR by using an inexpensive, hand-held flow meter at home while documenting their symptoms in a diary. This approach allows correlation of the patient's symptoms with an objective measure of airflow. Other measurements of pulmonary function may be helpful in distinguishing asthma from other causes of increased resistance to airflow. For example, the single-breath diffusing capacity is normal in asthma but low in emphysema. Flow-volume loops can be important in ruling out upper airway obstruction, which can mimic asthma.

Bronchoprovocational testing of airway responsiveness to methacholine, histamine, or exercise is sometimes useful in supporting the diagnosis. As the patient inhales increasing doses of either histamine or methacholine, serial FEV_1 measurements are obtained. A 20 percent decrement in the FEV_1 (PD_{20}) at a dose of 8.0 μmol methacholine or 16 mg/mL histamine indicates airway hyperresponsiveness. To evaluate exercise-induced bronchospasm, serial measurements of FEV_1 are performed prior to, during, and after exercise in order to determine whether the patient experiences an exercise-induced increase in airflow resistance. A decrease in the FEV_1 by 20 percent with exercise is considered a positive test.

Chest X-Ray

During the acute attack of asthma, the chest radiograph usually reveals hyperinflation of the lungs in association with a small, elongated cardiac silhouette. More importantly, the chest radiograph is helpful in evaluating suspected complications of acute asthma, such as rib fractures from protracted coughing, pneumomediastinum, atelectasis, or pneumonia. It can also be helpful in patients with upper airway obstruction rather than asthma in whom wheezing and dyspnea are due to foreign bodies or extrinsic compression of the trachea by tumor or goiter, or in making the diagnosis of CHF.

Other Tests

Differential white blood counts frequently reveal eosinophilia (5 to 15 percent) in patients with asthma. However, absolute eosinophilia (greater than 3000 cells per cubic millimeter) suggests alternative diagnoses—e.g., Loeffler's syndrome, idiopathic hypereosinophilia syndrome, allergic bronchopulmonary aspergillosis, drug reactions, chronic myelogenous leukemia, Churg-Strauss syndrome, or parasitic infections.

Total serum IgE levels are often high in allergic asthma and are not useful for characterizing the severity of the disease. Normal skin tests as well as normal total serum IgE levels suggest alternative diagnoses; however, nonatopic patients with asthma may also have negative tests.

Differential Diagnosis

Table 8-1 lists entities frequently confused with asthma.

NATURAL HISTORY AND OUTCOME

The natural history of asthma is not well characterized. Childhood asthma often persists into adulthood and the prognosis of children with asthma appears to be related to the age of onset of respiratory symptoms, history of exposure to cigarette smoke, magnitude of the decrease in the FEV_1 while asymptomatic, airway hyperreactivity (as demonstrated by inhalational challenge), as well as degree of atopy at presentation. Some patients who are severely hyperresponsive to methacholine as children have been found to develop irreversible airflow obstruction as adults despite "adequate" treatment of their asthma with corticosteroids. Further studies aimed at identifying risk factors for the development of irreversible bronchoconstriction in asthma are needed in order to better understand this progression.

Although asthma is generally regarded as a benign disease and deaths due to asthma are uncommon, mortality due to asthma has been rising. Most of

TABLE 8-1 Differential Diagnosis of Asthma

Mass lesions
  Endobronchial or intratracheal tumor
  Extrinsic compression of the trachea (e.g., goiter)
  Foreign body
Inflammatory or immunologic
  Anaphylaxis or anaphylactoid reactions
  Laryngeal edema or laryngospasm
  Epiglottitis
  Endobronchial sarcoidosis
  Amyloidosis
  Vasculitis (e.g., Wegener's granulomatosis)
  Pulmonary embolus (mediator release)
Airway edema
  Congestive heart failure
Psychological
  Hysterical vocal cord dysfunction

these deaths occur outside the hospital and the mortality for hospitalized asthmatics remains less than 1 percent. Factors related to increased asthma mortality are shown in Table 8-2.

In approximately 10 percent of asthmatics, airflow obstruction can be partially irreversible. The precise causes of irreversible airflow obstruction in asthma remain unknown. Histopathologically, severe asthmatics manifest epithelial desquamation, mucous gland hypertropy and hyperplasia, airway smooth muscle hypertrophy and hyperplasia, and increased numbers of blood vessels as well as subbasement membrane fibrosis. Collectively, these findings have been described as "airway remodeling." Whether airway remodeling causes irreversible airflow obstruction in asthma remains controversial. To date, no medication abrogates airway remodeling.

Treatment

Successful treatment of the patient with asthma requires the appropriate choice of medication as well as an emphasis on patient education. The goals of patient education include avoidance strategies for specific trigger events as well as treatment strategies for exacerbations. Studies have clearly shown that frequent contact between the physician and asthmatic can play a major role in decreasing the severity of episodes.

The pharmacotherapy of asthma is focused mainly on bronchodilation and on reducing inflammation within the airways. Bronchodilators, acting

TABLE 8-2 Circumstances Associated with Fatal Asthma
in the United States

Demographics
  Occurs more frequently in urban African Americans
History
  Prior history of intubation or admission to an intensive care unit for asthma
  Two or more hospitalizations for asthma in the past year
  Serious psychiatric disease or psychosocial problems
Other
  Patients with large diurnal variations in airflow are at greatest risk
  Usually associated with inadequate assessment and treatment

primarily on smooth muscle to effect relaxation, include beta-adrenergic agents, anticholinergic agents, and theophylline.

Anti-inflammatory agents include inhaled steroids, systemic steroids, and leukotriene-modifier agents. Other agents such as cromolyn sodium are more difficult to classify.

While the use of inhaled beta agonists may cause a prompt increase in airway caliber and thus make the patient feel better, it does not treat the airway inflammation and hyperresponsiveness that characterize the late phase of asthma. For these reasons as well as because recent studies have demonstrated excess mortality in patients treated with long-acting or regularly scheduled beta agonists, combination therapy with beta agonists and anti-inflammatory drugs (e.g., inhaled steroids and/or leukotriene modifiers) is considered to be the most appropriate approach for most patients.

Beta-Adrenergic Agents

These agents act to increase cAMP within airway smooth muscle and cause a decrease in force production leading to a widening of the airway. They are available both as oral and inhalational agents (and intravenous in rare cases). Inhaled beta-adrenergic agents have a wider therapeutic index than oral adrenergic agents. Table 8-3 summarizes the currently recommended use of inhaled bronchodilators in asthma.

Theophyllines

Theophylline preparations are prescribed frequently for asthma, though their role in therapy is declining. The mechanism of action of theophylline is still unclear, though the major therapeutic effect is relaxation of airway smooth muscle. The dosing of theophylline is confounded by erratic absorption, unpredictable excretion kinetics, and a narrow therapeutic range. Despite serum levels in the therapeutic range, many patients experience anxiety, tremor, palpitations, and gastrointestinal symptoms. In addition, aminophylline affects only a slight further increase in indices of airflow than that achieved by inhaled beta agonists. Currently, theophylline preparations are generally reserved for those patients who cannot be adequately treated with beta agonists. For those patients receiving theophylline, the target concentration in the

TABLE 8-3 Aerosolized Beta-Adrenergic Agents

Drug	β_2-Specific	Onset of action (min)	Peak effect (min)	Duration (h)	Aerosol dose by nebulizer[a]	Aerosol dose by metered dose inhaler
Isoproterenol	No	5	15	1	2.5–5 mg	250 mg/2 puffs
Isoetharine	Yes	10	30	2–3	5 mg	680 mg/2 puffs
Metaproterenol	Yes	10	45	3–6	15 mg	1300 mg/2 puffs
Albuterol	Yes	10	60	4–6	2.5–5 mg	180 mg/2 puffs
Terbutaline	Yes	10	60	4–6		400 mg/2 puffs
Pirbuterol	Yes	10	60	4–6		400 mg/2 puffs
Bitolterol[b]	Yes	10	60	3–8		1050 mg/3 puffs
Fenoterol[b]	Yes	10	60	4–8		400 mg/2 puffs
Salmeterol	Yes	10	60	8–10		50 mg/puff
Formoterol[b]	Yes	10	60	8–10		12 mg/puff

[a]Aerosol dose by nebulizer diluted in 3 mL saline.
[b]Not available in the United States.

blood is 10 to 20 μg/mL. A variety of drugs affect theophylline metabolism through interaction with the hepatic P450 enzyme system; concurrent use of these drugs necessitates that the dose of theophylline be adjusted according to measured blood levels.

Anticholinergics

Ipratropium bromide acts to block muscarinic receptors in the airways leading to a modest bronchodilation. Though inhaled anticholinergic therapy is as effective as beta-agonist therapy in patients with COPD, the same is not true in asthma. Thus, the role of ipratropium in asthma remains as a second-line therapy to beta agonists.

Steroids

Corticosteroids, unlike bronchodilators, act to treat the consequences of airway inflammation, which include cellular infiltration, edema, and mediator release. Corticosteroids have no acute effects on airway caliber and exert their effects only after a delay of 3 to 6 h. The most significant recent advance in the use of steroids in asthma has been the introduction of inhaled corticosteroids that achieve an anti-inflammatory effect localized to the airways, without significant systemic side effects. The agents that are currently available in the United States include beclomethasone diproprionate, triamcinolone acetonide, flunisolide, fluticasone, and budesonide. Some inhaled steroids are given by a metered-dose inhaler (MDI); as with beta agonists, the patient must learn the effective use of an inhaler to assure delivery of the drug to the airways. The use of dry-powder inhaled steroids such as fluticasone and budesonide has greatly enhanced patient adherence. Although inhaled steroids at currently approved doses are free from systemic side effects, delivery of a significant amount of the steroid to the oropharynx may result in symptomatic candidal infections. Such infections may be prevented by proper MDI technique, the use of a spacer, by gargling after each dose of the inhaled steroid, or by using a dry-powder formulation.

Systemic Steroids

Systemic steroids play an important role in the management of acute and chronic asthma, as they represent the most effective anti-inflammatory therapy available. In acute exacerbations of asthma, short courses of prednisone or methylprednisolone (iv or po) may be necessary in patients already taking inhaled steroids or too sick to use them. There is little evidence that doses higher than 40 to 60 mg of prednisone four times a day result in further improvement of airway obstruction. Despite the well-known complications of chronic steroid use, short courses of even high-dose corticosteroids are generally well tolerated. Hyperkalemia, hyperglycemia, muscle weakness, and alterations in mental status can occur but usually resolve promptly. The optimal method to taper steroids is unclear. Patients are usually switched from parenteral methylprednisolone to either oval prednisone or methylprednisolone once symptoms and airflow are clearly improving. Dosing frequency is cut to either once or twice daily and the patient is tapered to a target of 20 mg/day over 10 to 14 days. In many patients, inhaled steroids can fully replace this dose of prednisone and the oral steroids can be discontinued.

Cromolyn

Cromolyn, which inhibits mast cell degranulation, can inhibit both the early and late phases of allergen-induced bronchoconstriction. It is most effective when used as prophylaxis in patients with exercise-induced asthma. Cromolyn is not a bronchodilator, and it is ineffective in treating acute asthma and adults with chronic severe asthma.

Leukotriene Inhibitors

Leukotrienes are potent bronchoconstrictor molecules secreted by mast cells and by eosinophils in asthmatic airways. Leukotriene-receptor antagonist medications such as montelukast or zafirlukast or 5-lipoxygenase inhibitors such as zileuton are effective in chronic asthma. These therapeutic agents are administered orally and therefore foster improved patient adherence. Whether these drugs also promote bronchodilation is controversial, since increases in FEV_1 after taking these medications can occur within 60 min of administration. Collectively, these agents are less effective than inhaled steroids but are very effective "add-on" therapy that enables the physician to decrease the dose of inhaled steroids.

Experimental Agents

A number of therapeutic agents useful in some patients with asthma are at various stages of investigation. Investigational bronchodilators include calcium-channel blockers, potassium-channel agonists, intravenous magnesium, and inhaled diuretics.

The immune modulatory effects of low-dose methotrexate and cyclosporine have been disappointing as steroid-sparing agents in patients requiring chronic high-dose systemic steroids. Although both agents appear to be able to decrease the required daily dose of steroids, their use is limited by substantial toxicity. Some agents, such as the macrolide antibiotics troleandomycin (TAO) and erythromycin, also appear to be "steroid-sparing" in some patients.

BIBLIOGRAPHY

Barnes PJ: Inhaled glucocorticoids for asthma. *N Engl J Med* 332:868–875, 1995.

Busse WW, Lemanske RF: Asthma. *N Engl J Med* 344:350–362, 2001.

McFadden ER Jr: Asthma: Acute and chronic therapy, in Fishman AP (ed): *Pulmonary Diseases and Disorders,* 2d ed., New York, McGraw-Hill, 1988, p 1311.

Murray RK, Panettieri RA: Management of asthma: The changing approach, in Fishman AP (ed): *Update: Pulmonary Diseases and Disorders,* New York, McGraw-Hill, 1992, pp 67–82.

9 | Aspirin- and Exercise-Induced Asthma*

Jack A. Elias

ASPIRIN-INDUCED ASTHMA

Introduction

Aspirin-induced asthma (AIA) was first reported in 1902. More than 60 years later, the association between aspirin sensitivity, asthma, and nasal polyps was recognized. The prevalence of aspirin sensitivity in asthmatics was subsequently noted to range between 5 and 30 percent, depending on the characteristics of the asthmatics being studied (severity increases risk) and the criteria applied to make the diagnosis. Drug reactions cause asthma exacerbations in 10.5 percent of patients. Aspirin is responsible for approximately 50 percent of these reactions.

Clinical Presentation

Reactions to aspirin can take two distinct forms: *cutaneous,* leading to urticaria and angioedema, and *respiratory,* resulting in rhinoconjunctivitis and bronchospasm.[1] In the former, a subpopulation of patients with established urticaria experience cutaneous flares of hives with or without angioedema after ingesting nonsteroidal anti-inflammatory drugs (NSAIDs). Almost all of these patients were able to ingest the same NSAIDs before the development of urticaria, suggesting that the NSAIDs interact with an underlying urticarial process but do not directly and independently cause the hives.

In contrast to classic atopic asthma, which usually presents before the age of 20, AIA generally occurs in people in the fourth decade of life. In general, these patients do not have a history of sensitivity to NSAIDs or a family history of the disorder. Men and women are affected equally. Aeroallergen skin testing of these patients is usually negative, IgE levels are normal, and blood eosinophilia is not noted after aspirin challenge.

The upper (nasal) and lower (asthma) respiratory manifestations of these patients are generally linked, although sometimes upper respiratory symptoms precede the development of asthmatic reactions to these agents. These patients usually develop a virus-like upper respiratory tract illness. This is associated with chronic eosinophilic inflammation of the nasal mucosa and paranasal sinuses. Although nasal polyps are noted as part of the classic triad, it is becoming increasingly evident that polyps are at times *absent,* while virtually all patients present with sinusitis.[1]

The typical reaction after aspirin ingestion by these patients is the slow development (within one-half to 4 h; mean 50 min) of nasal congestion with

*Edited from Chap. 49, "Aspirin- and Exercise-Induced Asthma," by Geba GP. In: *Fishman's Pulmonary Diseases and Disorders,* 3d ed., edited by Fishman AP, Elias JA, Fishman JA, Grippi MA, Kaiser LR, Senior RM. New York, McGraw-Hill, 1998, pp 745–756. For fuller discussion of topics dealt with in this chapter, the reader is referred to the original text, as noted above.

profuse rhinorrhea, cutaneous flushing of the head and neck, mild conjunctivitis, and bronchial obstruction, usually manifest as wheezing. In severe reactions, headache, nausea and vomiting, and acute hypercarbic respiratory failure culminating in death can occur. Life-threatening responses with faster kinetics have been reported with systemically administered NSAIDs. Combined cutaneous and respiratory reactions (i.e., true urticarial eruptions in association with asthma) occur in less than 3 percent of cases.

Cross-Reactivity

Cross-reactivity of aspirin with other NSAIDs is well recognized. A partial list of NSAIDs reported to provoke asthma is provided in Table 9-1. A number of analgesics have long been thought to be well tolerated in patients with AIA. They are also listed in Table 9-1. However, some analgesics formerly considered safe for use by these patients have been shown to be capable of provoking bronchospasm if given in large doses. For example, in doses of 600 to 1000 mg, acetaminophen can provoke significant declines in FEV_1 in some aspirin-sensitive asthmatics.

Although it was initially believed that tartrazine dyes were capable of provoking asthma exacerbations in patients with AIA, this has not been confirmed on further study.[2] This supports the view that tartrazine intolerance is extremely rare and that true cross-reactivity with aspirin probably does not exist. Similar conclusions can be drawn regarding the cross-reactivity of other FD&C dyes, sodium benzoate, other benzoic acid derivatives, monosodium glutamate, and sodium and potassium sulfites. An interesting association

---

TABLE 9-1   NSAIDs in Aspirin-Induced Asthma

NSAIDs that can provoke airway narrowing in AIA

Carboxylic acids
  Salicylates
    Acetylsalicylic acid (aspirin, Easpirin, Zorpin)
  Acetic acids
    Indomethacin (Indocin)
    Sulindac (Clinoril)
    Tolmentin (Tolectin)
    Diclofenac (Voltaren)
    Ketorolac (Toradol)
    Zomepirac (Zomax)
Propionic acids
    Ibuprofen (Motrin, Advil, Nuprin)
    Naproxen (Naprosyn)
Fenamates
    Meclofenamate (Meclomen)
    Mefenamic acid (Ponstel)
Enolic acids
    Piroxicam (Feldene)

NSAIDs and analgesics that appear to be well tolerated in AIA

Sodium salicylate
Choline salicylate
Salicylamide
Dextropropoxyphene
Acetaminophen in low doses

between AIA and sensitivity to hydrocortisone has also been reported.[3] Reactions to prednisolone, betamethasone, and dexamethasone have not, however, been noted in these individuals.[4]

Pathogenesis

Alterations in arachidonic acid metabolism may play a central role in AIA. Arachidonic acid is derived from membrane phospholipids by phospholipase A_2. It is then metabolized via the cyclooxygenase pathway to prostaglandins and thromboxanes or via the lipoxygenase pathway to sulfidopeptide (cysteinyl) leukotrienes. The leukotrienes have a variety of effects, including the induction of contraction of bronchial smooth muscle. In contrast, the prostaglandins, in particular PGE_2, act as bronchodilators and may inhibit T cell–mediated inflammatory responses in the lung. Aspirin and the other NSAIDs that cause AIA inhibit cyclooxygenase activity. A shift occurs after the administration of aspirin or appropriate doses of cross-reacting agents, shunting approximately 90 percent of the arachidonic acid metabolism to the 5-lipoxygenase pathway, decreasing prostaglandin and thromboxane production, and increasing leukotriene generation. In comparison to normal persons, patients with AIA generate leukotrienes in exaggerated quantities after aspirin challenge. They may also be more sensitive than normal subjects to the bronchoconstrictor properties of leukotrienes (particularly LTE_4) and more susceptible to the loss of the bronchodilating and potentially antiinflammatory effects of PGE_2. Other theories of AIA pathogenesis suggest that basophils, mast cells, and/or platelets from AIA patients also release enhanced quantities of histamine, serotonin, and other mediators after aspirin ingestion.[1,5] Although complement activation has been proposed to be important in AIA, alterations in CH50 and C4 levels after aspirin ingestion have not been documented.

Diagnosis

AIA is diagnosed historically and, when required, confirmed with placebo-controlled oral aspirin challenges (Table 9-2). This testing can be performed according to published protocols using single- or double-blind approaches. These protocols generally begin with 3-mg doses of aspirin, with the dosage of aspirin increased to a maximum of 650 mg over a 3-day period. Spirometry is serially monitored during the challenge to assess the degree of bronchial obstruction. Airway reactivity to methacholine is not a viable surrogate for spirometry, since aspirin does not consistently alter methacholine sensitivity. This challenge procedure should probably be reserved for use in research centers experienced in its application and adverse effects. An alternative to oral challenge, used in some centers in Europe for the diagnosis of AIA, is the inhalation of stabilized lysine-aspirin.

Treatment

Treatment of AIA depends on the correct diagnosis and avoidance of aspirin and other cyclooxygenase inhibitors that induce symptoms. Patients should be instructed that many over-the-counter medications contain aspirin or other NSAIDs; they should carefully read package inserts before using any medication. Currently there appears to be no clear role for systemic corticosteroids or theophylline in the prevention of AIA. Treatment of symptoms after acute

TABLE 9-2 Diagnosis of Aspirin-Induced Asthma: Aspirin (ASA) Challenge Protocols

Single-blind oral 3-day aspirin challenge

Time	Test days 1	2	3
0	Placebo	ASA 3 or 30 mg	ASA 150 mg
+3 h	Placebo	ASA 60 mg	ASA 325 mg
+6 h	Placebo	ASA 100 mg	ASA 600 mg

Double-blind oral aspirin challenge

Both tester and patient are blinded to eliminate potential bias.

Bronchial challenge with lysine-aspirin

Time (minutes)	Challenge (lysine-aspirin in mg/mL)
0	Placebo
45	Placebo
90	11.25
135	22.5
180	45
225	90
270	180
315	360
350	360 (10 breaths)

Patients receive four breaths of all doses of lysine-aspirin unless otherwise indicated.

SOURCE: Data from Stevenson and Simon[1] and from Phillips GD, Foord R, Holgate ST: Inhaled lysine-aspirin as a bronchoprovocation procedure in aspirin-sensitive asthma: Its repeatibility, absence of a late-phase reaction, and the role of histamine. *J Allergy Clin Immunol* 84:232–241, 1989.

ingestion relies mainly on beta-adrenergic agonists to reverse bronchospasm and topical vasoconstrictors for both nasal congestion and eye symptoms. Some investigators have found that antihistamines such as clemastine and mast cell stabilizers such as ketotifen and cromolyn can have prophylactic efficacy. However, not all subjects on these drugs are protected against bronchoconstriction after aspirin challenge. Leukotriene regulators have, however, shown remarkable efficacy and may be the first line of therapy for patients with this disorder.

In cases where aspirin (or cross-reacting NSAIDs) cannot be avoided or the efficacy of prophylactic measures cannot be assured, aspirin "desensitization" can be considered. Protocols are available for selected patients.[6] These methods can effectively protect many patients from experiencing symptoms on exposure to aspirin or other NSAIDs and will maintain this level of desensitization as long as aspirin is ingested indefinitely at doses of 325 to 650 mg a day.

The presence of sinusitis and nasal polyps must be considered and effectively treated in patients with AIA. High-dose topical intranasal corticosteroids can shrink polyp tissue and prevent obstruction of nasal passageways. In the setting of chronic sinusitis, standard approaches—including topical vasoconstrictors, antihistamines, and antibiotics—should also be utilized. Surgery to drain sinuses and remove polyps has been shown to be effective in the short term. However, polyps can regrow and the sinusitis often recurs.

EXERCISE-INDUCED ASTHMA

Introduction

Exercise-induced asthma (EIA) can be defined as a condition in which vigorous physical activity triggers acute airway narrowing in persons with heightened airway reactivity.[8] EIA is always associated with an asthmatic diathesis, although it can be seen before other characteristic features of asthma emerge. EIA is seen in 50 to 90 percent of asthmatics and 40 percent of patients with allergic rhinitis without known asthma.[9] Some have suggested that all asthmatics can be shown to manifest airway narrowing to thermal provocations of sufficient intensity. Other susceptible persons are first-degree relatives of asthmatics, atopic "nonasthmatics," and patients with cystic fibrosis.

Clinical Presentation

Normal persons and asthmatics generally first respond to exercise by bronchodilation. This response is short-lived, peaking at midexercise, and is followed by a return of normal baseline airway tone at the end of exercise. In patients with EIA, the transient bronchodilation and reversal are followed by bronchoconstriction coincident with the symptoms of cough, wheezing, dyspnea, and chest tightness typical of asthmatic attacks. Typically, when patients are provoked with a brief, intense exercise period in the laboratory, maximal bronchoconstriction occurs 5 to 10 min after the cessation of exercise and lasts for 30 to 60 min. Rarely does this form of bronchoconstriction result in ventilatory failure, although it can limit the performance of trained athletes.

In addition to asthma after exercise, many athletes describe dyspnea during exercise. If these athletes are able to continue to exercise despite the initial airway obstruction, especially if they are able to increase their level of activity, relief of bronchoconstriction often occurs. This is associated with a symptomatic improvement with time described as "running through the attack." This has been taken as evidence that airway function during exercise reflects a balance between bronchoconstrictor and protective bronchodilator influences and that this balance can be influenced by rapid changes in exercise intensity.

The exercise intensity, the temperature and humidity of the inspired air, and the patient's baseline airway reactivity are fundamental in determining whether exercise will lead to bronchoconstriction. If asthma is better controlled at baseline, EIA may be more difficult to provoke. If climatic conditions vary, even though asthma is not well controlled, EIA may fail to develop. For a fixed minute ventilation, cold, dry air inspired during exercise is more likely to provoke EIA than warm, humid air. Thus, EIA is more likely to occur with jogging during the winter than with swimming indoors. About 50 percent of patients with EIA will not manifest a bronchoconstrictor response after exercise if rechallenged with the same stimulus within 60 min. After 3 h, even patients who were refractory to repeated challenge will again respond to exercise with bronchoconstriction.

Pathophysiology

Despite intense scrutiny, the pathophysiology of EIA is still a subject of considerable debate. Three principal, non–mutually exclusive potential pathogenetic schema have emerged from these studies. These hypotheses focus on the roles of (1) heat exchange, water loss, and airway warming; (2) airway inflammation; and (3) leukotriene mediators in the airway.

Differential Diagnosis

The diagnosis of EIA is accomplished most accurately by well-established exercise protocols coupled with pulmonary function testing. However, patients are commonly given a presumptive diagnosis based on their history and physical examination. Important points in the history include the level and type of exercise that provokes asthma, the timing of symptom onset, situations that modify symptom onset, and the precise symptoms experienced. Many of the symptoms of EIA can mimic other conditions that would require an entirely different therapeutic approach (Table 9-3). For example, chest tightness with exercise should be unequivocally distinguished from coronary ischemia. Other cardiac disorders that can mimic EIA are arrhythmias, cardiomyopathies, atrial myxoma, and mitral valve prolapse, all of which can manifest with dyspnea and wheezing. Exercise-induced anaphylaxis can also mimic EIA but will generally exhibit skin manifestations (urticaria), and respiratory symptoms will be less prominent. Nearly all patients with EIA cough with provocation. However, EIA can also need to be differentiated from exercise-induced cough that is not associated with bronchospasm. EIA can also be mimicked by fixed glottal and tracheal obstruction, which become noticeable with the increased ventilation of exercise and exercise-induced vocal cord/arytenoid dysfunction that is not present at rest. Last, panic disorders and the excessive tachypnea associated with deconditioning can be confused with EIA, especially in atopic or asthmatic subjects.[9] In contrast to EIA, symptoms due to these other conditions generally are greatest *during* exercise provocation rather than afterward, when airflow limitation due to EIA usually reaches its peak.

Physiologic Documentation

To formally diagnose EIA, the clinician must document airflow obstruction that reaches a peak just after provocation, during the recovery period. Two basic methods of provocation have been used, exercise and the inhalation of dry air (isocapnic hyperventilation, or ISH). The latter is an acceptable surrogate for exercise, since the bronchoconstriction it induces is similar to that induced by exercise in terms of magnitude, time course, and refractory period. However, significant differences exist between the two provocation techniques.

TABLE 9-3 Differential Diagnosis of Exercise-Induced Asthma

Cardiac disease	Functional abnormalities
Coronary ischemia Mitral valve prolapse Atrial myxoma Cardiomyopathy Arrhythmias	Vocal cord dysfunction Panic disorders
Lung disease	General deconditioning
Fixed airway obstruction Interstitial lung disease Exercise-induced cough	Anemia

Exercise provocation, whether performed on an ergometer or a treadmill, leads to significantly greater increases in heart rate, metabolic rate, and oxygen consumption. In addition, the bronchodilatory response that characterizes exercise is provoked by exercise but not by ISH. ISH does, however, have a number of advantages over exercise. The first relates to the ease with which the ISH protocol can be standardized. The other relates to the finding that oxygen consumption and heart rate are not increased with ISH. As a result, ISH is useful in differentiating EIA from occult cardiac disease and is especially valuable when elderly or cardiac patients are being evaluated.

The most commonly used protocol for the diagnosis of EIA in the United States is that published by O'Byrne and colleagues[10] and modified by Philips and coworkers.[11] This is accomplished by registering changes in pulmonary function in response to varying rates of ventilation using dry air with a fixed CO_2 content of 4.9 percent to maintain isocapnia. Each ventilatory challenge is performed for 3 min, with spirometry performed at intervals thereafter. Serial increases in hyperventilation are performed until maximal voluntary ventilation is reached. If the FEV_1 falls 10 to 20 percent after provocation, the test is considered positive, confirming the diagnosis of EIA. Although some have pointed out that it is not necessary to condition air to subfreezing temperatures in order to perform the test, Scandinavian investigators showed that assessing bronchoconstrictor responses to whole-body exposure to very cold air resulted in a significant increase in the number of asthmatic patients who experienced bronchoconstriction. To maximize yields, it is also important that all drugs that can potentially attenuate bronchoconstrictor responses be discontinued for a sufficient period before the evaluation.

Treatment

The treatment of EIA depends in part on the treatment of the underlying asthma, since, in general, patients with more severe baseline asthma are most inconvenienced by EIA. Prophylactic measures to prevent EIA include avoiding exercises that expose the patient to cold, dry air while favoring those that expose the patient to humid air during exercise. Patients can reduce the severity of their EIA by breathing through the nose rather than through the mouth during exercise. Face masks can be used by the many people who find it impossible to breathe through the nose during intense exercise. It is still unclear whether physical training and improvement in work capacity can relieve symptoms of EIA. A series of repeated short sprints has been shown to be effective in inducing the refractory state, which might then allow the athlete to exercise maximally without developing EIA.[12] A warm-up period to induce the refractory period has been advocated by some to improve performance in the competitive athlete. However, this effect may not last longer than 40 min.[8]

Several classes of drugs have been shown to prevent EIA if administered just before (10 to 20 min) exercise. The list includes beta-adrenergic agonists, leukotriene regulators, cromolyn sodium, anticholinergics, and possibly rapid-release theophylline. Beta-adrenergic agonists are very effective drugs for use against EIA. They are especially useful if the patient has some reversible airway obstruction, since they also improve lung function before exercise. Longer-acting beta-adrenergic agonists, such as salmeterol, have also been found to be effective in preventing EIA and can confer protection that lasts 10 h. Recently, leukotriene regulators have been shown to be effective and safe prophylactic agents for this disorder.

Cromolyn sodium (and related agents) have also been shown to attenuate bronchoconstriction in patients with EIA. This medication will not be effective in those who seek reversal of preexercise bronchoconstriction, since it is not a direct bronchodilator. Importantly, it does not contribute to tachycardia and is therefore useful in elderly patients or patients with cardiac compromise.

Anticholinergics, such as ipratropium bromide, prevent airway narrowing after exercise in a high percentage of patients with EIA. Theophylline—with its weak bronchodilatory effects, unfavorable side-effect profile, and slow onset of action—is not recommended for routine use as pretreatment for EIA. However, it has been shown to confer protection against EIA if 100 to 200 mg is taken 2 h before exercise. Other orally administered drugs that are not commonly used but have the potential to be helpful in preventing EIA are terbutaline, albuterol (2 h before exercise), some alpha-adrenergic agonists, verapamil, and sublingual nifedipine (the last two if taken one-half hour before exercise). Beneficial effects have also been reported with the inhaled antihistamine clemastine and the diuretic furosemide. For the elite athlete, it is important to remember that only a few of these drugs are approved for use in competition by international sporting regulatory authorities.

REFERENCES

1. Stevenson DD, Simon RA: Aspirin sensitivity: Respiratory and cutaneous manifestations, in Middleton E Jr, Reed CE, Ellis EF, et al (eds): *Allergy: Principles and Practice.* St. Louis, Mosby, 1993, pp 1747–1767.
2. Sladek K, Dworski R, Soja J, et al: Eicosanoids in bronchoalveolar lavage fluid of aspirin-intolerant patients with asthma after aspirin challenge. *Am J Respir Crit Care Med* 149:940–946, 1994.
3. Dajani BM, Sliman NA, Shubair KS, Hamzeh YS: Bronchospasm induced by intravenous hydrocortisone sodium succinate (Solu-Cortef) in aspirin-sensitive asthmatics. *J Allergy Clin Immunol* 68:201–206, 1981.
4. Szczelik A, Nizankowska E, Czerniawska-Mysik G, Sek S: Hydrocortisone and airflow impairment in aspirin-induced asthma. *J Allergy Clin Immunol* 76:530–536, 1985.
5. Ameisen JC, Capron A, Joseph M, et al: Aspirin-sensitive asthma: Abnormal platelet response to drugs inducing asthma attacks: Diagnostic and pathophysiological implications. *Int Arch Allergy Appl Immunol* 78:438–448, 1985.
6. Pleskow WW, Stevenson DD, Mathison DA, et al: Aspirin desensitization in aspirin-sensitive asthmatic patients: Clinical manifestations and characterization of the refractory period. *J Allergy Clin Immunol* 69:11–19, 1982.
7. Slavin RG: Nasal polyps and sinusitis, in Middleton E Jr, Reed CE, Ellis EF, et al (eds): *Allergy: Principles and Practice.* St. Louis, Mosby, 1993, p 1459.
8. McFadden ER Jr: Exercise-induced airway obstruction. *Clin Chest Med* 16:671–682, 1995.
9. Cycar D, Lemanske RF Jr: Asthma and exercise. *Clin Chest Med* 15:351–368, 1994.
10. O'Byrne PM, Ramsdale EH, Hargreave FE: Isocapnic hyperventilation for measuring airway hyperresponsiveness in asthma and chronic obstructive pulmonary disease. *Am Rev Respir Dis* 143:1444–1445, 1991.
11. Philips YY, Jaeger JJ, Laube BL, Rosenthal RR: Eucapnic voluntary hyperventilation of compressed gas mixture: A simple method for bronchial challenge by respiratory heat loss. *Am Rev Respir Dis* 131:31–35, 1985.
12. Schnall RP, Landau LI: Protective effects of repeated short sprints in exercise-induced asthma. *Thorax* 3:828–832, 1980.

10 | Allergic Bronchopulmonary Aspergillosis and Hypersensitivity Reactions to Fungi*

Jack A. Elias

DEFINITION OF ALLERGIC BRONCHOPULMONARY ASPERGILLOSIS (ABPA)

ABPA is a disease in which the fungus *Aspergillus fumigatus* colonizes sputum plugs in the bronchi of asthmatics with little or no tissue invasion by the organism. Antigens released from the fungus stimulate a hypersensitivity reaction in the host, resulting in the production of IgE, IgG, and IgA antibodies against the organism, intense production of nonspecific IgE, and prominent tissue inflammation. If the disease goes undetected and untreated, damage to bronchial mucosa and pulmonary tissue will occur and fibrosis can be seen.

The full-blown picture of ABPA consists of asthma, peripheral blood eosinophilia, sputum eosinophilia, fleeting pulmonary infiltrates, golden-brown sputum plugs with hyphae in the sputum, and positive sputum cultures for *A. fumigatus.* ABPA can also be seen when asthma is mild, in the absence of eosinophilia and infiltrates, and in patients presenting with atelectasis or pulmonary fibrosis. This full-blown picture of ABPA is also masked by treatment with corticosteroids, which control the asthma, diminish fungal growth, suppress tissue inflammation, induce the resolution of chest x-ray infiltrates, and may prevent progression to end-stage pulmonary fibrosis.

CLASSIFICATION AND STAGING

The stages of ABPA are outlined in Table 10-1.[1] In the acute phase (stage I), all of the typical findings of ABPA may be present and improve with prednisone therapy. This includes the resolution of pulmonary infiltrates, decline in total serum IgE (by at least 35 percent), and alleviation or disappearance of eosinophilia. However, the precipitating antibody and IgE and IgG antibody indices may remain positive for months or even years.

After control of the acute phase, the patient enters the remission phase (stage II), which may persist for months or years. Once in this state, there may be recurrent exacerbations (stage III), characterized by respiratory symptoms, a doubling (at least) of total serum IgE, and often pulmonary infiltrates.

---

*Edited from Chap. 51, "Allergic Bronchopulmonary Aspergillosis and Hypersensitivity Reactions to Fungi," by Patterson R. In: *Fishman's Pulmonary Diseases and Disorders,* 3d ed., edited by Fishman AP, Elias JA, Fishman JA, Grippi MA, Kaiser LR, Senior RM. New York, McGraw-Hill, 1998, pp 777–782. For fuller discussion of topics dealt with in this chapter, the reader is referred to the original text, as noted above.

TABLE 10-1 Classification and Staging of ABPA

Classification	Stage	Description
Acute	I	Findings at time of diagnosis, usually including pulmonary infiltrates, eosinophilia, asthma in varying degrees, with positive serology
Remission	II	Follows treatment with prednisone with clearing of radiograph (if infiltrates are present), decline in eosinophilia and total serum IgE, and disappearance of asthma; remission may persist for months or years
Recurrent exacerbation	III	Manifestations of acute phase reappear and total serum IgE rises; reversal of all manifestations occurs with prednisone therapy
Corticosteroid-dependent asthma	IV	Patient requires corticosteroids for control of asthma—systemic or topical, irrespective of whether ABPA is stage I, II, or III
Fibrotic end-stage disease	V	Severe fibrotic lung disease
Other Useful Classifications		
Serologic ABPA		Patient with positive serology and no other manifestations of ABPA; patient at risk for progression of ABPA; observation is required
Central bronchiectasis		Present or absent in stages I–IV; always present in stage V; demonstrates structural damage to bronchi

In stage IV ABPA, corticosteroids (inhaled and/or systemic) are required to control the patient's asthma. Patients with stage V disease have end-stage fibrotic lung disease. In any patient, the acute stage (stage I) may be followed by stages II, III, or IV. When the diagnosis of the acute stage is made, it is impossible to predict which stage will follow. With appropriate therapy, progression from the earlier stages to stage V disease is not commonly noted. This suggests that timely diagnosis and treatment of ABPA can prevent pulmonary fibrosis.

DIAGNOSIS

The diagnosis of ABPA is easily made in a patient presenting with the typical constellation of findings: asthma, fleeting pulmonary infiltrates, eosinophilia, *A. fumigatus* in sputum cultures, increase in total serum IgE and rapid clearing of clinical symptoms and radiographic lesions, and decrease in total serum IgE in response to prednisone therapy. In contrast, low-grade, indolent ABPA with mild asthma and a normal chest radiograph may be overlooked unless every patient with asthma or cystic fibrosis is evaluated to exclude ABPA. This is accomplished by skin testing for immediate-type hypersensitivity to *A. fumigatus*. This initially entails a skin-prick test to *A. fumigatus*. If this is negative, an intradermal test with *A. fumigatus* is done. If the skin tests are negative, ABPA has been ruled out. If either skin test is positive, ABPA must be excluded with appropriate serologic tests performed by a qualified laboratory.[2] Four serologic tests are necessary (Table 10-2). The diagnosis of ABPA is supported by the following criteria: total serum IgE greater than 1000 ng/mL, IgE and IgG indices more than twice the prick test–positive asthma control pool (see below), and precipitins against *A. fumigatus.* If three of four tests are positive, ABPA is likely. If two of four tests are positive, the serologic tests should be repeated 3 to 6 months later. A positive serologic result should prompt evaluation for central bronchiectasis to determine whether damage to bronchi has occurred.

The IgE and IgG antibody indices are calculated with the enzyme-linked immunosorbent assay (ELISA). Initially, a reading is obtained for an IgE antibody activity against *A. fumigatus* antigen in the test serum. A similar reading is obtained for an aliquot from a pool of serum samples from patients who are skin test–positive to *A. fumigatus* but in whom ABPA has been excluded (asthma pool). A patient:pool IgE ratio greater than 2 is consistent with ABPA. A similar process is carried out for IgG antibody activity; again, a reading greater than 2 is consistent with ABPA. Of the serologic tests for ABPA, the most variable is the total serum IgE, which decreases in response to prednisone therapy. The diagnosis of serologic (S) ABPA is made in patients with asthma with positive ABPA skin tests and serologies that have no other features of ABPA.

Once the diagnosis of ABPA has been established, subsequent evaluation should focus on the extent of lung damage. Chest x-rays and pulmonary function tests both before and after therapy are helpful. High-resolution computed tomography (HRCT) is also needed to rule out central bronchiectasis.[3,4]

MANAGEMENT

In the acute stage (stage I) and during exacerbations (stage III), prednisone at a dose of 0.50 mg/kg daily for 2 to 4 weeks is required. The prednisone is then switched to an alternate-day regimen, gradually reduced thereafter, and then terminated. In the course of treatment, the IgE level will drop at least 35 percent before reaching a plateau, which varies from patient to patient. The dose and duration of prednisone therapy should be adjusted to achieve this plateau, not to normalize the IgE level. Attempts to normalize IgE can cause overtreatment, inducing significant steroid side effects. After the

TABLE 10-2 Serologic Studies of Value in Diagnosis of ABPA

Serologic Test[a]	Positive
Total serum IgE	>1000 ng/mL
Precipitation test	Precipitin band present
IgE antibody index	>2 compared with asthma pool
IgG antibody index	>2 compared with asthma pool

[a]Four results positive, diagnostic of ABPA; three results positive, consistent with ABPA; two results positive, possible ABPA—repeat serology in 3 to 6 months; all negative or one positive, ABPA excluded.

diagnosis of ABPA and initiation of prednisone therapy, IgE levels are determined monthly until the plateau is documented and every 3 months over the ensuing year. These intervals may be extended if the patient's condition remains stable and the disease is in remission.

In stage IV (the corticosteroid-dependent asthma stage), chronic administration of corticosteroids is required to control the asthma. In this stage, exacerbations may take the form of bouts of asthma or recurrences of ABPA, manifest by a doubling of the IgE level.

Treatment of stage V ABPA often does not require high-dose prednisone, since the inflammatory process in the lungs of these patients may not be active. Instead, the primary goal of therapy is the management of recurrent respiratory infections (which are usually bacterial) and supportive management of fibrotic lung disease. Severe central bronchiectasis generally accounts for the recurrent respiratory infections. These patients are often colonized with the same organisms seen in patients with cystic fibrosis.

The natural history of patients with serologic (S) ABPA is poorly defined and, as a result, the optimal treatment for these patients has not been established. They may be at risk for the development of active ABPA. Thus, a treatment regimen comparable with that used for stage I ABPA has been proposed.

RADIOGRAPHIC STUDIES

The infiltrates in acute ABPA can be fleeting or persistent and can occur in the presence or absence of respiratory symptoms. Cavitation and mucoid impaction with obstruction of first-, second-, or third-order bronchi with plugs containing mucus, hyphae, and cellular debris can also be seen. These obstructions can be fleeting or persistent and may be associated with local atelectasis. Less common than in previous years are manifestations of pulmonary fibrosis: scarring, volume loss, and local retraction. HRCT is the optimal way to document the central bronchiectasis with normal peripheral airways seen in this disorder.

OTHER ALLERGIC BRONCHOPULMONARY MYCOSES

ABPA-like syndromes can also be caused by a variety of non-*Aspergillus* fungal species. This occurs most commonly with *Candida, Curvularia,* and *Helminthosporium.*[5] In these patients, all serologic tests to demonstrate antibody against aspergillosis are negative and identification of the offending fungus can be difficult. Nevertheless, these patients respond to the corticosteroid regimen used for ABPA.

CYSTIC FIBROSIS AND ABPA

Aspergillus species are often found in the respiratory secretions of patients with cystic fibrosis. In some of these patients, the complete spectrum of the ABPA syndrome is seen.[6] Treatment with prednisone, as in the asthma patient with ABPA, results in remission of the ABPA process.

HYPERSENSITIVITY REACTIONS TO FUNGI

Inhaled fungi also cause hypersensitivity pneumonitis and immediate-type hypersensitivity reactions in the respiratory tract. Patients with hypersensitivity pneumonitis due to mold spores (for example, *Aspergillus flavus*) have pulmonary infiltrates that are not due to infection, a decreased diffusing capacity, positive IgG antibody titers, and a granulomatous lung biopsy with or without bronchiolitis obliterans.

IgE antibody–mediated reactions to fungi are a common cause of allergic rhinitis, conjunctivitis, and asthma. Skin test reactivity and atmospheric surveys suggest that *Aspergillus, Alternaria, Cladosporium,* and *Penicillium* are the most important fungal precipitants of these disorders. The diagnosis of IgE-mediated rhinitis and asthma due to mold spores is based on the physical examination and the presence of symptoms during mold season, when pollens are not prevalent. IgE antibody against mold antigens can be demonstrated by immediate-type skin tests using appropriate antigens. Positive skin tests and perennial symptoms that are exacerbated during mold seasons suggest mold allergy. Negative skin tests exclude the evaluated fungal antigens as triggers of these IgE-mediated reactions. The treatment of mold allergy is based on pharmacologic control of rhinitis and asthma. When other aeroallergens are part of the stimulus to the allergic response, immunotherapy, including mold allergens, may be a reasonable approach.

REFERENCES

1. Patterson R, Greenberger PA, Radin RC, Roberts M: Allergic bronchopulmonary aspergillosis: Staging as an aid to management. *Ann Intern Med* 96:286–291, 1982.
2. Roberts M, Greenberger PA: Serologic analysis of allergic bronchopulmonary aspergillosis, in Patterson R, Greenberger PA, Roberts ML (eds): *Allergic Bronchopulmonary Aspergillosis.* Providence, RI, Oceanside Publications, 1995, pp 11–15.
3. Angus RM, Davies M-L, Cowan MD, et al: Computed tomographic scanning of the lung in patients with allergic bronchopulmonary aspergillosis and in asthmatic patients with a positive skin test to *Aspergillus fumigatus. Thorax* 49:586–589, 1994.
4. Panchal N, Pant C, Bhagat R, Shah A: Central bronchiectasis in allergic bronchopulmonary aspergillosis: Comparative evaluation of computed tomography of the thorax with bronchography. *Eur Respir J* 7:1290–1293, 1994.
5. Hogan MB: Other allergic bronchopulmonary mycoses, in Patterson R, Greenberger PA, Roberts ML (eds): *Allergic Bronchopulmonary Aspergillosis.* Providence, RI, Oceanside Publications, 1995, pp 57–59.
6. Ditto AM, Patterson R, Sider L: Allergic bronchopulmonary aspergillosis, idiopathic anaphylaxis and cystic fibrosis in a 9-year-old: A case report. *Pediatr Asthma Allergy Immunol* 9:107–115, 1995.

OTHER OBSTRUCTIVE DISORDERS

11 | Upper Airway Obstruction*

Michael A. Grippi

INTRODUCTION

The upper airway comprises the conducting airways between the nose or mouth and main carina; it includes the oral cavity, nose, pharynx, larynx, and trachea. Historically important causes of upper airway obstruction (UAO) include syphilis, diphtheria, croup, and aspirated foreign bodies. Smoking-related airway malignancies, trauma, and use of endotracheal and tracheostomy tubes for mechanical ventilation are now common etiologies.

DIAGNOSIS

Symptoms and signs of UAO may be acute or chronic. With acute obstruction, asphyxia and death may arise within minutes. With chronic development of UAO, slowly progressive dyspnea, bleeding, change in vocal quality, respiratory failure, or symptoms of progression of malignancy may be observed. Significant obstruction may antedate symptoms. Exertional dyspnea occurs with an airway diameter of 8 mm, and dyspnea at rest is seen with an airway diameter of 5 mm, coinciding with the onset of *stridor,* which is a musical inspiratory sound of constant pitch, usually heard loudest in the neck (wheezing, which characterizes diffuse lower airway narrowing, occurs predominantly during expiration). When the obstructing lesion is below the thoracic inlet, both inspiratory and expiratory stridor may be heard. Laryngeal lesions producing upper airway obstruction may be accompanied by hoarseness. Muffling of the voice without hoarseness may be observed with a supraglottic lesion.

Routine spirometry may be useful in diagnosing UAO. The peak expiratory flow rate (PEFR) may be reduced disproportionately to the FEV_1. A ratio of $FIF_{25-75\%}$ to $FEF_{25-75\%}$ of less than 1 and an FEV_1 that is decreased to the same degree as the $FEF_{25-75\%}$ are also suggestive findings. A maximal voluntary ventilation (MVV) less than 35 to 40 times the FEV_1 suggests the

*Edited from Chap. 52, "Upper Airway Obstruction," by Braman SS, Gaissert HA. In: *Pulmonary Diseases and Disorders,* 3d ed., edited by Fishman AP, Elias JA, Fishman JA, Grippi MA, Kaiser LR, Senior RM. New York, McGraw-Hill, 1998, pp 783–802. For fuller discussion of topics dealt with in this chapter, the reader is referred to the original text, as noted above.

165

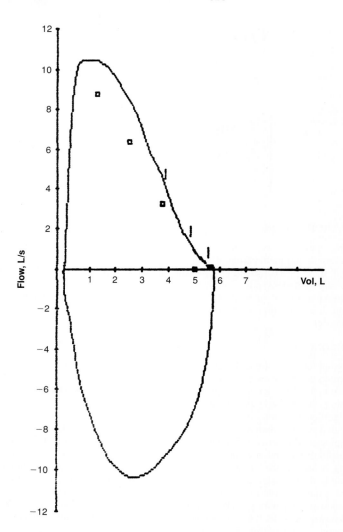

FIG. 11-1 Normal flow-volume loop following maximal expiratory (*above*) and inspiratory (*below*) effort. Small vertical lines denote seconds.

possibility of UAO. In addition, whenever the MVV is reduced in the presence of a normal FEV_1, a diagnosis of UAO should be considered.

The flow-volume loop (FVL) is an important test in the diagnosis of UAO (Fig. 11-1), although the airway must be narrowed by 80 percent to produce abnormalities. Characteristic changes may be seen with obstructions above or below the thoracic outlet (Table 11-1).

TABLE 11-1 Physiologic Classification of Upper Airway Obstruction

Type	Clinical Examples	Flow Characteristics	$FEF_{50\%}/FIF_{50\%}$
Variable extrathoracic	Vocal cord paralysis, glottic stricture, tumors	Forced inspiration increases obstruction and causes decrease in inspiratory flow. Forced expiration decreases the obstruction.	>2
Variable intrathoracic	Malignant tumors, tracheomalacia	During forced expiration, positive pleural pressure causes decrease in airway diameter and increases obstruction. During inspiration, the negative pleural pressure decreases obstruction.	Very low (~0.3)
Fixed extra- or intrathoracic	Goiter, postintubation stricture	No change in airway diameter; fixed flow with inspiration and expiration.	~1

A *fixed obstruction,* which may be intra- or extrathoracic, is defined as an obstruction whose cross-sectional area does not change with the phases of respiration. Both inspiratory and expiratory limbs of the FVL are flattened (Fig. 11-2A). The ratio of $FEF_{50\%}$ to $FIF_{50\%}$ is normal (approximately 1). Disorders that may cause a fixed upper airway obstruction include strictures from prolonged endotracheal intubation, large goiters, posttracheostomy tracheal stenosis, and benign and malignant tracheal tumors.

A *variable obstruction* is one whose cross-sectional area changes with the phases of the respiratory cycle. With a *variable extrathoracic obstruction*, the inspiratory limb is flattened while expiratory flow is relatively preserved (Fig. 11-2B). The ratio of $FEF_{50\%}$ to $FIF_{50\%}$ is increased (e.g., greater than 2). Causes include vocal cord paralysis, epiglottitis, and tumors. With a *variable intrathoracic obstruction,* maximal expiratory flow is reduced because of dynamic compression of the intrathoracic airways (Fig. 11-2C); maximal inspiratory flow is preserved. The ratio of $FEF_{50\%}$ to $FIF_{50\%}$ is low. While the flow ratio in UAO is similar to that in COPD and chronic asthma, the configuration of the FVL in the latter disorders is different. The expiratory curve seen in COPD and asthma is altered mainly in the effort-independent portion of the curve, leading to a characteristic shape—unlike the plateau configuration of an UAO.

CAUSES

UAO has many etiologies.

Infection

Acute *epiglottitis* occurs in children and, less commonly, in adults. Most pediatric cases occur after age 2 years. The disease is more common in winter.

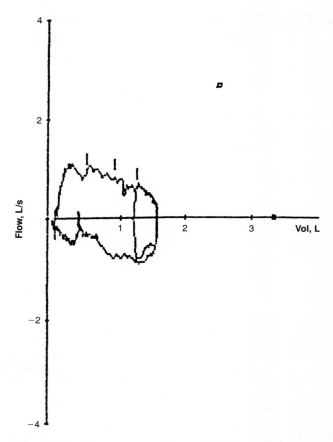

FIG. 11-2A.   Flow-volume loop in fixed upper airway obstruction (e.g., due to tracheal stenosis). The loop demonstrates flattening of inspiratory and expiratory limbs; the $FEF_{50\%}/FIF_{50\%}$ ratio is approximately 1.

In children, symptoms and signs include dysphagia, dysphonia, respiratory distress, drooling, stridor, and fever. In adults, symptoms usually develop over 24 h and include fever, sore throat, and dysphagia. Up to 50 percent develop respiratory difficulties.

In children, direct inspection of the upper airway may precipitate acute airway obstruction and should be avoided. Direct laryngoscopy under general anesthesia is advised; emergency tracheostomy may be necessary. In adults, fiberoptic laryngoscopy through the nose is not likely to provoke laryngospasm. Multiple sites in the larynx and oropharynx may also be involved (*supraglottitis*), with the epiglottis least affected. Lateral neck radiographs are abnormal in about two-thirds of cases. *Haemophilus influenzae* is the most common cause.

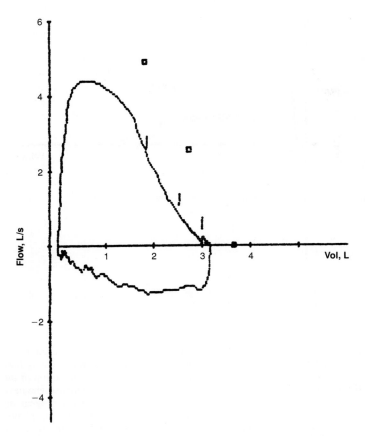

FIG. 11-2*B.* Variable extrathoracic obstruction. Flow-volume loop shows flattening of the inspiratory limb. $FEF_{50\%}/FIF_{50\%}$ is increased.

Additional pathogens in adults include *Streptococcus pneumoniae,* group A or F streptococcus, *Staphylococcus aureus,* and *Streptococcus viridans.* Due to ampicillin-resistant strains of *H. influenzae,* third-generation cephalosporins and the second-generation cephalosporin cefuroxime are the antimicrobials of choice. Corticosteroids are of no proven benefit. Nebulized racemic epinephrine may be helpful.

Laryngotracheobronchitis (croup) is characterized by subglottic tracheal narrowing; symptoms include inspiratory stridor, barking cough, and hoarseness, which usually begin several days after onset of a cold in a child under 4 years of age. Causative agents include parainfluenza virus, respiratory syncytial virus, adenovirus, and influenza A and B viruses. Acute *tonsillitis* and *pharyngitis* (usually caused by beta-hemolytic streptococci), with or without retropharyngeal abscess, acute uvulitis, acute

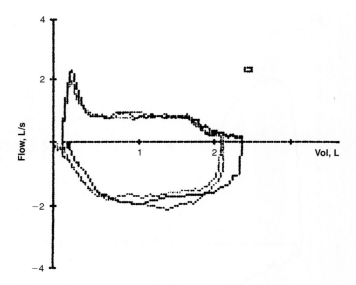

FIG. 11-2C. Variable intrathoracic obstruction. The expiratory limb is flattened. $FEF_{50\%}/FIF_{50\%}$ is 0.4.

lingular cellulitis, suppurative parotitis (most commonly caused by *S. aureus*), bacterial tracheitis (caused by *S. aureus*), and tuberculosis may lead to acute UAO. *Ludwig's angina* is a potentially lethal infection of the floor of the mouth and submandibular space occurring in patients who have a history of dental disease, external facial trauma, or oropharyngeal instrumentation. Neck swelling, pain, sore throat, drooling, and dysphagia are seen; acute UAO may occur. Soft-tissue radiographs of the neck are usually helpful in showing the extent of the bilateral cellulitis. Antibiotics, maintenance of the airway, and, frequently, surgical drainage are the mainstays of therapy.

Angioedema

Angieodema—characterized by swelling of the face, lips, tongue, and mucous membranes of the nose, mouth, and throat—may produce UAO. Causes include common allergens—such as drugs, chemical additives, and insect bites—and reactions to histamine-releasing drugs (e.g., narcotics and radiocontrast materials), aspirin and other nonsteroidal anti-inflammatory drugs, and angiotensin converting enzyme (ACE) inhibitors. Rarely, C1 esterase inhibitor deficiency is the cause. Physical stimuli (cold, heat, stress) and circulating immune complex diseases (e.g., serum sickness, systemic lupus erythematosus) are also triggers.

Angioneurotic edema following ingestion of ACE inhibitors occurs in 0.1 to 0.2 percent of patients and usually begins within hours or at most within 1 week. Onset is not dose-related; findings resolve spontaneously within hours after discontinuation of the drug. Subcutaneous epinephrine and intravenous or intramuscular diphenhydramine are effective immediately; corticosteroids are useful for associated late-phase reactions. Patients with idiopathic angioedema should probably avoid ACE inhibitors.

Hereditary angioedema, an autosomal dominant disorder characterized by painless nonpitting edema of the face and upper airway beginning in childhood, is due to a deficiency in production or function of C1 esterase inhibitor and resultant activation of complement, fibrinolytic, and kinin pathways. Swelling progresses over many hours and then resolves over 1 to 3 days. Blood levels of C4 are low during and between attacks. If the C4 level is low, a C1 esterase inhibitor level should be measured; 85 percent of patients have levels below 30 percent of normal (type I disease), while the remainder have abnormal functional assays (type II disease). An acquired form has been reported in patients with a B-cell proliferative disorder. Although epinephrine, antihistamines, and corticosteroids appear to have little efficacy in treating hereditary angiodema, they are often used. Airway protection is key. Infusion of C1 inhibitor concentrate may resolve the attack within hours. The attenuated androgens stanozolol and danazol, which may increase C1 production by the liver, are used for prophylaxis.

Tumors

Benign or malignant tumors of the pharynx, larynx, trachea, or bronchi may produce UAO. Examples include adenoid cystic carcinoma and squamous cell carcinoma. Pharyngeal tumors ordinarily interfere with swallowing before causing airflow limitation. Secondary tracheal involvement occurs with local advancement of bronchogenic, laryngeal, esophageal, and thyroid carcinomas or Hodgkin's lymphoma.

Trauma

Either blunt or penetrating trauma to the face, neck, or chest may cause UAO. Motor vehicle accidents are the most common cause of blunt injury. Laryngeal injury may occur with hyperextension of the neck. Laryngeal and tracheal compression against the spine results in fractures of the laryngeal cartilage and laceration of the mucosa. Symptoms include dyspnea, stridor, dysphonia or aphonia, neck pain, cough, aspiration, hemoptysis, and dysphagia. The laryngeal prominence is lost, and the contour of the neck is flat. Subcutaneous emphysema may develop. Deep soft-tissue infection in the neck may occur from contamination with oropharyngeal organisms.

Physical examination includes assessment of quiet respiration and speech. Cervical spine x-rays and computed tomography are useful in ruling out a fracture, and laryngoscopy is key in evaluation of the laryngeal lumen and glottic function. With laryngeal injury, translaryngeal intubation should be performed only under direct vision by an experienced physician.

Segments of the tracheobronchial tree within 2 cm of the carina are most susceptible to laceration from blunt trauma, followed by the cervical trachea and main-stem bronchi. Presenting findings include subcutaneous emphysema and hemoptysis. Ten percent of tracheobronchial lacerations are located in the cervical trachea, 22 percent in the thoracic trachea, 27 percent in the right main bronchus, 17 percent in the left main bronchus, and 16 percent in a lobar bronchus. The chest radiograph demonstrates unilateral or bilateral pneumothorax and pneumomediastinum. Airway obstruction may occur with complete transection of the trachea above the carina. Laceration of the tracheobronchial tree is diagnosed with bronchoscopy; a rigid bronchoscope should be used if the airway is not secure.

Inhalation Injuries

Fires in closed spaces, inhalation of irritant gases—such as aldehydes, ammonia, and hydrochloride acid—and heat result in severe tracheobronchitis and mucosal sloughing. If the airway's basal membrane is destroyed, granulation tissue formation, scarring, and stenosis may develop. Diagnosis of acute inhalation injury is based on history and the presence of oropharyngeal soot, hoarseness, or stridor. Bronchoscopy is very useful. Major airway complications develop in 25 to 30 percent of patients with severe inhalation injury and tracheostomy. Late strictures of larynx and trachea are common following inhalation injury, particularly after long-term intubation.

Vascular Causes

Narrowing of the upper airway in adults may occur uncommonly as a result of enlarging aneurysms of the thoracic aorta. In children, vascular compression of the airway arises in infancy or childhood as a developmental disorder. The *innominate artery syndrome* is caused by pressure of the innominate artery on the anterior wall of the trachea. An intrinsic weakness of the tracheal wall and tracheomalacia may be operative. Most children get better without therapy. Cyanotic spells, with apnea, bradycardia, or even cardiac arrest, may occur during bottle feeding and are an indication for surgical intervention. In the *double aortic arch* anomaly, the smaller left aortic arch passes anterior to the trachea, with the descending aorta usually located on the left side. The tightness of the ring determines the severity of symptoms (stridor, recurrent pneumonia, and dysphagia) and the time of presentation. Surgical correction involves division of the anterior left arch and of the ligamentum arteriosum. With the *aberrant left pulmonary artery sling,* the left pulmonary artery arises from the right pulmonary artery and passes behind the trachea to the left hilum; congenital tracheal stenosis coexists in approximately 50 percent of cases.

Foreign-Body Aspiration

Aspiration of food, toys, or dental appliances may produce acute UAO. Risk factors include advanced age, altered state of consciousness, poor dentition, and neurologic disorders. *Café coronary syndrome* is sudden aspiration of food (usually meat) into the hypopharynx and upper portion of the larynx. Respiratory embarrassment and inability to talk occur. Emergency measures using a food extractor or the Heimlich maneuver may be lifesaving. A large foreign body lodged in the esophagus may also cause UAO by compressing the trachea.

Neuromuscular Disorders

Neuromuscular disorders affecting the bulbar muscles may produce UAO. In children, vocal cord paralysis may be a complication of Dandy-Walker syndrome or Arnold-Chiari malformation. In adults, causes include familial bulbar spinal muscle atrophy, postpoliomyelitis syndrome, Parkinson's disease, multiple sclerosis, acute poliomyelitis, amyotrophic lateral sclerosis, Guillain-Barré syndrome, brainstem stroke, and large stroke of the cerebral hemisphere. Other causes of UAO include laryngeal nerve injury following neck surgery, endotracheal intubation-related injury, laryngeal trauma, infection, and thoracic aortic aneurysm. Dystonic extrapyramidal reactions due to neuroleptic medications (e.g., haloperidol) may cause significant UAO. Laryngeal-pharyngeal dystonia can be associated with severe upper airway dysfunction. If not reversed, symptoms can last for days or lead to respiratory arrest.

The FVL often shows evidence of a variable extrathoracic upper airway obstruction, with or without flow oscillations during inspiration ("sawtooth pattern"). This abnormal flow pattern, first noted in patients with sleep apnea, is commonly seen with extrapyramidal disorders (where the flow oscillations correspond to vocal cord tremor), myasthenia gravis, and motoneuron disease (where muscle denervation causes irregular muscle fasciculations and resulting tremor of the upper airway muscles). It is also observed in patients who have functional stridor and wheezing (see below).

Iatrogenic Causes

Among the most common iatrogenic causes of UAO are laryngeal or tracheal complications resulting from prolonged endotracheal intubation. Pressure-related damage to the vocal cords typically regresses within 2 to 3 months. The more serious complication of stenosis at the posterior glottic commissure correlates with the duration of intubation. UAO may also arise acutely from postextubation glottic edema or laryngospasm.

Complications from tracheostomy may lead to acute airway obstruction soon after the procedure, as well as delayed obstruction months or years afterward. Tracheal stenosis typically occurs at the tracheostomy tube cuff site, 1.0 to 3.5 cm below the stoma. Use of high-volume, low-pressure cuffs has decreased the incidence. Cuff overinflation remains a cause of tracheal strictures. Stenosis at the level of the stoma is caused by an excessively large stoma or excess traction on the tracheostomy tube. Stenosis of the subglottic trachea may also occur, usually from a stoma placed too high. Tracheomalacia due to thinning of the tracheal cartilage may occur by itself or in combination with tracheal stricture and may lead to UAO.

Vocal Cord Dysfunction

Vocal cord dysfunction ("laryngeal asthma") refers to paradoxical closure of the cords intermittently during inspiration (normally, the glottic opening widens during inspiration and narrows during expiration). Psychogenic mechanisms appear to be operative. Signs and symptoms resemble those of laryngeal edema, laryngospasm, vocal cord paralysis, or asthma. Some patients have concurrent asthma; many have been previously misdiagnosed as having asthma. Frequent emergency room visits, hospitalizations, and endotracheal intubations are the rule. Psychiatric disorders and a history of sexual and physical abuse are commonly discovered. A high index of suspicion should be present for a patient with wheezing, stridor, or both in whom the adventitious sounds are heard loudest over the neck. Despite their respiratory distress, patients often have little difficulty completing full sentences or holding their breath. The laryngeal-induced sounds are eliminated during a panting maneuver.

Pulmonary function testing shows an increase in the ratio of $FEF_{50\%}$ to $FIF_{50\%}$; the FVL demonstrates a variable extrathoracic obstruction. The inspiratory limb may show "sawtoothing" or fluttering, representing fluctuations in the abnormal cord motion. Multiple attempts at the FVL maneuver often give variable results. Direct visualization of the vocal cords during an attack reveals inspiratory anterior vocal cord closure with a posterior glottic chink. Treatment includes speech therapy or psychotherapy.

Miscellaneous Causes

Relapsing polychondritis (excessive airway flaccidity and collapse), Sjögren's syndrome (compressing mediastinal lymph nodes), Wegener's granulomatosis (tracheal stenosis due to inflammation), rheumatoid arthritis (midline fixation of the arytenoid cartilages at their articulations with the cricoid cartilage), and ankylosing spondylitis (hyperostosis of the cervical spine) are uncommon causes of UAO. Tracheobronchiomegaly, a rare familial disorder associated with marked dilatation of the respiratory tract and bronchiectasis, is characterized by increased tracheal compliance and an irregular, corrugated appearance of the trachea seen on chest radiography. Occasionally, the coronal diameter of the trachea is markedly reduced and the sagittal diameter is correspondingly increased (so-called *saber sheath trachea*). *Tracheobronchopathia osteochondroplastica,* a degenerative disease of the trachea and bronchi in older men, is characterized by submucosal cartilagenous and bony nodules that may narrow the airway lumen.

NONCARDIOGENIC PULMONARY EDEMA AS A COMPLICATION OF ACUTE UPPER AIRWAY OBSTRUCTION

Noncardiogenic pulmonary edema as a complication of UAO was first recognized in children following acute epiglottitis and foreign-body aspiration. It has since been reported as a result of hanging, strangulation, goiter, hypothyroidism, upper airway tumors, acromegaly, mediastinal tumors, and insertion of a peroral dental prosthesis. The most common cause in adults is postanesthetic laryngospasm. Risk factors include an anatomically difficult intubation, nasal or laryngeal surgery, obesity, short neck, and obstructive sleep apnea.

The mechanism appears to be multifaceted and may include an acquired defect in alveolar-capillary permeability and change in hydrostatic forces due to generation of negative intrathoracic and transpulmonary pressures from attempted inspiration against an obstructed airway. Most patients have a relatively benign course and experience rapid improvement with supportive care and supplemental oxygen. Vigorous diuresis can be deleterious and lead to hypotension. Noninvasive ventilatory support with nasal ventilation can be helpful when the pulmonary edema is more severe and profound hypoxemia occurs.

ACUTE MANAGEMENT OF UPPER AIRWAY OBSTRUCTION

Rapid, careful assessment of the patient is critical to correct management. Unless respiratory arrest is imminent, diagnostic evaluation should be pursued, as time permits. Humidified, oxygen-enriched air should be administered to the upright patient. Racemic epinephrine and a helium-oxygen mixture may be helpful in treating laryngeal edema. Corticosteroids appear useful in treating croup. Corticosteroids are indicated for allergic, IgE-mediated angioedema. Their efficacy in acute epiglottitis, hereditary angioedema, or postextubation laryngeal edema has not been demonstrated.

With oropharyngeal obstruction, secretions should be suctioned and an oropharyngeal airway inserted while implementing jaw-thrust and chin-lift maneuvers. If an airway cannot be established with these maneuvers and laryngoscopy fails to visualize the vocal cords, a tracheostomy should be performed. Laryngeal obstruction is approached in a similar manner. Pharmacologic muscle relaxation should be avoided in order to maintain spontaneous breathing. For lesions located above the cricoid cartilage, the inability to intubate indicates the need for tracheostomy. For tracheal lesions, either emergent intubation using a small (5-mm) endotracheal tube or, under more controlled circumstances, rigid bronchoscopy, is preferred. When cricothyroidotomy is performed as an emergency procedure for UAO, a 2-cm transverse incision is made over the cricothyroid membrane. A scalpel or, more appropriately, a 7-mm endotracheal (or tracheostomy) tube is inserted. A formal tracheostomy is then performed after 24 to 48 h to prevent damage to the subglottic space and cricoid cartilage.

BIBLIOGRAPHY

Crapo RO: Causes of respiratory injury, in Haponik EF, Munster AM (eds): *Respiratory Injury: Smoke Inhalation and Burns.* New York, McGraw-Hill, 1990, pp 47–60.

Dark A, Armstrong T: Severe postoperative laryngeal edema causing total airway obstruction immediately on extubation. *Br J Anaesth* 82:644–646, 1999.

Frantz TD, Rasgon BM, Quesenberry CP: Acute epiglottitis in adults. *JAMA* 272:1358–1360, 1994.

Israili ZH, Hall WD: Cough and angioneurotic edema associated with angiotensin-converting enzyme inhibitor therapy. *Ann Intern Med* 117:234–242, 1992.

Kharasch M, Graff J: Emergency management of the airway. *Crit Care Clin* 11:53–66, 1995.

Kollef MH, Pluss J: Noncardiogenic pulmonary edema following upper airway obstruction: 7 cases and a review. *Medicine (Baltimore)* 70:91–98, 1991.

Lewis RJ: Tracheostomies: Indications, timing and complications. *Clin Chest Med* 13:137–149,1992.

McGee DL, Wald DA, Hinchliffe S: Helium-oxygen therapy in the emergency department, *J Emerg Med* 15:291–296, 1997.

Mehta AC, Dasgupta A: Airway stents, *Clin Chest Med* 20:139–151, 1999.

Newman KB, Mason UG III, Schmaling KB: Clinical features of vocal cord dysfunction. *Am J Respir Crit Care Med* 152:1382–1386, 1995.

Symbas PN, Justicz AG, Ricketts RR: Rupture of the airways from blunt trauma: Treatment of complex injuries. *Ann Thorac Surg* 54:177–183, 1992.

12 | Cystic Fibrosis*

Lisa M. Bellini and Michael A. Grippi

INTRODUCTION

Cystic fibrosis (CF) is a heritable disorder demonstrating an autosomal recessive pattern. In the United States, the incidence in Caucasians is approximately 1 in 3300 live births; in African Americans, it is 1 in 15,300. The frequency of unaffected heterozygote carriers in persons of northern European ancestry is 1 in 25. The disorder affects all exocrine glands; symptoms due to lung and pancreatic involvement usually dominate the clinical picture.

GENETICS

CF is caused by mutations in a single gene—the *cystic fibrosis transmembrane conductance regulator* (CFTR)—which can be detected in a variety of tissues, including lungs, pancreas, and sweat glands. The most common (and first described) CF mutation is the deletion of phenylalanine from position 508 (ΔF508) of the CFTR glycoprotein.

CFTR is an integral membrane glycoprotein that functions as an apical chloride channel and is expressed in epithelial cells of affected organs. CFTR mutations have been grouped into several classes based on the effect of the mutation on the expression, processing, and function of the protein. ΔF508, which represents 66 percent of CF mutations, is a processing mutation in which very little of the mutant protein reaches the apical surface. More than 600 CF mutations have been reported; the list continues to grow. Benign sequence variations also have been described. The large number of mutations makes accurate detection of a satisfactory percentage of carriers extremely difficult. Testing for 32 of the most common mutations is commercially available and detects approximately 90 percent of carriers in Caucasians of northern European descent. In families with an affected individual and known mutations, prenatal diagnosis and carrier testing using direct mutation detection are accurate. In families with a member diagnosed as having CF but with undetected mutations, use of restriction fragment length polymorphism analysis using linked DNA markers can be informative in a high percentage of cases.

Numerous attempts have been made, with limited success, to characterize phenotype on the basis of genotype. In general, homozygotes for ΔF508 have pancreatic insufficiency. A direct association of a particular genotype with progression of the pulmonary disease has not been found. A CF-associated mutation has been identified in approximately 35 percent of males with congenital bilateral absence of the vas deferens (CBAVD). These patients lack a

---

*Edited from Chap. 53, "Cystic Fibrosis," by Robinson C, Scanlin TF. In: *Fishman's Pulmonary Diseases and Disorders,* 3d ed., edited by Fishman AP, Elias JA, Fishman JA, Grippi MA, Kaiser LR, Senior RM. New York, McGraw-Hill, 1998, pp 803–824. For fuller discussion of the topics dealt with in this chapter, the reader is referred to the original text, as noted above.

TABLE 12-1 Complications and Presenting Symptoms of Cystic Fibrosis by Age Group

Infancy	Childhood	Adolescence/Adulthood
Meconium ileus	Pulmonary infections with *Staphylococcus* and *Pseudomonas*	Chronic bronchitis
Obstructive jaundice	Malnutrition with steatorrhea and pancreatic insufficiency	Pansinusitis
Edema with hypoproteinemia, anemia/hypoprothrombinemia	Heat prostration with hypoelectrolytemia and metabolic alkalosis	Hemoptysis
Failure to thrive	"Atypical asthma" with clubbing and/or bronchiectasis	Chronic abdominal pain
Intussusception	Esophageal varices	Delayed sexual development
Volvulus	Hypersplenism	Obstructive aspermia
Rectal prolapse	Nasal polyps	
Recurrent pneumonia/bronchiolitis		

vas deferens, but they are otherwise healthy and have normal sweat test results (see below). Certain alleles associated with CF are associated with nasal polyposis and bronchiectasis but normal sweat test results.

CLINICAL MANIFESTATIONS

In cystic fibrosis, all exocrine glands appear to be affected, and the range of symptoms and complications is broad (Table 12-1).

Pulmonary

In the lungs, hypersecretion of viscid mucus and chronic bacterial infection produce progressive airway obstruction, eventually leading to diffuse, severe bronchiectasis. The most common pathogens are *Staphylococcus aureus* and *Pseudomonas aeruginosa.* Less common are mucoid *Escherichia coli, Klebsiella,* and *Haemophilus influenzae.* In later stages of the disease, *Pseudomonas* usually predominates. By adulthood, more than 80 percent of patients are colonized with *P. aeruginosa.*

Respiratory secretions increase when a patient with CF, already chronically colonized with *Pseudomonas,* develops an increased bacterial burden in the airways. The resultant increase in secretions leads to worsening cough and sputum production, increase in respiratory rate, retraction of the chest during inspiration, and diffuse, coarse inspiratory crackles. Fever and leukocytosis are common. The chest radiograph demonstrates worsening hyperinflation, increased peribronchial thickening, and worsening nodular or cystic densities. Decreases in the forced vital capacity (FVC), forced expiratory volume in 1 s (FEV_1), and forced expiratory flow between 25 and 75 percent of the exhaled vital capacity ($FEF_{25-75\%}$) and an increase in residual volume (RV) are seen. Treatment (see below) generally restores most indices of pulmonary function to, or almost to, baseline. However, despite the return to baseline, the cumulative effect of repeated episodes is progressive bronchiectasis, atelectasis, and an irreversible decrease in pulmonary function.

Gastrointestinal

Thick, viscous secretions from the exocrine portion of the pancreas progressively obstruct the pancreatic ducts, resulting in pancreatic autodestruction by its own enzymes. In advanced stages, pancreatic fibrosis may obliterate the islets of Langerhans and cause diabetes mellitus.

Obstruction of the biliary tract by viscid secretions may produce focal biliary cirrhosis, sometimes evident in early infancy. Some newborns develop *inspissated bile syndrome,* characterized by prolonged obstructive jaundice starting at 2 to 8 weeks of age. The jaundice often clears without therapy. Compared with age-matched controls, the risks of cholelithiasis and cholecystitis are increased in adults with CF.

In the intestines, hyperplasia of the mucous glands and globlet cells is seen. Abnormalities in intestinal mucins may contribute to malabsorption, most of which in CF can be corrected by administration of pancreatic enzymes. However, the abnormal mucins may decrease intestinal transit time, which, in conjunction with maldigestion, may cause fecal impaction in the terminal ileum—*meconium ileus equivalent* or distal intestinal obstruction syndrome. Volvulus or intussusception may further complicate the picture.

Reproductive Tract

Except for an increase in viscosity and an abnormal midcycle ferning pattern in cervical mucus, no consistent pathologic changes occur in the female reproductive tract. In males, the vas deferens is either atretic or absent at birth. Viscous secretions may contribute to obstruction in utero, followed by failure of development of the vas deferens. More than 97 percent of males with CF are aspermic.

Sweat Glands

The sweat glands in CF show no distinctive histologic changes. Nonetheless, their function is abnormal. The precursor solution secreted by the sweat glands, as in normals, is isotonic to plasma. Normally, as sweat flows along the duct of the gland, sodium and chloride are reabsorbed and sweat at the skin surface is hypotonic with respect to both sodium and chloride. In CF, the relative impermeability of the ducts to chloride ions is thought to be responsible for the characteristic increase in potential differences across isolated, perfused sweat glands and respiratory epithelial cells.

DIAGNOSIS

Diagnosis is based on demonstration of elevated sweat sodium and chloride levels in a patient with a consistent history. The most prominent clinical features are those of chronic pulmonary disease and pancreatic insufficiency. A positive family history of CF, particularly in a sibling, supports the diagnosis. With the appropriate clinical or family history, two clearly positive sweat tests using the quantitative pilocarpine iontophoresis method permit establishment of the diagnosis with assurance.

In children, concentrations of sodium and chloride of less than 40 meq/L are usually regarded as normal. However, the averages for sodium and chloride concentrations are about 20 meq/L for normal subjects and 95 meq/L for those with CF. In children, values between 40 and 60 meq/L are borderline elevated; such values call for repetition of the sweat test until a clear pattern emerges. The concentration of sodium and chloride in sweat increases gradually with age. Conditions other than CF in which the concentrations of sodium and chloride in sweat are abnormally high include malnutrition, adrenal insufficiency, hereditary nephrogenic diabetes insipidus, ectodermal dysplasia, and fucosidosis.

Genetic analysis can be used to confirm the diagnosis of CF. In patients with minimal symptoms, the diagnosis of CF can be made with certainty if two CF-associated alleles are present. Screening for 32 of the most common alleles yields an overall sensitivity of 90 percent due to undetected alleles.

CLINICAL ASSESSMENT

Clinical evaluation of the patient with known or suspected CF is multifaceted.

Radiography

Early chest radiographic findings include mild hyperinflation and minimal peribronchial thickening. With disease progression, peribronchial thickening, perhaps first isolated to the upper lobes, develops and extends to affect all lobes. In advanced disease, ring shadows, cystic lesions, nodular densities, bronchiectases, and atelectasis are seen. High-resolution computed tomography (HRCT) scans are more sensitive than plain radiographs and commonly demonstrate "ground glass" opacities. Early bronchiectasis may be seen on the CT scan before the chest radiograph becomes abnormal.

Pulmonary Function Testing

All of the pulmonary function abnormalities seen in chronic bronchitis, emphysema, and asthma may be seen in CF; however, it is the bronchiectasis that modifies pulmonary performance. Bronchiectatic airways are excessively compliant and collapse during rapid expirations or cough. In addition, the small airways are vulnerable to obstruction early in the course of CF.

Spirometry shows an obstructive pattern (see Chap. 11). Increases in residual volume (RV) and, subsequently, in functional residual capacity (FRC) and total lung capacity (TLC) are also seen. Widening of the alveolar-arterial oxygen gradient and an increase in the ratio of dead space to tidal volume (V_D/V_T) occur. The diffusing capacity for carbon monoxide ($D_{L_{CO}}$) is low at rest and does not increase normally during exercise. Hypoxemia develops, and pulmonary hypertension, cor pulmonale, and right ventricular failure follow in turn. Late in the course of the disease, hypercapnia and respiratory acidosis contribute to the final picture of respiratory failure.

Pulmonary function testing in CF allows tracking of the natural history of the disease and assessment of the value of therapeutic interventions. Up to age 6 years, determination of arterial oxygenation can be used as a measure of overall pulmonary function, both in the stable state and during an intercurrent infection. After age 6 years, pulmonary function tests may be performed reliably.

Sputum Analysis

In many patients with CF, *P. aeruginosa* and *S. aureus* are found alone or in combination in the sputum. Rarely are the organisms (especially *Pseudomonas*) eradicated, even with prolonged administration of antibiotics. Although these organisms are sometimes found in sputum from patients with pulmonary disorders other than CF, their isolation should raise suspicion of the disease.

Pancreatic Function

Ninety percent of patients with CF have pancreatic insufficiency. In infants, the hallmark is often failure to thrive. In older children, a history of bulky, foul, malodorous stools may be elicited. Fat malabsorption may be quanitifed and is usually substantial in CF.

Direct assessment of pancreatic function includes a serum immunoreactive assay for trypsin (abnormally high in CF, usually reflecting ongoing destruction of the pancreas) in infants, determination of trypsin or chymotrypsin activity in stool, and the secretin stimulation test. Endocrine function of the pancreas is usually preserved in children, but approximately 50 percent of adults are overtly diabetic by age 30 years.

Liver Function

In infants and children with CF, serum bilirubin and transaminases, while sometimes transiently increased, are usually normal. The prothrombin time is occasionally prolonged due to malabsorption and decreased hepatic synthesis of clotting factors. Rarely, patients present with bleeding esophageal varices from advanced cirrhosis.

Semen Analysis

Occasionally, a man who is found to have aspermia during the course of an evaluation for infertility is found to have CF. In men with known CF, a complete semen analysis is part of the evaluation. Azoospermia is found in more than 97 percent.

ATYPICAL PRESENTATIONS

Atypical clinical presentations confound the diagnosis, and a high index of suspicion is required. Approximately 6 percent of patients are diagnosed after age 18 years. Recovery of unusual gram-negative organisms, mucoid *Pseudomonas* species, or *S. aureus* from sputum of asthmatics with persistent sputum production, chest radiographic abnormalities, or clubbing should prompt referral for sweat testing. Recurrent sinusitis and nasal polyposis may be the only manifestations of CF in a mildly affected person. Isolation of *P. aeruginosa* from deep nasal cultures should raise suspicion. Sweat testing and referral to a CF center should be considered for men with azoospermia or CBAVD.

MANAGEMENT

Comprehensive, multidisciplinary CF treatment programs have led to a dramatic increase in the median age of survival of affected patients.

Chest Physical Therapy

More than 90 percent of CF patients die from pulmonary complications. Strategies to clear pulmonary secretions in order to prevent complications arising from airway plugging by viscous secretions are paramount in management. Chest physiotherapy—i.e., "percussion and postural drainage"— performed regularly is the most widely prescribed method. All patients with CF should maintain a regular (e.g., twice daily) chest physiotherapy regimen. More frequent chest physiotherapy should be applied during an exacerbation of chronic pulmonary infection. Use of autogenic drainage and a small pipe- like device (the Flutter valve) that produces an oscillating resistance during a forced expiratory maneuver have been employed as well.

Antibiotics

Antibiotic administration must balance the dangers of overzealous admin- istration against progressive airway damage and bronchiectasis resulting from untreated infection. The most useful approach is based on sputum cul- ture at the time of diagnosis and at regular intervals thereafter. When signs and symptoms herald worsening of the pulmonary infection (i.e., increased cough or sputum production) or new abnormalities on the physical exami- nation, the chest radiograph, or pulmonary function tests, use of percussion and postural drainage should be increased and appropriate oral antibiotics given.

Antibiotic choices are directed at staphylococcal and pseudomonal infections. Early in the course of the pulmonary disease, a small fraction of *Pseudomonas* strains may be sensitive to tetracycline, trimethoprim/sul- famethoxazole, or chloramphenicol. Occasionally, even *Pseudomonas* strains considered resistant according to laboratory sensitivity tests appar- ently respond to these antibiotics. Ciprofloxacin, a quinolone derivative that can be given orally, is initially effective against many strains of *Pseudomonas* and has gained widespread use in the outpatient manage- ment of CF; however, resistance often develops after a few courses of treatment. For treatment of a pulmonary exacerbation of CF caused by *Pseudomonas,* a combination of an aminoglycoside given intravenously and a semisynthetic penicillin is generally used. In order to achieve high levels of antibiotics in the airways and in secretions, the aminoglycoside is generally administered in higher doses and more often than usual. The resulting concentrations in serum are monitored to achieve a serum level of 8 to 10 μg/mL. Although many patients begin to show improvement af- ter 5 to 7 days, most CF centers continue antibiotics intravenously for at least 2 weeks in order to decrease the relapse rate and to avoid a decrease in the interval between exacerbations.

In the occasional hospitalized patient who experiences a relapse or mani- fests an increase in symptoms shortly after administration of intravenous antibiotics is stopped, long-term intravenous administration of an aminogly- coside can be continued with outpatient infusion therapy. Antibiotics admin- istered via the inhalational route have also been advocated in those infected with *Pseudomonas.* Although it has been argued that inhalation will not deliver effective concentrations to diseased portions of the lungs because of interference with ventilation by local airway obstruction, inhaled antibiotics are helpful in patients who have been hospitalized repeatedly for exacerbations of pulmonary symptoms that recur at increasing frequency and after shorter intervals between exacerbations. Often, if inhalation therapy is started after completion of a course of intravenous antibiotics, the interval before the next exacerbation is prolonged. The most commonly used preparation is inhaled tobramycin (TOBI), administered at a dose of 300 mg twice daily on an every-other-month basis.

Mucolytics

Pulmozyme, a DNA-cleaving enzyme and effective mucolytic agent, decreases sputum viscosity in CF. Pulmozyme has been shown to result in approximately a 6 percent improvement in FEV_1, as well as a decreased incidence of exacerbations requiring antibiotics and hospitalizations. N-acetylcysteine is no longer used, given its complications of bronchospasm and tracheitis. Other agents employed include inhaled amiloride. Amiloride effects changes in mucous viscosity by altering electrolyte concentrations in the sputum of patients with CF.

Bronchodilators and Anti-inflammatory Agents

Bronchodilators are often used in treating the pulmonary manifestations of CF. Their use should follow objective and quantitative measurement of bronchodilator effectiveness. Corticosteroids have been used with good results in infants with severe obstructive airway disease that does not respond to antibiotics and bronchodilators as well as in patients in whom the pulmonary disease is complicated by severe asthma or allergic bronchopulmonary aspergillosis. Patients with moderately severe obstructive airway disease and those with chronic *Pseudomonas* infection may benefit from steroid treatment for periods of less than 1 year. Other anti-inflammatory agents have been tried, including high doses of ibuprofen.

Nutritional Supplementation

The mainstay of management of pancreatic insufficiency in CF is use of pancreatic enzyme preparations, currently available as enteric-coated capsules containing coated microspheres. Dosage is adjusted to ensure a relatively normal pattern of bowel movements, adequate weight gain or maintenance of ideal weight for height, and decrease in bowel symptoms such as cramping and flatulence. Despite the use of pancreatic enzyme replacement, correction of pancreatic insufficiency is incomplete; accordingly, patients require more than 100 percent of their recommended caloric intake. In some, an even greater caloric intake is necessary because of increased energy expenditure due to increased work of breathing secondary to chronic pulmonary infection.

As a rule, patients with CF are advised to consume a double dose of a multivitamin preparation and a vitamin E supplement each day. Infants, those in whom the prothrombin time is prolonged, and those who take antibiotics uninterruptedly require supplemental vitamin K. Vitamin A supplementation is required in children with significant fat malabsorption and failure to thrive; however, care must be taken to avoid hypervitaminosis A.

Supplemental salt is needed by patients in order to prevent electrolyte depletion, metabolic alkalosis, and heat prostration. For infants, 1 to 2 g of salt per day is added to the feeding formula; children and adults are encouraged to salt their foods liberally and to take salt-containing liquids and snacks during hot weather.

Management of Selected Pulmonary and Infectious Disease-Related Issues

Recurrent pneumothorax is common in CF, particularly in older patients; tension physiology occurs in up to 30 percent. Tube thoracostomy is indicated when the pneumothorax occupies more than 10 percent of the area of the hemithorax seen on the posteroanterior chest radiograph. A high rate of recurrence warrants attempts at chemical or surgical pleurodesis; the latter is more effective and is no longer considered a contraindication to lung transplantation.

Minor hemoptysis is common in CF and is generally managed by intensifying home therapy for pulmonary infection. Expectoration of more than 30 to 60 mL of fresh blood should prompt hospitalization, even with an unchanged chest radiograph. While massive hemoptysis (greater than 300 mL) is uncommon, it represents a potentially life-threatening situation. While surgical intervention may be required to control the hemorrhage, bronchial artery embolization has been used successfully and is the treatment of choice when a physician experienced in the procedure is available.

Management of the patient with CF with respiratory failure is challenging. As a rule, patients with CF do not respond as well to mechanical ventilation and have more complications than do those with other forms of chronic obstructive airway disease. When respiratory failure marks the end of a chronic course of progressive pulmonary insufficiency, despite adequate medical therapy, mechanical ventilation is usually unhelpful. Noninvasive mechanical ventilation using bilevel positive airway pressure has been used successfully in relatively stable, end-stage patients, most of whom have been evaluated and listed for lung transplantation.

Many acute exacerbations of CF are caused by infections, including those due to unusual organisms. In the last 25 years, the importance of *Burkholderia cepacia* (formerly *Pseudomonas cepacia*) has been recognized. This gram-negative, oxidase-positive rod is frequently panresistant. *B. cepacia* colonization has been associated with septicemia, which is very rarely seen with *P. aeruginosa*. The clinical course after acquisition of *B. cepacia* may be fulminant, with death occurring in a matter of months. However, most patients' disease follows a more benign course. The combination of a poor clinical course after acquisition of *B. cepacia* and evidence supporting epidemic transmission has led to cohorting or isolation of infected patients. Other gram-negative, oxidase-positive organisms of clinical importance in CF include *S. maltophilia, F. oryzihabitans,* and *A. xylosidans.* Antibiotic therapy should be directed toward these bacteria when they are isolated from a patient experiencing an acute exacerbation.

Aspergillus and atypical mycobacteria may colonize the airways of patients with CF; eradication of these organisms from the airways is virtually impossible. Therapy is directed toward verifying that the organisms are resulting in worsening of the disease and controlling the infection rather than effecting a microbiologic cure.

Patients with CF should be screened for *Mycobacterium tuberculosis* infection with yearly PPD skin tests. Prophylaxis and treatment of *M. tuberculosis* in CF are the same as for patients without CF. A decision about therapy for isolation of atypical mycobacteria is based on the likelihood that the organism is contributing to airway infection and a decline in pulmonary function.

Approximately 5 to 15 percent of patients have allergic bronchopulmonary aspergillosis (ABPA). The diagnosis of ABPA in CF is difficult because of overlapping symptoms between the two disorders. ABPA in CF is treated with corticosteroids despite colonization of the lower airways with pathogenic bacteria.

Lung Transplantation

Lung transplantation has emerged as an option for patients with end-stage CF. Despite initial concerns about immunosuppression in suppurative lung disease, the outcome for those with CF who undergo lung transplantation is among the best reported (4-year survival about 50 percent). However, because CF is a multisystem disorder, both management and proper selection of patients for transplantation are more complicated than for other diseases. Colonization with multidrug-resistant *B. cepacia* has been associated with a poor clinical outcome. Patients with CF metabolize drugs differently from those without CF, complicating the dosing of medications, including cyclosporine. The difficulties in achieving an optimal drug dose may be related to malabsorption or enhanced excretion of the drug.

Nutritional issues also complicate the posttransplantation management of patients with CF. About 50 percent of all patients with CF over 30 years of age are overtly diabetic, and administration of corticosteroids induces diabetes in another 10 percent. Maintenance of proper nutrition is important in CF, especially for rapid postoperative recovery. The importance of nutrition is underscored by the fact that if patients are less than 75 percent of their ideal body weight, they are not listed for transplantation.

Psychosocial Support

Careful attention to the emotional, social, and financial well-being of the patient with CF and his or her family has considerable value in favorably influencing the course of the disease. At the time of diagnosis, it is important to strike an optimistic note while educating the patient about the illness and its management. As the disease runs its course, counseling and feedback about disease progression are essential. Managing a chronic illness becomes more complicated when patients must also begin to manage their independence and make life decisions regarding education, marriage, children, careers, insurance, and self-care. At the stage when medical therapy is of no further avail, however, the patient and family require considerable emotional support to accept the inevitable. In recent years, many CF centers have allowed patients to die at home rather than in the hospital.

Reproductive Issues

More than 97 percent of male patients with CF are sterile, secondary to bilateral absence of the vas deferens. Microsurgical epididymal sperm aspiration (MESA) coupled with in vitro fertilization has been successful in producing pregnancies in a few carefully selected patients. Since not all males with CF are sterile, they should be offered sperm analysis.

Pregnancy for women with CF is increasingly common, and several important issues remain unresolved. Maternal clinical status before pregnancy is the most important sign of maternal outcome. More severely affected women suffer an irreversible decline in clinical status during pregnancy. Recommendations about pregnancy for women who are either mildly affected or severely affected are straightforward. For the woman with moderately compromised pulmonary status (i.e., FVC under 50 to 60 percent of predicted), an overall assessment of the clinical situation is recommended, although no firm guidelines can be given. Increased incidence of fetal prematurity is noted in women with a pregravid FVC below 50 percent of predicted. Frequent use of antibiotics is unavoidable, and the teratogenic risk of many antibiotics is unknown. Despite this theoretical risk, good maternal and fetal health depend on aggressive management of pulmonary exacerbations, including use of antibiotics. Management of the gravid patient with CF is best accomplished in a CF center that has a program in high-risk obstetrics.

For men with CF who opt for MESA and for women with CF who are contemplating pregnancy, most offspring are obligate heterozygotes for CF. These offspring need to be counseled that their risk of having a child with CF is about 1 in 50 if the genotype of the spouse is not known. Although genetic testing of children from affected parents is not recommended, they should receive genetic counseling on reaching adolescence. Parents with CF also need to consider the ethical issues of a premature parental death and its effect on the family.

Discovery of the CF gene in 1989 led to the hope that prenatal diagnosis would eventually decrease the incidence of the disease. However, affected families are choosing either not to test at-risk pregnancies or, if tested and found to be affected, to continue the pregnancy.

PROGNOSIS

A comprehensive treatment program for CF has unequivocally improved the overall survival of patients. Thirty years ago, the median survival was only a few years of age; currently, it is about 30 years. The average duration of life seems to be approaching a plateau. An important determinant of the natural history of CF is the severity of the pulmonary disease and the rate at which it progresses.

In the future, pharmacologic approaches to the basic defect in CF may offer treatment alternatives or additional benefit to the anticipated use of directed gene therapy. For example, methylxanthine derivatives, amrinone, and milrinone have been shown to increase the chloride conductance of cells with the ΔF508 mutation by increasing intracellular levels of cAMP. Further understanding of the processing and function of CFTR should lead to additional, potentially useful therapies. Finally, since inflammation plays a critical role in the pulmonary pathophysiology of the disease, efforts have been directed at decreasing airway inflammation. The approaches are both pharmacologic (e.g., use of ibuprofen and prednisone) and physiologic (e.g., prevention of *Pseudomonas* binding to airway cells and immunization against *Pseudomonas*).

Improvements in gene transfer technology represent an important future direction in CF. Because the disease is inherited as an autosomal recessive trait, only one normal copy of the gene needs to be provided to cells for correction.

Progress toward cure of CF will require a multidisciplinary approach. The momentum gained from recent improvements in our understanding of basic pathogenetic mechanisms provides a basis for realistic optimism that specific therapy will result in better outcomes for patients with CF.

186   PART TWO   OBSTRUCTIVE LUNG DISEASES

BIBLIOGRAPHY

Albelda SM, Wiewrodt R, Zuckerman JB: Gene therapy for lung disease: hype or hope? *Ann Intern Med* 132:649–60, 2000.

Fuchs HJ, Borowitz DS, Christiansen DH, et al: Effect of aerosolized recombinant human DNase on exacerbations of respiratory symptoms and on pulmonary function in patients with cystic fibrosis. *N Engl J Med* 331:637–673, 1994.

Kerem E, Reisman J, Corey M, et al: Prediction of mortality in patients with cystic fibrosis. *N Engl J Med* 326:1187–1191, 1992.

Kotloff RM, Zuckerman JB: Lung transplantation for cystic fibrosis: Special considerations. *Chest* 109:787–798, 1996.

Ramsey BW: Management of pulmonary disease in patients with cystic fibrosis. *N Engl J Med* 335:179–188, 1996.

Riordan JR, Rommens JM, Kerem B, et al: Identification of the cystic fibrosis gene: Cloning and characterization of the complementary DNA. *Science* 245:1066–1073, 1989.

Rosenfeld MA, Collins FS: Gene therapy for cystic fibrosis. *Chest* 109:241–252, 1996.

Rubim BK: Emerging therapies for cystic fibrosis lung disease. *Chest* 115:1120–1126, 1999.

Wine JJ: The genesis of cystic fibrosis lung disease. *J Clin Invert* 103:309–312, 1999.

13 | Bronchiolitis*

Lisa M. Bellini and Michael A. Grippi

INTRODUCTION

Bronchiolitis is an inflammatory reaction that follows damage to the bronchiolar epithelium of the small conducting airways. Subsequent healing leads to excessive proliferation of granulation tissue within the airway walls, lumen, or both. Depending on disease stage, the repair process may cause narrowing and distortion of the small airways (constrictive bronchiolitis) or complete obliteration (bronchiolitis obliterans).

CLASSIFICATION

Bronchiolitis refers to a broad spectrum of histopathologic processes. *Bronchiolitis obliterans* is characterized by polypoid obliteration of the lumen of bronchioles without involvement of the distal lung parenchyma by inflammation or organizing pneumonia—i.e., constrictive bronchiolitis. *Bronchiolitis obliterans organizing pneumonia* (BOOP) is characterized by intraluminal polyps in the respiratory bronchioles, alveolar ducts, and alveolar spaces accompanied by organizing pneumonia in the more distal parenchyma—i.e., a "proliferative" bronchiolitis. Idiopathic BOOP is also referred to as *cryptogenic organizing pneumonia*. Clinical and histopathologic classification schemes are useful in defining cases of bronchiolitis (Table 13-1).

PATHOGENESIS

A similar sequence of events may lead to both histopathologic patterns of bronchiolitis. Differences appear to relate to type, extent, and severity of the initial insult and predominant site of the injury (bronchioles, alveolar ducts, or both). In some diseases associated with bronchiolitis, varying degrees of both proliferative and constrictive bronchiolitis are found.

In general, "proliferative" bronchiolitis appears to be a common "early" lesion that may resolve completely or partly. An initial alveolitis is seen, followed by fibroblast proliferation and formation of Masson bodies, polypoid buds, and extracellular matrix projecting into the lumina of respiratory bronchioles, alveolar ducts, and alveoli. In constrictive bronchiolitis, airway epithelial injury and destruction are followed by neutrophil-rich inflammation. Persistence of injury may lead to progression to a less reversible state, manifest by intramural and intraluminal fibrosis. Repair results in the characteristic obliterative bronchiolar lesions.

---

*Edited from Chap. 54, "Bronchiolitis," by King TE Jr. In: *Fishman's Pulmonary Diseases and Disorders,* 3d ed., edited by Fishman AP, Elias JA, Fishman JA, Grippi MA, Kaiser LR, Senior RM. New York, McGraw-Hill, 1998, pp 825–848. For fuller discussion of topics dealt with in this chapter, the reader is referred to the original text, as noted above.

TABLE 13-1 Comparison of Key Pathologic, Radiologic, and Physiologic Features in Proliferative and Constrictive Bronchiolitis

Feature	Proliferative Bronchiolitis	Constrictive Bronchiolitis
Histopathologic manifestations	Common finding Nonspecific reparative reaction to bronchiolar injury Organizing intraluminal exudate Most prominent in alveolar ducts Inflammatory changes in surrounding alveolar walls Foamy macrophages in alveoli	Very uncommon finding Obliterans not a constant feature Variety of histologic changes: bronchiolar inflammation to progressive concentric fibrosis; smooth-muscle hyperplasia, bronchioloectasia with mucous stasis; distortion and fibrosis of small airway walls with bronchial metaplasia extending onto peribronchiolar alveolar septa Follicular bronchitis (lymphoid hyperplasia) Cellular bronchiolitis Diffuse panbronchiolitis
Radiographic abnormalities	Bilateral patchy airspace opacities Interstitial opacities Small rounded opacities Opacities may be recurrent and migratory	May be normal Progressive increase in lung volume on serial radiographs HRCT scan may show marked heterogeneity of lung density
Pulmonary function	Restrictive defect (a mixed pattern may be seen)	Obstructive defect with hyperinflation
Clinical syndromes	Cryptogenic organizing pneumonia (idiopathic BOOP) Collagen vascular disease (e.g., rheumatoid arthritis, dermatomyositis, SLE) Organizing acute infection (especially influenza or *Nocardia asteroides*, *Mycoplasma*, *Pneumocystis carinii*, *Legionella pneumophila*, cytomegalovirus, or HIV infection) Chronic eosinophilic pneumonia	Allograft recipients (bone marrow, heart-lung, lung) Collagen vascular disease (especially rheumatoid arthritis) Postinfectious (especially respiratory syncytial virus, adenovirus, influenza, parainfluenza, *Mycoplasma*) Inhaled toxins (e.g., nitrogen dioxide, sulfur dioxide, ammonia, chlorine, phosgene)

	Hypersensitivity pneumonitis	Drugs (e.g., penicillamine, lomustine)
	Organizing diffuse alveolar damage/ARDS	Cigarette smoke
	Vasculitides, especially Wegener's	Mineral dust airway disease (asbestosis, silica,
	granulomatosis	iron oxide, aluminum oxide, talc, mica, and coal)
	Organ transplantation (rare)	Idiopathic
	Drug-induced reactions (hexamethonium,	Hypersensitivity reactions
	L-tryptophan, busulfan, free-base cocaine, gold,	
	cephalosporin,sulfasalazine, amiodarone,	
	acebutolol, sulindac)	
	Other uncommon associations: chronic	
	thyroiditis, ulcerative colitis, irradiation	
	pneumonitis, aspiration pneumonitis, distal to	
	bronchial obstruction, "obstructive pneumonitis,"	
	chronic heart or renal failure, common variable	
	immunodeficiency syndrome	
Natural history	Corticosteroid-responsive and usually reversible	Relatively corticosteroid-unresponsive and
		usually progressive with the development of
		irreversible airflow obstruction and air trapping

KEY: HRCT, high-resolution computed tomography; BOOP, bronchiolitis obliterans organizing pneumonia; SLE, systemic lupus erythematosus; ARDS, adult respiratory distress syndrome.
SOURCE: King TE Jr: Bronchiolitis. *Clin Chest Med* 14:607–772, 1993.

ETIOLOGIES

Etiologic categories of bronchiolitis syndromes include inhalational injuries, infections, connective tissue disorders, complications of organ transplantation, and idiopathic causes.

Inhalational Injury

Toxic gas inhalation rarely causes bronchiolitis, with or without obliterans. The concentration of the agent, duration and route of exposure, pattern of breathing, solubility and biologic reactivity of the agent, and biologic susceptibility of the individual determine the distribution and extent of the lung injury. Oxides of nitrogen are the most common and best-described etiologic agents. *Silo filler's disease* is caused by exposure to nitrogen dioxide (NO_2) and nitrogen tetroxide. NO_2 is relatively insoluble. After inhalation, the gas reaches the periphery of the lung, where it combines with water to form nitric and nitrous acids and nitric oxide—powerful oxidants capable of causing severe tissue injury.

During milder but acute exposures, upper airway and visual disturbances, cough, dyspnea, fatigue, cyanosis, vomiting, hemoptysis, hypoxemia, vertigo, somnolence, headache, emotional difficulties, and loss of consciousness are observed. Findings typically resolve within hours, but they may persist for several weeks; complete recovery without obvious sequelae is usually observed. At higher concentrations of exposure, pulmonary edema may arise. Patients may be asymptomatic at the time of exposure, only later (in 3 to 30 h) to develop the clinical picture of severe acute respiratory distress syndrome (ARDS). Recovery without long-term sequelae is usual, but death may occur at this stage. In the acute phase, methemoglobinemia is sometimes seen.

Occasionally, 2 to 6 weeks following exposure, a new onset of clinical illness may be seen. Progressive dyspnea, cough, tachypnea, crackles, and mild hypoxemia are noted. Widespread proliferative bronchiolitis is found, especially in those with preceding pulmonary edema; however, these findings may occur as the initial manifestation of previous exposure. Restrictive or obstructive pulmonary function abnormalities may be seen. The radiographic pattern ranges from a normal to a miliary or discretely nodular pattern characteristic of bronchiolitis obliterans. Occasionally, only pulmonary hyperinflation is seen.

Treatment of patients exposed to NO_2 (or other toxic gases) includes observation in the hospital for 48 h, followed by weekly or biweekly evaluations for 6 to 8 weeks. If respiratory dysfunction occurs, treatment with corticosteroids is started immediately and continued for at least 8 weeks. Corticosteroids are useful in the management of both acute (pulmonary edema) and late (bronchiolitis obliterans) phases. Bronchodilators are occasionally helpful; methemoglobinemia is treated using methylene blue. The prognosis is generally good.

Sulfur dioxide, chlorine gas, "smoke inhalation" or inhalation burns, hydrogen chloride, ammonia, phosgene, and chloropicrin produce a disease with clinical, physiologic, and radiographic manifestations similar to those described for NO_2 exposure.

Respiratory bronchiolitis may be found secondary to exposure to inorganic mineral dusts, including asbestos, silica, iron oxide, aluminum oxide, several different sheet silicates, and coal. The development of an obstructive rather than restrictive pattern is increasingly recognized in subjects with inorganic mineral dust exposure. Pathologically, these lesions are characterized by fibrosis in small airway walls and occasionally in alveolar ducts. Abnormalities are seen in nonsmokers but occur most commonly in heavily exposed workers who are cigarette smokers. The pathogenesis is unclear, but a synergistic role for cigarette smoking appears likely.

Bronchiolar lesions are seen in essentially all cases of hypersensitivity pneumonitis. The bronchioles contain granulomas within their walls or lumina, or they show tufts of granulation tissue, as seen in bronchiolitis obliterans. A reversible restrictive process is the most common physiologic abnormality. However, small airway dysfunction may be present in patients with early hypersensitivity pneumonitis. As the disease progresses, either obstructive or restrictive physiology may arise, depending on the predominant histopathologic process present.

Infection

Infection is the most common cause of acute bronchiolitis, although infectious causes are more frequent in children than adults. Acute viral bronchiolitis is common in infants and young children. Pathogens include respiratory syncytial virus (approximately one-third of cases); parainfluenza virus types 1, 2, and 3 (approximately one-third of cases); adenoviruses; influenza A and B; *Mycoplasma pneumoniae;* measles; and whooping cough (*Bordetella pertussis*).

The usual presentation is mild coryza and sneezing followed in several days by cough, dyspnea, tachypnea, tachycardia, fever, chest wall retractions, sibilant and sonorous rales, expiratory wheezing, and, in severe cases, cyanosis. The chest radiograph may be normal or show hyperinflation with increased bronchial markings. Subsegmental consolidation and collapse may be seen. A pattern similar to that of diffuse interstitial pneumonia, often in association with hyperinflation, is seen. Some patients demonstrate a diffuse nodular or reticulonodular pattern, whereas others may show patchy alveolar or ground-glass opacities. High-resolution computed tomography (HRCT) is useful in ruling out other diagnoses, especially bronchiectasis. Tests of lung function may be normal. However, obstructive changes with air trapping can often be documented. Resting hypoxemia is frequently present. Open lung biopsy is the "gold standard" for diagnosis; depending on the stage at which the biopsy is obtained, findings consistent with proliferative bronchiolitis ("early"), constrictive bronchiolitis ("late"), or both may be seen. Treatment includes supplemental oxygen, adequate hydration, bronchodilators, antibiotics, antiviral agents, and corticosteroids; mechanical ventilation is rarely required.

Recovery in a few days or weeks is usual. Whether or not bronchiolitis in infancy predisposes to asthma or chronic obstructive pulmonary disease (COPD) is unproved. *Swyer-James* (MacLeod) *syndrome*—unilateral hyperlucent lung—is a long-term complication of bronchiolitis in children, especially after adenoviral infection occurring in infancy. The chest radiograph demonstrates lobar or unilateral hyperlucent lung; normal or reduced volume of the affected lung is noted on full inspiration. Severe airway obstruction occurs during expiration. HRCT is the procedure of choice for identifying the characteristic changes in Swyer-James syndrome. The syndrome should be distinguished from congenital absence of the pulmonary artery, pulmonary artery occlusion, partial obstruction of a lobar or main bronchus, and congenital lobar emphysema.

Acute bronchiolitis in older children and young adults has been associated primarily with *M. pneumoniae;* however, a number of other viruses (e.g., respiratory syncytial virus, especially in the elderly) and bacterial agents have been implicated. Most patients have a history of an upper respiratory tract illness that precedes the onset of dyspnea with exertion, cough, tachypnea, fever, and wheezing. A number of adults have developed an acute or subacute diffuse ventilatory obstruction that has occasionally been fatal.

Connective Tissue Disorders

The clinical manifestations of bronchiolitis complicating connective tissue disorders are varied.

In rheumatoid arthritis, three bronchiolar syndromes have been observed: constrictive bronchiolitis, BOOP, and follicular bronchiolitis.

Constrictive bronchiolitis affects primarily middle-aged women with long-standing seropositive disease. Clinical findings include abrupt onset of dyspnea and dry cough, inspiratory crackles, and a midinspiratory "squeak." The chest radiograph is typically normal. HRCT usually excludes the presence of bronchiectasis. Pulmonary function studies reveal airflow obstruction and normal pulmonary compliance. Hypoxemia and respiratory alkalosis are observed. The rapid progression of obstruction is atypical for COPD. Treatment with antibiotics and bronchodilators is ineffective. Corticosteroid therapy appears effective in some patients. Intravenous cyclophosphamide and oral prednisone have been suggested. The prognosis is poor, with early deaths reported.

In some patients with bronchiolar disease complicating rheumatoid arthritis, BOOP is the predominant finding. The prognosis may be worse than for those with constrictive bronchiolitis; some patients develop a rapidly progressive, fatal form of pneumonia. In others, "follicular bronchitis" may be seen. This entity also occurs in Sjögren's syndrome, juvenile rheumatoid arthritis, immunodeficiency syndromes, familial lung disorders, chronic infection, and a heterogeneous group of patients with a hypersensitivity-type reaction. A positive rheumatoid factor is present, often in high titers (1:640 to 1:2560). The chest film shows bilateral reticulonodular opacities. Hypoxemia, hypocapnia, and a widened alveolar-arterial oxygen gradient are seen. Both obstructive and restrictive patterns have been identified by spirometry; the latter predominates. In almost all cases, a concentric inflammatory infiltrate of lymphocytes and plasma cells surrounds the bronchiole. The bronchiolar lumen is often compressed into a slit-like or fish-mouth shape. Some have suggested that follicular bronchiolitis may be the precursor of interstitial lymphoid pneumonia or pseudolymphoma. Treatment with corticosteroids has yielded variable results.

The role of penicillamine therapy in producing bronchiolitis obliterans in patients with rheumatoid arthritis is unclear. Most patients with penicillamine-associated bronchiolitis are women who never smoked. Breathlessness and cough begin within 3 to 14 months after initiation of the drug. Radiographic abnormalities are unusual except for mild hyperinflation. Pulmonary function abnormalities are characteristically obstructive. Lung biopsy reveals a concentric, constrictive form of bronchiolar obstruction. Death from progressive respiratory failure occurs in one-third of patients. Bronchiolitis obliterans has not been reported in other diseases treated with penicillamine. Although conclusive proof of an association between bronchiolitis obliterans and penicillamine therapy is lacking, when confronted with a dyspneic patient with rheumatoid arthritis on penicillamine therapy, one should stop the drug, consider open lung biopsy, and then administer corticosteroids to prevent disease progression.

Bronchiolitis in the other connective tissue disorders is uncommon. Secondary BOOP has been reported as a rare complication of Sjögren's syndrome. There have been few reports of obliterative bronchiolitis and BOOP complicating systemic lupus erythematosus. Clinically significant small airway disease is not frequently found in nonsmokers with progressive systemic sclerosis, even in the presence of interstitial pulmonary involvement; however, focal lymphoid hyperplasia (follicular bronchiolitis) may be seen. BOOP may occur de novo in patients with polymyositis or dermatomyositis. The pulmonary lesion is responsive to corticosteroid therapy.

Organ Transplantation

Progressive airflow obstruction secondary to bronchiolitis obliterans is one of the most frequent noninfectious posttransplant respiratory complications.

Following allogeneic bone marrow transplantation, cases of bronchiolitis obliterans appear after the first 100 days, usually in the setting of chronic graft-versus-host disease (GVHD). Cough, dyspnea, scattered wheezes, and expiratory "squeaks" are noted. The chest radiograph may show diffuse interstitial infiltrates or hyperinflation. In approximately 80 percent of cases, the lung fields are normal. Pneumothoraces may complicate the course of advanced disease. HRCT can reveal lobular or segmental areas of lung attenuation associated with narrowing of pulmonary vessels. The attenuation is presumed to represent areas of air trapping and oligemia. Pulmonary function testing shows a new, largely irreversible obstructive pattern. The diffusing capacity is reduced; hypoxemia is common. The appropriate treatment of bronchiolitis obliterans associated with bone marrow transplantation is questionable. In most cases, bronchodilators and corticosteroids have not improved airflow limitation. Furthermore, use of immunosuppressive agents for the treatment of chronic GVHD has had no consistent beneficial effect on pulmonary function. The prognosis is variable. A significant number of reported patients have had progressive or persistent disease; many have died secondary to respiratory failure (40 to 65 percent of subjects). Increasing recognition, early treatment, and the introduction of cyclosporine have resulted in a reduction of the incidence of posttransplant obstructive airway disease.

Bronchiolitis obliterans not uncommonly complicates both heart-lung and lung transplantation. The incidence ranges from 60 to 70 percent at greater than 5 years and is similar among all patients groups—i.e., heart-lung, single lung, and bilateral lung transplants. The major risk factor is frequent or severe episodes of acute rejection. Other risks include HLA-mismatching, cytomegalovirus (CMV) infection, and initial airway ischemia. Patients develop cough productive of mucopurulent sputum and progressive dyspnea. Transbronchial lung biopsies rarely aid in diagnosis, which rests on clinical criteria. *Bronchiolitis obliterans syndrome* (BOS) is defined as an otherwise unspecified fall in the FEV_1 below 80 percent of peak posttransplant values. No clearly useful treatment protocol has been established. Efforts at preventing repeated episodes of rejection seem most important. Prompt diagnosis and treatment of acute rejection and any infectious complications are paramount. Management of chronic rejection includes augmentation of immunosuppression acutely using cytolytic therapy (ATGAM, OKT3) or pulse steroids, and chronically by converting from cyclosporine to tacrolimus. However, evidence suggests that this merely slows the rate of decline in lung function and rarely results in its recovery. The only definitive therapy is retransplantation. This option should be reserved for fully ambulatory, nutritionally replete candidates, given the serious ethical concerns about retransplanation in an era of severe organ shortage.

Idiopathic Causes

Cryptogenic adult bronchiolitis is an uncommon syndrome of unclear pathogenesis. The disorder is diagnosed largely by exclusion and requires a high index of suspicion. Most patients are middle-aged women with nonproductive cough and dyspnea evolving over 6 to 24 months. A history of cigarette smoking, chronic sputum production, frequent chest infections, wheezing, known connective-tissue disorder, and immunoglobulin deficiency are absent. Physical findings are generally unremarkable, and chest radiographic findings are normal or nonspecific. Hyperinflation may be the only abnormality noted. HRCT scanning is normal or shows airway dilatation. Pulmonary function testing usually demonstrates increased lung volumes, airflow limitation, and reduced diffusing capacity. Resting hypoxemia may be present. Exercise testing shows gas exchange abnormalities and elevated V_D/V_T. Early treatment with corticosteroids may be beneficial.

Respiratory bronchiolitis–interstitial lung disease (RB-ILD) has been recognized as a distinct clinical syndrome found in current or previous cigarette smokers. This disease may be confused with chronic diffuse interstitial fibrosis, desquamative interstitial pneumonia, and eosinophilic granuloma of the lung (pulmonary histiocytosis X). The last two disorders also develop almost exclusively in male cigarette smokers in their third or fourth decade of life. The average exposure is more than 30 pack-years of cigarette smoking. Dyspnea and cough are the usual symptoms. The chest radiograph shows diffuse fine reticulonodular infiltrates. Diffuse or patchy ground-glass opacities or fine nodules are found on HRCT. Pulmonary function may be normal; however, a mixed obstructive-restrictive pattern is most commonly found; a normal or slightly reduced $D_{L_{CO}}$ is frequently present. Hypoxemia may be present at rest or with exercise. Inflammation in the membranous and respiratory bronchioles is characteristic, and tan-brown pigmented macrophages within respiratory bronchioles, neighboring alveolar ducts, and alveoli dominate the pathologic findings [a desquamative interstitial pneumonia (DIP)-like reaction]. Treatment centers on smoking cessation; corticosteroids appear to be useful.

Cryptogenic organizing pneumonia (COP) or idiopathic BOOP occurs equally in males and females, with onset usually in the fifth or sixth decade. Cigarette smoking is not a precipitating factor. Nonproductive cough and dyspnea follow a flu-like illness, with fever, malaise, and fatigue. Significant weight loss may be observed. Physical examination reveals inspiratory crackles; wheezing is rare and is usually present in conjunction with crackles. Clubbing is rare. Leukocytosis is seen in approximately half of patients; the erythrocyte sedimentation rate is elevated. Autoantibodies are usually negative or only slightly positive. The chest radiograph shows bilateral, diffuse alveolar opacities in the presence of normal lung volumes; the distribution of the opacities may be peripheral and similar to that in chronic eosinophilic pneumonia. Honeycombing may be seen as a late manifestation in the few patients who have progressive disease. CT shows patchy airspace consolidation, ground-glass opacities, small nodular opacities, and bronchial wall thickening and dilation. The patchy opacities occur more frequently in the periphery of the lung and are often in the lower lung zones. Pulmonary function testing usually shows a restrictive defect, although lung function is occasionally normal. Gas exchange abnormalities and exercise-related hypoxemia are common. The histopathologic lesion characteristic of COP is proliferative bronchiolitis with organizing pneumonia. An open or thoracoscopic lung biopsy is recommended to confirm COP and rule out other disorders. Once the characteristic findings of proliferative bronchiolitis are confirmed, the clinician must ensure that a thorough search has been performed to rule out the many other diagnostic considerations, including bacterial pneumonia, hypersensitivity pneumonitis, chronic eosinophilic pneumonia, viral infection, drug reactions, and connective-tissue disorders. COP is a diagnosis of exclusion.

Treatment of COP consists of high-dose oral corticosteroid therapy—e.g., prednisone at 1 to 1.5 mg/kg per day, not to exceed 100 mg daily. (High-dose parenteral corticosteroid therapy—e.g., methylprednisolone, 125 to 250 mg intravenously every 6 h for 3 to 5 days, has been recommended as initial treatment for patients with rapidly progressive COP.) After 4 to 8 weeks of treatment, if the patient's condition is stable or improved, the dose is gradually tapered to 0.5 to 1 mg/kg per day for the ensuing 4 to 6 weeks. The prednisone is then gradually tapered off after 3 to 6 months. Therapy is reinstituted aggressively with any sign of recurrence. If the patient's condition deteriorates despite corticosteroid therapy, the addition of a cytotoxic agent should be considered while low-dose (0.25 mg/kg per day) therapy with prednisone is continued. Cyclophosphamide in a single daily dose of 1 to 2 mg/kg has been used, although the optimal dose in COP is unknown. A daily dose of 50 mg may be used at the start of treatment; the dose is slowly increased over 2 to 4 weeks. Maximal dose should not exceed 150 mg per day. A trial of at least 3 to 6 months is needed to ensure an adequate opportunity for clinical response. Complete clinical recovery, physiologic improvement, and normalization of the chest film are seen in two-thirds of patients. Approximately one-third demonstrate persistent disease. In general, clinical improvement is rapid, within several days or a few weeks. Occasionally, recovery is quite dramatic. Relapses occur commonly when corticosteroids are withdrawn after 1 to 3 months. Most patients who relapse show improvement when re-treated with corticosteroids.

DIFFUSE PANBRONCHIOLITIS

Diffuse panbronchiolitis is relatively common in Japan, China, and Korea but appears to be rare in other parts of the world. A familial occurrence has been described. Environmental factors also appear important, since the disorder is very uncommon in persons of Asian ancestry living abroad. The male-to-female ratio is 2:1; peak incidence is between the fourth and seventh decades. Chronic sinusitis is present in 75 to 100 percent of cases, and sinus symptoms may precede chest symptoms by years or decades. Cough, purulent sputum production, exertional dyspnea, wheezing, and crackles are the most common clinical manifestations. Cigarette smoking or occupational exposures have not been shown to be predisposing factors.

A persistent, marked elevation of serum cold agglutinins has been observed; mycoplasmal antibody titers are negative. Rheumatoid factor may be elevated. The chest radiograph often reveals diffuse, small nodular opacities up to 2 mm in diameter. Hyperinflation may also be present. On HRCT, the nodular shadows are distributed in a centrilobular fashion. Inhomogeneity in lung density may be apparent as a result of peripheral air trapping. Bronchiectasis may be prominent in advanced disease. Pulmonary function tests reveal marked obstruction; rarely, a restrictive ventilatory defect is present. Arterial blood gases show hypoxemia, with or without hypercapnia. The diffusing capacity is variably reduced. Lung biopsy reveals thickening of the walls of the respiratory bronchiole, infiltration with lymphocytes, plasma cells, and histiocytes and extension of the inflammatory changes into peribronchiolar tissue.

Optimal therapy is unclear. Low-dose erythromycin (200 to 600 mg a day) is adequate for most patients. Corticosteroids are utilized commonly in treatment regimens, but there is no evidence supporting their efficacy. Nonsteroidal anti-inflammatory drugs, by altering airway epithelial ion and water transport, may have a role in controlling the bronchorrhea associated with this disease. Routine use of bronchodilators and treatment of coexisting sinus disease may be helpful. The disease progresses insidiously, and the prognosis is often poor, with fatalities because of repeated respiratory infections (especially due to *Pseudomonas aeruginosa*).

PRIMARY DIFFUSE HYPERPLASIA OF PULMONARY NEUROENDOCRINE CELLS

Primary diffuse hyperplasia of pulmonary neuroendocrine cells is characterized by diffuse hyperplasia and dysplasia of neuroendocrine cells of the distal bronchi and bronchioles. The disorder is seen primarily in women in their fifth or sixth decade. Clinical findings include nonproductive cough and longstanding dyspnea (usually of more than 10 years' duration). All reported cases are in never-smokers. The chest examination is unrevealing. Chest radiographs show diffuse reticulonodular opacities in most cases; multiple nodules are seen in a few cases. HRCT demonstrates diffuse small airway thickening, with patchy areas of hyperlucency suggesting air trapping. The most common physiologic abnormality is irreversible airflow obstruction. Open or thoracoscopic lung biopsy is required for diagnosis. Histopathologic changes include diffuse hyperplasia and dysplasia of neuroendocrine cells, numerous neuroepithelial bodies, prominent carcinoid tumorlets, and even typical carcinoid tumors in the distal bronchi and bronchioles. The pathogenesis, treatment, and prognosis of the syndrome are unknown. Most patients have a relatively benign course characterized by many years of symptoms.

BIBLIOGRAPHY

Alasaly K, Muller N, Ostrow D, et al: Cryptogenic organizing pneumonia: A report of 25 cases and a review of the literature. *Medicine* 74:201–211, 1995.

Clark JG, Crawford SW, Madtes DK, Sullivan KM: Obstructive lung disease after allogeneic marrow transplantation: Clinical presentation and course. *Ann Intern Med* 111:368–376, 1989.

Colby TV, Myers JL: The clinical and histologic spectrum of bronchiolitis obliterans including bronchiolitis obliterans organizing pneumonia (BOOP). *Semin Respir Med* 13:119–133, 1992.

Epler GR, Colby TV, McLoud TC, et al: Bronchiolitis obliterans organizing pneumonia. *N Engl J Med* 312:152–158, 1985.

Izumi T, Kitaichi M, Nishimura K, Nagai S: Bronchiolitis obliterans organizing pneumonia: Clinical features and differential diagnosis. *Chest* 102:715–719, 1992.

Katzenstein AL, Myers JL: Nonspecific interstitial pneumonia and the other idiopathic interstitial pneumonias: Classification and diagnostic criteria. *Am J Surg Pathol* 24:1–3, 2000.

Lazor R, Vandevenne A, Pelletier A, et al: Cryptogenic organizing pneumonia. Characteristics of relapses in a series of 48 patients. The Groupe d'Etudes et de Recherche sur les Maladles "Orphelines" Pulmonaires (GERM"O"P). *Am J Respir Crit Care Med* 162 (Part 1):571–577, 2000.

Verleden GM: Bronchiolitis obliterans syndrome after lung transplantation: Medical treatment. *Monaldi Arch Chest Dis* 55:140–145, 2000.

14 | Bullous Diseases of the Lung*

Lisa M. Bellini and Michael A. Grippi

INTRODUCTION

A *bulla* is a large, air-containing space within the lung parenchyma resulting from destruction, dilatation, and confluence of airspaces distal to terminal bronchioles. Bullae are larger than 1 cm in diameter and are composed of attenuated and compressed parenchyma. They are seen in emphysema ("bullous emphysema"), usually of the acinar (paraseptal) variety; in pulmonary fibrosis complicating the late stages of sarcoidosis or pneumoconiosis; and in "vanishing lung" syndrome. *Bullous lung disease* refers to multiple bullae in otherwise normal lungs; its pathogenesis is distinct from that of chronic obstructive pulmonary disease (COPD) complicated by bullae.

Bullae are distinguished from blebs and cysts (Table 14-1). A *bleb* is an accumulation of air between the layers of the visceral pleura. The thin covering of a bleb predisposes to rupture and entry of air into the pleural space. *Cysts* are epithelium lined cavities that resemble bullae radiographically.

CLASSIFICATION

Bullae are classified into three main types. The thin-walled *type I bulla,* which predominates in the apices (presumably due to greater mechanical stresses and more negative intrapleural pressure at the apices) and along the lingula and middle lobe edges, is characterized by a narrow neck that connects the bulla with the pulmonary parenchyma. Type I bullae may be caused by overinflation of a region of abnormal lung parenchyma and often occur in association with paraseptal emphysema. The *type II bulla* arises from the

TABLE 14-1 Characteristics of Blebs, Bullae, and Cysts

	Bleb	Bulla	Cyst
Site	Within visceral pleura	Arises within secondary lobule	Lung parenchyma or mediastinum
Size	1–2 cm	1 cm to >75% of a lung	2–10 cm
Lining	Elastic laminae of the pleura	Connective tissue septa	Epithelium
Associated condition	Spontaneous pneumothorax		Respiratory infection

*Edited from Chap. 55, "Bullous Diseases of the Lung," by Murphy DM, Fishman AP. In: *Fishman's Pulmonary Diseases and Disorders,* 3d ed., edited by Fishman AP, Elias JA, Fishman JA, Grippi MA, Kaiser LR, Senior RM. McGraw-Hill, New York, 1998, pp 849–866. For fuller discussion of topics dealt with in this chapter, the reader is referred to the original text, as noted above.

subpleural parenchyma and is characterized by a neck of panacinar emphysematous lung tissue. Its interior consists of emphysematous lung in which blood vessels are still present, and its outer walls are formed by pleura covered with intact mesothelial cells. Type II bullae predominate in the upper lobe, along the anterior surface of the middle lobe, and over the diaphragm. The *type III bulla* consists of slightly hyperinflated lung connected to the rest of the lung by a broad base that extends deep into the parenchyma. Type III bullae are believed to represent an atrophic form of emphysema.

PATHOGENESIS

Bullae originate in conjunction with emphysema of distal acini; cigarette smoking; scar formation, which traps areas of normal lung or enlarges airspaces by traction on surrounding intact alveoli or by retraction or shrinkage of the intact walls of adherent alveoli; intravenous drug use; chronic inflammation and destructive changes in the terminal and first-order respiratory bronchioles, causing overdistention of airspaces; and alpha$_1$-antitrypsin deficiency.

The most popular hypotheses regarding the development of bullous disease is that underlying paraseptal emphysema results in destruction of alveoli adjacent to connective tissue septa or the pleura, with small "bubbles" developing along the edges of the lung. Small bullae may be evident on computed tomography. Previously asymptomatic bullae may rupture, leading to spontaneous pneumothorax. Large bullae also cause lung parenchymal crowding. Very large airspaces can expand across the midline or even extend into the neck.

CLINICAL MANIFESTATIONS

Bullae may be asymptomatic or give rise to progressive dyspnea or chest pain. Marked dyspnea may occur with spontaneous pneumothorax or a sudden increase in the size of a bulla due to air trapping. Further reductions in expiratory flow can make chronic dyspnea worse. Physical findings usually reflect the underlying lung disease. Only infrequently do giant bullae become large enough to cause a localized decrease in or absence of breath sounds and the associated increase in resonance to percussion over the bulla.

Onset of fatigue and increased cough and sputum production herald infection in a bulla. Pleuritic chest pain is occasionally seen. Fever and leukocytosis are often not prominent, and Gram's stain of the sputum often shows only mixed flora without a predominant organism. An air-fluid level is usually seen on the chest radiograph. On occasion, infection of a bulla causes the bulla to disappear completely; more often, the air-fluid level persists for weeks or months after the infection has cleared.

RADIOLOGY

Routine chest radiography identifies only about 15 percent of bullae observed at autopsy. Bullae appear as areas of increased radiolucency sharply delineated by fine radiopaque lines that define their walls. These "hairline shadows" are composed of compressed and fused interlobular septa or pleura. The hairline shadows of bullae are to be distinguished from the thicker, sometimes irregular walls of a cavity. Distinction between bullae and cysts is more difficult; the presence of other radiologic signs of emphysema or fibrotic lung disorders favors the diagnosis of bullae over cysts.

The radiographic differential diagnosis of a localized air-fluid level includes an infected bulla, abscess, cavitary tuberculosis, fungal infection, cavitary lung carcinoma, hemorrhage within a bulla, and carcinoma arising from a bulla. If a bulla is located subpleurally, the presence of a fluid level occasionally prompts the mistaken diagnosis of a loculated hydropneumothorax. Computed tomography may be helpful in making the distinction. When locules within the bulla fill with fluid, the bulla shows characteristic strands or septa, sometimes in a "stepladder" configuration; in contrast, a loculated hydrothorax shows no septa.

A chest radiograph taken during forced expiration may accentuate the presence of bullae because of air trapping, resulting in lack of decrease in size as the surrounding lung empties.

On computed tomography, bullae are identified as areas of hyperlucency that usually do not contain blood vessels and are confined by visible walls. High-resolution computed tomography shows that bullous emphysema occurs with both distal acinar (paraseptal) and centriacinar emphysema. Computed tomography has also shown that when bullae occur in the context of general emphysema, the main determinant of respiratory function is the severity of emphysema in the bulla-free parts of the lung.

Ventilation-perfusion lung scanning shows the crowded distribution of the pulmonary vasculature, as well as absence of, or marked diminution in, ventilation of bullae. A continuous ventilation scan often shows slow filling and emptying of bullae. Complete lack of communication between the airways and bullae is reflected in the absence of filling during all phases of the continuous ventilation scan.

PATHOPHYSIOLOGY

Patients with localized bullous disease may be good candidates for thoracic surgery, while those with bullae complicating obstructive airway disease are generally poor candidates owing to impaired pulmonary function. Hence, distinction of the two conditions is important.

Pulmonary function is generally normal as long as bullae occupy one-third or less of the volume of the lung. Expansion of a large bulla that crowds intervening normal lung may produce a restrictive pattern. The volume of air in the lungs can be estimated by computed tomography, body plethysmography, and closed-(helium dilution) or open-(nitrogen washout) circuit methods. The volume of air trapped in bullae is determined as the difference between the functional residual capacities determined plethysmographically and by open- or by closed-circuit methods (in which the inert gas fails to enter bullae).

As large bullae distend, they cause adjacent lung tissue to relax, followed by lung compression. The relaxation decreases airway radial traction and increases airway resistance. Bullectomy sometimes increases the lung's static recoil pressure and decreases airway resistance; in other instances, bullectomy decreases the lung's elastic recoil pressure.

In patients with a few circumscribed bullae but otherwise normal lungs, exercise testing (see Chap. 2) demonstrates a normal Pa_{O_2}, alveolar-arterial difference in P_{O_2}, V_D/V_T ratio, and $D_{L_{CO}}$. In patients in whom bullae are associated with panacinar emphysema, the alveolar-arterial difference in P_{O_2} is widened, both at rest and during exercise, and arterial hypoxemia occurs during exercise. Pa_{CO_2} tends to hover around the upper limits of normal at rest and during exercise. The V_D/V_T ratio is higher, and the steady-state diffusing capacity is reduced. Patients in whom bullae are associated with chronic bronchitis show a widened alveolar-arterial difference in P_{O_2} and an increased V_D/V_T ratio at rest. However, the decrease in arterial P_{O_2} during exercise is only modest, even though arterial Pa_{CO_2} at rest is abnormally high and increases further during exercise, indicating progressive alveolar hypoventilation. Findings consistent with widespread emphysema should discourage surgical consideration.

As a rule, pulmonary arterial pressure and blood flow at rest are within normal limits in bullous disease (the bullae act like "amputated" lung segments). However, during exercise, the volume of the vascular bed available for recruitment as cardiac output increases is limited, and pulmonary artery pressure may increase. When the extent of the pulmonary vascular bed has been severely limited by widespread bullous disease, pulmonary arterial pressure may be elevated both at rest and during exercise. Underlying pulmonary disease exaggerates the increment in pulmonary arterial pressure during exercise.

COMPLICATIONS

Complications of bullous disease include infection of the bulla, chest pain, hemorrhage, spontaneous pneumothorax, and lung cancer.

Infected bullae are rare. In most bullae, air-fluid levels are the result of peribullous pneumonitis. Airspace fluid is usually sterile and is often reabsorbed in association with shrinkage and complete resolution of the bulla. Chest pain is attributed to the overdistention of bullae; it may be retrosternal and angina-like. Hemoptysis may be massive and results from rupture of blood vessels within the walls of bullae. Pneumothorax can severely compromise the patient's ventilatory reserve in the setting of generalized emphysema. Risk of recurrence is generally higher (incidence of 50 percent) with pneumothorax due to rupture of a bulla than to rupture of a bleb. Patients with pneumothoraces due to ruptured bullae also tend to have prolonged air leaks and increased pleural and parenchymal infections.

Primary lung cancer has been reported to be associated with bullous lung disease. The higher incidence may be due to the more frequent occurrence of lung cancers in scars, which predispose to the development of bullae. Dystrophic changes in the lung parenchyma caused by bullous disease or persistence of potential inhaled carcinogens in poorly ventilated spaces may play pathogenetic roles.

MANAGEMENT

Asymptomatic bullae are managed expectantly. Smoking cessation is encouraged. Activities that could potentially result in the rupture of bullae (e.g., contact sports and scuba diving) are proscribed. Concurrent chronic bronchitis, asthma, and emphysema are managed accordingly.

Management of an infected bulla includes antibiotics chosen on the basis of sputum culture and Gram's stain results. Fiberoptic bronchoscopy may be helpful in obtaining microbiologic specimens. Direct sampling of fluid from within the bulla is rarely useful. Chest physiotherapy plays an adjunctive role. Treatment is prolonged, since poor drainage is associated with slow resolution. Most infected bullae eventually respond to medical therapy, although infected bullae with large amounts of fluid may require surgical intervention because of the risk of fluid "decanting" into the contralateral lung.

In general, patients with bullae complicating obstructive or fibrotic lung disease do not benefit from bullectomy and have a higher surgical mortality. However, in some patients with localized bullous disease who have well-preserved pulmonary function, surgical intervention may provide symptomatic relief, better exercise tolerance, and improved results on pulmonary function tests. The surgical outcome depends on the size and number of resected bullae, condition of the compressed lung, and status of the contralateral lung. Ventilation/perfusion scans and computed tomography can be helpful in preoperative assessment of the compressed lung.

Resection of bullae in bullous lung disease ought to be considered when the bullae are large enough to cause dyspnea or compress surrounding lung tissue, cause recurrent pneumothoraces, are infected and fail to respond to medical treatment, or cause acute respiratory insufficiency. In addition, bullae that become acutely distended, cause severe chest pain due to increasing size, or are associated with primary lung cancer ought to be considered for resection. Median sternotomy results in less postoperative morbidity than does standard thoracotomy and is appropriate for bilateral upper lobe bullae. As a rule, small wedge excisions or plications of large bullae have produced greater increments in expiratory flow than has lobectomy. Surgical approaches include laser ablation.

The size of a bulla is an important selection criterion in determining the outcome of surgery, as the best functional improvement occurs when the bulla constitutes 50 to 100 percent of the hemithorax. In such patients, postoperative increments in FEV_1 range from 50 to 200 percent. Good results are expected when the affected lung contributes little to overall ventilation, large volumes of trapped air exist, and there is crowding of normal lung parenchyma. Overall surgical mortality is about 1.5 percent; infection and respiratory failure are the most common causes of death. Sudden development of a contralateral pneumothorax or herniation of a bulla across the mediastinum are occasionally seen. Postoperative complication rates range between 14 and 44 percent. Not surprisingly, persistent air leaks and pleuropulmonary infections have been the major complications. The benefit usually lasts for about 5 years; there is no evidence that bullectomy hastens progression of the underlying emphysematous process.

BIBLIOGRAPHY

Champion JK, McKernan JB: Bilateral thoracoscopic stapled volume reduction for bullous vs. diffuse emphysema. *Surg Endosc* 12:338–41, 1998.

CIBA Guest Symposium: Terminology, definitions and classifications of chronic pulmonary emphysema and related conditions. *Thorax* 14:286, 1959.

Daniel TM, Wyatt, DA: Pneumothorax and bullous disease, in Kaiser LR, Daniel TM (eds), *Thoracoscopic Surgery*. Boston, Little, Brown, 1993, pp 85–96.

De Giacomo T, Venuta F, Rendina EA, et al. Video-assisted thoracoscopic treatment of giant bullae associated with emphysema. *Eur J Cardiothorac Surg.* 15:753–757, 1999.

DesLauriers J, Leblanc P: Management of bullous disease. *Chest Surg Clin North Am* 4:539, 1994.

Gould GA, Redpath AT, Ryan M, et al: Parenchymal emphysema measured by CT lung density correlates with lung functions in patients with bullous disease. *Eur Respir J* 6:698, 1993.

Klingman RR, Angelillo VA, DeMasters TR: Cystic and bullous lung disease. *Ann Thorac Surg* 52:576, 1991.

Nickoladze GD: Functional results of surgery for bullous emphysema. *Chest* 101:119, 1992.

Part Three | # OCCUPATIONAL AND ENVIRONMENTAL DISORDERS

15 | Occupational Lung Disorders: General Principles and Approaches*

Lynn T. Tanoue

CLASSIFICATION OF OCCUPATIONAL AND ENVIRONMENTAL LUNG DISEASE

Environmentally induced lung diseases can be classified according to several schemes. A given exposure (asbestos, cobalt, etc.) can cause more than a single disorder. It can also be helpful to classify occupational lung diseases by types of exposures that can cause lung disease, such as mineral dusts (asbestos, silica, coal), biologic factors (animal exposures, microbial agents), metals (beryllium, nickel, cobalt, aluminum), or inorganic gases (carbon monoxide, chlorine, nitrogen oxides). Additionally, identification of the type of industry potentially associated with respiratory diseases—such as mining, agriculture, forestry, or welding—may be important. Table 15-1 outlines classification by clinical presentation or disease.

While occupational and environmental exposures play an important role in many lung disorders, accurate estimates of the contribution of such factors to specific lung diseases are difficult to find. It is generally believed that underrecognition and underreporting of occupational lung diseases are widespread.[1] Although historically the pneumoconioses have been the most commonly diagnosed occupational lung diseases, occupational asthma has become the most prevalent occupational lung disease in developed countries.[2,3] Worldwide, silicosis remains the most common occupational lung disease.[4] In a few instances, such as the rare tumor mesothelioma, most cases can be attributed to occupational exposure to asbestos. However, the contribution of occupational and environmental factors to most other lung diseases is much harder to determine. For example, estimates of the proportion of lung cancers attributable to occupational exposures have ranged from 1 percent to over 40 percent,[5,6] and estimates of the prevalence of occupational asthma in adult asthmatics have ranged from 2 percent to over 20 percent.[7–9]

*Edited from Chap. 56, "Occupational Lung Disorders: General Principles and Approaches," by Redlich CA. In: *Fishman's Pulmonary Diseases and Disorders,* 3d ed., edited by Fishman AP, Elias JA, Fishman JA, Grippi MA, Kaiser LR, Senior RM. New York, McGraw-Hill, 1998, pp 867–876. For fuller discussion of the topics dealt with in this chapter, the reader is referred to the original text, as noted above.

TABLE 15-1 Classification of Occupational Lung Disorders

Major disease category	Representative causative agents
Upper respiratory tract irritation	Irritant gases, solvents
Airway disorders	
Occupational asthma	
Sensitization	
Low molecular weight	Diisocyanates, anhydrides, wood dusts
High molecular weight	Animal-derived allergens, latex
Irritant-induced, RADS	Irritant gases
Byssinosis	Cotton dust
Grain dust effects	Grain
Chronic bronchitis/COPD	Mineral dusts, coal
Acute inhalation injury	
Toxic pneumonitis	Irritant gases, metals
Metal fume fever	Metal oxides: zinc, copper
Polymer fume fever	Plastics
Smoke inhalation	Combustion products
Hypersensitivity pneumonitis	Bacteria, fungi, animal proteins
Infectious disorders	Tuberculosis, viruses, bacteria
Pneumoconioses	Asbestos, silica, coal, beryllium, cobalt
Malignancies	
Sinonasal cancer	Wood dust
Lung cancer	Asbestos, radon
Mesothelioma	Asbestos

KEY: RADS, reactive airway dysfunction syndrome; COPD, chronic obstructive pulmonary disease.

BASIC PRINCIPLES OF OCCUPATIONAL AND ENVIRONMENTAL LUNG DISEASE

Certain principles apply broadly to the full range of respiratory disorders caused by inhalational exposure to agents in the workplace or environment:

1. Most environmental and occupational lung diseases are difficult to distinguish from disorders of nonenvironmental origin. Few present with pathognomonic features. Since most lung disorders can be caused or exacerbated by environmental or occupational exposures, such triggers must be constantly sought in the evaluation and management of pulmonary disorders.
2. A given substance in the workplace or environment can cause more than one clinical or pathologic entity.
3. The etiology of many lung diseases may be multifactorial, and occupational factors may interact with other factors. For example, the risk of developing lung cancer in asbestos-exposed workers who smoke is much greater than that in those exposed to either asbestos or cigarettes alone.
4. The dose of exposure is an important determinant of the proportion of people affected or the severity of disease. Higher doses of exposure usually result in more affected individuals or greater disease severity. Dose generally correlates with severity in patients experiencing nonimmunologic direct toxicity, such as chemical toxic pneumonitis, asbestosis, or silicosis. In those with malignant or immune-mediated disorders, dose more commonly affects incidence than severity.

5. Individual differences in susceptibility to exposures do exist. Adverse effects may occur in some persons, while others with similar exposure are spared. Host factors that determine susceptibility to environmental agents are poorly understood but probably include both inherited, genetic factors and acquired factors such as diet and the presence of other lung diseases and other exposures.[10,11] Occupational diseases, especially immune-mediated processes such as chronic beryllium disease or low-molecular-weight occupational asthma, can occur or progress at low levels of exposure, even those below government-set exposure standards.[3,12]

6. The effects of a given occupational or environmental lung exposure occur after the exposure with a predictable latency interval. For acute diseases such as toxic pneumonitis, there is a short and usually predictable period between exposure and resultant clinical manifestations. This brief interval facilitates the recognition of a causal relationship between the exposure and the disease. When symptoms or signs are recurrent with repeated exposures, as with occupational asthma, this temporal relationship can help establish the diagnosis. For chronic diseases such as cancer or most pneumoconioses, long latency periods between the first exposure and subsequent clinical manifestations are common. Consequently, the patient's exposure to the offending agent(s) may have ceased long before the onset of disease, making the diagnosis of such diseases more challenging.

There are several compelling reasons to pursue the search for an occupational or environmental cause in all cases of pulmonary disease. First, knowledge of cause may affect patient management and prognosis and may prevent further disease progression in the affected person. Second, establishment of cause may have significant legal, financial, and social implications for the patient. Third, occupational and environmental lung diseases can also serve as important disease models. Fourth, the recognition of occupational and environmental risk factors can also have important public health and policy consequences.

ESTABLISHING A CAUSE

Diagnostic Criteria

To establish whether a lung disease has an occupational or environmental origin, it must first be defined and characterized; then the degree to which occupational or environmental exposures are causative or contributory must be determined. The following criteria are used to determine whether a disease is caused or exacerbated by agents in the workplace or environment:

1. The clinical presentation and workup are consistent with the diagnosis.
2. A causal relationship between the exposure and the diagnosed condition has been previously established or strongly suggested in the medical, epidemiologic, or toxicologic literature. Case series and disease cluster reports often play an important role in identifying potential occupational causes of lung disease. Such reports may provide impetus to proceed to more extensive epidemiologic studies focusing on establishing association and/or causality.[13]
3. There is sufficient exposure to cause the disease. Human data relating to toxic exposures are often limited. In such situations animal toxicologic studies can be helpful in determining the relationship between occupational

exposure and disease.[14] While extrapolation of the results of animal studies to human disease may be imperfect, important information about adverse medical effects related to exposures, dose-response relationships, and primary organ sites of toxicity can be obtained.
4. The details of the particular case, such as the temporal relationship between exposure and disease, are consistent with known information about the exposure-disease association.
5. There is no other more likely diagnosis.

In addition, for acute diseases such as occupational asthma, improvement away from the exposure and reproduction of the disease manifestations by reexposure to the suspected agent may provide compelling evidence to support the diagnosis.

CLINICAL APPROACH TO THE PATIENT

As noted above, there are two important phases in the workup of any patient with a potential occupational or environmental lung disease. First, as with any patient presenting with a potential disorder of the respiratory tract, its nature and extent must be defined and characterized regardless of the suspected origin. Although knowledge of exposures may guide the order of the diagnostic workup, it is crucial to establish the basic disorder before proceeding to investigate the etiology of the process. Second, the extent to which the disease or symptom complex is caused or exacerbated by an exposure at work or in the environment must be determined.

The initial approach to all such patients includes a detailed history, review of prior medical records, physical examination, appropriate laboratory testing, chest radiograph, and pulmonary function testing (PFT). Initial exposure information can be used to direct the sequence of the workup and to obviate unnecessary procedures when the diagnosis is fairly straightforward. If the initial evaluation does not fully explain the patient's symptoms, other tests are available to better characterize the nature and extent of the respiratory disorder, including computed chest tomography, cardiopulmonary exercise studies, nonspecific inhalation challenge, bronchoscopy, open lung biopsy, and various immunologic studies. However, few are specific for any given occupational or environmental diagnosis.

The Occupational and Environmental History

The occupational and environmental history is the single most useful tool in determining whether a respiratory problem may be related to an exposure.[8,15,16] A detailed occupational history includes a chronologic list of all jobs, including job title, a description of job activities, potential toxins at each job, and an assessment of the extent and duration of exposure, and is outlined in Table 15-2. Focus should be directed at the jobs and exposures of greatest concern. Such an approach can provide key information on whether exposure to one or more environmental agents has occurred, the magnitude and extent of the exposure, and the timing of the exposure in relationship to symptoms or the disease. A thorough description of the job process or work done is key. The length of time (hours to years) of exposure to the agent, the nature and use of personal protective equipment such as respirators, and a description of the ventilation and overall hygiene are all helpful in attempting to quantify exposure from the patient's history.

TABLE 15-2 Taking an Occupational and Environmental History

General health history
 Does the patient think symptoms/problems are related to anything at work?
 When was the onset of symptoms, and how are they related to work?
 Has patient missed days of work, and why?
 Prior pulmonary problems
 Medications
 Cigarette use
Current or most relevant employment
 Job/process: title and description
 Type of industry and specific work
 Name of employer
 Years employed
Exposure information
 General description of job process and overall hygiene
 Materials used by worker and others
 Ventilation/exhaust system
 Use of respiratory protection
 Are other workers affected?
 Industrial hygiene samples/OSHA data
Environmental nonoccupational factors
 Cigarettes
 Diet
 Hobbies
 Pets
Specific workplace exposures
 Fumes/dusts/fibers
 Gases
 Metals
 Solvents
 Other chemicals: plastics, pesticides, corrosive agents
 Infectious agents
 Organic dusts: cotton, wood
 Physical factors
  Noise
  Repetitive trauma
 Radiation
 Emotional factors, stress
Past employment
 List jobs in chronologic order
 Job title
 Exposures
 Military service

Patients should be asked whether they think their problem is related to anything in the environment. The presence of similar symptoms among coworkers should be determined. Information about potential exposures outside the workplace, such as in the home or with hobbies, should also be obtained.

Diagnostic Evaluation

Chest Radiography

The chest radiograph is the most important diagnostic test for occupational pneumoconioses. It is critical that radiographs of high technical quality be obtained. In some situations, the chest radiograph can be highly suggestive of an occupational disorder and may be sufficient, along with an appropriate exposure history, to establish a diagnosis. For example, silicosis, coal workers' pneumoconiosis, and asbestosis with pleural disease all have characteristic radiographic findings strongly suggestive of the specific occupational diagnosis. The finding of small rounded opacities, progressive massive fibrotic lesions in the upper zones, and "eggshell" calcification is highly suggestive of silicosis. Similarly, the finding of bilateral pleural plaques and diffuse small irregular linear opacities in the lower lung zones is highly suggestive of asbestosis. However, radiographic findings can also be nonspecific, as with asbestosis without pleural plaques, hard-metal disease, or beryllium disease. Furthermore, chest radiographs can be normal in patients with symptomatic pneumoconiosis.[17]

The International Labour Office (ILO) in Geneva, Switzerland has established a uniform classification system to evaluate chest radiographs for epidemiologic studies, clinical evaluation, and screening.[18] The evaluation requires a posteroanterior radiograph with comparison to a standard set of radiographs and must be performed by a qualified reader. Classification is based on the presence of parenchymal opacities, which are then further classified according to shape, size, extent, and concentration. The ILO classification is outlined in Table 15-3.

Computed Tomography

Computed tomography (CT) scanning has an increasing role in the evaluation of patients with occupational interstitial lung disease, primarily asbestosis.[19,20] This has arisen because conventional chest radiography is insensitive, missing as many as 10 to 15 percent of cases with pathologically documented disease.[21] Conventional CT scanning (8- to 10-mm-thick slices) and high-resolution computed tomographic (HRCT) scanning (1- to 3-mm-thick slices) can be used to better evaluate pleural and parenchymal abnormalities. Conventional CT scanning can also be helpful in distinguishing subpleural fat from pleural fibrosis. HRCT scanning is most useful in allowing improved visualization of the lung parenchyma, particularly in the setting of patients with asbestosis and other interstitial diseases. Conventional or HRCT scanning is not a necessary part of evaluation in all patients. If the diagnosis of an interstitial lung disease is clear on the basis of the chest radiograph, HRCT scanning is probably not indicated. In patients with suspected interstitial lung disease because of unexplained dyspnea or abnormal physiologic testing but with normal chest radiographs, HRCT may be helpful in identifying occult parenchymal abnormalities. The specific features and distribution of the HRCT changes may occasionally be suggestive of a specific cause and help narrow the differential diagnosis.

Physiologic Testing

Resting PFTs—including spirometry, lung volumes, and diffusing capacity—are the most important tool to assess functional respiratory status in patients with occupational lung disease, especially interstitial processes.[6,8] PFT findings are generally not specific for a particular cause but are important for evaluating dyspnea, differentiating obstructive from restrictive airway defects, and assessing the degree of pulmonary impairment. Other tests may be useful in the diagnosis of obstructive airway disorders. When spirometry is normal, methacholine challenge testing may demonstrate the presence of

TABLE 15-3 International Labor Office (ILO) Classification of Parenchymal Abnormalities

Small opacities (≤10 mm diameter)
 Rounded opacities
  p   diameter ≤1.5 mm
  q   diameter >1.5–3.0 mm
  r   diameter >3.0–10.0 mm
 Irregular opacities
  s   diameter ≤1.5 mm
  t   diameter >1.5–3.0 mm
  u   diameter >3.0–10.0 mm

Large opacities (>10 mm diameter)
 A   diameter <10–50 mm or
   multiple opacities, each >10 mm in diameter with combined diameters ≤50 mm
 B   diameter ≥50 mm or
   multiple opacities with combined diameters ≤ area of right upper lobe
 C   a single opacity or several large opacities > area of right upper lobe

Profusion of small opacities

Category	Description
0	small opacities absent or less profuse than in category 1
1	small opacities present but few in number, normal lung markings not obscured
2	numerous small opacities, normal lung markings usually partly obscured
3	very numerous small opacities, normal lung markings more obscured

Profusion scale

0/-	0/0	0/1
1/0	1/1	1/2
2/1	2/2	2/3
3/2	3/3	3/+

The 12-point profusion scale allows recognition of a continuum of changes. The first number represents the category chosen. The second number represents an alternative category seriously considered.

hyperreactive airways. For the diagnosis of occupational asthma, demonstration of airflow limitation on exposure to the suspected agent and of improvement with removal is key. This can be accomplished by obtaining preshift and postshift FEV_1 measurements, serial measurements of peak expiratory flow rates, or specific inhalation challenge.[7,22,23] Specific challenge testing with the suspected agent(s) is considered the "gold standard" for diagnosing occupational asthma.[3,7] A 20 percent fall in FEV_1 after exposure to the offending agent is diagnostic of occupational asthma. However, such testing requires a specialized chamber, carries certain risks, is time-consuming, is not widely available, and can produce false negatives. Specific challenge is not necessary for the diagnosis of most cases of occupational asthma. Cardiopulmonary exercise testing is being used increasingly to assess functional impairment and disease progression in patients with certain occupational respiratory disorders.[6] Exercise testing can help distinguish among cardiac, pulmonary, and deconditioning causes of dyspnea. Cardiopulmonary exercise testing is particularly helpful in evaluating a select group of patients with dyspnea and normal pulmonary function tests, or dyspnea that appears out of proportion to the changes in lung function. However, it is not helpful in determining the specific origin of the pulmonary disease.

Bronchoscopy

Bronchoscopy with transbronchial biopsy and bronchoalveolar lavage (BAL) may occasionally be helpful diagnostically in the evaluation of occupational lung disease.[24] Transbronchial biopsies yield small tissue samples that may be adequate to document interstitial fibrosis but are often unable to shed light on the reason for the pathology noted. Transbronchial biopsies are most helpful in diagnosing granulomatous interstitial processes such as sarcoidosis, beryllium disease, hypersensitivity pneumonitis, or diffuse malignant processes. Sufficient tissue is usually not obtained for performance of extensive analyses for dust content. BAL can also be diagnostically helpful. A predominance of lymphocytes suggests certain diagnoses such as sarcoidosis, hypersensitivity pneumonitis, or beryllium disease but is not by itself diagnostic. The diagnosis of beryllium disease can be established with the finding of a positive lymphocyte transformation test in the BAL cells of exposed patients. Characteristic multinucleated giant cells may be seen in the BAL cells of patients with hard-metal lung disease. Cells obtained from BAL may also contain dust particles, which may reflect current and possibly also past exposures.

Pathologic Examination of Tissues

Thoracoscopic and open lung biopsy techniques are usually not needed to make a diagnosis of occupational interstitial lung disease. They can be useful when there is no clear cause or exposure history in establishing the diagnosis and can rule in or out certain nonoccupational causes of lung disease, such as pulmonary vascular disease, infection, or bronchiolitis obliterans.[25] Both surgical biopsy techniques obtain more tissue for histologic and mineralogic analysis than does transbronchial biopsy. A number of methods have been used to analyze the dust content of lung tissue.[25] Light microscopic evaluation with polarization is widely available and can provide a qualitative assessment of the presence of dust particles and ferruginous bodies. More definitive identification and quantification of minerals and dusts requires bulk and microanalytic techniques. These include radiographic fluorescence scanning, electron microscopy, and energy dispersion radiographic spectroscopy. When a patient with interstitial lung disease in whom an occupational or environmental cause is being considered or a patient with an unclear occupational history undergoes surgical lung biopsy, more extensive particle analysis should be considered if light microscopic histologic examination is not diagnostic. However, there remain several serious diagnostic limitations. First, only particulates that are insoluble and retained in tissue at sufficient concentration will be detected. More soluble agents, such as cobalt, can be underestimated. Second, these analytic methods can be tedious, and there can be significant differences in results from different laboratories. Most important, a positive finding documents biologically detectable exposure but does not establish a causal relationship with disease.

Sources of Exposure Information

As noted above, the occupational and environmental exposure history is frequently the best and only source of information regarding exposures. However, it is frequently helpful to obtain additional exposure information. A number of sources are available.[8,26] In the United States, employers are required by federal law to provide employees with information about the potential toxicity of all materials used in the workplace, called Material Safety Data Sheets (MSDS).[15,27] Your patient can and should obtain an MSDS on any substance of concern for your review. For recent or current exposures, a site visit by a trained industrial hygienist or other environmental professional is usually most helpful in providing information about the nature and extent of potential exposures and other exposed workers. A number of methods and sampling strategies exist to measure particular exposures in either the work or home environment. They include personal or work-site sampling devices that absorb the contaminants, direct air sampling devices, and direct monitoring devices. When such data are reviewed, it should be remembered that sampling variability and analytic errors can occur and that the exposure information obtained usually reflects only the narrow window of time during which monitoring was performed. Employers are required to make available to patients any available information about exposure dose, such as the results of air sampling. Exposure information can also be obtained from results of inspections by health and regulatory agencies such as the Occupational Safety and Health Administration (OSHA), unions, insurance groups, and community groups.

Recently there has been great interest in developing biologic markers that attempt to more accurately identify and quantify exposure(s), or an early effect of the exposure, such as sensitization to a specific antigen. Such markers can be measured in the target organ, such as the lung or BAL fluid, or in blood or urine. Examples of possible markers of exposure include the radioallergosorbent test (RAST) or skin tests to a specific antigen or tissue mineralogic analysis. However, at present such markers have relatively limited use in clinical practice.

Once the available information is obtained, the clinician must make a final determination about whether occupational or environmental exposures are causing or contributing to the patient's disease process. Although some diagnoses such as asbestosis are fairly straightforward, others may be diagnostically more challenging and easily overlooked. The degree of uncertainty in diagnosing occupational illnesses is generally significantly greater than in other medical settings—a source of uneasiness for many clinicians. In the United States, for most workers' compensation systems, a disease is considered occupational if "more probably than not" (greater than 50 percent chance) it is work related. Thus, occupational or environmental diseases are diagnosed even in the presence of a significant degree of uncertainty.

PREVENTION AND REGULATORY ISSUES

It is important for the clinician to remember that making the diagnosis of an occupational or environmental respiratory disease almost invariably has important social, economic, legal, and public health considerations. For the individual patient, such a diagnosis can have a profound impact on the patient's work, income, and social situation. When one is evaluating a patient with a suspected occupational or environmental lung disease, it is extremely helpful to determine the patient's agenda and the agenda of others (such as referring physician, employer, attorney, insurance companies) engaged in the patient's care. In addition, related broader public health issues may be concerned, such as prevention of disease among other exposed workers. In the United States, a number of federal and state laws and agencies regulate hazardous substances in the environment and workplace, including the Environmental Protection Agency and OSHA, which was established in 1970 by the Occupational Safety and Health Act to reduce the risk of injury and illness to workers. The National Institute for Occupational Safety and Health, also established in 1970, is charged with performing research and teaching, and evaluating occupational safety and health hazards. Some states require reporting of occupational diseases and have ongoing surveillance programs. The Americans with Disabilities Act prohibits discrimination in employment if the worker has a physical or mental disability, and it can affect physician decision making regarding employability.

The United States workers' compensation system consists of a series of state and federal laws that establish "no-fault" insurance to provide medical, lost-work-time, and other benefits for workers with work-related injuries and illnesses. Physicians are obligated to diagnose and treat work-related illness, to inform the patient of such an illness, and to assist with documentation.[28]

Prevention is central to the practice of occupational and environmental medicine. There are two main strategies for prevention: primary prevention, which entails removal or modification of the hazardous risk or exposure before disease has occurred, and secondary prevention, aimed at early detection and prompt treatment after some adverse effect of the exposure has occurred. Physicians can play important roles in prevention through (1) monitoring of patients to detect early abnormalities, (2) early diagnosis and removal from further exposures, and (3) modification of potential disease complications.

Respirators

The best strategy for reducing inhalational exposures is to prevent or contain the exposure or substitute a less harmful material for a toxic one. Respiratory protective devices (respirators) are used to provide protection from exposure by inhalation when adequate engineering control of airborne contaminants is not feasible or in an emergency or temporary situation. There are two main types of respirators: air-purifying respirators, which remove contaminants from the air using filters or chemical absorbents, and atmosphere supply respirators, which supply breathable air from another source, such as an air cylinder. The choice of respirator depends on characteristics of both the exposure (i.e., type of chemical or dust) and the workplace (i.e., the ventilation system and oxygen supply).[29,30]

Respirators are effective only if the proper device is chosen, it fits properly and is maintained properly, and the worker has been trained in its use. Respirators do not provide absolute protection; rather, they serve to reduce exposure. In the United States, federal regulations set by OSHA include specific rules for respirator use, and they require the employer to provide an acceptable respirator protection program, including fit testing, correct choice of respirator, and worker education and training.

Physicians may be asked to determine a worker's fitness for respirator use.[21,29] OSHA regulations mandate that a worker performing a job requiring use of a respirator must be able to perform the work with a respirator. No spirometric or other specific criteria exist to determine respirator fitness. The physician must use clinical judgment in determining whether a worker is able to use a respirator, keeping in mind that respirators can increase the work of breathing and can interfere with the worker's ability to perform the job by reducing vision, range of motion, and hearing. Factors that can limit respirator use include facial hair, inability to tolerate the respirator, claustrophobic reactions, and particular medical conditions, such as pulmonary or cardio-vascular disease. Reassessment after a brief trial of respirator use is indicated if the patient is having problems or concerns.

REFERENCES

1. Schwartz DA, Wakefield DS, Fieselmann JF, et al: The occupational history in the primary care setting. *Am J Med* 990:315–319, 1991.
2. Chan-Yeung M, Malo JL: Aetiological agents in occupational asthma. *Eur Respir J* 7:346–371, 1994.
3. Chan-Yeung M, Malo JL: Occupational asthma. *N Engl J Med* 333:107–112, 1995.
4. Cullen MR, Cherniack MG, Rosenstock L: Medical progress: Occupational medicine. *N Engl J Med* 322:594–601, 675–683, 1990.
5. Doll R, Peto R: The causes of cancer: Quantitative estimates of avoidable risks of cancer in the United States today. *J Natl Cancer Inst* 66:1192–1308, 1981.
6. Weiderman HP: Evaluating pulmonary impairment: Appropriate use of pulmonary function and exercise tests. *Cleve Clinic J Med* 58:148–152, 1991.
7. Bernstein IL, Chan-Yeung M, Malo J-L, et al (eds): *Asthma in the Workplace.* New York, Marcel Dekker, 1993.
8. Harber P, Schenker M, Balmes J (eds): *Occupational and Environmental Respiratory Disease.* St. Louis, Mosby–Year Book, 1995.
9. U.S. Code of Federal Regulations, Title 29, Part 1910, 134(A) (1), Respiratory Protection.
10. Cullen MR, Redlich CA: Significance of individual sensitivity to chemicals: Elucidation of host susceptibility by use of biomarkers in environmental health research. *Clin Chem* 41:1809–1813, 1995.
11. Vineis P, Lorenzo S: Proportion of lung and bladder cancers in males resulting from occupation: A systemic approach. *Arch Environ Health* 46:6–15, 1991.
12. Cullen MR, Kominsky JR, Rossman MD, et al: Chronic beryllium disease in a precious metal refinery: Clinical epidemiologic and immunologic evidence for continuing risk from exposure to low level beryllium fume. *Am Rev Respir Dis* 135:201–208, 1987.
13. Fleming LE, Ducatman AM, Shalat SL: Disease clusters: A central and ongoing role in occupational health. *J Occup Med* 33:818–825, 1991.
14. Klaassen CD (ed): *Casarett and Doull's Toxicology: The Basic Science of Poisons,* 5th ed. New York, McGraw-Hill, 1996.
15. Newman LS: Occupational illness. *N Engl J Med* 333:1128–1134, 1995.
16. Timmer S, Rosenman K. Occurrence of occupational asthma. *Chest* 104:816–820, 1993.
17. Epler GR: Normal chest roentgenograms in chronic diffuse infiltrative lung disease. *N Engl J Med* 27:934–939, 1978.
18. International Labour Office: Guidelines for the use of ILO International Classification of Radiographs of Pneumoconioses. *Occupational Safety and Health Series,* no 22 (revised). Geneva, ILO, 1980.
19. Begin R: Computed tomography in the early detection of asbestosis. *Br J Ind Med* 50:689–698, 1993.
20. Padley S, Gleeson F, Flower CDR: Current indications for high resolution computed tomography scanning of the lungs. *Br J Radiol* 68:105–109, 1995.

21. Parkes WR: *Occupational Lung Disorders.* Oxford, Butterworth-Heinemann, 1994.
22. Burge PS: Use of serial measurements of peak flow in the diagnosis of occupational asthma. *Occup Med* 8:279–294, 1993.
23. Moscato G, Godnic-Cvar J, Maestrelli P, et al: Statement on self-monitoring of peak expiratory flows in the investigation of occupational asthma. *Eur Respir J* 8:1605–1610, 1995.
24. Kreiss K, Miller F, Newman LS, et al: Chronic beryllium disease—From the workplace to cellular immunology, molecular immunogenetics, and back. *Clin Immunol Immunopathol* 71:123–129, 1994.
25. Churg A, Green FHY (eds): *Pathology of Occupational Lung Disease.* New York, Igaku-Shoin, 1988.
26. Rosenstock L, Rest KM, Benson JA Jr, et al: Occupational and environmental medicine: Meeting the growing need for clinical services. *N Engl J Med* 325:924–927, 1991.
27. Himmelstein JS, Frumkin H: The right to know about toxic exposures: Implications for physicians. *N Engl J Med* 312:687–690, 1985.
28. American College of Physicians: Occupational and environmental medicine: The internist's role. *Ann Intern Med* 113:974–982, 1990.
29. Beckett WS: Certifying the worker for respirator use. *Semin Occup Med* 1:119–124, 1986.
30. *NIOSH Guide to the Selection and Use of Particulate Respirators.* DHHS (NIOS) Publication no 96-101, January 1996.

16 | Asbestos-Related Lung Disease*

Lynn T. Tanoue

Asbestos is a fibrous hydrated magnesium silicate which, owing to its indestructible nature, fire resistance, and spinnability, has more than 3000 commercial uses. Beginning in the late nineteenth century, asbestos was widely used in fireproof textiles and as insulation for boilers and pipes. Asbestos has also been used in yarn, felt, paper, millboard, shingles, paints, cloth, tape, filters, and wire insulation. More recently, asbestos has been used in cement pipes for potable water, in gaskets, friction materials including brake linings, and roofing and floor products. Asbestos was extensively used for ship construction during World War II. World consumption of asbestos declined in the 1990s to approximately 50 percent of the peak in 1973. In 1994, approximately 2.7 million tons were produced, with the United States consuming less than 27,000 metric tons.

Approximately 98 percent of the asbestos used in the United States has been chrysotile, a serpentine form of asbestos. Other asbestos types are the amphiboles—notably amosite and crocidolite. These asbestos fiber types have strikingly different physical characteristics: chrysotile tends to be wavy and long, occuring in bundles; crocidolite is needle-shaped with many long fibers; and amosite is similar to crocidolite but generally thicker. At present, the U.S. Occupational Safety and Health Administration (OSHA) regulates the usage of all types of asbestos fibers. Industrial hygiene efforts to control exposure have focused on engineering controls, including enclosure of the process lines, especially all sites where asbestos is introduced into a system; increasing ventilation; and the use of wet manufacturing methods. Personal respirators are used as a last resort in achieving control of exposure in the workplace. Most of the insulation-manufacturing industry has switched to alternative materials, especially fibrous glass, rock and slag wool, and refractory ceramic fibers. Animal experiments have generally shown these asbestos substitutes to be safe except that refractory ceramic fibers were able to produce mesotheliomas in hamsters. Asbestosis and asbestos-related cancers may occur at increased rates in the future owing to the increased use of asbestos in developing countries.

TYPES OF EXPOSURE

Asbestos exposure has occurred in a variety of settings. Primary exposures occurred in miners and millers. Secondary exposures occurred in manufacturing plants using asbestos in the production of textiles, friction materials, tiles, and insulation materials. Epidemiologic studies focused on cohorts in

*Edited from Chap. 57, "Asbestos-Related Lung Disease," by Rom WT. In: *Fishman's Pulmonary Diseases and Disorders,* 3d ed., edited by Fishman AP, Elias JA, Fishman JA, Grippi MA, Kaiser LR, Senior RM. New York, McGraw-Hill, 1998, pp 877–892. For fuller discussion of the topics dealt with in this chapter, the reader is referred to the original text, as noted above.

these plants, since asbestos fiber type was often specified and dust measurements were obtained. These studies demonstrated that the intensity and duration of exposure play important roles in the prevalence of asbestos-related disease. In a study of 1584 insulation workers and 1330 sheet-metal workers, 83.5 percent of the insulators had abnormal chest radiographs (55 percent with parenchymal opacities), whereas 42 percent of the sheet-metal workers had abnormal chest radiographs (17 percent with parenchymal opacities).[1] Significant exposures have also occurred in the construction trades. These have included asbestos insulators (called "laggers" in the United Kingdom), who mixed asbestos cement on site to insulate joints and elbows on pipes; boilermakers and sheet-metal workers, who worked adjacent to the asbestos workers; and electricians, carpenters, plumbers, and others who worked in the vicinity of work requiring asbestos. These exposures were mainly to chrysotile asbestos, since practically no crocidolite was imported into the United States, and only small amounts of amosite were admixed.

Asbestos workers and other construction workers wore their asbestos-covered clothes home, so their spouses and children were often also exposed. These household contact exposures are often referred to as *indirect exposures,* and those exposed while working near asbestos workers are called *bystander exposures.* In the United States, approximately 14 million persons who were exposed to asbestos in the workplace between 1940 and 1979 were alive in 1980. From this cohort, estimates have been projected for the late 1990s of a peak incidence of approximately 3000 mesothelioma deaths and 5000 asbestos-related lung cancer deaths. Pleural fibrosis remains a relatively common finding among asbestos-exposed workers, whereas asbestosis is becoming increasingly uncommon.

NONMALIGNANT PLEURAL MANIFESTATIONS

Pleural Plaques

Pleural plaques are the most common manifestation of asbestos exposure. They are focal, irregular, raised white lesions found on the parietal and, rarely, the visceral pleura. The plaques may be small or extensive; commonly they occur in the lateral and posterior midlung zones, where they may follow rib contours and the diaphragm. They commonly enter lobar fissures and can invade the mediastinum or pericardium; rarely, they invade the apices or costophrenic sulci. Histologically, asbestos-related pleural plaques are characterized by a paucity of cells, extensive collagen fibrils arranged in a basket-weave pattern, and a thin covering of mesothelial cells. The parietal pleura is uniformly involved, with minimal thickening of the visceral pleura. The two pleural surfaces are free of adhesions. Pleural calcifications frequently develop in these fibrohyaline lesions as the length of time from exposure increases. Exposure to asbestos is the most frequent cause of pleural plaques. These plaques, although typical of asbestos, are not specific for asbestos exposure.

The proposed pathogenesis of pleural plaques is based on the direct effects of fibers that reach the pleural space.[2] Asbestos fibers—the short, thin ones in particular—have been shown to be transported by subpleural lymphatics to the pleural space. There, it is believed that they scratch, injure, and irritate the pleural surface, leading to hemorrhage, inflammation, and eventually fibrosis.

In the 1960s, hyaline and calcified pleural plaques were noted to be an index of exposure to asbestos. In shipyard workers, the frequency of pleural abnormalities was approximately 10 times that of parenchymal disease. The greater the exposure, the more likely the worker was to have extensive calcified pleural plaques as well as parenchymal fibrosis. The intensity of the exposure has been noted to be an important determinant of the prevalence of these abnormalities. For example, among British shipyard workers, 36 percent of those with continuous exposure as laggers developed pleural plaques, while extensive pleural thickening and pulmonary fibrosis were seen in 5 and 7 percent, respectively.[3] In contrast, those with intermittent exposure had a 6 percent prevalence of plaques and no pulmonary fibrosis. On average, the latency time for the appearance of plaques is 30 years, but the time can vary greatly. This variation can also be appreciated from studies of British shipyard workers, in whom the prevalence of pleural plaques increased from 17 percent at 10 years after the first exposure to 70 percent at 30 years among those with continuous exposure; for those with intermittent exposures, the prevalence increased from 1 percent at 10 years to 16 percent at 30 years.

All asbestos fibers are equally capable of inducing pleural plaques, which have been found in American insulators or shipyard workers exposed to chrysotile or amosite as well as miners in western Australia who were exposed to crocidolite. Circumscribed pleural plaques are not associated with pleural effusions. They increase in size slowly, usually over decades, and rarely if ever give rise to diffuse malignant mesothelioma. In addition to occupational exposures, domestic and residential exposures have, on rare occasions, been implicated in the production of pleural plaques. Evidence for the latter is the remarkably high rates of pleural calcification (up to 30 percent) in some rural areas of Greece, Bulgaria, and Turkey.

Clinical, Physiologic, and Radiographic Features

Pleural plaques are usually picked up as asymptomatic incidental findings on chest radiographs. Pleural disease, both plaques and diffuse pleural fibrosis, can be associated with a restrictive ventilatory defect. In nonsmoking asbestos workers with circumscribed or diaphragmatic pleural plaques, decrements in FVC but not FEV_1/FVC are well described.[4,5] The visualization of plaques on routine chest radiography depends on their thickness and location and the orientation of the radiographic beam. As a result, they can be viewed in profile along the lateral chest wall or on en face with a rolled or holly-leaf pattern, especially if calcified. Only a modest proportion of plaques detected at autopsy can be seen on the standard posteroanterior (PA) chest radiograph. Oblique views and computed tomographic (CT) scanning increase plaque detection, recognizing them at a much earlier and less well defined state than the conventional chest radiograph. The CT scan is particularly useful for perivertebral and pericardiac plaques, and high-resolution CT scanning (HRCT) can help to establish the presence of diaphragmatic lesions. In all cases, the CT scan can help to differentiate plaques from extrapleural fat pads and can detect concomitant parenchymal abnormalities that may be difficult or impossible to see on the PA chest radiograph.

Pleural plaques due to asbestos exposure are usually bilateral (80 percent of the time). Unilateral pleural plaques should suggest other etiologies. The lesions are usually stable and will remain the same size for months. This helps to differentiate plaques from pleural tumors. Histologic tissue examination is usually not necessary for diagnosis. No specific treatment is required for asbestos pleural plaques. Since they are markers of asbestos exposure and identify patients at risk for other asbestos-related disorders,[6] medical surveillance, including periodic chest radiographs, is recommended.

Diffuse Pleural Thickening

Diffuse pleural fibrosis occurs most commonly as part of a fibrotic process of the visceral pleura and subadjacent interstitium. It may, however, occur in patients with minimal pulmonary parenchymal fibrosis and can be quite severe. On routine chest radiographs, diffuse pleural fibrosis presents as a continuous pleural opacity extending over more than 25 percent of the pleural surface of a lung, often blunting the costophrenic angle. The fibrotic responses can be localized or diffuse and either unilateral or bilateral, varying in thickness from a whitish discoloration of the lung surface to a thick white peel that can encase significant pulmonary structures. In 90 percent of the patients, it affects the costophrenic angle. The most common pathogenic mechanism is thought to be the fibrotic resolution of a benign pleural effusion, producing diffuse pleural thickening. Additionally, confluence of large pleural plaques or the extension of subpleural fibrosis to the visceral pleura can result in pleural fibrosis.

Clinical, Physiologic, and Radiographic Features

Diffuse pleural fibrosis most often occurs long after short-term heavy exposure to asbestos. When mild, diffuse pulmonary fibrosis can be asymptomatic and discovered as an incidental finding on a chest radiograph obtained for another reason. The diffuse nature of the lesion, however, often leads to pulmonary symptoms, including dyspnea on exertion, chronic dry cough, and chest pain. Diffuse pleural thickening can cause a restrictive physiologic abnormality, the severity of which varies with the degree of fibrotic response. On rare occasions, in patients with severe bilateral disease, respiratory insufficiency and death have occurred.

The diagnosis of diffuse pleural fibrosis is usually based on the clinical presentation and chest radiograph. In more than 30 percent of cases, a history of asbestos-related pleuritis can be obtained. Diffuse pleural fibrosis is not unique to asbestos-exposed persons and can represent old inflammatory reactions from tuberculosis, thoracic surgery, hemorrhagic chest trauma, or drug reactions. Differentiation among these causes is frequently based on a careful clinical history. Radiographic patterns are also helpful, since bilateral interstitial changes in the lower lung zones in association with pleural plaques or calcifications strongly support a diagnosis of asbestos exposure. A biopsy may be required when the thoracic lesion is progressing or when malignancy is in the differential. There are no specific therapies for asbestos-related diffuse pleural fibrosis. Medical surveillance is required to detect disease progression and observe for other asbestos-related disorders. In the rare extremely severe case, pleurectomy may be required.

Rounded Atelectasis

Rounded atelectasis is a rare complication of asbestos-induced pleural disease. It is caused by scarring of the visceral and parietal pleura and the adjacent lung, with the pleural reaction folding over on itself. The pleural surfaces then fuse to one another, trapping the underlying lung and leading to atelectasis. As a result of this alteration, a mass lesion that can mimic lung cancer can be seen on the chest radiograph. This lesion is most easily appreciated with use of conventional or HRCT scanning, which may demonstrate continuity to areas of diffuse pleural thickening, evidence of volume loss in the adjacent lung, or a characteristic "comet tail" of vessels and bronchi sweeping into a wedge-shaped mass. CT scanning can also demonstrate stability over time (from months to years), which supports the diagnosis of a benign lesion, and pleural plaques or parenchymal changes, which support a diagnosis of asbestos exposure. If the benign nature of the lesion cannot be assured by radiographic techniques, the patient may require biopsy to rule out a malignant process.

Acute Benign Pleural Effusions

Acute benign pleural effusions are common pleural manifestations in asbestos-exposed persons between 20 and 40 years of age. The latency period for these effusions is shorter than for pleural plaques, malignant mesotheliomas, or pulmonary malignancies, generally occurring 12 to 15 years after the first asbestos exposure. However, benign effusions can also occur as long as 30 years after first exposure.[7] The effusions may be small to moderate in size or may be manifest as an increase in the extent or severity of an existing pleural reaction. They may persist for 6 months or more. They frequently clear spontaneously, only to recur on the contralateral side.

About 50 percent of the patients with acute benign pleural effusions are asymptomatic. When symptomatic, the manifestations may be those of pleurisy (chest pain, chest tightness, dyspnea, cough, and fever). Physical examination reveals the signs of a pleural effusion; a pleural friction rub may be heard. The effusions are exudative and often bloody, with normal glucose concentrations. Cellular analysis demonstrates mesothelial cells in about 50 percent and eosinophils in about 25 percent of patients. Asbestos bodies are rarely found.

Benign asbestos pleural effusions do not presage the development of malignant mesotheliomas. However, a benign asbestos pleural effusion is a risk factor for the development of pleural thickening, especially diffuse pleural fibrosis. The diagnosis is one of exclusion. Thoracentesis is essential and pleural biopsy is frequently required to rule out other causes of pleural effusions, including mesothelioma. Long-term follow-up is also a diagnostic requirement, since the diagnosis of a benign pleural effusion cannot be fully established until a 3-year tumor-free period has passed.[8]

ASBESTOSIS

Asbestosis is the interstitial pneumonitis and fibrosis caused by exposure to asbestos fibers. Early lesions are characterized by discrete areas of fibrosis in the walls of respiratory bronchioles. In addition to the peribronchiolar fibrosis, there is an intense peribronchiolar cellular reaction that may narrow and obstruct the airway lumen. Initially, the disease usually involves first-order bronchioles; subsequently, second- and third-order bronchioles are affected. As the disease progresses, the fibrosis becomes diffuse, the architecture of the lung undergoes extensive remodeling, and honeycombing supervenes. In contrast to other pneumoconioses, lymph node enlargement and progressive massive fibrosis do not occur. Pathologically, the alterations seen in asbestosis cannot be differentiated from many other interstitial fibrotic disorders except for the presence of asbestos bodies and uncoated asbestos fibers.

Asbestos fibers are deposited at airway bifurcations and in respiratory bronchioles and alveoli by impaction, sedimentation, and interception. Incomplete clearance of fibers by macrophages can result in pulmonary fibrosis. The degree of fibrosis in asbestosis relates, in general, to the lung's dust burden. If the dust load is small, the tissue reaction may be limited and the disease may be mild and not progress. If the retained dust load is great, tissue reaction and macrophage alveolitis are proportionately more intense, greater injury occurs, and chronic and progressive lung disease can develop. A dose-response relationship is evident in asbestos workers. The prevalence of parenchymal asbestosis increases with duration and intensity of exposure.

Asbestosis becomes evident only after an appreciable latent period. Because work sites around the world increasingly meet recommended control levels, high-level exposure to asbestos is now uncommon and clinical asbestosis is becoming a less severe disease that manifests after a longer latent interval. However, even low-level exposure can result in disease, but this may not become evident for decades.[9] Once established, radiographic asbestosis may remain static or progress. Rarely has regression been recorded. The factors that determine the outcome are poorly understood, though level and duration of exposure (i.e., cumulative exposure) appear to be prognostic factors. Progression is also considerably more common in persons who already have radiographic abnormalities. This fact provides the basis for the advice that further exposure is to be avoided once the diagnosis of parenchymal asbestosis has been made.

Cigarette smoking can affect the expression of asbestosis. Smokers without dust exposure may have a few irregular radiographic opacities, probably representing acute or chronic bronchitis or bronchiectatic changes in the lung parenchyma. Both smokers and ex-smokers have a higher frequency of asbestos-related irregular opacities on their chest radiographs than do their nonsmoking colleagues.[10] Smoking does not appear to influence asbestos-induced pleural fibrosis. The effects of smoking on asbestosis may be clinically important, since the mortality from asbestosis is higher in asbestos workers who have smoked than in their nonsmoking coworkers. This risk declines if the worker quits smoking.

Clinical, Physiologic, and Radiographic Features

Dyspnea on exertion is the earliest, most consistently reported, and frequently the most distressing symptom of asbestosis. Dyspnea may be accompanied by a persistent cough, sputum production, chest tightness, and wheezing. In a cross-sectional survey of 816 asbestos-exposed workers using the respiratory symptom questionnaire of the American Thoracic Society, cough, phlegm, wheeze, and dyspnea were inversely related to pulmonary function.[11]

Rales are a distinctive feature of asbestosis. They are usually bilateral, late to paninspiratory in timing, heard best at the posterior lung bases, and not cleared by coughing. In prevalence surveys, approximately 83 percent of patients with higher radiographic categories of asbestosis have bilateral rales.[12] It is important to appreciate that the clinical features of asbestosis and the findings on physical examination are not unique to this disorder and resemble those of a variety of other diffuse interstitial inflammatory and fibrotic processes.

In years past, asbestosis-induced respiratory failure was a frequent cause of death in patients with this disorder. In recent years, as the severity of asbestosis appears to have attenuated, cancer has become an increasingly common terminal event.

Prospective measurements of lung function are useful as part of medical surveillance for asbestos-exposed persons. The characteristic pulmonary function changes of asbestosis are a restrictive impairment, with a reduction in lung volumes and diffusing capacity ($D_{L_{CO}}$), and arterial hypoxemia.[13,14] Large airway function, as reflected in the FEV_1/FVC ratio, is generally well preserved. In a large cohort of 2611 asbestos insulators, the FVC percent predicted decreased as the profusion of irregular opacities on the chest radiograph increased; pleural thickening exaggerated the decrease for each category of profusion.[13]

Mild airway obstruction can also be seen in nonsmokers with asbestosis, superimposed on a restrictive pattern of lung function.[15] Open lung biopsies from a limited number of these patients suggest that these obstructive findings may be due to peribronchiolar fibrosis, since they revealed peribronchiolar infiltrates with macrophages and fibrosis that extended into the adjacent interstitium. Therefore it is not surprising that lesser grades of asbestosis can show a mixed restrictive and obstructive abnormality.

In asbestosis, the standard PA chest radiograph reveals bilateral diffuse reticulonodular opacities, predominantly in the lower lung zones. According to the ILO classification (see Chap. 15), category 1 chest radiographs are consistent with mild asbestosis. Moderate asbestosis and advanced asbestosis are defined as category 2 and 3 chest radiographs, respectively. As duration from onset and intensity of exposure increase, there is an increase in prevalence and severity of asbestosis as reflected in the chest radiograph.

CT scanning has improved the sensitivity for detecting asbestos-related lesions. Five HRCT features of asbestosis have been identified: curvilinear subpleural lines, increased intralobular septa, dependent opacities, parenchymal bands and interlobular core structures, and honeycombing.[16] In asbestos-exposed workers, abnormal HRCT has been shown to correlate with restrictive physiologic abnormalities and abnormal diffusing capacities.[17] HRCT is also extremely sensitive in documenting asbestos-related pleural abnormalities. The presence of pleural plaques (particularly if they are bilateral) provides useful evidence that the parenchymal process is asbestos-related. Hilar node enlargement is not a feature of asbestosis, and progressive massive fibrosis is also uncommon.

Diagnosis

Asbestosis is defined as parenchymal fibrosis, with or without pleural thickening, usually associated with dyspnea, bibasilar rales, and pulmonary function changes.[18] To diagnose this disorder, one must establish the presence of pulmonary fibrosis and determine whether exposure has occurred of a duration and intensity sufficient to put the person at risk for developing this syndrome. The PA chest radiograph and its interpretation are the most important factors in the former. When radiographic or lung function changes are marginal, CT scanning can reveal characteristic parenchymal abnormalities as well as pleural plaques and/or pleural fibrosis.

The diagnosis of asbestosis requires an appropriate exposure history defining the duration, onset, type, and intensity of exposure. Convincing occupational exposures include the manufacturing of asbestos products, asbestos mining and milling, construction trade work (insulator, sheet-metal worker, electrician, plumber, pipe fitter, carpenter), power plant work, boilermaking, and shipyard work. Exposures over 10 to 20 years are usually necessary. However, it is important to keep in mind that intensity of exposure can be heavy even if duration of exposure is short. For example, heavy exposures were experienced by shipyard workers engaged in insulation application or removal in contained areas for brief periods aboard ship and by asbestos insulators during their apprenticeship when they unloaded asbestos sacks into troughs and mixed asbestos cement. Short, intense exposures of this sort, which lasted from several months to 1 or 2 years, can be sufficient to cause asbestosis. The timing of the exposure is also relevant. Industrial hygiene controls in the 1950s and 1960s, especially in the construction trades, were not widely applied or enforced. Thus, workers exposed during these periods may have received a heavy asbestos load. Time since onset of exposure is also crucial. Latency is an important factor, with the prevalence of asbestosis increasing with time since the onset of exposure.

Diagnostic difficulty can occur in patients with other underlying lung diseases, usually cigarette-smoking history and concurrent emphysema. In the absence of an adequate exposure history or in the presence of a confusing clinical presentation, biopsy material may be helpful in identifying the nature of the disease. It allows histologic evaluation of the interstitial process, including examination for the presence of asbestos materials. Bare, uncoated asbestos fibers in the lung are visible only on electron microscopy. Coated fibers or asbestos bodies are visible by light microscopy. The presence of asbestos bodies or fibers is considered the hallmark of exposure, past or current. The presence of more than one coated fiber has been cited as a necessary criterion for the pathologic diagnosis of asbestosis. However, cases have been described in which the load of uncoated fibers was high in the absence of asbestos bodies, and asbestos bodies have been noted in the tissues of people without significant asbestos exposure. Thus, the absence of asbestos bodies should not exclude the diagnosis of asbestosis.

Major causes of morbidity and mortality in patients with asbestosis include progressive lung disease with accelerated loss of pulmonary function, the development of lung cancers, and malignant mesotheliomas.[8,19] At present, there is no established treatment for asbestosis. Because of the risk of lung cancer and mesothelioma, medical surveillance is recommended.

MALIGNANT MESOTHELIOMA

Most instances of mesothelioma occur in persons who have been exposed to asbestos fibers. In its early stage, the mesothelioma appears as multiple small, grayish nodules on the visceral and parietal pleura that then become locally invasive, spreading along the pleural wall and invading the lung, mediastinal lymph nodes, and other thoracic and nearby structures. Distant metastases can also occur in up to 50 to 80 percent of patients. These tumors then invade thoracic and other structures by direct extension, causing the morbidity and mortality of disease. Fewer than 25 percent of malignant mesotheliomas are peritoneal in origin. Mesotheliomas are conventionally classified into three histologic patterns: epithelial, sarcomatous, and mixed or biphasic; these patterns account for 50, 20, and 30 percent, respectively. The epithelial variant is most easily confused with metastatic adenocarcinoma; thus the pathologic diagnosis of malignant mesothelioma may be difficult.

Epidemiology

In 1960, Wagner and colleagues published a landmark paper demonstrating an association between malignant mesothelioma and asbestos exposure.[20] They reported on 33 patients from South Africa, 28 of whom were exposed in the crocidolite mining region and 4 of whom were exposed in asbestos factories. They observed that mesotheliomas occurred 20 to 40 years after exposure to asbestos dust and found asbestos bodies in lung tissue from 8 of 10 patients from whom lung tissue was available for study. Subsequently, the importance of direct asbestos exposure was confirmed and the potential importance of indirect exposure to asbestos recognized.[21,22]

Evaluations of asbestos fiber content have shown a clear association between asbestos exposure and the occurrence of mesothelioma.[23] Epidemiologic studies have shown that crocidolite may be the more potent fiber type among asbestos miners. Most mesotheliomas have occurred from chrysotile-amphibole mixtures, since chrysotile is the most common fiber in commercial use.[24] Few controversies in medicine are as intense as the disagreements concerning the relation between asbestos fiber type and carcinogenic risk.[25] Nonetheless, associations between malignant mesothelioma and other (non-crocidolite) fiber types have been reported.

The incidence of mesothelioma is increasing because of the cohort exposed to asbestos between 1940 and 1970. Incidence rates vary from a low of 11 to 13 per million per year in the United States to 33 per million per year in South Africa and to 66 per million per year in western Australia. These rates reflect mining and manufacturing industries and the location of crocidolite mines. Although the peak incidence in the United States may have passed, since imports decreased after 1945, imports of asbestos in the United Kingdom reached their peak in the 1960s to 1970s. Thus, the peak of mesothelioma deaths in the United Kingdom is expected to occur in 2020, when up to 1 percent may die of the disease. Chrysotile was the major asbestos import to the United Kingdom, and half of this material went into the construction industry. Amosite was the leading amphibole import, and most of it went into insulation board. Thus, workers in the construction industry in the United Kingdom seem to be at greatest risk.[24]

It is universally accepted, however, that mesothelioma is not associated with cigarette smoke per se. Cigarette smoking is a confounding variable in studies that relate asbestos-exposed persons to cancer risk. The contribution that cigarettes make to the risk of lung cancer is impressive (see below).

Clinical and Radiographic Features

Pleural mesotheliomas are found mainly in males (ratio, between 3 and 4 to 1) and are most commonly diagnosed in patients between 50 and 70 years of age. Symptoms are related to invasion of the pleura, lung, and thoracic structures. Chest pain is the most common symptom experienced by patients with mesotheliomas. Dyspnea is next in frequency, followed by cough, weight loss, and fever. The presence of asbestosis or of pleural plaques on the opposite side can assist in establishing the diagnosis. A pleural effusion is usually present and can be massive. The effusion is an exudate, can be hemorrhagic, and may have high levels of hyaluronic acid. Metastases are less common but can give rise to symptoms due to tumor in the diaphragm, heart, liver, spleen, adrenals, gastrointestinal tract, bone, pancreas, and kidneys. Clubbing is rare. Thrombocytosis is common, and can lead to thromboembolic complications. Ascites and weight loss are characteristic features of peritoneal mesothelioma.

Radiographic abnormalities include a thick pleural peel along the lateral chest wall that can extend to the apex with an irregular nodular surface, multiple pleural nodules or masses, plaquelike opacities, and pleural effusion(s). As the disease progresses, the lung parenchyma may be involved, the affected hemithorax may decrease in size, and the mediastinum or hilar nodes may be invaded. Pericardial thickening or effusion, abdominal extension, and chest wall invasion are common.

Diagnosis and Treatment

The diagnosis of malignant mesothelioma requires cytologic or histologic validation. Obtaining a cytologic diagnosis from the pleural exudate is difficult because reactive mesothelial cells and malignant cells are not easy to distinguish; thus biopsy is usually required. Thoracoscopy is probably the procedure of choice, with diagnostic rates greater than 80 percent. It should be noted that mesothelioma can invade the biopsy tract. Local radiation after biopsy can significantly reduce such spread.

The prognosis of malignant mesothelioma is poor, with median survival time approximately 8 to 12 months. Overall, fewer than 20 percent of patients are alive at 2 years. Pleurectomy or pneumonectomy, combined with radiation therapy, has failed to significantly influence survival rates. Chemotherapy with doxorubicin has shown variable responses without prolonging survival. Interventions, such as gene therapy or the use of cytokines, for the treatment of malignant mesothelioma are currently being investigated.

LUNG CANCER

The association between asbestos exposure and the development of lung cancer is based on a number of successive epidemiologic investigations. Case reports of lung cancer and asbestos deaths occurred as early as 1935. Series of patients with asbestosis who went to autopsy were reported by 1947. In 1955, an epidemiologic cohort study of 113 men exposed to asbestos for 20 years disclosed 11 deaths due to cancer (compared with 0.8 expected), all of which had evidence of asbestosis.[26] In 1964, a retrospective cohort study in two asbestos insulator unions in the United States reported that deaths from lung cancer were 6.8 times the expected rate and that the incidence of lung cancer increased with time after exposure.[22] In 1968, a follow-up of men in this cohort demonstrated an important synergy between asbestos exposure and cigarette smoking, since the risk of lung cancer was almost entirely borne by those who had a history of cigarette smoking.[27]

The largest survey of asbestos-related deaths looked at a North American asbestos insulator cohort.[28] This study demonstrated a threefold excess of cancer deaths that were due primarily to pulmonary malignancies. Comparatively few of these excess deaths were observed among those less than 25 years after the start of exposure. Lung cancer peaked at 40 years from exposure and mesothelioma at 45 years. In contrast, death rates from asbestosis increased progressively with time. This study confirmed the multiplicative effect of smoking plus asbestos exposure on the risk of lung cancer. Moreover, it showed that deaths from lung cancer dropped by almost two-thirds for asbestos insulators who subsequently stopped smoking. Such studies have documented several important findings: (1) a latency period of about 20 years is usually observed before the increase in cancer occurs; (2) the greater the cumulative asbestos exposure, the greater the risk of developing lung cancer; and (3) the greater the dose or exposure time, the shorter the latency period before the tumor develops. Malignancies have also been noted in the spouses and children of these workers who were exposed to asbestos in the household, primarily on work clothes. Studies of a variety of other cohorts have confirmed the increased incidence of lung cancer. Asbestos-exposed populations have also demonstrated an increased frequency of digestive cancers and cancer of the larynx. [21,29–31]

Clinical and Radiographic Features

Asbestos-related lung cancers are not distinctive in presentation. The patterns of presentation of lung cancer among asbestos workers are similar to those of all patients with lung cancer. Cough, chest pain, dyspnea, hemoptysis, recurrent bouts of pneumonia, and localized wheezing are major pulmonary symptoms that bring patients to medical attention. However, patients can also be asymptomatic at the time of initial discovery, the abnormality being noted on a routine or screening chest radiograph. All histologic types of lung cancer occur with increased frequency, but adenocarcinoma has the highest incidence. In the vast majority of patients, histologic evidence of asbestosis and/or asbestos bodies are found.

Whether asbestos-related lung cancers occur in the absence of asbestosis is debatable. One of the most vexing questions in asbestos-related lung cancers is the relationship between the lung cancer and asbestosis. Asbestosis can be detected radiographically or histologically in the vast majority of patients with asbestos-related lung cancer. However, it is clear that not all cases of asbestosis can be detected by chest radiograph and that radiographic evidence of asbestosis cannot be detected in all patients with asbestos-related lung cancer. Furthermore, the radiographic manifestations of asbestos-induced lung cancers do not differ, per se, from those of lung cancers associated with other carcinogens. Mass lesions, atelectasis, postobstructive pneumonia, and pleural effusions are all seen, frequently superimposed on a background of asbestosis or asbestos-induced pleural abnormalities. Pleural plaques or rounded atelectasis can usually be distinguished from cancer by stability over time.

Diagnosis and Treatment

The principles employed in the diagnosis of lung cancer in asbestos workers are identical to those in the diagnosis of pulmonary malignancies in other patients exposed to other carcinogenic agents, with the exception that evidence of asbestos exposure by light or electron microscopy may specifically be pursued. Similarly, therapeutic approaches parallel those employed for lung cancers in general. The impact of other asbestos-related pulmonary processes must always be taken into account. For example, severe asbestosis may limit operability, and diffuse pleural thickening may make surgical intervention problematic.

REFERENCES

1. Lilis R, Miller A, Godbold J, et al: Comparative quantitative evaluation of pleural fibrosis and its effects on pulmonary function in two large asbestos-exposed occupational groups—Insulators and sheet metal workers. *Environ Res* 59:49–66, 1992.
2. Rom WN, Travis WD, Brody AR: Cellular and molecular basis of the asbestos-related diseases: State of the art. *Am Rev Respir Dis* 143:408–422, 1991.
3. Sheers G, Templeton AR: Effect of asbestos on dockyard workers. *Br Med J* 3:574–579, 1968.
4. Lilis R, Miller A, Godbold J, et al: Pulmonary function and pleural fibrosis: Quantitative relationships with an integrative index of pleural abnormalities. *Am J Ind Med* 20:145–161, 1991.
5. Schwartz DA, Galvin JR, Yagla SJ, et al: Restrictive lung function and asbestos-induced pleural fibrosis. *J Clin Invest* 91:2685–2692, 1993.
6. Hillerdal G: Pleural plaques and risk for bronchial carcinoma and mesothelioma. *Chest* 105:144–150, 1994.
7. Hillerdal G, Ozesmi M: Benign asbestos pleural effusion: 73 exudates in 60 patients. *Eur J Respir Dis* 71:113–121, 1987.
8. Bégin R, Samet JM, Shaikh RA: Asbestos, in Harber P, Schenker MB, Balmes JR (eds): *Occupational and Environmental Respiratory Disease.* St. Louis, Mosby–Year Book, 1996, pp 293–321.
9. Ehrlich R, Lilis R, Chan E, et al: Long-term radiological effects of short-term exposure to amosite asbestos among factory workers. *Br J Ind Med* 49:268–275, 1992.
10. Lilis R, Selikoff IJ, Lerman Y, et al: Asbestosis: Interstitial pulmonary fibrosis and pleural fibrosis in a cohort of asbestos insulation workers: Influence of cigarette smoking. *Am J Ind Med* 10:459–470, 1986.
11. Brodkin CA, Barnhart S, Anderson G, et al: Correlation between respiratory symptoms and pulmonary function in asbestos-exposed workers. *Am Rev Respir Dis* 148:32–37, 1993.
12. Murphy RLH, Gaensler EA, Holford SK, et al: Crackles in the early detection of asbestosis. *Am Rev Respir Dis* 129:375–379, 1984.
13. Miller A, Lilis R, Godbold J, et al: Relationship of pulmonary function to radiographic interstitial fibrosis in 2611 long-term asbestos insulators. *Am Rev Respir Dis* 145:263–270, 1992.
14. Rosenstock L, Barnhart S, Heyer NJ, et al: The relation among pulmonary function, chest roentgenographic abnormalities, and smoking status in an asbestos-exposed cohort. *Am Rev Respir Dis* 138:272–277, 1988.
15. Bégin R, Cantin A, Berthiaume Y, et al: Airway function in lifetime-nonsmoking older asbestos workers. *Am J Med* 75:631–638, 1983.
16. Gamsu G, Salmon CJ, Warnock ML, Blanc PD: CT quantification of interstitial fibrosis in patients with asbestosis: A comparison of two methods. *AJR* 164:63–68, 1995.
17. Staples CA, Gamsu G, Ray CS, Webb NR: High resolution computed tomography and lung function in asbestos-exposed workers with normal chest radiographs. *Am Rev Respir Dis* 139:1502–1508, 1989.
18. American Thoracic Society: The diagnosis of nonmalignant diseases related to asbestos. *Am Rev Respir Dis* 134:363–368, 1986.
19. Rom WN: Accelerated loss of lung function and alveolitis in a longitudinal study of non-smoking individuals with occupational exposure to asbestos. *Am J Ind Med* 21:835–844, 1992.
20. Wagner JC, Sleggs CA, Marchand P: Diffuse pleural mesothelioma and asbestos exposure in the northwestern Cape province. *Br J Ind Med* 17:260–271, 1960.
21. Newhouse ML, Berry G, Wagner JC: Mortality of factory workers in east London, 1933–80. *Br J Ind Med* 42:4–11, 1980.
22. Selikoff IJ, Churg J, Hammond EC: Asbestos exposure and neoplasia. *JAMA* 188:22–26, 1964.

23. Whitwell F, Scott J, Grimshaw M: Relationship between occupations and asbestos fibre content of the lungs in patients with pleural mesothelioma, lung cancer, and other disease. *Thorax* 32:377–386, 1977.

24. Peto J, Hodgson JT, Matthews FE, Jones JR: Continuing increase in mesothelioma mortality in Britain. *Lancet* 345:535–539, 1995.

25. Mossman BT, Gee JBL: Asbestos-related diseases. *N Engl J Med* 320:1721–1730, 1989.

26. Doll R: Mortality from lung cancer in asbestos workers. *Br J Ind Med* 12:81–86, 1955.

27. Selikoff IJ, Lee DH: Asbestos and its distribution: Historical background, in Selikoff IJ, Lee DH (eds): *Asbestos and Disease* (Environmental Science Series). New York, Academic Press, 1978, pp 3–3.

28. Selikoff IJ, Seidman H: Asbestos-associated deaths among workers in the United States and Canada, 1967–1987. *Ann NY Acad Sci* 643:1–14, 1991.

29. Dement JM, Harris RL, Symons MJ, Shy CM: Exposures and mortality among chrysotile asbestos workers: Part II. Mortality. *Am J Ind Med* 4:421–433, 1983.

30. Finkelstein MM: Mortality among employees of an Ontario asbestos cement factory. *Am Rev Respir Dis* 129:754–761, 1984.

31. Hughes JM, Weill H, Hammad YY: Mortality of workers employed in the asbestos cement manufacturing plants. *Br J Ind Med* 44:161–174, 1987.

17 | Chronic Beryllium and Hard-Metal Lung Disease*

Lynn T. Tanoue

CHRONIC BERYLLIUM DISEASE

History

Beryllium is the lightest metal. The commercial uses of beryllium stem from its light weight, thermal and electrical conductivity, high melting point, and tensile strength. Industrial use of beryllium began after World War I, when it was used as an alloy, first with aluminum and later with copper, nickel, and cobalt. The industry grew in the 1930s because of the increased use of beryllium-copper products during World War II and the use of beryllium oxide in the refractory and fluorescent lamp industries. More recently, beryllium has been used in the nuclear industry because of its ability to function as a neutron multiplier. As a result, beryllium is used both for civilian nuclear reactors and for military weapons.

Beryllium-related disease was first noted in the 1930s.[1] Acute beryllium disease is a toxic, dose-related injury syndrome that commonly affects the upper respiratory tract. With high-level exposure, chemical pneumonitis may ensue, with involvement of both airways and alveoli. Since the implementation of industrial hygiene standards, acute beryllium disease would now be seen only if there were serious lapses in these standards or with severe accidents such as plant explosions. In contrast to acute beryllium disease, chronic beryllium disease, which is the result of a hypersensitivity reaction to beryllium, is an ongoing hazard facing beryllium workers.

Chronic Beryllium Disease

Chronic beryllium disease (CBD) is primarily a pulmonary granulomatous disorder. Although involvement of other organ systems has been reported (e.g., lymph nodes, skin, and liver), the lungs are the principal organ affected. Early CBD may be asymptomatic. Radiologic abnormalities on routine chest radiographs and diffusing capacity abnormalities on pulmonary function tests may trigger further evaluation.[2] Blood proliferative response to beryllium at this stage would be evidence for beryllium hypersensitivity.[3] Symptomatic disease usually begins with exertional dyspnea and cough. As the disease progresses, symptoms characteristic of interstitial lung disease develop, including nonproductive cough, substernal chest discomfort, and exertional dyspnea. At this stage, dry bibasilar crackles are often observed on physical examination. With progressive disease, weakness, easy fatigability, dyspnea

---

*Edited from Chap. 58, "Chronic Beryllium and Hard-Metal Lung Disease," by Rossman MD and Edelman JD. In: *Fishman's Pulmonary Diseases and Disorders,* 3d ed., edited by Fishman AP, Elias JA, Fishman JA, Grippi MA, Kaiser LR, Senior RM. New York, McGraw-Hill, 1998, pp 893–900. For fuller discussion of the topics dealt with in this chapter, the reader is referred to the original text, as noted above.

at rest, anorexia, and weight loss may occur. Acrocyanosis, clubbing, and physical signs of cor pulmonale may be seen. Fever may be seen but is unusual. Hypercalcemia, nephrocalcinosis, joint pains, and severe cachexia have been described. Mild abnormalities of liver function tests have been noted to occur in the setting of liver granulomas. Skin involvement occurs in 10 to 30 percent of cases and frequently manifests itself as small granulomatous nodules on the hands, arms, and chest.

The radiographic changes seen with CBD are nonspecific. The most common radiographic abnormalities are diffuse round and/or reticular abnormalities.[4] These opacities are usually present diffusely throughout the lung but may be confined to the upper lobes. Hilar adenopathy is seen in up to 50 percent of cases. This may present similarly to the adenopathy seen in sarcoidosis, but in large "potato-type" node involvement. As disease advances, radiologic evidence of scarring can be seen, with hilar retraction, conglomerate masses, and emphysematous bullae. Gross architectural distortion can occur from severe fibrosis. Pleural thickening can be seen in the presence of long-standing disease.

Immunopathogenesis

Three important characteristics of chronic beryllium disease should be noted. First, disease occurs only after an industrial exposure to beryllium. Persons directly engaged in the heating, grinding, abrading, or handling of beryllium metals, alloys, salts, or oxides as well as workers indirectly exposed from processes occurring near them are at risk for disease. Current industrial hygiene practices include efforts to prevent beryllium from becoming airborne by removal at the source, thereby limiting the number of workers with potential exposure. Rarely, disease has been seen in nonindustrial workers who were exposed to beryllium airborne emissions from beryllium plants or by exposure to contaminated work clothes.

Second, chronic beryllium disease is characterized by a long interval or latency between initial exposure and the onset of disease. The average time to the onset of clinical symptoms is 10 years.[5] This fact, combined with the lack of a clear-cut dose-response relationship to CBD, has hampered efforts to determine a safe level of beryllium. It is uncertain whether the peak exposure level or a total accumulated dose is more important for the development of CBD. At present, standards set by the Occupational Safety and Health Administration (OSHA) preclude exposure to levels greater than $2 \ \mu g/m^3$ per 8-h shift as a threshold weighted average.

Third, only 1 to 5 percent of exposed workers will develop the disease. Despite intensive efforts by industry to reduce the potential for exposure, this percentage has remained stable. The tendency for CBD to occur in only a subgroup of exposed people raises the question of the role of predisposing factors. Of interest, certain human leukocyte antigen (HLA) motifs have been shown to be strongly associated with CBD.[6] These findings imply that a genetic predisposition may be required in the acquisition of the disorder.

CBD is the result of a cell-mediated immune response to beryllium. Peripheral blood cells from a large percentage of patients with CBD demonstrate positive proliferative responses to beryllium.[7,8] Examination of cells obtained by bronchoalveolar lavage (BAL) from patients with CBD has been particularly helpful in defining pathogenesis. BAL $CD4^+$ T lymphocytes from patients with CBD demonstrate positive proliferative responses to beryllium.[9–11] In contrast, BAL lymphocytes from beryllium workers with non-beryllium-related lung disease, from patients with lung disease without beryllium exposure, or from normal volunteers have no response to beryllium. The positive response in lymphocytes from patients with CBD can be blocked by antibodies against the T-cell interleukin-2 receptor or against major histocompatibility MHC class II molecules.[12] These observations suggest that the beryllium-induced lymphocyte proliferative response in these patients is a normal immunologic response, since the T-cell receptor on $CD4^+$ T cells recognizes antigen in the context of MHC class II molecules. It also appears to be antigen-driven, since the beryllium-sensitive T cells from these patients can be cloned and shown to retain their specific reactivity for beryllium but not for other antigens. In contrast, when other antigen-sensitive cells from the same patients were cloned, these cells did not react to beryllium.

Thus, the following model for the pathogenesis of chronic beryllium disease has been proposed. Beryllium is inhaled and deposited in the periphery of the lung. In predisposed persons beryllium, acting as a hapten, combines with a normal lung protein(s), causing it to be recognized as a foreign antigen (sensitization). The beryllium protein is poorly digestible and cannot be removed by the immune response. The host response to this antigen leads to persistent inflammation and to granuloma formation, which results in tissue destruction and fibrosis.

Diagnosis

A diagnosis of CBD requires the demonstration of a granulomatous reaction and beryllium hypersensitivity. The former requires biopsy material; the latter can be most convincingly demonstrated by testing the proliferative response of bronchoalveolar cells to beryllium. If BAL cells cannot be easily or safely obtained, assessing the proliferative response of blood cells to beryllium is a reasonable alternative.

Assessments of blood lymphocyte proliferative responses to beryllium constitute the most sensitive screening test for CBD.[3,13] The major drawback to the use of this assessment as a screening tool is the number of positive responses seen in asymptomatic, otherwise normal subjects. It is not known whether these represent false-positive responses or early CBD. It is also not known whether all persons with a positive blood response to beryllium will develop CBD. Until the natural course of the blood lymphocyte proliferative responses to beryllium is characterized, it will be difficult to establish definitive recommendations for screening workers. Nevertheless, because the risk of developing CBD is not temporally limited, lifelong surveillance may be necessary for all workers with exposure to beryllium or beryllium sensitivity.

Differential Diagnosis

The differential diagnosis of CBD includes sarcoidosis and other granulomatous diseases (Table 17-1). The confusion of CBD and sarcoidosis is not surprising, since many of the radiographic and clinical manifestations of the diseases are similar (Table 17-2). Most cases of CBD that are misdiagnosed are diagnosed as sarcoidosis because either the exposure to beryllium was not known by the patient or the physician failed to elicit an occupational history. Differentiation between CBD, sarcoidosis, and other disorders often depends on the result of in vitro beryllium proliferation testing. Patients with sarcoidosis and other lung disorders do not manifest a blood proliferative

TABLE 17-1 Differential Diagnosis of Chronic Beryllium Disease

Sarcoidosis
Hypersensitivity pneumonitis
Tuberculosis
Histoplasmosis
Silicosis
Talc granulomatosis
Eosinophilic granuloma
Idiopathic pulmonary fibrosis

response to beryllium, while CBD patients do. Sarcoidosis and other granulomatous disorders can be diagnosed in beryllium workers in this manner. Caution should always be exercised, however, and repeated assessments of the blood and lung cell proliferative responses to beryllium should always be obtained before granulomatous lung disease in a beryllium worker is diagnosed as a disorder other than CBD.

Treatment

The long-term prognosis for CBD is uncertain. Follow-up of cases that were diagnosed in the 1940s and 1950s suggests that the mortality of the disease might be as high as 30 percent.[2] Diagnostic techniques using cellular proliferation to beryllium now allow the diseases to be detected earlier. However, the natural history of the disease detected at the presymptomatic stage is unknown. We do not know whether this early disease is inevitably progressive or whether it may be reversible with treatment.

Corticosteroids are the first line of therapy for patients with CBD. In early disease, complete resolution of radiographic abnormalities can occur with treatment. Complete spontaneous disappearance of the radiographic lesions of CBD has not been observed. Corticosteroids should be tapered to the lowest dose that controls signs of active disease. Patients should be monitored with chest radiographs and pulmonary function tests. In some cases, exercise testing or serial measurement of serum angiotensin converting enzyme levels may be helpful. Most cases of CBD will be arrested with corticosteroid treatment. However, recurrences are common as corticosteroids are tapered.

TABLE 17-2 Comparison of Chronic Beryllium Disease and Sarcoidosis

Manifestations	Sarcoidosis	Chronic beryllium disease
Erythema nodosum	10–20%	Absent
Hilar adenopathy	50–75%	<50%
Peripheral adenopathy	Occasional	Rare
Hypercalcemia	Occasional	Rare
Nephrocalcinosis	Rare	Rare
Bone changes	In chronic disease	Absent
Parotid involvement	Occasional	Absent
Posterior uveitis	Occasional	Absent
Liver involvement	Common	Frequent
Splenomegaly	Rare	Rare
Skin	Uncommon	Unusual
Central nervous system	Occasional	Absent
Response to steroids	Only active disease	Only active disease

In cases of treatment failure with progression to end-stage disease, lung transplantation may be a reasonable consideration.

Beryllium and Lung Cancer

Animal studies have clearly indicated that beryllium is carcinogenic.[14] Whether beryllium is carcinogenic in humans is not clear. The most recent study undertaken by the National Institute for Occupational Safety and Health (NIOSH) suggests that a small increase in lung cancer [standardized mortality ratio (SMR) = 1.26] may occur in beryllium workers.[15] This finding has been challenged, however, because of potential confounding issues related to cigarette smoking.[16] This issue will remain controversial until additional studies are performed.

HARD-METAL LUNG DISEASE

Hard metal is a sintered alloy containing mainly tungsten carbide and cobalt, with smaller amounts of chromium, molybdenum, nickel, niobium, tantalum, titanium, and vanadium. These components are milled to a fine powder, mixed together, pressed into the desired shape, and heated under pressure to between 800 and 1000°C, yielding a product with a chalk-like consistency. The material may then undergo additional machining before being baked at 1500°C, which is above the melting point of cobalt and leads to the formation of an alloy that is 90 to 95 percent as hard as a diamond. Because of this property, hard metal is an important component in cutting tools, drill bits, armor plate, and jet engine parts. The industrial processes associated with hard-metal lung disease produce respirable fine metallic dust particles. They also produce metallic ions that accumulate in the coolants used in the metalworking procedure and are absorbed through the skin or inhaled in vaporized coolant fluids.

Hard metal was developed in the 1920s, and interstitial lung disease was first reported in hard-metal workers in 1940. Lung disease has been noted to occur in those working in both the initial production of hard metal and the machining and maintenance of hard-metal tool components. In addition, although hard metal is not used in the diamond-polishing industry, a similar spectrum of disease has been reported in diamond polishers using steel polishing disks whose cutting surfaces consist of microdiamonds cemented into a fine cobalt mesh. In contrast, workers in the cobalt-producing industry, who are more likely to be exposed to cobalt alone, may develop occupational asthma but appear to be much less likely to develop interstitial lung disease.

Interstitial Lung Disease (Hard-Metal Disease)

Interstitial lung disease has been seen in hard-metal workers and diamond polishers. In recent studies, the prevalence of fibrosis in hard-metal workers has ranged up to 2.6 percent. Although interstitial lung disease may occur after a short duration and low levels of exposure, longer duration or higher levels of exposure are associated with increased risk.[17] Nonsmokers and former smokers also appear to be at higher risk.[18] Interstitial disease is more common in workers engaged in the grinding of hard metal, where there is exposure to ionized cobalt in the grinding coolants in addition to hard-metal dust.[17] It is possible that ionized cobalt, which is highly protein-bound, acts as a hapten in this setting.

In some patients, hard-metal disease presents as a hypersensitivity pneumonitis or allergic alveolitis. These patients manifest fever, anorexia, cough, dyspnea, inspiratory crackles, and fine reticulonodular infiltrates on the chest radiograph. Pulmonary function testing typically shows a restrictive pattern, with a reduced $D_{L_{CO}}$. Symptoms may resolve when exposure is discontinued but may recur with reexposure. Over time, progressive dyspnea, lung function impairment, and interstitial fibrosis may develop. Fibrosis may also occur in the absence of antecedent symptoms. Patients with advanced disease exhibit weight loss, hypoxemia, digital clubbing, pulmonary hypertension, and cor pulmonale. Patients with alveolitis or fibrosis related to cobalt often have positive skin patch tests to cobalt.

The histopathologic manifestations of the interstitial disease in these patients can be varied, with findings consistent with bronchiolitis, desquamative interstitial pneumonitis, usual interstitial fibrosis, and giant-cell interstitial pneumonitis (GIP). Granuloma formation does not occur. Lung biopsies may show heterogeneous patchy involvement, with foci of active alveolitis, fibrosis, and normal parenchyma. Bronchiolitis may be seen in areas with and without active alveolitis. GIP is characterized by lymphoplasmocytic infiltration, epithelial desquamation, and the presence of numerous multinucleated giant cells in the alveolar spaces.[19] These giant cells are formed by both actively phagocytic alveolar macrophages and type II pneumocytes.[4] Infiltration with eosinophils has also been described. Analysis of BAL fluid may demonstrate hypercellularity, with increased numbers of macrophages and giant cells. A relative or absolute increase in the number of lymphocytes—with a reduced CD4/CD8 ratio as well as increased numbers of neutrophils, eosinophils, and mast cells—may also be seen.[20]

Electron microscopy with energy-dispersive x-ray analysis (EDAX) of the particulate material present in biopsy specimens may demonstrate the presence of the elements used to form hard metal. Because of its high solubility, significant amounts of cobalt may not always be present.[18] Neutron activation analysis of BAL fluid yields similar results.[21] Such findings in clinical specimens are suggestive of hard-metal exposure but do not necessarily indicate disease.

Treatment for this disease consists of discontinuation of exposure and administration of systemic corticosteroids. Although no clinical trials have been performed, dosage and duration of treatment similar to those used in other forms of active alveolitis or fibrosis should be considered. Patients with active alveolitis may show a dramatic response to steroids, whereas patients with more prominent fibrosis may show minimal response despite prolonged steroid treatment.[22] GIP has been observed to recur after lung transplantation despite cessation of occupational exposure.[23]

OCCUPATIONAL ASTHMA

The reported prevalence of asthma or wheezing related to cobalt or hard-metal exposure ranges from less than 1 percent to 10.9 percent. This variation may be attributed to different levels of exposure and the criteria used by various authors to define occupational asthma. As with other forms of occupational asthma, patients may note cough, wheezing, dyspnea, chest tightness, conjunctivitis, and rhinitis. Throughout the workday, symptoms may increase in severity, and a progressive decline in peak flow may be demonstrated. Symptoms usually abate during weekends or vacations and often resolve when exposure is discontinued. Upper airway symptoms may result from either direct airway irritation or atopic responses.

The diagnosis of occupational asthma relies heavily on the demonstration of an association between workplace exposure and symptoms. The diagnosis may be confirmed by bronchoprovocation testing (BPT) with cobalt or cobalt salts, but such testing should be strictly limited to laboratories with experience in such testing. A positive radioimmunosorbent test (RAST) to cobalt-conjugated human serum albumin has also been reported in some patients, suggesting a type I allergic response.[24] Patients with hard-metal asthma may have positive RAST and BPT responses to both nickel and cobalt.[25] Skin patch testing with cobalt salts does not appear to be of use in diagnosing hard-metal asthma.

The dose-response relationship between heavy-metal or cobalt exposure and asthma has been looked at in a number of studies. A twofold increase in the relative odds ratio for work-related wheezing was noted when cobalt exposure exceeded the current allowance standard of 0.05 mg/m^3.[17] Recent studies have also demonstrated statistically significant reductions in FEV_1 and FVC values in situations where cobalt levels were well below 0.05 mg/m^3, suggesting that the current exposure limit may not protect all workers against the development of cobalt-induced asthma.[26,27] Because of such findings, baseline and screening evaluations should be performed in workers exposed to hard-metal dust. In patients with symptoms or findings suggestive of occupational asthma, peak flow monitoring during working and nonworking hours should be performed and other causes of pulmonary function deterioration ruled out. Specific BPT and RAST results may provide additional positive criteria for diagnosis. Personal employee air sampling and measurement of urinary cobalt levels can provide information about ongoing exposure. The workplace should also be examined for levels of cobalt exposure and employee protective practices.

Treatment for occupational asthma related to cobalt includes control of exposure as well as usual medical therapy for asthma. Systemic corticosteroid treatment is usually not required.

LUNG CANCER

Cobalt and cobalt-containing compounds have been shown to cause cancer in rats after local injection and intratracheal instillation. The International Agency for Research on Cancer reviewed the evidence for the carcinogenicity of cobalt in 1991 and concluded that although there was sufficient evidence for the carcinogenicity of cobalt metal powder and cobalt oxide in experimental animals, there was inadequate evidence for the carcinogenicity of cobalt and cobalt compounds in humans.[28] Controversy continues with regard to whether there is an association between cobalt or hard metal and the development of lung cancer in humans.

REFERENCES

1. Van Ordstrand HS, Hughes R, Carmody MG: Chemical pneumonia in workers extracting beryllium oxide: Report of three cases. *Cleve Clin Q* 10:10–18, 1943.
2. Stoeckle SD, Hardy HL, Weber AL: Chronic beryllium disease. *Am J Med* 46:545–561, 1969.
3. Kreiss K, Mroz MM, Zhen B, et al: Epidemiology of beryllium sensitization and disease in nuclear workers. *Am Rev Respir Dis* 148:985–991, 1993.
4. Aronchick JM, Rossman MD, Miller WT: Chronic beryllium disease: Diagnosis, radiographic findings and correlation with pulmonary function tests. *Radiology* 163:677–682, 1987.

5. Eisenbud M, Lisson J: Epidemiological aspects of beryllium-induced nonmalignant lung disease: A 30 year update. *J Occup Med* 25:196–202, 1983.
6. Richeldi L, Sorrentino R, Saltini C: HLA-DPB1 glutamate 69: A genetic marker of beryllium disease. *Science* 262:242–244, 1993.
7. Deodhar SD, Barna B, Van Ordstrand HS: A study of the immunologic aspects of chronic berylliosis. *Chest* 63:309–313, 1973.
8. Marx JJ Jr, Burrell R: Delayed hypersensitivity to beryllium compounds. *J Immunol* 111:590–598, 1973.
9. Cullen MR, Kominsky JR, Rossman MD, et al: Chronic beryllium disease in a precious metal refinery: Clinical epidemiologic and immunologic evidence for continuing risk from exposure to low level beryllium fume. *Am Rev Respir Dis* 135:201–209, 1987.
10. Epstein PE, Dauber JH, Rossman MD, Daniele RP: Bronchoalveolar lavage in a patient with chronic berylliosis: Evidence for hypersensitivity pneumonitis. *Ann Intern Med* 97:213–216, 1982.
11. Rossman MD, Kern JA, Elias JA, et al: Proliferative response of bronchoalveolar lymphocytes to beryllium. *Ann Intern Med* 108:687–693, 1988.
12. Saltini C, Winestock D, Kirby M, et al: Maintenance of alveolitis in patients with chronic beryllium disease by beryllium-specific T cells. *N Engl J Med* 320:1103–1109, 1989.
13. Kreiss K, Wasserman S, Mroz MM, Newman LS: Beryllium disease screening in the ceramics industry. *J Occup Med* 35:267–274, 1993.
14. Groth DH: Carcinogenicity of beryllium: Review of the literature. *Environ Res* 21:56–62, 1980.
15. Ward E, Okun A, Ruder A, et al: A mortality study of workers at seven beryllium processing plants. *Am J Ind Med* 22:885–904, 1992.
16. MacMahon B: The epidemiological evidence on the carcinogenicity of beryllium in humans. *J Occup Med* 36:15–24. 1994.
17. Sprince NL, Oliver LC, Eisen EA, et al: Cobalt exposure and lung disease in tungsten carbide production. *Am Rev Respir Dis* 138:1220–1226, 1988.
18. Antila S, Sutinen S, Paananen M, et al: Hard metal lung disease: A clinical, histological, ultrastructural and x-ray microanalytical study. *Eur J Respir Dis* 69:83–94, 1986.
19. Ohori NP, Sciurba FC, Owens GR, et al: Giant-cell interstitial pneumonia and hard metal pneumoconiosis. *Am J Surg Pathol* 13:581–587, 1989.
20. Forni A: Bronchoalveolar lavage in the diagnosis of hard metal disease. *Sci Total Environ* 150:69–76, 1994.
21. Rizzato G, Fraioli P, Sabbioni E, et al: The differential diagnosis of hard metal lung disease. *Sci Total Environ* 150:77–83, 1994.
22. Cugell DW: The hard metal diseases. *Clin Chest Med* 13:269–279, 1992.
23. Frost AE, Keller CA, Brown RW, et al: Giant cell interstitial pneumonitis disease recurrence in the transplanted lung. *Am Rev Respir Dis* 148:1401–1404, 1993.
24. Shirakawa T, Kusaka Y, Fujimura N, et al: Occupational asthma from cobalt sensitivity in workers exposed to hard metal dust. *Chest* 95:29–37, 1989.
25. Shirakawa T, Kusaka Y, Fujimura N, et al: Hard metal asthma: Cross immunological and respiratory reactivity between cobalt and nickel? *Thorax* 45:266–271, 1990.
26. Kennedy SM, Chan-Yeung M, Marion S, et al: Maintenance of stellite and tungsten carbide saw tips: Respiratory health and exposure-response evaluations. *Occup Environ Med* 52:185–191, 1995.
27. Nemery B, Casier P, Roosels D, et al: Survey of cobalt exposure and respiratory health in diamond polishers. *Am Rev Respir Dis* 145:610–616, 1992.
28. International Agency for Research on Cancer: Chlorinated drinking water, chlorination by-products, some other halogenated compounds. *IARC Monographs on the Evaluation of Carcinogenic Risks to Humans,* vol 52., Lyon, France, World Health Organization, IARC, 1991.

18 | Coal Workers' Lung Diseases and Silicosis*

Lynn T. Tanoue

COAL WORKERS' LUNG DISEASES

Coal miners are at risk for developing several distinct clinical illnesses in relation to their occupational exposures. Coal workers' pneumoconiosis (CWP) is the parenchymal lung disease that results from the inhalation and deposition of coal mine dust and the tissue's reaction to its presence. Exposure to coal mine dust also increases a miner's risk of developing chronic bronchitis and emphysema and accelerates loss of ventilatory lung function.

Coal and Coal Mining

Coal is not a pure mineral. It is a conglomeration of carbonaceous rocks derived from the accumulation of vegetation sedimented under swampy conditions and subjected to extreme pressure over long periods. Coals are characterized by rank (which relates to geologic age), hardness, carbon content, and the amount of heat released (BTUs) when burned. Peat is the lowest-ranked (softest) and geologically newest type of coal, while anthracite is the highest-ranked (hardest) and oldest coal.

Coal can be found in outcroppings and seams only a few feet below the surface. From such sites, coal can be obtained by simply scraping off the surface, or overburden, and mining with large earth-moving equipment (strip mining). Occasionally, surface mining is also performed by boring into coal outcrops with an auger. Coal seams may also be buried deep within the earth's crust. In these cases it is not feasible simply to strip away the overburden. The only practical way of mining the coal is to sink shafts from the surface to the coal seam and then follow the seam with a series of horizontal tunnels. In the past, most coal mines were of this type. At present, strip mining accounts for somewhat more than half of the coal mined in the United States.

Not all coal-mining jobs are equally exposed to respiratory hazards.[1,2] In underground mines, airborne dust concentrations are highest at the coal cutting face, where coal is removed from the intact seams. Face jobs include the loading of coal into transportation vehicles and, depending on the techniques used in the mine, operation of continuous or long wall-mining machines. Exposure to crystalline silica—and thus the risk of silicosis—also occurs in underground mines, particularly to miners engaged in roof support (roof bolting) or drilling operations and in motormen who operate underground coal trains and use sand for traction on the rails. Dust levels in the air at surface mines are generally considerably lower than those in underground mines. However, miners in some exclusively aboveground coal-mining operations may also

*Edited from Chap. 59, "Coal Workers' Lung Diseases and Silicosis," by Parker JE, Petsonk EL. In: *Fishman's Pulmonary Diseases and Disorders,* 3d ed., edited by Fishman AP, Elias JA, Fishman JA, Grippi MA, Kaiser LR, Senior RM. New York, McGraw-Hill, 1998, pp 901–914. For fuller discussion of the topics dealt with in this chapter, the reader is referred to the original text, as noted above.

have important exposure to dusts. These include workers at tipples and preparation plants, where crushing, sizing, washing, and blending of coal are done
and coal is stored and loaded into ships, railroad cars, or river barges. Workers at surface coal mines who operate the drilling rigs (drillers)—to make
holes into which explosives are placed—are exposed to silica and at risk for
the development of silicosis.

Epidemiology

The first major survey of the health of American coal workers was conducted
by the U.S. Public Health Service (USPHS) from 1969 to 1971, evaluating
symptoms, lung function, and chest radiographic findings.[3] This study included more than 9000 miners at 2 anthracite and 29 bituminous mines.
Radiographic data showed an overall prevalence of simple and complicated
CWP of nearly 30 percent. There was variation by region of the country and
the type (rank) of coal mined. Among eastern Pennsylvania anthracite (high-
rank) coal miners, 46 percent had simple and 14 percent complicated CWP.
In contrast, among miners in the western plateau of Colorado and Utah, mining a lower-rank coal, only 5 percent had simple CWP and none had the complicated form. Among underground miners, those working at the coal face
and exposed to higher concentrations of coal mine dust had higher preva-
lences of CWP than surface workers or those whose jobs caused them to enter the face area only intermittently.

Enforcement of compliance with dust control measures dates to 1969. Since
then, a decline in the prevalence of CWP in active U.S. miners[4] has been
demonstrated in periodic chest radiograph surveillance programs in U.S. miners. In 1970–73, CWP was found in 28 percent of participants with 25 years
or more underground. By 1992–95, fewer than 10 percent showed radiographic evidence of CWP.[4] It appears that both the attack rate in miners without CWP as well as the risk of disease progression in miners with simple
CWP have decreased because of mandated dust standards limiting the mass
of respirable dust to which a miner is exposed.[5,6] However, the latter is not
true for the complicated form of CWP—progressive massive fibrosis (PMF).
Once a person has inhaled sufficient coal mine dust into the lungs for the
chest radiograph to be classified with at least ILO category 2 pneumoconiosis, the probability of its progressing to the complicated form appears to be
independent of any further dust exposure. The rate of progression to PMF
appears to be influenced chiefly by the age at which the miner begins to show
radiographic changes of CWP.

Pathology of Coal Miners' Lung Diseases

The coal macule is the primary pathologic lesion of simple CWP, consisting
of a focal collection of coal dust in pigment-laden macrophages around respiratory bronchioles, tapering off toward the alveolar duct.[7] A fine network
of reticulin is present in the early lesion. Macules may also contain a small
amount of collagen. Centriacinar emphysema is also observed with increased
prevalence in the lungs of coal miners. The severity of this lesion is proportional to the miner's cumulative dust exposure and retention. Focal emphysema is the form of centriacinar emphysema that is seen as an integral part
of the lesion of simple CWP. It is characterized by enlargement of the airspaces immediately adjacent to the dust macule. Muscular thickening of
pulmonary arteries can be observed in both simple and complicated CWP.

Pathologic changes in the airways consistent with chronic bronchitis, including enlargement of mucous glands, have also been noted in miners' lungs.

With increasing dust exposure, coal-induced lesions increase in size and number owing to the overwhelming of normal lung clearance mechanisms. These larger fibrotic lesions are called *coal nodules* and are palpable in gross lung specimens. Palpable coal nodules are classified as micronodular up to 7 mm in diameter and macronodular if they are 7 mm or larger. The diagnosis of complicated CWP or PMF is made when one or more nodules in a lung specimen are noted to attain a size of 2 cm or greater in diameter.[7] Radiographically, PMF is said to be present when coal-induced radiographic shadows are at least 1 cm in diameter. These lesions are solid, heavily pigmented, and rubbery to hard; they occur most commonly in the apical posterior portions of upper lobes or the superior segments of lower lobes. They tend to occur symmetrically, but they may be asymmetrical and cavitate. Airways and vessels adjacent to the lesions may be distorted; within the lesions, they are destroyed. PMF generally occurs in association with background pathologic changes of simple CWP.

Clinical Features of Coal Workers' Lung Diseases

Many coal-exposed workers, even those with simple pneumoconiosis, have no symptoms. Others experience a variety of respiratory problems, with chronic cough and sputum production being the most common. The symptoms are probably related to bronchitic changes in the large airways, including thickening of the airway wall, mucous gland enlargement, and hypersecretion, which are more common with increasing dust exposure. Continued inhalation of dust particles presents a chronic burden to the mucociliary escalator. With worsened pneumoconiosis or in the presence of more severe airflow obstruction, dyspnea, cough, and sputum production are more frequent. Complicated or advanced CWP can result in edema of the lower extremities with cor pulmonale. Melanoptysis (expectoration of black sputum) has also been reported; it is due to the excavation of lesions of PMF.

Clubbing is not a feature of coal miners' lung diseases; if noted, it should prompt further studies. In contrast to silicosis, CWP has not been associated with an increased risk for mycobacterial infection. It should be kept in mind, however, that in autopsy studies, the lungs of 12 percent of miners show classic silicotic nodules.[8] Thus, the appearance of a cavity in PMF should prompt examination of the sputum for typical and atypical mycobacteria.

Radiology and Diagnosis of CWP

The diagnosis of CWP can be made with confidence, without histologic confirmation, in the presence of an adequate history (at least 5 to 10 years) of coal mine dust exposure and a characteristic chest radiograph. The radiograph in simple pneumoconiosis shows small opacities, ranging in size from a pinhead up to 1 cm in diameter. Rounded nodules predominate and tend to appear first in the upper zones and involving middle and lower zones as the number of opacities increase. Progressive massive fibrosis is characterized by one or more large opacities greater than 1 cm in diameter, usually with an upper lobe predominance. The 1980 radiographic classification of the International Labour Office (ILO) is the most widely accepted classification of pneumoconiosis and is outlined in Chap.15.[9] A profusion reading of category 1/0 indicates the definite presence of opacities consistent with pneumoconiosis.

Complicated CWP (PMF) is divided into categories A, B, and C, based on the size of large opacities. Lower lobe emphysema is also commonly noted in coal workers. HRCT scanning appears to be the most sensitive radiologic technique in coal workers, since it can demonstrate parenchymal nodules and emphysema when standard radiographs are normal.[10]

Lung Function and Respiratory Impairment in Coal Miners

Coal mine exposures may result in several pathologic processes, including simple and complicated CWP, chronic bronchitis, emphysema, and dust-related airflow limitation, each of which may have adverse physiologic consequences. In an individual miner, the pattern and severity of impairment will be related to such recognized factors as the intensity and duration of respirable dust exposure, geologic factors (e.g., coal rank, silica content), residence time of dust in the lung, and exposure to other respiratory hazards (e.g., tobacco smoke). In miners with airway hyperresponsiveness, greater functional deficits and an increased risk of symptoms may be expected.[11]

Pulmonary Function

Miners with complicated CWP in general consistently show important defects in lung function. These can be restrictive or obstructive, depending on the contributions of fibrosis and bronchitis, respectively. A number of studies have evaluated lung function in miners with respect to cumulative dust exposure.[12,13] Miners demonstrate a progressively greater risk of lung function loss with increasing dust exposure, which is independent of the chest radiographic findings of CWP.[12] Subgroups of miners may experience more severe effects. Loss of FEV_1 is most severe in those who work for many years at the dustiest jobs. In one study evaluating the lung function of 1072 miners over an 11-year period, work at coal face jobs resulted in lung function losses essentially similar to those due to smoking.[12]

Among smoking miners, the effects of tobacco smoke appear to be additive to the dust effect.[14] It has also been noted that miners experience a more rapid loss of lung function over their first few years of mining, with slower dust-related declines after that time.[15] Although, on average, functional losses associated with dust are small, it is estimated that 35 years of work at the current dust limit will cause a clinically important FEV_1 loss in 8 percent of nonsmoking coal miners.[16] The mild obstructive abnormalities seen in nonsmokers with simple CWP are frequently the result of small airway dysfunction—a finding that correlates nicely with the pathologic features of dust deposition in this disorder.[17]

When large opacities of complicated CWP are present, DL_{CO} is often reduced. Cardiopulmonary exercise testing in coal miners with or without CWP is a field that continues to be investigated. Current reports have been based largely on patients referred for disability evaluations, and thus suffer from ill-defined selection biases. Patients with complicated CWP or airflow obstruction may demonstrate exertional hypoxia, pulmonary arterial hypertension, and excess ventilation.[18,19]

Caplan's Syndrome

In 1953, Anthony Caplan described an association between distinctive nodular opacities in the lungs of Welsh coal miners and rheumatoid arthritis.[20]

The pulmonary nodules were 0.5 to 5 cm in diameter, bilateral, and located peripherally. They often developed rapidly (over weeks) in the presence of a mild pneumoconiosis and could cavitate or calcify. In many cases, the pulmonary opacities preceded the onset of the arthritis by months to years. In others, the pulmonary nodules and arthritis appeared coincidentally or the pulmonary lesions appeared only after the arthritis was full-blown. In its early stages, the opacities of Caplan's syndrome and progressive massive fibrosis are readily distinguishable. They are not mutually exclusive, however: Caplan's lesions and PMF lesions have been found in the same subjects. The definition of Caplan's syndrome has since been broadened to include patients with rheumatoid arthritis, similar radiographic abnormalities, and a variety of pneumoconioses, including silicosis and asbestosis.

The potential role of immunologic factors in the pathogenesis of mineral dust pneumoconioses was first noted with the description of Caplan's syndrome. A Caplan's-like syndrome has been noted in miners without arthritis but with circulating rheumatoid factor (RF). Patients with CWP have a high prevalence of autoantibodies, with RF and antinuclear antibody (ANA) evaluations being positive in 9 to 10 percent and 17 to 34 percent of patients, respectively.[21,22] Of note, the prevalence of these autoantibodies varies with the stage of CWP, with a positive ANA or RF being detected in 13 percent of patients with simple CWP and 45 percent of patients with stage C CWP.[21–23]

Management of Coal Workers' Lung Diseases

There is no specific therapy for CWP. Management is directed at prevention, early recognition, and treatment of complications. Primary prevention of lung disease in miners includes continuing efforts at reducing exposure to coal mine dust. Improved mining methods appear to be reducing exposure and the number of new cases of both simple and complicated pneumoconiosis. Medical surveillance programs, using chest radiographs, allow early recognition of workers with simple pneumoconiosis. Workers with simple pneumoconiosis should be encouraged to exercise transfer rights to low-dust jobs. Any worker found to have PMF should be strongly advised about the hazards of further dust exposures.

Workers presenting with respiratory symptoms should have more extensive evaluation. The history, physical examination, and chest radiograph should be supplemented by pulmonary function testing. If indicated, an evaluation of bronchodilator responsiveness and resting arterial blood gas measurement can be made. A thorough baseline evaluation allows accurate assessment of the worker's respiratory health over time and may be important in assessing response to therapy or progression of disease.

Mortality

As a group, miners experience increased mortality attributable to pneumoconiosis, emphysema, and chronic bronchitis. Complicated CWP (i.e., PMF) is consistently associated with higher mortality, especially in categories B and C. Among miners with simple CWP, decreases in survival are significantly smaller.[24,25] The major clinical challenges are the recognition and management of airflow obstruction, respiratory infection, hypoxemia, respiratory failure, cor pulmonale, arrhythmias, and pneumothorax. Factors that should heighten suspicion of the potential for increased risk of a clinically significant dust effect are a history of prolonged exposures in dusty jobs, exposures to higher-rank coals, a younger age at first employment, and the finding of radiographic changes of CWP.

Symptomatic airflow obstruction may benefit from usual treatment for reversible airflow obstruction. When it is an issue, smoking cessation should be strongly encouraged. Patients with significant airflow obstruction or PMF should receive appropriate immunization with influenza and pneumococcal vaccines. Bacterial and viral episodes of bronchitis or pneumonia should be promptly recognized and appropriately treated. Hypoxemia can be a serious complication in advanced, complicated pneumoconiosis. As with situations of chronic hypoxemia, additional complications including polycythemia, pulmonary hypertension, cor pulmonale, and cerebral dysfunction can occur.

Patients with complicated CWP, especially those who have been exposed to silica as well as coal dust, deserve special attention with regard to mycobacterial infection. Any patient suspected of bacterial infection should be promptly investigated with a chest radiograph and sputum AFB examination. Occasionally, fiberoptic bronchoscopy with brushings and washings is required to establish the diagnosis. Active tuberculosis in patients with CWP can usually be successfully treated with the usual drug regimens provided that rifampin is one of the drugs employed.[26] In coal miners with a significant history of concurrent silica exposure (such as motormen, roof bolters, and shaft development workers), some authorities suggest that the treatment for tuberculosis should be more aggressive (see "Silicosis," below). Long-term follow-up is also indicated in view of several reports of recurrent pulmonary tuberculosis in patients with PMF after completion of apparently adequate therapy.[27]

The clinician may also be presented with the diagnostic dilemma of distinguishing a primary or metastatic neoplasm from an unusual presentation of progressive massive fibrosis or Caplan's syndrome. When typical large opacities of PMF occur symmetrically and bilaterally on a background of simple CWP, one can be confident that the lesions are unlikely to represent neoplastic disease. Prior radiographs from medical screening programs are often obtainable and can help confirm stability or progression over a long time. If the background of simple CWP is sparse or absent, the lesion is unilateral, or there are multiple peripherally situated nodules (Caplan's syndrome), the differentiation from a neoplasm may indeed be impossible without a biopsy.

SILICOSIS

Silica, or silicon dioxide, is the predominant component of the earth's crust. It is particularly important in sandstone, granite, and slate, as it makes up 20 to 100 percent of these rock formations. When the earth's crust is disturbed or silica-containing rock is used or processed, there are potential respiratory risks for workers. Occupational exposure to silica particles of respirable size (aerodynamic diameter of 0.5 to 5 μm) is associated with mining, quarrying, drilling, tunneling, and abrasive blasting with quartz-containing materials (sandblasting). Silica exposure also poses a hazard to stonecutters and to pottery, foundry, ground silica, and refractory workers. The silicon dioxide that is inhaled is usually crystalline and most often quartz. Cristobalite and tridymite are other crystalline forms of silica. These three crystalline forms are also called "free silica" to distinguish them from silicates, such as asbestos and talc.

Silicosis is a fibrotic disease of the lungs caused by the inhalation, retention, and reaction to crystalline silica. This serious and potentially fatal occupational lung disease remains prevalent throughout the world. The development and progression of silicosis frequently occur after exposure has ceased. Crystalline silica exposure is widespread. Silica sand is such an inexpensive and versatile component of so many manufacturing processes that millions of workers throughout the world, including workers in developed countries, are at risk of the disease.[2,28,29]

Forms of Silicosis

Chronic (or Classic) Silicosis

Chronic silicosis may be asymptomatic or result in insidiously progressive exertional dyspnea or cough. A latency of 15 years or more since onset of exposure is common. Radiographically, it presents with small (less than 10-mm) rounded opacities, predominantly in the upper lung zones. The pathologic hallmark is the silicotic nodule, which is characterized by a cell-free central area of concentrically arranged whorled, hyalinized collagen fibers, surrounded by cellular connective tissue with reticulin fibers. Under polarized light, birefringent particles are typically seen most prominently in the periphery of the silicotic nodule. Silicotic nodules can also be seen in the visceral pleura and in regional lymph nodes.

Progressive massive fibrosis (PMF) or conglomerate silicosis occurs when one or more groups of the small nodules in the lungs of a patient with chronic silicosis coalesce to form larger (over 10-mm) shadows on the chest radiograph. Progressive illness may occur even after exposure to silica-containing dust has ceased. Symptoms of exertional dyspnea and reduced functional status usually accompany diminished $D_{L_{CO}}$ and reduced arterial oxygen tension at rest or with exercise with a demonstrable restrictive pattern on pulmonary function evaluation. Concomitant dust-induced bronchitis or distortion of the bronchial tree may also result in productive cough or airflow obstruction. Recurrent bacterial infections may be seen. Weight loss and cavitation of the large opacities should prompt concern for tuberculosis or other mycobacterial infections. Pneumothorax may be a life-threatening complication, since the fibrotic lung may be difficult to reexpand. Hypoxemic respiratory failure with cor pulmonale and congestive heart failure can be terminal findings.

Accelerated Silicosis

Accelerated silicosis results from exposures that are more intense and of shorter (5 to 10 years) duration than in the chronic form. The symptoms, radiographic findings, physiologic measurements, and lung pathology of chronic and accelerated silicosis are quite similar. However, rate of disease progression is more rapid for accelerated silicosis. Workers with accelerated disease are at risk for superimposed mycobacterial infection. Findings consistent with autoimmune diseases such as scleroderma are also more frequent in the accelerated form of silicosis.

Acute Silicosis

Acute silicosis develops within a few months up to about 5 years after a massive inhalation of silica.[2] Dramatic dyspnea, weakness, and weight loss are often presenting symptoms. The radiographic findings differ from those in the more chronic forms of silicosis and are dominated by a diffuse alveolar filling pattern with a predominance in the lower lung zone. Air bronchograms may be present. Histologic findings similar to those of pulmonary alveolar proteinosis have been described, and extrapulmonary (renal and hepatic) abnormalities are occasionally reported. The usual clinical course of this rare form of silicosis is rapid progression to severe hypoxemic ventilatory failure and death.

Other Disorders

Even in the absence of radiographic silicosis, silica-exposed workers may develop chronic bronchitis and emphysema from their occupational dust exposure. Progressive declines in lung function have also been documented in workers exposed to silica and other occupational mineral dusts.

Association with Tuberculosis

The propensity for people with silicosis to get tuberculosis has been recognized for nearly a century.[30] Tuberculosis can complicate all forms of silicosis. Patients with the acute and accelerated forms of the disease appear to be at the highest risk of infection. Vigilance for infectious complications cannot be overemphasized. New onset or a change in cough, hemoptysis, fever, or weight loss should trigger evaluation. Silica exposure alone, even without silicosis, may predispose to this infection.

Mycobacterium tuberculosis is the usual organism, but atypical mycobacteria (and, less often, *Nocardia asteroides*) can also be seen. The mechanism of this susceptibility is poorly understood but may be related to the toxic effects of silica on alveolar macrophages.

The diagnosis of active tuberculosis infection in patients with silicosis can be difficult. Clinical symptoms of weight loss, fever, sweats, and malaise should prompt radiographic evaluation, sputum acid-fast stains for bacilli, and cultures. Radiographic changes with infection may be subtle and atypical. Enlargement and cavitation in conglomerate lesions or nodular opacities are of particular concern. Bacteriologic studies on expectorated sputum may not always be reliable in silicotuberculosis. Fiberoptic bronchoscopy for additional specimens for culture and study may be helpful in establishing a diagnosis of active disease. The use of multidrug therapy for suspected active disease in patients with silicosis is justified at a lower level of suspicion than in the nonsilicotic subject owing to the difficulty in firmly establishing evidence for active infection. To obtain satisfactory results in the presence of silicosis, antituberculous treatment must be more prolonged, with regimens lasting at least 8 months.

Clinical Manifestations of Silicosis

Patients with silicosis can be asymptomatic and present with abnormal chest radiographs. They can also be minimally symptomatic in spite of advanced radiographic abnormalities. When silicosis is symptomatic, the primary symptom is usually exertional dyspnea. Productive cough is often present secondary to chronic bronchitis from occupational dust exposure, tobacco use, or both. Cough may at times also be attributed to pressure from large masses of silicotic lymph nodes on the trachea or main-stem bronchi. Other chest symptoms are less common. Wheeze and chest tightness may occur as part of associated obstructive airway disease or bronchitis. Chest pain and finger clubbing are not features of silicosis. Hemoptysis and systemic symptoms such as fever and weight loss should suggest complicating infection or neo-plastic disease. Advanced forms of silicosis are associated with progressive respiratory failure with or without cor pulmonale.

Radiographic Patterns in Silicosis

In silicosis, rounded opacities of ILO "q" and "r" type are the earliest radio-graphic signs of uncomplicated silicosis (see Table 15-3).[9] Other patterns have also been described, including linear or irregular shadows. They are usu-ally found to predominate initially in the upper lung zones and may progress to invade other zones. Hilar lymphadenopathy may also be noted. Eggshell calcification of the lymph nodes, while rare, is strongly suggestive of silicosis.

PMF is characterized by the formation of large opacities that are usually in the upper lung zones. These lesions tend to contract, leaving areas of com-pensatory emphysema at their margins and in the lung bases. As a result of this process, small rounded opacities that previously were evident on the radiograph may become less visible or at times disappear. Pleural abnormal-ities are uncommon but do occur, particularly in association with conglom-erate lesions. Although ischemic necrosis may occur in large silicotic lesions, the onset of cavitation or a rapid change in the radiographic appearance should prompt a search for active mycobacterial disease.

Lung Function Abnormalities in Silicosis

No specific or characteristic pattern of ventilatory impairment is present in silicosis. Spirometry may be normal; when it is abnormal, the tracings may show obstruction, restriction, or a mixed pattern depending on whether fibrotic or bronchitic processes coexist. Obstruction may indeed be the more common finding. Silica and mixed dust exposures[31] may lead to clinically significant airflow limitation independent of radiographic abnormality.[16] In general, workers experience lung function loss proportionate to the du-ration and intensity of silica dust exposure. While functional changes tend to be more marked with advanced radiologic findings, no good correlation exists between radiographic abnormalities and ventilatory impairment. Im-pairment of diffusing capacity may also occur in the absence of ventilatory impairment.

Complications and Special Diagnostic Issues in Silicosis

With a history of exposure and a characteristic radiograph, the diagnosis of silicosis is generally not difficult to establish. Challenges arise only when the radiologic features are unusual or the history of exposure is not recognized. Lung biopsy is rarely required to establish the diagnosis. However, tissue samples are helpful in some clinical settings when complications are present or the differential diagnosis includes tuberculosis, neoplasm, or PMF. Biopsy material should be sent for culture; in research settings, dust analysis may be a useful additional measure. When tissue is required, open or thoraco-scopic lung biopsies are generally necessary to obtain adequate material for examination.

Lung Cancer and Silicosis

Substantial concern and interest about the relationship between silica exposure, silicosis, and cancer of the lung continue to stimulate debate. The

International Agency for Research on Cancer[32] has classified crystalline silica as a 2A carcinogen on the basis of "sufficient" evidence of carcinogenicity in experimental animals and "limited" evidence of carcinogenicity in humans. This issue may be particularly problematic because the radiographic distinction between PMF lesions and lung neoplasm may be difficult.

Prevention of Silicosis

Prevention remains the principal goal in dealing with this occupational lung disease. Exposures can be reduced through the use of improved ventilation and local exhaust, process enclosure, wet abrasive techniques, personal protection (including the proper selection of respirators), and, when possible, substitution of industrial agents less hazardous than silica. The education of workers and employers regarding the hazards of silica dust exposure and measures to control exposure are also important.

If silicosis is recognized in a worker, termination of exposure is advisable. Unfortunately, the disease can progress even without further silica exposure. Additionally, the finding of a case of silicosis, especially in the acute or accelerated form, should prompt a thorough evaluation of workplace exposures and industrial hygiene measures, with the goal of recognizing the hazardous operation and protecting other workers who may be at risk.

Workers exposed to silica and other mineral dusts should undergo periodic screening for adverse health effects as a supplement to dust exposure control but not a substitute for it. Such screening commonly includes evaluations for respiratory symptoms, spirometric abnormalities, radiographic changes, and neoplastic disease. Evaluation for tuberculosis infection with intradermal skin testing should be performed on a yearly basis. Workers with latent TB infection should receive chemoprophylaxis.

Therapy, Management of Complications, and Control of Silicosis

There is no specific therapy for silicosis. Treatment is directed largely at complications of the disease, including management of airflow obstruction, infection, pneumothorax, hypoxemia, and respiratory failure. For workers with a diagnosis of silicosis, further exposure to silica-containing dusts is undesirable. If the disease is advanced or has occurred after a relatively short exposure (less than 15 years), further dust exposure should be assiduously avoided. Advice on job reassignment should be considered in the context of the worker's age, symptoms, functional status, the current working conditions, and measured silica exposures.

Acute silicosis may rapidly progress to respiratory failure. No specific therapy for this aggressive form of silicosis is available, though whole-lung lavage under general anesthesia as well as glucocorticoid therapy have been described.[33] The rare young patient with end-stage silicosis may be considered a candidate for lung or heart-lung transplantation.

The lack of a specific therapy for silicosis emphasizes the crucial role of primary prevention in our approach to this disorder. The control of silicosis ultimately depends on the control of workplace dust exposures, which can be accomplished by rigorous and conscientious application of fundamental occupational hygiene and engineering principles and a commitment to the preservation of worker health.

REFERENCES

1. Amandus HE, Petersen MR, Richards TB: Health status of anthracite surface coal miners. *Arch Environ Health* 44:75–81, 1989.
2. Banks DE, Bauer MA, Castellan RM, Lapp NL: Silicosis in surface coalmine drillers. *Thorax* 38:275–278, 1983.
3. Morgan WKC, Burgess DB, Jacobsen G, et al: The prevalence of coal workers' pneumoconiosis in U.S. coal miners. *Arch Environ Health* 27:221–226, 1973.
4. CDC/NIOSH: *Criteria for a Recommended Standard, Occupational Exposure to Respirable Coal Mine Dust.* DHHS (NIOSH) Publication No. 95-106, September 1995.
5. Attfield MD, Seixas NS: Prevalence of pneumoconiosis and its relationship to dust exposure in a cohort of U.S. bituminous coal miners and ex-miners. *Am J Ind Med* 27:137–151, 1995.
6. Jacobsen M, Rae S, Walton WH, Rogan JM: The relation between pneumoconiosis and dust exposure in British coal mines, in Walton WH (ed), *Inhaled Particles,* vol III. Woking, Surrey, Unwin Brothers, 1971, pp 903–917.
7. Kleinerman J, Green F, Lacquer W, et al: Pathology standards for coal workers' pneumoconiosis. *Arch Pathol Lab Med* 103:374–432, 1979.
8. Green FHY, Althouse R, Weber KC: Prevalence of silicosis at death in underground coal miners. *Am J Ind Med* 16:605–615, 1989.
9. International Labour Office: *Guidelines for the Use of ILO International Classification of Radiographs of Pneumoconiosis,* rev ed. Geneva, International Labour Office, 1980.
10. Collins LC, Willing S, Bretz R, et al: High-resolution CT in simple coal workers' pneumoconiosis: Lack of correlation with pulmonary function tests and arterial blood gas values. *Chest* 104:1156–1162, 1993.
11. Petsonk EL, Daniloff EM, Mannino DM, et al: Airway responsiveness and job selection: A study in coal miners and non-mining controls. *Occup Environ Med* 52:745–749, 1995.
12. Attfield MD, Hodous TK: Pulmonary function of U.S. coal miners related to dust exposure estimates. *Am Rev Respir Dis* 145:605–609, 1992.
13. Marine WM, Gurr D, Jacobsen M: Clinically important respiratory effects of dust exposure and smoking in British coal miners. *Am Rev Respir Dis* 137:106–112, 1988.
14. Attfield MD, Hodous TK: Does regression analysis of lung function data obtained from occupational epidemiologic studies lead to misleading inferences regarding the true effect of smoking? *Am J Ind Med* 27:281–291, 1995.
15. Seixas NS, Robins TG, Attfield MD, Moulton LH: Longitudinal and cross sectional analyses of exposure to coal mine dust and pulmonary function in new miners. *Br J Ind Med* 50:929–937, 1993.
16. Oxman AD, Muir DC, Shannon HS, et al: Occupational dust exposure and chronic obstructive pulmonary disease. A systematic overview of the evidence (see comments). *Am Rev Respir Dis* 148:38–48, 1993.
17. Wright JL, Cagle P, Churg A, et al: State of the art: Diseases of the small airways. *Am Rev Respir Dis* 146:240–262, 1992.
18. Lapp NL, Seaton A, Kaplan KC, et al: Pulmonary hemodynamics in symptomatic coal miners. *Am Rev Respir Dis* 104:418–426, 1971.
19. Nemery B, Veriter C, Brasseur L, Frans A: Impairment of ventilatory function and pulmonary gas exchange in non-smoking coalminers. *Lancet* 2:1427–1430, 1987.
20. Caplan A: Certain unusual radiological appearances in the chest of coal miners suffering from rheumatoid arthritis. *Thorax* 8:29–37, 1953.
21. Lippmann M, Eckert HL, Hahon N, Morgan WKC: Circulating antinuclear and rheumatoid factors in United States coal miners. *Ann Intern Med* 79:807–811, 1973.
22. Soutar CA, Turner-Warwick M, Parkes WR: Circulating antinuclear antibody and rheumatoid factor in coal pneumoconiosis. *Br Med J* 3:145–147, 1974.

23. Wagner JC, McCormick JN: Immunological investigations of coalworkers' disease. *J R Coll Physicians Lond* 2:49–56, 1967.
24. Kuempel ED, Stayner LT, Attfield MD, Buncher CR: Exposure-response analysis of mortality among coal miners in the United States. *Am J Ind Med* 28:167–184, 1995.
25. Miller BG, Jacobsen M: Dust exposure, pneumoconiosis, and mortality of coalminers. *Br J Ind Med* 42:723–733, 1985.
26. Dubois P, Gyselen A, Prignot J: Rifampicin-combined chemotherapy in coal worker's pneumoconio-tuberculosis. *Am Rev Respir Dis* 115:221–228, 1977.
27. Morgan EJ: Silicosis and tuberculosis. *Chest* 75:202–203, 1979.
28. CDC: Silicosis: Cluster in sandblasters—Texas, and Occupational Surveillance for Silicosis. *MMWR* 39:433–437, 1990.
29. Wagner GR: The inexcusable persistence of silicosis (editorial). *Am J Public Health* 85:1346–1347, 1995.
30. Snider DE: The relationship between tuberculosis and silicosis. *Am Rev Respir Dis* 118:455–460, 1978.
31. Becklake MR: Chronic airflow limitation: Its relationship to work in dusty occupations. *Chest* 88:608–617, 1985.
32. International Agency for Research on Cancer: *IARC Monographs on the Evaluation of the Carcinogenic Risk of Chemicals to Humans: Silica and Some Silicates,* vol 42. Lyon, France, World Health Organization, IARC, 1987, pp 49, 51, 73–111.
33. Wilt JL, Banks DE, Weissman DN, et al: Reduction of lung dust burden in pneumoconiosis by whole lung lavage. *J Occup Environ Med* 38:619–624, 1996.

Occupational Asthma, Byssinosis, and Industrial Bronchitis*

Lynn T. Tanoue

INDUSTRIAL BRONCHITIS

Byssinosis

There are over 800,000 textile workers in the United States.[1] These are the individuals who are primarily at risk for developing chronic bronchitis due to inhalation of cotton dust, termed *byssinosis*. Flax and hemp workers are also at risk for developing the problem. Clinical studies suggest that approximately 65 percent of the general population will react significantly on de novo inhalation of components of cotton dust. Therefore the majority of those who begin employment involved with cotton, flax, or hemp processing are at risk for developing respiratory symptoms. Clinical studies have reported prevalence rates of chronic bronchitis in cotton mill workers of 4.5 to 26 percent.[2,3]

Certain jobs in the textile mill are associated with a higher risk for development of bronchitis. Ginning, opening, or carding work carry a higher degree of risk.[4] Workers who clean out or maintain the various machines that divide up and clean the cotton are also prone to develop symptoms. These are particularly high-risk jobs because of the high levels of cotton dust generated during the cleaning procedure. Strippers and grinders, who maintain the carding machinery that cleans and aligns the cotton, are also particularly at risk for development of symptoms. In fact, byssinosis has been termed "strippers' asthma" in the past.

Clinical Presentation, Pathogenesis, and Treatment

Shortness of breath often occurs on the day back to work after several days of absence, as on a Monday after being off work over the weekend ("Monday-morning fever"). Subsequently, workers can develop more persistent symptoms. It has been established that workers with more symptoms tend to have a more rapid decline in pulmonary function.[5] Length of employment in a cotton mill and dust exposure level correlate with the development of byssinosis. Tobacco smoking has also been shown to be synergistic with cotton dust exposure for producing chronic bronchitis.[6] Although it is debatable whether cotton dust exposure results in chronic pulmonary disability in the absence of cigarette smoking, it appears that 7 percent of exposed individuals will develop irreversible airway obstruction that cannot be explained by smoking.[7]

Byssinosis is associated with a reduction in the forced vital capacity (FVC) and forced expiratory volume in 1 s (FEV_1) characteristically seen on the day

---

*Edited from Chap. 60, "Occupational Asthma, Byssinosis, and Industrial Bronchitis," by Cooper JAD Jr. In: *Fishman's Pulmonary Diseases and Disorders,* 3d ed., edited by Fishman AP, Elias JA, Fishman JA, Grippi MA, Kaiser LR, Senior RM. New York, McGraw-Hill, 1998, pp 915–924. For fuller discussion of the topics dealt with in this chapter, the reader is referred to the original text, as noted above.

of return to work after an absence. The degree of reduction in these parameters increases over the workday. This change will generally be more severe on the first day of work after an absence than on subsequent days.[1] The mechanism by which this developed tolerance occurs is unknown. Whether subjects with byssinosis have airways that are hyperreactive to methacholine challenge is controversial.

The histopathology of byssinosis appears to be similar to that associated with tobacco smoke–induced bronchitis, with mucous gland hyperplasia and polymorphonuclear neutrophil infiltration into bronchi.[1]

A large amount of information points to a lipopolysaccharide (endotoxin) produced by bacterial contaminants of cotton as the causative agent of byssinosis. The most compelling study examining this issue was presented by Castellan and colleagues,[8] who demonstrated that ambient concentrations of endotoxin in a simulated carding room correlated with reduction in airway flow rates in a time frame similar to that occurring after exposure to cotton dust at the workplace.[3] The acquired tolerance over the work week displayed in patients with byssinosis can be simulated with multiple aerosols of endotoxin in animals. Because airborne levels of endotoxin appear to be directly related to the pathogenesis of byssinosis, mechanisms to control this and other airborne components of cotton dust have been implemented in the textile industry. This has met with success in controlling industrial bronchitis due to cotton dust.

The most important treatment for byssinosis is removal of the individual from the offending work environment. Screening pulmonary function testing at the workplace is important to identify individuals who exhibit airflow abnormalities. In addition, since the 1970s, measures have been taken in developed countries to control cotton dust levels in textile mills. In 1970, Burlington Industries began a program for dust control and annual medical surveillance, resulting in a fall in the incidence of symptoms of byssinosis from 4.5 percent in 1970 to 0.6 percent in 1979.[3]

Grain Dust–Induced Industrial Bronchitis

Exposure to grain dust can also result in the development of chronic bronchitis. Between 4 and 11 percent of grain workers show a reduction in FEV_1 of 10 percent or greater over the work shift. This reduction in flow rates is directly related to the amount of dust in the air. Studies have suggested that the component of grain dust responsible for causing airway symptoms is endotoxin,[9] the apparent active component of cotton dust (see above). Grain dust extract, possibly its endotoxin contaminant, can activate complement, and this may be a mechanism by which grain dust induces inflammation in bronchi. However, in contrast to cotton dust, grain dust can, in sensitive individuals, also precipitate an acute drop in airway flow rates rather than only a slow reduction in flow rates. This finding suggests that airway reactions to grain dust may be heterogeneous. Grain dust also tends to produce skin abnormalities in affected individuals, in contrast to cotton dust, which generally does not cause skin reactions.

OCCUPATIONAL ASTHMA

Occupational asthma is characterized by variable airway obstruction resulting from exposure to ambient dusts, vapors, gases, or fumes incidentally present at a workplace.[10–12] Bronchial hyperresponsiveness to agents such as methacholine or histamine is usually present. In this setting, asthma may be caused de novo by the offending agent, as in the case of isocyanate-induced asthma, or underlying asthma may be exacerbated by the offending agent. The subcommittee on occupational allergy of the European Academy of Allergology and Clinical Immunology has proposed five steps in the diagnosis of this disorder: (1) a history supporting the reaction, (2) evidence of variable obstructive airway disease, (3) confirmation of bronchoconstriction at the workplace, (4) documentation of bronchial sensitization to the suspected agent, and (5) establishment of a causal connection by bronchial challenge with the agent.[13] Bronchial challenge should be performed only by experienced clinicians in a controlled setting. This usually entails the use of an environmental chamber or comparable facility for the challenge.

Agents that have been associated with induction of occupational asthma can be conveniently grouped into categories of high- and low-molecular-weight (MW) compounds (Table 19-1). All of these agents tend to sensitize the individual, so that low ambient concentrations of the substance can ultimately cause significant bronchoconstriction. In addition, certain agents can cause direct irritant-related bronchoconstriction and airway hyperreactivity.

Atopy appears to be the major risk factor for developing occupational asthma, particularly when the inciting agent is a high-MW compound.[12] Family or personal history of atopy appears to put the subject at risk. Because low-MW agents can induce asthma through nonallergic as well as allergic mechanisms, atopy may not be as important. Smoking is also a risk factor for the development of occupational asthma. There have been several studies documenting that workers who smoke have a higher incidence of asthmatic reactions to specific airborne agents, possibly due to overall higher IgE levels in smokers as compared with nonsmokers.[14]

Clinical Presentations

Occupational asthma presents in a similar manner as other forms of asthma. If the physician does not maintain a high index of suspicion, symptoms will be treated but the inciting agent will not be identified.

Two general forms of occupational asthma have been identified[12]:

1. Occupational asthma with latency: Most commonly patients who develop occupational asthma do so after a period of exposure to the inciting agent. Agents that induce this sort of pattern include high- and low-MW molecules. Subjects usually are exposed to the agent for weeks to months prior to development of symptoms. With the appearance of symptoms, nonspecific airway hyperreactivity, determined by methacholine or histamine challenge, is present. Also with appearance of symptoms, the subject is hypersensitive to low ambient concentrations of the implicated agent. Therefore exposure to very low concentrations of the material at the workplace can precipitate severe bronchoconstriction. Controlled exposure with the offending agent will elicit bronchoconstriction in patients with this syndrome, especially when asthma is due to a high-MW molecule.
2. Occupational asthma without latency: This syndrome is less common. Symptoms develop within hours of the exposure. Agents that commonly cause this syndrome are irritant gases or fumes such as chlorine or ammonia. In addition, certain agents such as acid anhydrides and isocyanates can cause occupational asthma with and without latency.

TABLE 19-1 Categories of Agents That Commonly Cause
Occupational Asthma

Categories	Occupations at risk	Major putative component
High-MW compounds		
Animal products	Animal handlers Veterinarians	Pelt or urinary proteins
Seafoods	Crab or prawn processors Oyster farmers	Water-extractable proteins
Insects	Entomologists Grain workers Laboratory workers River workers Flight crews	Insect proteins
Plants	Grain handlers Bakers Tea workers Brewery chemists Tobacco manufacturers	Extractable plant proteins
Biologic enzymes	Detergent industry workers Pharmaceutical workers Bakers	*Bacillus subtilis,* trypsin, pancreatin, papain, pepsin
Latex	Health care workers Doll manufacturers Glove makers	Latex rubber extract
Gums	Printers Gum manufacturers	Gum acacia Gum tragacanth
Low-MW compounds		
Diisocyanates	Polyurethane workers Plastic workers Foundry workers Spray painters	Isocyanate-protein complex
Anhydrides	Epoxy resin workers Plastics workers	Phthalic anhydride-protein complexes
Wood dust	Carpenters Sawmill workers	Plicatic acid (western red cedar) Wood dust extracts
Fluxes	Aluminum solderers Electronics workers	Aminoethylethanolamine
Pharmaceuticals	Pharmaceutical manufacturers	Antibiotics, psyllium, piperazine
Fixatives	Hospital workers	Formaldehyde, glutaraldehyde

Mechanisms and Pathology

Most commonly, high-MW compounds, usually proteins, produced at the workplace induce asthma through IgE-dependent classic immediate hypersensitivity reactions. Specific serum IgE antibodies to the protein can usually be demonstrated, which trigger most cell degranulation. Skin tests using extracts of the substance show positive results. Atopic individuals are at higher risk for developing the syndrome. The latent period for developing the reaction is usually long, sometimes several months or years. Low-MW compounds can also cause IgE-dependent bronchoconstriction. However, in contrast to higher-MW agents, specific IgE or IgG antibodies produced in these individuals are directed at the low-MW compound coupled to a protein within the serum. There is also some evidence that low-MW compounds induce asthma through IgE-independent mechanisms, possibly by affecting T lymphocytes directly. Evidence for this mechanism exists for cobalt and nickel salts as well as isocyanates.[12] Certain low-MW compounds can also directly affect chemical pathways that are involved in airway tone. For example, organophosphates have been shown to induce bronchoconstriction through anticholinergic effects.[15] Other agents may cause asthma simply through irritation of the airways.

Diagnostic Evaluation

A high index of suspicion must always be present when patients with new-onset asthma are being evaluated. Because asthma can be induced by remote exposure to a substance, the current and previous occupational history is very important. The history should include documentation of specific jobs for the individual as well as potential exposures during performance of those jobs. The history can be verified through the use of material safety data sheets, industrial hygiene data, and employee health records from the workplace. Historical factors that suggest occupation-related asthma include symptoms that occur at work and improve when the patient is away from work for a period of time, as during vacations. The duration of symptoms prior to removal from the offending environment is important for predicting prognosis. Those subjects who have had symptoms for a longer period of time are more likely to develop chronic symptoms that do not remit after exposure has been discontinued.[12] It should be noted that many compounds induce a late reaction, several hours after exposure. Therefore the relationship between the exposure and symptoms may not be entirely apparent to the patient. The history should also be directed at nonoccupational causes of airway obstruction, including tobacco use, family history, and whether respiratory symptoms preceded beginning a particular job.

General atopy appears to be a risk factor for developing certain forms of occupational asthma when it is due to high-MW compounds. Therefore routine skin testing, using a panel of allergens, for wheal-and-flare reactions can be useful. In addition, extracts of a compound that is suspected to cause occupational asthma in a particular patient can be used for skin testing. Extracts from flour, animal by-products, coffee, and other sources have been used for skin testing in various studies.[11] Specific IgE antibodies to extracts containing high-MW compounds or to low-MW compounds coupled to a serum protein, such as albumin, can also be detected by the radioallergosorbent test (RAST) or enzyme-linked immunosorbent assay (ELISA). In addition, specific IgE antibodies to low-MW compounds have been detected in patients with asthma due to these compounds. However, positive results in all of these tests do not necessarily indicate that disease is due to the specific agent; they simply suggest sensitization. All of these tests must be evaluated in the context of the individual patient.

Patients with workplace-induced asthma may present with normal pulmonary function tests when they are away from the inciting agent. Thus, pulmonary function tests should temporally be assessed with exposure.

Pulmonary function tests before and after work can be very helpful in objectively evaluating respiratory function in relation to work.

Peak flow monitors are useful in the assessment of workplace-related symptoms because they can be used on the job. Initially, peak flow measurements should be determined at least four times per day: on awakening, at the beginning and end of work, and before bed.[16] Similarly timed measurements should also be performed on days that the subject is off work. Three measurements at each time period should be made and recorded; two of these should be within 20 L/min of each other to demonstrate reproducibility. Measurements should be performed each day over a 3- to 4-week period. If peak flow measurements suggest that there is an airway reaction to a substance at the workplace, a technician with a portable spirometer can be sent to the workplace to measure FVC and FEV_1 at suitable intervals during work to more accurately document changes in air flow obstruction. Because peak flow measurements are very effort-dependent, they should be supplemented by other methods for assessing the degree of impairment. It is always important to document that patients who are being evaluated for occupational asthma are not malingering to obtain compensation for their disorder.

Bronchial provocation tests may be useful in the evaluation of occupational asthma. Patients who develop occupational asthma invariably develop bronchial hyperreactivity to nonspecific agents such as methacholine and histamine. In fact, in those patients with normal spirograms at presentation, a bronchial challenge with either of these agents may be necessary for diagnosis.

Specific bronchoprovocation with a particular agent can be a valuable tool to determine whether a subject's symptoms are due to that agent. Bronchial challenge should be performed only by experienced clinicians in a controlled setting, which requires the use of an environmental chamber or comparable facility.

Management

Once it has been determined that an individual has developed asthma due to workplace exposure, he or she should be removed from the offending environment. Once the individual is sensitized, very low concentrations of the specific agent can induce bronchospasm.[17] Because it is sometimes difficult to convince a patient to change jobs, an alternative to this is the use of a protective mask to prevent airway exposure to the offending agent. The inciting agent dictates the type of protective headgear employed. For example, subjects working with low-MW compounds require helmet respirators with an isolated air source to prevent exposure. If the subject continues to work in the implicated environment, pulmonary function tests should be done frequently to rule out progressive physiologic impairment.

Specific examples of occupations that carry risk for the development of asthma, and the putative agents responsible, are listed in Table 19-1.

Disability Determination

Documentation of impairment associated with objective physiologic changes occurring primarily at the workplace suggests an occupation-related disorder. Patients with asthma due to an occupational exposure should be referred to the appropriate compensation or review board. The American Thoracic Society[18] has developed guidelines for the evaluation of impairment and disability due to this disorder. Determination of initial impairment should be made after optimal treatment of the asthma has been given. Impairment should be assessed using lung function tests, measurements of airway hyperresponsiveness using methacholine or histamine, documentation of the type and amount of medication required to treat the patient, and observation of the effect of the disease on the patient's lifestyle.

REFERENCES

1. Spencer H: *Pathology of the Lung,* 2d ed. New York, Pergamon Press, 1968.
2. Beck GJ, Schachter EN, Maunder LR, Schilling RSF: A prospective study of chronic lung disease in cotton textile workers. *Ann Intern Med* 97:645–651, 1982.
3. Rylander R: Diseases associated with exposure to plant dusts: Focus on cotton dust. *Tubercle Lung Dis* 73:21–26, 1992.
4. Schilling RSF, Goodman N: Cardiovascular disease and cotton workers: Part I. *Br J Ind Med* 8:77–82, 1951.
5. Kamat SR, Kamat GR, Salpekar VY, Lobo E: Distinguishing byssinosis from chronic obstructive pulmonary disease: Results of a prospective 5 year study of cotton mill workers in India. *Am Rev Respir Dis* 124:31–40, 1981.
6. Schacter EN: Occupational airway disease. *Mt Sinai J Med* 58:483–493, 1991.
7. Bouhuys A, Schoenberg JB, Beck GJ, Schilling RSF: Epidemiology of chronic lung disease in a cotton mill community. *Lung* 154:167–187, 1977.
8. Castellan RM, Olenchock SA, Kinsley KB, Hankinson JL: Inhaled endotoxin and decreased spirometric values. *N Engl J Med* 317:605–610, 1987.
9. Cooper JAD Jr, Buck MG, Gee JBL: Vegetable dust and airway disease: Inflammatory mechanisms. *Environ Health Perspect* 66:7–15, 1986.
10. Bardana EJ Jr: Occupational asthma and related respiratory disorders. *Dis Mon* 41:143–199, 1995.
11. Chan-Yeung M, Lam S: Occupational asthma. *Am Rev Respir Dis* 133:686–703, 1986.
12. Chan-Yeung M, Malo J-L: Occupational asthma. *N Engl J Med* 333:107–112, 1995.
13. Subcommittee on "Occupational Allergy" of the European Academy of Allergology and Clinical Immunology: Guidelines for the diagnosis of occupational asthma. *Clin Exp Allergy* 22:103–108, 1992.
14. Zetterstrom O, Ostermann K, Machado L: Another smoking hazard: Raised serum IgE concentrations and increased risk of occupational allergy. *Br Med J* 283:1215–1217, 1981.
15. Weiner A: Bronchial asthma due to organic phosphate insecticide. *Ann Allergy* 19:397–401, 1961.
16. Chan-Yeung M, Brooks SM, Alberts WM, et al: Assessment of asthma in the workplace. *Chest* 108:1084–1117, 1995.
17. Fine JM, Balmes JR: Airway inflammation and occupational asthma. *Clin Chest Med* 9:577–590, 1988.
18. American Thoracic Society Ad Hoc Committee on Impairment/Disability Evaluation in Subjects with Asthma: Guidelines for the evaluation of impairment/disability in patients with asthma. *Am Rev Respir Dis* 147:1056–1061, 1993.

20 | Toxic Inhalations*

Lynn T. Tanoue

Many fumes, gases, vapors, dusts, and other inhaled substances have potentially toxic effects that are manifest by pulmonary as well as extrapulmonary injury. Exposure by inhalation occurs in industrial settings as well as in the home, public places, and other environments.

IRRITANT-INDUCED PULMONARY INJURY

General categories of inhaled toxins include gases, vapors, fumes, aerosols, and smoke. Tables 20-1 and 20-2 summarize the physical properties of these inhalants. The initial pathologic responses to a harmful inhaled agent depend on a number of factors, including the concentration of the substance in the ambient air, the pH of the inhaled substance, the presence and size of particles, the relative water-solubility of the inhaled agent, the duration of exposure, and whether the exposure occurs in an enclosed space or in an area with adequate ventilation and free circulation of fresh air. In addition, an undetermined number of host factors—including age, smoking status, the presence of preexisting pulmonary or extrapulmonary disease, and the use of respirators or other protective breathing apparatus—all affect a person's response to the inhalation of a toxic substance.[1,2]

Inhaled gases with potential irritant effects manifest their actions at different anatomic locations in the respiratory system. In general, substances that are highly water-soluble—such as ammonia, sulfur dioxide, and hydrogen chloride—can cause immediate irritant injury to the upper airway. The acute

TABLE 20-1 Definitions of Types of Inhaled Substances

Gas:	A formless state of matter in which molecules move freely about and completely occupy the space of enclosure
Aerosol:	A relatively stable suspension of liquid droplets or solid particles in a gaseous medium
Vapor:	The gaseous form of a substance that normally exists as a liquid or solid and generally can be changed back to a liquid or solid by either an increase in ambient pressure or a decrease in temperature
Fume:	An aerosol of solid particles generally less than 0.1 μm in size that arises from a chemical reaction or condensation of vapors, usually after volatilization from molten materials
Smoke:	The volatilized gaseous and particulate products of combustion whose particles are generally less than 0.5 μm in size and do not settle readily

SOURCE: Adapted from Kizer.[1]

*Edited from Chap. 61, "Toxic Inhalations," by Schwartz DA, Blaski CA. In: *Fishman's Pulmonary Diseases and Disorders,* 3d ed., edited by Fishman AP, Elias JA, Fishman JA, Grippi MA, Kaiser LR, Senior RM. New York, McGraw-Hill, 1998, pp 925–940. For fuller discussion of the topics dealt with in this chapter, the reader is referred to the original text, as noted above.

TABLE 20-2 Physical Properties and Mechanisms of Lung Injury of Gaseous Respiratory Irritants

Irritant gas	Water solubility	Mechanism of injury
Ammonia	High	Alkali burns
Chlorine	Intermediate	Acid burns, reactive oxygen species
Hydrogen chloride	High	Acid burns
Oxides of nitrogen	Low	Acid burns, reactive oxygen species
Ozone	Low	Reactive oxygen species
Phosgene	Low	Acid burns
Sulfur dioxide	High	Acid burns

SOURCE: Adapted from Schwartz.[2]

effects of highly water-soluble irritants on the upper airway, exposed skin, and other mucous membranes often produce such unpleasant symptoms that exposed persons quickly leave the area of exposure and avoid continued inhalation of the harmful toxins. In contrast, inhaled toxins that have low water-solubility—such as phosgene, ozone, and oxides of nitrogen—often have little or no acute effect on the upper airway and instead produce irritant effects at the level of the terminal bronchiole and alveolus. Because agents of low water-solubility do not produce immediately noticeable upper airway irritation (except in episodes of massive acute exposure), exposed persons may inadvertently remain in the area of exposure and thus increase their duration of exposure to harmful inhalants. Agents that exhibit intermediate water-solubility, such as chlorine, can have pathologic effects throughout the respiratory system. However, extreme exposure to any one of these irritants may result in upper and lower respiratory tract involvement. Absorption of any one of these irritants on particulate matter may also alter the area of involvement.

In addition to solubility, the size of inhaled particles is important in the pathogenesis of the toxic inhalation injury.[1] Aerosols, dusts, fumes, and smoke can produce upper airway injury as well as parenchymal damage. The location and extent of injury depend on the size of the inhaled particles as well as the intensity of the exposure. Particles that are 5.0 μm or less in diameter have the ability to penetrate into the lower respiratory tract and often produce significant injury at the level of the terminal bronchioles and alveoli. The particles themselves may have direct toxic effects, or they may serve as vehicles for adsorbed gaseous agents that are carried more distally into the lungs and do harm when they interact with terminal bronchioles and alveolar cells.

Irritants directly injure cells through non-immunologically-mediated mechanisms of injury and inflammation. Cell injury involves the deposition or formation of an acid (chlorine, hydrogen, chloride, oxides of nitrogen, phosgene, and sulfur dioxide), alkali (ammonia), or reactive oxygen species (ozone, oxides of nitrogen, and possibly chlorine).[2,3] The primary injury is localized in airway epithelial tissues, but extensive damage may also occur in subepithelial and alveolar regions. Acid injury results in coagulation of the underlying tissue, while acute injury due to alkali results in liquefaction of the mucosa and deep penetrating lesions in the airways. Reactive oxygen species include oxygen-derived metabolites (such as hydrogen peroxide and hydrochlorous acid) and oxygen-derived free radicals (such as superoxide anions and hydroxyl radicals). These reactive oxygen species may injure tissues and cells through lipid peroxidation, which can directly injure cells and lead to elaboration of inflammatory mediators that can perpetuate the initial damage.[3] Regardless of the initial mechanism of irritant injury, inflammatory mechanisms that involve networks of proinflammatory cytokines may subsequently be initiated. The resultant inflammation may be important with regard to perpetuation of the acute injury as well as long-term sequelae. In addition, disruption and eventual repair of the airway epithelia may decrease the host's ability to defend against future inhaled infectious or irritant substances.

Upper Airway

Acute Injury

The potential for an inhaled substance to acutely injure the upper airway depends largely on that substance's irritant qualities. Water-solubility and particle size as well as duration and intensity of exposure influence the host response to a specific exposure.

Persons exposed to irritants that injure the upper airway often have associated injury to exposed mucous membranes and skin. Clinical presentations include burns of exposed skin and corneas, rhinitis, conjunctivitis, tracheobronchitis, and oral mucositis. Persons exposed to upper airway irritants may experience burning sensations of the eyes, nasal passages, and throat; profuse lacrimation and copious sputum production may also occur. Coughing and sneezing may be prominent symptoms. Upper airway injury from irritant inhalants is generally acute and self-limited. Life-threatening upper airway obstruction due to mucosal edema, large amounts of secretions and sloughed epithelial cells, or laryngospasm can occur in cases of massive acute exposure. Hoarseness or stridor may warn of impending airway compromise; patients presenting with either of these physical findings must be carefully observed and may require emergency management of acute upper airway obstruction.

Treatment for most inhaled substances is not specific; instead, it addresses removal of the patient from the exposure. Basic principles of airway management are paramount, because the most likely acute life-threatening manifestation of this injury is upper airway obstruction due to a combination of tissue edema, thick secretions, and laryngospasm. Frequent suctioning of secretions is often required. Provision of adequate supplemental oxygen is necessary if there is evidence of hypoxemia. Inhaled racemic epinephrine may be useful for patients susceptible to upper airway obstruction, but it should not be employed as a substitute for emergency airway management by endotracheal intubation or tracheotomy if that is necessary. Corticosteroids have not been conclusively shown to influence outcome, but they are suggested in cases of extensive upper airway edema. Toxic substances that remain on the skin or mucosal surfaces should be removed by irrigation with large amounts of water. Basic principles of burn management should be applied to burns on skin and mucosal surfaces. Ophthalmologic consultation is recommended for management of injuries to the corneas or other eye structures.

Conducting Airways

Acute Injury

Inhaled irritants that penetrate to the conducting airways are capable of inducing immediate as well as long-lasting injury through a variety of mechanisms. Disruption of the airway epithelium by irritant inhalation may result in edema and inflammation, leading to exposure of submucosal structures (nerves, vessels, and muscle), direct-muscle contraction, and stimulation of neuronal afferent receptors.

Damage to the airway epithelium, particularly at tight junctions, renders the respiratory mucosa permeable to other inhaled substances, which are then able to penetrate the subepithelial mucosal region. These agents may directly interact with effector cells in subepithelial mucosa, causing smooth-muscle bronchoconstrictive effects. They may also stimulate parasympathetic sensory afferent nerve endings, resulting in extensive bronchoconstriction. Airway hyperresponsiveness caused by localized inflammatory response may ensue.[4]

Damage to the airway epithelium and inflammation of the subepithelial mucosa may contribute to the development of airway disease in persons exposed to irritant gases and aerosols. Inhaled agents, either allergens or irritants, may cause mucosal inflammation that subsequently results in increased epithelial permeability. The altered epithelial permeability exposes subepithelial irritant receptors, which are subsequently at risk of being stimulated by a variety of agents, including cold air, changes in humidity and temperature (exercise), and cigarette smoke. Damage to the airway epithelium from cigarette smoke is associated with increased epithelial permeability and an inflammatory reaction characterized by mucosal edema and infiltration of neutrophils.[5] In addition, direct damage to the airway epithelium may result in decreased production of epithelium-derived bronchodilating substances and neutral endopeptidases that would normally serve to reduce the effects of bronchoconstricting agents.[5]

The inflammatory response in the epithelial and subepithelial regions can result in chronic remodeling of the underlying airway architecture. For example, striking inflammatory changes are seen in transbronchial biopsy specimens obtained from asthmatic persons following aerosol challenges.[6] Chronic bronchitis is strongly associated with airway hyperresponsiveness and has been demonstrated in animals after exposure to irritant gases.[2]

Changes in the structure of the airways may significantly enhance the development of airway reactivity and contribute to the development of respiratory symptoms. Baseline airway caliber appears to be an important determinant of airway hyperresponsiveness.[26] The airway caliber can be influenced by a variety of factors, including the tone of the airway smooth muscle and the overall thickness of the subepithelial region. Inflammation and edema of the submucosal region may not only decrease airway caliber but may also alter airway smooth-muscle mechanics, resulting in maximal contraction following stimulation of the airway smooth muscle. Similarly, chronic changes in the architecture of the basement membrane may also alter smooth-muscle length-tension relations.

Lower airway injury resulting from irritant toxic inhalation can be manifest as transient or long-lasting intrathoracic airflow obstruction, presumably via inflammatory mechanisms. Cigarette smokers or persons with preexisting airway obstruction may be at increased risk for the persistence of toxin-induced airflow obstruction. Lower airway injury may not be immediately recognizable, but symptoms may develop and worsen over the first 24 to 48 h after exposure. Hospitalization for observation is indicated for initially asymptomatic exposed subjects with any objective evidence of respiratory compromise (decreased airflow, abnormalities of gas exchange, spirometric abnormalities, or an abnormal chest radiograph) or whose exposure history is suggestive of an intense exposure. In addition, persons who report respiratory symptoms including dyspnea or chest tightness should be hospitalized, followed closely with objective measures of pulmonary function, and treated symptomatically, even in the absence of objective abnormalities. For persons without significant decrements in airflow but with symptomatic chest tightness or wheezing, inhaled steroids are essential and bronchodilators may be useful. In cases that demonstrate airflow obstruction (FEV_1 of 80 percent or less than predicted, or 10 percent or less than the patient's initial baseline), a short course of systemic corticosteroids may be beneficial in addition to the use of inhaled steroids and bronchodilators. However, there is no definitive evidence that treatment with parenteral corticosteroids substantially relieves the airflow obstruction or prevents the onset of bronchiolitis obliterans.

Chronic Injury

Obstructive airway disease Previously healthy people who experience acute toxic inhalation may go on to develop clinical and pathologic features of chronic obstructive pulmonary disease (COPD). The inhaled irritants most often implicated in the development of chronic bronchitis, emphysema, or reversible airflow obstruction are chlorine[8] and sulfur dioxide.[9] However, definitive evidence that demonstrates a causal relationship between a toxic exposure and resultant chronic respiratory disease is at times difficult to elicit. This is often because of the frequent concomitant presence of potentially confounding factors, most prominently cigarette smoking, that independently increase risk for the development of COPD. Nevertheless, there is some evidence that acute exposure to a number of inhaled irritants may produce conditions in the conducting airways that lead to a complex interaction of inflammation, smooth-muscle activity, and neuronal inputs, resulting in varying degrees of fixed and reversible airflow obstruction.

The development of irritant-induced COPD appears to depend on the intensity of the exposure. In addition, underlying host factors, including cigarette smoking and preexisting pulmonary disease, may increase a person's likelihood of developing COPD. It is extremely difficult to accurately assess the potential contribution of acute irritant inhalation to chronic lung disease in cigarette smokers. Baseline measures of pulmonary function can help determine the presence of preexisting disease, but unfortunately this information is often unavailable, especially in cases of accidental acute exposure. Evaluation of possible irritant-induced COPD includes a thorough history, physical examination, radiographic evaluation, and objective measures of pulmonary function, including spirometry, measurement of lung volumes, determination of diffusing capacity, and assessment of gas exchange. Frequent measurement of spirometry may help determine progression or regression of airflow abnormalities. Treatment is as for COPD due to causes other than acute irritant exposure and includes bronchodilators, corticosteroids, smoking cessation, and, if necessary, supplemental oxygen.

Reactive airway dysfunction syndrome The persistence of airway reactivity after acute exposure to respiratory irritants has been termed reactive airway dysfunction syndrome (RADS).[10] A variety of inhaled irritants have been associated with this syndrome, including sulfuric acid, chlorine, ammonia, household cleaners, and smoke. Most often, the initial inhalation injury is due to a single acute, high-intensity exposure. Symptoms of airflow obstruction—including cough, dyspnea, and wheezing—are reported immediately or several hours after the end of the exposure and may persist for months to years. Previous exposure or sensitization to the toxic agent does not appear to be necessary. By definition, persons who develop RADS have no history of respiratory illness. Pulmonary function test results may be normal, or they may demonstrate airflow obstruction. Persons with RADS have persistent positive responses to methacholine challenge testing even in the presence of normal pulmonary function test results. Nonspecific bronchial reactivity may persist for months to years after the initial inhalation injury.

Treatment of RADS includes the use of corticosteroids to help minimize inflammatory mechanisms and bronchodilators to reverse bronchospasm. There is limited, mostly anecdotal, evidence for the efficacy of corticosteroids. Bronchodilators may only partly alleviate airflow obstruction—especially in later, chronic stages of the syndrome.[11] Despite treatment with corticosteroids and bronchodilators, many exposed persons may be left with persistent asthma-like symptoms, airflow obstruction, and nonspecific bronchial hyperreactivity.

Pulmonary Parenchyma

Acute Injury

Toxic inhaled agents that have relatively low water solubilities—such as phosgene, ozone, and nitrogen oxides—produce most of their irritant damage distal to the upper airway. Because of the relatively low solubilities of these substances, inhalation does not typically result in upper airway irritation and its associated symptoms. As a result, subjects may endure continued exposure to the toxic gases and thus increase the total time and amount of exposure. In addition, massive acute inhalation of gases and aerosols that have intermediate (chlorine) or high water solubilities (ammonia, sulfur dioxide) can overwhelm the absorptive capacity of the upper airway and injure more distal structures. Damage may be particularly severe when particulates form part of the inhaled substance, perhaps because particle deposition in the alveoli provides a nidus for ongoing inflammation. Respirable particles with diameters in the range of 0.3 to 0.5 μm can bypass the upper airways and can be deposited in the more distal airways and alveoli.[1] The clinical consequences of these injuries include diffuse bronchiolar inflammation and obstruction as well as alveolar filling (pulmonary edema). Atelectasis may result from destruction or disruption of the surfactant layer. Persons who have sustained an initial toxic insult to the lower airways and lung parenchyma may be more susceptible to subsequent pulmonary infections because of damage to inflammatory cells, including alveolar macrophages, that provide host defense against infectious agents.

The lower respiratory tract and alveoli are susceptible to injury from many inhaled toxins. In general, the extent and severity of acute lung injury due to a toxic inhalant appear to be dose-related. Pulmonary parenchymal injury that results from inhalation of irritant substances runs the spectrum of acute lung injury and includes pneumonitis, pulmonary edema, and adult respiratory distress syndrome (ARDS). Unlike some focal processes that progress to ARDS, toxin inhalation is more likely to produce a diffuse, relatively homogeneous acute lung injury. Pneumonitis is the most frequent parenchymal manifestation of inhalation injury. Clinical features include dyspnea, productive or dry cough, hypoxemia, mild restriction of ventilation, decreased alveolar gas diffusion, and diffuse bilateral infiltrates on the chest radiograph. Generally, pneumonitis caused by toxic inhalation is a self-limited process, with clinical improvement mirrored by rapid clearing of infiltrates seen on the chest radiograph. Treatment is supportive, usually includes supplemental oxygen, and may require mechanical ventilation. The use of corticosteroids has not been shown to be of significant benefit in the treatment of pneumonitis secondary to the inhalation of irritant gases such as chlorine, ozone, and phosgene but may be indicated in cases of known inhalation of fumes from some metals, such as mercury, cadmium and zinc, which have been reported to progress to severe and sometimes fatal acute lung injury. As it is for toxic pneumonitis, the treatment of toxin-induced pulmonary edema and ARDS remains largely supportive and may include hemodynamic monitoring and mechanical ventilation.

Chronic Injury

Bronchiolitis obliterans Bronchiolitis obliterans can occur as a late consequence of the inhalation of several toxins. Exposures to ammonia, mercury, oxides of nitrogen, and sulfur dioxide have been associated with bronchiolitis obliterans.[12–15] High-intensity inhalation exposures can be followed by acute pulmonary edema and ARDS. Survivors of the acute lung injury may experience a relatively asymptomatic period that is followed by the development of irreversible airflow obstruction, which often presents 1 to 3 weeks after the initial injury. Early inspiratory crackles are a characteristic finding on physical examination. The appearance of the chest radiograph is variable and may demonstrate the degree of clinical severity. Patients with mild cases can have normal chest radiographs, while more severely affected persons may demonstrate hyperinflation. Infiltrates are generally absent. Pulmonary function tests typically demonstrate airflow obstruction that may in some cases also be associated with restrictive defects. The histologic picture is characterized by the presence of granulation tissue plugs within the lumina of small airways and occasionally alveolar ducts as well as by the destruction of small airways with obliterative fibrous scarring. The process may not respond to treatment with corticosteroids; however, a 6-month trial of corticosteroids should be given. Bronchodilators may be efficacious in some symptomatic patients, although clear-cut evidence of this potential benefit is not available.

Bronchiolitis obliterans–organizing pneumonia Bronchiolitis obliterans–organizing pneumonia (BOOP) may also be a late or delayed consequence of the inhalation of toxic substances.[16,17] The clinical presentation is characterized by a persistent, nonproductive cough, fever, sore throat, and malaise. The lung examination typically reveals late inspiratory crackles but no wheezes; many patients have no abnormalities on physical examination. The characteristic findings on the chest radiograph include bilateral, patchy, "ground-glass" densities, which start as focal lesions but may coalesce with time. In contrast to patients with bronchiolitis obliterans, those with BOOP present with restrictive ventilatory physiology and decreased diffusing capacity.

The histology of BOOP includes the presence of granulation tissue in the small airways and alveolar ducts, as in bronchiolitis obliterans. In addition, however, the granulation tissue extends into the alveoli and may result in interstitial scarring. This distinction between the histologic features of BOOP and those of "pure" bronchiolitis obliterans (without organizing pneumonia) may reflect different host responses to similar inhaled toxins.[16]

Treatment of BOOP with corticosteroids often results in dramatic clinical improvement. Pulmonary function abnormalities can lessen considerably and in some cases may resolve rapidly. Duration of therapy is generally at least 6 months but should be guided by the rate and completion of the clinical response. The radiographic abnormalities also clear rapidly. A small number of patients may not respond to corticosteroid therapy and may develop progressive fibrosis.

EFFECTS OF SPECIFIC INHALED TOXINS ON THE RESPIRATORY SYSTEM

The following sections specifically address the pulmonary effects of a number of inhaled toxins. Table 20-3 summarizes the acute and long-term manifestations.

Ammonia

Ammonia is a highly water-soluble substance that is extensively used in the manufacturing, chemical, and agricultural industries. Most inhalation exposures are the result of accidental releases, including tank leaks and transportation mishaps.[15,18,19] Ammonia is highly water-soluble and reacts with water that is present on mucosal surfaces to form ammonium hydroxide, which in turn forms hydroxyl ions. Exposure to ammonia gas or vapors causes immediate irritation of the mucosal surfaces. Thermal burns, chemical injury, and alkali burns may result in injury to the eyes, skin, nose, oropharynx, larynx, and trachea.

The severity of ammonia-induced injury depends on the concentration and duration of exposure. Lower airway and pulmonary parenchymal injury can occur acutely with high-intensity exposures, resulting in pulmonary edema, hemorrhage, and atelectasis. A biphasic pattern of pulmonary response to

TABLE 20-3 Pulmonary Manifestations of Toxin Inhalation

	Acute Clinical Manifestations			Chronic Clinical Manifestations		
Substance	Onset	Upper airway irritation	Pneumonitis, ARDS	Bronchiolitis obliterans, BOOP	Obstructive lung disease	RADS
Irritant Gases						
Ammonia	Minutes	Severe	+	+	+	+
Chlorine	Minutes to hours	Moderate	+	−	+	+
Hydrogen chloride	Minutes	Severe	+	−	−	−
Oxides of nitrogen	Hours	Mild	+	+	+	+
Ozone	Minutes to hours	Mild	+	−	−	−
Phosgene	Hours	Mild	+	−	+	−
Sulfur dioxide	Minutes	Severe	+	+	+	+
Metals						
Cadmium	Hours	Mild	+	−	+	−
Mercury	Hours	Mild	+	+	−	−
Zinc chloride	Minutes	Mild	+	−	−	−
Zinc oxide	Hours	Mild	+	−	−	−

KEY: +, exposure reported to be associated with clinical entity; −, exposure as yet not reported to be associated with clinical entity.

ammonia inhalation has been reported, characterized by initial, acute pneumonitis that may clear over the next 2 to 3 days, followed in some patients by the gradual development of airway obstruction and respiratory failure.[18] Bronchopneumonia due to superinfection with bacterial organisms is common. Bronchiectasis and focal bronchiolitis obliterans have been associated with this late phase.

Initial treatment of persons exposed to ammonia gas or vapors includes immediate irrigation of all exposed surfaces, especially the eyes, with copious amounts of water. The airway must be secured; in some persons, emergency tracheotomy is necessary. Evidence of lower airway and pulmonary parenchymal injury is best assessed initially by physical examination. The presence of rales determines the subsequent hospital course, even in the absence of hypoxemia and abnormalities on the chest radiograph.[18] Treatment of pulmonary impairment is supportive and includes supplemental oxygen and mechanical ventilation with positive pressure if indicated. The use of corticosteroids is controversial, and prophylactic antibiotics have not been shown to clearly improve outcome.

Chlorine, Chloramine, and Hydrochloric Acid

Chlorine (Cl_2) is a highly reactive gas that is widely found in industrial, environmental, and home settings. Episodes of toxic inhalation exposure are most often the result of transportation accidents, industrial mishaps, and accidental spills or releases at swimming pools and sewage treatment facilities.[20,21] Chlorine reacts with water to form hydrochloric acid (HCl) and hypochlorous acid (HOCl). These products, as well as elemental chlorine itself, exert various irritative effects on the respiratory system. Chlorine has intermediate water solubility, and its inhalation can therefore result in irritation of both the upper and lower respiratory tracts. Its mechanism of cellular injury appears to entail the generation of oxygen free radicals as well as HCl and HOCl.

A significant number of toxic inhalation exposures result from the mixing of chlorine compounds and other substances. Many of these exposures are to household cleaning agents.[22] Chloramine gas is formed when chlorine or hypochlorous acid is mixed with ammonia. Chloramine gas, in turn, decomposes to ammonia and HOCl or HCl when it comes into contact with water. Ammonia, HOCl, and HCl are all highly water-soluble and therefore have primarily upper respiratory tract irritative effects. Household bleach (which contains HOCl, or hypochlorite) reacts to form chlorine gas when it is mixed with phosphoric acid or HCl. The resultant chlorine gas subsequently produces irritative symptoms throughout the respiratory tract.

Chlorine gas was one of several chemical warfare agents used in World War I. Several follow-up studies of exposed military personnel report long-lasting pulmonary impairments, including chronic bronchitis and airflow obstruction, in some victims. Others, however, apparently made full recoveries from similar degrees of chlorine gas exposure. The total amount of exposure is probably the most significant determinant of long-term adverse respiratory effects following acute chlorine inhalation, although host factors that are currently not well defined may also contribute to chronic debility.[8]

Sulfur Dioxide

Sulfur dioxide is a heavy, colorless gas that is widely used in many industrial processes including mining, ore smelting, sugar refining, and the bleaching of wool and wood pulp. Persons who experience acute, high-intensity exposure report the immediate onset of symptoms that include burning of the eyes, nose, and throat, rhinorrhea, tearing of the eyes, dyspnea, chest tightness, and cough. Sulfur dioxide is highly water-soluble and hydrolyzes to sulfuric acid upon contact with water on mucous membranes. Extremely high-intensity, acute exposures can lead to death within minutes from respiratory failure due to a combination of alveolar hemorrhage and edema, possible reflex vagal stimulation, and the asphyxiating effect of high concentrations of sulfur dioxide.[9] Less intense acute exposures can produce a broad range of upper and lower respiratory tract injuries that appear to occur in a dose-dependent manner. Acute pneumonitis can progress to ARDS. Survivors of the acute lung injury may experience a relatively asymptomatic period that is followed several weeks later by the onset of irreversible airflow obstruction due to bronchiolitis obliterans.[23] Other victims may demonstrate immediate, persistent airflow obstruction and nonspecific bronchial hyperreactivity consistent with RADS.[10]

Treatment of inhalation injury due to sulfur dioxide and sulfuric acid is supportive and includes supplemental oxygen, maintenance of a patent airway, and, if necessary, mechanical ventilation. Corticosteroids have not been shown to positively influence the course of ARDS due to this toxic inhalation, and they rarely provide significant benefit for patients who have developed bronchiolitis obliterans. However, a trial course of corticosteroids is not unreasonable. Bronchodilators may be helpful for patients with symptomatic airflow obstruction, but this has not been systematically studied. Prevention of acute exposure can be problematic because many serious exposures occur as industrial accidents. Persons working with or near sulfur dioxide or sulfuric acid should be aware of the potential for serious inhalation injury, should recognize initial symptoms of the irritant injury, and should have appropriate respiratory protective equipment.

Nitrogen Oxides

Nitrogen oxides are major components of air pollution. In addition, accidental releases of nitrogen oxide gases can occur in occupational settings and result in high-intensity exposures. Oxides of nitrogen are present in a number of industrial settings, including mining, acetylene welding, and explosives manufacturing. These gases can also be present in closed or poorly ventilated areas in which engines are operated. Perhaps the best-recognized occupational exposure to nitrogen oxides occurs in agricultural workers ("silo-filler's disease") who are exposed to silo gas that is formed by the decomposition of organic matter.[24] Clinical manifestations of toxicity include signs and symptoms of a chemical pneumonitis, the severity of which is dose-dependent and is influenced by both the time and concentration of the exposure. Severe cases can rapidly progress to ARDS and sometimes lethal acute lung injury, whereas less severe cases can completely resolve or result in varying degrees of chronic airway obstruction and RADS. Bronchiolitis obliterans can be a late cause of death and may develop following a relatively asymptomatic period after the resolution of ARDS.

The treatment of the acute lung injury is supportive and includes supplemental oxygen and mechanical ventilation. In addition, awareness of the potential for the development of obstructive lung disease, including bronchiolitis obliterans, several weeks after initial apparent recovery is important. Persons who survive the acute lung injury are at risk for these later complications and should be followed closely with serial assessment of pulmonary mechanics and gas exchange. Asymptomatic hypoxemia or decrements in airflow should be closely monitored, since these patients may develop bronchiolitis obliterans. Corticosteroids may be helpful in preventing or decreasing the severity of progressive airflow obstruction and should be considered in asymptomatic subjects who demonstrate spirometric or gas exchange abnormalities. Prevention of exposure includes the provision of adequate ventilation and appropriate respiratory protective equipment in all environments in which nitrogen oxides may be encountered.

Phosgene

Phosgene, another gaseous toxin that has relatively low water solubility, is perhaps most notorious for its role as a war gas. Its use in World War I reportedly led to as many as 80 percent of all the gas deaths during that conflict. Its contemporary industrial uses include roles in the production of polyurethane resin, toluene diisocyanate, pesticides, pharmaceutical products, and dyes. In addition, it is produced from the heat decomposition of various solvents, paint removers, dry-cleaning fluids, and methylene chloride.[25]

Like other inhaled toxins that have low water solubilities, phosgene produces its most recognized clinical effects through injury to the lower airway and lung parenchyma. The duration of the latent period is inversely proportional to the severity of exposure and is also thought to be inversely proportional to the subsequent severity of disease. A clinical picture of pneumonitis that can progress to ARDS results. Clinical manifestations of the lower airway and parenchymal effects include dyspnea, chest tightness, cough, and increasing respiratory distress. Physical examination may reveal cyanosis and rales. Chest radiographs can show diffuse bilateral infiltrates consistent with pulmonary edema. Hypoxia and decreased vital capacity are observed. Treatment is supportive and may include mechanical ventilation with positive pressure, supplemental oxygenation, and hemodynamic monitoring. Persons who survive the acute injury can be left with chronic bronchitis or emphysema, although others may experience no long-lasting adverse clinical sequelae.[25]

Ozone

Ozone is recognized as a major constituent of environmental smog and is also present as a naturally occurring gas in the upper atmosphere, where it has a protective effect against ultraviolet radiation from the sun. It has relatively low water solubility. Chronic and acute adverse health effects from the concentrations of ozone (0.05 to 0.8 ppm) that are commonly found in ambient air have been well described and include a myriad of respiratory symptoms as well as evidence of upper and lower airway irritation, inflammation, and airflow obstruction.[26] In the occupational setting, ozone has been implicated as a toxic inhalant in airplane cabins during high-altitude flight, in industries where it is used as an oxidizing agent, and in arc welding, where it can occur in association with oxides of nitrogen.[27]

Cadmium

Cadmium is a highly corrosion-resistant metal that has many industrial applications. Toxic inhalation exposures may be encountered by workers who do soldering, brazing, smelting, and refining. Plumbers, coppersmiths, and electronic equipment assemblers may be exposed, as may persons who engage in hobbies that include working with sheet metal.[28]

Heating of cadmium-containing materials can release vapors and cadmium oxide fumes. Most toxic exposures have been reported following exposure to cadmium vapors in enclosed spaces or poorly ventilated areas. The typical clinical presentation is similar to that for metal fume fever, and includes an initial asymptomatic period that lasts several hours and is followed by fevers, chills, and myalgias. These constitutional symptoms are often accompanied or soon followed by respiratory distress, including cough, chest tightness, and dyspnea. The chest radiograph reveals bilateral infiltrates consistent with pneumonitis. Initial pulmonary function tests can show a restrictive ventilatory defect and decreased diffusion. Fatal cases have been remarkable for initial pneumonitis that relentlessly progresses to ARDS and eventual death from respiratory failure.[29] Victims who survive the acute lung injury may be left with persistent ventilatory restriction.

Treatment of acute lung injury due to the inhalation of cadmium fumes is supportive and similar to treatment for other forms of acute lung injury and ARDS. Corticosteroids may help improve outcome, but their efficacy is not well established. Elevated blood and urine cadmium levels may help establish cadmium as the likely etiologic agent in cases in which the nature of the exposure is not clear. Blood levels may reflect acute exposure, while urine levels better reflect the total body burden. Monitoring of blood or urine levels during treatment has not been shown to influence the clinical outcome.[28]

Mercury

Acute mercury vapor inhalation occurs in occupational settings, including metal reclamation processing, fur and felt hat making, and dentistry. Exposures in the home have been reported during amateur attempts to extract precious metals from amalgams that also contain mercury.[30,31] Common to episodes of toxic mercury inhalation is vapor generation in closed spaces or poorly ventilated areas.

Mercury vapor has little or no immediate upper airway or mucosal surface irritant effects; as a result, exposed persons may unknowingly remain in an area where the harmful vapors are present. Typical clinical presentations include symptoms of cough, dyspnea, and respiratory distress that develop 12 to 24 h after exposure. These initial symptoms are sometimes accompanied by fever, nausea, vomiting, diarrhea, and a metallic taste in the mouth, similar to what is often experienced by patients with metal fume fever and associated transient pneumonitis. In fact, mercury vapor inhalation can be mistaken for metal fume fever or influenza. Symptoms of mercury vapor inhalation do not, however, spontaneously resolve in a pattern similar to that for metal fume fever. Instead, the pneumonitis may progress to ARDS. Death due to progressive respiratory failure may ensue; pneumothorax has been reported to be a preterminal event in several cases. The severity of the injury appears to depend on the intensity of exposure and possibly the size and age of the exposed person. Children and small household pets seem especially vulnerable to life-threatening acute lung injury after the inhalation of mercury, but death due to respiratory failure has also been reported in exposed adults.[31] Adults who survive the acute lung injury usually experience resolution of their symptoms 2 to 7 days after onset, although longer courses of resolution have been reported for those who have sustained more severe injury.

The acute effects of inhaled mercury are usually confined to the respiratory system, although renal impairment with acute tubular necrosis has been reported.[13] The acute gastrointestinal and renal injuries that are seen after mercury ingestion are not typical of acute inhalation exposure. Chronic, low-intensity inhalation exposure may be associated with central nervous system and systemic symptoms and injury similar to that observed after ingestion. Treatment of mercury inhalation is supportive and addresses the acute lung injury. Corticosteroids have no proven benefit. Chelating agents, such as dimercaprol and penicillamine, which are frequently used to increase the rate of mercury excretion after ingestion, have not been shown to affect the outcome of the acute lung injury.[31]

Zinc Chloride Smoke Bombs

Oxides and chlorides of zinc and chloride are formed by the ignition of hexachloroethane, zinc oxide, and calcium chloride and are produced by some of the smoke-generating devices used by the military, in firefighter training, and for the generation of special effects in the entertainment industry.[32,33] Toxic inhalations have occurred when people have breathed in smoke in confined spaces. The smoke effect tends to contribute to the duration of exposure by obscuring vision, sometimes resulting in directional disorientation and the inability to escape quickly from the area of exposure.

Zinc chloride ($ZnCl_2$) is a hygroscopic, caustic salt that forms HCl and zinc oxychloride upon contact with water on mucous membranes and other surfaces. The severity of injury appears to be related to the intensity of the exposure and depends both on the duration of exposure and the concentration of zinc chloride in the smoke. $ZnCl_2$ is also present in particulate form, the average particle size being 0.1 μm. This size makes it possible for relatively large amounts of the inhaled hexite to penetrate into the lower respiratory tract, and as much as 20 percent of the total may reach beyond the level of the respiratory bronchioles. Deposition of particles in the lungs and subsequent formation of HCl may be primarily responsible for the diffuse lung injury.[33]

Signs and symptoms of tracheobronchitis and pneumonitis are common after inhalation of smoke that contains $ZnCl_2$. Initial chest radiographs can be normal but can also show diffuse bilateral infiltrates that are consistent with pneumonitis. Hypoxemia may not be present initially but can develop over the course of several days after the exposure as signs and symptoms of pneumonitis become more predominant. Progression to ARDS following an initial period of clinical stabilization or partial resolution has been reported. Pneumothorax is a frequent complication of the acute lung injury due to subpleural emphysema.

The treatment of $ZnCl_2$ inhalation includes oxygen supplementation and mechanical ventilatory support with positive pressure if indicated. Corticosteroids have been used, but it is unclear whether they significantly alter the clinical course. N-Acetylcysteine may minimize oxidant-induced lung injury, but it is not clear whether this influences the clinical outcome.[32] Exposed persons who survive may have persistent ventilatory and diffusion defects.

SYSTEMIC ILLNESS FROM INHALED TOXINS

A number of inhaled substances can cause extrapulmonary illness and injury. Metal fumes, fumes composed of heat-degraded fluorocarbons, and organic dusts have been implicated as causative agents in self-limited systemic syndromes (metal fume fever, polymer fume fever, and the organic dust toxic syndrome) that are notable for influenza-like illness with complete resolution within hours to days of exposure.[34–36] While some exposed persons experience only constitutional symptoms, there appears to be a continuum of illness that extends to include significant pulmonary parenchymal injury in others.

Metal Fume Fever

Metal fume fever is a self-limited syndrome characterized by the delayed onset of fever, chills, myalgias, and generalized malaise after exposure to fumes that contain metal oxides. Welders are the workers most often reported to experience metal fume fever, although a variety of other metalworking occupations—including soldering, brazing, cutting, metallizing, forging, melting, and casting—have been associated with exposures to metal fumes that are responsible for the syndrome. A common scenario is that of exposure to metal oxide fumes generated by welding in a closed space or poorly ventilated area. Zinc oxide is often implicated as the toxic agent responsible for metal fume fever; however, fumes composed of oxides of copper, cadmium, mercury, aluminum, antimony, selenium, iron, magnesium, nickel, silver, and tin have also been implicated.[34]

Constitutional symptoms are often preceded or accompanied by complaints of dry throat and a sweet or metallic taste in the mouth. The characteristic fever, chills, and myalgias—which are sometimes accompanied by headache and nausea—usually develop 4 to 8 h after exposure to metal fumes and spontaneously resolve over the next 24 to 48 h. Tachyphylaxis appears to occur in some people who are repeatedly exposed to metal oxide fumes, usually in occupational settings. These workers often report recurrent "Monday-morning fever" after returning to the workplace following weekend or vacation absences. Metal fume fever has been mistaken for influenza, atypical or community-acquired pneumonia, and a malaria-like illness because of overlapping presenting symptoms.

Some but not all affected subjects also complain of chest tightness, cough (usually nonproductive), and varying degrees of dyspnea. The chest radiograph is typically normal, but a radiographic picture consistent with pneumonitis has been reported in persons with respiratory symptoms. Pulmonary function is usually normal, although in those with symptomatic and radiographic evidence of pneumonitis, there have been reports of obstructive and restrictive defects as well as abnormalities of diffusion. There appears to be a continuum of clinical severity that ranges from the classic, self-resolving, constitutional symptoms of metal fume fever to transient pulmonary impairment and to more severe, sometimes even life-threatening pulmonary injury. The predisposition to developing these more serious manifestations of metal fume exposure appears to be related to the duration and concentration of the inhalation exposure and is most frequently reported after inhalation of fumes from zinc, mercury, and cadmium. The treatment of metal fume fever is supportive and includes antipyretics and analgesics. Prevention includes provision of adequate ventilation, fume-removal devices, and respiratory protection for workers in environments where metal oxide fumes are generated.

Polymer Fume Fever

Polymer fume fever is a syndrome with many clinical similarities to metal fume fever. It results from the inhalation of pyrolosis products of fluoropolymers, the most often reported of which is polytetrafluoroethylene (PTFE, or Teflon).[35] In addition to their popularly recognized use as nonstick coatings on cooking equipment, fluorocarbon polymers are widely used in industrial settings as mold-release sprays, lubricants, and fabric or leather treatments. Heating of fluoropolymers to high temperatures results in the production of fumes composed of a vapor phase that can contain or ultimately produce carbonyl fluoride, perfluorinated alkanes, hydrofluoric acid, and carbon dioxide. Respirable particles may also contribute to the toxic elements in the heat-generated fumes.[35] The fumes produced may lead to the systemic and pulmonary toxicities through mechanisms that are not well understood.

The clinical presentation of polymer fume fever includes initial, sometimes immediate, symptoms of upper airway irritation: dry throat, rhinitis, chest tightness, and conjunctivitis. Typically, constitutional symptoms consisting of fever, chills, and myalgias occur 4 to 8 h after exposure and spontaneously resolve over the next 24 h. No consistent pattern is seen in pulmonary function studies. However, persons with preexisting obstructive lung disease may experience worsening obstruction after recurrent exposures to polymer fumes. Cough and dyspnea that are associated with wheezing, and sometimes radiographic evidence of parenchymal consolidation are common. Pneumonitis accompanies constitutional symptoms more often than is reported in cases of metal fume fever. The reasons for this difference are unknown but may relate to the release of hydrofluoric acid. Unlike the decline in the severity of symptoms of metal fume fever that is observed with frequent, repeated exposures to metal fumes, tolerance does not appear to develop in people repeatedly exposed to pyrolized fluoropolymers, implying possible qualitative differences in the mechanisms of injury and host response in these two syndromes.[35] It is interesting to note that many workers who experience symptoms consistent with polymer fume fever are cigarette smokers, some of whom have reported the abrupt onset of symptoms immediately after smoking tobacco products that they have carried into the work environment. Several reports have suggested that these workers may have directly contaminated their smoking products with inert fluoropolymers that are subsequently pyrolized and inhaled in concentrated form along with the tobacco smoke. Alternatively, cigarette smoking may independently predispose persons to the development of polymer fume fever and associated acute lung injury.

Treatment of polymer fume fever is supportive and similar to that for metal fume fever. Prevention includes provision of adequate ventilation. In addition, workers should adhere to strict handwashing habits after handling products containing fluoropolymers; should not eat, drink, or smoke in the work environment; and should not carry smoking materials into work.

Organic Dust Toxic Syndrome

Organic dust toxic syndrome (ODTS)—also referred to as silo unloader's syndrome, atypical farmer's lung, or pulmonary mycotoxicosis—is a self-limited illness characterized by fever, chills, myalgias, dry cough, headache, and dyspnea that occurs 4 to 8 h after exposure to large amounts of organic dusts.[36] These symptoms usually resolve spontaneously with no long-term adverse sequelae over the next 36 to 48 h. The etiologic agents are probably substances that are present in moldy organic material. Agricultural workers as well as others who are exposed to environments where large amounts of grains, hay, straw, or wood chips are present can develop this syndrome.

The physical examination in patients with ODTS is usually normal but can show the presence of bibasilar crackles and scattered wheezes. Mild hypoxemia and infiltrates on the chest radiograph have been reported. The initial symptoms of ODTS are sometimes confused with those of hypersensitivity pneumonitis. However, unlike hypersensitivity pneumonitis, ODTS is transient, can occur in previously unexposed persons, and requires a relatively intense exposure. In contrast to what is often found in cases of hypersensitivity pneumonitis, serum allergic precipitins are usually negative in persons with ODTS.[36]

The course of ODTS is benign, with spontaneous resolution of symptoms as well as laboratory and radiographic abnormalities within days of the exposure. Treatment is symptomatic. Long-term sequelae of repeated high-intensity exposures that lead to recurrent episodes of ODTS may be associated with chronic bronchitis and decrements in airflow, but these have not been clearly established. Prevention requires education of agricultural workers and other potentially exposed subjects regarding practices related to the handling of moldy hay, grains, and other organic materials. In addition, people who engage in activities known to produce large quantities of potentially harmful airborne organic substances—such as weighing of swine and the intense handling of moldy grain, hay, straw, or wood chips—should be advised to wear respiratory protection.

REFERENCES

1. Kizer KW: Toxic inhalations. *Emerg Clin North Am* 2:649–666, 1984.
2. Schwartz DA: Acute inhalational injury, in Rosenstock L (ed), *Occupational Medicine: Occupational Pulmonary Disease,* vol 2, no. 2. Philadelphia, Hanley & Belfus, 1987, pp 297–318.
3. Barnes PJ: Reactive oxygen species and airway inflammation. *Free Radic Biol Med* 9:235–243, 1990.
4. Metzger WJ, Richerson HB, Worden K, et al: Bronchoalveolar lavage of allergic asthmatic patients following allergen provocation. *Chest* 89:477–483, 1986.
5. Hay DWP, Muccitelli RM, Wilson KA, et al: Agonist specificity in the effects of epithelium removal on contractions of the guinea pig trachea produced by leukotrienes, 5-hydroxytryptamine, and U-44069. *Pharmacologist* 28:141–148, 1986.
6. Beasley R, Roche WR, Roberts JA, Holgate, ST: Cellular events in the bronchi in mild asthma and after bronchial provocation. *Am Rev Respir Dis* 139: 806–817, 1989.
7. O'Connor G, Sparrow D, Tayler D, et al: Analysis of dose-response curves to methacholine. *Am Rev Respir Dis* 136:1412–1417, 1987.
8. Moore BB, Sherman M: Chronic reactive airway disease following acute chlorine gas exposure in an asymptomatic atopic patient. *Chest* 100:855–856, 1991.
9. Charan NB, Myers CG, Lakshminarayan S, Spencer TM: Pulmonary injuries associated with acute sulfur dioxide inhalation. *Am Rev Respir Dis* 119:555–560, 1979.
10. Brooks SM, Weiss MA, Bernstein IL: Reactive airways dysfunction syndrome (RADS). *Chest* 88:376–384, 1985.
11. Gautrin D, Boulet L-P, Boutet M, et al: Is reactive airways dysfunction syndrome a variant of occupational asthma? *J Allergy Clin Immunol* 93:12–22, 1994.
12. Galea M: Fatal sulfur dioxide inhalation. *Can Med Assoc J* 91:345–347, 1964.

13. Kanluen S, Gottlieb CA: A clinical pathologic study of four adult cases of acute mercury inhalation toxicity. *Arch Pathol Lab Med* 115:56–60, 1991.
14. McAdams AJ, Krop S: Injury and death from red fuming nitric acid. *JAMA* 158:1022–1024, 1955.
15. Price SK, Hughes JE, Morrison SC, Potgieter PD: Fatal ammonia inhalation: A case report with autopsy findings. *S Afr Med J* 64:952–955, 1993.
16. Epler GR, Colby TV, McLoud TC, et al: Bronchiolitis obliterans organizing pneumonia. *N Engl J Med* 312:152–158, 1985.
17. Epler GR: Bronchiolitis obliterans organizing pneumonia: Definition and clinical features. *Chest* 102:2S–6S, 1992.
18. Arwood R, Hammond J, Ward GG: Ammonia inhalation. *J Trauma* 25:444–447, 1985.
19. Montague TJ, Macneil AR: Mass ammonia inhalation. *Chest* 77:496–498, 1980.
20. Das R, Blanc PD: Chlorine gas exposure and the lung: A review. *Toxicol Ind Health* 9:439–455, 1993.
21. Sabonya R: Fatal anhydrous ammonia inhalation. *Hum Pathol* 8:293–299, 1977.
22. Reisz GR, Gammon RS: Toxic pneumonitis from mixing household cleaners. *Chest* 89:49–52, 1986.
23. Woodford DM, Coutu RE, Gaensler EA: Obstructive lung disease from acute sulfur dioxide exposure. *Respiration* 38:238–245, 1979.
24. NIOSH: *Criteria for a Recommended Standard: Occupational Exposure to Oxides of Nitrogen (Nitrogen Dioxide and Nitric Oxide).* Cincinnati, OH: U.S. Dept. of Health, Education and Welfare, 1976.
25. Bradley BL, Unger KM: Phosgene inhalation: A case report. *Texas Med* 78:51–53, 1982.
26. Menzel DB: Ozone: An overview of its toxicity in man and animals. *J Toxicol Environ Health* 13:183–204, 1984.
27. Tashkin DP, Coulson AH, Simmons MS, Spivey GH: Respiratory symptoms of flight attendants during high-altitude flight: Possible relation to cabin ozone exposure. *Int Arch Occup Environ Health* 52:117–137, 1983.
28. Barnhart S, Rosenstock L: Cadmium chemical pneumonitis. *Chest* 86:789–791, 1984.
29. Patwardhan JR, Finckh ES: Fatal cadmium-fume pneumonitis. *Med J Aust* 1:962–966, 1976.
30. Moutinho ME, Tompkins AL, Rowland TW, et al: Acute mercury vapor poisoning. *Am J Dis Child* 135:42–44, 1981.
31. Rowens B, Guerrero-Betancourt D, Gottlieb CA, et al: Respiratory failure and death following acute inhalation of mercury vapor: A clinical and histologic perspective. *Chest* 99:185–190, 1991.
32. Hjortso E, Qvist J, Bud MI, et al: ARDS after accidental inhalation of zinc chloride smoke. *Intens Care Med* 14:17–24, 1988.
33. Homma S, Jones R, Qvist J, et al: Pulmonary vascular lesions in the adult respiratory distress syndrome caused by inhalation of zinc chloride smoke: A morphometric study. *Hum Pathol* 23:45–50, 1992.
34. Gordon T, Fine JM: Metal fume fever. *Occup Med* 8:505–517, 1993.
35. Shusterman DJ: Polymer fume fever and other fluorocarbon pyrolysis–related syndromes. *Occup Med* 8:519–531, 1993.
36. Von Essen S, Robbins RA, Thompson AB, Rennard SI: Organic dust toxic syndrome: An acute febrile reaction to organic dust exposure distinct from hypersensitivity pneumonitis. *J Toxicol Clin Toxicol* 28:389–420, 1990.

21 | Indoor and Outdoor
Air Pollution*

Lisa M. Bellini and Michael A. Grippi

INTRODUCTION

Adverse effects of air pollution may be acute and dramatic or subtle and chronic. Biologic and clinical responses reflect the exposure and delivery of the injurious agent to the target site within the respiratory tract.

PRINCIPLES

Indoor and outdoor atmospheric pollutants exist in both gaseous and particulate forms. Respiratory tract penetration and retention of toxic gases depend on the physical properties of the gas (e.g., solubility), concentration of gas in inspired air, rate and depth of ventilation, and extent to which the material is reactive. Highly water-soluble gases, such as sulfur dioxide (SO_2), are almost completely extracted by the upper airways during brief exposures at rest. Less water-soluble gases, such as nitrous oxide (NO_2) or ozone (O_3), may penetrate to the airways and alveoli. Carbon monoxide (CO) is poorly soluble in water and is not removed in the upper airways. On reaching the lung, CO diffuses across the alveolar-capillary membrane and binds avidly to hemoglobin. Exercise greatly augments penetration of gases and the total dose of pollutants delivered to the airway. The switch from nasal to oral breathing during moderate to heavy exercise results in less efficient pollutant removal.

Inhalational deposition of particles suspended in aerosols depends on many factors, including the aerodynamic properties of the particle (primarily size), airway anatomy, and breathing pattern. Particles larger than 10 μm are effectively filtered out in the nose and nasopharynx through impaction against surfaces and gravitational forces. Particles less than 10 μm in aerodynamic diameter (PM_{10}) may be deposited in the tracheobronchial tree; deposition in the lung's alveoli is maximal for particles 1 to 2 μm in diameter. Particles smaller than 0.5 μm move by diffusion to the alveolar level, where they collide with gas molecules by Brownian movement and impact on alveolar surfaces. Removal of particles from the larger airways by the mucociliary apparatus is efficient and occurs within hours of deposition; clearance by alveolar macrophages requires days to months.

*Edited from Chap. 62, "Indoor and Outdoor Air Pollution," by Samet JM, Utell MJ., In *Fishman's Pulmonary Diseases and Disorders,* 3d ed., edited by Fishman AP, Elias JA, Fishman JA, Grippi MA, Kaiser LR, Senior RM. New York, McGraw-Hill, 1998, pp 941–964. For fuller discussion of topics dealt with in this chapter, the reader is referred to the original text, as noted above.

The mechanisms by which inhaled gases and particles injure the lung are diverse. Oxidant gases, e.g., O_3 and NO_2, cause inflammation of the respiratory epithelium, presumably through production of toxic oxidant species and release of potent mediators. SO_2 is also an irritant gas. Acidic compounds on particles may dissolve into tissue fluids and induce inflammation. Organic materials on particles may also produce inflammation or act as initiators or carcinogens.

Concentration refers to the amount of material present in air. *Exposure* constitutes contact with a material at a portal of entry into the body—the respiratory tract, the gastrointestinal tract, and the skin. Exposure is the unit of concentration multiplied by time. *Dose* refers to the amount of material that enters the body, while *biologically effective dose* is the amount reaching target sites for injury—e.g., the mass of respirable particles delivered to the small airways. For most inhaled pollutants, dose varies with activity and level of minute ventilation.

Total personal exposure to a pollutant is the time-weighted average pollutant concentration in an individual's "microenvironments." Microenvironments are locations having relatively constant concentrations of the pollutant during the time spent there (e.g., an office where smoking is allowed, an urban home where time is spent both outdoors and indoors). Indoor microenvironments can contribute to exposures to pollutants typically considered outdoor pollutants, such as particles and CO.

Toxicologic studies help characterize the hazards of air pollutants. *Epidemiologic studies* provide an assessment of the adverse effects of pollution exposures under the circumstances of "real world" exposure and have direct public health and regulatory relevance. *Risk assessment* requires review of all relevant data and mathematical modeling to characterize the risk. The findings of risk assessment guide *risk management,* the process by which decisions are made about the need for risk reduction and the approaches to be implemented to reduce risks. Risk management involves choosing among the options to control risk and balancing risk reduction, costs, and technologic capability for reducing exposure.

OUTDOOR AIR POLLUTION

In the United States, the Clean Air Act identifies two sets of outdoor air pollutants: *criteria pollutants* (Table 21-1) and *toxic air pollutants*. Criteria pollutants include combustion-related pollutants (SO_2, NO_2, CO, and particles), O_3, and lead. Toxic pollutants are predominantly carcinogens, which principally comprise industrial emissions and waste products (e.g., benzene, chlordane, ethylene oxide, hydrochloric acid, methane, parathion, propylene oxide, toluene, and vinyl chloride).

For criteria pollutants, National Ambient Air Quality Standards (NAAQS) are set after extensive review of all relevant evidence; the standards must afford protection to the entire population, including those with heightened susceptibility, and they must offer an "adequate margin of safety." The hazardous pollutants are predominantly carcinogens, such as asbestos and radionuclides; standards for maximum concentrations are also intended to provide a margin of safety. In spite of existing federal standards for ambient air quality, excesses are common in many areas of the country, particularly for O_3.

TABLE 21-1 Criteria Pollutants, Sources, and National Ambient Air Quality Standards (NAAQS)

Pollutant	Sources	Primary Standards	Averaging Time
Sulfur dioxide	Coal and petroleum combustion, smelting and other manufacturing	0.14 ppm (365 μg/m^3) 0.03 ppm (80 μg/m^3)	24 h Annual (arithmetic mean)
PM$_{10}$	Coal and petroleum combustion, vehicles, industry surface dust	150 μg/m^3 50 μg/m^3	24 h Annual (arithmetic mean)
Nitrogen dioxide	Coal and petroleum combustion, vehicles, industry	0.053 ppm (100 μg/m^3)	Annual (arithmetic mean)
Carbon monoxide	Coal and petroleum combustion, vehicles	35 ppm (40 μg/m^3) 9 ppm (10 μg/m^3)	1 h 8 h
Ozone	Secondary formation from NO$_2$ and hydrocarbons	0.12 ppm (235 μg/m^3)	Maximum daily 1-h average
Lead	Gasoline, lead-containing dust	1.5 mg/m^3	Maximum quarterly average

Sulfur Dioxide

Sulfur oxides are produced by combustion of sulfur-containing fuels, e.g., coal and crude petroleum. Smelting of ores containing sulfur is an important source in the southwestern United States. Previously, regulatory concern over sulfur oxides was directed primarily at the health effects of sulfur dioxide (SO$_2$), the criteria pollutant regulated by the Environmental Protection Administration (EPA). SO$_2$ is a water-soluble gas that is effectively scrubbed from inspired air by the upper airway; exercise, however, may increase the inhaled dose. This pollutant has been shown to have adverse effects without concomitant exposures to other pollutants.

Exposures to SO$_2$ in outdoor air occur primarily with simultaneous exposures to other combustion-related pollutants, including nitrogen oxides and particles. Heavy industry and coal-burning power plants are predominant sources. Power plant smokestacks release sulfur oxides and nitrogen oxides high into the atmosphere, where residence time is prolonged. Sulfur oxides and nitrogen oxides form acidic sulfate and nitrate particles, which may undergo long-range transport. Acidic particles represent a regional air pollution problem, particularly evident in the central and northeastern United States and portions of Canada.

Asthmatics are particularly susceptible to SO$_2$. Acute exposures at concentrations under 1.0 ppm cause bronchoconstriction after only 5 min in asthmatics, whereas inhalation of concentrations in excess of 5 ppm causes only small decrements in airway function in normals. Lung function responses to SO$_2$ in asthmatics are greater when SO$_2$ exposure is accompanied by increased ventilation, usually stimulated by exercise. Inhalation of SO$_2$ produces an immediate response and does not provoke delayed reactions or repetitive nocturnal attacks. The bronchoconstriction resolves within an hour, and peak bronchoconstrictor responses may lessen on repeated challenge after a short recovery period. The response can be ameliorated by anticholinergic agents, cromolyn, or beta agonists.

Nitrogen Dioxide

Nitrogen oxides, like sulfur oxides, are produced by combustion and contribute to formation of acid aerosols. Even though nitrogen dioxide (NO_2) is regulated by the EPA as a criteria pollutant, most personal exposure in the United States occurs indoors with use of unvented gas stoves and space heaters. The principal outdoor source is motor vehicle emissions; power plants and industrial sources may also contribute. The health effects of NO_2 released into outdoor air probably arise principally from the formation of secondary pollutants, such as O_3, and acidic nitrate particles.

NO_2, an oxidant gas of low solubility that penetrates to the small airways and alveoli, may impair lung defenses against respiratory pathogens and cause airway inflammation. Risk for respiratory infections, respiratory symptoms, reduced lung function, and exacerbation of chronic respiratory diseases may be increased; however, limited epidemiologic data are available. Epidemiologic studies on the acute effects of NO_2 in asthma are inconclusive. Patients with chronic obstructive pulmonary disease (COPD) may have increased susceptibility to short-term exposure to NO_2 outdoors.

Particles

Particles in outdoor air have natural and human-made sources; the latter include power plants, industry, and motor vehicles. Diesel-powered vehicles emit particles in the inhalable size range. Large populations in the United States and other industrialized countries are exposed to acid aerosols arising from primary combustion pollutants. Release of SO_2, NO_2, and particles from tall smokestacks results in transformation to acid particles containing sulfates and nitrates. These acid aerosols predominantly affect the central and eastern United States and adjacent portions of Canada.

Recent studies have shown a statistically significant association between particle concentration and daily mortality counts for some regions in the United States, suggesting that the present NAAQS for particulate matter may not protect against adverse health effects with the "adequate margin of safety" mandated by the Clean Air Act. However, the toxicologic mechanisms by which inhaled particulate matter might lead to cardiopulmonary morbidity and mortality are not yet established. Epidemiologic data indicate associations of acid aerosol levels with mortality and respiratory symptoms in children. Asthmatics also appear to be sensitive to acid aerosols. Persons considered at greatest risk are those working outdoors and, consequently, highly exposed, and those with increased airway responsiveness or asthma.

Carbon Monoxide

Carbon monoxide (CO) is an invisible gas formed by incomplete combustion of fossil fuels and other organic materials. The most prominent outdoor source is vehicle exhaust; indoor sources include cooking stoves and tobacco smoke. Urban locations with high traffic density tend to have the highest concentrations.

The current U.S. standard for CO levels in outdoor air (Table 21-1) is intended to protect susceptible persons with coronary artery disease. Inhaled CO binds avidly to hemoglobin. Depending on ambient levels of CO, level of activity, and lung function, the half-life of CO in the body ranges from about 2.5 to 4 h. Formation of carboxyhemoglobin (COHb) reduces oxygen transport. Persons with cardiovascular disease are considered to be at greatest risk from CO exposure. Federal standards for outdoor air were selected to prevent COHb levels from rising above 1.5 percent.

Ozone

Photochemical pollution or *smog* is a complex oxidant mixture produced by the action of sunlight on hydrocarbons and nitrogen oxides in vehicle exhaust. Ozone (O_3) is invariably present in photochemical pollution, and its concentration serves as an index of the level of this mixture. In animals, low-level exposures cause small airway damage. Volunteers exposed to O_3 at concentrations in the range of the current standard (often present during pollution episodes) experience transient reductions of lung function; normal subjects have a range of responses that is wide but reproducible. Hence, the potential exists for chronic effects from repeated inhalation. Surprisingly, in clinical studies, asthmatics have not been shown to have a greater susceptibility to O_3 than do nonasthmatics. Relevant epidemiologic data are suggestive of chronic effects of O_3, but these data are not definitive.

Toxins

The toxic air pollutants are predominantly carcinogens, but they are also responsible for other adverse health effects. Approximately 200 hazardous pollutants are listed as air toxins in the 1990 Clean Air Act amendments. Examples include asbestos, benzene, cadmium compounds, chlorine, formaldehyde, and nickel. Although the sources are diverse, emission releases tend to be localized, often at industrial sites or from municipal incinerators or waste sites.

Only a small proportion of lung cancers can be attributed to air pollution. Exposure to diesel exhaust for years may result in a small excess risk of lung cancer. However, given the difficulties of measuring exposure along with confounding variables related to cigarette smoking and occupational exposures, it is difficult to reach any definitive conclusion about the role of diesel exhaust in causing lung cancer in the general population.

INDOOR AIR POLLUTION

Sources of indoor air pollution include gas cooking stoves, burning cigarettes, fireplaces, wood stoves, and unvented space heaters. Evaporation of *volatile organic compounds* from a variety of materials and products leads to contamination by these agents. Other indoor pollutants include asbestos, biologic agents, radon, and penetrating outdoor air pollutants. The concentration of an indoor contaminant depends on the strength of its source, the rate of removal, the volume of the space, and the rate of exchange of air between the space and outdoors.

Carbon Monoxide

The biologic effects of carbon monoxide were discussed previously. Indoors, carbon monoxide (CO) is released by cooking and heating devices and by smoking. Residential concentrations are typically low, ranging from 2 to 4 ppm during the winter, when windows of homes are generally closed and the homes heated. People living in homes with gas cooking ranges and those living with smokers have slightly higher levels of exposure. Measurements of CO in commercial and institutional buildings show concentrations in the same range as in residences. The CO in residences and public buildings without combustion sources primarily reflects entry of motor vehicle exhaust from outdoor air. About 900 accidental deaths in the United States are attributed annually to asphyxiation by CO inhalation.

Unexposed nonsmokers have COHb levels of approximately 0.5 percent. This endogenous COHb comes from catabolism of hemoglobin and heme-containing enzymes of the liver. In comparison, COHb levels of cigarette smokers average about 4 percent and may be much higher. Headache and dizziness, early symptoms of CO poisoning, have been associated with COHb levels greater than 10 percent. Frank CO poisoning (headache, loss of motor control, and coma) generally occurs with COHb levels above 20 percent.

Nitrogen Dioxide

Unvented gas cooking stoves and kerosene space heaters are the major sources of indoor nitrogen dioxide (NO_2). Levels increase when homes are closed for heating or air conditioning purposes. During cooking, concentrations may reach 1000 ppb while a stove is in use, resulting in substantial exposures for persons near the stove. A wide variety of health effects of NO_2 are of potential concern, including reduced host defense mechanisms, exacerbation of asthma and chronic obstructive pulmonary disease, and respiratory tract inflammation. In spite of extensive investigation using laboratory and epidemiologic approaches, the evidence still remains inconclusive in regard to each of these health outcomes.

Environmental Tobacco Smoke

Environmental tobacco smoke (ETS) refers to the combination of *sidestream smoke* released from the cigarette's burning end and *mainstream smoke* exhaled by the smoker. Hundreds of chemical compounds have been identified in cigarette smoke. Markers of ETS are *respirable suspended particles* (RSP), which are particles of mean aerodynamic diameter of less than 2.5 μm, CO, and nicotine (in the vapor phase). Smoking in the home approximately doubles the 24-h average indoor RSP concentration.

ETS causes both malignant and nonmalignant diseases in nonsmokers. Maternal smoking increases the risk of infants for lower respiratory tract illnesses. Smoking by household members, particularly the mother, increases the incidence of chronic respiratory symptoms and reduces the rate of lung growth in children. Children with asthma whose parents smoke have heightened airway responsiveness and increased morbidity. Exposure to ETS is also a suspect cause of asthma; infants of smoking parents have increased airway responsiveness shortly after birth. Epidemiologic studies show that parental smoking is associated with persistent middle-ear effusions.

Exposure of never-smokers to ETS has been linked to lung cancer. Numerous epidemiologic studies show a positive association between living with a smoker and risk of lung cancer. Meta-analysis demonstrates an increased risk of lung cancer (increase of 20 percent) for never-smoking women married to smokers. The EPA classifies ETS as a class A carcinogen, a designation applied to agents causally linked to cancer.

A number of epidemiologic studies have shown that marriage to a smoker increases risk for ischemic heart disease. The American Heart Association has concluded that ETS exposure is a major preventable cause of cardiovascular disease and death. Mechanisms may include promotion of atherosclerosis, increased platelet aggregation, endothelial cell damage, and the consequences of CO exposure. ETS exposure at home and in the workplace has been linked to reduced lung function. Other proposed associations of ETS with disease are increased risk for cancers at sites other than the lung, younger age at menopause, increased risk for sudden infant death syndrome, reduced birth weight, and worsening of cystic fibrosis.

Wood Smoke

Indoor wood smoke includes particles, organic compounds, and CO. Available data suggest that the routine operation of a properly installed and maintained wood stove does not directly affect indoor air quality. Outdoor air contaminated with wood smoke can enter homes without wood stoves. Although the toxicology of some components of wood smoke—such as benzo[a]pyrene, other polycyclic organic compounds, and nitrogen oxides—has been extensively studied, little research exists on the toxicology of wood smoke as a complex mixture.

Organic Compounds

Organic compounds are released indoors from furnishings, equipment, construction materials, and consumer and office products. They include volatile, semivolatile, and particulate components. The volatile and semivolatile components are most relevant to human health. Volatile organic compounds exist as vapors over the normal range of air temperatures and pressures, whereas semivolatile organic compounds are liquids or solids; they also evaporate.

Formaldehyde, an extensively used organic compound, is a key component in urea and phenol-formaldehyde resins, used in the manufacture of laminated wood products and particle board. The health risks of organic compounds include carcinogenesis and mutagenesis (e.g., benzene). Irritant effects (e.g., formaldehyde and terpenes) and neurotoxicity (e.g., aromatic compounds) have also been described. However, few studies have shown specific exposure-disease associations, largely because of the difficulty of characterizing exposures and identifying effects of components of complex mixtures in indoor air. Irritation of mucosal surfaces and neurotoxic effects may contribute to the symptom complex widely referred to as the *sick-building syndrome.*

Radon

Radon 222, a noble gas, is in the decay chain of naturally occurring uranium 238. Its decay produces progeny that release alpha particles thought to damage cellular DNA and produce lung cancer. The principal source of radon in buildings derives from naturally occurring gas in soil. The driving pressure for entry of soil gas into a building is the pressure gradient established by a structure across the soil. The soil gas enters through openings such as sump pump wells, drains, cracks, and utility access holes.

The average value for radon concentration for homes in the United States is about 1.5 picocuries per liter (pCi/L). Homes with high concentrations have been identified in all states, although the proportion exceeding the EPA's action guideline of 4 pCi/L is variable among the states. Radon is present in most homes and can reach high concentrations—as high as those in underground mines—with a documented excess of lung cancer. It is believed that radon causes an estimated 10,000 to 20,000 cases of lung cancer annually in the United States. The burden of radon-related lung cancer in the general population reflects in part the synergism between radon and cigarette smoking.

The EPA-conducted radon reduction program in the United States calls for voluntary measurement of radon levels in single-family homes and modification if the annual concentration exceeds the agency's guideline level of 4 pCi/L. Two types of passive measurement devices for radon are available: short-term devices, which make measurements over a few days, and long-term devices, which make measurements for periods of months up to a year. The short-term devices, primarily charcoal canisters, are often used when a measurement is needed quickly during a real estate transaction; the longer-term devices incorporate a piece of plastic that is etched by alpha particles released by radon progeny. Radon concentrations can be lowered by sealing basement cracks and sump holes, ventilating the basement to the outside, and, for homes built on concrete slabs, providing a system to exhaust soil gas from beneath the slab.

Asbestos and Synthetic Fibers

Asbestos has high tensile strength and protective thermal properties and has been extensively used in building materials since the beginning of the twentieth century. Asbestos fibers may be released from acoustic ceiling tiles, vinyl floor tiles, paints, wall and ceiling plaster, pipe coatings, boiler linings, and coatings on structural steel beams. More recently, synthetic mineral fibers have been used in building materials; principal types include glass fibers (glass wool and glass filaments), rock wool, and slag wool and ceramic fibers. Fiber glass and glass wool are silica-based vitreous fibers which, because of their fibrous nature, have generated concern about the same health effects as for asbestos.

Exposures to airborne asbestos fibers, rather than the presence of asbestos-containing materials in a building, determine occupant risk. The risks for exposed office workers and visitors are principally mesothelioma and lung cancer; asbestosis is not a significant threat based on the level of exposure for building occupants. The risks of indoor asbestos for the general population have been estimated by extrapolation of risks for occupationally exposed persons, and uncertainty is inherent in this approach. Because of the morphologic and toxicologic comparability of asbestos and synthetic mineral fibers, there has been concern that exposure to synthetic mineral fibers could produce the same diseases caused by asbestos; however, to date there are no data to support this conclusion.

Biologic Substances

Indoor levels of allergens and microbes are increased by accumulation of human and animal dander and growth of fungi and bacteria on interior surfaces or in air-conditioning systems. Indoor pollen is derived almost entirely from outdoor sources; fungal spores from outdoors may also enter indoors on air infiltration or inadvertently on people, animals, or objects.

Significant indoor biologic pollution may arise from growth of microorganisms on interior surfaces that are wet and moist. High relative humidity (>70 percent) promotes condensation on interior surfaces (e.g., cool exterior walls or windowsills). Humidifiers, vaporizers, and air conditioners may become contaminated and distribute fungal fragments, spores, and dissolved allergens into room air. Factors such as aerodynamic behavior, respirability, solubility, and cross-reactivity with other allergens are important in immunologic sensitization and development of allergic disease.

Dust mites (*Dermatophagoides pteronyssinus, D. farinae,* and *Euroglyphus maynei*) are commonly found in houses and are important sources of allergens, particularly for persons with asthma. These mites live in carpets, upholstered furniture, mattresses, and bedding, where they eat skin scales. Two major dust mite allergens have been identified, *Der p* I and *Der p* II. These proteins are derived from digestive enzymes in the gut of the mite and are found in high concentrations in the fecal pellets.

Domestic cockroaches are commonly found indoors and represent another source of allergen in residences, particularly in infested inner-city housing. Fecal material and saliva contain large amounts of the allergens *Bla g* I and *Bla g* II.

Cats and dogs are common allergen sources. *Fel d* I is the most significant allergen associated with cats, and high levels of this protein are found in cat dander and fur as well as in saliva and urine. The presence of the allergen in the dust of homes and buildings in which cats are not kept suggests that the allergen can be transported on clothing. The major dog allergen, *Can f* I, is present in dog fur and saliva and is a relatively stable protein that may persist in dust for a long time.

Fungi are present in the air of virtually all homes and public buildings. Commonly isolated genera include *Cladosporium, Penicillium, Alternaria, Epicoccum, Aspergillus,* and *Drechslera.*

Biologic agents in indoor air may cause direct toxicity, infections, or immune hyperresponsiveness. Home dampness and mold have been associated with upper respiratory symptoms and eye irritation. Allergic rhinitis ("hay fever") affects approximately 20 percent of adults in the United States. Identification of the specific indoor allergen associated with the symptoms may be accomplished by skin testing and in vitro measurement of antibody [radioallergosorbent test (RAST)]. Many persons with asthma are sensitive to specific antigens from pollens, animal fur, fungi spores, and house dust. Avian proteins are present in bird excreta (e.g., the droppings of pet birds such as parakeets), and fungal spores of thermophilic actinomycetes, *Aspergillus, Penicillium,* and *Aureobasidium* species may contaminate the indoor environment and cause hypersensitivity pneumonitis. A careful review of symptom pattern in relation to home and work environments and site evaluation may be needed to identify the source of exposure.

CONTROL STRATEGIES

Limiting time outside and vigorous exercise outdoors during episodes of air pollution represents an effective strategy in controlling exposure. Susceptible patients should be counseled, including those with asthma, emphysema, coronary artery disease (and, possibly, peripheral vascular disease), infants, the elderly, and children with chronic pulmonary disease (e.g., cystic fibrosis or bronchopulmonary dysplasia).

Respiratory protective equipment developed for the workplace may increase the work of breathing and is usually not well tolerated by patients with respiratory disease. Generally, respiratory protective equipment should not be suggested as a method for reducing the risks of air pollution. Similarly, air cleaners have not been shown to have health benefits.

During times of increased air pollution, the EPA issues *health advisories* or *cautionary statements* (the Pollutant Standards Index for criteria pollutants) regarding outdoor air quality. These statements prompt actions to be taken by the public when certain "alert levels" are reached. The EPA's advice is intended for use by local air pollution agencies in preparing daily air quality summaries to be disseminated to the media.

BIBLIOGRAPHY

American Thoracic Society, Committee of the Environmental and Occupational Health Assembly: Health effects of outdoor air pollution. Part 1. *Am J Respir Crit Care Med* 153:3–50, 1996.

American Thoracic Society, Committee of the Environmental and Occupational Health Assembly: Health effects of outdoor air pollution. Part 2. *Am J Respir Crit Care Med* 153:477–498, 1996.

American Thoracic Society: Environmental controls and lung disease. *Am Rev Respir Dis* 142:915–939, 1990.

Darby SC, Samet JM: Radon, in Samet JM (ed), *Epidemiology of Lung Cancer.* New York, Marcel Dekker, 1994.

Heinrich J, Hoelscher B, Wichmann HE: Decline of ambient air pollution and respiratory symptoms in children. *Am J Respir Crit Care Med* 161:1930–1936, 2000.

MacNee W, Donaldson K: Exacerbations of COPD: Environmental mechanisms. *Chest* 117(suppl 2):390S–397S, 2000.

Pershagen G: Passive smoking and lung cancer, in Samet JM (ed), *Epidemiology of Lung Cancer.* New York, Marcel Dekker, 1994.

Smith KR, Samet JM, Romieu I, Bruce N: Indoor air pollution in developing countries and acute lower respiratory infections in children. *Thorax* 55:518–532, 2000.

Stone V: Environmental air pollution. *Am J Respir Crit Care Med* 162(part 2):S44–S47, 2000.

22 | Pulmonary Disorders Related to High Altitude*

Lisa M. Bellini and Michael A. Grippi

INTRODUCTION

The body's responses to ascent and dwelling at high altitude are clinically important. A variety of disorders may arise when ascent is so rapid as to preclude physiologic adaptations or when the adaptations are incomplete. Several important clinical disorders associated with high altitude are discussed below.

ADAPTATIONS TO HIGH ALTITUDE

A number of important physiologic adaptations to high altitude have been well described.

Respiratory Control Mechanisms

The peripheral chemoreceptors, located in the carotid and aortic bodies, determine the ventilatory response to hypoxia. Type I cells in the carotid body trigger an increase in ventilation in response to hypoxia and hypercapnia. The response to acute hypoxia is not sustained; the increased ventilation abates somewhat after about a minute. With sustained hypoxia, ventilation continues to increase further over several hours or days, a process known as *ventilatory acclimatization.* During acclimatization, alveolar P_{CO_2} decreases as alveolar P_{O_2} diminishes with ascent. The carotid bodies are essential for ventilatory acclimatization to hypoxia. Upon returning to sea level, a significant decrease in ventilation occurs immediately, but a similar time-dependent decrease in ventilation also occurs.

Control of Pulmonary Vascular Tone

Although pulmonary blood vessels are supplied extensively with fibers from the autonomic nervous system, regulation of pulmonary vasomotor tone is largely mediated by local effects of P_{O_2} and P_{CO_2}. Normally, regional hypoxia (e.g., due to bronchiole obstruction), constricts blood vessels and shunts blood away from the hypoxic area. Local CO_2 accumulation leads to a decline in pH, which, in turn, leads to vasoconstriction. Similarly, at high altitude, generalized hypoxia induces widespread pulmonary vasoconstriction; over time, muscularization of the pulmonary arteries and pulmonary hypertension (systolic and diastolic) are observed. The magnitude of the pulmonary hypertension is accentuated by exercise. Relief of hypoxia permits regression

---

*Edited from Chap. 63, "Pulmonary Adaptation and Clinical Disorders Related to High Altitude," by Lahiri S, Milledge JS. In: *Fishman's Pulmonary Diseases and Disorders,* 3d ed., edited by Fishman AP, Elias JA, Fishman JA, Grippi MA, Kaiser LR, Senior RM. New York, McGraw-Hill, 1998, pp 965–978. For fuller discussion of topics dealt with in this chapter, the reader is referred to the original text, as noted above.

of the histologic changes, pulmonary hypertension, and resultant right ventricular hypertrophy.

Exercise

During steady-state exercise at sea level, ventilation increases in proportion to oxygen uptake, so that alveolar P_{CO_2} remains essentially unchanged. During heavy exercise, lactic acid generation stimulates ventilation further, so that alveolar P_{CO_2} falls. With ascent to altitude, the resulting decrease in inspired P_{O_2} stimulates resting ventilation, determining the "set point" for the increase in ventilation during exercise. The mechanism by which alveolar P_{CO_2} is maintained constant during exercise is not clear.

At sea level, the low-pressure pulmonary circulation accommodates the increased blood flow easily, with a small rise in pulmonary artery pressure and vascular resistance with progressive exercise. During hypoxia, the relationship between pulmonary blood flow and pulmonary artery pressure is altered. With chronic hypoxia, including that due to high altitude, structural remodeling of pulmonary arterioles results in increases in resting pulmonary arterial pressure and resistance, resulting in a parallel, upward shift of the pulmonary arterial pressure-flow relationship, presumably due to increased resistance in the microcirculation. Thus, altitude resets the regulation of the pulmonary circulation by way of structural remodeling of the lungs.

Sleep

During normal sleep at sea level, alveolar P_{O_2} decreases and alveolar P_{CO_2} increases. At altitude, these changes become critically important, stimulating breathing. This then increases P_{O_2} and decreases P_{CO_2}, which, in turn, decreases ventilation, triggering periodic breathing. At an altitude above 3000 m, normal people manifest periodic breathing during sleep. The quality of both rapid-eye-movement (REM) and non-REM sleep becomes impaired. With acclimatization, the sleep pattern tends to become more normal, but periodic breathing during non-REM sleep continues. Periodic breathing and apnea with ascent to high altitude disappear with administration of acetazolamide, which stimulates central chemoreceptors through a rise in central CO_2. Similarly, high-altitude natives with blunted hypoxic drives seldom manifest periodic breathing and apnea.

Circulatory Volume

Hypoxia-induced increases in levels of erythropoietin lead to increased numbers of erythrocytes. In addition, the normal response to ascent to high altitude is a diuresis that persists during the stay at high altitude. The diuresis is accompanied by suppression of voluntary sodium and water intake. Peripheral arterial chemoreflexes may play a role. Lung edema, cerebral edema, and peripheral edema may be seen (see below), with elevated levels of aldosterone and antidiuretic hormone.

CLINICAL MANIFESTATIONS OF MALADAPTION TO HIGH ALTITUDE

Clinically important disorders reflective of maladaptation to ascent to high altitude include acute mountain sickness, high-altitude pulmonary edema, and high-altitude cerebral edema. The likelihood of developing symptoms depends on the speed of ascent, elevation, length of stay at altitude, and individual susceptibility. With long-term high-altitude dwelling, chronic mountain sickness may be observed.

Acute Mountain Sickness

Acute mountain sickness (AMS) affects previously healthy individuals who ascend rapidly to high altitude. The incidence, which depends upon the altitude and rate of ascent, is approximately 9 percent at 2850 m, 13 percent at 3050 m, 34 percent at 3650 m, and 53 percent at 4559 m. Symptoms develop a few hours to 2 days after ascent and include headache (usually frontal), nausea, vomiting, irritability, malaise, insomnia, and poor climbing performance. The milder form of the condition is self-limiting, lasting 3 to 5 days. The disorder does not recur at the altitude at which it appears, although it may develop if the subject goes to a higher altitude. Severe forms of AMS (see below) may be seen, including high-altitude pulmonary edema (HAPE), high-altitude cerebral edema (HACE), or a mixed form of these two disorders. If not treated, these conditions are frequently fatal in a matter of hours.

Hypoxia of more than a few hours' duration is necessary for development of AMS. Susceptibility among individuals ascending to high altitude is variable and cannot be predicted; however, past performance at altitude may be a marker. People of all ages and either sex seem to be equally affected. Fitness is no protection; indeed, the fit are likely to ascend faster and therefore may be at greater risk. Any respiratory infection is probably a risk factor and may account for illness in the subject who has previously acclimatized well. High-altitude dwellers who have a blunted hypoxic ventilatory response are less prone to develop AMS than are lowlanders. A brisk pulmonary artery pressor response to hypoxia may be a risk factor for HAPE.

Symptoms are delayed by several hours after ascent and are likely due to some degree of cerebral edema (and often subclinical pulmonary edema). Frequently, dependent or periorbital edema exists as well, suggesting altered capillary permeability throughout the body. Changes in minute ventilation may play a role in the development of AMS. Exercise is thought to be a risk factor. Prolonged exercise performed by mountaineers causes retention of sodium and water through activation of the renin-aldosterone system, which may place subjects at risk for AMS.

A slow rate of ascent is the best way to prevent AMS. In general, above 300 m (10,000 ft), ascent should be no more than 300 m (1000 ft) per day, with a rest day every 3 days, during which no further ascent is made. If symptoms of AMS develop, the individual should go no higher. If symptoms become severe, the individual should descend to lower altitude. Use of the carbonic acid anhydrase inhibitor acetazolamide reduces the risk of AMS. Acetazolamide probably acts as a respiratory stimulant, increasing Pa_{O_2} and decreasing Pa_{CO_2}. The recommended dose is 250 mg or 125 mg twice daily, with the first dose administered at least 24 h prior to a major ascent. Side effects include a mild diuresis that tends to decrease if the drug is continued; paresthesias of the fingers and toes are almost universal. Flushing, thirst, headache, rash, and blood dyscrasias have been described but are rare. Finally, beer and all carbonated beverages taste flat. Of course, AMS, and even HAPE or HACE, are still possible while taking the drug. Dexamethasone has been shown to be an effective prophylactic drug, but most would consider it unjustified for this purpose.

Simple or benign AMS is self-limiting and usually lasts about 3 days; treatment is not essential. Aspirin may be used to relieve headache, but it is not very efficacious. In a placebo-controlled trial, ibuprofen has been shown to be effective. If the condition progresses to HAPE or HACE, treatment is urgent.

High-Altitude Pulmonary Edema

The potentially lethal condition of *high-altitude pulmonary edema* (HAPE) is less common than AMS. The incidence depends on the rate of ascent and the population examined. An incidence of 0.5 to 2.0 percent has been reported. Individuals with a previous history of HAPE are at greater risk of developing the syndrome. Both lowlanders and high-altitude residents who reascend to altitude are susceptible. Young males appear to be particularly at risk; athletic fitness affords no protection.

Onset is heralded by dyspnea and cough, which is initially dry. Subsequently, frothy white sputum, which may become blood-tinged, develops. Chest discomfort may be noted. The pulse and respiratory rate are increased; crackles at the lung bases, peripheral edema, increased jugular venous pressure, a right ventricular heave, and accentuated pulmonary second heart sound may be observed. Over a few hours, cyanosis develops.

The chest radiograph typically shows asymmetrical, patchy pulmonary edema. A neutrophil-predominant leukocytosis is present. Arterial blood gases show a reduced P_{O_2} compared with those of fit individuals at the same altitude. The P_{CO_2} is variable, but it is not significantly different from values in unaffected individuals. The electrocardiogram reveals tachycardia and changes consistent with pulmonary hypertension. Cardiac catheterization confirms the presence of high pulmonary artery and normal pulmonary artery occlusion pressures. The cardiac output is normal. Pulmonary edema fluid has a high protein content. Necropsy shows edematous lungs; the edema is patchy and hemorrhagic in areas. Thrombi are seen in small arteries and veins. The alveoli contain fluid, red blood cells, polymorphonuclear leukocytes, and macrophages; hyaline membrane formation may be noted.

The mechanism of HAPE is not clear. Susceptible subjects appear to have a brisk hypoxic pulmonary artery pressor response and demonstrate nonhomogeneous areas of vasoconstriction throughout the lung. Greatly increased blood flow through less vasoconstricted areas of the lung may cause capillary damage and resultant patchy pulmonary edema in the setting of pulmonary hypertension.

The most important intervention in HAPE is evacuation of the patient to a lower altitude. A reduction in altitude of as little as 300 m (1000 ft) may result in significant clinical improvement. Supplemental oxygen should be administered to all patients. A portable, lightweight, rubberized canvas hyperbaric chamber (Gamow bag) is commercially available for the treatment of HAPE. The patient can be placed in the chamber and its pressure increased by 2 psi using a foot pump. Use of this device effectively reduces the patient's altitude by almost 2000 m (6000 ft). Cases have been reported in which dramatic clinical improvement in HAPE (and HACE) has been observed with use of the chamber. Considerable effort is required to maintain pumping if limited help is available. The device may result in sufficient patient improvement to allow unaided descent.

Since pulmonary vasoconstriction is thought to be important in the genesis of HAPE, vasodilators have been tried as therapy. The calcium-channel blocker nifedipine has been shown to be beneficial. A slow-release oral dose of 20 mg has been used. Diuretics have been used but are losing favor among those who see many cases of HAPE. Similarly, morphine and digoxin have been tried, but evidence from controlled trials to support their use is lacking.

Patients who survive a bout of HAPE should be cautious with reascent since they are at greater risk for recurrence.

High-Altitude Cerebral Edema

Another serious form of AMS is *high-altitude cerebral edema* (HACE). Its incidence is lower than that of HAPE. In its early stages, HACE is indistinguishable from simple AMS; symptoms include headache, nausea, and vomiting. When ataxia occurs, HACE is present. Truncal ataxia, hallucinations, clouding of consciousness, and a variety of neurologic signs, including extensor plantar reflexes and papilledema, may follow. Signs of pulmonary edema are often present as well. The patient may become unconscious and die if not treated. As with HAPE, both lowlanders and highlanders as well as men and women of any age may be victims. The mechanism of HACE is presumably the same as that underlying simple AMS. In the few cases of HACE in which postmortem examination has been conducted, evidence of cerebral edema, increased intracranial pressure, and petechial hemorrhages has been noted. Venous thrombi have also been reported.

Treatment for HACE is similar to that for HAPE. The most important measure is descent to lower altitude. While awaiting evacuation, administration of supplemental oxygen and use of a pressure bag may help, but the beneficial effect may be slower to develop than in HAPE, especially in more severe cases. Dexamethasone, 4 mg intramuscularly in severe cases or orally in milder cases, helps reduce cerebral edema and should be used while awaiting patient evacuation. As in HAPE, descent often leads to rapid improvement in HACE. In some cases, however, recovery is delayed for several days. Permanent or long-lasting neurologic defects may be observed.

Chronic Mountain Sickness

Monge's disease, or *chronic mountain sickness* (CMS), is quite different from AMS. This disorder is more common in males and develops in middle and later life. CMS is found most often in the Andes, where it was first described. Patients have vague neuropsychological complaints, including headache, dizziness, somnolence, fatigue, difficulty in concentration, and loss of mental acuity. Irritability, depression, and hallucinations may be present. Dyspnea on exertion is not a common complaint, but poor exercise tolerance is frequent. Patients may also gain weight. A characteristic feature of CMS is that symptoms disappear with descent to sea level, only to reappear upon return to altitude.

Due to their high hemoglobin concentration and low oxygen saturation, patients with CMS are very cyanotic. In Andean natives—the population with the greatest incidence of CMS—additional signs may be florid. The conjunctivae are congested and the fingers may be clubbed. In Caucasians at lower altitudes—e.g., Leadville, Colorado (3100 m)—the appearance is less striking. These people look similar to patients with polycythemia secondary to hypoxic lung disease at sea level. Some with CMS have few clinical signs of disease.

Although hypoxemia is the crucial factor in the development of CMS, modulating factors include the altitude above sea level (higher the altitude, greater the incidence), lung function, hypoxic ventilatory response, age (increased incidence with age), gender (females appear protected, perhaps by respiratory-stimulating effects of female sex hormones and menstrual blood loss), and hyperventilation or apneas during sleep.

The red blood cell count, hemoglobin concentration, and packed red cell volume are increased; hemoglobin values as high as 28 g/dL and hematocrits as high as 83 percent have been recorded. White blood cell counts are not increased. Arterial blood-gas values, compared with those of healthy individuals as controls at the same altitude, show a higher Pa_{CO_2} and lower Pa_{O_2}. The lower Pa_{O_2} is partly due to hypoventilation, as indicated by the increased Pa_{CO_2}. In many cases, the alveolar-arterial oxygen gradient is increased. In some cases, standard pulmonary function tests show abnormalities consistent with obstructive or restrictive defects, suggesting that patients have coexisting chronic lung disease.

The very high hematocrit increases the blood viscosity. Systemic blood pressure may be moderately elevated, and the pulmonary artery pressure is significantly higher than in healthy high-altitude residents. Cardiac output is not significantly changed; calculated pulmonary vascular resistance is high. The hemodynamic alterations lead to right ventricular hypertrophy and associated electrocardiographic changes.

Symptoms and signs of CMS clear with descent to sea level. By lowering the hematocrit, phlebotomy improves many of the neuropsychological symptoms, pulmonary gas exchange, and exercise performance. Long-term use of the respiratory stimulant medroxyprogesterone has been used with some success, but side effects, including loss of libido, are a limitation.

The diagnosis of CMS is based on the hemoglobin. A value of 23 g/dL has been used, but for practical purposes a value of two standard deviations above the mean for the altitude can be considered the cutoff for "normal." An important diagnostic problem is how to address individuals with coexisting lung disease. Most clinicians are content to apply the diagnosis of CMS to any patient with a hemoglobin higher than 23 g/dL, with or without overt lung disease.

PREPARATION FOR ASCENT TO HIGH ALTITUDE

The effect of any condition that interferes with oxygen transport is exaggerated by altitude. As a general rule, individuals should be as fit as possible before leaving for a trip to high altitude. The ability to ascend to altitude safely depends more on degree of fitness than age, although rapid ascent and undue exertion place more strain on older individuals. Fitness is, however, no protection from acute mountain sickness.

Nasal polyps or a deviated nasal septum that interferes with breathing should be treated prior to ascent. Patients with perennial rhinitis and sinusitis should have adequate supplies of their usual medications.

Many asthmatic patients have less trouble at altitude than at home, possibly because of freedom from inhaled allergens. The importance of taking a sufficient supply of asthma medication and using it regularly must be stressed. No evidence exists that asthmatics are at greater risk of acute mountain sickness than nonasthmatics, although it must be presumed that poorly controlled patients may be at some risk. Acetazolamide helps to prevent acute mountain sickness in asthmatic patients.

With chronic obstructive pulmonary disease (COPD) and interstitial lung disease, ventilatory capacity may be reduced and oxygen uptake impaired. If patients are short of breath with exercise at sea level, they will certainly be worse at altitude. These patients should probably be advised to avoid trips to high altitude. In all but the mildest cases, patients with cystic fibrosis should be advised against ascending to high altitude.

BIBLIOGRAPHY

Gibbs JS: Pulmonary hemodynamics: Implications for high altitude pulmonary edema (HAPE). A review. *Adv Exp Med Biol* 474:81–91, 1999.

Hackett PH: High altitude cerebral edema and acute mountain sickness. A pathophysiological update. *Adv Exp Med Biol* 474:23–45, 1999.

Heath D, Williams D: *High Altitude Medicine and Pathology,* 4th ed. Oxford, UK, Oxford Medical Publishers, 1995.

Houston CS, Dickenson J: Cerebral form of high-altitude illness. *Lancet* 2:758–761, 1985.

Hurtado A: Chronic mountain sickness. *JAMA* 120:1278–1282, 1941.

Leon-Velarde F, Reeves JT: International consensus group on chronic mountain sickness. *Adv Exp Med Biol* 474:351–353, 1999.

Schoene RB: Lung disease at high altitude. *Adv Exp Med Biol* 474:47–56, 1999.

Winslow RM, Monge CC: *Hypoxia, Polycythermia, and Chronic Mountain Sickness.* Baltimore, Johns Hopkins University Press, 1987.

23 | Diving Injuries and Air Embolism*

Lisa M. Bellini and Michael A. Grippi

INTRODUCTION

Pulmonary barotrauma and decompression sickness represent two clinically important adverse effects of diving on the lung and other vital organs. The average fatality rate from these injuries is approximately 90 cases annually.

BAROTRAUMA

Descent while breath-holding results in compression of gas within a diver's lungs. The volume of the gas is inversely proportional to the increasing pressure. To prevent lung collapse to below residual volume and resultant tearing of lung parenchyma and blood vessels, the diver must breathe an oxygen-containing gas mixture at a pressure equal to that of the surrounding water. Conversely, during ascent to atmospheric pressure, the diver must continuously exhale in order to allow expanding compressed gas within the lungs to escape. The greatest danger of alveolar rupture occurs within the last 33 ft of ascent to the surface, as the relative gas volume doubles during that period. Theoretically, a critical threshold for alveolar rupture could be reached by ascent from as shallow a depth as 4 ft (1.2 m) if a full inspiration occurs at that depth. Fatal arterial gas embolism has been reported following ascent from a depth of 7 ft (2 m).

Clinical Manifestations

Following rupture of alveolar septa, expanding gas enters the interstitial spaces and dissects along perivascular sheaths to enter the mediastinum (mediastinal emphysema). Gas may also enter the pleural space, causing a pneumothorax. Mediastinal gas may further dissect into the pericardial sac, the retroperitoneal space, or the subcutaneous tissues of the neck. Gas entering the vasculature to form gas emboli constitutes another potentially life-threatening form of barotrauma.

Mediastinal emphysema is often associated with mild substernal aching or tightness, exacerbated by deep inspiration, coughing, or swallowing; the pain may radiate to the shoulders, neck, or back. Unless extensive, mediastinal emphysema is usually not associated with dyspnea, tachypnea, or other signs of respiratory distress. Subcutaneous emphysema causes swelling and crepitance in the neck and supraclavicular fossae. These signs may be associated with sore throat, dysphagia, or a change in voice. Subcutaneous gas can also be demonstrated radiographically. Recompression therapy is not needed for

---

*Edited from Chap. 64, "Diving Injuries and Air Embolism," by Clark JM. In: *Fishman's Pulmonary Diseases and Disorders,* 3d ed., edited by Fishman AP, Elias JA, Fishman JA, Grippi MA, Kaiser LR, Senior RM. New York, McGraw-Hill, 1998, pp 979–988. For fuller discussion of topics dealt with in this chapter, the reader is referred to the original text, as noted above.

uncomplicated cases of mediastinal or subcutaneous emphysema. If symptoms are bothersome, resolution of gas can be hastened by breathing 100% oxygen at normal atmospheric pressure. Gas volumes within the pericardial sac or retroperitoneal space are seldom large enough to be clinically significant.

Pneumothorax is an infrequent complication of pulmonary barotrauma. Recompression of an individual with a pneumothorax should be avoided in the absence of neurologic symptoms or other manifestations of arterial gas embolism. Conversion from a simple to a tension pneumothorax will occur if a tear in the visceral pleura remains open during descent, thereby allowing compressed gas to enter the pleural space. The tear then becomes effectively sealed, and upon decompression, the gas in the pleural space expands, compressing the lung and interfering with venous return. Severe dyspnea, cyanosis, and hypotension may occur, requiring immediate recompression and insertion of a chest tube before decompression is resumed.

If expanding extraalveolar gas enters the septal vessels and pulmonary veins, it will eventually traverse the left atrium and left ventricle before entering the systemic circulation as *gas emboli*. These emboli lodge in arteries and arterioles and create direct endothelial damage. Circulatory arrest and distal ischemia ensue. With the body in the head-up, erect position, most of the embolic air travels to the brain; coronary vessels are embolized more frequently with the body in a feet-up, inverted posture. Some affected divers develop apnea, unconsciousness, and cardiac arrest during ascent or immediately after surfacing from a dive; most die even when recompression is initiated within minutes. Some of these catastrophes may be caused by direct embolization of the coronary arteries. Most with diving-related arterial gas embolism present with stable hemodynamics, along with neurologic signs and symptoms that occur during ascent or within minutes after surfacing. Focal signs such as monoparesis or discrete sensory deficits or diffuse brain dysfunction as indicated by confusion, stupor, or coma may be observed. In response to prompt recompression, most patients undergo complete resolution of all neurologic deficits; some fail to respond completely or experience initial improvement followed by recurrence of the presenting signs and symptoms. The probability of an incomplete response or recurrence is increased as the time between onset of symptoms and initiation of definitive therapy is prolonged.

Iatrogenic arterial gas embolism is a serious and sometimes lethal complication of many procedures, including cardiovascular, pulmonary, neurologic, or head and neck surgery; use of intravenous catheters (especially central venous catheters); hemodialysis; arteriography; mechanical ventilation; abdominal or retroperitoneal gas insufflation; liver transplantation; and uterine catheterization or insufflation. Focal or diffuse manifestations of brain ischemia are observed, which are often misdiagnosed or recognized only after a delay of several hours. In many patients, hyperbaric oxygen therapy, if administered promptly, completely reverses all neurologic deficits.

DECOMPRESSION SICKNESS

Decompression sickness occurs when ambient pressure is reduced too rapidly to allow the inert gas dissolved in blood and body tissues to remain in physical solution. Usually seen in the diver who is inadequately decompressed from prolonged exposure to increased ambient pressures, the disorder can also occur in the aviator or astronaut with blood and body tissues that are saturated with inert gas at normal atmospheric pressure who is exposed to high altitude or space. Both extravascular and intravascular bubbles have been found (the latter more likely formed in veins than in arteries). Primary effects include obstruction of blood vessels and the mechanical disruption of tissue. Secondary effects include tissue reactions to intravascular or extravascular bubbles, such as activation of leukocytes, platelets, and the complement, coagulation, and kinin systems.

Clinical Manifestations

Principal clinical manifestations are musculoskeletal, neurologic, and pulmonary.

Musculoskeletal pain in one or more extremities is the most common symptom of decompression sickness in professional divers, while neurologic symptoms predominate in sport divers. The difference may reflect professional divers' reluctance to report neurologic symptoms because of potential occupational penalties and the tendency of many recreational divers to delay seeking medical assistance until neurologic symptoms occur.

Among divers who present with neurologic involvement, half are symptomatic within 10 min of surfacing; over 90 percent are symptomatic within 3 h. About 90 percent of divers who present with musculoskeletal pain only develop symptoms within 6 h after the dive. Onset of decompression sickness 36 h or more after the dive has been reported, but delays exceeding 24 h are extremely rare. Relatively long delays prior to symptom onset sometimes occur during flights in commercial aircraft that are not pressurized to 1.0 atm and may have cabin altitudes as high as 8000 ft. It is generally recommended that flying be delayed for at least 24 h after diving.

Clinical manifestations of neurologic decompression sickness usually reflect involvement of the spinal cord at the lower thoracic or upper lumbar levels. Paresthesias and sensory deficits may occur with or without associated weakness or paralysis. Transient or persistent abdominal pain may be present. Bladder or bowel dysfunction may occur alone or with associated signs. A form of decompression sickness that is characterized by vestibular involvement may present with the sudden onset of vertigo and severe impairment of balance. Associated symptoms often include nausea, vomiting, nystagmus, tinnitus, and sometimes hearing loss. Vestibular decompression sickness, as manifest by a slow or incomplete response to aggressive hyperbaric oxygen therapy, can be unusually difficult to treat.

Pulmonary decompression sickness (the "chokes") is manifest by substernal pain, cough, dyspnea, and malaise and occurs most frequently after short, deep dives or altitude decompressions. Symptoms occur within minutes of decompression but may be delayed for several hours. In some instances, the only finding is mild chest "tightness" that resolves spontaneously. Severe untreated cases may terminate in asphyxia, shock, and death. Pathogenesis, which is poorly understood, apparently involves pulmonary accumulation of embolic bubbles along with entrapped aggregates of platelets, fibrin, leukocytes, and erythrocytes. The occurrence of acute respiratory distress syndrome (ARDS) following accidental venous air embolism has been reported.

MANAGEMENT

Although little additional oxygen can be combined with hemoglobin at normal arterial P_{O_2}, the quantity of physically dissolved oxygen increases linearly with arterial P_{O_2} (about 2.4 mL O_2 per 100 mL blood per atmosphere of inspired P_{O_2}). Under hyperbaric conditions, the increment in arterial oxygen content is associated with a much larger elevation of the oxygen partial pressure gradient from capillary blood to metabolizing cell, thereby improving oxygen delivery.

Arterial gas embolism and decompression sickness have different etiologies and clinical presentations. However, similar therapeutic principles can be applied to both conditions: reduction in bubble size, acceleration of bubble resolution, and maintenance of tissue oxygenation. Initially, patients are compressed to 165 ft, effecting a reduction in bubble size to one-sixth of original volume; some of these smaller bubbles traverse capillaries and enter the venous circulation to be trapped in the lung. Administration of 50% oxygen throughout this phase provides hyperoxygenation at a level slightly greater than that afforded by breathing 100% oxygen at 60 ft. Oxygen is administered intermittently throughout the remainder of the therapy to accelerate bubble resolution and maintain tissue oxygenation while avoiding oxygen toxicity. Hyperbaric oxygen therapy of decompression sickness, which seldom involves cerebral gas embolism, is usually performed by compressing directly to 60 ft without prior pressurization to 165 ft.

ADDITIONAL USES OF HYPERBARIC OXYGEN

Hyperbaric oxygen therapy has been used in a variety of other disorders (Table 23-1). In clostridial myonecrosis (gas gangrene), high oxygen concentrations inhibit multiplication of the anaerobic organisms and prevent formation of lecithinase, which causes necrotizing myositis. Furthermore, the antibacterial actions of polymorphonuclear leukocytes, which are decreased under hypoxic conditions, are improved when oxygen tension is elevated.

High-dose radiation therapy in cancer treatment causes a delayed-injury response in nonmalignant irradiated tissues, apparently caused by progressive destruction of the microcirculation from obliterative endarteritis. The resultant radiation necrosis in bone and soft tissues, delayed or arrested

---

TABLE 23-1 Current Indications for Hyperbaric Oxygen Therapy Approved by the Hyperbaric Oxygen Committee of the Undersea and Hyperbaric Medical Society

---

Gas lesion diseases
  Decompression sickness
  Gas embolism
Infections
  Clostridial myonecrosis
  Necrotizing soft tissue infections
  Chronic refractory osteomyelitis
Vascular insufficiency states
  Radiation necrosis of bone or soft tissue
  Healing enhancement in problem wounds
  Compromised skin grafts or flaps
  Acute traumatic ischemias
  Thermal burns
Postischemic reperfusion injury
  Carbon monoxide poisoning

SOURCE: Clark JM: Hyperbaric oxygen therapy, in Crystal RG, West JB, Weibel ER, Barnes PJ (eds), *The Lung: Scientific Foundations,* 2nd ed. Philadelphia, Lippincott-Raven, 1997, pp 2667–2676.

healing in response to accidental or surgical trauma, fistula formation, and pathological fractures can be avoided or ameliorated by the adjunctive use of hyperbaric oxygen (which increases fibroblast activity and induces capillary angiogenesis in the irradiated tissues).

Nonhealing foot wounds in diabetic patients who have significant microvascular impairment with little or no large vessel disease often respond favorably to hyperbaric oxygen therapy. As a component in the comprehensive care of thermal burns, adjunctive hyperbaric oxygen therapy can significantly reduce morbidity and mortality, decrease the required number of surgical procedures, and reduce the length of hospitalization. Potential mechanisms for these beneficial effects include increased capillary angiogenesis and rate of epithelialization, edema reduction, decreased extravasation of fluid, and reduced incidence of infection.

In carbon monoxide poisoning, hyperbaric oxygenation reduces the half-time for carboxy-hemoglobin dissociation from about 90 min on 100% O_2 at 1.0 atm to about 23 min on O_2 at 3.0 atm. It may also oppose CO effects on the cytochrome chain. However, any therapeutic advantage is frequently lost due to the time required to transport a patient from the CO exposure site to a hyperbaric chamber. Nevertheless, patients with CO poisoning without loss of consciousness appear to have a decreased incidence of delayed neuropsychological sequelae when treated with hyperbaric oxygen compared to those treated with oxygen at 1.0 atm.

OXYGEN TOXICITY

During oxygen breathing at increased ambient pressures, the toxicity increases progressively in proportion to inspired P_{O_2}. Pulmonary manifestations of oxygen toxicity limit the duration of oxygen exposure at 1.0 to 2.0 atm. At oxygen pressures of 3.0 atm or higher, visual impairment and convulsions usually occur before development of prominent pulmonary intoxication. Although the toxic effects of oxygen are numerous, they can be avoided when hyperbaric oxygen therapy is used appropriately. Early stages of intoxication, even when associated with symptoms and detectable functional alterations, are fully reversible upon termination of exposure. The onset of toxic effects is delayed effectively by periodic interruption of oxygen exposure with scheduled "air breaks."

BIBLIOGRAPHY

Clark JM: Hyperbaric oxygen therapy, in Crystal RG, West JB, Weibel ER, Barnes PJ (eds), *The Lung: Scientific Foundations,* 2d ed. Philadelphia, Lippincott-Raven, 1997, pp 2667–2676.

Clark JM, Lambertsen, CJ: Pulmonary oxygen toxicity: A review. *Pharmacol Rev* 23:37–133, 1971.

Elliott DH, Harrison JAB, Barnard EEP: Clinical and radiological features of 88 cases of decompression barotrauma, in Shilling CW, Beckett MW (eds), *Underwater Physiology,* vol 6. Bethesda, MD, FASEB, 1978, pp 527–535.

Elliott DH, Moon RE: Manifestations of the decompression disorders, in Bennett PB, Elliott DH (eds): *The Physiology and Medicine of Diving,* 4th ed. Philadelphia, Saunders, 1993, pp 481–505.

Moon RE: Treatment of diving emergencies. *Crit Care Clin* 15:429–456, 1999.

Moon RE, de Lisle Dear G, Stolp BW: Treatment of decompression illness and iatrogenic gas embolism. *Respir Care Clin North Am* 5:93–135, 1999.

Thom SR: Hyperbaric oxygen therapy. *J Intens Care Med* 4:58–74, 1989.

24 | Thermal Lung Injury and Acute Smoke Inhalation*

Jack A. Elias

Smoke inhalation can trigger a wide variety of clinical manifestations that range from minor exacerbations of preexisting asthma or bronchitis following transient smoke exposure to tragic and lethal respiratory failure. The degree of pulmonary injury from acute smoke inhalation depends on the magnitude of the smoke and thermal exposure. The fire environment is also a major variable, since, in addition to heat and smoke, fires produce a variety of toxic gases and particulates.

THE FIRE AND FIRE ENVIRONMENT

Smoke is a suspension of visible particles and toxic gases. If significant quantities of hydrocarbon-containing materials are consumed, the smoke is black in the initial stages of the fire. White smoke can indicate the combustion of plastic polymers; yellow flame the combustion of cloth, wood, and paper; red flame the combination of flammable liquids and hydrocarbon by-products. Blue flame is produced by alcohol and natural gas. A large number of toxic gases and chemicals can be generated in the fire environment[1,2] (Table 24-1), including carbon monoxide, hydrogen chloride, isocyanates, cyanide, ammonia, oxides of nitrogen, acrolein, sulfur dioxide, hydrogen bromide and chlorine gases.[3] Since the materials that are burning differ from fire to fire, the toxic gases, fumes, and hazardous chemicals produced differ in each fire setting. These agents also differ in their water solubility. Highly water-soluble agents (e.g., ammonia, sulfur dioxide, hydrogen fluoride, and acrolein) have a propensity to injure proximal airways. Since they are quite noxious, the irritation they cause is usually noted by fire victims. In contrast, agents with low levels of water solubility (e.g., chlorine, phosgene, and nitrogen oxide) are more likely to cause insidious injury and thus delayed and severe respiratory damage.[4]

Fire consumes oxygen, placing fire victims into hypoxic environments. This is striking during the flashover phase of a fire (when a room bursts into flame), during which inspired oxygen concentrations can decrease to 10 to 15%.[5] Motor coordination is impaired when the ambient air oxygen concentration is approximately 17%. Faulty judgment and fatigue occur when the oxygen concentration is 10 to 14% and unconsciousness and death result when the oxygen concentration is 6 to 10%.

Carbon Monoxide

Carbon monoxide is the most dangerous gas produced at fires. It is odorless and colorless and competes with oxygen for binding sites on the hemoglobin

---

*Edited from Chap. 65, "Thermal Lung Injury and Acute Smoke Inhalation," by Loke JS. In: *Fishman's Pulmonary Diseases and Disorders,* 3d ed., edited by Fishman AP, Elias JA, Fishman JA, Grippi MA, Kaiser LR, Senior RM. New York, McGraw-Hill, 1998, pp 989–1002. For fuller discussion of topics dealt with in this chapter, the reader is referred to the original text, as noted above.

TABLE 24-1 Features of Fire and the Fire Environment

Smoke
Particulates
Organic acids
Aldehydes
Hydrocarbon material

Flame
Yellow color—due to combustion of cloth, wood, paper
Red color—due to combustion of flammable liquids and hydrocarbon by-products
Blue color—due to combustion of alcohol or natural gas

Heat
Gases/chemicals
Carbon monoxide
Cyanide
Hydrogen chloride
Chlorine
Phosgene
Ammonia
Isocyanates
Oxides of nitrogen
Hydrogen fluoride
Hydrogen bromide
Sulfur dioxide
Benzene

Decreased inspired oxygen concentration

molecule. As a result, it decreases tissue oxygen release, causing tissue hypoxia. Carbon monoxide poisoning manifests itself most frequently in the central nervous system (CNS) and, to a lesser extent, in the cardiovascular system. Dizziness, psychomotor impairment, behavioral abnormalities, and decreased vision can be seen. Headache, confusion, and collapse occur when the blood carboxyhemoglobin (COHb) level is 40 to 50%, and unconsciousness, convulsions, respiratory failure, and death can occur at levels greater than 60%. Decreased exercise tolerance, increased myocardial ischemia, and complex arrhythmias have been noted in patients with coronary artery disease with mild carbon monoxide poisoning. Chest pain and myocardial infarctions occur in patients with coronary disease and severe poisoning.[6] Carbon monoxide poisoning can also cause skin blisters, retinal hemorrhages, disseminated intravascular coagulation, myonecrosis, hyperglycemia, and diabetes insipidus.

Hydrogen Cyanide

Hydrogen cyanide is a colorless gas with the odor of bitter almonds, which, unfortunately, is difficult to detect at a fire scene. It interferes with cellular utilization of oxygen and inhibits cytochrome-c oxidase in mitochondria, causing anaerobic metabolism and lactic acidosis.[7] Poisoning initially stimulates respiration by causing hypoxia of the CNS. Later on it causes CNS depression. Flushing and tachycardia occur when the blood cyanide level is 0.5 to 1.0 mg/L. Patients with severe poisoning (blood levels $\geq$2.5 mg/L) may be obtunded and hypotensive, with slow, labored breathing and dilated pupils. Their faces and nail beds are often pink and their venous blood is bright red despite poor oxygen utilization. There may also be a severe anion gap metabolic lactic acidosis. Dyspnea and tachycardia are frequently noted. At times, pulmonary edema is seen, followed by bradycardia, apnea, coma, and death. Hydrogen cyanide and carbon monoxide interact to depress the CNS, preventing fire victims from escaping. The half-life of cyanide is 1 h. The cyanide antidote should be given if cyanide poisoning is suspected clinically.

Hydrogen Chloride

Combustion of the polyvinyl chloride in plastic polymers produces hydrogen chloride, which forms an aerosol of hydrochloric acid when combined with water. Hydrochloric acid is a mucosal irritant that can produce severe and even fatal alterations of the mucous membranes of the eyes, nose, and respiratory tract.

Aldehydes

The aldehydes—formaldehyde, acetaldehyde, and acrolein—are dermal and mucosal irritants that affect the skin, eyes, nose, and mucous membranes of the lung. They cause airways obstruction when present in modest quantities and can be associated with pulmonary edema and death at high concentrations.

THERMAL INHALATION LUNG INJURY

Although smoke and toxic gases are the leading causes of respiratory morbidity and mortality in fire victims, heat and flames can also cause thermal injury to the airways.[4,8] These lesions are usually limited to the upper airways because the trachea and upper airways are an efficient heat sink that protects the lower respiratory tract. There are, however, a number of settings in which burns of the subglottic airways or lung parenchyma should be suspected. They include overwhelming heat exposures, the inhalation of steam, aspiration of hot liquids, and burns caused by the inhalation of the ignited vehicle used with crack cocaine. Thermal injury occurs most commonly in victims who were exposed in an enclosed environment or were close to the flames or heat. These patients commonly note shortness of breath, hoarseness, wheezing, carbonaceous sputum, and/or burns of the face and oropharyngeal area.

PATHOPHYSIOLOGY OF ACUTE SMOKE INHALATION AND THERMAL INHALATION INJURY

Burn patients can manifest metabolic alterations, changes in the surface barrier of the skin, complex pathophysiologic alterations in respiratory structure and function, and, in some cases, a systemic dysfunction of a variety of visceral organs—including the lung, liver, and kidney—referred to as the systemic inflammatory response syndrome (SIRS). The metabolic alterations include a hypermetabolic and hypercatabolic state with fever; increased levels of plasma catecholamines, glucagon, cortisol, and growth hormone; increased oxygen consumption; and hyperglycemia. The increase in catecholamines leads to systemic vasoconstriction and an increase in systemic vascular resistance. In severe second- and third-degree burns, heightened evaporative heat loss, the third-spacing of bodily fluids, and—when the lesions are severe—hypothermia and/or hypotension can be seen.

Acute smoke inhalation and thermal injury have a number of important effects in the lung, including (1) impairment of mucociliary function; (2) hypersecretion of mucus; (3) tissue inflammation with tracheobronchitis, bronchitis, laryngitis, and/or pneumonitis; (4) epithelial sloughing; (5) surfactant inactivation; (6) increased vascular permeability with bronchorrhea and pulmonary edema; and (7) bronchoconstriction.[9] The injuries to the ciliated epithelium compromise particulate clearance and contribute to the high frequency of respiratory infection experienced by victims of smoke inhalation. The alterations in the permeability of the lower respiratory tract and surfactant inactivation lead to atelectasis, restrictive physiologic alterations, and, when severe, respiratory failure due to the adult respiratory distress syndrome (ARDS). Studies of tissues and investigations using bronchoalveolar lavage (BAL) have demonstrated a granulocyte and macrophage–predominant inflammatory response and the augmented release of cytokine mediators [such as tumor necrosis factor (TNF), interleukins-1, -6, and -8] and the activation of complement in these patients.

Enhanced bronchomotor tone, edema, hypersecretion of mucus, bronchorrhea, and mucosal sloughing can contribute to the bronchoconstriction and enhanced airway resistance seen in burn patients. The bronchospasm and bronchorrhea may be due to the direct effects of the smoke- or irritation-induced reflex responses. Bronchoconstrictive mediators, including histamine and thromboxane A_2, are also produced at these sites of injury. In the initial phases of acute smoke inhalation, the major sites of obstruction are the large airways. Subsequently large or small airway dysfunction can be present. Airway and alveolar injuries, carbon monoxide poisoning, and cyanide toxicity all contribute to the arterial hypoxemia in smoke and thermal inhalation injury victims.

SPECTRUM OF CLINICAL MANIFESTATIONS

The respiratory tract injuries and alterations noted in fire victims can be most easily thought of as those affecting the nervous system, upper airway, lower airways, and lung parenchyma. Syndromes associated with specific toxins must also be kept in mind. The neurologic manifestations include altered sensorium, obtundation, and coma, with associated alveolar hypoventilation and compromised protection of the upper airway. In the lung, airway injuries are more common than parenchymal injuries and upper airway lesions are more common than lower airway lesions. The types of injuries can be classified as

TABLE 24-2 Acute Respiratory Complications of Smoke Inhalation and Thermal Injury

Site/Type	Description
Neurologic	Altered sensorium, obtundation, coma
	Alveolar hypoventilation
	Compromised ability to protect upper airway
Toxic	Carbon monoxide intoxication
	Cyanide intoxication
Upper airway obstruction	Oropharyngeal and laryngeal edema, mucosal sloughing
Airway obstruction	Bronchitis
	Bronchospasm
	Airway inflammation/edema
	Atelectasis
Alveolar	Capillary membrane permeability alterations
	Pulmonary edema, ARDS[a]

[a]Adult respiratory distress syndrome.

TABLE 24-3 Risk Factors for Significant Smoke Inhalation or Thermal Injury

Exposure in closed spaces
Victim entrapment
Unconsciousness or other neurologic alterations
Facial or cervical burns
Respiratory signs or symptoms

those that are acute (occurring within the first 24 to 48 h of fire exposure) and those that occur in a subacute or chronic fashion.

Acute Manifestations

The major acute manifestations of smoke inhalation and thermal injury (Table 24-2) are upper airway obstruction due to pharyngeal edema, laryngeal edema, and, rarely, mucosal sloughing. Airway obstruction due to bronchitis and/or bronchospasm and pulmonary edema due to alterations in alveolar permeability or myocardial injury can also be seen. The risk factors for these manifestations are outlined in Table 24-3. The presence of facial burns, stridor, sore throat, painful swallowing, and carbonaceous sputum are of major concern.

Subacute/Chronic Manifestations

The subacute and chronic complications experienced by fire-exposed subjects may represent delayed manifestations of the initial injury, dysregulated healing, or complications of patient management (Table 24-4). Important manifestations of the initial injury include delayed-onset upper airway obstruction, delayed lower airway obstruction, and ARDS. The upper airway obstruction is caused most commonly by airway edema that occurs after aggressive fluid resuscitation and less commonly by mucosal sloughing 3 to 4 days after the original

TABLE 24-4 Subacute/Chronic Pulmonary Manifestations of Smoke Inhalation and Thermal Injury

Delayed manifestations of initial injury

Upper airway edema/mucosal sloughing
Pulmonary edema, ARDS[a]
Airway obstruction/bronchospasm
Bronchitis
Atelectasis

Manifestations of abnormal repair

Pulmonary fibrosis
Bronchiolitis obliterans
Bronchiectasis
Endobronchial polyposis
Hyperactivity of the airways, asthma

Complications of patient management

Pneumonia
Pulmonary embolus
Tracheal stenosis

[a]Adult respiratory distress syndrome.

injury. The lower airway obstruction can be the result of airway inflammation and edema, epithelial injury, and associated hyperreactivity of the airways.[9] Over time, an asthma-like syndrome can be seen. The ARDS can be due to irritant gas exposure, hypotension, superimposed sepsis, or diffuse pneumonia.

In the vast majority of cases, acute fire-induced injuries to the upper airway, tracheobronchial tree, and parenchyma heal with minimal sequelae. In a minority of cases, pulmonary fibrosis, bronchiolitis obliterans, bronchiectasis, coagulative necrosis of alveoli, and/or endobronchial polyposis are seen.

CLINICAL EVALUATION

Patients can present with trivial exposures and minimal injury or with complicated multiorgan dysfunction. Their clinical picture can be further complicated by traumatic injuries experienced at the fire scene and/or alcohol and illicit drug use that triggered the fire in the first place. Proper evaluation must shed light on the extent and severity of the patient's injury. The history should elicit details regarding the fire, the fire environment (see Table 24-1), and the patient's exposure. This includes the patient's location, duration of exposure, entrapment, state of consciousness, and the use or lack of use of protective clothing and breathing devices. The history should also define the patient's respiratory symptomatology. Dyspnea, cough, chest pain, the expectoration of carbonaceous sputum, an increase in nasal and oral secretions, headache, and dizziness are frequently noted. Hemoptysis is seen less frequently. Hoarseness, a change in voice quality, and dysphagia raise the possibility of severe upper airway injury and stridor; quiet or forced breathing suggests critical pharyngeal edema. Rales generally reflect severe lung injury; bronchospasm in a nonasthmatic subject suggests significant respiratory exposure; and facial burns are frequently associated with clinically significant respiratory damage (Table 24-4).

Depending on the patient's presentation and available resources, arterial blood-gas evaluations, carbon monoxide and cyanide determinations, chest radiographs, and pulmonary function testing (including serial flow-volume loop studies) may be required to provide information about the anatomy and severity of the injury. When clinically appropriate, alcohol levels and drug toxicology screens should be performed.

Chest X-ray

Most chest radiographs of fire victims are normal on initial presentation. When abnormalities are noted, a spectrum of alterations can be seen, including focal atelectasis, diffuse interstitial changes, and alveolar filling processes such as pulmonary edema.[10] Patients with smoke inhalation and thermal injury may manifest focal and patchy lung infiltrates as late as 24 to 48 h after smoke inhalation,[11] and diffuse alveolar infiltrates may be seen as late as 96 h after presentation. Thus, a normal chest radiograph immediately after exposure does not accurately predict a lack of inhalation injury.

Quantification of Toxic Gases

In all but patients with the most trivial of smoke exposures, COHb levels should be measured, since these levels cannot be inferred reliably from clinical signs or symptoms. In patients with arterial hypoxemia and a severe metabolic acidosis, significant carbon monoxide or cyanide poisoning should be suspected. Cyanide and thiocyanide levels should be measured when cyanide poisoning is suspected. Interpretation of arterial blood gases can be difficult in patients with an increase in COHb. In these patients, a normal Pa_{O_2} and a normal calculated oxygen saturation may be seen in the presence of a reduced measured arterial oxygen saturation and arterial oxygen content. Serial measurements of actual arterial oxygen saturation are especially useful in monitoring patients with significant carbon monoxide poisoning.

Anatomic Evaluation of the Airways

Unrecognized, untreated upper airway injury can lead to severe and sudden airway obstruction with catastrophic results. Unfortunately, clinical evaluations do not rule out significant upper airway injury with sufficient accuracy. Thus, the anatomic definition of upper (and at times lower) airway injury is frequently required. In patients with very mild smoke exposure and no other significant injury, simple oropharyngeal and nasal inspection may suffice. In all patients in whom serious injury is an issue, more extensive evaluation is required. This is most readily accomplished with laryngoscopy[4] or fiberoptic bronchoscopy.[8] The spectrum of findings ranges from mild erythema to the documentation of soot, carbonaceous materials, secretions, blisters, hemorrhage, ulcers, dynamic airway abnormalities (laryngospasm), and ischemia and edema of the hypopharyngeal, supraglottic, and glottic areas. In rare cases, large bronchial casts composed of sloughed necrotic mucosa, inflammatory exudate, and carbon particles are noted.[8] These casts may have to be removed with a rigid bronchoscope, since dislodgment may result in potentially life-threatening acute airway obstruction.

Physiologic Evaluation

The airways are the major site of injury in patients with smoke inhalation and thermal injury. Thus, obstructive ventilatory defects characterized by reduced expiratory volumes and flow rates and a reduced FEV_1/FVC ratio are the major findings in these patients. When pulmonary edema, atelectasis, pneumonia, or other major parenchymal abnormalities occur or large surface burns are present, restrictive ventilatory defects with decreased lung volumes can be superimposed.

Maximal inspiratory and expiratory flow-volume curves are used to evaluate upper airway lesions. Studies of these curves have demonstrated a number of characteristic flow-volume loop abnormalities. They include patterns compatible with variable extrathoracic obstruction (a predominant reduction in inspiratory flow rates or a plateau pattern in the inspiratory loop), fixed upper airway obstruction (reductions in expiratory and inspiratory flow rates), variable intrathoracic obstruction (reduction in expiratory flow rates), and sawtoothing of normally smooth curves, reflecting upper airway instability. Serial flow-volume curves are useful in the detection of delayed-onset upper airway obstruction and late-onset subglottic stenosis in fire victims.

TREATMENT

The treatment of fire injury victims must include the management of respiratory dysfunction and associated medical and traumatic problems. This treatment focuses on the maintenance of airway patency, ventilation, and oxygenation and on fluid replacement, nutritional supplementation, and burn wound management. Specific therapies directed against asphyxiant gas exposures (carbon monoxide/cyanide), bronchospasm, and infection may also be required. Empiric antibiotic therapy is not recommended.

Airway Patency and Ventilation

Altered neurologic function can cause fire victims to hypoventilate and diminish their ability to protect their airways. Patients may also experience upper airway obstruction, which can present as a medical emergency or arise insidiously over time. Patients with hypoventilation, poorly protected airways, severe hypoxemia, and/or carbon dioxide retention should be intubated and ventilated initially with 100% oxygen. A low threshold for intubation is also warranted for patients with established or evolving upper airway obstruction, stridor, respiratory distress, or facial burns and those with respiratory failure and coexisting chronic obstructive pulmonary disease (COPD). In patients with upper airway dysfunction that is not immediately life-threatening, the status of the upper airway can be assessed with serial flow-volume studies, laryngoscopy, or fiberoptic bronchoscopy. In addition, inhaled racemic epinephrine (1% solution) may be useful in decreasing upper airway edema.

Carbon Monoxide Toxicity

Carbon monoxide poisoning must be considered in all patients with smoke inhalation. The prognosis in carbon monoxide poisoning depends on the level of COHb, rapidity of therapeutic intervention, nature of the therapeutic intervention (100% O_2 alone versus hyperbaric hyperoxia), and spectrum of end-organ consequences experienced by the patient. When possible, all fire victims with significant exposure should be resuscitated with and transported on 100% oxygen. In hospitals in which hyperbaric oxygen therapy is available, it is the treatment of choice for severe carbon monoxide poisoning. By hastening the clearance of carbon monoxide, it decreases the acute toxic effects and may decrease the late onset neuropsychiatric manifestations caused by carbon monoxide.[12] The alternative treatment is the continued administration of 100% oxygen. This may require elective intubation and mechanical ventilation. These interventions should be undertaken in all patients with elevated COHb levels and evidence of end-organ toxicity or in those with COHb levels greater than 40% even without obvious symptoms. In comatose patients with severe arterial hypoxemia and metabolic acidosis, emergency endotracheal intubation and mechanical ventilation with 100% oxygen should be initiated before the results of the COHb measurement are available.

Cyanide Toxicity

In patients with cyanide poisoning, specific antidotes (Lilly Cyanide Antidote Kit) with inhaled amyl nitrite pearls, 10% sodium nitrite, and 25% sodium thiosulfate solutions are given.[13]

Bronchodilators

A variety of bronchodilators—including oral and intravenous theophylline, inhaled beta$_2$ sympathomimetics, and anticholinergic agents—have been administered to patients with smoke- or thermal injury–induced acute or chronic airway obstruction. In wheezing and burned patients with a history of COPD or asthma, these agents have well-documented efficacy. These therapies may also be useful in patients without preexisting obstructive lung disease.

Corticosteroids

Corticosteroid therapy is not indicated for fire victims with dermal burns and thermal inhalation injury.[8] Although controversial, corticosteroid therapy is also not routinely recommended in acute isolated smoke inhalation injuries. Corticosteroids are, however, useful in patients with underlying asthma, severe bronchospastic responses, smoke inhalation–induced bronchiolitis obliterans, or upper airway edema.

REFERENCES

1. Hartzell GE, Packham SC, Switzer WG: Toxic products from fires. *Am Ind Hyg Assoc J* 44:248–255, 1983.
2. Lowry WT, Juarez L, Petty CS, Roberts B: Studies of toxic gas production during actual structural fires in the Dallas area. *J Forens Sci* 30:59–72, 1985.
3. Lowry WT, Peterson J, Petty CS, Badgett J: Free radical production from controlled low-energy fires: Toxicity considerations. *J Forens Sci* 30:73–85, 1985.
4. Haponik EF: Clinical smoke inhalation injury: Pulmonary effects. *Occup Med* 8:431–468, 1993.
5. Crapo RO: Some inhalation injuries. *JAMA* 246:1694–1696, 1981.
6. Sheps DS, Herbst MC, Hinderliter AL, et al: Production of arrhythmias by elevated carboxyhemoglobin in patients with coronary artery disease. *Ann Intern Med* 113:343–351, 1990.
7. Graham DL, Lawson D, Theodore J, Robin ED: Acute cyanide poisoning complicated by lactic acidosis and pulmonary edema. *Arch Intern Med* 137:1051–1055, 1977.
8. Shirani KZ, Moylan JA, Pruitt BA Jr: Diagnosis and treatment of inhalation injury in burn patients, in Loke J (ed), *Pathophysiology and Treatment of Inhalation Injuries.* vol 34. New York, Marcel Dekker, 1988, pp 239–280.
9. Loke J, Matthay RA, Walker Smith GJ: The toxic environment and its medical implications with special emphasis on smoke inhalation, in Loke J (ed), *Lung Biology in Health and Disease: Pathophysiology and Treatment of Inhalation Injuries,* vol 34. New York, Marcel Dekker, 1988, pp 453–504.
10. Putman CE, Loke J, Matthay RA, Ravin CE: Radiographic manifestations of acute smoke inhalation. *Am J Roentgenol* 129:865–870, 1977.
11. Chiles C, Hedlund LW, Putman CE: Diagnostic imaging in inhalation lung injury, in Jacob L (ed), *Lung Biology in Health and Disease: Pathophysiology and Treatment of Inhalation Injuries,* vol 34. New York, Marcel Dekker, 1988, pp 187–206.
12. Thom SR, Taber RL, Mendiguren II, et al: Delayed neuropsychologic sequelae after carbon monoxide poisoning: Prevention by treatment with hyperbaric oxygen. *Ann Emerg Med* 25:474–480, 1995.
13. Hall AH, Rumack BH: Clinical toxicology of cyanide. *Ann Emerg Med* 15:1067–1074, 1986.

Part Four | **DRUG-INDUCED LUNG DISEASES**

25 | Drug-Induced Lung Disease due to Nonchemotherapeutic Agents*

Lynn T. Tanoue

CLINICAL SYNDROMES IN DRUG-INDUCED PULMONARY DISORDERS

The clinical presentations of patients with drug-induced lung diseases typically fall into a fairly small group of syndromes outlined in Table 25-1. None are drug-specific, however, since all are frequently caused by processes other than drug toxicity. Despite this lack of specificity, it is important to summarize these syndromes because drug toxicity must be carefully considered whenever these constellations of signs and symptoms are encountered. The diagnosis of drug-induced pulmonary toxicity rests on the exclusion of a variety of other pathologic conditions, including neoplasm, infection, pulmonary thromboembolism, and congestive heart failure. Drug toxicity can also be difficult to distinguish from progression of the underlying disease for which the patient was originally treated. Furthermore, agents that cause pulmonary toxicity are commonly used in multidrug regimens or in combination with toxic concentrations of oxygen or lung-damaging radiation.

Interstitial Lung Disease

Interstitial disorders are the most common and best-recognized form of pulmonary drug toxicity. These disorders fall into two general patterns. The first is a subacute to chronic form of interstitial disease that resembles idiopathic pulmonary fibrosis, designated *chronic alveolitis/fibrosis syndrome.* The second pattern, termed *hypersensitivity lung disease,* has a more acute presentation and is often associated with peripheral or tissue eosinophilia. In both syndromes, chest radiographs reveal interstitial or mixed interstitial-alveolar infiltrates. Pulmonary function studies show a restrictive ventilatory defect, with decreased diffusing capacity.

Acute Noncardiogenic Pulmonary Edema

A variety of drugs can cause alterations in pulmonary vascular permeability. In all cases, widespread bilateral alveolar or alveolar-interstitial infiltrates are noted. The severity and outcome of these cases are quite variable. Most often the pulmonary edema is rapidly reversible. In some patients, however, severe lung injury occurs, and the clinical course progresses to the point where the case fulfills criteria for adult respiratory distress syndrome (ARDS).

*Edited from Chap. 67, "Drug-Induced Lung Disease due to Nonchemotherapeutic Agents," by Zitnik RJ. In: *Fishman's Pulmonary Diseases and Disorders,* 3d ed., edited by Fishman AP, Elias JA, Fishman JA, Grippi MA, Kaiser LR, Senior RM. New York, McGraw-Hill,1998, pp 1017–1036. For fuller discussion of the topics dealt with in this chapter, the reader is referred to the original text, as noted above.

309

TABLE 25-1 Major Clinical Syndromes Associated with Pulmonary Drug Toxicity

Interstitial lung disease
  Chronic alveolitis/fibrosis
    Amiodarone
    Gold
    Nitrofurantoin
    Methotrexate
    Mexiletine
    Penicillamine
    Tocainide
  Hypersensitivity lung disease
    Beta-lactam and sulfa antibiotics
    Carbamazepine
    Diphenylhydantoin
    Gold
    Methotrexate
    Nitrofurantoin
    NSAIDs
    Penicillamine
Noncardiogenic pulmonary edema
  Amiodarone
  Aspirin and NSAID overdose
  Opiate and sedative/hypnotic agent overdose
  Tocolytic therapy
    Terbutaline
    Isoxuprine
    Ritodrine
Alveolar hypoventilation
  Aminoglycosides
  Polymyxins
  Opiates and sedative-hypnotic agents
Bronchospasm
  Adenosine and dipyridamole
  Aspirin and NSAIDs
  Beta-adrenoreceptor antagonists
  Sotalol
Drug-induced SLE
  Hydralazine
  Isoniazid
  Procainamide
  Quinidine
Bronchiolitis obliterans
  Gold
  Penicillamine
Alveolar hemorrhage
  Cocaine
  Penicillamine
Pulmonary infiltrates with eosinophilia
  Beta-lactam antibiotics
  Sulfa antibiotics
  Fluoroquinolones
  Tetracycline and derivatives
  Erythromycin and derivatives
  Nitrofurantoin
  Anti-TB medications (isoniazid, PAS, ethambutol)
  NSAIDs
Isolated cough
  ACE inhibitors

KEY: NSAID, nonsteroidal anti-inflammatory drug; SLE, systemic lupus erythematosus; PAS, para-aminosalicylic acid; ACE, angiotensin converting enzyme.

Alveolar Hypoventilation

Respiratory depression is a well-known side effect of many centrally acting therapeutic agents, particularly sedatives and opiates. Alveolar hypoventilation can also be caused by drugs that impede neuromuscular transmission or diaphragmatic muscle function. Usually, the effects of these agents are clinically insignificant. However, these drugs can cause hypercarbic respiratory failure in normal persons and can be particularly problematic in patients with underlying pulmonary or neuromuscular disease.

Bronchospasm

Drug-induced wheezing and bronchospasm can occur as a direct pharmacologic effect of the drug, as in the case of beta-adrenergic receptor–blocking agents. Other mechanisms can also be operative, as exemplified by aspirin-induced bronchospasm in asthmatics and the bronchospasm that can be caused by adenosine and protamine.

Drug-Induced Systemic Lupus Erythematosus

A disorder that exhibits many of the features of idiopathic systemic lupus erythematosus can be caused by a wide variety of drugs. Patients with this toxicity frequently experience arthralgias, arthritis, fever, and/or pericarditis. The most common pulmonary manifestations are pleurisy and pleural effusions, which are sometimes associated with parenchymal infiltrates.

Bronchiolitis Obliterans

A number of drugs have been reported to produce bronchiolitis obliterans without pathologic features of organizing pneumonia. Patients with this reaction manifest severe, progressive, fixed obstructive ventilatory defects. Drug-induced bronchiolitis obliterans often occurs during treatment for rheumatoid arthritis, a disease that itself can be complicated by bronchiolitis obliterans as a systemic manifestation. Thus, the distinction between collagen vascular and drug-associated bronchiolitis is sometimes difficult.

Alveolar Hemorrhage

Both acute and recurrent alveolar hemorrhage has been reported to occur in response to some drugs. Patients present with hemoptysis and, on chest radiographs, with alveolar infiltrates. In some cases, the alveolar hemorrhage occurs as part of a pulmonary-renal syndrome that is very similar to Goodpasture's disease.

Pulmonary Infiltrates with Eosinophilia

Eosinophilic infiltration is a well-documented manifestation of a variety of pulmonary drug toxicities. These eosinophilic syndromes can resemble acute or chronic eosinophilic pneumonia. Most commonly, a Loeffler's syndrome is noted, with dyspnea, cough, blood eosinophilia, and transient pulmonary infiltrates.

DRUGS USED TO TREAT CARDIOVASCULAR DISORDERS

The evaluation and treatment of drug-induced pulmonary dysfunction in patients with cardiovascular disease present a number of specific challenges. First, fever and hypoxemia associated with drug toxicity are very poorly tolerated in patients with coronary artery disease and left ventricular dysfunction. Many of the deaths ascribed to drug toxicity in this population are caused by secondary cardiac ischemia or arrhythmias rather than primary respiratory failure. Second, the worsening cough and pulmonary infiltrates seen in these patients can be misattributed to congestive heart failure rather than drug toxicity. Similarly, since obstructive airway disease and cardiovascular disease often coexist, drug-induced bronchospastic exacerbations may not be appropriately recognized. Third, patients with congestive heart failure, angina, or claudication often become sedentary. This can mask pulmonary symptoms; it also increases the risk of developing venous thrombosis and pulmonary embolism, which can further confound diagnosis. Finally, even after drug toxicity is determined to be the cause of the patient's respiratory problem, immediate withdrawal of the causative agent is not always possible. This is especially true with medications used in the treatment of life-threatening disorders such as ventricular arrhythmias. Often a second antiarrhythmic medication must be started before the offending drug is withdrawn.

Adenosine

Adverse effects to adenosine occur in 30 to 60 percent of patients. The most common pulmonary side effect is acute dyspnea during the infusion, which occurs in 5 to 10 percent of patients. Much less commonly, adenosine infusions can precipitate acute bronchospasm in patients with a history of asthma or chronic obstructive pulmonary disease (COPD). Inhaled adenosine causes a dose-dependent drop in FEV_1 in asthmatics. Adenosine-induced bronchospasm typically responds quickly to intravenous aminophylline. In this setting, aminophylline probably acts as a direct adenosine receptor antagonist. A history of COPD or asthma is not an absolute contraindication to the use of intravenous adenosine; however, it should be administered with extreme caution.

Amiodarone

Amiodarone can cause ophthalmic, cutaneous, hepatic, and thyroid toxicities. Pulmonary toxicity occurs with an incidence of approximately 5 percent, with case fatality rates in the range of 10 to 20 percent.[1] Elimination half-life is long, approximately 30 to 60 days. Thus, even after amiodarone is discontinued, measurable serum levels and a continued antiarrhythmic effect can persist for weeks to months. Amiodarone pulmonary toxicity has several clinical manifestations. The most common is a subacute or chronic alveolitis/fibrosis syndrome. The chronic form occurs in about two-thirds of patients and is characterized by the insidious onset of cough, dyspnea, and weight loss. These symptoms are associated with bilateral interstitial infiltrates and a restrictive ventilatory defect. The more acute form presents with fever, chest pain, and alveolar or mixed alveolar-interstitial infiltrates on the chest radiograph. This presentation occurs in the remaining one-third of patients and may mimic an infectious process. A peripheral leukocytosis and elevated erythrocyte sedimentation rate are features of both presentations. Peripheral eosinophilia is uncommon. Several less common radiographic manifestations have also been described, including isolated pleural effusions, pleural-based or parenchymal mass lesions, solitary nodules, and lobar or segmental infiltrates.

Amiodarone use has been associated with episodes of acute noncardiogenic pulmonary edema typically occurring after pulmonary angiography and several types of cardiac and noncardiac surgery. There is frequently a 24- to 48-h lag between the onset of ARDS and the procedure. At present, it is unclear whether the reports represent a true clinical syndrome or the coincidental occurrence of ARDS after surgery in severely ill patients. However, a recent retrospective series noted a much higher incidence of ARDS in patients on amiodarone than in very similar control groups undergoing identical cardiac surgical procedures. In addition, a prospective, randomized study of amiodarone in the treatment of postpneumonectomy atrial arrhythmias was prematurely terminated because of a substantial increase in the incidence of ARDS among patients treated with the drug postoperatively.[2]

The risk factors for amiodarone pulmonary toxicity are not well defined. While a daily amiodarone dose of less than 400 mg appears to be associated with a lower risk, pulmonary toxicity can occur at lower doses, and higher doses are often well tolerated. Total cumulative dose and serum levels of amiodarone and its metabolite, desethylamiodarone, do not reliably presage toxicity. Whether baseline pulmonary function or radiographic abnormalities portend subsequent toxicity is also very controversial. Finally, several prospective studies of patients treated with amiodarone have shown that a decrement in diffusing capacity is a poor indicator of toxicity. Thus, a decreased diffusing capacity is not by itself reason to discontinue the drug in the absence of clinical signs and symptoms or a worsening chest radiograph. Computed tomography (CT) during episodes of toxicity may show both localized and diffuse areas of very high CT attenuation. These regions correspond pathologically to areas of focal accumulation of macrophage inclusion bodies filled with phospholipids ("foamy macrophages"). These cells contain large amounts of amiodarone, which is 37 percent iodine by weight, accounting for the high CT attenuation. Foamy macrophages are seen in the lungs of all patients taking amiodarone. The presence of foamy macrophages or high-attenuation areas on CT are not diagnostic of toxicity. Scanning with gallium 67 is positive in most cases of toxicity and typically reverts to negative after clinical resolution. Gallium scanning cannot differentiate amiodarone toxicity from other causes of lung inflammation or congestive heart failure. However, a positive scan along with other supportive clinical evidence may be helpful in excluding other diagnostic entities.

The diagnosis of amiodarone toxicity can often be made clinically. Bronchoscopy may sometimes be necessary to exclude infection. Once the diagnosis of amiodarone toxicity is established, the drug should be discontinued and a new antiarrhythmic agent begun. Although there are no controlled studies to support the use of corticosteroids, they are frequently initiated. Responses are well documented, and a recrudescence of symptoms can occur during corticosteroid tapering. Courses of treatment longer than 6 months in duration are sometimes necessary.

Angiotensin-Converting Enzyme Inhibitors

The major adverse pulmonary effect of angiotensin-converting enzyme (ACE) inhibitors is a chronic nonproductive cough. Nonproductive cough occurs to an approximately equal extent with all ACE inhibitors. The incidence of cough varies widely, but in most studies it has been noted to occur in 5 to 15 percent of patients. The cough typically begins after 1 to 2 months, but it can occur up to 1 year after the initiation of treatment. After drug withdrawal, improvement typically occurs within 1 to 2 weeks. Patients without a history of asthma who develop a cough are slightly more sensitive to methacholine challenge than those who do not. However, ACE inhibitors do not reproducibly diminish airflow, and known asthmatics are not at increased risk for developing ACE inhibitor–induced cough. The cough recurs with rechallenge, and patients who develop a cough in response to one ACE inhibitor also cough when "cross-challenged" with other ACE inhibitors. In most cases, the occurrence of ACE inhibitor–induced cough is an indication to withdraw the drug. In patients for whom no alternative therapy is practical, one can "treat through" the cough. In these cases, the cough will occasionally resolve spontaneously despite continued exposure. ACE inhibitor–induced cough can also be treated with inhaled cromolyn sodium.

ACE inhibitors also cause angioneurotic edema, a rare side effect characterized by transient edema of the skin, lips, tongue, and upper airway. The episodes are usually self-limited and respond to epinephrine and steroid treatment. When severe, they can cause airway obstruction resulting in respiratory failure and death.

Beta-Adrenergic Receptor Blockers

Beta-adrenergic receptor blockers commonly precipitate bronchospastic exacerbations in patients with asthma or worsen chronic airway obstruction in patients with COPD. They have been implicated as a very rare cause of pulmonary fibrosis and drug-induced systemic lupus erythematosus (SLE). In asthma and COPD patients with chronic stable hypertension, nonselective beta blockers such as propranolol cause substantial dose-dependent decreases in FEV_1. They often precipitate episodes of clinically significant bronchospasm. While $beta_1$-receptor-selective blockers, drugs with intrinsic sympathomimetic effect, and the mixed alpha/beta antagonist labetolol are better tolerated, these agents are still capable of causing severe bronchospasm and should be used carefully if at all. In contrast, esmolol, an intravenous beta blocker often used in intensive care units (ICUs), is well tolerated in most asthma and COPD patients because its "ultrashort" half-life allows treatment to be immediately withdrawn in case of a significant reaction. It is currently the agent of choice when beta blockade is required in patients with a history of asthma or COPD.

Dipyridamole

In the evaluation of patients with suspected coronary artery disease who are not capable of performing standard treadmill exercise tests, cardiac nuclear imaging with thallium 201 is often carried out after infusion of intravenous dipyridamole. Dipyridamole induces tachycardia and acts as a coronary vasodilator, thereby simulating the effect of exercise on the heart. Its mechanism of action is to prevent cellular reuptake of adenosine. This increases adenosine concentrations within the lung and other organs in a manner similar to a direct adenosine infusion. Dipyridamole-thallium stress testing precipitates acute bronchospasm in about 0.15 percent of patients. Most of these patients have a history of asthma. As is the case in bronchospastic exacerbations caused directly by adenosine, dipyridamole-induced bronchospasm responds to intravenous aminophylline. While a history of obstructive airway disease is not an absolute contraindication to dipyridamole stress testing, the study should be performed with extreme caution.

Hydralazine

Hydralazine causes drug-induced SLE in approximately 5 percent of patients when used in antihypertensive doses and in up to 15 percent of patients when used at higher vasodilator doses. As with procainamide, "slow" acetylation status may be a risk factor for the occurrence of drug toxicity. The clinical presentation is similar to that seen in SLE caused by other drugs, although renal disease occurs more commonly. Pleural disease is the most common pulmonary manifestation. Parenchymal infiltrates occur in only 3 percent of patients.

Mexiletine

Mexiletine can rarely cause an alveolitis/fibrosis syndrome with reticulonodular infiltrates on chest radiograph. The prognosis is usually good, though respiratory failure has been reported. Mexiletine also interferes with theophylline metabolism and can cause serum theophylline concentrations to rise to toxic levels. Theophylline levels should be adjusted during the initiation of mexiletine therapy.

Procainamide

Procainamide is commonly implicated as a cause of drug-induced SLE. Remarkably, between 50 and 90 percent of patients taking procainamide for more than 2 months develop serum antinuclear antibodies (ANAs). Some 10 to 20 percent of these ANA-positive patients will develop symptomatic drug-induced SLE, and 40 to 80 percent of them will have pulmonary manifestations. As in other types of drug-induced SLE, the ANA is positive in a homogeneous or diffuse pattern, and antihistone antibodies are present. Anti–double-stranded DNA antibodies are absent. Procainamide, hydralazine, and isoniazid all have the capacity to cause drug-induced SLE, and all are metabolized by acetylation. The rate at which acetylation occurs is genetically determined, and there is evidence that "slow acetylators" develop ANAs and clinical SLE more rapidly than "fast acetylators."

Clinically, arthralgias and fever are common presenting symptoms, while renal and central nervous system (CNS) impairments are rare. Pleural effusions and pleuritic chest pain are the most common pulmonary findings. Parenchymal pulmonary infiltrates are seen in up to 40 percent of patients with pulmonary impairment. In contrast, parenchymal infiltrates are unusual in SLE caused by drugs other than procainamide. Other pulmonary manifestations of idiopathic SLE—such as chronic interstitial fibrosis, alveolar hemorrhage, and progressive atelectasis—are quite rare in drug-induced SLE.

Procainamide therapy does not need to be discontinued in patients who develop an isolated positive ANA. The development of rheumatologic symptoms should, however, prompt drug withdrawal. The response after discontinuation of the drug is rapid, and symptoms frequently resolve within 2 to 3 weeks. When corticosteroids are added, the improvement is even more rapid, sometimes occurring within days. Despite rapid clinical resolution, the ANA can remain positive for months to several years after drug withdrawal. Once the drug is withdrawn, persistent or relapsing rheumatologic symptoms do not occur.

Protamine

Protamine neutralizes heparin and is frequently given intravenously to reverse anticoagulation during cardiac catheterization and cardiopulmonary bypass.

Transient, mild pulmonary hypertension and systemic hypotension occur during approximately 5 percent of infusions. Systemic anaphylaxis, urticaria, angioedema, and bronchospasm occur in 0.2 percent of patients, usually within 1 h of infusion. In rare cases, protamine causes a severe delayed reaction, with progressive and refractory pulmonary hypertension, cor pulmonale, and systemic hypotension. This syndrome carries a 30 percent mortality rate.

Several purported risk factors for protamine toxicity have been described. Insulin-dependent diabetics often develop antiprotamine antibodies as a result of exposure to the protamine present in NPH insulin preparations. Similarly, since protamine is prepared from the testicular tissue of fish, patients with fish allergies and those who have undergone vasectomy may develop immunologic cross reactivity to the agent. While no large retrospective study has confirmed that these patients are at increased risk, protamine should be used with caution in such cases. Treatment of protamine toxicity is supportive, including H_1 and H_2 histamine receptor blockers, fluid resuscitation, and inotropic agents.

Quinidine

Quinidine causes pulmonary toxicity only rarely. It has most commonly been implicated as a cause of drug-induced SLE. The most common pulmonary manifestations are pleuritis and pleural effusions. Drug withdrawal and corticosteroid treatment usually result in prompt improvement.

Sotalol

Sotalol causes respiratory symptoms in up to 2 percent of patients. Most commonly, it exacerbates bronchospasm in patients with preexisting obstructive airway disease. Because of this problem, the use of sotalol should be avoided in patients with asthma and COPD.

Tocainide

Tocainide causes adverse nonpulmonary effects in up to 50 percent of patients. Pulmonary toxicity occurs far less frequently. The most common respiratory side effect is an interstitial pneumonitis/fibrosis syndrome, which occurs in approximately 0.3 percent of patients. Radiographically, interstitial infiltrates are seen, while high-resolution CT scanning shows interstitial septal thickening and patchy airspace disease. In most reported cases, the prognosis after drug withdrawal and treatment with steroids is good, although deaths have been reported.

TOPICAL OPHTHALMIC AGENTS

In addition to their use in cardiovascular diseases, beta blockers are used in the treatment of open-angle glaucoma. When applied to the corneal surface, they can be absorbed across mucosal membranes. This can result in substantial serum levels and systemic beta blockade. Significant decreases in FEV_1 occur even in asymptomatic patients. Severe bronchospastic exacerbations with sporadic fatalities have been reported in asthmatics using these agents. Most of these exacerbations have been attributed to the nonselective agent timolol. The cardioselective agent betaxolol is purported to be better tolerated. The presence of asthma is a strong relative contraindication to the use of either drug.

TOCOLYTIC AGENTS

Beta-adrenergic agonists suppress uterine contractions and are used therapeutically to delay premature delivery. Terbutaline is the most commonly employed agent. Acute pulmonary edema occurs during tocolytic therapy with
an incidence of up to 4.4 percent. Most commonly, the pulmonary edema occurs approximately 2 days into the course of therapy but can be delayed for
up to 12 h after the tocolytic agent is discontinued. The pathogenesis of this
disorder is not known.

Clinically, patients with tocolytic-induced pulmonary edema present with
acute-onset chest pain, dyspnea, cough, and the expectoration of frothy pink
sputum. These symptoms are associated with tachypnea, tachycardia, hypoxemia, and bilateral alveolar infiltrates on the chest radiograph. The differential
diagnosis of acute respiratory compromise in the peripartum period includes
pulmonary thromboembolism, gastric aspiration, amniotic fluid embolism, peripartum cardiomyopathy, and Valsalva-induced pneumomediastinum. In most
cases the syndrome is mild, with only 3 to 10 percent of patients requiring
intubation and mechanical ventilation. The pulmonary edema usually resolves
quickly with diuresis and discontinuation of the tocolytic.

ANTIBIOTICS

Antibiotic-Induced Hypersensitivity Lung Disease

Hypersensitivity reactions caused by antibiotics typically present as -
pulmonary infiltrates with eosinophilia, or "PIE" syndromes. These reactions
are idiosyncratic and fairly uncommon. In some cases, toxic responses are
severe or prolonged and resemble either acute or chronic eosinophilic pneumonia.[3] The most common antibiotic-associated PIE syndrome is simple pulmonary eosinophilia, or *Loeffler's syndrome.* Beta-lactam and sulfa antibiotics (including antimalarials) are most often associated with this type of
reaction. Fluoroquinolones, tetracycline and erythromycin derivatives, and nitrofurantoin can also cause this syndrome. The antituberculosis drugs isoniazid, para-aminosalicylic acid, and ethambutol have also been implicated.
Loeffler's syndrome is characterized by dyspnea, cough, fever, and peripheral
blood eosinophilia with transient, patchy pulmonary infiltrates. It is usually
acute in onset and from 1 to 4 weeks in duration. In general, patients are not
very ill and respiratory symptoms are mild. Spontaneous resolution often
occurs when the drug is withdrawn, and the response to a brief course of
corticosteroids is usually excellent.

Nitrofurantoin Pulmonary Toxicity

Nitrofurantoin has been used in the treatment of both acute urinary tract infections and asymptomatic bacteriuria. Although ARDS and alveolar hemorrhage have been reported, most cases of nitrofurantoin toxicity fall into one
of two distinct categories: an acute form, which typically fits the pattern of
hypersensitivity lung disease, and a chronic alveolitis/fibrosis syndrome.[4]

Acute Nitrofurantoin Toxicity

The onset of acute nitrofurantoin toxicity occurs less than 1 month after the
first dose in 86 percent of cases and recurs with rechallenge. The acute
syndrome is characterized by fever, dyspnea, cough, chest pain, and a maculopapular rash. An elevated erythrocyte sedimentation rate is common, and

peripheral blood eosinophilia occurs in 83 percent. Radiographically, mixed interstitial and alveolar infiltrates are seen. Pleural effusions are observed in approximately 16 percent of patients. The chest radiograph may be normal in up to 18 percent of patients. Pulmonary function testing reveals a restrictive ventilatory defect with decreased diffusing capacity. Although infectious causes must be ruled out, in most cases the diagnosis can be made clinically. Drug withdrawal alone usually results in rapid improvement. Corticosteroid treatment is sometimes necessary. In general, the prognosis is good, although some patients develop respiratory failure and ARDS. Most patients will experience either full normalization or at least improvement in the chest radiograph and pulmonary function parameters with alleviation of symptoms. The mortality in acute nitrofurantoin pulmonary toxicity is 0.5 percent.

Chronic Nitrofurantoin Toxicity

Chronic nitrofurantoin toxicity usually occurs in elderly patients undergoing chronic oral suppression therapy for bacteriuria. As in the acute form, cyanosis, dyspnea, and cough are seen. However, fever and rash are less common as presenting symptoms, while fatigue, weight loss, and other constitutional symptoms are often observed. Peripheral blood eosinophilia occurs but is less common than in the acute form. Low-level positive titers of ANAs and rheumatoid factor and elevated serum gamma globulins have also been noted. The chest radiograph usually shows bilateral, predominantly interstitial infiltrates. Pleural effusions are uncommon. In most cases a clinical diagnosis can be made, although BAL and occasionally lung biopsy may be necessary. The prognosis is substantially worse than that for patients with acute toxicity. Most patients (73 percent) either fail to improve at all or show significant residual chest radiograph or pulmonary function testing abnormalities. The overall mortality in patients with chronic nitrofurantoin toxicity is approximately 8 percent.

Isoniazid-Induced Systemic Lupus Erythematosus

While a large number of patients taking isoniazid will develop ANAs, most patients will not progress to clinically significant SLE. SLE is caused less frequently by isoniazid than by hydralazine or procainamide. The typical clinical presentation of isoniazid-induced SLE includes fever, anemia, rash, arthralgias, and arthritis. Pleuritis and pericarditis with associated pleural and pericardial effusions are the most common chest findings. Renal, CNS, and parenchymal pulmonary impairments are unusual. In patients on isoniazid, a tuberculous effusion may be difficult to differentiate from isoniazid-induced SLE with pleuritis. The presence of a positive ANA and antihistone antibodies is helpful diagnostically. Thoracentesis and even pleural biopsy may be necessary for TB to be adequately excluded. Withdrawal of isoniazid results in the rapid resolution of symptoms. Improvement can be hastened by corticosteroids.

Antibiotic-Induced Alveolar Hypoventilation

Antibiotics can induce alveolar hypoventilation and precipitate acute hypercarbic respiratory failure by either causing or potentiating neuromuscular blockade.[5] This form of toxicity occurs in four major clinical scenarios: First, patients can have postoperative and postanesthetic respiratory dysfunction. This is often manifest as an unexplained inability to be extubated postoperatively, an enhancement of the normal effects of neuromuscular blocking agents given during anesthesia, or delayed-onset postoperative respiratory depression in patients who have already recovered from the effects of anesthesia (the "recurarization phenomenon"). Second, patients with underlying, previously unrecognized myasthenia gravis can have their myasthenia "unmasked" by neuromuscular blockade due to antibiotics. Third, patients with known myasthenia gravis can have an acute "myasthenic crisis" precipitated by antibiotics. Finally, acute weakness and respiratory failure can, in rare instances, occur as part of a "myasthenia-like syndrome" in normal patients.

Aminoglycosides are the class of antibiotics that most commonly cause neuromuscular blockade. Respiratory failure has been reported after intraperitoneal lavage with aminoglycosides during laparotomy and can also occur after intravenous or intramuscular administration. Toxicity is potentiated by conditions, such as renal insufficiency, that decrease aminoglycoside clearance, and by concomitant treatment with other neuromuscular blocking agents. Polymyxins, tetracyclines, ampicillin, and fluoroquinolones have rarely been reported to cause this type of toxicity. Treatment is mainly supportive but should include specific treatment for myasthenia if appropriate.

ANTICONVULSANTS

Diphenylhydantoin

Diphenylhydantoin (DPH) causes several forms of pulmonary toxicity. A generalized *dilantin hypersensitivity syndrome* has been described that is often accompanied by substantial life-threatening pulmonary disease. This syndrome is rare and there are no established risk factors for its occurrence. Symptoms typically occur within 1 month after beginning the drug. They are heralded by the onset of fever, lymphadenopathy, skin rash, and peripheral eosinophilia. A multiorgan-system reaction often ensues, including hepatitis, acute renal failure, myositis, aseptic meningitis, and granulocytopenia. Pulmonary manifestations include the acute onset of wheezing, dyspnea, and interstitial or mixed alveolar-interstitial radiographic infiltrates. They can be of sufficient severity to cause either hypoxemic or hypercarbic respiratory failure. A subgroup of patients with DPH hypersensitivity reactions develop a systemic vasculitis affecting the skin and visceral organs, including the lung. A spectrum of pathologic features have been noted in these patients, including lesions consistent with polyarteritis nodosum and hypersensitivity vasculitis. Although a rapid response to drug withdrawal and steroids is typical in cases of DPH hypersensitivity, the clinical course may continue to worsen for many days before improvement is seen. Fatalities are common, especially in cases that manifest the systemic vasculitis.

Based on isolated case reports, DPH has also been associated with an interstitial lung disease resembling lymphocytic interstitial pneumonitis. Patients with this presentation have interstitial chest radiographic abnormalities without fever or peripheral eosinophilia. DPH may also cause a "pseudolymphoma" syndrome, which mimics malignant lymphoma clinically and pathologically. DPH-induced pseudolymphoma can occur as an isolated entity but more often presents at the same time as a systemic DPH hypersensitivity reaction. Patients manifest fever, skin rash, diffuse peripheral lymphadenopathy, hepatosplenomegaly, and, in many cases, radiographic evidence of hilar and mediastinal lymphadenopathy. DPH-induced pseudolymphoma recurs with rechallenge; anecdotally, it responds well to drug withdrawal and steroid treatment.

Carbamazepine

Carbamazepine causes an acute hypersensitivity syndrome similar to that induced by DPH. Fever, peripheral eosinophilia, exfoliative dermatitis, hepatitis, and generalized lymphadenopathy occur in association with interstitial pulmonary infiltrates. The syndrome recurs with rechallenge and cross challenge with other agents, including both diphenylhydantoin and phenobarbital.

NONSTEROIDAL ANTI-INFLAMMATORY AGENTS

Aspirin

Aspirin-Induced Asthma

Aspirin sensitivity occurs in approximately 5 percent of a general population of asthmatics. In asthmatics who have nasal polyposis and chronic sinusitis, or "Sampter's triad," the incidence of aspirin and other NSAIDs sensitivity approaches 30 percent.[6] Episodes of asthma exacerbation induced by aspirin usually occur 30 min to 2 h after ingestion. In addition to bronchospasm, profuse rhinorrhea, facial flushing, angioedema, and gastrointestinal symptoms can be observed. The diagnosis is made from a careful exposure history. Unfortunately, a history of aspirin use may be difficult to elicit because many over-the-counter aspirin-containing medications are not clearly labeled. Occasionally, a controlled diagnostic aspirin challenge is required to establish the diagnosis.

In aspirin-sensitive asthmatics, symptoms of nasal polyposis are managed with inhaled corticosteroids, and episodes of acute sinusitis are treated with antibiotics. Surgical excision of the polyps may also be necessary to obtain symptomatic control. The most important aspect of management is aspirin avoidance. For patients with rheumatologic disorders or other conditions that necessitate the use of aspirin or NSAIDs, symptoms can sometimes be managed with the 5-lipoxygenase inhibitor zileuton. In addition, choline magnesium trisalicylate and salicylsalicylic acid are much weaker inhibitors of cyclooxygenase and are safe in all but the most sensitive patients.

Salicylate-Induced Pulmonary Edema

Aspirin can induce pulmonary edema. Several reports of adult patients with salicylate toxicity have established that pulmonary edema complicates approximately 10 to 15 percent of severe salicylate overdoses. Such overdoses may be purposeful during suicide attempts, but older patients on chronic salicylate therapy may overdose inadvertently.

Salicylate-induced pulmonary edema is usually apparent on presentation, but it can be delayed by up to 24 h. In addition to dyspnea and tachypnea, mental status alterations are very common. A simple respiratory alkalosis or a mixed anion gap metabolic acidosis and respiratory alkalosis are seen in almost all patients. Significant proteinuria with an otherwise unremarkable urinary sediment is another common feature. Although there is no clear relationship between the serum salicylate level and the development of pulmonary edema, this complication is unusual in patients with levels below 40 mg/dL. The chest radiographs of these patients show bilateral perihilar alveolar infiltrates, usually without pleural effusion or cardiomegaly. Left ventricular filling pressures and systolic function are normal.

Treatment includes supportive measures. Alkaline diuresis decreases the free salicylate level by increasing its albumin binding, and also increases renal salicylate excretion. In young and otherwise healthy patients, with prompt recognition of the overdose, mortality is 1 to 2 percent or less. Conversely, older patients with numerous medical problems in whom the diagnosis is delayed suffer death rates as high as 25 percent.

Other NSAIDs

Like salicylates, other NSAIDs can induce noncardiogenic pulmonary edema after overdose. They can also exacerbate bronchospasm in aspirin-sensitive asthmatics. NSAIDs can also cause a PIE syndrome and virtually all currently available NSAIDs can cause acute pulmonary hypersensitivity reactions.[7] This rare form of toxicity is idiosyncratic, and there are no clear risk factors or predisposing conditions for its occurrence. NSAID-induced PIE syndromes can recur with controlled or inadvertent rechallenge as well as cross challenge with a second NSAID.

The onset of NSAID toxicity is variable, occurring in some cases after less than 1 week and in others up to 3 years after first exposure to the drug. Patients with this syndrome experience cough, dyspnea, fever, chest pain, and rash. These symptoms are accompanied by peripheral blood and bronchoalveolar lavage (BAL) eosinophilia and an elevated erythrocyte sedimentation rate. Bilateral interstitial infiltrates are the most common radiographic manifestation. Patchy alveolar infiltrates, dense peripheral infiltrates with central sparing ("radiographic-negative pulmonary edema"), pleural effusions, and hilar adenopathy are noted less frequently. Gallium-67 lung scans are typically positive during the acute illness and become negative after clinical resolution. It is interesting that the scan becomes positive once again with PIE syndrome recurrence after NSAID rechallenge.

The symptoms and radiographic abnormalities of these patients resolve rapidly after discontinuation of the NSAID. Treatment with corticosteroid is usually not needed. In rare cases, a severe reaction including acute respiratory distress syndrome and multiorgan system failure may ensue.

Methotrexate

Pulmonary toxicity due to methotrexate was initially found only after high-dose regimens given during cancer chemotherapy. As the drug came into wider use for the treatment of rheumatoid arthritis, it became clear that toxicity also occurred during low-dose oral therapy in an outpatient setting. Pulmonary toxicity has been reported to complicate the treatment of asthma, psoriasis, primary biliary cirrhosis, and most other disorders for which methotrexate has been used. Methotrexate pulmonary toxicity occurs in 1 to 5 percent of patients with rheumatoid arthritis and as many as 14 percent of patients treated for primary biliary cirrhosis.[8] A number of factors have been proposed to increase risk for the development of pulmonary toxicity, including higher daily and cumulative doses, renal insufficiency, concomitant high-dose NSAID therapy, and preexisting lung disease. None of these risk factors have been definitively established.

The typical clinical presentation of methotrexate pulmonary toxicity is subacute, occurring 1 to 5 months into therapy. Fever, cough, dyspnea, and inspiratory rales are noted. They are accompanied by hypoxemia and a peripheral leukocytosis. Peripheral eosinophilia is seen in one-third to one-half of the patients experiencing this complication. Radiographically, a bilateral interstitial or mixed interstitial-alveolar pattern occurs, in some cases accompanied by a pleural effusion or hilar adenopathy. Pulmonary function studies reveal a restrictive ventilatory defect with decreased diffusing capacity.

Patients taking low-dose methotrexate are at increased risk for opportunistic infections. It is interesting to note that there is an especially high frequency of infectious complications in rheumatoid arthritis patients taking methotrexate compared to rheumatoid patients on other immunosuppressive regimens. *Pneumocystis carinii* pneumonia is the most common complication. Disseminated histoplasmosis, herpes zoster, and a variety of other infections can occur. Exclusion of opportunistic pathogens is especially important in the differential diagnosis of methotrexate pneumonitis.

The treatment of methotrexate pneumonitis includes withdrawal of the drug and supportive care. Corticosteroids may also be useful and are generally initiated after infection has been excluded. However, there are no clear guidelines for the optimal dose or duration of therapy. Although fatalities can occur, the outcome is generally favorable.

Gold

Gold-induced pulmonary toxicity has been reported during the treatment of rheumatoid arthritis, asthma, osteoarthritis, and pemphigus. Gold typically causes an interstitial pneumonitis. A few cases of bronchiolitis obliterans have also been noted. However, the association between bronchiolitis obliterans and gold use is much more tenuous than that with penicillamine therapy. Clinically, gold toxicity usually occurs after 2 to 4 months of therapy. Patients with this toxicity present with dyspnea, cough, fever, skin rash, and peripheral eosinophilia. Radiographically, the most common pattern is a diffuse interstitial infiltrate. The mainstays of treatment of gold toxicity include drug withdrawal and corticosteroids. Improvement without steroid treatment is rare. Since relapse is sometimes observed after rapid steroid withdrawal, a treatment duration of at least 1 to 3 months is recommended.

Penicillamine

Penicillamine has been documented to cause a wide variety of systemic toxicities, including membranous glomerulonephritis, a myasthenia gravis–like syndrome, and drug-induced systemic lupus erythematosus. The pulmonary manifestations of penicillamine toxicity include interstitial lung disease, bronchiolitis obliterans, and alveolar hemorrhage occurring as part of a pulmonary-renal syndrome.[7]

Interstitial lung disease has been reported only in patients being treated for rheumatoid arthritis. Patients usually have nonspecific respiratory complaints. They also manifest a restrictive ventilatory defect with decreased diffusing capacity and chest radiographs with diffuse interstitial infiltrates. In the subgroup of patients with hypersensitivity reactions, elevated serum IgE levels and peripheral eosinophilia are observed. This form of toxicity is characterized by a favorable response to corticosteroids, a lack of residual pulmonary function derangements, and a low mortality.

Penicillamine-induced bronchiolitis obliterans is rare. There are no clearly defined risk factors that contribute to the frequency of this toxic response. Patients note the subacute onset of cough, wheeze, and dyspnea. On auscultation, severe expiratory wheezes and a high-pitched "midinspiratory squeak" are often appreciated. Chest radiographs reveal increased lung volumes in the absence of pulmonary infiltrates. PFTs show an obstructive ventilatory defect, markedly increased lung volumes due to air trapping, and a normal diffusing capacity when corrected for alveolar volume. Drug withdrawal and supportive therapy are the mainstays of treatment for penicillamine-induced bronchiolitis obliterans. Corticosteroids, azathioprine, and cyclophosphamide have also been used, but whether any of these agents have a substantial impact on outcome is unclear. Unfortunately, the prognosis of this form of penicillamine toxicity is poor. Approximately 50 percent of reported cases have had a fatal outcome, and in patients who survive, severe residual obstructive impairment is common.

Penicillamine can also cause a pulmonary-renal syndrome with features similar to those of Goodpasture's syndrome. This complication is rare with fewer than a dozen cases reported. Patients experience the rapid onset of cough, dyspnea, hemoptysis, and hematuria associated with acute renal failure and severe hypoxemia. Progressive respiratory failure requiring mechanical ventilatory support is common. Chest radiographs show diffuse alveolar infiltrates without cardiomegaly or pleural effusions. Circulating anti–glomerular basement membrane (GBM) antibodies have been reported only rarely. Serum antinuclear antibodies are often present at high titer, but anti–double-stranded DNA antibodies are negative and complement levels are normal. In contrast to the linear anti-GBM immunofluorescence seen in idiopathic Goodpasture's syndrome, complement and immunoglobulin deposits with a "lumpy" appearance are noted in glomerular regions. BAL in these patients reveals red blood cells and hemosiderin-laden macrophages. Open lung biopsies show alveolar hemorrhage in the absence of linear anti-GBM staining or pulmonary vasculitis.

The prognosis of this complication of penicillamine therapy is poor, with a mortality of about 50 percent and a high incidence of progression to chronic renal insufficiency and dialysis. In patients who recover, a residual restrictive ventilatory defect with decreased diffusing capacity is common. Drug withdrawal and high-dose steroids are always employed in treatment. Cyclophosphamide or azathioprine have been used as adjunctive immunosuppressive agents, though there are no controlled trials that demonstrate their efficacy.

COMPLICATIONS OF ILLICIT DRUG USE

The use of illicit drugs can result in a variety of pulmonary complications (Table 25-2). These include the ability of sedative and hypnotic agents to diminish respiratory drive, resulting in alveolar hypoventilation and, when severe, hypercarbic respiratory failure. Patients are at high risk for gastric aspiration and aspiration pneumonia. In addition, intravenous injections can cause right heart endocarditis and other endovascular infections, which may result in septic pulmonary emboli and pulmonary infarction. Since the incidence of HIV infection is high in this population, HIV-associated opportunistic pulmonary infections are a concern. Finally, intravenous drug abusers are at high risk for community-acquired pneumonia as well as both drug-sensitive and multidrug-resistant tuberculosis.

TABLE 25-2 Complications of Illicit Drug Use

Alveolar hypoventilation, hypercarbic respiratory failure
Gastric aspiration, aspiration pneumonia
Endocarditis, intravascular infections, septic emboli
HIV-associated infections
Tuberculosis
Complications of central cannulation
  Pneumothorax
  Intravascular infections
  Soft tissue infections
  Arterial aneurysm and/or dissection
Foreign-body granulomatosis
Opiate-induced pulmonary edema
Cocaine "crack" lung
  Bronchospasm
  Pneumothorax, pneumomediastinum, pneumopericardium
  Airway burns
  Noncardiac pulmonary edema
  Pulmonary infiltrates with eosinophilia
  Acute alveolar hemorrhage syndrome

Complications of Central Venous Cannulation

Intravenous drug users who have destroyed the peripheral vessels of their extremities will often attempt to obtain vascular access by using their internal jugular and subclavian veins. They will attempt to cannulate these vessels themselves or with the help of others, who are paid to perform the injections. These attempts can be complicated by symptomatic pneumothoraces, sometimes requiring chest tube drainage. The incidence of pleural space infection is surprisingly low in these patients. In contrast, soft tissue and endovascular infections occur quite commonly. In addition, aneurysms and dissections following inadvertent arterial cannulation are well documented.

Foreign-Body Granulomatosis

Foreign-body granulomatosis results from the injection of insoluble material during intravenous drug abuse. It can be caused by particulate contaminants used to "cut" street heroin or by the injection of crushed tablets that contain filler substances such as talc and methylcellulose. The injected material lodges in pulmonary arterioles and initiates a thrombogenic as well as granulomatous inflammatory response, causing chronic pulmonary vascular and parenchymal destruction.

Foreign-body granulomatosis can result in relentlessly progressive dyspnea. During the early phase, chest radiographs show nodular interstitial infiltrates. Over several years, these nodules can coalesce to form large infiltrates resembling the progressive massive fibrosis syndrome that sometimes complicates inhalational silicosis. These large fibrotic masses are surrounded by cystic and bullous spaces, which can rupture, producing pneumothoraces. The early phase is characterized by a mild obstructive ventilatory defect. As the disorder progresses, the bullous and cystic changes are accompanied by worsening airflow obstruction, air trapping, and a markedly decreased diffusing capacity. Eventually, pulmonary hypertension, parenchymal destruction, and extreme scarring may ultimately result in respiratory failure and cor pulmonale. Corticosteroids have little effect on the poor outcome seen in most cases of foreign-body granulomatosis.

Opiate-Induced Pulmonary Edema

Acute noncardiogenic pulmonary edema is a common complication of serious heroin overdoses. Pulmonary edema has been seen following inadvertent and intentional overdoses with a wide variety of oral and intravenous narcotics in addition to heroin. Opiate antagonists such as naloxone are also capable of causing pulmonary edema, often paradoxically when they are used during the treatment of an overdose or intoxication. In addition, pulmonary edema occurs after overdoses with nonopiate sedative and hypnotic agents such as ethchlorvynol and chlordiazepoxide. Pulmonary edema is usually apparent on presentation, but it can occur up to 24 h after the initial episode of intoxication. Patients experience dyspnea and appear cyanotic. These symptoms are accompanied by a typical perihilar alveolar infiltrate on the chest radiograph. In some cases, a depressed sensorium caused by the CNS effects of the opiate may mask the dyspnea. In addition, the clinical picture can be clouded by the presence of fever, especially when gastric aspiration has occurred. In some cases, opiate-induced pulmonary edema progresses to ARDS. Such patients have a more protracted course, with a longer duration of mechanical ventilation. However, if ARDS, pneumonia, or other complications of intravenous drug abuse do not supervene, the pulmonary edema usually resolves with supportive care over 48 to 72 h.

Pulmonary Complications of Cocaine Use

Cocaine hydrochloride can be injected intravenously. The pulmonary toxicities of intravenous cocaine are similar to those of intravenous opiates. Freebase cocaine smoking causes a distinct spectrum of pulmonary disorders often referred to as "crack lung."[9] Complaints of cough, chest pain, dyspnea, hemoptysis, wheezing and expectoration of soot are typical among cocaine smokers. Other common sequelae are thermal burns of the upper airway and trachea and pneumothorax, pneumomediastinum, or pneumopericardium caused by strong Valsalva maneuvers during the act of smoking. Crack smoking is also associated with acute pulmonary edema, pulmonary infiltrates with eosinophilia, and acute alveolar hemorrhage. Cocaine-induced pulmonary edema is usually noncardiogenic and often culminates in hypoxemic respiratory failure. A cardiogenic component to the edema may also be present owing to cocaine-induced myocardial infarction or severe systemic hypertension. In most uncomplicated cases, the infiltrates and hypoxemia resolve within 24 to 48 h.

An acute pulmonary hemorrhage syndrome with chest pain, hemoptysis, and fleeting interstitial or alveolar infiltrates is also commonly noted in cocaine abusers. The clinical presentation ranges in severity from recurrent low-grade hemoptysis, resulting in iron deficiency anemia, to massive hemoptysis and fatal asphyxiation. Pathologic evidence of pulmonary hemorrhage is found coincidentally at autopsy in up to 70 percent of free-base cocaine smokers regardless of the direct cause of death. Some patients with cocaine-induced pulmonary hemorrhage develop severe disease with fatal respiratory failure. In most cases, however, the outcome is favorable, with radiographic and clinical resolution in 2 to 5 days.

REFERENCES

1. Dusman RE, Stanton MS, Miles WM, et al: Clinical features of amiodarone-induced pulmonary toxicity. *Circulation* 82:51–59, 1990.
2. Van Mieghem W, Coolen L, Malysse I, et al: Amiodarone and the development of ARDS after lung surgery. *Chest* 105:1642–1645, 1994.
3. Allen JN, Davis WB: Eosinophilic lung diseases. *Am J Respir Crit Care Med* 150:1423–1438, 1994.
4. Holmberg L, Boman G: Pulmonary reactions to nitrofurantoin. *Eur J Respir Dis* 62:180–189, 1981.
5. Argov Z, Mastaglia FL: Disorders of neuromuscular transmission caused by drugs. *N Engl J Med* 301:409–413, 1979.
6. Fischer AR, Israel E: Identifying and treating aspirin-induced asthma. *J Respir Dis* 16:304–317, 1995.
7. Zitnik RJ, Cooper JAD: Pulmonary disease due to antirheumatic agents. *Clin Chest Med* 11:139–150, 1990.
8. Barrera P, Laan RFJM, van Riel PLCM, et al: Methotrexate-related pulmonary complications in rheumatoid arthritis. *Ann Rheum Dis* 53:434–439, 1994.
9. Kissner DG, Dwayne LW, Selias JE, Flint A: Crack lung: Pulmonary disease caused by cocaine abuse. *Am Rev Respir Dis* 136:1250–1252, 1987.

26 | Pulmonary Toxicity Associated with Chemotherapeutic Agents*

Lynn T. Tanoue

The diagnosis of lung disease caused by chemotherapeutic agents poses a particular challenge to the clinician. An estimated 5 to 10 percent of patients undergoing chemotherapy ultimately develop therapy-related pulmonary disease.[1] Diagnosis of pulmonary toxicity in the oncologic patient population is made more complicated by several factors. First, treatment may be given in multidrug regimens or in combination with other modalities, such as radiation therapy or bone marrow transplantation. Assigning pulmonary toxicity to a single drug within such a regimen is often impossible. Moreover, the combined toxicity of two or more drugs or a single drug with radiation therapy may exceed the individual toxicities of those drugs. Second, patients undergoing chemotherapy are often immunosuppressed and therefore susceptible to opportunistic infections, which may be mimicked by drug toxicity. Infection is still the most common pulmonary complication in the immunocompromised host, with the lung the most common site of serious infection. A relative minority (5 to 30 percent) of pulmonary complications in the immunocompromised host are actually due to drug toxicity.[1] Third, cancers themselves may mimic lung disease. This is particularly true when there is lymphangitic tumor spread or metastasis to the parenchyma or pleura. Fourth, pulmonary toxicity due to a single chemotherapeutic agent may present with several different syndromes that vary clinically, radiographically, and temporally. Toxicity due to some chemotherapeutic agents may appear months to years after the treatment. Last, toxicity from some drugs appears to be related to cumulative dosage levels. However, adverse reactions may occur even with a low cumulative dose, when clinical suspicion for toxicity is low.

Recognizing these diagnostic challenges, awareness of potential iatrogenic complications related to drug therapy is essential. The major pulmonary toxicities associated with chemotherapeutic agents are reviewed below.

CYTOTOXIC ANTIBIOTICS

Bleomycin

Bleomycin is a cytotoxic antibiotic. The drug is concentrated in skin and lung. Limitation of its use usually hinges on its potential for pulmonary toxicity. The overall incidence of bleomycin-induced lung injury varies from 3 to 40 percent.[2] The clinical presentation of bleomycin toxicity is usually

*Edited from Chap. 66, "Pulmonary Toxicity Associated with Chemotherapeutic Agents," Tanoue LT. In: *Fishman's Pulmonary Diseases and Disorders,* 3d ed., edited by Fishman AP, Elias JA, Fishman JA, Grippi MA, Kaiser LR, Senior RM. New York, McGraw-Hill,1998, pp 1003–1016. For fuller discussion of topics dealt with in this chapter, the reader is referred to the original text, as noted above.

subacute and insidious, occurring within a few weeks to 6 months after treatment. A more fulminant presentation with acute respiratory failure does occur but is less common. Patients generally present with dyspnea, nonproductive cough, and low-grade fever. Substernal or pleuritic chest pain occurs but is infrequent. Up to 20 percent of patients are asymptomatic. Chest radiographs usually show bilateral reticular or fine nodular infiltrates with a basilar predominance, often beginning at the costophrenic angles. Various radiographic patterns—including alveolar infiltrates, lobar consolidation, asymmetric lung involvement, and even lung nodules—have been described. Computed tomographic scanning appears to be more sensitive in the evaluation of radiographic abnormalities and may be useful in patients who have spirometric or clinical evidence of toxicity but negative chest radiographs.

Risk factors for the development of bleomycin-induced pulmonary toxicity include the following: (1) *Total dose*. Toxicity appears to correlate with higher cumulative dosages, the risk escalating significantly when total doses exceed 400 U. However, pulmonary injury has been observed after administration of as little as 20 U. (2) *Oxygen*. Oxygen is clearly a synergistic toxin in patients with prior bleomycin therapy. (3) *Radiation*. Thoracic irradiation before, during, or after bleomycin administration has been associated with an increase in toxicity. This injury may extend beyond the original port of irradiation. This "radiation recall" effect may last for years after bleomycin therapy. (4) *Renal function*. Abnormal renal function is a risk factor for pulmonary toxicity. Bleomycin is excreted by the kidneys. Drug half-life increases when creatinine clearance decreases below 35 mL/min. (5) *Age*. Older persons, especially those over 70, appear to be more susceptible to toxicity. (6) *Concurrent use of other cytotoxic agents*. The possibility has been raised that concurrent use of other chemotherapeutic agents can confer synergistic toxicity. Drugs implicated have included doxorubicin, cyclophosphamide, vincristine, and methotrexate. However, this synergistic effect has not been consistently reproducible.

Bleomycin has also caused an acute syndrome of dyspnea, cough, and rash immediately after administration of the drug. Lung biopsy in these cases has shown eosinophilic infiltration and changes consistent with a hypersensitivity response. Rechallenge with drug has not consistently caused recurrence of the syndrome, suggesting that this syndrome is not a true immune reaction. Bleomycin toxicity may also present with acute chest pain concurrent with bleomycin infusion in approximately 3 percent of patients.

The overall mortality due to drug toxicity in patients receiving bleomycin is 1 to 2 percent.[1,3] In patients who develop pulmonary toxicity, mortality varies from 10 to 83 percent.[2,3] In patients with mild toxicity, stopping the drug may suffice to reverse the abnormalities. However, corticosteroids are generally recommended for patients with clinically significant bleomycin-induced toxicity. Doses of corticosteroids are usually in the range of 60 to 100 mg of prednisone per day; tapering is done slowly, according to the clinical stability of the patient. When improvement does occur, it generally does so within weeks. Complete resolution may take up to 2 years. Some patients will be left with residual radiographic or physiologic abnormalities.

Mitomycin

Mitomycin is an alkylating cytotoxic antibiotic. The incidence of pulmonary toxicity due to mitomycin is variably reported as between 3 and 39 percent.

This variation may be due in part to two factors. First, the drug is rarely given alone, and toxicity seems dependent to some extent on concurrent administration of other agents or therapies. Although agreement about synergistic toxicity is not universal, pulmonary toxicity may be potentiated when mitomycin is used in conjunction with bleomycin, vinca alkaloids, cisplatin, 5-fluorouracil, cyclophosphamide, and doxorubicin. Therapeutic thoracic irradiation and oxygen may also be cotoxins. Second, mitomycin-induced lung injury presents with at least three clinically distinct syndromes: an interstitial pneumonitis with fibrosis, an acute lung syndrome with bronchospasm, and a hemolytic-uremic syndrome.

The most common form of mitomycin-induced lung toxicity is a chronic pneumonitis with pulmonary fibrosis similar to that seen with bleomycin. Toxicity is believed to be potentiated by oxygen supplementation and therapeutic radiation. Toxicity does not appear to be dose related. Pulmonary toxicity usually occurs after 2 to 12 months of therapy but may occur after a single dose.[2] Clinically, patients present with a subacute syndrome of cough and progressive dyspnea, often with fatigue and sometimes with pleuritic chest pain. Fever is less common. Chest radiographs usually show bilateral interstitial infiltrates, occasionally with alveolar or fine nodular patterns. Histologically, biopsy specimens show mononuclear cell infiltration, alveolar lining cell hypertrophy, collagen deposition, and alveolar septal thickening. Type II pneumocyte enlargement and lymphocytic or eosinophilic infiltration have also been seen. Patients develop a clinical picture of interstitial pneumonitis and fibrosis. This syndrome generally responds to discontinuation of drug and institution of corticosteroids.

The second syndrome of mitomycin-induced pulmonary toxicity is seen in patients who have also received vinca alkaloids. While drugs of the latter category confer little risk of pulmonary toxicity when used as single agents, vinblastine and vindesine given along with mitomycin or after its administration have been reported to precipitate a syndrome of acute pulmonary toxicity. Clinically, patients experience onset of dyspnea or bronchospasm within hours after administration of a vinca alkaloid. Pulmonary symptoms may be associated with hypoxia and bilateral interstitial infiltrates on the chest radiograph. In a series of 126 patients, 6 percent developed this syndrome.[4] A smaller number may develop respiratory failure and noncardiogenic pulmonary edema. While the acute dyspnea syndrome usually subsides with supportive care, withdrawal of drug, and administration of corticosteroids, long-term impairment of clinical and physiologic parameters may persist. Rechallenge with a vinca alkaloid causes recurrence of symptoms in most patients.

The third syndrome associated with mitomycin toxicity is a hemolytic uremic syndrome, which consists of microangiopathic-hemolytic anemia, thrombocytopenia, and renal failure. Approximately half of these patients develop noncardiogenic pulmonary edema. Pulmonary alveolar hemorrhage is another manifestation of mitomycin toxicity. The mechanism of toxicity appears related to pulmonary vascular endothelial injury. The prognosis for patients with this syndrome is poor. In a series of 39 patients, overall mortality was 72 percent.[5] In patients who also developed pulmonary edema, mortality increased to 95 percent. A variety of therapies have been tried in attempts to reverse this toxicity, including the administration of corticosteroids, plasmapheresis, heparin, and cytotoxic agents. None have had clear benefit.

Dactinomycin

Dactinomycin is an antitumor antibiotic that can occasionally be associated with pulmonary toxicity, usually presenting as an interstitial pneumonitis with pulmonary fibrosis. Like bleomycin and mitomycin, dactinomycin may exacerbate radiation-induced injury. This radiosensitizing effect may be long-standing.

ALKYLATING AGENTS

Busulfan

Busulfan is used in the treatment of chronic myeloproliferative disorders. Because of the nature of these hematologic malignancies, patients may require therapy for months to years. Cumulative dosage is therefore of concern, although a threshold dose for toxicity has not been evident. Busulfan is usually well tolerated. Histologically, up to 46 percent of patients treated with busulfan may have evidence of pulmonary fibrosis; most have no clinical symptoms.

Symptoms of busulfan lung injury usually present insidiously, often weeks to even years after initiation of therapy. Symptoms include cough, fever, fatigue, weight loss, and progressive dyspnea. Chest radiographs usually show bilateral interstitial infiltrates with basilar predominance. Pathologic findings are consistent with other cytotoxic drug–induced pulmonary injury syndromes, with an interstitial pneumonitis, type II pneumocyte hyperplasia, dysplasia, and desquamation into alveolar spaces. Fibroblast proliferation, collagen deposition, and fibrosis are usually evident. Scattered cases of pulmonary ossification and pulmonary alveolar proteinosis have also been reported.

When clinically evident busulfan-induced pulmonary toxicity does occur, prognosis for recovery is poor. The overall mortality is estimated at 50 to 80 percent.[6] Corticosteroids have anecdotally been reported to be of benefit.

Cyclophosphamide

Cyclophosphamide is widely used in the treatment of a variety of malignancies as well as in the treatment of nonneoplastic inflammatory disorders. The incidence of pulmonary toxicity is reported to be less than 1 percent. Clinically, the onset of cyclophosphamide-induced pulmonary toxicity is usually insidious, with symptoms of cough and progressive dyspnea, often accompanied by fever. The timing of the onset of pulmonary toxicity is exceedingly variable, occurring 2 weeks to 13 years after initiation of treatment. However, most patients develop symptoms soon after exposure to the drug. No definite dose-response relationship has been established for cyclophosphamide. Chest radiographs usually show an interstitial pattern with basilar predominance. In patients who present with very late onset of lung fibrosis, the upper zones may be predominantly affected.[2] Histologic findings are similar to those seen with toxicity from other cytotoxic drugs.

Cyclophosphamide-induced lung injury carries significant morbidity. When cyclophosphamide is used to treat nonneoplastic lung disease, the underlying pulmonary process may be compounded by superimposed drug toxicity. The distinction between the two processes may be difficult to delineate. When cyclophosphamide is used as a chemotherapeutic agent, its identification as the specific cause of lung injury may be difficult, since it is seldom used alone. As with all multidrug or multimodality regimens, pinpointing specific toxicity to a single agent may be impossible. Moreover, it is recognized that cyclophosphamide appears to have synergistic toxicity with therapeutic thoracic radiation as well as with other chemotherapeutic agents. The prognosis of a patient with symptomatic drug toxicity ascribed to cyclophosphamide is poor; mortality is approximately 50 percent.[2] Most authors recommend treatment with corticosteroids even though there is no definitive evidence that cyclophosphamide toxicity is reversed by this intervention.

Other Alkylating Agents

Chlorambucil and melphalan are slow-acting nitrogen mustards. Like cyclophosphamide, chlorambucil has also been used in the treatment of nonneoplastic diseases, including sarcoidosis. Pulmonary toxicity occurs in less than 5 percent of patients.[1] As with busulfan, treatment may encompass long time spans. Pulmonary toxicity may appear months to years after initiation of therapy and may be related to cumulative dosage. Clinical and histologic manifestations of drug toxicity are similar to those seen with other alkylating agents.

Melphalan-induced pulmonary toxicity is rare and resembles that caused by other cytotoxic drugs with respect to clinical, radiographic, and pathologic findings. Of note is that radiographic findings of predominantly upper lobe infiltrates in melphalan toxicity contrast with the more typical bibasilar pattern seen with most of the other cytotoxic drug–induced pulmonary disorders.

ANTIMETABOLITES

Methotrexate

Methotrexate is a folate antagonist used as a chemotherapeutic agent as well as for the treatment of nonneoplastic inflammatory diseases. When the agent is used in high doses for the treatment of cancers, the incidence of pulmonary toxicity is estimated at 7 percent.[6] Toxicity does not appear to have dose-dependency but may be related to frequency of administration. In one study, daily or weekly treatment carried more risk of pulmonary injury than did treatment every 2 to 4 weeks.[7] Synergistic toxicity has been reported with combination therapy using cyclophosphamide. Tapering of corticosteroid therapy or adrenalectomy may also increase the risk of methotrexate-induced toxicity.

Methotrexate-induced toxicity presents with several syndromes. The most common of these is characterized by fever, dyspnea, cough, malaise, and myalgias, usually within weeks of the initiation of therapy. Chest radiographs usually show diffuse interstitial infiltrates. Occasionally, chest radiographs may show unilateral or bilateral effusions or a nodular appearance; they may even look normal. Skin rash is present in up to 17 percent of patients, and peripheral blood eosinophilia is noted in up to 40 percent.

Methotrexate-induced pulmonary disease may resolve even though the drug is continued. Rechallenge does not necessarily result in relapse. These findings suggest that the disorder is not due to an immune mechanism of injury. This presentation of methotrexate-induced pulmonary toxicity parallels the hypersensitivity-type syndrome that is sometimes observed with bleomycin. Since some patients will go on to develop chronic pneumonitis and pulmonary fibrosis, the drug is generally withdrawn when toxicity occurs.

Pulmonary toxicity from methotrexate may also present as a more insidious subacute syndrome of interstitial lung disease. Symptoms—including cough, fever, dyspnea, headache, and malaise—typically occur within 4 months after the initiation of treatment. Radiographically and clinically, this syndrome more closely resembles the type of chronic pneumonitis seen with other cytotoxic drugs and has been described as complicating all routes of methotrexate administration (oral, intravenous, intrathecal). In contrast to that from many other chemotherapeutic agents, the pneumonitis caused by methotrexate appears in general to be responsive to corticosteroids.

Methotrexate-induced lung injury may also appear as an acute syndrome with pleuritis and pleural effusion. Respiratory distress progressing to non-cardiogenic pulmonary edema has been seen after intrathecal administration of drug and may be neurogenic.

The prognosis with methotrexate-associated lung toxicity is generally favorable. As noted above, symptoms and radiographic abnormalities may resolve despite continuation of treatment. The use of corticosteroids is generally recommended, although prospective trials of this treatment are not available. The overall mortality with methotrexate-induced pneumonitis is approximately 10 percent.

Cytosine Arabinoside

Cytosine arabinoside, or cytarabine (ara-C), is a pyrimidine nucleoside analog that rapidly inhibits DNA synthesis. Pulmonary toxicity parallels intensity of treatment. High-dose regimens have been associated with a 5 to 44 percent incidence of acute or subacute respiratory insufficiency.[1,2] Symptoms include fever, cough, dyspnea, and tachypnea and may either coincide with the chemotherapeutic treatment or be delayed for up to several weeks after treatment is initiated. Hypoxemia may be present. Chest radiographs generally show a diffuse interstitial or alveolar pattern.

Treatment for ara-C lung toxicity is standard supportive care for noncardiogenic pulmonary edema. Administration of corticosteroids has been recommended by some authors, but this form of therapy is of uncertain benefit. Clinical and radiographic resolution may take 7 to 21 days. Overall mortality associated with ara-C–induced pulmonary toxicity ranges from 6 to 13 percent.[2]

Fludarabine

Fludarabine phosphate is a purine nucleoside analog used in the treatment of chronic lymphoproliferative disorders. As the drug is generally used after failure of standard alkylating agent therapy, experience with toxicities has been limited and sometimes difficult to evaluate because of prior treatment with other drugs. Both a hypersensitivity-type pulmonary reaction and interstitial pneumonitis have been reported after fludarabine administration. It should be noted that therapy with fludarabine has been associated with a high incidence of opportunistic infections, including *Pneumocystis carinii* pneumonia. The drug is immunosuppressive, and its effects may persist for months after initiation of treatment. The risk of opportunistic infection appears to be increased by the use of corticosteroids before, during, or after fludarabine administration.

Azathioprine/Mercaptopurine

Azathioprine is used as an immunosuppressive agent in the treatment of nonneoplastic diseases and in the medical management of organ transplantation. Its metabolic product, mercaptopurine, is used as an antineoplastic agent. These drugs are rarely associated with pulmonary toxicity. Interstitial pneumonitis, eosinophilic pneumonitis, and fibrosis have been reported. In one series of seven renal transplant patients, a more fulminant course of respiratory toxicity associated with diffuse alveolar damage was described.[8]

NITROSOUREAS

Carmustine

Of the nitrosoureas, carmustine (BCNU) has been most extensively studied. The onset of symptoms related to BCNU pulmonary toxicity is highly variable, occurring from a few days to up to 17 years after the initiation of chemotherapy. A number of factors that increase the risk of BCNU pulmonary toxicity have been delineated, including the total cumulative dose of BCNU, the duration of treatment, and a history of preexisting lung disease. As a result, it is recommended that the cumulative dose of BCNU be limited to 1400 mg/m^2 and that frequent pulmonary physiologic testing be done during treatment. It has also been recommended that BCNU be excluded from use in patients with preexisting symptomatic pulmonary disease or with baseline pulmonary physiologic abnormalities, particularly an abnormal vital capacity or $D_{L_{CO}}$.

The clinical presentation of BCNU-induced lung toxicity is variable. It may present fulminantly as acute respiratory failure; more commonly, however, it presents insidiously with asymptomatic physiologic abnormalities or radiographic evidence of pulmonary fibrosis. Symptoms of the latter, subacute course include cough, fatigue, and progressive dyspnea. The chest radiograph is rarely normal in symptomatic patients, usually showing bilateral interstitial infiltrates with a basilar predominance. Patients with an acute presentation may present with confluent alveolar infiltrates. Pneumothorax may occur and may be bilateral. A pulmonary function test (PFT) generally shows a restrictive ventilatory defect with diffusion abnormalities and eventually hypoxia. As with bleomycin, $D_{L_{CO}}$ may decrease without radiographic or clinical evidence of disease. While it has been suggested that a decrease in $D_{L_{CO}}$ may be the earliest sign of pulmonary toxicity, prospective evaluations of screening pulmonary function studies in the diagnosis of BCNU-induced lung toxicity are not yet available. Pathologic changes in the lung resemble those seen with other cytotoxic agents. The cardinal feature of BCNU-induced lung toxicity appears to be interstitial fibrosis, which may be patchy and often occurs without clinical evidence of inflammation. Angiocentric necrotizing granulomatous inflammation has been noted in some patients.

The prognosis for patients with BCNU-induced lung injury is poor. Estimates of mortality range as high as 90 percent.[6] Administration of corticosteroids simultaneously with BCNU does not appear to prevent pulmonary toxicity. Likewise, institution of corticosteroid therapy after the onset of symptoms does not consistently result in improvement. The primary approach to BCNU toxicity is to withdraw the drug immediately as soon as signs of toxicity appear. Long-term treatment remains supportive. In light of the long latent period that can exist between treatment and the onset of signs of toxicity, long-term follow-up is also warranted.

Other Nitrosoureas

The other nitrosoureas used as chemotherapeutic agents—lomustine (CCNU), semustine (methyl CCNU), and chlorozotocin—have also been associated with pulmonary toxicity. In general, these drugs have been less widely used than BCNU, and in smaller cumulative doses. As with BCNU, toxicity tends to become manifest insidiously with interstitial pneumonitis and pulmonary fibrosis.

BIOLOGIC RESPONSE MODIFIERS

Retinoic Acid

All-trans retinoic acid is a biologically active agent that has proven benefit in the treatment of acute promyelocytic leukemia. In contrast to conventional cytotoxic chemotherapy, activity of this drug occurs through the promotion of the differentiation of malignant into mature neutrophils. In up to 25 percent of treated patients, this therapy has been associated with a constellation of symptoms termed the *retinoic acid syndrome,*[9] characterized by fever, dyspnea, and pleural or pericardial effusions, often in association with hypertension or renal insufficiency. Chest radiographs show interstitial infiltrates and pleural effusions. Leukocytosis, which is common during treatment, is often, though not invariably, associated with the syndrome. In a series of 35 patients treated with all-trans retinoic acid, 9 developed the retinoic acid syndrome.[9] More than 50 percent of these patients required mechanical ventilation, and 33 percent died of complications related to the syndrome. The cause of the syndrome is unclear, but it must be linked to the differentiation process induced by the drug.

Recent reports indicate that the severity of the retinoic acid syndrome may be decreased by treatment with corticosteroids. However, in patients who develop leukocytosis and therefore appear to be at increased risk of retinoic acid syndrome, management is unclear. Full-dose cytotoxic chemotherapy has been suggested as a therapeutic strategy in this circumstance, although this approach remains uncertain on two accounts: fewer than half of the patients who develop leukocytosis will develop retinoic acid syndrome, and cytotoxic chemotherapy has inherent risks. At present, regimens using all-trans retinoic acid should also include corticosteroids.

Interleukin-2

Interleukin 2 (IL-2) is a glycoprotein secreted by activated lymphocytes. IL-2 therapy, alone or in conjunction with lymphokine-activated killer (LAK) cells, has proved beneficial in patients with metastatic renal cell carcinoma or melanoma. However, significant treatment-related pulmonary toxicities have been observed. In a series of 54 patients who received high-dose IL-2 and LAK therapy, 80 percent were noted to have focal or diffuse parenchymal lung opacities.[10] Pleural effusions were also common. The spectrum of pulmonary toxicities ranges from subclinical restrictive and obstructive physiologic abnormalities, often associated with a decline in the $D_{L_{CO}}$, to more severe clinically evident respiratory insufficiency. The latter generally presents as a syndrome of noncardiogenic pulmonary edema and may be associated with hypotension and renal insufficiency. IL-2 appears to have a cumulative dose-dependent lung toxicity, which seems to be compounded by LAK cell administration. Lung toxicity does appear to be reversible. In most cases, clinical and radiographic abnormalities will resolve within several days after cessation of therapy.

MISCELLANEOUS AGENTS

Doxorubicin

The use of the anthracycline doxorubicin is usually limited by cardiac toxicity. While direct pulmonary toxicity has not been described for this drug, the combination of the drug and therapeutic thoracic radiation, either during or preceding doxorubicin therapy, increases the incidence of radiation pneumonitis in 10 percent of patients. In severe cases, a capillary leak syndrome and noncardiogenic pulmonary edema may develop. Of note is that in contrast to conventional radiation-induced lung injury, radiographic abnormalities in cases of combined doxorubicin and radiation therapy may be observed outside the ports of radiation—a situation similar to that seen with bleomycin.

Procarbazine

Procarbazine has been associated with a hypersensitivity type of pneumonitis as well as with the more usual cytotoxic drug–induced interstitial pneumonitis. The incidence of pulmonary toxicity with procarbazine appears to be low.

Vinca Alkaloids

The vinca alkaloids given as sole agents are generally not associated with pulmonary toxicity. However, the combination of vinblastine or vindesine with mitomycin has been reported to be associated with noncardiogenic pulmonary edema, interstitial pneumonitis, and bronchospasm. This synergistic toxicity is discussed in more detail in a preceding section on cytotoxic antibiotics.

Paclitaxel

Paclitaxel (Taxol) was the first of a new class of anticancer agents known as taxanes. The incidence of major hypersensitivity reactions—including dyspnea, bronchospasm, urticaria, and hypotension—is high (25 to 30 percent). The administration of histamine (H_1 and H_2) antagonists and corticosteroids before treatment with paclitaxel has reduced the incidence of such reactions to a more acceptable 1 to 2 percent. Paclitaxel has not been associated with any specific syndromes of lung injury. This may not be the case with other drugs of this group. Docetaxel, like paclitaxel, is associated with hypersensitivity reactions. Unlike paclitaxel, docetaxel is also associated with cumulative pulmonary toxicity, including a syndrome of noncardiogenic pulmonary edema.

REFERENCES

1. Rosenow EC III: Drug-induced pulmonary disease. *Dis Mon* 40:253–310, 1994.
2. Zitnik RJ: Drug-induced lung disease: Cancer chemotherapy agents. *J Respir Dis* 16:855–865, 1995.

3. Jules-Elysee K, White DA: Bleomycin-induced pulmonary toxicity. *Clin Chest Med* 11:1–20, 1990.

4. Kris MG, Pablo D, Graller J, et al: Dyspnea following vinblastine or vindesine administration in patients receiving mitomycin plus vinca alkaloid combination therapy. *Cancer Treat Rep* 68:1029–1031, 1984.

5. Sheldon R, Slaughter D: A syndrome of microangiopathic hemolytic anemia, renal impairment, and pulmonary edema in chemotherapy-treated patients with adenocarcinoma. *Cancer* 58:1428–1436, 1986.

6. Cooper JAD Jr, White DA, Matthay RA: Drug-induced pulmonary disease. Part 1: Cytotoxic drugs. *Am Rev Respir Dis* 133:321–340, 1986.

7. Ginsberg SJ, Comis RL: The pulmonary toxicity of antineoplastic agents. *Semin Oncol* 9:34–51, 1982.

8. Bedrossian CWM, Sussman J, Conklin RH, Kahan B: Azathioprine-associated interstitial pneumonitis. *Am J Clin Pathol* 82:148–154, 1984.

9. Frankel SR, Eardley A, Lauwers G, et al: The "retinoic acid syndrome" in acute promyelocytic leukemia. *Ann Intern Med* 117:292–296, 1992.

10. Saxon RR, Klein JSB, Bar MH, et al: Pathogenesis of pulmonary edema during interleukin-2 therapy: Correlation of chest radiographic and clinical findings in 54 patients. *Am J Radiol* 156:281–285, 1991.

Part Five | **INTERSTITIAL AND INFLAMMATORY LUNG DISEASES**

27 | Interstitial Lung Disease: A Clinical Overview and General Approach*

Lynn T. Tanoue

The interstitial lung diseases (ILDs) are several acute and chronic lung disorders with variable degrees of pulmonary fibrosis. In the immunocompetent host, any of this heterogeneous group of diseases can present with the following common clinical features: (1) exertional dyspnea; (2) bilateral diffuse infiltrates on chest radiographs; (3) physiologic abnormalities with a restrictive lung defect, decreased diffusing capacity ($D_{L_{CO}}$), and abnormal alveolar–arterial oxygen gradient ($P_{A_{O_2}}$–Pa_{O_2}) at rest or with exertion; and (4) absence of pulmonary infection and neoplasm; and (5) histopathology with varying degrees of fibrosis and inflammation, with or without evidence of granulomatous or secondary vascular changes in the pulmonary parenchyma. Idiopathic pulmonary fibrosis (IPF), a distinct clinical entity, is considered the prototypic ILD. Since there are no pathognomonic features for IPF, it is often diagnosed by careful elimination of other interstitial disorders. The term has also been used to describe ILDs in general. The term *cryptogenic fibrosing alveolitis* [(CFA)—"cryptogenic," meaning hidden] is synonymous with IPF.

In some ILDs, the small airways—the respiratory and terminal bronchioles—are primarily affected. Respiratory bronchiolitis–associated interstitial lung disease (RBILD), is an idiopathic inflammatory condition of respiratory bronchioles and adjacent alveolar structures occurring almost exclusively in cigarette smokers. RBILD is physiologically characterized by a restrictive lung defect with or without coexisting airflow obstruction. In contrast, bronchiolitis obliterans (BO), also referred to as obliterative bronchiolitis, is a disorder localized to the walls of the small airways and is physiologically characterized by obstructive airflow defect. BO may occur as an idiopathic entity, as a result of toxic gas exposure or viral infection, as a complication of bone marrow or lung transplantation, or in association with collagen vascular diseases (especially rheumatoid arthritis). Since there is no alveolar inflammation in BO, it should not be confused with bronchiolitis obliterans

*Edited from Chap. 68, "Interstitial Lung Disease: A Clinical Overview and General Approach," by Raghu G. In: *Fishman's Pulmonary Diseases and Disorders,* 3d ed., edited by Fishman AP, Elias JA, Fishman JA, Grippi MA, Kaiser LR, Senior RM. New York, McGraw-Hill, 1998, pp 1037–1055. For fuller discussion of the topics dealt with in this chapter, the reader is referred to the original text, as noted above.

organizing pneumonia (BOOP), characterized by a restrictive lung defect. Histologically BOOP appears as an organizing noninfectious pneumonia associated with an inflammatory exudative and fibrotic process within the small airways. Bronchiolitis obliterans syndrome (BOS), a distinct clinical entity occurring in the transplanted lung, also involves the small airways primarily and should not be confused with BO or BOOP, which occur in non-transplant situations. BOOP can manifest in several clinical situations, including pulmonary disorders associated with collagen vascular diseases and drug and environmental causes. The term *cryptogenic organizing pneumonia* (COP) has also been used to describe BOOP.

In thinking of the ILDs, it is important to differentiate terms used to define clinical entities and terms describing the pathologic lesions of these disorders. IPF, CFA, lone CFA, idiopathic BOOP/lone COP, RBILD, BO, BOS, and acute interstitial pneumonia of unknown origin (probably the previously described Hamman-Rich syndrome) are descriptions of clinical syndromes. Pathologic descriptions include usual interstitial pneumonia, desquamative interstitial pneumonia, lymphocytic interstitial pneumonia, giant-cell interstitial pneumonitis, diffuse alveolar damage, nonclassifiable interstitial pneumonia, and BOOP. Identical pathologic lesions can be seen in a variety of clinical syndromes, and a variety of pathologic entities can be seen in a single lung biopsy. In addition, the boundaries between these clinical and pathologic entities are not always clear. For example, desquamative interstitial pneumonia, originally thought to represent the early cellular stage of IPF, is known to aptly describe RBILD. In contrast, usual interstitial pneumonia, initially described as the late fibrotic phase of IPF, remains a characteristic histologic feature of this disorder. Nevertheless, these clinical and pathologic terms have informational features in their own right. Each is useful as long as its relationship to other entities is appropriately acknowledged.

CLINICAL APPROACH AND DIFFERENTIAL DIAGNOSIS

The clinician confronted with a patient with possible ILD must first determine if the patient truly has ILD. This requires the appropriate consideration of a variety of other pathologic processes that can mimic the interstitial disorders. This is particularly important in the setting of acquired immunosuppression (drug- or virus-induced) and transplantation, where opportunistic lung infection and transplant-related immunologic problems need to be primarily addressed. Similarly, diffuse neoplasia, congestive heart failure, pulmonary infection, occupational exposure, and pulmonary vascular disorders must be suspected in appropriate clinical settings. Second, the physician must also be aware of at least 150 other clinical entities and situations associated with ILD. Third, owing to the broad differential diagnoses and the availability of various ever-evolving invasive and noninvasive diagnostic techniques, the best approach to use to establish a specific diagnosis is frequently difficult to determine. Fourth, in a significant portion of patients, a conclusive cause cannot be ascertained even when the most invasive diagnostic pathways are taken. Finally, even when a specific diagnosis is made, an effective therapeutic regimen is not available for many patients with ILD.

The diagnostic process should start with a very thorough medical history that must include a review of environmental factors, occupational exposures, medication and drug usage, and family medical history. The patient's age, cigarette-smoking status, and sex may provide useful clues. IPF is almost always an adult disorder, typically occurring in patients beyond 50 years of age. Pulmonary sarcoidosis is more common in young adults and middle-aged people. Langerhans' cell granulomatosis (also known as pulmonary histiocytosis X and eosinophilic granuloma) typically occurs in young cigarette-smoking males. RBILD is seen almost exclusively in cigarette smokers. Lymphangioleiomyomatosis is a very rare disorder occurring exclusively in women of childbearing age. An occupational history is also essential, as it may lead to a specific inhalation cause for ILD. The clinician's index of suspicion for the diagnosis of hypersensitivity pneumonitis is generally raised by a history of at-risk employment (such as farming) or exposure to known causes of hypersensitivity pneumonitis.

The history should also include a careful review of medication and therapeutic interventions to identify iatrogenic causes of ILD. Many drugs are well known to cause ILD. Any new medication that the patient may have taken before the onset of ILD must be considered as a potentially attributable cause. Use of over-the-counter medications and "alternative medicines" must not be overlooked.

The presenting illness of a patient with ILD should be characterized with particular attention to the onset and duration of symptoms, rate of disease progression, and association with hemoptysis, fever, and extrathoracic symptoms. Symptoms lasting 4 weeks or less and the presence of fever suggest BOOP, drug-induced pulmonary injury, and hypersensitivity pneumonitis. This acute presentation is atypical in IPF, pulmonary histiocytosis X, and ILD associated with connective tissue disease. Patients with sarcoidosis and Lofgren's syndrome may also present with a brief illness, fever, erythema nodosum, and arthritis.

A number of extrapulmonary symptoms provide useful clues in the differential diagnosis of ILD. A history of aspiration or dysphagia suggests aspiration pneumonia, scleroderma, or mixed connective tissue disease; arthritis suggests a collagen vascular disease or sarcoidosis; recurrent sinusitis suggests Wegener's granulomatosis; pneumothorax can be seen with a variety of interstitial lung diseases, particularly eosinophilic granuloma and lymphangioleiomyomatosis; muscle and skin symptoms suggest polymyositis or dermatomyositis; dry and gritty eyes and dry mouth (sicca syndrome) suggest sarcoidosis, Sjögren's syndrome, or other collagen vascular disorders; and hemoptysis suggests alveolar hemorrhage syndromes such as Goodpasture's syndrome, Wegener's granulomatosis, pulmonary capillaritis, and systemic lupus erythematosus. When present, these symptoms will direct the clinician to appropriate laboratory tests that may lead to a specific diagnosis other than IPF.

Physical examination of the respiratory system is rarely helpful in the diagnostic evaluation of ILD. In contrast, extrathoracic findings can provide insight. For example, skin abnormalities, peripheral lymphadenopathy, and hepatosplenomegaly are commonly associated with sarcoidosis. Characteristic skin rashes and lesions also occur in collagen vascular diseases, disseminated histiocytosis X, tuberous sclerosis, and neurofibromatosis. Muscle tenderness and proximal muscle weakness raise the possibility of coexisting polymyositis. Signs of arthritis may be associated with sarcoidosis or collagen vascular disease. Patients with IPF also often have arthralgias. However, they rarely show active synovitis or arthritis on physical examination. Sclerodactyly, Raynaud's phenomenon, and telangiectatic lesions are characteristic features of scleroderma and CREST syndrome. Iridocyclitis, uveitis, or conjunctivitis may be associated with sarcoidosis and collagen vascular syndromes. Abnormalities of the central nervous system suggest the diagnosis of sarcoidosis (cranial nerve abnormalities, diabetes insipidus, anterior pituitary dysfunction), Langerhans cell granulomatosis (diabetes insipidus), and tuberous sclerosis (epilepsy, mental retardation).

Routine laboratory tests should include complete blood count, leukocyte differential, erythrocyte sedimentation rate, chemistry profile (calcium, liver function tests, electrolytes, renal function tests), screening for collagen vascular diseases, and urinalysis. When appropriate, creatinine kinase, aldolase, and levels of angiotensin converting enzyme should be measured.

Chest Radiographic Patterns

The pulmonary clinician should make every effort to obtain all previous chest radiographs for review. This makes it possible to ascertain the onset, progression, chronicity, and stability of the patient's disease. A rare patient with ILD will present with a normal chest radiograph. When radiographic abnormalities are noted, their distribution and appearance are useful in narrowing the differential diagnosis of the ILD. A pattern of upper-lobe/zone predominance suggests sarcoidosis, berylliosis, Langerhans' cell granulomatosis (eosinophilic granuloma), cystic fibrosis, silicosis, and ankylosing spondylitis. In contrast, the abnormalities of lymphangitic carcinomatosis, subacute eosinophilic pneumonias, IPF, asbestosis, and pulmonary fibrosis associated with rheumatoid arthritis or scleroderma are predominantly concentrated in the middle and lower lung zones.

The presence and the pattern of adenopathy may provide additional clues. The coexistence of paratracheal and symmetrical bilateral hilar adenopathy strongly suggests sarcoidosis. This pattern may, however, be seen in metastatic tumor and lymphoma as well. The presence of eggshell calcification suggests sarcoidosis or silicosis. Kerley B lines and ILD in association with a normal heart size suggest lymphangitic carcinomatosis. However, if concomitant radiographic evidence of pulmonary hypertension is present in the same setting, pulmonary venoocclusive disease must be considered.

The pattern of peripherally located pulmonary infiltrates in the upper and middle zones with relatively clear perihilar or central zones (often described as "photographic negative of pulmonary edema") is highly suggestive of chronic eosinophilic pneumonia. Bilateral infiltrates that recur in the same anatomic location raise the possibility of BOOP, chronic eosinophilic pneumonia, drug-induced ILD, or a relapse/recall radiation pneumonitis. In contrast, fleeting or migratory infiltrates suggest Churg-Strauss syndrome (allergic angiitis and granulomatosis), allergic bronchopulmonary aspergillosis (ABPA), BOOP, tropical eosinophilic pneumonia, or Loeffler's syndrome.

The presence of pleural plaques or localized thickening in the setting of ILD predominantly affecting the lower lobes suggest asbestosis. Diffuse pleural thickening can result from asbestos pleurisy, rheumatoid arthritis, scleroderma, or malignancy. The coexistence of pleural effusion raises the possibility of rheumatoid arthritis, systemic lupus erythematosus, a drug reaction, asbestos-related lung diseases, amyloidosis, lymphangioleiomyomatosis, or lymphangitic carcinomatosis. Apparently normal (preserved lung volume) and increased lung volumes on the chest radiograph in the context of ILD suggest the coexistence of an obstructive airflow defect and a few specific disease entities, including lymphangioleiomyomatosis, eosinophilic granuloma, hypersensitivity pneumonitis, tuberous sclerosis, and sarcoidosis. In interpreting these findings, it is important to realize that the chest radiograph provides only a semiquantitative assessment of lung volume and often correlates poorly with estimates of histologic and functional impairment. Despite these limitations, when the clues provided by the chest radiograph are combined with those from the history, physical examination, laboratory tests, and pulmonary function evaluation, the clinician is often able to narrow the differential diagnoses to a few possibilities.

Pulmonary Physiology Testing

Regardless of the cause, a restrictive lung defect and decreased diffusing capacity ($D_{L_{CO}}$) are the predominant physiologic abnormalities seen in ILD. The forced expiratory volume in 1 s (FEV_1) and forced vital capacity (FVC) are decreased proportionally, so the ratio of the two remains normal. The total lung capacity and lung volumes are reduced. The $P_{A_{O_2}}$–$P_{a_{O_2}}$ difference, at rest or with exercise, may be normal or increased, depending on disease severity. Similarly, the $D_{L_{CO}}$, corrected for hemoglobin concentration, may be normal or low. The $D_{L_{CO}}$, though highly nonspecific, is believed to be a relatively sensitive parameter in detecting the presence of pulmonary dysfunction and may be the only abnormality seen in early stages of interstitial lung disease. Additionally, it can be useful in the monitoring of disease progression or response to therapy. Significant changes in FVC, $D_{L_{CO}}$, and resting $P_{A_{O_2}}$–$P_{a_{O_2}}$ difference at the end of 1 year correlate with survival.[1,2]

Typically, static pulmonary function tests identify the presence of clinically significant restrictive physiology and quantify the severity of impairment, but do not aid in the differential diagnosis. However, a number of patterns can be seen that are of diagnostic utility. Diseases such as polymyositis, scleroderma, and systemic lupus erythematosus should come to mind when tests performed on a cooperative patient demonstrate reproducibly a decrease in the maximal voluntary ventilation out of proportion to the decrease in FEV_1 and a decrease in maximal inspiratory pressures in association with respiratory muscle weakness. When an obstructive airflow abnormality is present, the diagnostic possibilities are also narrowed. A mixed pattern of obstructive and restrictive abnormalities may be present when ILD coexists with chronic obstructive pulmonary disease, asthma or bronchiectasis. ILDs associated with asthma or recurrent bronchospasm include Churg-Strauss syndrome, ABPA, sarcoidosis (endobronchial), and tropical pulmonary interstitial eosinophilia.

The functional assessment of physiologic impairment by single or serial evaluations during exercise can play an important role in the management of patients with ILD. The degree of arterial hypoxemia induced by exercise and the alveolar-arterial difference in P_{O_2} (the "A–a O_2 gradient") correlate well with the degree of pulmonary fibrosis.[3,4] Exercise also affords the most sensitive diagnostic and physiologic test for ILD, since in some patients with biopsy-proven ILD the physiologic responses to exercise are distinctly abnormal even though static pulmonary function tests, chest radiographs, and high-resolution computed tomography (HRCT) scans are all normal. Exercise-induced physiologic abnormalities in ILD[5] include a decrease in work rate and maximal oxygen consumption, abnormally high minute ventilations at submaximal work rates (high ventilatory equivalents), decreased peak minute ventilations, failure of tidal volumes to increase at submaximal levels of work while respiratory rates increase disproportionately, increased heart rates, low O_2 pulses, progressive arterial hypoxemia and widening of the $P_{A_{O_2}}$–$P_{a_{O_2}}$ difference, and persistent respiratory alkalosis. In advanced pulmonary fibrosis, progressive exercise may be associated with an initial failure of $P_{a_{CO_2}}$ to decrease, followed by progressive increase in $P_{a_{CO_2}}$ in the terminal stages of exercise. As the level of exercise increases progressively, in patients with advanced pulmonary fibrosis, the physiologic dead space remains elevated and a low O_2 pulse (oxygen uptake/heart rate) may be present.

Computed Tomography and High-Resolution CT Images

CT and HRCT scans are more sensitive and have a greater ability to detect anatomic abnormalities than do chest radiographs.[6] While a normal HRCT does not exclude the presence of microscopic ILD in patients with a high pretest probability of the disorder, it is clear that pathology can be demonstrated by CT which it is not appreciated on chest radiograph. CT-based evaluations have also shown that hilar and mediastinal adenopathy may be present in IPF and the ILD that accompany collagen vascular diseases. The ability of these scans to be useful in staging and diagnosis of ILD comes from their perceived ability to differentiate between predominantly active and reversible versus fibrotic and irreversible disease. Enthusiasm has been increasing about the utility of HRCT in identifying "active inflammation" in ILD. It has been proposed that ground-glass attenuation on HRCT represents histologically "active" and reversible pulmonary inflammation. Unfortunately, increasing experience has shown that ground-glass attenuation is not as specific as was hoped. In a recent study, ground-glass attenuation corresponded to inflammation in only 65 percent of patients with ILD and to fibrosis in as many as 54 percent.[7] Another study, in patients with sarcoidosis, showed no correlation between ground-glass attenuation and active alveolitis. On the other hand, the presence of traction bronchiectasis and bronchiolectasis on HRCT does correlate with tissue fibrosis. Thus, diagnostic or treatment decisions should not be made solely on the basis of the presence or absence of ground-glass attenuation on HRCT. The current strength of HRCT lies in its ability to give an overall assessment on the severity of honeycombing and fibrotic changes that are, in general, irreversible. Extensive "fibrotic" changes suggest advanced stage disease with limited potential for therapeutic response. Findings of this sort might preclude an invasive diagnostic approach or a prolonged therapeutic trial that could be toxic, particularly in elderly patients with comorbid disease.

A number of HRCT patterns are suggestive of specific interstitial disorders. HRCT images provide valuable information on the fine architecture of pulmonary secondary lobules. As a result, HRCT has the potential for differentiating sarcoidosis, lymphangitic carcinomatosis, and bronchiolitis. The presence of cysts within the parenchyma raises the possibilities of three major "cystic" ILDs: lymphangioleiomyomatosis, tuberous sclerosis, and Langerhans' cell granulomatosis. In lymphangioleiomyomatosis and tuberous sclerosis, the cysts are numerous, thin-walled, typically less than 2 cm in diameter, and distributed throughout the pulmonary parenchyma. In Langerhans' cell granulomatosis, by contrast, cysts are distributed predominantly in the upper lobes and tend to be bizarrely shaped. In acute hypersensitivity pneumonitis, a frequent diagnostic clue is a markedly abnormal HRCT with multifocal ground-glass attenuation despite a normal chest radiograph and significant clinical symptoms. Similarly, smokers with symptomatic RBILD typically have patchy ground-glass attenuation on HRCT in the setting of bilateral interstitial radiographic infiltrates and normal lung volumes. Finally, IPF is characterized by patchy subpleural and basilar fibrosis.

Perhaps the most important aspect of HRCT is its potential utility in determining the most appropriate sites for obtaining lung biopsies. It is believed that HRCT will increase the probability of making a definitive diagnosis by helping the surgeon sample relatively unaffected, actively inflamed, and densely fibrotic areas of the lung.[8] Although the cost-effectiveness of the routine use of HRCT in diagnostic evaluation has not been established, it seems appropriate and justifiable, for the sake of selecting the optimal sites for biopsy, to obtain an HRCT scan of the chest before a patient is subjected to lung biopsy.

Bronchoscopy with Bronchoalveolar Lavage and Transbronchial Biopsy

The role of bronchoalveolar lavage (BAL) in the diagnosis and staging of ILD has been the subject of intense study. The results indicate that BAL can be diagnostic if an infectious agent or neoplastic cell is present in the specimen. Occasionally, special stains for Langerhans' cells and surfactant material may also reveal sufficient abnormalities in the BAL specimen to enable the diagnosis of Langerhans' cell granulomatosis or pulmonary alveolar proteinosis, respectively. In the absence of infection, an increase in T lymphocytes with an increased CD4:CD8 ratio (in the absence of an increase in neutrophils and eosinophils) is suggestive of sarcoidosis. However, the CD4:CD8 ratio can be highly variable in sarcoidosis, and other diseases are associated with similar BAL findings.

Bronchoscopy with transbronchial lung biopsy may provide additional information in some patients with ILD, especially when tissue abnormalities tend to be distributed in peribronchovascular areas. For instance, sarcoidosis, lymphangioleiomyomatosis, and lymphangitic carcinomatosis are typically bronchocentric disorders in that their infiltrative lesions tend to be located along the peribronchovascular bundles. Transbronchial lung biopsies may disclose certain distinctive abnormalities (e.g., the tight, uniform, well-formed, noncaseating granulomas of sarcoidosis; the smooth muscle proliferation of lymphangioleiomyomatosis; or the lymphatic metastasis of malignant cells). The presence of giant-cell granulomas is suggestive of hard-metal pneumoconiosis.

A transbronchial lung biopsy specimen is diagnostic if an infectious agent or malignancy is detected. In an appropriate clinical setting, a transbronchial lung biopsy that reveals granulomas without mycobacteria or fungi can support a diagnosis of sarcoidosis or hypersensitivity pneumonitis. At times, the diagnosis of Langerhans' cell granulomatosis or lymphangioleiomyomatosis may be made if characteristic microscopic features are present in the transbronchial lung biopsy. However, a lack of these findings in such specimens does not necessarily exclude these diseases, since the possibility of sampling error poses a problem. Thus, when transbronchial lung biopsies or bronchoalveolar lung specimens fail to confirm the clinically suspected disease, the ultimate diagnostic step—thoracoscopic or open lung biopsy—may be necessary to obtain a larger and more representative lung biopsy to clarify or confirm the diagnosis.

Surgical Lung Biopsy: Thoracoscopy-Guided and Open Lung Biopsy

As noted above, despite a thorough clinical evaluation and detailed analysis of the specimens obtained by transbronchial lung biopsy, the specific diagnosis for a patient with ILD often remains unclear. Thoracoscopy-guided lung biopsy (TGLB) or open lung biopsies merit consideration as the final diagnostic step. One may then ask which patients are suitable candidates for these procedures. Unexplained dyspnea on exertion or abnormal results on pulmonary function testing favor such interventions. Normal chest radiographs or HRCT scans do not, in themselves, negate the need for tissue diagnosis. On the other hand, not all patients with typical clinical features compatible with IPF require surgical lung biopsy for definitive diagnosis.[8] In selected patients, such as those who are elderly with comorbidity, it may be appropriate to make a clinical diagnosis of IPF after a thorough clinical, radiographic, and HRCT assessment even though bronchoscopy with BAL and transbronchial biopsies have proved nondiagnostic. The same approach merits consideration in patients more than 65 years of age with typical and long-standing chest radiographic findings (i.e., stable or slow progression of bibasilar interstitial abnormalities over several years, fibrotic changes in the lower zones, small lung volumes despite adequate inspiratory effort, absence of hilar or mediastinal adenopathy, and pleural abnormalities) who also have one of the following: (1) no other explanation for exertional dyspnea; (2) lack of extrapulmonary manifestations (except finger clubbing); (3) documented collagen vascular disease; (4) typical HRCT evidence of IPF; and (5) typical physiologic abnormalities (restrictive lung defect, decreased $D_{L_{CO}}$, with or without hypoxemia at rest). Among younger patients (under 65 years of age), however, surgical lung biopsy is indicated in the functionally impaired patient when the diagnosis is unclear despite thorough clinical evaluation (inclusive of bronchoscopic assessment). This is especially so when clinical features are suggestive of a diagnosis other than IPF or in addition to it. In the following associated clinical situations, histologic clarification by surgical lung biopsy is desirable to ascertain a specific diagnosis: (1) history of fever, weight loss, sweats, and hemoptysis; (2) family history of apparent familial ILD and IPF; (3) history of pneumothorax; (4) symptoms and signs of peripheral vasculitis; (5) atypical radiographic features of IPF (inclusive of normal chest radiographs); (6) unexplained extrapulmonary manifestations; (7) unexplained pulmonary hypertension; (8) unexplained cardiomegaly at the time of presentation; (9) rapidly progressive disease; or (10) rapid deterioration or new symptoms with new radiographic abnormalities in focal areas superimposed on long-standing "stable" diffuse radiographic changes.

The current clinical practice for subjecting patients with ILD to surgical lung biopsy is highly variable. This is understandable because the ILDs are a diverse group of diseases, each with a variable natural course. In addition, the therapies for these disorders vary in effectiveness and potential toxicity. Some diseases may respond promptly to intervention, whereas others respond minimally if at all. Studies are needed to determine whether surgical lung biopsy is indeed essential to make the diagnosis of diseases such as IPF before treatment is started in all symptomatic or functionally impaired patients who manifest typical clinical features but whose clinical assessment yields otherwise negative results.

Once the decision for surgical lung biopsy is made, the options are open lung biopsy and TGLB. There is increasing evidence supporting the routine use of TGLB, since it entails a less morbid surgical procedure. Adequate TGLB specimens are readily obtained by experienced surgeons. A concerted interaction of the pulmonary clinician, thoracic surgeon, and pathologist is needed, since several appropriately chosen biopsies should be obtained and the handling and processing of the lung specimens must be coordinated to maximize and optimize the diagnostic yield.

Treatment

The therapeutic regimens used for patients with ILD should to be tailored to the patient's specific disease process. Prognosis is variable with or without treatment depending on the underlying disease, again underscoring the need to make an exact diagnosis whenever possible.

REFERENCES

1. Hanson D, Winterbauer RH, Kirtland SH, Wu R: Changes in pulmonary function test results after 1 year of therapy as predictors of survival in patients with idiopathic pulmonary fibrosis. *Chest* 108:305–310, 1995.
2. Raghu G, Cain K, Hammer S, Winterbauer R: Improved forced vital capacity (FVC), $DLCO_{SB}$ and resting $P[A-a]O_2$ measurements at one year predict long term survival in idiopathic pulmonary fibrosis (IPF) (abstr). *Am Rev Respir Dis* 143:A57, 1991.
3. Cherniack RM, Colby TV, Flint A, et al: Correlation of structure and function in idiopathic pulmonary fibrosis. *Am J Respir Crit Care Med* 151:1180–1188, 1995.
4. Fulmer JD, Roberts WC, von Gal ER, Crystal RG: Morphologic-physiologic correlates of the severity of fibrosis and degree of cellularity in idiopathic pulmonary fibrosis. *J Clin Invest* 63:665–676, 1979.
5. Hansen JE, Wasserman K: Pathophysiology of activity limitation in patients with interstitial lung disease. *Chest* 109:1566–1576, 1996.
6. Padley SPG, Hansell DM, Flower CDR, Jennings P: Comparative accuracy of high resolution computed tomography and chest radiography in the diagnosis of chronic diffuse infiltrative lung disease. *Clin Radiol* 44:222–226, 1991.
7. Remy-Jardin M, Giraud F, Remy J, et al: Importance of ground-glass attenuation in chronic diffuse infiltrative lung disease: Pathologic-CT correlation. *Radiology* 189:693–698, 1993.
8. Raghu G: Interstitial lung disease: A diagnostic approach. Are CT scan and lung biopsy indicated in every patient? *Am J Respir Crit Care Med* 151:909–914, 1995.

28 | Systemic Sarcoidosis*

Lynn T. Tanoue

Sarcoidosis is a multisystem granulomatous disorder of unknown origin characterized by activation of T lymphocytes and mononuclear phagocytes at sites of disease. Although any organ can be involved, the disease most commonly affects the lungs and intrathoracic lymph nodes. Eye and skin involvement is seen in approximately 20 percent of patients; symptomatic involvement of other organs occurs less frequently. Since the cause of sarcoidosis is unknown, a diagnosis is most securely established from a compatible clinical history together with histologic evidence of widespread, noncaseating granulomas in more than one organ and the absence of a competing diagnosis, such as tuberculosis, fungal disease, or malignancy. Clinical, epidemiologic, and family studies support the hypothesis that sarcoidosis is caused by exposure to an environmental, possibly infectious, agent and that there may be genetic susceptibility to the disease. Corticosteroids remain the mainstay of treatment when patients need to be treated because of threatened organ failure or chronic progressive disease.

Despite the tools of modern medicine, the cause of sarcoidosis remains unknown. Extensive efforts directed at evaluating multiple infectious agents including mycobacteria, viruses, and other organisms have not yielded reproducible evidence for a single pathogen. Although direct demonstration of an infectious origin remains unproven, support for an infectious or environmental cause derives from several epidemiologic studies that demonstrate seasonal, time-space, or occupational clusters of sarcoidosis cases. The absence of convincing evidence for a primary infectious agent in sarcoidosis has led to the hypothesis that sarcoidosis is the result of an aberrant or autoimmune response to a persistent infectious or environmental agent or an autoantigen. The presence of antinuclear antibodies, rheumatoid factor, hypergammaglobulinemia, and immune complexes in sarcoidosis may reflect a generalized immune dysregulation that is consistent with this possibility.

Family studies support the concept that genetic factors may predispose to sarcoidosis or determine clinical expression of the disease.[1,2] One retrospective study reported that familial clustering of sarcoidosis occurred in 16 percent of African-American patients with sarcoidosis.[3] Familial clustering is seen less frequently in Caucasians. Monozygotic twins appear more likely to both have sarcoidosis than dizygotic twins, strongly suggesting a genetic component to the disease. However, the lack of a clear genetic pattern suggests that susceptibility to sarcoidosis is likely to be polygenic and associated with important environmental factors.

*Edited from Chap. 69, "Systemic Sarcoidosis," by Moller DR. In: *Fishman's pulmonary Diseases and Disorders,* 3d ed., edited by Fishman AP, Elias JA, Fishman JA, Grippi MA, Kaiser LR, Senior RM. New York, McGraw-Hill, 1998, pp 1055–1069. For fuller discussion of the topics dealt with in this chapter, the reader is referred to the original text, as noted above.

Kveim-Stilzbach Test

The hypothesis that sarcoidosis might be caused by an infectious agent led to attempts to develop skin tests similar to that for tuberculosis. The Kveim-Stilzbach test involves intradermal inoculation of a suspension of sarcoid tissue. In patients with sarcoidosis but not in normal controls, this results in the formation of firm papules in 1 to 14 weeks, which when biopsied contain sarcoid-like granulomas. Siltzbach and others demonstrated that a single, validated reagent was positive (showed a granuloma on biopsy 4 weeks after application) in up to 80 percent of patients with early sarcoidosis and manifested under 1 percent false-positive responses.[1,4,5] Unfortunately, the Kveim-Stilzbach test is not widely available due to limited access to the reagent.

PATHOLOGY

The pathologic hallmark of sarcoidosis is the presence of discrete, noncaseating epithelioid cell granulomas typically at different stages of development. In the lung, granulomas tend to form along perivascular and peribronchial regions, areas rich in lymphatic vessels. The dominant cell in the central core is the epithelioid cell (thought to be a differentiated form of a mononuclear phagocyte), which contains abundant eosinophilic cytoplasm and a pale staining nucleus. CD4+ lymphocytes and mature macrophages are typically interspersed throughout the epithelioid core, whereas both CD4+ and CD8+ lymphocytes may be seen in the periphery of the granuloma. Giant cells, often containing cytoplasmic inclusions such as calcium and iron-laden Schaumann bodies, are scattered throughout the inflammatory locus. These features are not specific for sarcoidosis, as similar histopathologic findings can be seen in beryllium disease, tuberculosis, leprosy, Crohn's disease, primary biliary cirrhosis, fungal disease, foreign-body material, and local "sarcoid reactions" that occur in lymph nodes near neoplastic or chronic inflammatory areas. Granulomas in sarcoidosis may resolve, leaving few residual changes, or may undergo fibrosis, leaving a stellate scar or hyalinized ghost of a former granuloma.

IMMUNOPATHOGENESIS

Granulomatous inflammation in sarcoidosis is regulated by a complex interplay of T cells, mononuclear phagocytes, fibroblasts, B cells, dendritic cells and other accessory cells.[6–9] Interactions among these cells are regulated in large part by cytokines and by direct cell-cell contact. The result is a tightly orchestrated granulomatous process that can damage local tissues. In some cases, it resolves with restoration of normal tissue architecture. In others, it leads to pulmonary fibrosis. T lymphocytes and macrophages play crucial roles in this response. The T cells that predominate at sites of tissue inflammation are activated and are predominately of the CD4+ phenotype. They express exaggerated amounts of the interleukin-2 (IL-2) receptor p55 subunit as well as a number of cytokines. The macrophages at these sites are also activated. They have a blood monocyte-like phenotype and produce exaggerated amounts of cytokines such as tumor necrosis factor (TNF) and IL-12. In contrast to the T cells and macrophages at these tissue sites, the peripheral blood of patients with sarcoidosis is characterized by circulating lymphopenia, demonstrating a degree of compartmentalization in this disorder.

Sarcoidosis is presumed to be an antigen-driven response. A current paradigm in immunology is that the nature of an immune response to an antigen stimulus is determined largely by the pattern of cytokines produced by CD4+ cells. T-helper 1 (Th1) cells express predominately interferon gamma (IFN-γ) and IL-12, cytokines important in macrophage activation and delayed-type sensitivity responses. T-helper 2 (Th2) cells express IL-4, IL-5 and IL-13, cytokines important in antibody-mediated responses and eosinophilia. There is now increasing evidence that granulomatous inflammation in sarcoidosis is characterized by a type I (or Th1) cytokine profile. It is not clear, however, why this Th1 response heals with scarring in some, but not all, patients with this disease.

Pulmonary Sarcoidosis

The clinical presentation and natural course of sarcoidosis vary greatly. Although almost any organ of the body can be affected, the lungs or intrathoracic lymph nodes are involved in more than 90 percent of patients with the disease. Up to two-thirds of patients are asymptomatic but have sarcoidosis diagnosed after an incidental radiographic finding of bilateral hilar adenopathy. Respiratory symptoms occur in 40 to 60 percent of patients. The most common symptoms are cough and shortness of breath, usually of a progressive, insidious nature. The cough is usually nonproductive and may be severe. Dyspnea is typically worse with exertion. Sputum production and hemoptysis are frequent in patients with fibrocystic sarcoidosis, a condition that is often associated with bronchiectasis and recurrent respiratory infections. Ill-defined chest pain is a frequent complaint, possibly caused by nerve irritation from inflammation, scarring, and lymph node enlargement in the chest. Chest tightness and wheezing are not uncommon, particularly with endobronchial disease or fibrocystic changes, but are rarely the only manifestation. These symptoms are usually poorly responsive to bronchodilators, except in a subgroup of patients with bronchial hyperresponsiveness and reversible airway obstruction. Segmental atelectasis and bronchial or tracheal stenosis are rare but have been reported. Pulmonary hypertension and cor pulmonale may be the result of chronic, severe fibrocystic sarcoidosis. Rarely, dyspnea from severe pulmonary hypertension occurs without extensive interstitial lung disease, presumably from granulomatous vasculitis of pulmonary vessels.

Löfgren's Syndrome

Sarcoidosis may present in patients with an acute onset of erythema nodosum and bilateral hilar adenopathy, usually associated with fevers, polyarthritis, and uveitis, known as Löfgren's syndrome. Erythema nodosum is characterized by tender reddish nodules several centimeters in diameter, usually located on the lower extremities. The polyarthritis is often severe and incapacitating. Typically the ankles, feet, knees, and occasionally wrists and elbows are affected. Approximately 10 percent of patients with this syndrome will have a normal chest radiograph. Löfgren's syndrome is more common in European and Caucasian populations than in African Americans.[2,10] The onset is usually abrupt, but the prognosis is excellent, with resolution of symptoms typically occurring within weeks to several months.

Extrapulmonary Sarcoidosis

Many patients have clinically important affliction of one or more organ systems with or without significant pulmonary disease (Table 28-1).[11,12]

TABLE 28-1 Major Clinical Manifestations of Sarcoidosis

Organ system	Clinical feature
Pulmonary	Restrictive and, less often, obstructive disease, fibrocystic disease, bronchiectasis, endobronchial granulomas, mycetomas, hemoptysis, lobar atelectasis
Upper airway	Hoarseness, laryngeal or tracheal obstruction, nasal congestion, sinusitis, saddle-nose deformity
Ocular	Anterior and posterior uveitis, chorioretinitis, conjunctivitis, optic neuritis, glaucoma, cataracts
Skin	Erythema nodosum, chronic nodules and plaques, lupus pernio, alopecia
Hepatic	Hepatomegaly, jaundice, cirrhosis
Cardiac	Arrhythmias, heart block, cardiomyopathy, sudden death
Central nervous	Facial and other cranial neuropathies (e.g., Bell's palsy), aseptic meningitis, brain mass, seizures, obstructing hydrocephalus, myelopathy, polyneuropathy, mono-neuritis multiplex
Salivary and lacrimal glands	Salivary, lacrimal, and parotid gland enlargement, sicca syndrome
Hematologic	Mediastinal, peripheral, and retroperitoneal lymphadenopathy, splenomegaly, hypersplenism, anemia, lymphopenia, thrombocytopenia
Joints and musculoskeletal	Polyarthritis, Achilles' tendinitis, heel pain, polydactylitis, bone cysts, myopathy
Endocrine	Hypercalciuria, hypercalcemia, hypopituitarism, diabetes insipidus, epididymitis
Renal	Renal calculi, nephrocalcinosis, renal failure

Systemic constitutional symptoms such as fever, malaise, fatigue, and weight loss are seen in about 20 percent of patients and may be disabling.

Sarcoidosis of the upper respiratory tract occurs in 5 to 10 percent of patients, usually in those with long-standing disease. Severe nasal congestion and chronic sinusitis may result in considerable morbidity. Typically, these symptoms are unresponsive to decongestants and inhaled steroids. Laryngeal sarcoidosis may present with severe hoarseness, stridor, and acute respiratory failure secondary to upper airway obstruction. Frequently, laryngeal sarcoidosis is associated with chronic skin lesions, particularly lupus pernio.

Uveitis is the most common eye lesion in sarcoidosis and may be the initial presenting manifestation. The uveitis is more commonly anterior, may be unilateral or bilateral, and is frequently associated with bilateral hilar adenopathy. Chronic uveitis occurs in as many as 20 percent of patients with chronic sarcoidosis and may be more frequent in African Americans. Severe chorioretinitis occurs uncommonly. Optic neuritis may present dramatically with blindness. Granulomatous conjunctivitis appears as a granular or cobblestone-like appearance of the conjunctivae.

Chronic sarcoidosis of the skin usually manifests as plaques and subcutaneous nodules typically located around the hairline, eyelids, ears, nose, mouth, and extensor surfaces of the arms and legs. Occasionally, the skin lesions are pruritic or tender and may be either hyper- or hypopigmented. Lupus pernio is a particularly disfiguring form of cutaneous sarcoidosis of the face, with violaceous plaques and nodules covering the nose, nasal alae, malar areas, and areas around the eyes. Chronic skin lesions are more common and severe in African Americans.

The liver is frequently affected in sarcoidosis, but hepatic involvement is rarely the sole manifestation of the disease.[13] Active hepatic inflammation may be associated with fever and tender hepatomegaly. Pruritus can be severe and disabling in a small number of patients. Characteristically, the serum alkaline phosphatase and gamma-glutamyltransferase are elevated proportionately higher than the transaminases or bilirubin, though all patterns can be seen. Elevated serum liver function frequently reverts to normal spontaneously or after treatment with corticosteroids. Progressive cirrhosis may occur if chronic granulomatous inflammation of the liver is not treated. Symptomatic gastrointestinal impairment in sarcoidosis is rare. Splenomegaly occurs in 10 to 20 percent of patients, often associated with hepatomegaly and, less frequently, hypercalcemia. Occasionally, splenic enlargement may be massive. Hypersplenism with anemia and thrombocytopenia occurs but is uncommon. Peripheral blood leukopenia is common in sarcoidosis, probably more often as a result of altered trafficking of lymphocytes than splenic trapping. Splenic rupture rarely occurs.

Myocardial sarcoidosis is clinically apparent in less than 5 percent of patients with sarcoidosis. However, it is an important cause of mortality in young adults with sarcoidosis.[14] Arrhythmia, heart block, or sudden death can result from granulomatous inflammation of the conduction system. Extensive involvement of the myocardium can lead to cardiomyopathy. Endomyocardial biopsy can establish the diagnosis but is positive in only 60 percent of cases. Holter monitoring or electrophysiologic testing may be indicated to evaluate arrhythmias. Echocardiography is useful in assessing structural abnormalities such as abnormal myocardial wall motion.

Neurologic symptoms occur in less than 5 percent of patients with sarcoidosis. The most common manifestation is cranial neuropathy, usually affecting the seventh and fifth nerves. Eighth nerve involvement may cause hearing loss and vestibular dysfunction. Central nervous system involvement can include mass lesions mimicking malignancy, aseptic meningitis, obstructive hydrocephalus, and hypothalamic or pituitary dysfunction. Seizures, headache, change in mental status, confusion, and diabetes insipidus may be presenting symptoms. Cerebrospinal fluid characteristically demonstrates nonspecific elevation in protein levels with a lymphocytic pleocytosis. Magnetic resonance imaging with gadolinium enhancement or contrast-enhanced computed tomography (CT) may demonstrate inflammatory lesions with a propensity for the leptomeningeal and periventricular areas. Peripheral neuropathies account for about 15 percent of cases of neurosarcoidosis, typically presenting as mononeuritis multiplex or a predominant sensory deficit.

Granulomatous inflammation of salivary, parotid, and lacrimal glands results in enlarged, tender glands and/or sicca syndrome with dry mouth and dry eyes in less than 5 percent of patients with sarcoidosis. The association of fever, parotid enlargement, facial palsy, and uveitis is known as uveoparotid fever, or Heerfordt's syndrome, and is usually accompanied by bilateral hilar adenopathy.

Peripheral lymph node enlargement is usually minimal in sarcoidosis and often regresses spontaneously. A pattern of bilateral, symmetrical lymphadenopathy in the cervical, supraclavicular, axillary, and epitrochlear nodes is most frequently seen.

Arthralgias are a frequent complaint in sarcoidosis. True joint disease is found in less than 5 percent of patients.[15] Signs of arthritis or synovitis of the knees, phalanges of the hands, shoulders, or ankles are most common.

Joint erosion is rare, but "punched out" bony lesions with cystic changes and loss of bony trabeculae may be seen on radiographs.

Abnormal calcium metabolism is found in sarcoidosis, with hypercalciuria more frequent than hypercalcemia. Evidence supports the concept that these abnormalities are due primarily to increased conversion of vitamin D metabolites to active $1,25(OH)_2$ vitamin D by tissue macrophages and epithelioid cells at sites of granulomatous inflammation.[16] Kidney stones are the most frequent manifestation of renal sarcoidosis, usually related to abnormal calcium metabolism. Renal failure due to nephrocalcinosis may result from chronic, often asymptomatic hypercalcemia or hypercalciuria.

CLINICAL ASSESSMENT

An initial evaluation routinely includes a comprehensive history and physical examination, chest radiograph, pulmonary function tests with lung volumes, spirometry and diffusing capacity, complete blood count, urinalysis, measurement of urinary calcium excretion, liver function tests, calcium level, electrocardiogram, and a purified protein derivative (PPD) skin test. An initial slit-lamp examination is recommended in all cases of sarcoidosis in order to exclude uveitis that may not be clinically apparent. Other tests may be indicated if the clinical history or physical examination suggests specific organ involvement. For example, a Holter monitor or echocardiogram may be indicated if cardiac sarcoidosis is suspected.

Chest Radiography

Chest radiographs are abnormal in more than 90 percent of cases and carry prognostic information.[10,17,18] By international convention, the chest radiograph is divided into stages or types (Table 28-2). Stage 0 chest radiographs are seen in 5 to 10 percent of patients who present with extrapulmonary sarcoidosis. Stage I chest radiographs demonstrate hilar adenopathy that is typically bilateral and symmetrical. Mediastinal adenopathy may also be present. Stage II chest radiographs display hilar adenopathy as well as pulmonary infiltrates. The parenchymal abnormalities are usually interstitial, with a predilection for the upper lobes, but they may also present in a nodular or miliary pattern. Stage III chest radiographs demonstrate pulmonary parenchymal abnormalities without adenopathy. Stage IV radiographs include those of patients with extensive scarring, usually with fibrobullous and cystic abnormalities with volume loss and retraction in a predominantly upper lobe distribution.

Pulmonary Function Tests

Pulmonary function may be normal even when the chest radiograph demonstrates pulmonary infiltrates.[17,19] However, restrictive impairment with

TABLE 28-2 Radiographic Staging of Sarcoidosis

Stage	Radiographic findings
0	Normal
I	Hilar/mediastinal adenopathy
II	Hilar/mediastinal adenopathy with parenchymal pulmonary abnormalities
III	Parenchymal pulmonary abnormalities without adenopathy
IV	Severe parenchymal abnormality with fibrobullous changes

reduction in lung volumes, FVC, and FEV_1 is common, particularly when pulmonary infiltrates are present on the chest radiograph. Reduction in diffusing capacity can be seen in association with restrictive impairment or as an isolated deficit. Obstructive impairment is common in advanced fibrocystic disease but can also be caused by endobronchial disease, laryngeal involvement, or tracheal and bronchial stenosis. A subgroup of patients have bronchial hyperresponsiveness to methacholine and airway obstruction, which may respond to bronchodilators. Resting hypoxemia and exercise oxygen desaturation are typical when there is severe obstructive or restrictive impairment. CO_2 retention is unusual except in advanced pulmonary disease.

Cutaneous Anergy

A well-recognized feature of sarcoidosis is the impaired cutaneous response to common antigens that elicit delayed-type hypersensitivity reactions, seen in 30 to 70 percent of patients.[1] Since anergy to PPD is common in sarcoidosis, active tuberculosis must be strongly considered in any patient who develops a positive tuberculin skin test. Postulated mechanisms underlying the cutaneous anergy include a redistribution of T cells to sites of inflammation and the presence of local inhibitors of delayed-type hypersensitivity reactions, though additional mechanisms are also likely to be important.

DIAGNOSTIC APPROACH

A diagnosis of sarcoidosis is established on the basis of a compatible clinical and radiographic picture, evidence of widespread noncaseating granulomas, and exclusion of other granulomatous disorders. Although histologic evidence is needed from only a single site, clinical involvement of more than one system is necessary to exclude local granulomatous reactions to foreign bodies, infections, or tumor.

In some instances, the clinical presentation alone may be highly suggestive of sarcoidosis. For example, the acute onset of erythema nodosum, fever, uveitis, and polyarthritis with bilateral hilar adenopathy is highly suggestive of Löfgren's syndrome. When the possibility of infections such as histoplasmosis is low, it may be reasonable to observe without biopsy confirmation. There is controversy over the need for tissue confirmation in persons presenting with isolated bilateral hilar adenopathy. In the absence of symptoms and with a negative physical examination, this presentation is almost always a manifestation of sarcoidosis, and a period of observation is often justified.[20] When the adenopathy is asymmetrical, massive, or located in the posterior or anterior mediastinum, or symptoms such as fever, chest pain, or constitutional symptoms are present, the increased risk of malignancy or infectious granulomatous disease favors biopsy. Some authorities recommend biopsy for all cases of bilateral hilar adenopathy to exclude malignancy.

In general, the easiest accessible biopsy site is used to confirm a diagnosis of sarcoidosis. Biopsy of a skin nodule, superficial lymph node, lacrimal gland, conjunctivae, or salivary gland can often help to establish a diagnosis but has a reasonable yield only if the tissue is grossly abnormal. A liver biopsy can support a diagnosis in the proper clinical context despite the nonspecificity of hepatic granulomas. A positive Kveim-Stilzbach test may be used to support a diagnosis of sarcoidosis in centers possessing validated reagent. Mediastinoscopy should be considered in cases in which lymphoma, metastatic disease, or infection cannot be reasonably excluded.

Fiberoptic bronchoscopy is frequently used to confirm a diagnosis of pulmonary sarcoidosis.[21] The yield of transbronchial biopsies approaches 90 percent when pulmonary infiltrates are seen radiographically and at least four biopsies are taken. When hilar adenopathy alone is present, the yield of transbronchial biopsy may still exceed 50 to 70 percent. Transbronchoscopic needle aspiration of lymph nodes can increase the probability of making a diagnosis when the location of the adenopathy makes the procedure technically feasible. Endobronchial biopsy of nodular or "cobblestoned" bronchial musoca may yield granuloma.

Serum angiotensin converting enzyme (ACE) levels are elevated in 30 to 80 percent of patients with clinically active disease.[22] However, elevated levels are seen in a variety of disorders, including infectious granulomatous diseases, lymphoma, hepatitis, and diabetes. The low specificity and wide variability of ACE levels argue against their use as a diagnostic marker. Although ACE levels tend to correlate with extent of granulomatous inflammation throughout the body, the marked variability of this test in different studies has made the clinical utility of ACE levels in disease monitoring uncertain.[23]

Gallium-67 scans almost always demonstrate enhanced uptake in the lungs or hilar or mediastinal regions in patients with active pulmonary sarcoidosis.[5,6] These findings correlate with active inflammation but are not specific. Extrapulmonary sites such as the parotid, salivary, and lacrimal glands ("panda" pattern) may also demonstrate positive uptake. Recent data from many centers suggest that routine use of gallium scanning is not warranted as a diagnostic aid or for clinical staging, owing to the lack of specificity, wide variability, expense, and radiation exposure of the test.

CLINICAL COURSE AND PROGNOSIS

Prognosis in sarcoidosis is strongly influenced by the initial disease presentation.[10,17,18,24–26] Patients with Löfgren's syndrome generally have an excellent prognosis, with symptoms regressing within weeks to months. Patients with asymptomatic hilar adenopathy also generally remain stable or experience complete spontaneous recovery within several years. Overall, 60 to 80 percent of patients presenting with a stage I chest radiograph undergo spontaneous remission or remain stable. When taken together with the large group of patients with unrecognized sarcoidosis who also have a high incidence of complete spontaneous remission, the prognosis for most patients with sarcoidosis is excellent.

Patients presenting with stage II chest radiographs have a somewhat poorer outcome, with spontaneous resolution or stability occurring approximately 40 to 60 percent of the time. When treated with corticosteroids, they usually respond promptly, though treatment may have to be continued for an extended interval to prevent progressive fibrosis. Patients with stage III chest radiographs undergo spontaneous remission infrequently and do not uniformly respond to corticosteroid therapy, though dramatic improvement can be noted in some cases. Progression to pulmonary insufficiency and cor pulmonale is particularly common in patients with advanced fibrocystic disease. This group of patients has a particularly poor prognosis, since all have irreversible lung damage that may progress despite treatment.

When extrathoracic impairment is symptomatic and severe on presentation, the disease tends to be persistent and usually requires treatment. The pattern of organ involvement typically declares itself during the first year of clinical disease and does not change with time. In general, pregnancy has little effect on the long-term course of sarcoidosis. Sometimes, spontaneous abatement of chronic sarcoidosis occurs in pregnant patients, allowing a temporary reduction in steroid dosage. After pregnancy, however, an exacerbation often occurs, requiring a return to the original maintenance dose.

Estimates from available hospital statistics suggest that sarcoidosis may be directly responsible for the death of 4 to 5 percent of persons with the disease.[10] Major causes of death include respiratory insufficiency and cor pulmonale, massive hemoptysis, cardiac arrest, and uremia from chronic renal failure. Several centers in the United States and Britain suggest that race is an important prognostic indicator, with African-American and West Indian patients being most likely to have chronic persistent disease and to suffer from the morbidity and mortality of the disorder.

TREATMENT

The need for treatment must be balanced against the overall excellent prognosis for most patients with sarcoidosis.[24] This is particularly true for patients with stage I disease, for whom systemic therapy is rarely required. Symptomatic or local therapy should be utilized whenever possible. Examples include analgesics and antipyretics for constitutional symptoms, topical steroids for anterior ocular lesions, and the avoidance of calcium and sunlight for patients with disordered calcium metabolism. Persistent symptomatic or progressive pulmonary disease is generally accepted to be an indication for a course of systemic corticosteroid therapy. Threatened organ failure such as severe ocular, central nervous system (CNS), or cardiac disease should also be treated with systemic corticosteroids. Similarly, persistent hypercalcemia, renal or hepatic dysfunction, posterior uveitis, or anterior uveitis not responding to local steroids, severe fatigue and weight loss, and disfiguring skin disease are other indications for treatment.

Corticosteroid Therapy

Corticosteroids are the mainstay of therapy for sarcoidosis. Although controversy exists regarding their overall effectiveness in altering the long-term course of the disease, there is no disagreement that corticosteroids can provide prompt symptomatic relief and often reverse organ dysfunction.[24,28–29] Furthermore, anecdotal experience from many centers around the world attests to the clinical impression that corticosteroids favorably affect the course of the disease, preventing or delaying progressive pulmonary fibrosis and organ dysfunction in chronic cases.[10,29]

Initial treatment of pulmonary and systemic sarcoidosis with corticosteroids usually does not require more than 40 mg per day of prednisone. Some have even proposed initiating therapy with an alternate-day regimen or lower daily doses of prednisone in patients without life- or organ-threatening diseases. An example of a reasonable regimen for treating pulmonary sarcoidosis with corticosteroids is outlined in Table 28-3.[24] Treatment should ordinarily be continued for a minimum of 6 to 12 months, since premature attempts to taper off steroids are likely to result in relapse of disease. A maintenance dose of 5 to 15 mg per day of prednisone is usually sufficient to suppress persistent pulmonary disease.

TABLE 28-3 Oral Drug Regimens for the Treatment
of Sarcoidosis

	Initial dose	Duration
Pulmonary and systemic sarcoidosis		
Prednisone:	40 mg/day	2 weeks
	30 mg/day	2 weeks
	25 mg/day	2 weeks
	20 mg/day	2 weeks
	15 mg/day	6–8 months
Taper 2.5 mg/day every 2–4 weeks; assess for relapse.		
Mucocutaneous sarcoidosis		
Chloroquine:	500 mg/day	2 weeks
	250 mg/day	5 1/2 months
	0 mg/day	6 months
Repeat as needed at 6-month intervals.		

Special Circumstances

High doses of oral corticosteroids or high-dose pulse intravenous therapy may be indicated for serious ocular or CNS disease. Anterior uveitis can usually be treated with topical ophthalmologic steroid drops; posterior uveitis and chronic eye disease usually need oral therapy. CNS sarcoidosis tends to be chronic, requiring long-term therapy.

Erythema nodosum (Löfgren's syndrome) is usually managed with bed rest and aspirin or nonsteroidal anti-inflammatory drugs. Corticosteroids are almost always immediately effective but are recommended only in cases in which symptoms are disabling and persistent. In this situation, corticosteroids are usually needed for only several weeks.

Chloroquine is efficacious in many patients with mucocutaneous sarcoidosis.[30] This drug is particularly useful in lupus pernio and severe nasal sarcoidosis, diseases that are often poorly responsive to corticosteroids. Hypercalcemia has also been reported to respond to this drug. Chloroquine may be useful in chronic laryngeal sarcoidosis, though steroids are usually used initially to reduce airway obstruction. Ocular toxicity has limited its use but is rare when low doses are employed. Hydroxychloroquine appears to be less effective, but its lower toxicity may make this agent a useful alternative to chloroquine. These drugs are generally not effective in pulmonary or systemic sarcoidosis.

Treatment of cardiac sarcoidosis consists of antiarrhythmic therapy, diuretics, and afterload-reducing agents for specific cardiac abnormalities. Automatic implantable defibrillators may prevent sudden death in patients with serious arrhythmias. In addition, corticosteroids in moderate doses are generally recommended, even when extensive myocardial fibrosis is present, in an attempt to reduce ongoing inflammation and prevent further fibrosis.

Fibrocystic sarcoidosis may be complicated by mycetomas, bronchiectasis, and recurrent, occasionally massive hemoptysis.[31] *Aspergillus fumigatus* is the usual organism to colonize preexisting cystic spaces. Spontaneous resolution of mycetomas may be seen. Antifungal agents are not recommended, since they are not effective and the fungi rarely cause invasive disease. Bronchiectasis is usually present in these patients and is often associated with chronic and acute bacterial infections and episodes of hemoptysis. Rotating chronic antibiotics and low-dose steroid therapy are often effective in treating symptoms. Massive hemoptysis may be life-threatening, requiring therapeutic embolization of the appropriate bronchial or collateral artery for control. Surgery is usually not feasible because of severe underlying restrictive lung disease.

Management of cor pulmonale includes supplemental oxygen, diuretics, and bronchodilators for obstructive impairment. Aggressive antibiotic treatment of bronchitis and bronchiectasis is indicated to reduce the frequency of infectious episodes. Corticosteroids in low to moderate doses are also indicated in an attempt to prevent progressive pulmonary insufficiency.

Alternative Agents

Methotrexate has been used to treat severe sarcoid skin disease with anecdotal success. Recently, methotrexate in low weekly doses has been proposed as an alternative therapy for refractory pulmonary and systemic sarcoidosis.[32] Experience with this drug in sarcoidosis is limited, however, and the long-term toxicity of the drug in these patients is not known. Clear advantages of methotrexate over low-dose corticosteroids in the routine management of pulmonary or systemic sarcoidosis have not been established. Other immunosuppressive agents—such as azathioprine, chlorambucil, and cyclophosphamide—have had anecdotal successes in treating progressive sarcoidosis refractory to corticosteroids, though the potential toxicity of these drugs has limited their usefulness. Clinical experience with cyclosporine, a drug known to inhibit T-cell activation, has proved disappointing.

Transplantation

Successful lung and heart-lung transplantations have been performed in a small number of patients with advanced pulmonary sarcoidosis and respiratory insufficiency. Although noncaseating granulomas have recurred in some transplanted lungs, it is not apparent that these findings portend a poor outcome. Indications for single- or double-lung transplantation in patients with advanced pulmonary sarcoidosis are still being debated, and as experience grows, it is likely that specific guidelines will emerge. Heart transplantation for end-stage sarcoid cardiomyopathy has also been successful in a small number of patients.

REFERENCES

1. Mitchell DN, Scadding JG: Sarcoidosis. *Am Rev Respir Dis* 110:774–802, 1974.
2. Teirstein AS, Lesser M: Worldwide distribution and epidemiology of sarcoidosis, in Fanburg BL (ed): *Sarcoidosis and Other Granulomatous Diseases of the Lung.* New York, Marcel Dekker, 1983.
3. Harrington DW, Major M, Rybicki B, et al: Familial sarcoidosis: Analysis of 91 families. *Sarcoidosis* 11:240–243, 1994.
4. Hirsch JG, Cohen ZA, Morse SI, et al: Evaluation of the Kveim reaction as a diagnostic test for sarcoidosis. *N Engl J Med* 265:827–830, 1961.
5. Johns CJ (ed): Tenth International Conference on Sarcoidosis and Other Granulomatous Disorders, Sept 17–22, 1984, Baltimore, MD. *Ann NY Acad Sci* 465:1–749, 1986.
6. Crystal RG, Roberts WC, Hunninghake GW, et al: Pulmonary sarcoidosis: A disease characterized and perpetuated by activated lung T-lymphoctyes. *Ann Intern Med* 94:73–94, 1981.
7. Daniele RP, Dauber JH, Rossman MD: Immunologic abnormalities in sarcoidosis. *Ann Intern Med* 92:406–416, 1980.
8. Semenzato G, Agostini C: Immunology in sarcoidosis, in Schwartz MI, King TE (eds), *Interstitial Lung Disease.* St. Louis, Mosby–Year Book, 1993.

9. Thomas PD, Hunninghake GW: Current concepts of the pathogenesis of sarcoidosis. *Am Rev Respir Dis* 135:747–760, 1987.

10. Siltzbach LE, James DG, Neville E, et al: Course and prognosis of sarcoidosis around the world. *Am J Med* 57:847–852, 1974.

11. Longcope WT, Freiman DG: A study of sarcoidosis: Based on a combined investigation of 160 cases including 30 autopsies from the Johns Hopkins Hospital and Massachusetts General Hospital. *Medicine* 31:1–132, 1952.

12. Mayock RL, Bertrand P, Morrison CE, Scott JH: Manifestations of sarcoidosis: Analysis of 145 patients with a review of nine series selected from the literature. *Am J Med* 35:67–89, 1963.

13. Maddrey WC, Johns CJ, Boitnott JK, Iber FL: Sarcoidosis and chronic hepatic disease: A clinical and pathological study of 20 cases. *Medicine* 49:375–395, 1970.

14. Roberts WC, McAllister HA Jr, Ferrans VJ: Sarcoidosis of the heart: A clinicopathologic study of 35 necropsy patients (group I) and review of 78 previously described necropsy patients (group II). *Am J Med* 63:86–108, 1977.

15. Gumpel JM, Johns CJ, Shulman LK: The joint disease of sarcoidosis. *Ann Rheum Dis* 26:194–205, 1967.

16. Bell NH, Stern PH, Pantzer E, et al: Evidence that increased circulating 1 α, 25-dihydroxyvitamin D is the probable cause for abnormal calcium metabolism in sarcoidosis. *J Clin Invest* 64:218–225, 1979.

17. DeRemee RA: The roentgenographic staging of sarcoidosis: Historic and contemporary perspectives. *Chest* 83:128–133, 1983.

18. Hillerdal G, Nou E, Osterman K, Schmekel B: Sarcoidosis: Epidemiology and prognosis, a 15-year European study. *Am Rev Respir Dis* 130:29–32, 1984.

19. Winterbauer RH, Hutchinson JF: Use of pulmonary function tests in sarcoidosis. *Chest* 78:640–647, 1980.

20. Winterbauer RH, Belic N, Moores KD: A clinical interpretation of bilateral hilar adenopathy. *Ann Intern Med* 78:65–71, 1973.

21. Koerner SK: Transbronchial lung biopsy for the diagnosis of sarcoidosis. *N Engl J Med* 293:268–270, 1975.

22. Lieberman J: Elevation of serum angiotensin-converting-enzyme (ACE) level in sarcoidosis. *Am J Med* 59:365–372, 1975.

23. Turner-Warwick M, McAllister W, Lawrence R, et al: Cortico-steroid treatment in pulmonary sarcoidosis: Do serial lavage lymphocyte counts, serum angiotensin converting enzyme measurements and gallium-67 scans help management? *Thorax* 41:903–913, 1986.

24. Bascom R, Johns CJ: The natural history and management of sarcoidosis. *Adv Intern Med* 31:213–241, 1986.

25. Neville E, Walker AN, James DG: Prognostic factors predicting the outcome of sarcoidosis: An analysis of 818 patients. *Q J Med* 208:525–533, 1983.

26. Sones M, Israel HL: Course and prognosis of sarcoidosis. *Am J Med* 29:84–93, 1960.

27. DeRemee RA: The present status of treatment of pulmonary sarcoidosis: A house divided. *Chest* 71:388–393, 1977.

28. Hunninghake GW, Gilbert S, Pueringer R: Outcome of the treatment of sarcoidosis. *Am J Respir Crit Care Med* 149:893–898, 1994.

29. Johns CJ, Zachary JB, Ball WC Jr: A 10-year study of corticosteroid treatment of pulmonary sarcoidosis. *Johns Hopkins Med J* 134:271–283, 1974.

30. Siltzbach LE, Teirstein AS: Chloroquine therapy in 43 patients with intrathoracic and cutaneous sarcoidosis. *Acta Med Scand* 425:S302–S308, 1964.

31. Johns CJ: Management of hemoptysis with pulmonary fungus balls in sarcoidosis. *Chest* 82:400–401, 1982.

32. Lower EE, Baughman RP: The use of low dose methotrexate in refractory sarcoidosis. *Am J Med Sci* 299:153–157, 1990.

29 | Idiopathic Pulmonary Fibrosis*

Lynn T. Tanoue

Idiopathic pulmonary fibrosis (IPF) is an inflammatory interstitial lung disease of unknown origin. *Cryptogenic fibrosing alveolitis* and *diffuse interstitial fibrosis* are synonymous terms. Although the etiologic factors responsible for the disorder have not been defined, its clinical features and course are sufficiently distinctive to represent a unique entity.

The prevalence of IPF is difficult to determine, as open lung biopsy, the "gold standard" for the diagnosis of IPF, is not performed in large population-based epidemiologic studies. In 1988, some 30,000 hospitalizations and 4851 deaths in the United States were attributed to interstitial pulmonary diseases.[1] By contrast, more than 665,000 patients are hospitalized annually for chronic obstructive lung disease. Studies cite varying prevalence rates ranging from 3 to 6 cases per 100,000 persons to as high as 27 to 29 cases per 100,000.[1,2] Most patients present after age 50, with a peak incidence in the seventh decade. IPF is slightly more common in males than in females. Inherited or familial IPF, while described, is rare.[3] Exposure to dusts, metals, or organic solvents; residence in agricultural or polluted urban areas; and a history of cigarette smoking are associated with an increased risk.[2] Up to 70 percent of patients with IPF are current or former smokers.[2,4,5] Workers at increased risk include painters, miners, metalworkers, woodworkers, laundry workers, beauticians, or those in occupations resulting in the inhalation of hazardous dusts or chemicals.[2]

Clinical Features

IPF usually presents insidiously, with the gradual onset of nonproductive cough and dyspnea.[6] Physical examination shows crackles on chest auscultation in more than 80 percent of patients. These are typically dry and end-inspiratory and are most prevalent in the lung bases. With progression of the disease, rales may extend to the apices. The presence of bronchial breath sounds may reflect alveolar consolidation. Digital clubbing is noted in 25 to 50 percent of patients. Cyanosis, cor pulmonale, an accentuated pulmonic second heart sound, right ventricular heave, and peripheral edema may be observed in the late phases of the disease.[6,7] Fever is rare and suggests an alternative diagnosis.

The differential diagnosis of IPF is extensive. Important considerations include congestive heart failure, lymphangitic carcinomatosis, sarcoidosis, hypersensitivity pneumonitis, pneumoconiosis, asbestosis, pulmonary alveolar proteinosis, bronchiolitis obliterans–organizing pneumonia, pulmonary

---

*Edited from Chap. 70, "Idiopathic Pulmonary Fibrosis," by Lynch JP III, Toews GB. In: *Fishman's Pulmonary Diseases and Disorders,* edited by Fishman AP, Elias JA, Fishman JA, Grippi MA, Kaiser LR, Senior RM. New York, McGraw-Hill, 1998, pp. 1069–1084. For fuller discussion of the topics dealt with in this chapter, the reader is referred to the original text, as noted above.

infection, malignancy, eosinophilic granuloma, and drug-induced interstitial lung disorders. Serologic studies are useful to exclude alternative diagnoses, particularly as pulmonary fibrosis indistinguishable from IPF may complicate collagen vascular diseases. High titers of antinuclear antibody may suggest an associated collagen vascular disease. Serum precipitating antibodies to *Aspergillus* species, *Thermoactinomyces* species, *Micropolyspora faeni,* or pigeon products may identify cases of hypersensitivity pneumonitis.[8] Angiotensin converting enzyme levels are not elevated in IPF.

Natural History and Prognosis

The natural history of IPF is characterized by a gradual but inexorable loss of lung function over months to years.[7,9–11] In rare cases the course is fulminant, progressing to fatal respiratory failure within 6 to 12 months. This variant has been termed *acute interstitial pneumonitis* or *Hamman-Rich syndrome.* Occasionally, the process stabilizes after an initial period of decline. Spontaneous resolution rarely occurs (fewer than 1 percent of cases). The 5-year mortality of IPF exceeds 40 percent, with the major cause of death being respiratory insufficiency. Lung cancer complicates IPF in 9 to 11 percent of patients. Severe derangements in pulmonary function, male sex, and low bronchoalveolar lavage (BAL) lymphocyte counts have been associated with a worse survival. A BAL lymphocytosis is associated with a higher rate of responsiveness to corticosteroids. Early institution of therapy may maximize the chances of averting progressive fibrosis and fatal respiratory insufficiency.

DIAGNOSTIC STUDIES

Chest Radiographs

Chest radiographs are abnormal in 95 percent of patients with IPF. The most common radiographic abnormalities are symmetrical bibasilar reticular or reticulonodular infiltrates with small lung volumes.[6,11] Strictly unilateral disease is rare. The infiltrates are distributed preferentially in the peripheral or subpleural regions of the lung.[3,12,13] With progression of disease, extension of the infiltrates to the apices and progressive shrinking of lung volumes occur. The presence of cystic radiolucencies ranging in size from 3 to 15 mm in diameter (honeycomb cysts) correlates with fibrosis, destruction of the alveolar architecture, and poor responsiveness to therapy.[3,13] Overlapping features—with areas of interstitial infiltrates, alveolar (ground-glass) opacities, and honeycomb cysts—may be present in individual patients. Pleural effusions are not a feature of IPF. Intrathoracic lymphadenopathy may be present but is uncommon. Conventional chest radiographs cannot reliably predict prognosis or responsiveness to corticosteroid therapy.[13] Asymptomatic patients with abnormal chest radiographs or mildly symptomatic patients with normal chest radiographs should raise the possibility of early and potentially treatable presentations of IPF.

High-Resolution Computed Tomographic Scanning

High-resolution computed tomographic (HRCT) scanning is more sensitive and specific for the detection of idiopathic pulmonary fibrosis than is plain chest radiography.[3,12–16] HRCT is noninvasive, does not require contrast, and can provide useful clinical and prognostic information. It has demonstrated that the pulmonary impairment in IPF is patchy and heterogeneous, tending to involve the peripheral (subpleural) and basilar regions of the lung in a disproportionate fashion. The characteristic features of IPF on HRCT include focal alveolar (ground-glass) opacifications, cystic airspaces, air bronchograms, ragged pleural surfaces, irregular or thickened bronchial walls or pulmonary vessels, and increased lung attenuation. Of these, the ground-glass, reticular, and honeycombing patterns appear to be the major abnormalities noted and are usually present in a mixed pattern.[12,16]

The HRCT abnormalities seen in IPF correlate with histopathologic manifestations of the disease. Areas of alveolar (ground-glass) opacification correlate with a cellular biopsy (active alveolitis). A reticular pattern, characterized by intersecting fine or coarse lines, reflects fibrosis, small (less than 5-mm) honeycomb cysts, or inflammation within alveolar septa, ducts, and airspaces. Air bronchograms (1 to 2 mm in diameter) on HRCT represent dilated peripheral airways surrounded by fibrotic lung tissue. Cystic lesions on HRCT greater than 5 mm in diameter correspond to macroscopic honeycombing on open lung biopsy. Pathologic and HRCT evaluations also reveal traction bronchiectasis, severe volume loss, anatomic distortion, and dilated pulmonary arteries in end-stage IPF. Zones of emphysema (particularly in the upper lobes) may be present concomitantly in smokers with IPF.

Though the predictive value of HRCT findings is uncertain, extensive ground-glass opacities and little honeycombing on HRCT appear to be associated with improvement in pulmonary functional parameters following corticosteroid therapy. By contrast, honeycomb cysts are seen in end-stage disease and predict minimal or no response to therapy. Reticular patterns are often associated with disease progression.

Pulmonary Function Tests/Exercise Tests

Pulmonary Function Testing

Characteristic physiologic aberrations in IPF include reductions in lung volumes, impaired single-breath diffusing capacity for carbon monoxide (D_{LCO}), and impaired oxygenation (either at rest or with exercise).[6,17,18] Expiratory flow rates are preserved, and the FEV_1/FVC ratio is usually normal or increased. Cigarette smoking can be associated with worsening gas exchange and increased lung volumes, reflecting a component of emphysema in addition to pulmonary fibrosis. Spirometry demonstrating reduced vital capacity and normal or supranormal expiratory flow should suggest the possibility of fibrosis. More sophisticated tests—including lung volumes, D_{LCO}, and cardiopulmonary exercise tests—are more sensitive than spirometry and may be helpful in monitoring the course of the disease. The D_{LCO} is an indirect measure of the pulmonary vasculature, with reductions reflecting destruction or loss of integrity of alveolar walls or capillary units. The D_{LCO} is the most sensitive of the static pulmonary functional parameters and may be reduced even when lung volumes are preserved. Severe impairment or a declining D_{LCO} has been associated with a higher mortality.[9,17,18] The 3-year mortality exceeds 50 percent when the D_{LCO} falls below 45 percent of predicted values.[11,17] Changes in total lung capacity do not correlate with histology, prognosis, or survival.[18] It should be noted that no physiologic parameter can distinguish alveolitis from fibrosis or predict responsiveness to therapy in individual patients.[7,10,18] Sequential evaluation of pulmonary function following institution of therapy is probably of most value. Failure to respond at 3 months implies a low likelihood of improvement with continued corticosteroid use.

Exercise Testing

Abnormal gas exchange is a hallmark of IPF.[10,18] The resting alveolar-arterial O_2 gradient ($P_{A_{O_2}}$–Pa_{O_2}) is increased in more than 85 percent of patients with IPF and invariably worsens with exercise. Exercise testing provides a reproducible and objective marker of extent of impairment.[18,19] Characteristic findings in patients with IPF include markedly limited exercise tolerance, widening $P_{A_{O_2}}$–Pa_{O_2} difference, respiratory alkalosis, reduced oxygen consumption, increased dead space (V_D/V_T), increased minute ventilation for the level of oxygen consumption, and low oxygen pulse.[18,20] Serial measurement of exercise gas exchange is the most sensitive physiologic indicator of disease course. However, exercise testing is expensive, requires considerable technical support, is modestly uncomfortable, and may be difficult in elderly or debilitated patients. Less formalized tests such as a 6-min walk test may be acceptable as a quantifiable index of disease progression (or regression).

Laboratory Tests

There are no laboratory or serologic tests specific for IPF. The erythrocyte sedimentation rate is elevated in 60 to 94 percent of cases, circulating antinuclear antibodies or rheumatoid factor is present in 10 to 20 percent, and circulating immune complexes are detected in 50 to 67 percent.[6,8] These various tests do not correlate with the extent or activity of the disease and do not predict therapeutic responsiveness.

Bronchoalveolar Lavage

Bronchoalveolar lavage (BAL) has been enormously helpful as a research tool in elucidating the key immune effector cells driving the inflammatory response in IPF.[21,22] Increases in polymorphonuclear neutrophils (PMNs), neutrophil products, activated alveolar macrophages, alveolar macrophage products, cytokines, growth factors, and immune complexes have been noted in patients with IPF. However, BAL has limited clinical usefulness.[23] Increases in the percentage of PMNs or eosinophils (or both) in BAL fluid are noted in 67 to 90 percent of patients with IPF. BAL lymphocytosis, found in fewer than 15 percent of patients with IPF, has been associated with a more cellular lung biopsy, less honeycombing, and a greater responsiveness to corticosteroid therapy.[5,22,24] Conversely, some studies have noted that patients with increased BAL eosinophils have a worse prognosis.[25] At present, BAL should be considered primarily an investigational tool.

Lung Biopsy

The optimal approach to biopsy in IPF is controversial. Surgical lung biopsies are considered the diagnostic gold standard. In some instances, transbronchial lung biopsies (TBB) may be acceptable provided that clinical, radiographic, and physiologic features are all consistent with IPF.[3,16,26] Transbronchial biopsies may also substantiate a variety of other specific diagnoses (eosinophilic granuloma, sarcoidosis, malignancy, hypersensitivity pneumonitis, infections, bronchiolitis obliterans, eosinophilic pneumonia, pulmonary alveolar proteinosis, etc.). Because of the small biopsy size (2 to 5 mm), TBBs cannot be used to determine the degree of fibrosis or inflammation or to assess prognosis in IPF.[27] A surgical lung biopsy (open or video-assisted thoracoscopic technique) can more accurately gauge the extent of inflammatory and fibrotic lesions.[15,28] Determining the degree of active alveolar inflammation (alveolitis) and end-stage fibrosis (honeycombing) has some prognostic value provided that representative samples are obtained from at least two sites in the lung. The most severely affected areas should generally be avoided. Biopsies of both moderately affected and grossly unaffected areas can yield information about the type and evolution of the disease process. Two or three biopsies from upper and lower lobes of the same side should be obtained. The tip of the lingula and middle lobe should be avoided, as nonspecific scarring or inflammation is frequently present in these regions.

Variability in the degree of cellularity and fibrosis from lobe to lobe (or even within the same lobe) within individual patients may cause problems in assessing the prognosis of IPF even when surgical lung biopsies are available.[3,27] Semiquantitative scoring systems and morphometric analytic techniques have been applied to more accurately assess degrees of fibrosis or inflammation. These sophisticated scoring systems grade the overall degrees of fibrosis and cellularity and quantify the nature and extent of the inflammatory and fibrotic processes within specific sites (alveolar walls, alveolar spaces, airways). Certain histologic features (alveolar wall metaplasia and smooth-muscle and vascular changes) correlate with honeycombing and fibrotic lesions. Distinguishing young connective tissue from end-stage fibrosis (honeycombing) has been advocated. Significant interobserver variability is a problem, even among experienced pathologists. No studies have determined whether the use of such complex scoring systems improves the prognostic value of a lung biopsy.

It should be recognized that surgical lung biopsy is performed in a minority of patients with chronic interstitial lung disease. This may reflect the low likelihood that lung biopsy will alter the course of treatment.[3,12,16] In the United Kingdom, transbronchial and open lung biopsies were performed in only 33 and 7.5 percent, respectively, of 200 patients with cryptogenic fibrosing alveolitis (CFA). The diagnosis of CFA was made on clinical grounds in most cases.[26] Clinical activities in the United States mirror this practice.[15] This reluctance to subject patients to open lung biopsy is most evident in older patients with "classic" clinical, radiographic, and physiologic features of IPF.

Thus, a flexible approach to biopsy is appropriate. The potential risks and cost associated with surgical lung biopsy must be balanced against the likelihood of altering the treatment plan or affecting efficacy. Ideally, a surgical biopsy should be performed in most patients. If positive, video-assisted thoracoscopic lung biopsy should be the preferred technique, as it is associated with less morbidity, less prolonged chest tube drainage, and reduced length of hospital stay than open lung biopsy.[28] Fiberoptic bronchoscopy with transbronchial lung biopsies may be acceptable for patients at increased risk for surgical complications (e.g., age greater than 70 years, extreme obesity, concomitant cardiac disease, extreme impairment in pulmonary function) when other features are classic for IPF.

PATHOLOGY

Histologic analysis of lung biopsies is critical to exclude alternative diagnoses and objectively quantify the extent of fibrosis and inflammation. The cardinal histologic features of IPF include varying degrees of alveolar septal (interstitial) and intraalveolar inflammation and fibrosis.[27] The presence of granulomas, vasculitis, minerals, or inorganic material should suggest diagnoses other than IPF. The pathologic abnormalities in IPF are heterogeneous and patchy, with a predilection for the peripheral (subpleural) regions of the lung. Some alveolar walls are usually spared, even within a heavily involved secondary lobule. Early in the course of the disease, the alveolar architecture is preserved, but the alveolar walls are expanded by edema and interstitial collections of inflammatory cells. Mononuclear cells predominate (e.g., lymphocytes, plasma cells, monocytes, or macrophages), but scattered PMNs and eosinophils are observed.

In the early phases of the disorder, focal aggregates of alveolar macrophages (termed *desquamative interstitial pneumonitis*) may be seen, which are absent in moderate or advanced disease. As the disease progresses, the chronic inflammatory infiltrates are less evident, and the alveolar structures are replaced by dense collagen. The alveolar walls are disrupted and destroyed, leading to dilated cystic airspaces (honeycombing). At this late phase, excessive lung collagen, extracellular matrix, and fibroblasts are apparent within the pulmonary interstitium, even though inflammatory cells may be sparse or absent. The alveolar epithelium also becomes hyperplastic, and squamous dysplasia may be observed in long-standing disease. Marked reactive smooth-muscle hyperplasia occurs in some patients, and enlarged pulmonary vessels and secondary pulmonary hypertensive changes may be present. Airspaces may also become distorted and give rise to "traction bronchiectasis." Emphysematous changes may be observed concomitantly in smokers with IPF. Emphysema is distinguished from honeycombing by the presence of fibrosis around the honeycomb cysts.

Diffuse alveolar damage is not a feature of early IPF but may be seen in patients with rapidly progressive disease or at necropsy in patients with fatal respiratory insufficiency. Hyaline membranes, fibrinous exudates, epithelial cell necrosis, and interstitial and intraalveolar edema may be prominent in this setting. As the process organizes and undergoes repair, type II cells proliferate along alveolar walls, hyaline membranes and airspace exudates resorb, and fibroblasts proliferate within the alveolar interstitium and alveolar space. This variant has been termed *acute interstitial pneumonitis* and is similar to pathologic descriptions originally cited by Hamman and Rich more than 50 years ago. These histologic features are not specific for IPF but may be seen with a large number of other disorders, including adult respiratory distress syndrome (ARDS); inhalation-, radiation-, or drug-induced injury; collagen vascular disorders, and infections.

Subgroups of patients have been characterized on the basis of their pathologic findings. Usual interstitial pneumonitis (UIP), the classic histopathologic variant observed in patients with IPF, is observed in the vast majority of cases. Defining features include a prominent fibrotic component, dense interstitial inflammatory infiltration, a minimal intraalveolar component, destruction of the alveolar architecture, and heterogeneous involvement.[27] UIP is characteristic of moderate to advanced disease and has been associated with a poor prognosis and low rate of responsiveness to corticosteroid therapy. By contrast, another histologic variant, desquamative interstitial pneumonitis (DIP), is associated with well-preserved alveolar architecture, minimal or absent fibrosis, a pronounced intraalveolar inflammatory component, and a striking uniformity throughout the lung architecture. The striking heterogeneity and peripheral distribution characteristic of UIP are lacking in DIP. DIP correlates with ground-glass opacities on chest radiographs or CT scans and a high rate of therapeutic responsiveness. The relationship of DIP to UIP is controversial. The fact that foci of both UIP and DIP may be observed within the same biopsy in individual patients suggests that DIP could be an early phase of IPF rather than a distinct disease. However, the remarkable dissimilarities in treatment-responsiveness and rate of disease progression argue that these disorders are distinct entities. The uniformity of the lung lesion in DIP suggests a reaction to an inhaled stimulus or agent.

Nonspecific interstitial pneumonia (NIP) is a third histopathologic variant of IPF.[29] Defining criteria include varying proportions of inflammation and fibrosis—which tend to be histologically uniform, suggesting that the lesions are of similar age and result from a single insult. The pathologic spectrum ranges from pure inflammation to dense fibrosis. The interstitial infiltrates contain primarily lymphocytes and plasma cells. Eosinophils and neutrophils are present in smaller numbers. The extent of fibrosis ranges from minimal to extensive, with honeycomb cysts. In its original description, scattered foci of bronchiolitis obliterans–organizing pneumonia were noted in 31 of the 64 patients with NIP and fibrosis. In addition, prominent accumulations of intraalveolar macrophages were noted in 19 and loosely formed granulomas in 5 of these patients. It is apparent that these histologic features overlap extensively with UIP and somewhat with DIP. The intraalveolar cellular component is patchy in nonspecific interstitial pneumonitis but uniform in DIP. The interstitial component is lacking in DIP and is overshadowed by the prominent intraalveolar collections of macrophages. The key feature distinguishing NIP from UIP is its histologic and presumed temporal uniformity. The clinical and radiographic features of NIP are similar to those of IPF, with bibasilar interstitial infiltrates, cough, dyspnea, and a subacute to chronic course. As with IPF, this histologic picture can also be seen in patients with collagen vascular disorders (10 of the 64 patients in the report providing its original description). The prognosis of NIP is considerably more favorable than that of UIP. In one series in which 48 patients were available for follow-up, 5 (11 percent) died of respiratory failure, while nearly half recovered completely.

The separation of pulmonary fibrotic disorders according to these histopathologic criteria is arbitrary. It is likely that UIP, DIP, and NIP represent stereotypical responses to diverse lung toxins or injuries. Additional studies assessing CT patterns, clinical features, and outcomes are required to determine the relationship between NIP and the other histologic variants.

THERAPY

Optimal therapy for IPF is a subject of contention. Treatment strategies are based on eliminating or suppressing the inflammatory component. Treatment options include corticosteroids, immunosuppressive/cytotoxic agents, and antifibrotic agents (colchicine or penicillamine), alone or in combination.[6,9,11,30–32] Only 10 to 30 percent of patients respond to existing therapies, and toxicity is substantial. Responses are usually partial and transient. Cures (sustained, complete remissions) are achieved in fewer than 5 percent of patients. Even among responders, relapses or progression of the disease following an *initial* response is common and suggests that these patients require prolonged treatment.[33]

Limited data exist regarding the determinants of responsiveness to treatment of IPF. Response rates may be higher when treatment is initiated early in the course of the disease, before irreversible fibrosis has developed. Factors associated with an improved prognosis and responsiveness to therapy include female sex, young age, less severe degrees of physiologic or radiographic impairment, a shorter duration of symptoms, a histologic pattern of desquamative interstitial pneumonitis on open lung biopsy, an increased percentage of lymphocytes on BAL, and ground-glass opacities on chest radiographs or CT studies.[11,16,19,25] Unfortunately, criteria for assessing disease activity and response to therapy have not been uniform. Changes in pulmonary function parameters have typically been used to identify response. However, increases of only 10 to 15 percent in even a single parameter of pulmonary function have in some cases been deemed favorable responses. Lack of change, or "stabilization," has also been considered to represent a response among patients previously exhibiting a rapid downhill course.

Patients being treated for IPF should be closely monitored for drug side effects and complications as well as for evidence of response to therapy. Patients should have a thorough evaluation 3, 6, and 12 months after diagnosis and initiation of therapy and at least annually thereafter. The assessment should include a careful history and physical examination, lung imaging (chest radiography or HRCT), pulmonary function testing (including diffusing capacity), and lung volume and gas exchange studies at rest and during exercise. Clinical deterioration is usually due to disease progression but may be caused by complications associated with IPF or adverse effects of therapy, including heart failure, pneumothorax, pulmonary infections, bronchogenic carcinoma, and thromboembolic disease. Identification of the cause of deterioration is important so that therapeutic interventions can be appropriately directed.

Corticosteroids

Despite a lack of prospective studies, corticosteroids have been the cornerstone of therapy for IPF for more than 3 decades. Unfortunately, only 10 to 30 percent of patients respond to therapy, and complete remissions are rare.[5,6,11,24,31] In the vast majority of patients, the disease worsens in spite of therapy. Most investigators initiate therapy with high-dose corticosteroids (40 to 80 mg daily of prednisone or prednisolone) for 2 to 4 months, with a subsequent gradual taper.[11,30,31] No studies have compared differing dosages or duration of corticosteroid therapy in matched patients. If responses occur with corticosteroids, improvement is usually noted within 2 to 3 months.

Maintenance corticosteroid therapy should be reserved for patients exhibiting *objective* improvement on pulmonary function testing or HRCT. Corticosteroid-responsive patients are maintained on prednisone chronically (sometimes indefinitely), but with a tapering dose. There are no prospective studies vigorously evaluating the optimal duration of the taper. However, dosage changes are generally done relatively slowly, aiming at a dose of 15 to 20 mg/day by 6 months. The dose of corticosteroid and rate of tapering should be guided by clinical and physiologic parameters. Since it is unlikely that corticosteroids completely eradicate the disease, treatment for a minimum of 1 to 2 years (and sometimes indefinitely) is reasonable for patients exhibiting unequivocal responses to therapy. Relapses or deterioration warrant an increase of the dose or the addition of an immunosuppressive agent.

High-dose intravenous "pulse" methylprednisolone (1 to 2 g once weekly or biweekly) has been used, but it has no proven advantage over oral corticosteroids. Patients failing to respond to corticosteroids may be candidates for immunosuppressive or cytotoxic agents.

Side effects of corticosteroid therapy are common and potentially disabling. Peptic ulcer disease, posterior capsular cataracts, and endocrine and metabolic alterations (hyperglycemia, hypokalemia, metabolic alkalosis, secondary renal insufficiency, impotence, menstrual irregularities, truncal obesity, and moon facies) can all occur. Musculoskeletal complications include osteoporosis, vertebral compression fractures, aseptic necrosis of femoral and humeral heads, and myopathy. Corticosteroid-induced myopathies may impair diaphragmatic strength and complicate the assessment of therapeutic efficacy. Psychiatric side effects include depression, psychoses, and inappropriate euphorias. These side effects occur especially in elderly patients. Finally, corticosteroid therapy suppresses immune and inflammatory responses to microbes and may render patients susceptible to opportunistic infection.

Immunosuppressive Agents

Immunosuppressive or cytotoxic agents (azathioprine or cyclophosphamide) should be considered as therapy for steroid nonresponders, patients experiencing serious adverse effects from corticosteroids, and those at high risk for corticosteroid complications (e.g., age over 70 years, poorly controlled diabetes mellitus or hypertension, severe osteoporosis, or peptic ulcer disease). Favorable responses have been noted with azathioprine or cyclophosphamide in 15 to 50 percent of cases.[9–11,30,34] However, few prospective or long-term studies have critically evaluated these agents.

Cyclophosphamide

Oral cyclophosphamide (Cytoxan, CTX) (1 to 2 mg/kg a day) has been associated with favorable responses in both idiopathic and collagen vascular–associated pulmonary fibrosis, even in patients previously not responding to corticosteroids.[11] However, data comparing cyclophosphamide with corticosteroids are limited. Neither of two randomized studies comparing the combination of cyclophosphamide and prednisone to prednisone alone demonstrated any long-term benefit of combination therapy over steroid alone.[30,35] Such studies do document that response to CTX is slower than with corticosteroids, with a delay of at least 3 months. Thus, a minimum of 4 to 6 months of therapy with CTX is required to judge efficacy.

Toxicity associated with CTX remains a major impediment to the routine use of this agent for IPF.[36] Hematologic monitoring is necessary, as leukopenia, anemia, and thrombocytopenia can all occur, necessitating adjustment of drug dose. Bacterial and opportunistic infections can also occur. Herpes zoster is frequently reported during cyclophosphamide therapy. Prophylaxis against *Pneumocystis carinii* infection with trimethoprim-sulfamethoxazole in patients receiving therapy with prednisone and CTX should be considered. Urologic complications include hemorrhagic cystitis and carcinoma of the bladder. Infertility may occur in males. Ovarian fibrosis, follicular destruction, ovarian failure, and amenorrhea are well documented complications in females. GI symptoms of stomatitis, nausea, and diarrhea may occur. Therapy with CTX also increases the risk of subsequent leukemias and other hematologic neoplasms.

Despite all of this, situations warranting the use of CTX in treatment for IPF are not infrequent. With adequate monitoring, consideration of CTX should be given, particularly in patients failing corticosteroids or experiencing adverse effects from corticosteroids.

Azathioprine

Azathioprine (Imuran) is a purine analog that inhibits DNA synthesis in a variety of cell lines and exhibits global immunosuppressive effects on both humoral and cellular immunity. Uncontrolled studies and case series have reported positive responses to azathioprine in the treatment of IPF. Only two prospective studies have evaluated azathioprine in combination with prednisone for IPF.[15,32] In one uncontrolled prospective study of 20 patients, 60 percent of patients responded favorably to a maintenance combination of azathioprine and low-dose prednisone.[32] However, a subsequent double-blind study failed to demonstrate any benefit of adding azathioprine to prednisone versus prednisone alone.[9]

Significant adverse drug reactions cause azathioprine to be discontinued in 20 to 30 percent of patients.[15] Nausea, vomiting, peptic ulcer disease, and diarrhea are the most frequent side effects. Leukopenia, anemia, thrombocytopenia, pure red cell aplasia, and pancytopenia also occur, and then hematologic monitoring is necessary. Elevation of hepatic enzymes occurs in approximately 5 percent of patients.

Thus, as with CTX, azathioprine should be considered as an alternative therapy in patients with progressive IPF that is refractory to corticosteroids or in patients experiencing the side effects of corticosteroids. An initial dose of 100 mg/day can be increased to a maximal dose of 200 mg/day as long as toxicity does not ensue. Blood counts should be monitored biweekly for the first 6 weeks and monthly thereafter. As with CTX, response to azathioprine may be delayed; accordingly, a 4- to 6-month trial is recommended.

Agents That Influence Collagen Synthesis or Fibrosis

Since therapeutic results achieved with immunosuppressive or anti-inflammatory agents have been disappointing, strategies employing antifibrotic agents (colchicine)[34] and penicillamine[36] have been advocated. However, the value of these interventions is unproven.

Colchicine inhibits collagen formation and modulates the extracellular milieu in vitro and in animal models. It suppresses the release of alveolar-macrophage–derived growth factor and fibronectin by alveolar macrophages from patients with sarcoidosis or IPF cultured in vitro and reduces the concentration of neutrophil elastase in BAL fluid from ex-smokers.[37] Data regarding colchicine as therapy for idiopathic or collagen vascular disease–associated pulmonary fibrosis are limited. However, side effects attributed to colchicine are rarely severe. As a result, oral colchicine (0.6 mg once or twice daily) may be considered as adjunctive therapy for patients refractory to corticosteroids, either alone or in combination with immunosuppressive and cytotoxic agents.

Penicillamine reduces collagen deposition in animal models of fibrosis and may have beneficial effects in rheumatoid arthritis and collagen vascular disorders.[31] Anecdotal responses to penicillamine have been noted in idiopathic pulmonary fibrosis and scleroderma-associated pulmonary fibrosis.[11,31] Penicillamine is toxic, and significant adverse effects (loss of taste, nausea, vomiting, stomatitis, nephrotoxicity, etc.) complicate its use in up to 50 percent of patients. In view of its toxicity and the lack of data affirming its efficacy, penicillamine has little value as therapy for idiopathic pulmonary fibrosis.

Other antifibrotic agents are currently being investigated for the treatment of pulmonary fibrosis. These include interferon gamma, interferon beta, and inhibitors of collagen production. Such agents are presently investigational.

Accepting that evidence for efficacy of any treatment is lacking, a recent international consensus statement by the American Thoracic Society and the European Respiratory Society recommended that patients who are deemed appropriate for treatment be offered combined therapy with the following initial regimen: (1) prednisone 0.5 mg/day for 4 weeks, with subsequent taper, plus (2) cyclophosphamide 25 to 50 mg/day, increasing to a maximum of 150 mg/day, or azathioprine 25 to 50 mg/day, increasing to a maximum of 150 mg/day.[38]

For recommendations regarding length of treatment and evaluation of response, the reader is referred to a more thorough discussion of this topic in the reference above.

Lung Transplantation

Single-lung transplantation is an important treatment option for certain patients with end-stage pulmonary fibrosis refractory to medical therapy.[39] The prognosis for patients with IPF who fail medical therapy is poor; many patients will die within 2 to 3 years. Severe derangements in pulmonary function (vital capacity or total lung capacity less than 60 percent predicted or diffusing capacity less than 40 percent predicted) and oxygen dependency have been associated with a 2-year mortality exceeding 50 percent. Unless specific contraindications exist, patients with severe functional impairment, oxygen dependency, and a deteriorating course should be considered for lung transplantation. Owing to limited donor availability, early listing is important, as waiting time for procuring a suitable donor organ may exceed 2 years. Unfortunately, patients with rapidly progressive or severe IPF may die while awaiting transplantation. Contraindications to lung transplantation include age over 60 to 65 years, unstable or inadequate psychosocial profile/stability, and significant extrapulmonary disorders (liver, renal, or cardiac dysfunction), which may negatively influence survival.

REFERENCES

1. Coultas DB, Zumwalt RE, Black WC, Sobonya RE: The epidemiology of interstitial lung diseases. *Am J Respir Crit Care Med* 150:967–972, 1994.
2. Iawai K, Mori T, Yamada N, et al: Idiopathic pulmonary fibrosis: Epidemiologic approaches to occupational exposure. *Am J Respir Crit Care Med* 150:670–675, 1994.
3. Raghu G: Interstitial lung disease: a diagnostic approach: Are CT scan and lung biopsy indicated in every patient? *Am J Respir Crit Care Med* 151:909–914, 1995.
4. Schwartz DA, Merchant RK, Helmers RA, et al: The influence of smoking on lung function in patients with idiopathic pulmonary fibrosis. *Am Rev Respir Dis* 144:504–506, 1991.
5. Schwartz DA, Van Fossen DS, Davis CS, et al: Determinants of progression in idiopathic pulmonary fibrosis. *Am J Respir Crit Care Med* 149:444–449, 1994.
6. Panos RJ, King TE Jr: Idiopathic pulmonary fibrosis, in Lynch JP III, DeRemee RA (eds): *Immunologically Mediated Pulmonary Diseases*. Philadelphia, Lippincott, 1991, pp 1–39.

7. Panos RJ, Mortenson RL, Niccoli SA, King GE Jr: Clinical deterioration in patients with idiopathic pulmonary fibrosis: causes and assessment. *Am J Med* 88:396–404, 1990.
8. Lynch JP III, Chavis AD: Chronic interstitial pulmonary disorders, in Victor L (ed): *Clinical Pulmonary Medicine.* Boston, Little, Brown, 1992, pp 193–264.
9. Raghu G, DePaso WJ, Cain K, et al: Azathioprine combined with prednisone in the treatment of idiopathic pulmonary fibrosis: A prospective, double-blind, randomized, placebo-controlled trial. *Am Rev Respir Dis* 144:291–296, 1991.
10. Raghu G, Hert R: Interstitial lung diseases: Genetic predisposition and inherited interstitial lung diseases. *Semin Respir Med* 14: 323–332, 1993.
11. Rudd RM, Haslam PL, Turner-Warwick M: Cryptogenic fibrosing alveolitis: Relationships of pulmonary physiology and bronchoalveolar lavage to response to treatment and prognosis. *Am Rev Respir Dis* 124:1–8, 1981.
12. Nishimura K, Kitaichi M, Izumi T, et al: Usual interstitial pneumonia: Histologic correlation with high-resolution CT. *Radiology* 182:337–342, 1992.
13. Terriff BA, Kwan SY, Chan-Yeung MM, Muller NL: Fibrosing alveolitis: Chest radiography and CT as predictors of clinical and functional impairment at follow-up in 26 patients. *Radiology* 184:445–449, 1992.
14. Grenier P, Chevret S, Beigelman C, et al: Chronic diffuse infiltrative lung disease: Determination of the diagnostic value of clinical data, chest radiography and CT with Bayesian analysis. *Radiology* 191:383–390, 1994.
15. Remy-Jardin M, Giraud F, Remy J, et al: Importance of ground-glass attenuation in chronic diffuse infiltrative lung disease: Pathologic-CT correlation. *Radiology* 189:693–698, 1993.
16. Wells AU, Rubens MB, du Bois RM, Hansell DM: Serial CT in fibrosing alveolitis: Prognostic significance of the initial patters. *Am J Roentgenol* 161:1159–1165, 1993.
17. Chinet T, Jaubert F, Dusser D, et al: Effects of inflammation and fibrosis on pulmonary function in diffuse lung fibrosis. *Thorax* 45:675–678, 1990.
18. Robertson HT: Clinical application of pulmonary function and exercise tests in the management of patients with interstitial lung disease. *Semin Respir Crit Care Med* 15:1–9, 1994.
19. Watters LC, King TE, Schwarz MI, et al: A clinical, radiographic and physiologic scoring system for the longitudinal assessment of patients with idiopathic pulmonary fibrosis. *Am Rev Respir Dis* 133:97–103, 1986.
20. Harris-Eze AO, Sridhar G, Clemens RE, et al: Oxygen improves maximal exercise performance in interstitial lung disease. *Am J Respir Crit Care Med* 150:1616–1622, 1994.
21. Lynch JP III, Standiford TJ, Rolfe MW, et al: Neutrophilic alveolitis in idiopathic pulmonary fibrosis: The role of interleukin-8. *Am Rev Respir Dis* 145:1433–1439, 1992.
22. Watters LC, Schwarz MI, Cherniak RM, et al: Idiopathic pulmonary fibrosis: Pretreatment bronchoalveolar lavage cellular constituents and their relationships to lung histopathology and clinical response to therapy. *Am Rev Respir Dis* 135:696–704, 1987.
23. Boomars KA, Wagenaar SS, Mulder PG, et al: Relationship between cells obtained by bronchoalveolar lavage and survival in idiopathic pulmonary fibrosis. *Thorax* 50:1087–1092, 1995.
24. Schwartz DA, Helmers RA, Galvin JR, et al: Determinants of progression in idiopathic pulmonary fibrosis. *Am J Respir Crit Care Med* 149:450–454, 1994.
25. van Oortegem K, Wallaert B, Marquette CH, et al: Determinants of response to immunosuppressive therapy in idiopathic pulmonary fibrosis. *Eur Respir J* 7:1950–1957, 1994.
26. Johnston ID, Gomm SA, Kalra A, et al: The management of cryptogenic fibrosing alveolitis in three regions of the United Kingdom. *Eur Respir J* 6:891–893, 1993.
27. Corrin B: Pathology of interstitial lung disease. *Semin Respir Crit Care Med* 15:61–76, 1994.

28. Bernsard DD, McIntyre RC, Simon JS, et al: Comparison of video thoracoscopic lung biopsy to open lung biopsy in the diagnosis of interstitial lung disease. *Chest* 103:765–770, 1993.
29. Katzenstein AA, Fiorelli RF: Nonspecific interstitial pneumonia/fibrosis: Histologic features and clinical significance. *Am J Surg Pathol* 18:136–147, 1994.
30. Johnson MA, Kwan S, Snell NJ, et al: Randomised controlled trial comparing prednisolone alone with cyclophosphamide and low dose prednisolone in combination with cryptogenic fibrosing alveolitis. *Thorax* 44:280–288, 1989.
31. Meier-Sydow J, Weiss SM, Buhl R, et al: Idiopathic pulmonary fibrosis: Current concepts and challenges in management. *Semin Respir Crit Care Med* 15:77–96, 1994.
32. Winterbauer RH, Hammar SP, Hallman KO, et al: Diffuse interstitial pneumonitis: Clinicopathological correlations in 20 patients treated with prednisone/azathioprine. *Am J Med* 65:661–672, 1978.
33. Hunninghake GW, Kalica AR: Approaches to the treatment of pulmonary fibrosis. *Am J Respir Crit Care Med* 151:915–918, 1995.
34. Peters SG, McDougall JC, Douglas WW, et al: Colchicine in the treatment of pulmonary fibrosis. *Chest* 103:101–104, 1993.
35. O'Donnell K, Keogh B, Cantin A, Crystal RG: Pharmacologic suppression of the neutrophil component of the alveolitis in idiopathic pulmonary fibrosis. *Am Rev Respir Dis* 136:288–292, 1987.
36. McCune WJ, Vallance DK, Lynch JP III: Immunosuppressive drug therapy. *Curr Opin Rheumatol* 6:262–272, 1994.
37. Rennard SI, Bitterman PB, Ozaki T, et al: Colchicine suppresses the release of fibroblast growth factors from alveolar macrophages in vitro: The basis of a possible therapeutic approach to the fibrotic disorders. *Am Rev Respir Dis* 137:181–185, 1988.
38. American Thoracic Society: Idiopathic pulmonary fibrosis: Diagnosis and treatment. *Am J Respir Crit Care Med* 161:646–664, 2000.
39. Hosenpud JD, Novick RJ, Breen TJ, Daily OP: The registry of the International Society for Heart and Lung Transplantation: Twelfth Official Report—1995. *J Heart Lung Transplant* 14:805–815, 1995.

30 | Hypersensitivity Pneumonitis*

Lynn T. Tanoue

A large number of agents cause hypersensitivity pneumonitis (HP). It is important to remember that there is a dynamic quality to the causes of HP. Some types of HP have apparently disappeared from their originally described clinical settings (e.g., bagassosis in Louisiana) but presumably exist in areas with similar agricultural or industrial settings. In addition, other forms of HP are being newly recognized (e.g., potato riddler's lung and machine operator's lung). Both the disappearance of previously described examples of HP and the appearance of new examples are due to changing agricultural or industrial practices that result in changes of exposure of subjects to antigenic material that can cause HP. At the present time, farmers' lung disease (FLD), bird fancier's disease (BFD), ventilator lung, and Japanese summer-type HP are the most commonly recognized forms. Drug reactions are sometimes described as representing HP, usually because certain bronchoalveolar lavage (BAL) fluid findings resemble those in HP. However, these are not HP, as the inciting agent is administered systemically and the pathogenetic mechanisms are probably different from those of HP.

Recognition of new examples of HP usually requires a cluster of new cases with a unifying exposure history. For example, introduction of a new metalworking fluid led to recognition of machine operator's lung in an auto parts manufacturing facility due to clustering of cases and a common unusual exposure (*Pseudomonas* in cooling fluid).[1] Since complete occupational and avocational histories are at times not obtained from patients with "pneumonia," it is likely that there are substantially more examples of HP that have not yet been recognized and described.

CLINICAL PRESENTATIONS: ACUTE AND CHRONIC

There are two different clinical presentations of HP.

In *acute HP,* dyspnea, nonproductive cough, myalgias, chills, diaphoresis, lassitude, headache, and malaise occur 2 to 9 h after a particular exposure. These symptoms typically peak between 6 and 24 h after exposure and resolve without specific treatment in 1 to 3 days (sometimes longer after a particularly intense exposure). Patients exhibit fever, tachypnea, bibasilar rales, and occasionally cyanosis. There is peripheral blood leukocytosis with neutrophilia and lymphopenia—but not eosinophilia—and BAL neutrophilia.

Chronic HP presents as progressively more severe dyspnea, nonproductive cough, weight loss, and often anorexia in a patient exposed to a recognized cause of HP. Symptoms are usually present for months to years. There is

---

*Edited from Chap. 71, "Hypersensitivity Pneumonitis," by Schuyler MR. In: *Fishman's Pulmonary Diseases and Disorders,* 3d ed., edited by Fishman AP, Elias JA, Fishman JA, Grippi MA, Kaiser LR, Senior RM. New York, McGraw-Hill, 1998, pp 1085–1098. For fuller discussion of the topics dealt with in this chapter, the reader is referred to the original text, as noted above.

typically no fever, but tachypnea and bibasilar dry rales are usually present. Symptoms and signs of cor pulmonale are not uncommon at presentation. In general, clubbing seldom occurs, although it has been reported in up to 50 percent of subjects with pigeon breeder's disease (PBD) in Mexico City. A proportion (20 to 40 percent) of patients with chronic HP present with symptoms of chronic bronchitis (e.g., chronic productive cough), some even without radiologic parenchymal densities on standard chest radiographs. Since most patients with HP are nonsmokers and have no other reason for the development of chronic bronchitis, these symptoms are probably a result of HP and may correlate with evidence of airway hyperreactivity in patients with chronic HP.

The reasons for the different clinical presentations (i.e., acute and chronic) of HP are not clear but could include differences of intensity and duration of exposure (low-intensity long-duration exposure tending to cause chronic HP; high-intensity short-duration exposure tending to cause acute HP). This is most clearly demonstrated in HP due to bird exposure. BFD (chronic exposure to low amounts of bird antigens) is associated with chronic HP. PBD can present as either acute or chronic HP. In the United States and Europe, pigeon breeders keep their animals in enclosures separate from human living areas. Exposure is then intermittent but relatively intense and is associated with acute disease.[2] In Mexico, birds are kept within human living quarters, so that exposure is at a low level but constant and is associated with chronic disease.[3] Therefore PBD in Mexico resembles BFD in the United States and Europe in type of exposure, clinical presentation, and prognosis. It differs greatly from the acute HP that characterizes PBD in the United States and Europe. Since the relevant antigens are similar in these two examples of bird-associated HP, it is likely that the type of exposure and not the antigen characteristics determines clinical presentation and prognosis.

Although the recognition of a new example of HP is usually associated with the acute form, most patients with well-recognized types of HP present with chronic disease. This might be related to the difficulties in establishing a link between chronic disease and chronic exposure as opposed to the relative ease in making the association of acute disease and acute exposure.

Thus HP, and particularly chronic HP, may be more prevalent than is readily apparent and may be confused with bronchitis or misdiagnosed as idiopathic pulmonary fibrosis (IPF). The latter may be particularly important because detailed histories are not always obtained from patients with IPF, the serum antibody levels to the agents responsible for HP tend to wane after cessation of exposure, and high-resolution computed tomography (HRCT) chest scans of chronic HP can resemble those of IPF.

RADIOLOGY

The chest radiographs of patients with acute and chronic HP differ significantly. In acute HP, chest radiographs demonstrate diffuse, poorly defined nodular radiodensities, at times with areas of ground-glass radiodensities or even consolidation. These radiodensities tend to occur in the lower lobes and spare the apices. Linear radiodensities (presumably representing areas of fibrosis from previous episodes of acute HP) may also be present. The nodular and ground-glass densities tend to disappear after cessation of exposure, so that chest radiographs may be normal after resolution of an acute episode of HP. HRCT scans often demonstrate ground-glass densities better than chest radiographs and at times reveal diffusely increased pulmonary radio-densities. They may also become normal after resolution of an acute episode. Pleural effusions or thickening, calcification, cavitation, atelectasis, localized radiodensities (coin lesions or masses), and intrathoracic lymphadenopathy are rare.

In chronic HP, chest radiographs are notable for diffuse linear and nodular radiodensities, with sparing of the bases, upper-lobe predominance, and volume loss. Pleural effusions and thickening are very unusual. HRCT scans of patients with chronic HP most commonly demonstrate multiple centrilobular nodules 2 to 4 mm in diameter throughout the lung fields, with some areas of ground-glass radiodensities, especially in the lower lobes.[4] Unlike sarcoidosis, the nodules are seldom attached to the pleura or bronchovascular bundles, and the border between the nodules and the surrounding lung is well demarcated. There are also well-delineated areas of increased radiolucency, which are presumably overinflated pulmonary lobules subserved by partly occluded bronchioles. The ground-glass densities and micronodules tend to resolve after cessation of exposure. Although these findings are suggestive of HP, they are found in only a subset (50 to 75 percent) of patients with HP. HRCT scans of the lungs of patients with HP can resemble those of patients with IPF.[4] A substantial prevalence of mild to moderate emphysema is also detectable by HRCT scans in nonsmoking patients with FLD. It is not clear if this represents lobular overinflation or emphysema.

EPIDEMIOLOGY

The prevalence of HP is quite variable in different populations, presumably because of differing intensity, frequency, and duration of inhalation exposure. Among pigeon breeders, 8 to 30 percent of members of pigeon-breeding clubs who participated in surveys exhibited PBD. Among farmers, 0.5 to 5 percent have symptoms compatible with FLD.[5] The prevalence of symptoms is lower in farms that use hay-drying methods that decrease exposure to the responsible antigens and increased after a wet summer season.

The population at risk and the season of exposure vary with the type of HP. For example, most cases of FLD occur in cold, damp climates in late winter and early spring, when farmers (usually male) use stored hay to feed their livestock. PBD occurs chiefly in men in Europe and the United States but predominantly in women in Mexico, owing to differing patterns of exposure.[2] BFD in Europe and the United States occurs in subjects who keep domestic birds and does not exhibit a predilection for either sex. Japanese summer-type HP occurs in June to September in warm, moist parts of the country, mostly in women without an occupation outside the home. HP demonstrates great variability of susceptibility among exposed populations and the apparent resistance to illness of most exposed persons. Possible reasons include differences of exposure or in host susceptibility.

In contrast to other pulmonary diseases, there is a remarkable predominance (80 to 95 percent) of nonsmokers in all examples of HP, which is substantially higher than the proportion of nonsmokers in similarly exposed subjects who are not ill. The mechanisms of this striking phenomenon are unknown but could include smoking-induced alterations of lung defense mechanisms or immunologic reactivity. This clinical finding indicates that the presence of active smoking is substantial evidence against the diagnosis of HP.

PATHOLOGY

Lung biopsies (almost always from patients with chronic HP) show chronic interstitial inflammation with infiltration of plasma cells, mast cells, macrophages, and lymphocytes, usually with poorly formed nonnecrotizing granulomas. There is often bronchiolitis and sometimes (in 25 to 50 percent of cases) bronchiolitis obliterans.[6] Organizing pneumonia is often also present, so that 15 to 25 percent of patients with HP have bronchiolitis obliterans with organizing pneumonia (BOOP). Conversely, patients with recognized BOOP may have HP as the cause of their BOOP. Varying degrees of interstitial fibrosis are also often present. The granulomatous interstitial inflammatory responses of HP and sarcoidosis can be difficult to differentiate. In contrast to sarcoidosis, however, the interstitial inflammatory cell infiltrate in HP occurs distal as well as proximal to the granulomas. The granulomas of HP also do not occur in groups and do not tend to occur near bronchi or in subpleural locations. Instead, they are usually adjacent to bronchioles and often single. Giant cells, at times with Schaumann's or asteroid bodies or cholesterol clefts, are present both within and outside the granulomas in patients with HP. When present, these specific histologic changes are quite helpful in making the diagnosis. However, the granulomas and respiratory bronchiolitis may not be present years after cessation of exposure, so only interstitial inflammation and fibrosis remain.

DIFFERENTIAL DIAGNOSIS

The symptoms, signs, and laboratory findings of acute HP can resemble those of many other lung diseases, including pulmonary edema, bronchoalveolar cell carcinoma, organic dust toxic syndrome, and some pneumoconioses. Acute HP is most often confused with infectious pneumonia (usually thought to be of viral or mycoplasmal origin and at times psittacosis in subjects exposed to birds). Chronic HP resembles IPF and in some instances is impossible to distinguish from it. The differential diagnosis also includes other causes of pulmonary fibrosis (chemotherapeutic agents, radiation, inhaled toxins, pneumoconiosis, etc.), granulomatous pneumonitis (sarcoidosis), and heart failure.

Organic dust toxic syndrome (ODTS) has been seen in some of the same populations exposed to materials that cause HP. ODTS can occur in a larger proportion of the exposed population than HP and is characterized by transient fever, dyspnea, nonproductive cough, peripheral blood leukocytosis, and BAL fluid neutrophilia; unlike HP, however, it is not associated with chest radiographic changes, permanent lung damage, or prior sensitization (as indicated by the absence of serum antibodies).[7] Patients presenting with ODTS tend to have more intense exposure of shorter duration than those who present with FLD.

A thorough and complete occupational and avocational history is essential to the diagnosis of both forms of HP. The history should seek to establish a link between a particular exposure (at work, at home, or elsewhere) and previous episodes of "pneumonia." Knowledge of other exposed persons with similar symptoms should be sought. If the history suggests a relationship between exposure and pulmonary symptoms, evidence of sensitization and the nature of the pulmonary inflammatory response should be determined. Sensitization is indicated by the presence of serum antibody to an agent known to cause HP.

Evidence of repetitive appropriate symptoms and laboratory and radiologic abnormalities associated with exposure to a particular environment is

TABLE 30-1 Major and Minor Criteria Used to Substantiate a Diagnosis of HP[a]

Major criteria for HP
    Evidence of exposure to appropriate antigen from history or detection of serum antibody
    Symptoms compatible with HP
    Findings compatible with HP on chest radiographs or high-resolution CT scan[b]
Minor criteria for HP
    Bibasilar rales
    Decreased diffusing capacity
    Arterial hypoxemia, either at rest or during exercise
    Pulmonary histologic changes compatible with HP
    Positive "natural challenge"
    BAL fluid lymphocytosis

[a]The diagnosis is confirmed if the patient fulfills all of the major criteria and at least four of the minor criteria and if all other diseases with similar symptoms are ruled out.
[b]Normal chest radiograph or HRCT acceptable if compatible pulmonary histologic changes are evident.

sufficient for a diagnosis of HP. In questionable instances, a "natural exposure" (i.e., documentation of appropriate symptoms and laboratory abnormalities after exposure to an environment suspected of causing HP) can be used to diagnose HP. A natural exposure challenge should not be considered positive unless there is objective evidence of a change in temperature, total peripheral white blood cell count, chest radiograph or HRCT scan, or increased A-a gradient as reflected by the development or worsening of decreased arterial P_{O_2}. A large proportion of lymphocytes in BAL fluid (usually over 40 percent) is suggestive of HP, although many other pulmonary processes can cause a BAL fluid lymphocytosis. In some patients, lung biopsy may be required to differentiate HP from other causes of diffuse pulmonary inflammation or fibrosis. Transbronchial lung biopsies often do not provide sufficient material to fully establish the presence and interrelationships of granulomas, bronchiolitis, and interstitial inflammation, so either open or thoracoscopically obtained lung biopsies are often required.

Clearly, a variety of lines of evidence are used to substantiate a diagnosis of HP. In patients in whom FLD is a question, major and minor diagnostic criteria have been proposed.[8] An adaptation of these criteria to HP in general is given in Table 30-1. The diagnosis is confirmed if the patient fulfills all of the major criteria and at least four of the minor criteria and if all other diseases with similar symptoms (e.g., sarcoidosis) are ruled out. A normal chest radiograph is acceptable if pulmonary histology is compatible with HP. A normal HRCT scan eliminates the possibility of active or chronic HP. However, it is possible to obtain such a scan between acute episodes, so a normal HRCT scan is acceptable if there are compatible pulmonary histologic changes.

LABORATORY FINDINGS

Despite the terms *hypersensitivity* and *allergic,* HP is not an atopic disease and is not associated with increased IgE or eosinophils. Patients with acute HP have a peripheral blood leukocytosis with neutrophilia. Nonspecific markers of inflammation, such as increased sedimentation rate and C-reactive protein, are often elevated during an acute episode of HP. There are a few reports of increased prevalence of rheumatoid factor in patients with HP. Antinuclear antibody or other autoantibodies are not present. There is increased uptake of gallium 67 in the lungs of patients with active HP, which declines with resolution of the disease. In contrast to sarcoidosis, the levels of serum angiotensin converting enzyme are usually not elevated. Prominent cellular abnormalities are also seen in the BAL fluid. At time points less than 48 h after exposure, the lavage is characterized by BAL fluid neutrophilia. At time points more than 5 days after the last exposure, a two- to fourfold increase in BAL fluid cell number and a BAL fluid lymphocytosis (typically 40 to 80 percent of total cells) are noted.

Virtually all patients with HP have easily demonstrable antibodies (typically IgG, IgM, and IgA) to the offending material in serum and often also in BAL fluid. A multitude of methods have been used to demonstrate these antibodies [simple agar diffusion ("Ouchterlony"), enzyme-linked immunosorbent assay (ELISA) and variants, indirect immunofluorescence, complement fixation, latex agglutination, counterimmunoelectrophoresis, radioimmunoassay, Western blot]. Unfortunately, antigen preparations are not standardized, and thus it is difficult to be confident of the meaning of a negative result unless the antigens have been tested against panels of sera from patients with and without HP. Even with this precaution, it is not always clear that the antigen used in the assay is the one the patient is reacting to. All in all, it is clear that reports of a negative "hypersensitivity pneumonitis panel" do not exclude the diagnosis of HP. The occurrence of serum antibody is also not consistently related to the intensity or duration of exposure. Further, serum antibody tends to wane after cessation of exposure, so patients with chronic HP who have not been exposed for some time may not have demonstrable antibody. For example, in FLD, approximately 50 percent of patients with initially positive serum antibody to *Mycobacterium faeni* (*Saccharopolyspora rectivirgula*) lose demonstrable antibody 6 years after cessation of exposure. Therefore, it is possible that patients with HP will have no detectable serum antibody owing to either use of an inappropriate antigen in the assay or the waning of antibody in time since the last exposure.

It should also be noted that serum antibody is also present in many exposed but not ill subjects in virtually the same amounts as in patients with HP. For example, in asymptomatic pigeon breeders without HP, the prevalence of antibody to pigeon antigens is 30 to 60 percent. Therefore, the presence of antibody indicates exposure and sensitization and not necessarily disease.

Skin tests (either immediate or delayed type) to detect sensitization to the suspected antigens are not useful, since extracts of agents that cause HP produce nonspecific reactions that do not indicate sensitization and do not discriminate between sensitized and nonsensitized subjects. In addition, preparations of antigens that cause HP are not readily commercially available. Tests designed to detect cell sensitization (most commonly antigen-induced lymphocyte proliferation or lymphokine secretion) are also not useful in the clinical diagnosis of HP, although they have been performed in specialized research settings. Patients with HP have depressed delayed-type skin reactivity to recall antigens, which is similar to that observed in patients with sarcoidosis.

Pulmonary function tests typically demonstrate a restrictive ventilatory defect with small lung volumes, normal or increased flow rates, increased lung elastic recoil, and usually decreased diffusing capacity. There is also the frequent occurrence of a mild obstructive defect and increased upstream airway resistance, probably related to either bronchiolitis or emphysema. Arterial hypoxemia with hypocapnia reflecting an increased A-a oxygen gradient either at rest or after exercise is common. Many patients with HP (20 to 40 percent) exhibit increased nonspecific airway reactivity, some (5 to 10 percent) also develop clinical asthma.[9] The increased airway reactivity and asthma tend to diminish after cessation of exposure.

PROGNOSIS AND TREATMENT

Prognosis varies considerably with the type of HP and even the geographic location. For example, FLD has a good prognosis in Quebec, even in farmers who continue to farm. However, FLD in Finland often results in significant physiologic impairment and even death. PBD has a good prognosis in the United States and Europe, whereas the same disease in Mexico has a 30 percent 5-year mortality. The reasons for these differences are not clear but probably include differences of the antigen and in the nature of the exposure.

Removal from exposure to the offending antigen(s) is usually sufficient to resolve symptoms and physiologic abnormalities within a few days for acute HP and within a month for chronic HP. In some patients, signs and symptoms of pulmonary fibrosis persist more than 6 months, suggesting a poor outcome.[2] Complete removal from exposure is most effective, but cleaning of the environment in situations when removal is impractical (for example in Japanese summer-type HP) can prevent further episodes of HP.

Systemic glucocorticosteroids are sometimes required to treat severe disease, although there is no formal evidence that such treatment is associated with long-term abatement of symptoms or radiologic or pulmonary function test abnormalities. The usual treatment is prednisone or prednisolone, 40 to 60 mg a day for 2 weeks, followed by a gradual decrease over 1 to 2 months. Patients with FLD treated with prednisolone demonstrated slightly more rapid resolution of some radiologic (ground-glass opacities) and some physiologic abnormalities than untreated patients (slight improvement of diffusing capacity, no difference in lung volumes or arterial P_{O_2}). However, there were no differences between the groups 6 months after the diagnosis of HP.[10] The above evidence suggests that systemic steroids may slightly increase the rate of resolution of acute pulmonary inflammation but have little or no effect on chronic residue of HP. Inhaled glucocorticosteroids, nonsteroidal anti-inflammatory drugs (e.g., cromolyn and nedocromil), or systemic immune modulators are not indicated in the treatment of HP.

If patients are removed from exposure before there are permanent radiologic or physiologic abnormalities, the prognosis is excellent, with little evidence of long-term ill effects. If removal from exposure is impossible, the use of an efficient mask during exposure can result in prevention of acute HP. If exposure persists, some patients (proportion unclear, but probably 10 to 30 percent) will progress to diffuse pulmonary fibrosis. Mortality from FLD is reported to be up to 20 percent and usually occurs after more than 5 years of recurrent symptoms, although there are a few case reports of death after acute massive exposure to the antigen. As noted above, the prognosis varies considerably with different types of HP. In general, long-term, relatively low-level exposure seems to be associated with poorer prognosis, whereas short-term, intermittent exposure is associated with a better prognosis.

Unfortunately, many patients with chronic HP present with pulmonary fibrosis and physiologic abnormalities that are only partly reversible after cessation of exposure.

REFERENCES

1. Bernstein DI, Lummus ZL, Santilli G, et al: Machine operator's lung: A hypersensitivity pneumonitis disorder associated with exposure to metalworking fluid aerosols. *Chest* 108:636–641, 1995.
2. Sansores R, Pérez-Padilla R, Paré PD, Selman M: Exponential analysis of the lung pressure-volume curve in patients with chronic pigeon-breeder's lung. *Chest* 101:1352–1356, 1992.
3. Craig TJ, Hershey J, Engler RJ, et al: Bird antigen persistence in the home environment after removal of the bird. *Ann Allergy* 69:510–512, 1992.
4. Lynch DA, Newell JD, Logan PM, et al: Can CT distinguish hypersensitivity pneumonitis from idiopathic pulmonary fibrosis? *Am J Roentgenol* 165:807–811, 1995.
5. Terho EO, Husman K, Vohlonen I: Prevalence and incidence of chronic bronchitis and farmer's lung with respect to age, sex, atopy, and smoking. *Eur J Respir Dis* 152(suppl):19–28, 1987.
6. Seal RM, Hapke EJ, Thomas GO, et al: The pathology of the acute and chronic stages of farmer's lung. *Thorax* 23:469–489, 1968.
7. doPico GA: Health effects of organic dusts in the farm environment: Report on diseases. *Am J Ind Med* 10:261–265, 1986.
8. Terho E: Diagnostic criteria for farmer's lung disease. *Am J Ind Med* 10:329–334, 1986.
9. Kokkarinen JI, Tukiainen HO, Terho EO: Recovery of pulmonary function in farmer's lung: A five-year follow-up study. *Am Rev Respir Dis* 147:793–796, 1993.
10. Mönkäre S, Haahtela T: Farmer's lung—A 5-year follow-up of eighty-six patients. *Clin Allergy* 17:143–151, 1987.

31 | Radiation Pneumonitis*

Lynn T. Tanoue

An estimated 65 percent of all cancer patients now receive radiotherapy at some point in the treatment of their malignancies. Radiotherapy seems destined to remain an important component of cancer treatment for the foreseeable future. In its early days radiotherapy was limited to poorly penetrating radiations, which delivered much higher doses of radiation to skin than to even relatively superficial tumors. As a result, severe early radiation reactions in the skin limited the doses of radiation that could be delivered to tumors. Advances in physics and engineering have led to the development of modern linear accelerators capable of delivering very high energy, deeply penetrating radiations, which can be used to deliver high radiation doses with great precision to tumors deep within the body. Precise systems for radiation dose measurement, or *dosimetry,* and precise algorithms for planning radiotherapy treatments have been developed. These advances have changed the dose-limiting radiation toxicities from painful early reactions in the skin to late reactions in the normal tissues surrounding the tumors. Radiation reactions in the lung therefore have acquired increasing importance with improvements in radiotherapy.

Many neoplasms involving the thorax are treated with regimens that include the use of radiotherapy to produce either cure or palliation. Radiotherapy is principally a localized and anatomically based modality. The success of radiotherapy hinges on delivering radiation selectively to the sites of malignant disease while sparing to the maximal extent possible the uninvolved normal tissues of the patient.[1] The radiation oncologist must consider the effects of radiation on the normal tissues within the treatment volumes. Many factors—including the radiation dose, the fractionation pattern of the radiotherapy, the volume of the tumor and involved margins, the prior or planned use of other therapies such as surgery or systemic chemotherapy, and the presence of other diseases—influence both the probability of controlling the neoplasm and that of producing toxic reactions. Optimal treatment frequently involves the use of multiple overlapping x-ray beams and possibly electron beams planned to encompass all of the cancer-containing tissues. Although treatments are carefully planned to include the smallest possible amount of healthy normal tissue, some normal tissue will necessarily be included in the radiation fields. The radiation sensitivity of the specific tissues in the irradiated fields and the acceptable level of risk for complications combine to limit the dose of radiation that can be administered. The planning of radiotherapy always involves a balance of benefit and risk, because the probabilities of controlling the malignant disease increase with increasing radiation dose, but the probabilities and severities of the potential complications increase with dose as well.

*Edited from Chap. 72, "Radiation Pneumonitis," by Rockwell S, Roberts KS. In: *Fishman's Pulmonary Diseases and Disorders,* 3d ed., edited by Fishman AP, Elias JA, Fishman JA, Grippi MA, Kaiser LR, Senior RM. New York, McGraw-Hill, 1998, pp 1099–1114. For fuller discussion of topics dealt with in this chapter, the reader is referred to the original text, as noted above.

The clinical course of lung injury related to radiotherapy includes a pneumonitic phase, developing weeks to months after radiation, followed by a fibrotic phase, developing months to years later. The current weight of evidence suggests that the pneumonitic and fibrotic processes are both manifestations of a common pathway of injury and response which begin on a cellular level within hours after large single doses of radiation. Histologically, one can recognize a typical sequence of events in the lung after large radiation doses. Within days to weeks, vascular congestion and intraalveolar edema and exudation occur, followed by infiltration of inflammatory cells and epithelial desquamation. Weeks later, collagen fibrils are deposited within areas of injury and interstitial edema, leading to a thickening of alveolar septa similar to that in hyaline membrane disease. The probability and severity of these changes are quite variable and depend on such factors as the radiation dose and treatment volume. The severity of the damage and volume of tissue affected determine whether a pneumonitic picture will be evident clinically. Resolution of inflammatory infiltrates and alveolar exudates, which can be improved by anti-inflammatory agents such as glucocorticoids, will correlate with symptomatic improvement and with resolution of radiographic opacities in the affected lung. These processes lead to pathologic changes that conform spatially to the areas where localized radiation was administered.

CONFOUNDING EFFECTS OF CHEMOTHERAPY

Many cytotoxic drugs employed as antineoplastic agents can produce pulmonary toxicity. Bleomycin, which kills cells by generating reactive free-radical species, can give rise to both pneumonitis and fibrosis. Mitomycin C and doxorubicin have also been associated with lung toxicity. As chemotherapy with high-dose alkylating agents is used more frequently in the setting of bone marrow or stem cell transplantation, agents such as cyclophosphamide, BCNU, and busulfan have been increasingly associated with clinically significant pneumonitis. The potential for pulmonary toxicity of these and other anticancer drugs raises concern for compounded toxicity related to treatment protocols combining systemic chemotherapy with lung irradiation.

Clinical experience suggests that regimens combining radiation with multidrug chemotherapy can result in significant risks of lung injury. However, it is often difficult to identify which of the drugs is responsible. For example, the administration of concurrent adriamycin or actinomycin D with thoracic radiotherapy should generally be avoided or, alternatively, the radiation doses should be significantly reduced. Sequential treatment with these drugs and radiation is less likely to produce lung injury. However, a phenomenon termed "radiation recall" has been well described, in which either of these two drugs given even several months after radiotherapy will produce an inflammatory reaction in the region corresponding to the radiation treatment fields. Although this reaction is best known in skin, it has also been well documented in the lungs. Radiation recall probably reflects the fact that the irradiated areas of the lung still retain residual, subclinical injury, which is exacerbated into clinical pneumonitis as a result of the additional injury from the drug. The biologic basis of the recall phenomenon is therefore analogous to that of the residual radiation injury, which decreases the ability of heavily irradiated lung tissue to tolerate a second course of radiotherapy delivered months or years later.[2]

CLINICAL SYNDROMES OF RADIATION-INDUCED PULMONARY TOXICITY

Acute Manifestations

It is relatively uncommon to observe acute pulmonary toxicity during the administration of fractionated radiotherapy. At relatively high therapeutic doses (50 to 60 Gy), however, acute radiation injuries to the tracheobronchial tree can be expected. Bronchoscopic examination of these patients is likely to reveal erythematous mucosa, with thickened secretions that can accumulate in and obstruct the airways. Although a majority of patients remain asymptomatic, occasional patients experience an irritative, dry cough. Antitussive agents such as codeine, adequate hydration, and reassurance are usually all that are required to manage this problem. Once the radiotherapy has been completed, the bronchial epithelium regenerates and heals over several weeks with a corresponding resolution of any symptoms.

Late Manifestations

Radiation Pneumonitis

A pneumonitic process frequently becomes evident 2 to 6 months following radiotherapy. At this time radiographs show alveolar opacities that generally conform to the treatment portals. The severity of radiation pneumonitis varies dramatically from patient to patient, even in those receiving identical therapeutic regimens. In most cases, the pneumonitis is asymptomatic, though radiologic abnormalities are quite common, having been found in some prospective studies in as many as 50 percent of patients. When symptomatic, this syndrome is often characterized by the abrupt onset of fever, cough, and dyspnea. The severity of symptoms depends on the extent of radiotherapy, increasing with the treated volume and the radiation dose. Symptoms in patients irradiated to limited lung volumes or to relatively low doses may consist of low-grade fever, cough, congestion, and chest fullness or discomfort. Any hemoptysis tends to be minimal. In more severe situations, dyspnea, high fever, and cough occur. When more than three-quarters of the total lung volume is irradiated to doses of 45 Gy—a situation, in fact, to be avoided—acute radiation pneumonitis is highly likely and can be extremely severe, producing respiratory distress.

It is important to distinguish radiation pneumonitis from infection, recurrent tumor, drug reactions, congestive heart failure, and other respiratory processes. Bacterial, fungal, viral, and *Pneumocystis carinii* pneumonias can be quite difficult to differentiate from injury induced by chemotherapy or radiation. The clinical course and the temporal relationship between therapy and the respiratory illness may aid in the differential diagnosis. The radiographic pattern of the infiltrate is very useful, with radiation pneumonitis often conforming to the outline of the sharply demarcated radiation portal. Bronchoscopy and lung biopsy can also be important diagnostic tools. Ruling out infection is particularly important, as treatment of symptomatic radiation pneumonitis relies on supportive care in conjunction with steroids, which would be relatively contraindicated with infection. Doses of gluco-corticoids generally can be tailored to the severity of the symptoms. Asymptomatic pneumonitis can be managed with close observation. Severe cases generally warrant treatment with 0.5 to 1.0 mg/kg per day of prednisone (or its equivalent) in divided doses. Response rates to steroid therapy between 20 and 100 percent have been reported, and dramatic clinical and radiographic improvement is not infrequently seen. Steroids should be tapered slowly after the patient is stabilized, because it is common to see a recrudescence of symptomatology when steroids are discontinued too rapidly. Failure to respond to steroid therapy carries the prospect of rapid disease progression.

Radiation Fibrosis

A more indolent fibrotic process can follow after either subclinical or symptomatic radiation pneumonitis.[1] This begins several months after radiotherapy and peaks in radiographic severity several years later. This fibrosis tends to occur in or adjacent to areas of prior pneumonitis, but can also occur in the absence of clinically overt radiation pneumonitis. Fibrotic changes and the retraction of the lung parenchyma from scarring occur in the irradiated regions. When the volume of lung irradiated is relatively small and the remaining lung parenchyma contains sufficient respiratory surface area, these changes tend to be asymptomatic. With increasing relative volumes of pulmonary fibrosis, a spectrum of symptomatology is possible, ranging from mild dyspnea on exertion to severe fibrosis with respiratory compromise, cyanosis, finger clubbing, and chronic cor pulmonale. At this end of the spectrum the syndrome can be life-threatening. In general, in the absence of other underlying lung disease, symptoms are mild when less than 25 to 30 percent of total lung parenchyma is involved.

Radiation-Induced Pleural Reactions

Pleuritis can also be seen 2 to 6 months following radiation. It can be associated with pleuritic chest pain, a pleural friction rub, and an exudative pleural effusion. Large effusions are, however, distinctly unusual and suggest other pathology. Like radiation pneumonitis, radiation-induced pleuritis can heal without significant residua or proceed through a fibrotic phase that generates pleural thickening.

DEFINING THE RADIATION TOLERANCE OF THE LUNGS

Whereas we customarily speak of radiation doses that can be delivered safely either to the whole body or to a particular organ, radiation tolerance is often defined as the dose that will yield a 5 percent risk of late radiation injury.[3] The tolerance of the lung varies with the volume of lung tissue irradiated. In addition, single-dose irradiations, fractionated irradiations, and irradiations given at low dose rates have different risks of injury and must be considered separately. Additional injury from surgery or chemotherapy or a prior course of radiotherapy must also be considered, as well as confounding effects of injury to lung tissue from coexisting cardiopulmonary disease and from the underlying malignancy.

Infections and immunologic reactions are also important. The clinical endpoints to define an index case of radiation pneumonitis also vary, because the severity of the lung injury spans a wide spectrum of diagnostic signs and clinical symptoms. Given the heterogeneity of clinical circumstances and biologic data in general, it is not surprising that the medical literature defining the risks for radiation pneumonitis and fibrosis is extremely complex and often difficult to interpret.

WHOLE-LUNG IRRADIATION

There are several circumstances in which the entire lung would be irradiated, including total-body irradiation (TBI) for hematopoietic transplantation, hemibody irradiation for palliation of widespread metastatic disease, and whole-lung irradiation electively or therapeutically for relatively radiosensitive tumors such as Wilms' tumor, Ewing's sarcoma, or Hodgkin's lymphoma. These are often circumstances in which chemotherapy is also being given. If administered as a single fraction, whole-lung irradiation, for instance in the setting of TBI for bone marrow transplantation (BMT), would result in an unacceptably high risk for pneumonitis. The most important factor in rendering TBI tolerable is that it is generally given at a low dose rate, so that the treatment is delivered over 1 to 2 hours. Still, in patients undergoing TBI for bone marrow transplantation, the incidence of pneumonitis is roughly 25 percent.[4] Fractionating the irradiation as well as delivering radiation at low-dose rate may also decrease the risk of lung injury.[5]

Pneumonitis in the BMT setting has a multifactorial etiology, reflecting not only the effects of radiation but also the effects of chemotherapy, graft-versus-host disease (GVHD), lung injury from tumor, opportunistic infections, and other risk factors. Cyclophosphamide is almost universally given with TBI, while the addition of other drugs is based on institutional treatment policies. Many anticancer drugs are known to injure the lung. BMT conditioning regimens that do not use TBI (which tend to use high-dose busulfan in place of radiation) in fact have rates of interstitial pneumonitis comparable to regimens including TBI. The presence of GVHD is also important, not only because it causes direct lung injury but also because the drugs used to control this disease can be toxic to the lung.

Historically, radiotherapy for Hodgkin's disease has utilized whole-lung treatment in situations where there is massive mediastinal adenopathy, hilar adenopathy, or overt pulmonary disease treated with chemotherapy. Risks of symptomatic pneumonitis ranging from 7 to 35 percent have been reported, with the risk highly dependent on the total radiation dose and the fractionation pattern.[6] When the whole lung is to be included, the available data suggest that the lungs should be treated through transmission blocks rather than with open fields. This reduces the total dose and the dose per fraction to the lungs, thereby reducing the risk of symptomatic pneumonitis to 4 to 7 percent over a broad range of total lung doses of 10 to 20 Gy. There is a suggestion that the addition of mediastinal irradiation to fractionated whole-lung radiotherapy increases the risk of pneumonitis. To many chemotherapists, the risk of radiation pneumonitis from such treatment seems too great. As a result, such patients are often treated primarily with chemotherapy (often with adjuvant low-dose radiotherapy), even though this, too, has significant risks for lung toxicity.

Lung radiotherapy using 12 to 14 Gy for pulmonary metastases in pediatric patients with Wilms' tumor (who also receive sequential doxorubicin and actinomycin D) is associated with a 10 percent incidence of pneumonitis.[7] Long-term follow-up in such children also shows restrictive lung disease, with total lung and vital capacities approximately 70 percent of the predicted values. In children receiving thoracic irradiation, inhibition of the normal growth and development of the lung parenchyma and bones from radiotherapy also produces significant morbidity. The effects of radiation on growth and development and the radiosensitivity of growing tissues raise special concerns in the treatment of pediatric patients.

PARTIAL-LUNG IRRADIATION

Assessment of Risk

Estimating the risks of radiation pneumonopathy for individual patients receiving fractionated external-beam radiotherapy is a daunting task because so many confounding factors must be considered. With lung cancer, the tumor size and location influence the volume of adjacent normal lung that must be irradiated. The volume irradiated should determine the number of capillary-alveolar units destroyed and therefore influence the risk of symptomatic radiation pneumonitis and fibrosis. This qualitative prediction is borne out by clinical experience, but quantifying the risks is not straightforward. The location irradiated is also important, because the upper lobe is less well perfused and therefore less important to gas exchange. Irradiation of this region produces less change in lung function than irradiation of areas lower in the lung. Treatment-related factors such as total dose, dose per fraction, and overall treatment time are also important.

Patients begin radiotherapy with a wide range of pulmonary functions, reflecting their age, smoking history, and the absence or presence of underlying cardiopulmonary disease. Because regional pulmonary fibrosis can be partially compensated by functional lung parenchyma, pretreatment lung status influences the severity of the symptoms. The clinical endpoints used to measure lung injury are quite varied and include symptom or quality-of-life scores, radiographic changes such as changes in lung density as assessed by computed tomography, pneumonitis, fibrosis, or other objective measures.

Pulmonary function tests are global organ measures that correlate quite crudely with symptomatology after partial-lung irradiation. A large tumor mass can cause localized obstructive or restrictive changes in lung function or phrenic nerve dysfunction, any of which may either improve or worsen as the tumor shrinks with treatment. These factors add to the variability produced by patient-to-patient differences in the treatment volume, dose, and fractionation. Thus the changes from radiotherapy in global lung function with regard to gas exchange, physiologic dead space, shunting, ventilation/perfusion ($\dot{V}/\dot{Q}$) mismatch, and respiratory surface area as measured by arterial blood gases, spirometry, and CO diffusing capacity ($D_{L_{CO}}$) are complex and highly individualized. Unfortunately, there are no firm tests or data to guide the development of tolerable regimens of radiotherapy for patients with borderline lung function; however, we know that treatment volumes should be minimized. If the initial FEV_1 is below 1.0 L or $D_{L_{CO}}$ is less than 50 percent of normal, large-volume radiotherapy (e.g., elective nodal irradiation for lung cancer) may well be excessively hazardous. Quantitative $\dot{V}/\dot{Q}$ scanning with superimposed radiation portals has been proposed as a potential prediagnostic tool but as yet is of limited utility. In selected patients, it may give a worst-case scenario to help the radiation oncologist decide on dose and volume of treatment.

TABLE 31-1 Dose Producing Clinically Apparent Radiation Pneumonitis after Conventionally Fractionated Radiotherapy

Lung volume irradiated	Dose (in Gy) producing pneumonitis	
	5% of Patients	50% of Patients
1/3	45	65
2/3	30	40
All	17.5	24.5

SOURCE: Data from Emami et al.[3] Doses are not corrected for heterogeneity in tissue density.

Clearly the most accurate and clinically relevant means to estimate risks for radiation pneumonopathy would be to study a large group of patients who receive a relatively standard dose and fractionation scheme for a given disease. As described above, the variability of the treatment volume for diseases such as lung cancer, as well as the frequent coexistence of other lung disease, especially chronic obstructive pulmonary disease (COPD) from tobacco use, makes this a difficult task. Nevertheless, one widely quoted expert consensus panel that reviewed the risks for late radiation toxicity using "conventionally" fractionated radiotherapy given in 1.8- to 2.0-Gy fractions developed the risk estimates depicted in Table 31-1 for radiation pneumonitis, stratifying by volume of lung irradiated.[3] These data reflect the incidence of clinically apparent radiation pneumonitis as defined by symptoms of cough and dyspnea as well as radiographic opacities corresponding to the treatment areas. Similar data regarding the incidence of radiation fibrosis are quite difficult to obtain, largely because of the wide spectrum of severity in symptomatology. Clinical experience would suggest that radiographic fibrosis is rare below 20 Gy and common above 40 to 50 Gy, with symptoms of respiratory insufficiency dependent on the volume of injured lung and on the presence of coexisting lung disease.

Local Tumor Boosting

In the treatment of lung and esophageal cancer, it is quite standard to boost the primary tumor and a small volume of the lung to total cumulative doses beyond 50 Gy and commonly to 60 to 65 Gy. Clinical data, notably the dose-escalation lung cancer trials of the Radiation Therapy Oncology Group, suggest that increasing doses to small volumes from ~50 to ~65 Gy is not associated with a significant increase in lung toxicity,[8] probably because the number of nonfunctional alveoli is not increased by this increase in dose. In most series of patients receiving radical thoracic radiotherapy, the risk of symptomatic radiation pneumonitis is usually around 5 to 10 percent, and some degree of radiographic fibrosis is almost universal.

Breast Cancer

Breast cancer radiotherapy, whether after lumpectomy or mastectomy, typically uses opposed tangential beams that irradiate a volume of lung anterolateral to a plane demarcating the midchest to the lateral axillary line to doses of 45 to 50 Gy in 23 to 25 fractions. The volume of the ipsilateral lung irradiated can be estimated for individual patients from the simulator films and is typically about 20 percent of the lung volume. If supraclavicular and axillary nodes are irradiated as well, the apex of the lung (roughly another 10 to 15 percent of ipsilateral lung volume) is also irradiated. The incidence of symptomatic pneumonitis from tangential fields alone is roughly 0.5 percent, with some series documenting an increased risk with increasing lung volume.[9] Nodal irradiation increases the risk for pneumonitis to 0.5 to 1.5 percent. Risk further increases to as high as 9 percent when chemotherapy is given concurrently. The risk of pneumonitis is much lower when chemotherapy and radiation are given sequentially.

Early-Stage Hodgkin's Disease

Radiotherapy for early-stage Hodgkin's lymphoma, using moderate doses (40 to 45 Gy in 1.5- to 2.0-Gy fractions) and large volumes to treat lymph node–bearing regions, has represented a remarkable success story in oncology. Because it now has produced very high cure rates in a young patient population, allowing for extended follow-up over several decades, this experience has also produced considerable data regarding late radiation toxicities. In these protocols, the chest is irradiated with treatment portals, generically called "mantle fields." With modern radiation techniques that use sequential shrinking fields, the incidence of symptomatic radiation pneumonitis is 3 to 4 percent. The risk of pneumonitis increases to roughly 10 percent when full doses of both chemotherapy (MOPP or ABVD-type combinations) and radiation to a mantle field are given sequentially. Studies on pulmonary function in Hodgkin's disease patients suggest that a transient reduction in FEV_1 and vital capacity, on the order of 5 to 20 percent, occurs 3 to 9 months after radiotherapy, corresponding to the period of pneumonitis.[10] There tends to be some recovery by roughly 1 year. Late follow-up of pulmonary function in Hodgkin's disease patients further suggests that mantle field radiotherapy is associated with small and for the most part clinically insignificant reductions in vital capacity and D_{LCO}. These decreases in pulmonary function tests are associated with minor or no symptomatology, even for treatment regimens that included sequential chemotherapy with doxorubicin or bleomycin. In the setting where lower-dose (20 to 25 Gy) involved-field radiotherapy is delivered after chemotherapy, the incidence of clinical pneumonitis is quite low, although small changes in spirometric and diffusion capacity parameters can still be detected in up to 50 percent of the patients.

REFERENCES

1. Marks LB: The pulmonary effects of thoracic irradiation. *Oncology* 8:89–104, 1994.
2. Casarett GW: *Radiation Histopathology.* Boca Raton, FL, CRC Press, 1980.
3. Emami B, Lyman J, Brown A, et al: Tolerance of normal tissue to therapeutic irradiation. *Int J Radiat Oncol Biol Phys* 21:109–122, 1991.
4. Shank B: Radiotherapeutic principles of bone marrow transplantation, in Forman S, Thomas ED, Blume K (eds): *Bone Marrow Transplantation.* Boston, Blackwell, 1994, pp 96–113.
5. Deeg HJ, Sullivan KM, Buckner CD, et al: Marrow transplantation for acute nonlymphoblastic leukemia in first remission: Toxicity and long-term follow-up of patients conditioned with single dose or fractionated total body irradiation. *Bone Marrow Transplant* 1:151–157, 1986.
6. Tarbell NJ, Thompson L, Mauch P: Thoracic irradiation in Hodgkin's disease: Disease control and long-term complications. *Int J Radiat Oncol Biol Phys* 18:275–281, 1990.

7. Green DM, Finklestein JZ, Tefft ME, Norkool P: Diffuse interstitial pneumonitis after pulmonary irradiation for metastatic Wilms' tumor. *Cancer*
63:450–453, 1989.
8. Cox JD, Azarnia N, Byhardt RW, et al: A randomized phase I/II trial of hyper-
fractionated radiation therapy with total doses of 60.0 Gy to 79.2 Gy: Possible
survival benefit with 69.6 Gy in favorable patients with Radiation Therapy
Oncology Group Stage III non-small cell lung carcinoma: Report of radiation
therapy oncology group 83-11. *J Clin Oncol* 8:1543–1555, 1990.
9. Lingos TI, Recht A, Vicini F, et al: Radiation pneumonitis in breast cancer patients treated with conservative surgery and radiation therapy. *Int J Radiat Oncol
Biol Phys* 21:355–360, 1991.
10. Horning SJ, Adhikari A, Rizk N, et al: Effect of treatment for Hodgkin's disease
on pulmonary function: Results of a prospective study. *J Clin Oncol* 12:297–305,
1994.

32 | Pulmonary Manifestations of the Collagen Vascular Diseases*

Lynn T. Tanoue

The pleuropulmonary complications associated with the collagen vascular diseases are frequent occurrences. It would be the exception rather than the rule for an individual to avoid one of these during the course of such an illness. These patients also experience an increased incidence of pneumonia, both community-acquired as well as associated with the immunosuppressive drugs employed for treatment. These cytotoxic drugs, particularly methotrexate and gold, can also induce various noninfectious interstitial reactions, which are often difficult to distinguish from a primary interstitial complication of a collagen vascular disease.

Although most pulmonary complications appear in an established case of a collagen vascular disease, in some situations the lung disease precedes the more typical manifestations. For example, in both rheumatoid arthritis and polymyositis-dermatomyositis, the interstitial lung disease may precede the joint and muscle disease for several months to several years. Pleuritis with or without effusion sometimes heralds the onset of rheumatoid arthritis or systemic lupus erythematosus.

The actual incidence of the pleuropulmonary complications (Table 32-1) is variable. It does appear that the incidence of interstitial lung disease is increasing for most of the collagen vascular diseases. This is primarily due to increased recognition, aided by the use of high-resolution computed tomography (HRCT) and bronchoalveolar lavage, as well as by the use of physiologic measures of gas exchange during exercise.

HISTOLOGIC SPECTRUM OF PARENCHYMAL REACTIONS IN COLLAGEN VASCULAR DISEASE

Interstitial Lung Disease

Interstitial involvement is a common respiratory manifestation of the collagen vascular disorders. It can present with diffuse alveolar damage and/or with one of a number of inflammatory responses. *Diffuse alveolar damage* is the underlying histologic lesion seen in the adult respiratory distress syndrome, idiopathic acute interstitial pneumonitis (Hamman-Rich syndrome), and cytotoxicity from some drugs. This damage consists of a mixed interstitial inflammatory infiltrate, interstitial edema and fibrin deposition, and characteristic intraalveolar hyaline membrane formation. An acute immunologic pneumonia in systemic lupus

*Edited from Chap. 73, "Pulmonary Manifestations of the Collagen Vascular Diseases," by Schwarz MI. In: *Fishman's Pulmonary Diseases and Disorders,* 3d ed., edited by Fishman AP, Elias JA, Fishman JA, Grippi MA, Kaiser LR, Senior RM. New York, McGraw-Hill, 1998, pp 1115–1132. For fuller discussion of topics dealt with in this chapter, the reader is referred to the original text, as noted above.

TABLE 32-1 Pulmonary Complications of the Collagen Vascular Diseases

Manifestation	Relative frequency (0–4)						
	SLE	RA	SS	PM-DM	MCTD	AS	Sjögren's
Respiratory muscle dysfunction	2	0	0	2	1	0	0
Aspiration pneumonia	0	0	3	3	2	0	2
Primary pulmonary hypertension	2	1	4	1	2	0	0
Vasculitis	2	2	0	1	1	0	0
Interstitial lung disease	2	3	4	3	2	1	3
Capillaritis+DAH	2	1	1	1	1	0	0
Bland DAH	2	0	0	0	1	0	0
Diffuse alveolar damage	2	0	0	2	1	0	0
Cellular interstitial pneumonitis	2	3	2	3	3	0	1
Lymphocytic interstitial pneumonitis	1	2	1	0	0	0	3
Usual interstitial pneumonitis	2	3	4	3	2	1	1
Honeycomb lung	1	2	4	3	2	1	1
Bronchiolitis obliterans–organizing pneumonia	1	3	1	3	2	0	1
Bronchiolitis	1	2	1	0	1	0	1
Obliterative bronchiolitis	0	2	0	0	0	0	1
Pleural effusion	2	3	1	0	2	0	1
Parenchymal nodules	0	2	0	0	0	0	1

KEY: SLE, systemic lupus erythematosus; RA, rheumatoid arthritis; SS, systemic sclerosis (scleroderma); PM-DM, polymyositis-dermatomyositis; MCTD, mixed connective tissue disease; AS, ankylosing spondylitis; Sjögren's, Sjögren's syndrome; DAH, diffuse alveolar hemorrhage.

erythematosus (acute lupus pneumonitis) and in polymyositis-dermatomyositis may demonstrate this underlying histologic appearance.

Cellular interstitial pneumonitis refers to a lymphoplasmacytic infiltration of the interstitium with minimal or no collagen deposition. This pneumonitis probably represents an early phase of usual interstitial pneumonitis (see below) and is most frequently seen with rheumatoid arthritis, polymyositis-dermatomyositis, and mixed connective tissue disease.

Lymphocytic interstitial pneumonitis refers to a monotonous infiltration of the interstitium by mature lymphocytes, which tend to form germinal centers within the interstitium. If unresponsive to treatment, lymphocytic interstitial pneumonitis can progress to usual interstitial pneumonitis and end-stage honeycomb lung. Among the collagen vascular diseases, this pneumonitis most commonly accompanies the primary form of Sjögren's syndrome as well as a secondary form of Sjögren's syndrome appearing with other collagen vascular diseases, particularly rheumatoid arthritis.

Usual interstitial pneumonitis is the underlying lesion of idiopathic pulmonary fibrosis and can also appear in all the collagen vascular diseases, thereby representing the most common interstitial reaction in this group of diseases. It consists of varying degrees of mononuclear cell infiltration and fibroblastic proliferation, leading to collagen deposition within the alveolar interstitium. With progression, this fibrotic reaction results in marked distortion of the lung architecture; what remains are 2- to 3-mm cystic spaces lined by metaplastic epithelium, the so-called honeycomb lung.

Bronchiolitis obliterans–organizing pneumonia (BOOP) is a distinctive histologic lesion that follows a variety of insults to the alveolar structures from drugs, infection, radiation, and idiopathic causes. BOOP can also complicate the collagen vascular diseases, particularly rheumatoid arthritis and polymyositis-dermatomyositis. BOOP has the potential for being a completely reversible lesion; however, with continuing injury, it may progress to usual interstitial pneumonia and honeycomb lung.

Pulmonary Vascular Disease

A form of idiopathic pulmonary hypertension that most commonly appears in patients with scleroderma is now being increasingly recognized in systemic lupus erythematosus, rheumatoid arthritis, and mixed connective tissue disease. It is histologically identical to the syndrome of primary pulmonary hypertension seen in young women without collagen vascular disease. This is a proliferative disorder (plexogenic arteriopathy) affecting the arterioles and small muscular pulmonary arteries. This form of pulmonary hypertension must be differentiated from secondary forms resulting from hypoxic vasoconstriction induced by interstitial lung disease, chronic thromboembolic disease, or vasculitis.[1]

Diffuse Alveolar Hemorrhage

Diffuse alveolar hemorrhage is recognized by the filling of the alveolar spaces with red blood cells. With recurrent episodes, intraalveolar and interstitial hemosiderin is deposited and the potential for interstitial fibrosis exists. There are two histologic appearances of diffuse alveolar hemorrhage. One is devoid of inflammation and is referred to as *bland hemorrhage,* which is similar in histologic appearance to idiopathic pulmonary hemosiderosis. The other, pulmonary capillaritis, is a unique neutrophilic infiltration of the alveolar interstitium which results in necrosis and loss of integrity of the alveolar-capillary basement membrane, capillary destruction and thrombosis, and an outpouring of red blood cells into the alveolar space. This lesion is most commonly seen in the systemic vasculitides, particularly Wegener's granulomatosis and microscopic polyangiitis, the small-vessel variant of polyarteritis nodosa. Of the collagen vascular diseases, both bland pulmonary hemorrhage and diffuse alveolar hemorrhage secondary to pulmonary capillaritis appear most frequently in systemic lupus erythematosus.[2] Cases of pulmonary capillaritis have also been reported to occur in rheumatoid arthritis, Sjögren's syndrome, polymyositis-dermatomyositis, and mixed connective tissue disease.

Bronchiolitis

Bronchiolitis refers to an inflammatory-fibrotic process involving the terminal and respiratory bronchioles and possibly the surrounding alveolar structures. Respiratory bronchiolitis is primarily seen in smokers with or without an associated collagen vascular disease. There is also a primary form of respiratory bronchiolitis that complicates the collagen vascular diseases, most often appearing in rheumatoid arthritis and Sjögren's syndrome. Histologically, there is a mononuclear cell infiltration of the wall of the bronchiole without impingement of the bronchiolar lumen. Bronchiolitis obliterans, or obliterative bronchiolitis, however, is a concentric fibrous obliteration of the bronchiolar lumen leading to a severe obstructive lung disease. Bronchiolitis obliterans is most often reported as a complication of rheumatoid arthritis.

Parenchymal Nodules

Noninfectious inflammatory parenchymal nodules occur in both rheumatoid arthritis and Sjögren's syndrome. In rheumatoid arthritis, the nodules are referred to as *necrobiotic* or *rheumatoid nodules.* This lesion is found both in the pleura and lung parenchyma and is identical in appearance to subcutaneous rheumatoid nodules. In the lung parenchyma, these nodules are located in the interlobular septa and in the subpleural parenchyma. The necrobiotic nodule is made up of palisading histiocytes, giant cells, and other mononuclear cells surrounding an area of fibrinoid debris. In Sjögren's syndrome, a rounded lesion known as pseudolymphoma can occasionally be detected on the chest radiograph. Pseudolymphoma is considered to be a localized form of lymphocytic interstitial pneumonia and is made up of a dense infiltrate of lymphocytes and histiocytes with occasional granuloma formation. It has potential for lymphomatous transformation.

CLINICAL FEATURES OF THE COLLAGEN VASCULAR DISEASES

Systemic Lupus Erythematosus

Systemic lupus erythematosus (SLE) is characterized by the production of antibodies against various cellular antigens derived from the nucleus, cytoplasm, and cell membrane. While a number of situations (Table 32-2) can cause an acute respiratory type illness, most patients with SLE who present with a febrile illness, cough, and new pulmonary infiltrates will have an infectious pneumonia. Infection can be community-acquired or result from immunosuppressive treatment. Infectious pneumonia represents the most common cause of pulmonary disease in SLE. Infections in general represent the most common reason for death (33 to 77 percent) in these patients.[3] Bronchoalveolar lavage can be extremely helpful in excluding an infectious pneumonia in the immunocompromised SLE patient.

Pulmonary embolization is another important consideration in an acutely dyspneic SLE patient, reportedly occurring in up to 25 percent and a significant cause of mortality.[4] The occurrence of thromboembolic disease correlates with the presence in the serum of acquired antiphospholipid antibodies (lupus anticoagulant and anticardiolipin). In large series, up to 34 percent of SLE patients have the antiphospholipid syndrome. Other clinical features associated with this syndrome are thrombocytopenia, recurrent venous thrombosis, hemolytic anemia, leg ulcers, and fetal loss.[5] Other causes for acute respiratory failure in SLE include a volume overload state due either to renal failure or to congestive heart failure secondary to myocarditis. Uremic pneumonitis with underlying diffuse alveolar damage is also a possible cause of an acutely dyspneic SLE patient.

TABLE 32-2 Acute Lung Syndromes in Systemic Lupus Erythematosus

Community-acquired or immunocompromised pneumonias
Pulmonary embolization
Uremic pneumonitis
Cardiogenic pulmonary edema
Acute reversible hypoxemia syndrome
Acute lupus pneumonitis
Diffuse alveolar hemorrhage
Pleurisy

A syndrome (acute reversible hypoxemia) occurring in acutely ill SLE patients who are experiencing systemic exacerbations has recently been described.[6] These patients have hypoxemia and a widened alveolar-arterial oxygen gradient, but both the chest radiograph and ventilation-perfusion lung scans are normal. It is postulated that there is complement-activated neutrophil aggregation in the pulmonary vasculature. With corticosteroid treatment of the acute exacerbation, the hypoxemia resolves.

Acute Lupus Pneumonitis

Acute lupus pneumonitis is a clinical syndrome whose underlying histology is diffuse alveolar damage, BOOP, cellular interstitial pneumonitis, or a combination of these. Acute lupus pneumonitis may be the presenting manifestation of SLE in up to 50 percent of cases who have this complication.[7] It also appears during a flare of the other systemic components of SLE—particularly pleuritis, pericarditis, arthritis, and nephritis—but is still a relatively uncommon complication (less than 5 percent). It is reportedly more common in the postpartum period.[8] This pneumonitis tends to recur, and cases have been documented that have progressed to a more chronic interstitial lung disease (usual interstitial pneumonia). The resultant acute respiratory failure often requires assisted mechanical ventilation. The chest radiograph demonstrates bilateral alveolar infiltrates, which can be patchy or densely consolidated and are often accompanied by pleural effusions and cardiomegaly due to underlying pericardial effusion or myocarditis. White blood cell counts and sedimentation rates are elevated, and serum complement is often low. Because of the difficulty in distinguishing acute lupus pneumonitis from an infectious pneumonia, a bronchoalveolar lavage and sometimes an open (thoracoscopic) lung biopsy are indicated prior to instituting anti-inflammatory and immunosuppressive therapy. Although recent data are not available, the mortality rate has been reported to be as high as 50 percent.[7]

Diffuse Alveolar Hemorrhage

In contrast to acute lupus pneumonitis, diffuse alveolar damage usually appears in well-documented cases of SLE, though it can occasionally be the presenting manifestation.[9] The underlying histopathology is either bland pulmonary hemorrhage or pulmonary capillaritis. The incidence of diffuse alveolar hemorrhage (approximately 5 percent) in a systemic lupus erythematosus population appears to be increasing.

Diffuse alveolar hemorrhage can present with symptoms reminiscent of an infectious pneumonia or acute lupus pneumonitis. The additional symptom of hemoptysis should raise the possibility of this diagnosis. However, not all patients with diffuse alveolar hemorrhage will have hemoptysis when first seen. A falling hematocrit, an elevated diffusing capacity due to the availability of hemoglobin to combine with carbon monoxide, or a serosanguineous bronchoalveolar lavage may be the first clue to this diagnosis. The chest radiograph shows diffuse alveolar infiltrates. Pleuritis and pericarditis are not prominent features as they are in acute lupus pneumonitis. The mortality rate is approximately 50 percent. Recurrence is the rule.

There are no controlled clinical trials for the treatment of either acute lupus pneumonitis or diffuse alveolar hemorrhage. Corticosteroids, azathioprine, cyclophosphamide, and plasmapheresis in various combinations have been employed. Once infection has been excluded, therapy can be instituted with intravenous methyl prednisolone (1 to 2 g daily in divided doses) for 3 to 4 days prior to tapering. Concomitantly, either oral or parenteral cyclophosphamide or azathioprine are administered. Cytoxan can be continued as oral therapy (2 to 3 mg/kg daily) or monthly intravenous therapy. Azathioprine is continued as oral therapy (2 to 3 mg/kg daily). Plasmapheresis and immune globulin therapy have no proven efficacy to date.

Lupus Pleuritis

Pleurisy and pleural effusion are the most common primary pulmonary complications of systemic lupus erythematosus, occurring in 50 to 80 percent.[10] Pleurisy and pleural effusion may also be the presenting and sole manifestations. Lupus pleuritis is usually recurrent and may accompany acute lupus pneumonitis. Patients complain of pleuritic pain, fever, and dyspnea. The chest radiograph may be normal (dry pleurisy) or demonstrate small to moderate pleural effusions, which are bilateral in 50 percent of patients. Massive effusions are rare.

The effusion is clear or serosanguineous, is an exudate, and contains increased concentrations of protein and lactic dehydrogenase. The white cell counts range from 5 to 10,000/mm^3. Early on, neutrophils predominate; with time, mononuclear cells appear. These characteristics are nonspecific. In distinction to rheumatoid arthritis, the pleural fluid glucose concentration is not reduced. As in rheumatoid pleural effusions, the rheumatoid factor may be positive, and the pleural fluid complement, both the total levels and the individual components, is reduced. A positive double-stranded pleural fluid DNA titer is nonspecific as opposed to the serum test, since it has been found in pleural effusions due to malignancy and tuberculosis. The most helpful measurement is the pleural fluid antinuclear antibody titer. Levels greater than 1:160 are very suggestive of lupus pleuritis. Corticosteroid treatment is effective for relief of pleural pain, but time to resolution of the pleural effusion is quite variable and probably unaffected by this treatment. In the unusual case, recurrent lupus pleuritis may result in massive pleural fibrosis and lung entrapment, necessitating a pleural stripping procedure.

Interstitial Lung Disease

It was previously held that clinically apparent interstitial lung disease occurred in a small percentage of patients with SLE. However, utilizing high-resolution computed tomography (HRCT) and physiologic testing of gas exchange with exercise, as many as 38 percent of patients with SLE have been found to have interstitial lung disease.[11,12]

In patients who develop the insidious form of interstitial lung disease, the diagnosis of SLE is present for several years, and no other pattern of organ involvement predicts its appearance. These patients have progressive dyspnea and cough with interstitial infiltration on the chest radiograph. HRCT indicates combinations of ground-glass attenuation, inter- and intralobular septal thickening, and honeycomb change. Pulmonary function tests reveal a restrictive pattern with reduction in the diffusing capacity and hypoxemia accentuated by exercise. Response to therapy, either corticosteroids alone or in combination with cyclophosphamide or azathioprine, depends upon the underlying histology. Those cases with underlying cellular interstitial pneumonitis or organizing pneumonia are more likely to respond to treatment than those who demonstrate excess collagen deposition and cystic honeycomb formation.

Pulmonary Vascular Disease

Idiopathic pulmonary hypertension due to plexogenic arteriopathy independent of interstitial lung disease is now being reported with increasing regularity. One study reported a 5 percent incidence.[13] This form of pulmonary hypertension is associated with Raynaud's phenomenon, digital vasculitis, serositis, antibodies to ribonucleoprotein, rheumatoid factor, antiphospholipid antibodies, and, most recently, antiendothelial cell antibodies. Patients complain of dyspnea and fatigue but have normal chest radiographs. In advanced cases, pulmonary arterial enlargement appears. Spirometry and lung volumes are normal, but there is often an isolated reduction of the diffusing capacity for carbon monoxide as well as gas exchange abnormalities. Ventilation/perfusion lung scanning and occasionally pulmonary arteriography are indicated, particularly in those patients with the antiphospholipid syndrome who have a potential for recurrent small pulmonary emboli. There is no effective treatment for idiopathic pulmonary hypertension, although oxygen and calcium-channel blockers possibly delay the onset of cor pulmonale. Continuous intravenous prostacyclin has recently been approved for patients with primary pulmonary hypertension as it appears to improve survival as well as functional status. It is likely that trials in pulmonary hypertension associated with collagen vascular disease are forthcoming.

Vasculitis in SLE is more likely to be discovered in lung biopsy specimens that demonstrate either diffuse alveolar hemorrhage or acute lupus pneumonitis as opposed to being an isolated finding. Autopsy series indicate small-vessel vasculitis in 20 percent of cases.

Bronchiolitis

BOOP with inflammatory polyps protruding into bronchiolar lumens is among the interstitial patterns that occur in acute lupus pneumonitis and in chronic interstitial lung disease in SLE. True concentric obliterative bronchiolitis has not been documented, as it has for rheumatoid arthritis.

Respiratory Muscle Dysfunction

It is estimated that weakness of the diaphragm and other respiratory muscles is found in 25 percent of patients with SLE and may be a cause of unexplained dyspnea. These patients have subsegmental atelectasis, an elevated diaphragm on chest radiograph, and restrictive physiology. This has been referred to as *unexplained dyspnea and shrinking lungs syndrome.* Although there is a reduction in static lung volumes, the diffusing capacity when corrected for alveolar volume remains normal, thereby distinguishing respiratory muscle dysfunction from interstitial lung disease. In patients with respiratory muscle weakness, no evidence for a generalized neuromuscular disease can be found. The pathogenesis of respiratory muscle dysfunction remains unexplained, although phrenic nerve conduction abnormalities have been excluded.[14] Progression of this restrictive process is unusual. Corticosteroids are generally not effective.

Rheumatoid Arthritis

Rheumatoid arthritis primarily affects the articular surfaces, but pleuropulmonary complications are responsible for an increased morbidity and mortality. A quoted 50 percent incidence for these complications likely underestimates their frequency. Pleuropulmonary complications are more apt to occur in patients with more severe chronic articular disease or high titers of rheumatoid factor and in patients who have subcutaneous nodules as well as other systemic complications such as cutaneous vasculitis, myocarditis, pericarditis, ocular inflammation, and Felty's syndrome. However, pleuropulmonary disease may appear in seronegative patients. Moreover, both methotrexate and gold compounds, commonly employed for treatment, can induce an interstitial lung disease, which is often difficult to distinguish from the primary forms complicating rheumatoid arthritis. Furthermore, interstitial lung disease, pleuritis, and occasionally obliterative bronchiolitis may be the first and only manifestation of the rheumatoid state, preceding the articular manifestations by months to years.

Pleurisy and Pleural Effusion

By autopsy, pleural disease occurs in 40 percent of patients with rheumatoid arthritis. Clinically apparent pleural disease occurs in approximately 20 percent, the majority of whom experience mild symptoms. Twenty percent of patients who develop pleural complications do so prior to the onset of articular disease. Pleural complications are more common in men and occur most frequently during episodes of active articular disease and in patients with subcutaneous rheumatoid nodules.

Pleural disease is often first discovered on routine chest radiographs. Both pleural fibrosis and effusions can be asymptomatic. Pleural effusion can be unilateral or bilateral and may coexist with interstitial lung disease or necrobiotic nodules. Symptomatic patients present with pleuritic pain, dyspnea, and occasionally fever. The effusion is an exudate by protein and lactic dehydrogenase criteria; if it is chronic, cholesterol concentrations are increased. Other characteristics include a low pleural fluid pH (less than 7.2) thought to be due to impaired carbon dioxide exit from the pleural space. The leukocyte counts can be as high as 15,000/mm^3 and consist of a mixture of neutrophils and mononuclear leukocytes. As in SLE, the total and individual complement components are low and the rheumatoid factor activity is increased. The presence of rheumatoid factor in pleural fluid is nonspecific and has also been reported with tuberculosis, malignancy, and other infectious diseases. A low pleural fluid glucose concentration, thought to be due to a defect in glucose transport, is characteristic of rheumatoid effusions. Up to 40 percent of patients have pleural fluid glucose levels less than 10 mg/dL, and 75 percent have levels under 50 mg/dL.[15] It has been stated that cytologic examination of the pleural fluid—which demonstrates a background of necrotic debris, spindle-shaped macrophages, and multinucleated histiocytes—is characteristic of a rheumatoid effusion. Necrobiotic nodules are thought to be involved in the pathogenesis of the pleural effusions, but transthoracic pleural biopsy will only occasionally demonstrate this finding rather than nonspecific acute and chronic inflammation.

Treatment is not indicated for asymptomatic cases; however, corticosteroids, when utilized for active articular disease, are also effective in hastening the resolution of the pleural effusion. Rarely is any other form of intervention such as intrapleural corticosteroids necessary for these patients. In the unusual case, pleural fibrosis with resultant lung entrapment occurs, requiring surgical intervention. Spontaneous pneumothorax due to rupture of a necrobiotic nodule, another uncommon complication, necessitates tube thoracostomy; with persistence of the bronchopleural fistula, surgical intervention is indicated.

Pulmonary Vascular Disease

In general, pulmonary vascular disease is the least common pleuropulmonary complication in rheumatoid arthritis. The fibroproliferative plexogenic arteriopathy typical of scleroderma and SLE is an infrequent complication, occurring in the setting of Raynaud's phenomenon. Small-vessel vasculitis in rheumatoid arthritis is a very rare event in rheumatoid arthritis but can occur in the setting of diffuse alveolar hemorrhage.

Necrobiotic (Rheumatoid) Nodule

Radiographically visible lung parenchymal rheumatoid nodules are infrequently seen in a rheumatoid population (less than 1 percent). When they do occur, they are more common in men with active articular disease and high rheumatoid factors and in those who have subcutaneous nodules.[16] Most nodules are asymptomatic. The major problem is differentiating the necrobiotic nodule from either malignant or infectious granulomatous diseases. Radiographically, the nodules can be single or multiple, with upper and midzone predilection; approximately 50 percent will undergo cavitation. Size is variable, with nodules up to 7 cm reported. Spontaneous resolution and recurrence are to be expected. Continuous growth can be seen but should prompt a more aggressive diagnostic approach. In most cases, no treatment is required.

Caplan's syndrome refers to a radiographic picture that developed in Welsh coal miners with rheumatoid arthritis.[17] It consists of the sudden appearance of discrete nodules primarily in the upper lobes that are histologically identical to the necrobiotic nodule. The incidence of necrobiotic nodules is higher in rheumatoid patients with underlying pneumoconiosis, including coal workers' pneumoconiosis, silicosis, and asbestosis, than it is in a general rheumatoid population.

Airway Disease

Upper airway involvement by the rheumatoid process is most likely to involve the cricoarytenoid joint, causing difficulty with inspiration and occasionally resulting in stridor. A sore throat, hoarseness, and fullness in the throat are other common complaints. The prevalence of this complication, although asymptomatic in the majority of cases, approaches 50 percent when screening by computed tomography is employed. Clinically significant disease can be detected by performing flow volume loops, which indicate a variable extrathoracic obstruction of the inspiratory loop.

Bronchiolitis obliterans or obliterative bronchiolitis is a well-recognized cause of progressive and often severe obstructive lung disease in patients with rheumatoid arthritis.[18] The onset of obliterative bronchiolitis is insidious, with patients complaining of progressive dyspnea and cough in the face of a normal or hyperinflated chest radiograph. Physical examination reveals a generalized reduction of breath sounds and occasionally an inspiratory squeak. Physiologic testing reveals varying degrees of airflow limitation and hyperinflation, with normal or reduced diffusing capacity. HRCT demonstrates adjacent areas of decreased and increased attenuation (geographic pattern). Some patients have responded to treatment with a combination of corticosteroids and cyclophosphamide, but the majority progress to hypercapnic respiratory failure.

Another form of bronchiolitis seen in rheumatoid arthritis is a respiratory or follicular bronchiolitis consisting of a dense infiltration of lymphocytes and plasma cells surrounding the terminal and respiratory bronchioles. These patients complain of cough and dyspnea. Chest radiographs are either normal or demonstrate a fine nodular pattern more predominant in the middle and lower lung zones. HRCT demonstrates centrilobular nodules and bronchiectasis. There is usually no physiologic evidence for airflow limitation or reduced lung volumes; rather, gas exchange abnormalities dominate the physiologic picture. Treatment with corticosteroids yields variable results.

Interstitial Lung Disease

Interstitial lung disease is a relatively common complication in patients with rheumatoid arthritis, occurring in 5 to 40 percent of patients, depending upon the methods of detection. It is likely that clinically important interstitial lung disease occurs in 5 to 10 percent of patients with rheumatoid arthritis, the most common form being usual interstitial pneumonitis with varying degrees of cellular interstitial pneumonitis. These patients are dyspneic and complain of cough. Physical examination reveals bibasilar crackles, clubbing of the digits in up to 75 percent, and evidence of cor pulmonale when pulmonary hypertension appears secondary to hypoxic vasoconstriction. The chest radiograph and CT scan demonstrate varying degrees of interstitial infiltrates with predilection for the lung bases and lung periphery. In advanced disease, the presence of honeycomb lung may be appreciated.

BOOP can present with identical symptoms to usual interstitial pneumonia and can also preempt onset of the articular disease. The chest radiograph and CT scan differ from that seen in usual interstitial pneumonia because the infiltrates are primarily alveolar and localized, patchy, or diffuse. Lymphocytic interstitial pneumonia may occur when rheumatoid arthritis is complicated by Sjögren's syndrome. In addition to dyspnea and cough, these patients complain of dry mouth and eyes (keratoconjunctivitis sicca and xerostomia). The chest radiograph indicates patchy alveolar infiltrates primarily seen at the lung bases. Patients with lymphocytic interstitial pneumonitis and BOOP are more treatment-responsive than those with usual interstitial pneumonitis. If the clinical assessment and imaging studies are not definitive, thoracoscopic or open lung biopsy should be considered. Treatment consists of corticosteroids with the addition of cytotoxic drugs in nonresponsive cases. Patients with BOOP associated with collagen vascular diseases are less responsive to treatment than patients with the idiopathic variety. Disease often recurs with tapering of the treatment regimen and can progress to usual interstitial pneumonitis.

Gold-induced pneumonitis must be differentiated from the primary forms of interstitial lung disease in rheumatoid arthritis patients, particularly since the underlying histology can be similar.[4] Dyspnea and cough usually begin 4 to 6 weeks following initiation of therapy, and peripheral eosinophilia occurs in a minority of cases. Occasionally, the chest radiograph will demonstrate upper- as opposed to lower-zone mixed alveolar interstitial infiltration. Differentiation from rheumatoid interstitial lung disease can only be made after withdrawal of the drug results in remission. In severe cases with marked gas exchange abnormalities, corticosteroid therapy will occasionally prompt reversal.

Methotrexate given in relatively low weekly doses (10 to 20 mg) is associated with the development of an interstitial disease in rheumatoid patients.[19] The incidence of methotrexate pneumonitis is 1 to 11 percent in patients with rheumatoid arthritis. The clinical onset is relatively acute, with cough, fever, dyspnea, and new mixed alveolar and interstitial pulmonary infiltrates on chest radiographs. Increased white blood cell counts with mild eosinophilia, elevated sedimentation rates, and increased serum lactic dehydrogenase are nonspecific findings. Bronchoalveolar lavage indicates lymphocytosis and should be performed to rule out an infectious etiology. Lung tissue reveals a cellular interstitial pneumonitis, organizing pneumonia, and granuloma formation reminiscent of a hypersensitivity pneumonitis. In patients who develop this clinical syndrome while on methotrexate, the drug should be discontinued, since progression to end-stage fibrosis occurs. With life-threatening respiratory failure, corticosteroids given intravenously are effective.

Scleroderma

Scleroderma or systemic sclerosis is an inflammatory-fibrotic disease that results in the laying down of excessive extracellular matrix in the skin and some internal organs. Pulmonary disease contributes significantly to both the morbidity and mortality of patients.

The lung is involved in the great majority of cases. Autopsy series indicate a 70 to 100 percent incidence.[20] Most patients with scleroderma develop dyspnea during the course of their illness due either to interstitial lung disease or to pulmonary hypertension. Although unusual, both of these complications can precede the dermatologic manifestations. Further, both bronchoalveolar lavage and HRCT scans in the face of normal chest radiographs have indicated interstitial lung disease in both symptomatic and asymptomatic patients.

Interstitial Lung Diseases

Usual interstitial pneumonitis progressing to honeycomb lung is the most common pulmonary complication of scleroderma, occurring in 30 to 100 percent of cases. The predominant underlying histology is usual interstitial pneumonia and honeycomb lung, similar to that found in idiopathic pulmonary fibrosis. Interestingly, the survival of scleroderma patients with usual interstitial pneumonia from time of onset of dyspnea far exceeds that for those with idiopathic pulmonary fibrosis.[21]

Usual interstitial pneumonitis is more likely to occur in the diffuse cutaneous forms of scleroderma, although it may also complicate limited cutaneous systemic sclerosis, formerly referred to as the "CREST" syndrome. As with other conditions associated with usual interstitial pneumonia, dyspnea with exertion and cough are the predominant symptoms. Bibasilar crackles are heard, but clubbing is unusual due to capillary destruction in the nail beds. Physical findings of cor pulmonale eventually appear. Bibasilar interstitial infiltrates followed by more diffuse changes, loss of lung volume, honeycomb cysts, and pulmonary hypertension are the typical radiographic features. Scleroderma was the first interstitial lung disease in which "scar carcinoma" (adenocarcinoma or alveolar cell carcinoma) was reported. Physiologic testing eventually reveals restrictive lung disease, preserved flow rates, and a reduced diffusing capacity. Early on, the aforementioned measurements may be normal, and hypoxemia and a widened alveolar-arterial oxygen gradient at rest and heightened by exercise may be the only physiologic abnormality. Lymphocytic interstitial pneumonitis in those cases associated with Sjögren's syndrome and rare cases of diffuse alveolar hemorrhage have also been reported.

Treatment is empiric, with beneficial effects in corticosteroid failures accorded to cyclophosphamide and penicillamine in a limited number of cases. Cases in which therapeutic effect is expected are those demonstrating ground-glass attenuation as compared to honeycomb change on HRCT, lymphocytic or even an eosinophilic predominance as opposed to neutrophil predominance on bronchoalveolar lavage, and cellular versus a fibrotic lung biopsy.

Pulmonary Vascular Disease

Idiopathic pulmonary hypertension due to a primary fibroproliferative process involving the pulmonary vessels occurs in approximately 10 percent of cases of scleroderma and is primarily seen in the limited cutaneous forms (CREST syndrome). In this form of scleroderma, idiopathic pulmonary hypertension may coexist with usual interstitial pneumonitis. Patients present with a gradual onset of dyspnea and increasing fatigue. Physical examination and chest radiograph may initially be normal, and, with disease progression, physical and radiographic signs of pulmonary hypertension appear. Lung volumes and airflow parameters are maintained unless there is concomitant interstitial lung disease. Typically there is an isolated reduction in the diffusing capacity as well as progressive hypoxemia. At present, treatment consists of supplemental oxygen, since the use of vasodilator compounds is generally unsuccessful. Survival past 5 years from the time of diagnosis is unusual.

Aspiration Pneumonia

There is a high incidence of esophageal dilatation and decreased peristalsis in patients with scleroderma, particularly in the limited cutaneous variety. This leads to dysphagia, heartburn, gastroesophageal reflux, and recurrent aspiration pneumonia. It has long been held that aspiration contributes to the development of interstitial lung disease. However, a definitive study has indicated that direct measurements of gastroesophageal reflux did not correlate with physiologic impairment (low lung volumes and diffusing capacity) in these patients.[22]

Polymyositis-Dermatomyositis

In polymyositis-dermatomyositis, pulmonary complications are common, are important causes of morbidity and mortality, and often predate or overshadow the muscle or skin manifestations. Pulmonary involvement has been reported in 40 percent of cases. In contrast to the other collagen vascular diseases, in polymyositis-dermatomyositis, primary involvement of the airways and pleura does not occur. Idiopathic pulmonary hypertension has been seen on only a few occasions, and in these cases crossover with scleroderma was suspected.

Aspiration Pneumonia

Aspiration pneumonia is probably the most common pulmonary complication in patients with polymyositis-dermatomyositis. Almost half of the patients complain of dysphagia as well.[23] This complication results from an inflammatory myositis affecting the striated muscle of the hypopharynx and upper esophagus. As a result, there is loss of normal swallowing function and failure to protect the airway. This complication is more likely in those patients with extensive skin or muscle involvement.

Respiratory Muscle Dysfunction

Fortunately, hypercapnic respiratory failure requiring assisted ventilation from extensive myositic involvement of the respiratory muscles is an uncommon event (less than 5 percent prevalence).[24] In fact, in a patient presenting with unexplained hypercapnic respiratory failure, this entity as well as other neuromuscular problems should be entertained. With less extensive involvement of these muscles, there is a reduction in cough generation with the potential for the development of hypostatic pneumonia and atelectasis due to mucous plugging. This weakness can also cause a restricted physiologic defect with resulting tachypnea and dyspnea in the face of a normal diffusing capacity, normoxemia, and hyperventilation. Respiratory muscle dysfunction as the cause of restrictive lung disease can best be demonstrated by measurement of the maximal pressure generated during both phases of the respiratory cycle. Pressures are reduced, and sequential measurements are useful for monitoring the disease course and response to treatment.

Interstitial Lung Disease

The prevalence of interstitial lung disease in polymyositis-dermatomyositis ranges from 5 to 30 percent. More recently, a much higher incidence (40 to 80 percent) has been reported related to the use of more sensitive screening techniques. Usual interstitial pneumonitis is the histologic type of interstitial lung disease in polymyositis-dermatomyositis. Diffuse alveolar damage, BOOP, and diffuse alveolar hemorrhage secondary to pulmonary capillaritis may also occur.[25–27] All forms of interstitial lung disease may precede, appear simultaneously with, or follow the muscle or skin manifestations. There is no relationship between interstitial lung disease and the extent of muscle or skin disease, the level of creatine phosphokinase elevation, or the presence of serum rheumatoid factor or antinuclear antibodies. There is, however, a relationship between interstitial lung disease and a serum antibody directed against the cellular enzyme histidyl-tRNA-synthetase, known as anti-Jo-1.[28] This antibody appears in 25 percent of patients with polymyositis-dermatomyositis, in 50 percent of patients with interstitial lung disease, and 13 percent of those who do not have this complication. In a patient thought to have idiopathic pulmonary fibrosis who is also positive for anti-Jo-1 antibody, there is a good chance that polymyositis-dermatomyositis will develop at a later date.

All forms of interstitial lung disease in this disorder are more common in women. The most common presentation is chronic cough and progressive dyspnea due to usual interstitial pneumonitis with varying degrees of cellular interstitial pneumonitis. Digital clubbing is rarely if ever seen. Chest radiographs demonstrate reticulonodular infiltrates; with disease progression there is a reduction of the lung volume and the development of radiographic honeycomb lung and pulmonary hypertension. Physiologic testing indicates a restrictive pattern with a low diffusing capacity. Response to treatment depends on the underlying histology, the more cellular disease being more responsive.

There is also an acute pulmonary presentation whose clinical and radiographic picture is reminiscent of a diffuse infectious pneumonia. Here the underlying lesion is diffuse alveolar damage.[27,29] Severe respiratory failure occurs, and recovery is unusual in spite of aggressive anti-inflammatory and immunosuppressive therapy. BOOP may have either an acute or subacute presentation. The differentiation from diffuse alveolar damage becomes important because of the marked disparity in treatment outcome and survival. In BOOP, corticosteroid responsiveness with or without an additional agent is the rule rather than the exception. The most recently described interstitial reaction reported in polymyositis-dermatomyositis is diffuse alveolar hemorrhage due to pulmonary capillaritis.[26] This complication appears simultaneously with the onset of the muscle disease. Although alveolar hemorrhage was present on histologic sections, hemoptysis did not occur. As with other forms of pulmonary capillaritis, these patients responded to corticosteroids and cyclophosphamide.

Mixed Connective Tissue Disease

Patients with mixed connective disease have features of SLE, polymyositis-dermatomyositis, and scleroderma. Mixed connective disease is characterized by elevated titers of a specific antinuclear antibody directed against nuclear ribonucleoprotein. Pleuropulmonary complications are frequent, occurring in 20 to 80 percent of cases.[30]

Pleural Disease

Pleurisy has been reported to occur in 40 percent of cases. An exudative pleural effusion appears in approximately 5 percent.[31]

Pulmonary Vascular Disease

Pulmonary hypertension may be caused by recurrent pulmonary emboli, hypoxic vasoconstriction secondary to interstitial lung disease, or idiopathic pulmonary hypertension due to a plexogenic arteriopathy as occurs in SLE and scleroderma. These patients, primarily women, present with dyspnea and fatigue, normal chest radiographs except for pulmonary arterial enlargement, and an isolated reduction in the diffusing capacity for carbon monoxide. Survival, as with this form of pulmonary hypertension in the other collagen vascular diseases, is rather dismal.

These patients may also have a circulating lupus anticoagulant (antiphospholipid syndrome), thereby making these women more susceptible to pulmonary embolism. Recurrent small pulmonary emboli may mimic the clinical picture of idiopathic pulmonary hypertension.[32]

Aspiration Pneumonia

In those patients with mixed connective tissue disease whose features resemble scleroderma or polymyositis-dermatomyositis, esophageal dysmotility and dilatation can be a significant problem, leading to reflux esophagitis and recurrent aspiration pneumonia. The incidence of abnormal esophageal manometry in one series was greater than 50 percent.[33]

Respiratory Muscle Dysfunction

In those patients with features of polymyositis-dermatomyositis, an inflammatory myositis with respiratory muscle involvement may lead to hypercapnic respiratory failure or a restrictive lung disease with the development of hypostatic pneumonia.[31]

Interstitial Lung Disease

As expected, the incidence of interstitial lung disease in the form of either cellular interstitial pneumonia and/or usual interstitial pneumonia which may progress to honeycomb lung is increased, particularly in those patients with the features of scleroderma. As with the other connective tissue diseases, this interstitial lung disease manifests as progressive dyspnea, bibasilar reticulonodular infiltrates on chest radiographs, and physiologic parameters indicating low lung volumes and a reduction in the diffusing capacity for carbon monoxide. Diffuse alveolar hemorrhage has been reported in a few cases of mixed connective tissue disease and is similar in presentation to this complication in SLE.

Sjögren's Syndrome

Sjögren's syndrome refers to a triad of keratoconjunctivitis sicca, xerostomia, and polyarthritis. This is an autoimmune exocrinopathy characterized by lymphocytic infiltration of the luminal and salivary glands. There is a primary form of this syndrome as well as a secondary form associated with one of the other collagen vascular diseases, most frequently rheumatoid arthritis. There is a strong female predominance (greater than 90 percent).[34] Positive rheumatoid factor (95 percent) and antinuclear antibodies in a speckled pattern (80 percent) are to be expected as well as positive tests for antibodies to extractable nuclear antigens (anti-SSA, anti-SSB) specific for the primary form of the syndrome.[35]

Airway Disease

Because of lymphoid infiltration of the mucous glands resulting in dessication of the tracheobronchial tree, these patients develop hoarseness, cough, inspissation of secretions resulting in atelectasis, recurrent pneumonias, and commonly bronchiectasis.[36] There is a high incidence of obstructive ventilatory dysfunction in these patients, and occasionally obliterative bronchiolitis occurs.

Interstitial Lung Disease

This occurs more often in the secondary forms of Sjögren's syndrome and most likely represents a complication of the associated collagen vascular disease. Usual interstitial pneumonia, however, is unusual in the primary isolated form of Sjögren's syndrome.[37]

Lymphoproliferation in the lung parenchyma can occur in two forms, lymphocytic interstitial pneumonitis and, less commonly, pseudolymphoma. Both of these lesions have the potential for lymphomatous conversion.[38] Lymphocytic interstitial pneumonitis is an interstitial lung disease; therefore cough, dyspnea, and a restrictive lung disease are to be expected. Because lymphocytes also infiltrate the alveolar spaces as well as the interstitium, the radiologic studies indicate mixed alveolar and interstitial infiltrates. The development of pleural effusion or the appearance of hilar or mediastinal adenopathy often but not always indicates the development of a lymphoma. Lymphocytic interstitial pneumonia is quite responsive to anti-inflammatory agents, occasionally requiring immunosuppressive therapy. Cyclosporine has also been recommended in corticosteroid-resistant cases.[39]

Pseudolymphoma is often difficult to distinguish from a malignant lymphoma. This tumor-like proliferation appears as single or multiple masses on chest radiographs. It has been suggested that pseudolymphoma, which is considered to be a localized form of lymphocytic interstitial pneumonitis, is a premalignant lesion. If associated with a monoclonal gammopathy, malignant conversion has probably occurred.[40]

Ankylosing Spondylitis

Ankylosing spondylitis is one of the seronegative spondyloarthropathies that may eventually result in fixation of the chest wall and a mild to moderate restrictive lung disease. Since there is no muscular involvement, diaphragmatic function is preserved, so respiratory failure on the basis of the chest wall fixation does not occur.[41]

The incidence of interstitial lung disease complicating ankylosing spondylitis is reportedly less than 2 percent.[3] In contrast to the other collagen vascular diseases, interstitial lung disease has a predilection for the upper lung zones, only appears late in the course of the chronic spondylitis, and never precedes interstitial lung disease. This complication often appears fibrocystic on the chest radiograph and is difficult to distinguish from tuberculosis. Histologically it is a fibrosing process with cystic formation. Progressive dyspnea and cough are the predominant symptoms; treatment with corticosteroids is ineffective and therefore not indicated. The most serious complication of this apical fibrocystic disease is infection with invasive *Aspergillus* species as well as atypical mycobacteria. Further, saprophytic colonization of the cysts by *Aspergillus* species (fungus balls) may induce life-threatening hemoptysis.[42]

REFERENCES

1. Brucato A, Baudo F, Barberis M, et al: Pulmonary hypertension secondary to thrombosis of the pulmonary vessels in a patient with the primary antiphospholipid syndrome. *J Rheumatol* 21:942–944, 1994.
2. Myers JL, Katzenstein AL: Microangiitis in lupus-induced pulmonary hemorrhage. *Am J Clin Pathol* 85:552–556, 1986.
3. Rosner S, Ginzler EM, Diamond HS, et al: A multicenter study of outcome in systemic lupus erythematosus: II. Causes of death. *Arthritis Rheum* 25:612–617, 1982.
4. Levinson ML, Lynch JP, Bower JS: Reversal of progressive gold hypersensitivity pneumonitis by corticosteroids. *Am J Med* 71:908–912, 1981.
5. Alarcon-Segovia D, Deleze M, Oria CV, et al: Antiphospholipid antibodies and the antiphospholipid syndrome in systemic lupus erythematosus: A prospective analysis of 500 consecutive patients. *Medicine* 89:353–365, 1989.
6. Abramson SB, Dobro J, Eberle MA, et al: Acute reversible hypoxemia in systemic lupus erythematosus. *Ann Intern Med* 114:941–947, 1991.
7. Matthay RA, Schwarz MI, Petty TL, et al: Pulmonary manifestations of systemic lupus erythematosus: Review of 12 cases of acute lupus pneumonitis. *Medicine* 54:397–409, 1975.
8. Wiedemann HP, Matthay RA: Pulmonary manifestations of systemic lupus erythematosus. *J Thorac Imaging* 7:1–18, 1992.
9. Byrd RB, Trunk G: Systemic lupus erythematosus presenting as pulmonary hemosiderosis. *Chest* 64:128–129, 1973.
10. Gross M, Esterley R, Earle RH: Pulmonary alterations in systemic lupus erythematosus. *Am Rev Respir Dis* 105:572–577, 1972.
11. Bankier AA, Kiener HP, Wiesmayr MN, et al: Discrete lung involvement in systemic lupus erythematosus: CT assessment. *Radiology* 196:835–840, 1995.
12. Boulware DW, Hedgpeth MT: Lupus pneumonitis and anti-SSA(Ro) antibodies. *J Rheumatol* 16:479–481, 1989.
13. Asherson RA, Higenbottam TW, Xuan D, et al: Pulmonary hypertension in a lupus clinic: Experience with 24 patients. *J Rheumatol* 17:1292–1298, 1990.

14. Wilcox PG, Stein HB, Clarke SD, et al: Phrenic nerve function in patients with diaphragmatic weakness and systemic lupus erythematosus. *Chest* 93:352–358, 1988.

15. Shannon TM, Gale ME: Non-cardiac manifestations of rheumatoid arthritis in the thorax. *J Thorac Imaging* 7:19–29, 1992.

16. Walker WC, Wright V: Pulmonary lesions and rheumatoid arthritis. *Medicine* 47:501–520, 1968.

17. Caplan A: Certain unusual radiographic appearances in the chest of coal miners suffering from rheumatoid arthritis. *Thorax* 8:19–37, 1953.

18. Geddes DM, Corrin B, Brewerton DA, et al: Progressive airway obliteration in adults and its association with rheumatoid disease. *Q J Med* 46:427–444, 1977.

19. Barrear P, Laan R, vanRiel P, et al: Methotrexate related pulmonary complications in rheumatoid arthritis. *Ann Rheum Dis* 53:434–439, 1994.

20. D'angelow W, Fries W, Masi A, et al: Pathologic observations in systemic sclerosis (scleroderma). *Am J Med* 46:428–440, 1969.

21. Wells AU, Cullinan P, Hansell DM, et al: Fibrosing alveolitis associated with systemic sclerosis has a better prognosis than lone cryptogenic fibrosing alveolitis. *Am J Respir Crit Care Med* 149:1583–1590, 1994.

22. Troshinsky MB, Kane GC, Varga J, et al: Pulmonary function and gastro-esophageal reflux in systemic sclerosis. *Ann Intern Med* 121:6–10, 1994.

23. Dickey BF, Myers AR: Pulmonary disease in polymyositis-dermatomyositis. *Semin Arthritis Rheum* 14:60–76, 1984.

24. Schwarz MI: Pulmonary and cardiac manifestations of polymyositis-dermatomyositis. *J Thorac Imaging* 7:46–54, 1992.

25. Schwarz MI, Matthay RA, Sahn SA, et al: Interstitial lung disease in polymyositis-dermatomyositis: Analysis of 6 cases and review of the literature. *Medicine* 55:89–104, 1976.

26. Schwarz MI, Sutarik JM, Nick J, et al: Pulmonary capillaritis and diffuse alveolar hemorrhage: A primary manifestation of polymyositis. *Am J Respir Crit Care Med* 151:2037–2040, 1995.

27. Tazelaar HD, Viggiano RW, Pickersgill J, Colby TV: Interstitial lung disease in polymyositis and dermatomyositis: Clinical features, and prognosis is correlated with histological findings. *Am Rev Respir Dis* 141:727–733, 1990.

28. Bernstein RM, Morgan SH, Chapman J, et al: Anti-Jo-1 antibody: A marker for myositis with interstitial lung disease. *Br Med J* 289:151–152, 1984.

29. Clawson K, Oddis CV: Adult respiratory distress syndrome in polymyositis patients with the anti-Jo-1 antibody. *Arthritis Rheum* 35:1519–1523, 1995.

30. Prakash UBS: Lungs in mixed connective tissue disease. *J Thorac Imaging* 7:55–61, 1992.

31. Sullivan WD, Hurst DJ, Harmen CE, et al: A prospective evaluation emphasizing pulmonary involvement in patients with mixed connective tissue disease. *Medicine* 63:92–107, 1984.

32. Hainaut P, Lavenne E, Magy JM, Lebacq EG: Circulating lupus type anticoagulant and pulmonary hypertension associated with mixed connective tissue disease. *Clin Rheumatol* 5:96–101, 1986.

33. Prakash UBS, Luthra HS, Divertie MB: Intrathoracic manifestations of mixed connective tissue disease. *Mayo Clin Proc* 60:813–821, 1985.

34. Block KG, Buchanan WW, Wohl MJ, et al: Sjögren's syndrome. *Medicine* 44:187–231, 1965.

35. Alspaugh MA, Tan EM: Antibodies to cellular antigen in Sjögren's syndrome. *J Clin Invest* 55:1067–1073, 1973.

36. Newball HH, Brahim SA: Chronic obstructive airway disease in patients with Sjögren's syndrome. *Am Rev Respir Dis* 115:295–304, 1977.

37. Kadota J, Kusano S, Kawakami K, et al: Usual interstitial pneumonia associated with primary Sjögren's syndrome. *Chest* 108:1756–1758, 1995.

38. Schuurman HJ, Gooszen HC, Tan IW: Low grade lymphoma of immature T-cell phenotype in a case of lymphocytic interstitial pneumonia and Sjögren's syndrome. *Histopathology* 11:1193–1204, 1987.

39. Moolman JA, Bardin PG, Rossouw DJ, Joubert JR: Cyclosporine as a treatment for interstitial lung disease of unknown etiology. *Thorax* 46:592–595, 1991.
40. Walters MT, Stevenson FK, Herbert A, et al: Urinary monoclonal free light chaining in primary Sjögren's syndrome: An aid to the diagnosis of malignant lymphoma. *Ann Rheum Dis* 45:210–219, 1986.
41. Fisher LR, Lawley MI, Holgate ST: Relation between chest expansion, pulmonary function and exercise tolerance in patients with ankylosing spondylitis. *J Rheum Dis* 49:921–925, 1990.
42. Tanoue L: Pulmonary involvement in collagen vascular disease: A review of the pulmonary manifestations of the Marfan syndrome, ankylosing spondylitis, Sjögren's syndrome, and relapsing polychondritis. *J Thorac Imaging* 7:62–77, 1992.

33 | The Eosinophilic Pneumonias*

Lynn T. Tanoue

The eosinophilic pneumonias are recognized as a heterogeneous group of disorders characterized by varying degrees of pulmonary parenchymal or blood eosinophilia. The spectrum of diseases that can be primarily or secondarily associated with blood or pulmonary eosinophilia is shown in Table 33-1. This chapter focuses on diseases in which eosinophilic infiltration of lung tissue is a characteristic feature.

EOSINOPHILIC PNEUMONIAS WITH ACUTE PRESENTATIONS

Loeffler's Syndrome (Simple Pulmonary Eosinophilia)

Loeffler's syndrome is characterized by mild respiratory symptoms, peripheral blood eosinophilia, and transient, migratory pulmonary infiltrates.[1] It may be induced by a variety of exposures, including parasite infections and drug exposures (Tables 33-2 and 33-3). Immune hypersensitivity to *Ascaris lumbricoides* has been recognized as the likely cause of most of the earliest reported cases, with pulmonary manifestations resulting from a hypersensitivity reaction to the *Ascaris* larvae as they migrate through the lung. During the pneumonic stage of the illness, *Ascaris* larvae may be identified in sputum or gastric aspirates. In keeping with the life cycle of *Ascaris,* stool examination for ova and parasites is typically negative until 8 weeks after the onset of the respiratory syndrome.

Loeffler's syndrome affects people of all ages. It is characterized clinically by the presence of low-grade fever, nonproductive cough, dyspnea (mild to severe), and occasionally hemoptysis. Symptoms are usually self-limited, typically resolving in 1 to 2 weeks. Laboratory examination of peripheral blood reveals moderate to extreme eosinophilia, the peak levels of which may be present as respiratory symptoms resolve. Expectorated sputum, if present, frequently contains eosinophils. Transient, migratory nonsegmental interstitial and alveolar infiltrates (often peripheral or pleural based) are evident on the chest radiograph. Pulmonary function evaluation typically reveals a mild to moderate restrictive ventilatory defect with a reduced diffusing capacity for carbon monoxide ($D_{L_{CO}}$). Histologic evaluation of lung tissue is usually not required for confirmation of the diagnosis. When tissue has been obtained, a characteristic and striking eosinophilic infiltration of interstitium and alveolar-capillary units is seen. Tissue necrosis and vasculitis are not features of the disorder. An identifiable etiologic agent may be lacking in up to one-third of patients.

*Edited from Chap. 74, "The Eosinophilic Pneumonias," by Rochester CL. In: *Fishman's Pulmonary Diseases and Disorders,* 3d ed., edited by Fishman AP, Elias JA, Fishman JA, Grippi MA, Kaiser LR, Senior RM. New York, McGraw-Hill, 1998, pp 1133–1150. For fuller discussion of topics dealt with in this chapter, the reader is referred to the original text, as noted above.

TABLE 33-1 Diseases Associated with Pulmonary Infiltrates and Eosinophilia

Asthma/allergy
Bronchocentric granulomatosis
Bronchiolitis obliterans–organizing pneumonia
Infections
 Parasitic
 Fungal (esp. coccidioidomycosis, *Aspergillus*)
 Tuberculosis
 Pneumocystis carinii
Interstitial lung disease
 Idiopathic pulmonary fibrosis
 Collagen-vascular disease–associated
 Sarcoidosis
 Eosinophilic granuloma (pulmonary histiocytosis X)
Malignancy
 Non-small-cell cancer of lung
 Non-Hodgkin's lymphoma
 Myeloblastic leukemia
Miscellaneous (e.g., ulcerative colitis)
Pulmonary eosinophilic syndromes
 Acute eosinophilic pneumonias (drugs, parasites, idiopathic, other)
 Tropical pulmonary eosinophilia
 Chronic eosinophilic pneumonia
 Allergic bronchopulmonary mycosis
 Churg-Strauss syndrome (allergic granulomatosis and angiitis)
 Idiopathic hypereosinophilic syndrome

TABLE 33-2 Drugs and Other Exposures Causing Eosinophilic Pneumonia

Ampicillin	Mephenesin carbamate
Acetaminophen	Methotrexate
Aluminum	Methylphenidate
Beclomethasone dipropionate	Minocycline
Bleomycin	Naproxen
Captopril	Nickel
Carbamazepine	Nitrofurantoin
Chlorpromazine	Para-aminosalicylic acid
Chlorpropamide	Penicillin
Clofibrate	Pentamidine (inhaled)
Cocaine (inhalation)	Phenytoin
Cromolyn (inhalation)	Piroxicam
Dapsone	Pyrimethamine
Desipramine	Rapeseed oil
Diclofenac	Red spider antigens
Ethambutol	Sulfonamides
Fenbarbamate	Sulindac
Fenbufen	Tamoxifen
GM-CSF[a]	Tetracycline
Heroin (inhalation)	Tolazamide
Ibuprofen	Tolfenamic acid
Iodinated contrast agents	L-Tryptophan

[a]Granulocyte-macrophage colony stimulating factor.

TABLE 33-3 Parasitic Infections Associated with Eosinophilic Pneumonia

Ancylostoma spp.	*Opisthorchis* spp.
Ascaris spp.	*Paragonimus westermani*
Brugia malayi	*Schistosoma* spp.
Clonorchis sinesis	*Strongyloides stercoralis*
Dirofilaria immitis	*Toxocara gondii*
Echinococcus spp.	*Trichinella spiralis*
Entamoeba coli	*Trichosporon terrestre*
Necator americanus	*Wuchereria bancrofti*

Parasitic Infections

In addition to *Ascaris* species, many other parasites may be associated with pulmonary infiltrates and blood or pulmonary eosinophilia (Table 33-3). *Strongyloides stercoralis, Toxocara canis,* and *Ancylostoma brasiliensis* are the parasitic agents most commonly associated with pulmonary eosinophilia in the United States.

Pulmonary eosinophilia occurs in association with *Strongyloides* infection when it is complicated by the "hyperinfection syndrome."[1] This usually occurs in persons with defects in cell-mediated immunity (e.g., lymphomas, HIV infection), after chronic corticosteroid use, and in persons with underlying gastrointestinal disease, but it may also occur in healthy persons. Respiratory manifestations include cough, dyspnea, chronic bronchitis, wheezing, hemoptysis, and pulmonary infiltrates in association with blood eosinophilia. The diagnosis of *Strongyloides* infection may be established by identification of larvae in sputum, bronchoalveolar lavage (BAL) fluid, bronchial brushings, or transbronchial biopsy specimens.

Ancylostomiasis is a nematodal infection endemic to the southeastern coastal regions of the United States. The organism is present in soil contaminated by stool from infected domestic animals. It penetrates human skin most commonly through the feet, resulting in the development of the "creeping eruption" lesion—a raised, erythematous, serpiginous, tunnel-like, and often itchy lesion on areas of exposed skin. A Loeffler's-like syndrome occurs in up to 50 percent of cases.

Infection with *T. canis* leads to the clinical syndrome of "visceral larva migrans," characterized by hepatomegaly, leukocytosis, fever, hypergammaglobulinemia, and persistent blood eosinophilia. Because the disease most commonly affects young children, a high degree of clinical suspicion is necessary to establish the diagnosis in adults. Respiratory symptoms, including cough and wheezing, may occur after ingestion of substantial numbers of larvae. Laboratory evaluation reveals peripheral blood and BAL eosinophilia, elevated serum levels of IgE, and poorly defined, diffuse nodular alveolar infiltrates on chest radiograph.

Drug-Induced Pulmonary Eosinophilic Syndromes

A vast number of drugs have been associated with the development of pulmonary infiltrates and blood or pulmonary eosinophilia. A partial list of these medications is given in Table 33-2. In general, drug-induced pulmonary eosinophilic syndromes have an acute onset and are not always related to either the cumulative dose of drug used or the duration of treatment.[2]

Respiratory symptoms vary widely in severity, from a mild Loeffler's-like illness with dyspnea, cough, and fever to severe fulminant respiratory failure. Interstitial or alveolar infiltrates are typically evident on chest radiographs. Elimination of exposure to the drug usually leads to resolution of symptoms, eosinophilia, and pulmonary infiltrates within a month. Residual radiographic abnormalities exist in fewer than 10 percent of cases several months after clinical recovery. Supplemental therapy with corticosteroids is not universally required, but it may hasten recovery in severely ill patients.

Idiopathic Acute Eosinophilic Pneumonia

In contrast to the generally benign Loeffler's syndrome, a more severe idiopathic form of eosinophilic pneumonia termed *acute eosinophilic pneumonia* (AEP) has been recognized as a distinct clinical entity.[3] AEP may affect persons of either sex and any age; it occurs commonly in previously healthy persons but has also been reported in persons with chronic myelogenous leukemia or HIV infection.

Idiopathic AEP presents as an acute illness with fever, myalgias, cough, dyspnea, pleuritic chest pain, and hypoxemia (P_{O_2} under 60 mmHg).[3,4] Patients often have diffuse crackles on chest auscultation. Overt respiratory failure requiring mechanical ventilation may develop. In contrast to other forms of acute eosinophilic pneumonia, blood eosinophilia is usually absent. Serum IgE levels may be moderately elevated in some cases. Early in the course of illness, the chest radiograph reveals subtle, patchy infiltrates with Kerley B lines. Bilateral, diffuse, symmetrical alveolar and interstitial infiltrates resembling adult respiratory distress syndrome (ARDS) with a ground-glass or micronodular appearance develop within 48 h. Small to moderate bilateral pleural effusions with a high pH and marked eosinophilia may also be present. Computed tomographic (CT) scanning confirms the presence of diffuse parenchymal infiltrates, with prominence along bronchovascular bundles and septa. Pulmonary function tests reveal a restrictive ventilatory defect, with a reduced $D_{L_{CO}}$. Striking eosinophilia (25 to 50 percent) is present in BAL fluid.[3] Light microscopic examination of lung tissue reveals prominent eosinophil infiltration in alveolar spaces, bronchial walls, and, to a lesser degree, the interstitium. There is no evidence of vasculitis or extrapulmonary involvement.

Idiopathic AEP is a diagnosis of exclusion. A careful search must be undertaken for other infectious, inflammatory, or neoplastic causes of pulmonary infiltrates. Most patients demonstrate a rapid, dramatic response to corticosteroid therapy, with abatement of fever and respiratory symptoms within hours and complete resolution of infiltrates within 1 to 2 weeks. The optimal steroid regimen for the treatment of AEP has not been determined. However, success has been noted with initial doses of methylprednisolone 60 to 125 mg administered every 6 h, followed by 40 to 60 mg of prednisone per day for 2 to 4 weeks and a subsequent taper over several weeks.[3] Spontaneous disease regression has been reported, and absence of clinical relapse is characteristic.

TROPICAL PULMONARY EOSINOPHILIA

Tropical pulmonary eosinophilia (TPE) is a syndrome caused by filarial infections and characterized by fevers, malaise, anorexia, weight loss, paroxysmal dry cough with dyspnea or wheezing, marked peripheral blood eosinophilia, and spontaneous resolution over several weeks' time.[5] The clinical features of TPE are believed to result from an intense hypersensitivity reaction to microfilarial antigens. Both human filariasis *(Wuchereria bancrofti)* and canine filarial forms (e.g., *Dirofilaria immitis*) have been implicated. Most adult patients with TPE manifest the disease between the age of 25 and 40 years. Typical symptoms include a 1- to 2-week period of low-grade fevers, weight loss, fatigue, malaise, and a paroxysmal nocturnal hacking cough. Dyspnea and wheezing, which can be severe, are common, and the clinical presentation may resemble status asthmaticus. Chest pain, muscle tenderness, and cardiac, pericardial, and central nervous system (CNS) involvement have also been reported. Physical examination of patients with TPE is notable for coarse rales or rhonchi and wheezing. Generalized lymphadenopathy and hepatosplenomegaly may be present, but they are less common in adults than in children.

Laboratory findings in TPE include extreme peripheral blood eosinophilia (up to 90 percent of the leukocyte differential; more than 3000 eosinophils per cubic millimeter) that persists for several weeks and marked elevation of total serum IgE (usually more than 1000 U/mL). Eosinophils may be identified in the sputum. High titers of filarial-specific IgE and IgG, measured by complement fixation and hemagglutination techniques, are the crucial diagnostic findings. Microfilariae are not found in blood or sputum but have been identified in lymph node tissue and lung. Examination of stool or urine for ova and parasites is typically unrewarding. Pulmonary function tests reveal an obstructive ventilatory defect in up to 30 percent of patients, particularly when symptoms have been present less than 1 month. A restrictive ventilatory defect and reduced $D_{L_{CO}}$ are more typical of long-standing disease. Ill-defined, diffuse reticulonodular infiltrates with a mottled appearance, usually in the mid to lower lung zones, are characteristic radiographic findings. Hilar adenopathy and pleural effusions have been reported occasionally. The chest radiograph may be normal at the time of presentation. Examination of BAL fluid demonstrates increased numbers of total cells and eosinophils (up to 50 percent of differential), elevated levels of total IgE, and filaria-specific IgG, IgM, and IgE.

The diagnosis of TPE is usually established on the basis of the clinical and laboratory findings described above. Lung biopsies are not typically required. The differential diagnosis includes Loeffler's syndrome, chronic eosinophilic pneumonia, allergic bronchopulmonary mycosis, drug reactions, other parasitic infections, hypereosinophilic syndrome, and lymphangitic spread of carcinoma. In nonendemic areas, the disease may also masquerade as asthma, atypical pneumonia, sarcoidosis, Churg-Strauss syndrome, Wegener's granulomatosis, or tuberculosis. Biopsy of enlarged lymph nodes may assist in establishing the diagnosis. A rapid treatment response to diethylcarbamazine may provide confirmatory evidence that the correct diagnosis has been made.

Acute relapses do occur, which often respond to additional treatment. Alternatively, mild, chronic inflammation may persist, causing chronic interstitial lung disease, with persistent respiratory symptoms, radiographic findings, and hematologic and serologic abnormalities. Persistent clinical symptoms have been reported over 2- to 5-year follow-up periods in up to 13 percent of patients with TPE treated with a standard course of therapy. BAL in these patients reveals a mild, persistent eosinophilia. Persons with symptoms of longer duration are less likely to have a favorable treatment response. Alternative antifilarial drugs (e.g., ivermectin) or a trial of corticosteroids may be useful therapies for the chronic variant of the disease.

CHRONIC EOSINOPHILIC PNEUMONIA

Chronic eosinophilic pneumonia (CEP) may develop in people of any age, with peak incidence occurring in persons 30 to 40 years of age. Women are affected approximately twice as often as men, and CEP has been reported during pregnancy. Most cases occur in Caucasians. There is no consistent association with a history of cigarette smoking, but approximately one-third to one-half of patients have antecedent atopy, allergic rhinitis, or nasal polyps. In addition, up to two-thirds have adult-onset asthma preceding (by several months) or arising concurrently with other pulmonary symptoms. In contrast to idiopathic AEP, CEP has a subacute presentation, with symptoms typically present for several months before diagnosis.[6] Common presenting complaints include low-grade fevers, drenching night sweats, and moderate (10- to 50-lb) weight loss. Cough, often dry initially and later productive of small amounts of mucoid sputum, is a virtually universal finding. Patients ultimately develop progressive dyspnea, which may be associated with wheezing in those with adult-onset asthma. Although a subacute presentation is typical, some patients with CEP may also have severe acute respiratory failure or ARDS. There are no major extrapulmonary manifestations of CEP. The majority of patients have peripheral blood eosinophilia, with eosinophils constituting more than 6 percent of their leukocyte differential.[6] Leukocyte differentials with up to 90 percent eosinophils have been noted in this disorder. However, a lack of peripheral blood eosinophilia does not rule out the diagnosis, since eosinophilia may be absent in one-third of cases. IgE levels are elevated in up to one-third of cases. The severity of pulmonary function abnormalities depends on the stage and severity of the disease. They typically reveal a moderately severe restrictive ventilatory defect, with reduced $D_{L_{CO}}$ and mildly elevated alveolar-arterial oxygen gradient. Persons with an asthmatic component may also have an obstructive defect.

Three radiographic features are characteristic for chronic eosinophilic pneumonia: (1) peripherally based, progressive dense infiltrates; (2) rapid resolution of infiltrates following corticosteroid treatment, with recurrences in identical locations; and (3) the appearance of infiltrates as the "photographic negative of pulmonary edema." In contrast to Loeffler's syndrome, the pulmonary infiltrates associated with CEP are nonmigratory and typically affect the outer two-thirds of the lung fields. The areas of consolidation are patchy and dense and can have ill-defined margins. They are frequently nonsegmental, subsegmental, or lobar in distribution and apposed to the pleura. Infiltrates are most commonly bilateral, are located in the mid- to upper lung zones, and may mimic loculated pleural fluid. The characteristic "photographic negative of pulmonary edema" appearance (which occurs in under 50 percent of cases) results if extensive infiltrates surround major portions of or the entire lung. Less typical radiographic findings include nodular infiltrates, a diffuse ground-glass alveolar filling pattern, linear oblique or vertical densities, and areas of fibrosis unassociated with anatomic divisions. Computed tomography (CT) scanning may be a useful diagnostic adjunct in cases in which CEP is suspected clinically but typical radiographic features are lacking. Various abnormalities have been identified, depending on the timing of the CT relative to the onset of symptoms. Typical areas of dense, peripherally located airspace consolidation are found in most cases within the first several weeks of disease onset. Streaky bandlike opacities may appear when symptoms have been present for more than 2 months. Mediastinal adenopathy may also be identified on CT scan.

The cause of CEP is unknown. The differential diagnosis of CEP includes infection (especially TB and fungal diseases like cryptococcosis), sarcoidosis, Loeffler's syndrome, desquamative interstitial pneumonitis, bronchiolitis obliterans–organizing pneumonia, chronic hypersensitivity pneumonitis, and eosinophilic granuloma. The diagnosis of CEP is based on clinical, radiographic, and BAL findings and on the exclusion of other diseases. Unfortunately, the clinical signs and symptoms of CEP are nonspecific, and blood eosinophilia and typical radiographic features may be absent in some cases. BAL eosinophilia of 30 to 50 percent is typical of CEP. In most reported series, open lung biopsy has been required only rarely to establish the diagnosis. Transbronchial biopsy, usually performed to rule out other diagnostic entities, may reveal eosinophil and mononuclear cell infiltrates. Because of the rapid and dramatic responsiveness of CEP to steroid treatment, a therapeutic trial of steroids is often useful in establishing the diagnosis. Failure to document rapid clinical improvement should alert the physician to consider other diagnoses.

Corticosteroids are the mainstay of therapy for CEP. Dramatic clinical, radiographic, and physiologic improvements typically follow steroid treatment. Even patients presenting with severe respiratory failure may respond well to steroid treatment. In most cases, treatment with prednisone leads to defervescence within 6 h, reduced dyspnea, cough, and blood eosinophilia within 24 to 48 h, resolution of hypoxia in 2 to 3 days, radiographic improvement within 1 to 2 weeks, complete resolution of symptoms within 2 to 3 weeks, and normalization of the chest radiograph within 2 months.[6]

The prognosis of CEP is generally favorable, but spontaneous remissions seldom occur in untreated patients. In steroid-treated patients (40 mg a day for 10 to 14 days, followed by tapering over 4 to 6 weeks), morbidity and mortality directly related to CEP are low. However, clinical, hematologic, or radiographic evidence of relapse occurs in most patients (58 to 80 percent) when steroids are tapered or discontinued. These relapses commonly occur in the exact anatomic distribution of the original disease. Patients may require 1 to 3 years of initial steroid treatment to control the disease, and up to 25 percent may require long-term maintenance treatment (2.5 to 10 mg prednisone a day) to remain disease-free. The lowest possible dose of steroid that suppresses disease activity should be used. Although no obvious factors exist to identify persons who are likely to relapse or require long-term steroids, relapses are more common in persons treated initially with a short course (1 to 3 months) of steroids. There may be multiple recurrences. The reinstitution of steroids generally leads to improvement during these relapses. In rare instances, patients develop pulmonary fibrosis and honeycombing.

ALLERGIC BRONCHOPULMONARY ASPERGILLOSIS (MYCOSIS)

Most cases of allergic bronchopulmonary aspergillosis (ABPA) entail hypersensitivity to *Aspergillus* species. However, the finding of a virtually identical clinical syndrome associated with immune sensitivity to other fungal species has led to the use of the term *allergic bronchopulmonary mycosis* to describe this syndrome. It is estimated that ABPA complicates approximately 1 to 2 percent of cases of chronic (often steroid-dependent) asthma and 10 to 15 percent of cases of cystic fibrosis. The disease has no predilection for either sex, and persons of any age may be affected. ABPA may have its onset in childhood or adolescence yet go unrecognized until adulthood. The peak age at disease recognition is in the third and fourth decades. Most patients have a history of atopy with rhinitis, history of drug allergy, asthma onset before age 20, and/or allergic conjunctivitis. Typical presenting complaints include dyspnea, wheezing, poor asthma control, cough (commonly productive of thick brown mucous plugs), malaise, low-grade fever, and hemoptysis.

The typical radiographic manifestations of ABPA include parenchymal infiltrates and bronchiectasis. The infiltrates are often irregular and transient (1 to 6 weeks) with a predilection for upper lobes. The bronchiectasis is classically cylindric and proximal (central), occurring within the proximal two-thirds of the lung. Less common radiographic findings include bullous changes, pneumothorax, and cavitating nodular lesions. High-resolution CT scanning is the most reliable noninvasive means of detecting proximal bronchiectasis.

A number of schema have been proposed for the diagnosis of ABPA. One is based on an appropriate clinical history, a positive immediate hypersensitivity skin test to *Aspergillus,* total IgE levels, and IgG and IgE antibody indices. Another is based on major and minor diagnostic criteria outlined in Table 33-4.[7] The major diagnostic criteria include (1) asthma (mild to severe), (2) peripheral blood eosinophilia, (3) serum IgG-precipitating antibody against *Aspergillus* (or other relevant fungus), (4) positive immediate hypersensitivity skin test to *Aspergillus,* (5) elevated serum total IgE, (6) history of pulmonary infiltrates, and (7) elevated serum *Aspergillus*–specific IgE and IgG. Radiographic evidence of proximal bronchiectasis is also considered a diagnostic criterion by some authors. However, its absence does not rule out the diagnosis, especially early in the course of the disease. Minor diagnostic criteria include the finding of brown mucous plugs, identification of *Aspergillus* in sputum, and dual (immediate and delayed) cutaneous reactions to challenge with *Aspergillus.* Rare cases lacking a history of asthma but meeting the other major diagnostic criteria have been reported.

The features of ABPA are believed to result from a complex immunologic reaction to chronic airway colonization by *Aspergillus* (or other relevant fungal) species. Five clinical stages of ABPA have been recognized. Stage I, the *acute* stage, is characterized by symptoms of asthma, elevated total IgE (typically more than 1000 ng/mL), positive immediate hypersensitivity skin reaction to *Aspergillus* challenge, infiltrate on chest radiograph (with or without proximal bronchiectasis), peripheral blood eosinophilia (frequently

TABLE 33-4 Diagnostic Criteria for Allergic Bronchopulmonary Aspergillosis

Major
 Asthma
 Peripheral blood eosinophilia
 Precipitating antibodies against *Aspergillus*
 Positive immediate hypersensitivity skin-prick test to *Aspergillus*
 Elevated total IgE
 Elevated serum *Aspergillus*–specific IgE, IgG
 History of pulmonary infiltrates (proximal bronchiectasis)
Minor
 Mucous plugs containing *Aspergillus*
 Dual cutaneous reaction to *Aspergillus*

greater than 2000/mm^3), and positive precipitating antibodies to *A. fumigatus* (up to fivefold concentration of serum may be required for detection of the precipitating antibodies). Treatment of stage I disease with corticosteroids typically results in decreased sputum production, improved control of bronchospasm, greater than 35 percent reduction in total IgE within 8 weeks, clearing of precipitating antibodies, and resolution of radiographic infiltrates. IgE levels typically do not completely normalize. Patients with stage II ABPA have disease that is in *remission*. This is characterized by the resolution of symptoms, radiographic clearing, and stabilization of total IgE levels. Remissions may last several months to years, and corticosteroid treatment can be tapered or discontinued. Patients with stage III ABPA have disease *exacerbations*. Their disease is characterized by the development of new pulmonary infiltrates or by a greater than 100 percent increase in total IgE. An isolated increase in severity of bronchospasm does not constitute an exacerbation. Disease exacerbation may occur in the presence or absence of a concomitant increase in symptoms. Since up to one-third of patients with radiographic infiltrates may be asymptomatic, evolving progressive lung damage may remain unrecognized. As such, total serum IgE levels should be monitored every 1 to 2 months for at least a year after diagnosis. IgE levels fluctuate with disease activity, and a normal IgE level in a symptomatic untreated person virtually excludes the diagnosis. *Aspergillus*-specific IgA levels may also be elevated in the acute or exacerbation stages of disease. Stage IV ABPA is defined as *steroid-dependent asthma*. In stage IV disease, total IgE, *Aspergillus* precipitins, and *Aspergillus*-specific IgE and IgG typically remain elevated despite chronic steroid therapy. Stage V is defined as *pulmonary fibrosis*. Stage V patients have prominent symptoms of dyspnea, are often steroid dependent because of persistent bronchospasm, frequently have chronic sputum production, recurrent respiratory infections, and gas exchange abnormalities, and may have cyanosis or clubbing. The serologic profile of patients with stage IV disease persists during stage V.

Analysis of BAL fluid from patients with ABPA reveals a moderate eosinophilia and increased levels of *Aspergillus*-specific IgE and IgA but not IgG. Mucoid impaction may be evident, and bronchial brushings may reveal mucus containing aggregates of eosinophils, fungal hyphae, and eosinophil-derived Charcot-Leyden crystals. Pulmonary function tests typically reveal an obstructive ventilatory defect (due to bronchospasm or mucous impaction of the bronchi) during stages I, III, IV, and often V. These pulmonary function findings often do not correlate with the duration of ABPA or asthma. Persons with stage V disease typically also have a restrictive ventilatory defect with a reduced $D_{L_{CO}}$.

The differential diagnosis of ABPA includes corticosteroid-dependent asthma without ABPA, TB, parasitic infections, hypersensitivity pneumonitis, Churg-Strauss syndrome, acute eosinophilic pneumonia, CEP, and cystic fibrosis (CF). The identification of ABPA in patients with mold-sensitive asthma and CF poses particular diagnostic difficulty. Serum precipitins to *Aspergillus* species may be present in up to 10 percent and positive immediate skin tests to *Aspergillus* in up to 25 percent of asthmatics. Persons with mold-sensitive asthma or ABPA can have peripheral blood eosinophilia and/or elevated serum total IgE levels. However, persons with ABPA have 2- to 20-fold higher serum levels of *Aspergillus*-specific IgE and total IgE than do mold-sensitive asthmatics without ABPA. In addition, proximal bronchiectasis is not seen in mold-sensitive asthma but is common in ABPA. Likewise, it is difficult to establish the diagnosis of ABPA in patients with CF, because patients with CF alone can manifest chronic airflow obstruction, recurrent infections, underlying bronchiectasis, pulmonary infiltrates, chronic sputum production, *Aspergillus* colonization of the airways, and positive serum precipitins. ABPA should be suspected in patients with CF who develop a greater than fourfold increase in total serum IgE (especially more than 500 U/mL) or who have positive *Aspergillus*-specific IgE or IgG. Patients with CF and ABPA may derive some symptomatic or functional improvement from steroid treatment. CF patients on steroids should, however, be followed closely for development of invasive aspergillosis. It is unclear whether the development of ABPA alters the course of CF disease progression.

Systemic corticosteroids are the mainstay of therapy for ABPA. Since, without treatment, ABPA can cause marked chronic lung impairment, initiation of appropriate treatment early in the course of disease is essential. Although there is no definitive proof that corticosteroid therapy prevents the development of bronchiectasis, retrospective studies have suggested that early therapeutic intervention with corticosteroids may prevent progression to lung fibrosis.[1] Therapy for stage I or III disease should include prednisone, 0.5 mg/kg a day for 2 weeks, followed by treatment every other day for 3 months. A subsequent taper (by 5 mg every 2 weeks) over the ensuing 3 months is advocated by some authors. A low maintenance dose (e.g., 7.5 mg a day) may be required for 1 year to prevent recurrence. Corticosteroid therapy leads to relief of symptoms and decreased airflow obstruction, decreased serum IgE, and resolution of pulmonary inflammation and infiltrates. Inhaled corticosteroids have occasionally been used as primary therapy and to minimize the dose of systemic steroid necessary to control symptomatic exacerbations. Bronchodilators and antibiotics also help control bronchospasm and secondary respiratory infections. Antifungal agents are generally ineffective in controlling ABPA. However, itraconazole had steroid-sparing effects in isolated case reports and an uncontrolled trial in six patients.

With appropriate treatment, long-term control of ABPA is feasible. Progression of stage IV disease to pulmonary fibrosis can be prevented if patients are maintained on low-dose steroids, and most patients with stage V disease have a stable course over several years' time. Persons with an FEV_1 persistently less than 0.8 L have a worse prognosis. In addition to severe airflow obstruction and pulmonary fibrosis, long-term complications of ABPA occasionally include the development of an aspergilloma, chronic or recurrent lobar atelectasis, allergic *Aspergillus* sinusitis, or limited *Aspergillus* tissue invasion.

CHURG-STRAUSS SYNDROME (ALLERGIC GRANULOMATOSIS AND ANGIITIS)

Churg-Strauss syndrome (CSS), is an uncommon systemic disease characterized by asthma, necrotizing vasculitis, eosinophilic tissue inflammation and extravascular granulomas, fever, and peripheral hypereosinophilia. CSS may occur in patients of any age, but it develops most commonly in patients age 38 to 50.[1,8] There is a slight male predominance (52 to 75 percent of patients in different series). In women, disease onset has been reported during pregnancy. CSS tends to follow a subacute course, with symptoms ranging over months to years. Three distinct clinical phases of the disease have been recognized: the prodromal phase, the eosinophilic phase, and the vasculitic phase. The prodromal phase is characterized by "late-onset" (usually after age 21) allergic disease in persons typically lacking a family history of atopy. Severe allergic rhinitis, sinusitis, drug sensitivity, and asthma are usually present 8 to 10 years (up to 30 years) before CSS disease recognition. The eosinophilic phase is typified by the development of marked peripheral blood eosinophilia and eosinophilic tissue infiltration, most commonly of the lung, GI tract, and skin. The onset of the vasculitic phase is often heralded by development of constitutional symptoms, including fever, malaise, weight loss, and increased allergic or asthmatic symptoms. Although the vasculitis tends to occur years after the onset of allergic manifestations of the disease, in some cases it develops within months of, or concomitant with, the onset of asthma. A short duration between the onset of asthma and vasculitis is associated with increased severity of vasculitis. During the vasculitic stage, the asthma symptoms may persist and worsen, or they may diminish. When asthma dissipates, it often flares later in the course of illness and may require prolonged steroid treatment. Although CSS typically affects multiple organ systems, more limited forms of disease have been described. Virtually every organ system may be affected, with the lungs, heart, skin, and nervous system being the most common.

Most of the respiratory manifestations of CSS occur in the prodromal and eosinophilic phases of the disease. All patients have asthma at some point in the illness. Upper airway allergic disease, including sinusitis, rhinitis, and polyposis, is seen in 75 to 85 percent of patients. The asthma and upper airway disease usually are long-standing and often require steroid therapy (systemic or inhaled) to control symptoms. Spirometry may reveal an obstructive ventilatory defect. In rare instances, recurrent respiratory infection leads to bronchiectasis. A Loeffler's-like syndrome with eosinophilic infiltration of the lung parenchyma is seen in 38 to 40 percent of patients. These patients may develop dyspnea, cough, and wheezing. Their chest radiographs have transient, migratory nonlobar, nonsegmental, often peripheral pulmonary infiltrates, with no regional predilection. Pulmonary function tests done in this setting may reveal a restrictive or obstructive ventilatory defect with a reduced $D_{L_{CO}}$. Up to 30 percent of patients develop pleural effusions, which may be associated with pleuritic chest pain. Less commonly, a radiographic pattern of diffuse nodularity or interstitial lung disease is seen. In contrast to Wegener's granulomatosis, the CSS nodules rarely cavitate. Hilar lymphadenopathy may be present, and occasionally the chest radiograph may be normal. High-resolution CT scanning has demonstrated patchy peribronchial thickening, pulmonary artery enlargement, irregular stellate configuration of some vessels, areas of septal thickening, and scattered patchy parenchymal opacities. These findings have been reported to correlate with pathologic findings evident on open lung biopsy.

Cardiac manifestations generally are not present on initial presentation of CSS. However, they typically occur during the vasculitic phase of the disease and are a major source of morbidity and the principal cause of death (in 33 to 48 percent of cases) from the disorder.[8] Progressive congestive heart failure (CHF) occurs in 47 percent of cases because of myocardial infiltration by eosinophils or ischemic cardiomyopathy resulting from necrotizing vasculitis of the coronary arteries. This coronary vasculitis is fatal up to 60 percent of the time. Pericarditis is present in approximately one-third of cases, and cardiac tamponade has been reported.

A wide array of neurologic manifestations may develop in CSS. Mono- or polyneuropathy (most notably mononeuritis multiplex) is present in 69 to

75 percent of cases. CNS manifestations occur in approximately two-thirds of patients and include cranial nerve impairment (especially optic neuritis), subarachnoid hemorrhage, and cerebral infarction. Skin, GI, renal, and other systemic alterations in CSS have been well described in CSS. Skin findings are present in 70 percent of cases and may develop in localized crops. They can manifest as nonthrombocytopenic purpura, tender cutaneous or subcutaneous nodules (which may ulcerate), urticaria, a maculopapular rash, or livedo reticularis. GI manifestations of CSS are present in up to 60 percent of cases. They can include diarrhea, abdominal pain, intestinal obstruction, cholecystitis, bleeding, abnormalities on liver function tests, and bowel perforation. They may relate to visceral eosinophilic tissue infiltration or to overt vasculitis. GI disease is the fourth leading cause of death in patients with CSS (after cardiac, CNS, and renal impairment). Renal insufficiency occurs in up to 50 percent of patients with CSS. Interstitial nephritis, focal glomerulonephritis, hematuria, and albuminuria are common. Severe, difficult-to-control hypertension is also a major sequela of CSS (in 25 to 75 percent of cases) and may be due to recurrent renal infarction. In contrast to Wegener's granulomatosis, overt renal failure is not commonly seen in CSS. Mild lymphadenopathy (in 30 to 40 percent), rheumatologic manifestations (migratory polyarthralgias, myalgias, temporal arteritis), urologic disease (ureteral, urethral, prostatic),[7] and ocular manifestations have also been described.

Laboratory studies of CSS are notable for a striking but fluctuating degree of peripheral blood eosinophilia (20 to 90 percent of the differential) in virtually all patients. The degree of eosinophilia may be suppressed by corticosteroid treatment of asthma. Serum total IgE levels are typically elevated (range, 500 to 1000 U/mL) and may parallel disease activity. Most patients have a normochromic, normocytic anemia and moderate elevation of their ESR. As many as 50 percent of patients have low titers of rheumatoid factor, and 50 to 70 percent of patients have positive pANCA. Circulating immune complexes, hypergammaglobulinemia, and elevated urinary levels of eosinophil-derived neurotoxin have been reported. Laboratory examination of pleural fluid reveals an acidotic eosinophilic exudate (pH under 3) with low glucose levels. BAL reveals an increased percentage of eosinophils, the magnitude of which is generally less than that seen with CEP or idiopathic hypereosinophilic syndrome.

The American College of Rheumatology has published diagnostic criteria for CSS.[9] The presence of at least four out of six of the following criteria yielded 85 percent sensitivity and 99.7 percent specificity in establishing the diagnosis: (1) asthma, (2) peripheral eosinophilia greater than 10 percent, (3) mono- or polyarthropathy, (4) migratory or transient pulmonary infiltrates, (5) paranasal sinus abnormality, and (6) extravascular eosinophils in a blood vessel on a biopsy specimen. The presence of asthma or allergy as well as more than 10 percent eosinophilia has been reported to carry 95 percent sensitivity and 99 percent specificity in distinguishing CSS among a subgroup of patients with well-documented systemic vasculitis. Open lung biopsy is the "gold standard" site for tissue biopsy. Biopsy of other sites (e.g., skin, pericardium, muscle, nerve, gut), with or without immunostaining, may assist in establishing the diagnosis in selected cases.

The pathogenesis of CSS is poorly understood. The differential diagnosis includes polyarteritis nodosa, Wegener's granulomatosis, CEP, idiopathic hypereosinophilic syndrome, Loeffler's syndrome, asthma, and disseminated fungal infection. The histopathologic hallmarks of CSS include tissue (inter-stitial, blood vessel, and alveolar) infiltration by eosinophils; necrotizing vasculitis of small arteries, arterioles, and, to a lesser extent, small veins, venules, and capillaries; and extravascular and interstitial eosinophilic gran-ulomas (typically microscopic). Both pulmonary and systemic vessels may be affected. The precise histopathology of vascular impairment depends on the stage of the lesion. Early lesions demonstrate eosinophilic infiltration of the vessels and perivascular region. Later lesions are characterized by necro-tizing arteritis or vessel obliteration and scarring. The extent of vascular impairment varies from mild, eosinophilic perivascular cuffing to severe trans-mural inflammation with necrotization. Lesions may be sparse or widespread.

Patients in whom CSS goes untreated have a poor prognosis, with up to 50 percent dying within 3 months after the onset of vasculitis. Efforts at early recognition and treatment are important. No large randomized, controlled trials exist comparing various treatment methods, largely because of the rarity of the disorder. Thus, it is difficult to define the optimal treatment for the dis-ease. Nevertheless, it is clear that corticosteroid treatment generally leads to dramatic clinical improvement, with disease stabilization or cure. Prednisone, 40 to 60 mg per day, is given for several weeks, aiming to eliminate consti-tutional symptoms and cardiac, renal, neurologic, or other vasculitic mani-festations. Higher doses are occasionally required. Severe hypertension and mononeuritis multiplex often require prolonged steroid treatment. Once the vasculitic phase is controlled, steroids may be tapered, with doses titrated to maintain disease control. Low-dose prednisone is often given every day or every other day for up to 1 year. Although relapses are uncommon, patients should be followed closely for evidence of clinical deterioration and should have periodic screening of total white blood cell (WBC) and differential, erythrocyte sedimentation rate, and IgE levels.

IDIOPATHIC HYPEREOSINOPHILIC SYNDROME

Idiopathic hypereosinophilic syndrome (IHS) is a rare disorder consist-ing of severe peripheral eosinophilia and diffuse organ infiltration with eosinophils.[10] IHS is now recognized as a clinically heterogeneous syndrome with a wide range of disease severity. Whereas some patients experience a mild, limited form of the disease with minimal involvement of noncritical organs (e.g., skin), others have life-threatening multiorgan dysfunction. IHS predominantly affects males, although the sex association is less prominent in older patients. Persons of any age may be affected but disease onset is most common between 20 and 50 years of age.

Symptoms vary according to the organ system(s) affected. Presenting complaints are often nonspecific and include weakness, fatigue, low-grade fevers, and myalgias. Involvement of virtually every organ system has been described. Cardiac disease occurs in most cases and is the major cause of morbidity and mortality. The most common cardiac manifestations are relentlessly progressive congestive heart failure (CHF), intracardiac thrombi, and endocardial fibrosis. Mitral regurgitation, restrictive cardiomyopathy, and bacterial endocarditis have also been noted. Involvement of the central or peripheral nervous system, which occurs in more than 60 percent of patients, is also a major cause of morbidity. Neurologic manifestations of IHS include neu-ropsychiatric dysfunction, gait disturbances, peripheral neuropathies, visual changes, and sequelae of thromboembolic events, including hemiparesis. The bone marrow is universally affected with a striking eosinophilia (up to 25 to 75 percent of the differential). Other hematologic manifestations are anemia, thrombocytopenia, elevated vitamin B_{12} levels, venous and arterial thromboembolism, hepatosplenomegaly, and lymphadenopathy (in 12 to 20 percent). GI (25 to 46 percent of patients), cutaneous (25 to 56 percent), renal (10 to 20 percent), musculoskeletal, ocular, and endocrine manifestations are all well described.

The respiratory system is affected in 40 to 60 percent of patients with IHS. Up to 60 percent of patients develop a predominantly nocturnal cough, which is either nonproductive or productive of small quantities of nonpurulent sputum. Wheezing and dyspnea are also common, without an obstructive ventilatory defect on spirometric examination. Pulmonary hypertension, ARDS, and pleural effusions (which may be due to CHF) have been reported. In patients with pulmonary manifestations, the chest radiograph may reveal transient focal or diffuse pulmonary infiltrates and/or pleural effusion(s). Histopathologic examination of affected lung specimens most commonly reveals intense interstitial infiltration with eosinophils. Less commonly, necrotic areas of parenchyma are found. These are believed to be due to pulmonary microemboli. In contrast to CSS, significant vasculitis is not present. Of interest is that whereas blood and BAL eosinophilia are both prominent in persons with pulmonary involvement, blood eosinophilia is present and BAL eosinophilia is absent in persons lacking pulmonary manifestations of the disease. This finding has raised the question whether BAL eosinophilia may serve as a marker for the development of pulmonary disease associated with IHS.

The differential diagnosis of IHS includes acute eosinophilic pneumonias, CEP, TPE, parasitic infection, tuberculous or fungal infection, allergic or autoimmune disease, and other lymphoproliferative disorders. The diagnosis of IHS is established by demonstrating multiorgan dysfunction, severe peripheral blood eosinophilia (greater than $1.5 \times 10^9/mm^3$) for at least 6 months (or with death before then), and an absence of any other known causes of peripheral blood eosinophilia. Occasionally, the disease presents with the incidental finding of blood eosinophilia before development of other complications.

The mainstay of therapy for IHS includes corticosteroids and the alkylating agent hydroxyurea. Median survival with treatment is more than 10 years. Persons with progressive organ dysfunction should receive prednisone (1 mg/kg per day) for several weeks, followed by a change to alternate-day dosing. Without therapy, average survival is 9 months, and 3- to 4-year survival is estimated at 10 to 12 percent. If the disease stabilizes or resolves, alternate-day corticosteroids should be continued for approximately 1 year at the minimal dose that effectively controls disease activity. Hydroxyurea (0.5 to 1.5 g per day) should be added to the regimen if there is evidence of further disease progression, with the aim of reducing the peripheral leukocyte count to the range of 5000 to 10,000. Vincristine has been used in patients with extremely high peripheral WBC counts. Etoposide and troleandomycin are effective alternative agents for cases that prove refractory to standard treatment. Interferon alpha, a mediator that suppresses eosinophil function in vitro, has been beneficial in the management of some cases of severe, refractory IHS. Allogeneic bone marrow transplantation has also been anecdotally reported to be successful in selected cases of IHS in which end-organ damage is potentially reversible.

APPROACH TO THE EVALUATION OF EOSINOPHILIC PNEUMONIAS

In approaching the patient with pulmonary infiltrates and eosinophilia, one must first establish whether the patient has one of the eosinophilic disorders described in this chapter or a disease process that is secondarily associated with eosinophilia (Table 33-1). It is crucial, whenever possible, to establish an accurate diagnosis. The importance of specific diagnosis results, in part, from the appreciation that the prognosis, dose, and duration of treatment and follow-up measures that these diseases require vary widely. Furthermore, chronic fibrotic lung disease may result from failure to accurately diagnose and treat some of these disorders in a timely fashion, and misdiagnosis with resultant inappropriate therapy (e.g., high-dose steroid treatment of invasive fungal infection masquerading as CEP) may be catastrophic.

REFERENCES

1. Allen JN, Davis WB: Eosinophilic lung diseases. *Am J Respir Crit Care Med* 150:1423–1438, 1994.
2. Cooper JAD, White DA, Matthay RA: Drug-induced pulmonary disease. Part 2: Noncytotoxic drugs. *Am Rev Respir Dis* 133:488–505, 1986.
3. Allen JN, Pacht ER, Gadek JE, Davis WB: Acute eosinophilic pneumonia as a reversible cause of noninfectious respiratory failure. *N Engl J Med* 321:569–574, 1989.
4. Hayakawa H, Sato A, Toyoshima M, et al: A clinical study of idiopathic eosinophilic pneumonia. *Chest* 105:1462–1466, 1994.
5. Spry CJF, Kumaraswami V: Tropical eosinophilia. *Semin Hematol* 19:107–115, 1982.
6. Jederlinic PJ, Sicilian L, Gaensler EA: Chronic eosinophilic pneumonia: A report of 19 cases and a review of the literature. *Medicine* 67:154–162, 1988.
7. Rosenberg M, Patterson R, Mintzer R, et al: Clinical and immunologic criteria for the diagnosis of allergic bronchopulmonary aspergillosis. *Ann Intern Med* 86:405–414, 1977.
8. Chumbley LC, Harrison EG Jr, DeRemee RA: Allergic granulomatosis and angiitis (Churg-Strauss syndrome): Report and analysis of 30 cases. *Mayo Clin Proc* 52:477–484, 1977.
9. Masi AT, Hunder GG, Lie JT, et al: The American College of Rheumatology 1990 criteria for the classification of Churg-Strauss syndrome (allergic granulomatosis and angiitis). *Arthritis Rheum* 33:1094–1100, 1990.
10. Fauci AS, Harley JB, Roberts WC, et al: The idiopathic hypereosinophilic syndrome: Clinical, pathophysiologic, and therapeutic considerations. *Ann Intern Med* 97:78–92, 1982.

34 | Pulmonary Histiocytosis X*

Jack A. Elias

INTRODUCTION

Primary pulmonary histiocytosis X is also called eosinophilic granuloma of the lung and pulmonary Langerhans' cell granulomatosis.[1] Like Letterer-Siwe disease and Hand-Schüller-Christian disease, it is characterized by abnormal organ infiltration by Langerhans' cells. These related disorders have been grouped under the classification of histiocytosis X. However, the three disorders are clinically distinct.

Letterer-Siwe disease is an acute, often fulminant disease of children less than 2 years of age characterized by widespread infiltration of the reticuloendothelial system, bones, and lungs. Hand-Schüller-Christian disease is a more indolent disorder of children and young adults that also typically affects the bones and the lungs. Diabetes insipidus, exophthalmos, and osteolytic skull lesions form the classic clinical triad associated with this disorder. There is some overlap of these diseases, since some children present with isolated pulmonary manifestations and some adults demonstrate more malignant-appearing, disseminated disease.

Primary pulmonary histiocytosis X is an uncommon, smoking-related interstitial lung disease that primarily affects young adults. Occasionally, solitary osteolytic bone lesions or multifocal disease approximating the pediatric histiocytoses are seen. Advanced disease may mimic idiopathic pulmonary fibrosis. However, it generally follows a more benign and protracted course.

EPIDEMIOLOGY

The true incidence and prevalence of pulmonary histiocytosis X are unknown. Despite this, pulmonary histiocytosis X is clearly an uncommon, if not rare, disease. No occupational or geographic predisposition has been reported. Higher-than-expected connections to farming, woodworking, and domestic exposure to animals have been reported. Nearly all affected persons report a prior smoking history. Thus, tobacco smoke is thought to be an etiologic factor.

Edited from Chap. 76, "Pulmonary Histiocytosis X," by King TE, Crausman RS. In: Fishman's Pulmonary Diseases and Disorders, 3d ed., edited by Fishman AP, Elias JA, Fishman JA, Grippi MA, Kaiser LR, Senior RM. New York, McGraw-Hill, 1998, pp 1163–1170. For fuller discussion of topics dealt with in this chapter, the reader is referred to the original text, as noted above.

Most patients present to medical attention in young adulthood (20 to 40 years of age). Pulmonary histiocytosis X can, however, present in any age group. The recent literature suggests an equal sex distribution. Caucasians are affected much more commonly than people of either African or Asian descent. Pulmonary histiocytosis X may be a premalignant lesion since it has been associated with a variety of bronchogenic and non-bronchogenic tumors and Hodgkins and non-Hodgkins lymphomas.[2] The contribution of cigarettes and histiocytosis X to the generation of these malignancies is difficult to discern.

NATURAL HISTORY AND CLINICAL PRESENTATION

Patients with pulmonary histiocytosis X can present to medical attention with an incidental abnormal chest radiograph, after pneumothorax, or with respiratory or constitutional symptoms.[3] When the patient is symptomatic, a nonproductive cough, dyspnea, rhinitis, chest pain, fatigue, weight loss, and fever can be noted.[4] Pleuritic pain and acute dyspnea with a spontaneous pneumothorax are recurrent problems in 25 percent of patients.[5] Pleural thickening or effusion is rarely seen in the absence of a history of pneumothorax. Hemoptysis is occasionally reported and should prompt consideration of superimposed infection (e.g., *Aspergillus*) or tumor.

Cystic bone lesions are present in 4 to 20 percent of patients with pulmonary histiocytosis X. They are usually solitary, involve flat bones, and produce localized pain or pathologic bone fractures. Skeletal involvement can be the sole symptomatic manifestation of pulmonary histiocytosis X and may precede the more typical pulmonary manifestations. Central nervous system involvement with diabetes insipidus is also seen in about 15 percent of patients and is thought to portend a poor prognosis.

The physical examination of patients with histiocytosis X is usually unremarkable. Crackles are not commonly found on chest examination.[6] Digital clubbing is uncommon.[4] Secondary pulmonary hypertension can occur and is probably underappreciated. Routine laboratory studies are usually unrevealing, and the peripheral eosinophil count is normal.

RADIOLOGY

Chest Radiograph

The radiographic appearance of pulmonary histiocytosis X can be very characteristic if not diagnostic. The combination of ill-defined or stellate nodules (2 to 10 mm in size), reticulonodular infiltrates, upper-zone cysts or honeycombing, preservation of lung volume, and costophrenic angle sparing are believed to be highly specific for this disorder.[7,8] Typically, the reticulonodular opacities are seen in the middle to upper zone, which parallels the pathology. The total lung volume is most often normal, although both hyperinflation and reduced volume have been described.[9] This puts histiocytosis on a list with a limited number of other disorders (Table 34-1).

Small cysts and nodules are the radiographic hallmark of pulmonary histiocytosis X. Occasionally, miliary disease is seen. Hilar or mediastinal adenopathy in pulmonary histiocytosis X is rare and should prompt consideration of malignancy as a secondary diagnosis. Pleural thickening is most often due to treated pneumothorax, as pleural involvement by the primary disease process is uncommon. Rare patients present with a solitary nodule that proves to be pulmonary histiocytosis X on biopsy.

TABLE 34-1 Interstitial Lung Diseases with Preserved or Increased Lung Volumes

Histiocytosis X
Lymphangioleiomyomatosis
Tuberous sclerosis
Chronic hypersensitivity pneumonitis
Stage III sarcoidosis
Constrictive bronchiolitis
Any interstitial disease in a patient with emphysema

Computed Tomography (CT) and Magnetic Resonance Imaging (MRI)

The combination of multiple mid-upper lung-zone-predominant cysts and nodules with interstitial thickening in a CT scan from a young smoker can be diagnostic of pulmonary histiocytosis X.[7] The nodules can be well or poorly defined and occasionally are large and bizarrely shaped. Honeycombing can be seen in advanced disease. Serial chest CT scanning suggests a progression from nodular to cavitary to cystic disease over time. The degree of cyst formation is often underappreciated with routine chest radiography. The role of MRI in pulmonary histiocytosis X is limited to the evaluation of bony and central nervous system (CNS) lesions.

PHYSIOLOGIC TESTING

Pulmonary Function

Pulmonary function testing of subjects with pulmonary histiocytosis X can yield normal results or obstructive, restrictive, or mixed abnormalities.[10,11] In general, total lung capacity is well preserved, with nearly normal airflow. The diffusing capacity is most often disproportionately reduced.[11] Restrictive disease with reduced lung volumes, reduced diffusing capacity, and increased elastic recoil is seen in some patients. Airflow limitation also occurs in a minority of patients and can sometimes be associated with reactive airways, with significant improvement after bronchodilator administration.[9] When present, reactive airways disease may reflect coexisting COPD. Classic asthma-like manifestations are unusual in this disorder. In general, the mean A-aP_{O_2} difference is abnormal at rest only in patients with severe disease. Thus, the resting arterial blood gas was a very insensitive indicator of disease.

Exercise Physiology

Patients with established pulmonary histiocytosis X generally demonstrate a limitation in activity and exercise intolerance that is out of proportion to their pulmonary function abnormalities. These patients manifest a markedly decreased exercise capacity and a maximal ventilatory response that is not limiting, and well below predicted ventilatory ceilings. Alveolar dead space to tidal volume ratio (V_D/V_T) is usually abnormally elevated or fails to decrease with exercise. Gas exchange abnormalities are reflected by increasing A-aP_{O_2} differences with increasing exercise. These findings suggest that exercise intolerance in subjects with pulmonary histiocytosis X is due to a combination of mechanical factors and pulmonary vascular involvement.[9]

HISTOPATHOLOGY

The histopathology of histiocytosis X is characterized by the enhanced accumulation of Langerhans' cells in a setting that includes tissue inflammation, tissue fibrosis, and cyst and cavity formation. The Langerhans' cell is a monocyte-macrophage–derived cell which, by electron microscopy, has classic pentalaminar cytoplasmic inclusions called Birbeck granules (X bodies). They are normally found in the dermis, reticuloendothelial system, and normal lung and pleura. They can also be found in lungs from cigarette smokers and at sites of other pulmonary pathologies such as idiopathic pulmonary fibrosis. In pulmonary histiocytosis X, the Langerhans' cells are characteristically found in clusters and outnumber those seen in other lung diseases.

The inflammatory response in early histiocytosis X has a bronchovascular distribution and is not granulomatous in nature. It usually contains lymphocytes and neutrophils. Although eosinophils are seen in some cases, they are most often not noted. Thus, the older term *eosinophilic granuloma* is a misnomer. Pseudodesquamative interstitial pneumonia, characterized by the accumulation of alveolar macrophages, and respiratory (smokers) bronchiolitis, with pigmented macrophages filling the lumina of bronchioles and alveoli, has also been described. Intraluminal fibrosis is also noted and may serve as a mechanism for alveolar collapse, with progression to interstitial fibrosis and lung remodeling in these patients.[3,11]

As histiocytosis X progresses, interstitial fibrosis and small cyst formation with a middle-upper-zone predominance occurs. In contrast, idiopathic pulmonary fibrosis generally has a lower lung zone predominance. More advanced lesions extend into the bronchovascular parenchyma producing "stellate" lesions.[11] Older lesions are relatively acellular and produce diffuse interstitial fibrotic pathologies that can be difficult to differentiate from other forms of end-stage pulmonary fibrosis.

PATHOGENESIS

The pathogenesis of pulmonary histiocytosis X is unknown. However, the nearly universal association with cigarette smoking strongly implies causation. The Bombesin hypothesis contends that increased levels of a Bombesin-like neuropeptide play a central role in the pathogenesis of this disorder. Although histiocytosis X is not a monoclonal disorder, the frequent association with cancer and lymphoma does suggest a relationship with malignancy.

DIAGNOSTIC EVALUATION

A diagnosis of histiocytosis X is based on clinical findings, radiographic studies, and in some cases, bronchoalveolar lavage (BAL) and histologic evaluations. Unfortunately, the signs and symptoms of pulmonary histiocytosis X are generally nonspecific and often point to other, more common pulmonary disorders, such as chronic obstructive pulmonary disease (COPD). When present, the history of recurrent pneumothorax, diabetes insipidus, or bone pain can be quite helpful. A chest x-ray showing preserved lung volumes with interstitial changes and cyst formation can also be highly suggestive. The chest CT, if classic, can be diagnostic and should be obtained from all suspected of having this disease. High-resolution CT studies as a prebiopsy step in the evaluation of any patient with diffuse interstitial lung disease suspected of having pulmonary histiocytosis X has been recommended and a characteristic chest CT in association with an appropriate history has been proposed to obviate the need for tissue confirmation. However, most chest CT scans in pulmonary histiocytosis X are not classic and can be confused with other disorders.

BAL can be of diagnostic value in cases of suspected histiocytosis X.[12] The total number of cells recovered is usually increased and a modest increase in the concentration of neutrophils and occasionally eosinophils is noted. In active disease, a decreased CD4:CD8 ratio has been reported, and increased Langerhans' cells are well documented. The Langerhans' cells are recognized by their characteristic staining for S-100 protein or peanut agglutination antigen. These cells are also OKT-6 (CD-1)-positive, react with monoclonal antibody (MT-1), [10] and contain characteristic Birbeck bodies on electron microscopy. Quantitative criteria for the definitive diagnosis of histiocytosis X based on BAL Langerhans' cell numbers have not been conclusively established. A BAL cell differential with more than 5% Langerhans' cells does, however, strongly suggest the diagnosis.[5,12]

When tissue confirmation is sought, transbronchial biopsy can be sufficient to make the diagnosis. Thoracoscopic or open lung biopsies are generally definitive and provide additional tissue for evaluation. Tissue immunostaining with monoclonal antibody against CD-1 distinguishes Langerhans' cells from other histiocytes and can be a useful adjunct in difficult cases. In cases of progressive disease with extensive fibrosis, the number of Langerhans' cells present in tissue specimen or BAL fluids decreases dramatically. Diagnosis at this stage can be difficult regardless of the laboratory methods used.

TREATMENT AND PROGNOSIS

The natural history of pulmonary histiocytosis X is extraordinarily variable, with some patients experiencing spontaneous remission of symptoms and others progressing to end-stage fibrotic lung disease. Most subjects demonstrate gradual progression with continued cigarette smoking and disease regression with smoking cessation.[13] It is therefore important to stress smoking cessation.

Corticosteroids have not been shown to be of any value in the treatment of histiocytosis X. Cytotoxic therapy, which may be of value in the treatment of disseminated disease, has not been shown to produce benefit in patients with histiocytosis X. Radiotherapy for symptomatic bone lesions can be palliative. Radiation is not useful in the treatment of the pulmonary manifestations. Lung transplantation has been successfully accomplished in a number of centers. It is a viable option for appropriate patients with end-stage disease.

REFERENCES

1. Hance AJ, Cadranel J, Soler P, Basset F: Pulmonary and extrapulmonary Langerhans' cell granulomatosis (histiocytosis X). *Semin Respir Med* 9:349–368, 1988.
2. Tomashefski JF, Khiyami A, Kleinerman J: Neoplasms associated with pulmonary eosinophilic granuloma. *Arch Pathol Lab Med* 115:499–506, 1991.
3. Basset F, Corrin B, Spencer H, et al: Pulmonary histiocytosis X. *Am Rev Respir Dis* 118:811–820, 1978.
4. Marcy TW, Reynolds HY: Pulmonary histiocytosis X. *Lung* 163:129–150, 1985.
5. Schwarz MI: Primary and unclassified interstitial lung diseases, in Schwarz MI, King TE Jr (eds): *Interstitial Lung Disease,* 2d ed. St Louis, Mosby–Year Book, 1993, pp 426–429.

6. Epler GR, Carrington CB, Gaensler EA: Crackles (rales) in the interstitial pulmonary diseases. *Chest* 73:333–339, 1978.
7. Kulwiec EL, Lynch DA, Aguayo SM, et al: Imaging of pulmonary histiocytosis X. *Radiographics* 12:515–526, 1992.
8. Lacronique J, Roth C, Battesti JP, et al: Chest radiological features of pulmonary histiocytosis X: A report based on 50 adult cases. *Thorax* 37:104–109, 1982.
9. Crausman RS, Jennings CA, Tuder R, et al: Pulmonary histiocytosis X: Pulmonary function and exercise pathophysiology. *Am J Respir Crit Care Med* 153:426–435, 1996.
10. Kahn HJ, Thorner PS: Monoclonal antibody MT1: A marker for Langerhans cell histiocytosis. *Pediatr Pathol* 10:375–384, 1990.
11. Travis WD, Borok Z, Roum JH, et al: Pulmonary Langerhans cell granulomatosis (histiocytosis X): A clinicopathologic study of 48 cases. *Am J Surg Pathol* 17:971–986, 1993.
12. Danel C, Israel-Biet D, Costabel U, et al: The clinical role of BAL in rare pulmonary diseases. *Eur Respir Rev* 2:83–88, 1991.
13. von Essen S, West W, Sitorius M, Rennard SI: Complete resolution of roentgenographic changes in a patient with pulmonary histiocytosis X. *Chest* 98:765–767, 1990.

Pulmonary Lymphangioleiomyomatosis and Tuberous Sclerosis*

Jack A. Elias

PULMONARY LYMPHANGIOLEIOMYOMATOSIS AND TUBEROUS SCLEROSIS

Epidemiology

Pulmonary lymphangioleiomyomatosis is a rare, idiopathic, diffuse, progressive interstitial lung disease. It presents almost exclusively in premenopausal women, with 70 percent of patients being 20 to 40 years of age at the time of symptoms or diagnosis and only 5 percent of cases occurring in women greater than 50 years of age.[1-4] The few reported cases occurring in postmenopausal women have most often been associated with estrogen replacement therapy.[1-11] Caucasians, and less commonly Asians, are afflicted more often than other racial groups.

Clinical Manifestations

At diagnosis, nearly all subjects complain of dyspnea.[4,12] Spontaneous pneumothorax is common and will occur in 50 percent of cases. It is often recurrent, can be bilateral,[6] and may necessitate pleurodesis for more definitive therapy. Barotrauma and cyst rupture can still occur after pleurodesis. This can manifest itself as pneumomediastinum, pneumoretroperitoneum, pneumoretropharynx, and subcutaneous emphysema. Treatment of these complications following pleurodesis is primarily observant, since they are only rarely associated with significant morbidity (i.e., tension pneumomediastinum or pneumopericardium, which requires surgical decompression). Chylothorax, due to obstruction of the thoracic duct or rupture of the lymphatics in the pleura or mediastinum by proliferating smooth muscle–like cells, is characteristic of this disorder but is present in only a minority of subjects at diagnosis. Chyloperitoneum (chylous ascites) occurs in approximately 10 percent of cases. More rarely, chyluria and chylopericardium are noted. Renal angioleiomyomata, a characteristic pathologic finding in tuberous sclerosis, are also common in lymphangioleiomyomatosis, being noted in as many as 50% of subjects.[7] They may grow to enormous size prior to clinical detection but only uncommonly affect renal function. Hemoptysis of mild to moderate severity is a well-described manifestation and may be life-threatening.

The physical examination can be unrevealing or may demonstrate end-expiratory rales (22 percent), hyperinflation, decreased or absent breath

*Edited from Chap. 77, "Pulmonary Lymphangioleiomyomatosis," by King TE Jr, Crausman RS. In: *Fishman's Pulmonary Diseases and Disorders*, 3d ed., edited by Fishman AP, Elias JA, Fishman JA, Grippi MA, Kaiser LR, Senior RM. New York, McGraw-Hill, 1998, pp 1171–1178. For fuller discussion of topics dealt with in this chapter, the reader is referred to the original text, as noted above.

sounds, ascites, and intraabdominal or adnexal masses. Clubbing is uncommon ($\leq$5 percent).[11]

Pathology

The pathology of lymphangioleiomyomatosis is characterized by (1) the exuberant proliferation of polyclonal, atypical, vascular smooth muscle–like cells in bronchovascular structures and the pulmonary interstitium and (2) the occurrence of diffuse, cystic dilatation of the terminal airspaces.[8,11]

Grossly and microscopically, the normal architecture is distorted by multiple small cysts ranging from 0.1 cm to several centimeters in diameter. The interstitium is thickened with evidence of smooth muscle–like cell proliferation around and within the pulmonary lymphatics, venules, and airways.[4,8] The lymphatic and venous vessels can also be quite tortuous and dilated. Hilar, mediastinal, and retroperitoneal lymph nodes are often involved and enlarged. The thoracic duct is frequently thickened and dilated. Extrapulmonary involvement with renal, retroperitoneal, intraabdominal, and pelvic angioleiomyomata commonly occurs.

Pathogenesis

The pathogenesis of the smooth muscle–like cell proliferation and cystic lung alterations in lymphangioleiomyomatosis is poorly understood. It is likely, however, that estrogen plays a central role, since the disease does not present prior to menarche and only rarely after menopause, accelerates during pregnancy, and abates after oophorectomy. Further, estrogen and progesterone receptors have been demonstrated in biopsy tissue.

Pulmonary Physiology

Lymphangioleiomyomatosis is one of the few interstitial lung diseases with reticulonodular opacities on chest radiographs, increased lung volumes, and an "obstructive" or "mixed" pattern on pulmonary function testing.[3,11,12] Lymphangioleiomyomatosis patients are often hyperinflated with an increased total lung volume (TLC), residual volume (RV), and RV/TLC ratio. Often there is evidence of airflow limitation with a decreased forced expiratory volume in 1 s (FEV_1) and FEV_1/FVC ratio. Studies of pulmonary mechanics show a decreased mean elastic recoil, and gas exchange studies reveal a markedly reduced diffusing capacity (DL_{CO}) and widened A-a gradient. In most patients, exercise evaluations reveal a diminished exercise performance, reduced oxygen consumption, low anaerobic threshold, and an abnormal and excessive ventilatory response with high respiratory rate, excessive minute ventilation, and reduced breathing reserve.

Radiology

Chest Radiograph

The chest radiograph findings in lymphangioleiomyomatosis are variable,[8,9,11] ranging from normal early in the course of the disease to severely emphysematous-like changes in advanced disease. Pneumothorax can be an early feature, and chylous pleural effusion can develop. Initial reports of lymphangioleiomyomatosis described a pseudoreticular or nodular pattern of irregular opacities. These opacities result from the compression of smooth muscle–rich interstitial tissue by more dilated cystic airspaces. Lymphatic obstruction with the development of Kerley B septal lines also contributes to the pattern. Cross-sectional studies show that 33 to 62 percent of individuals have hyperinflation with cystic dilatation of the airspaces, producing relatively radiolucent lung fields.[11,12]

Chest Computed Tomography

The high-resolution chest CT in lymphangioleiomyomatosis is more sensitive than the chest x-ray and characteristically reveals diffuse bilateral, homogenous, small (less than 1 cm in diameter), thin-walled cysts.[9,13] Ground-glass opacities (59%) and nodular opacities (5%) are noted less frequently; linear densities are not seen.[11] There is a close correlation between the extent of the cystic parenchymal replacement (as measured by quantitative high-resolution chest CT) and disease severity (as determined by spirometry, diffusing capacity, lung volume, or exercise performance).[9]

Diagnosis

Lymphangioleiomyomatosis can be readily diagnosed by its characteristic histologic findings on open lung or thoracoscopic biopsy. Often, transbronchial lung biopsy can yield an adequate sample for pathologic evaluation, especially when immunohistochemical stains specific for smooth muscle components; actin or desmin and more recently HMB-458 have been employed to improve diagnostic sensitivity and specificity. High-resolution chest CT can be characteristic enough to confirm the diagnosis and may obviate the need for tissue confirmation. The differential diagnosis includes emphysema, alpha$_1$-antitrypsin deficiency, asthma, chronic extrinsic allergic alveolitis, pulmonary histiocytosis X, cystic sarcoidosis, and panacinar emphysema due to intravenous drug use.

Prognosis

Lymphangioleiomyomatosis is an inexorably progressive disease with a median survival of 8 to 10 years from diagnosis. The prognosis is variable, with approximately 22 to 62 percent[11,12] succumbing to progressive respiratory failure after 8.5 years from diagnosis. Uncommonly, long-term survival 20 years after diagnosis has been reported. In the two most recent large case series,[11,12] there was an apparent improvement in survival. The rate of progression is quite variable and the disease can progress many years after diagnosis and after menopause.[12] Sudden onset of rapid deterioration is rare later in the course of the disease.[12] Pregnancy and the use of supplemental estrogen are known to accelerate the disease process. An elevated total lung capacity (percent predicted TLC), reduced FEV_1/FVC ratio, and a predominantly cystic versus muscular pattern of histopathology predict a worse prognosis.

Treatment

Treatment regimens have thus far been unsatisfactory. There is no role for either corticosteroids or cytotoxic agents. Alpha interferon has also been tried, but its utility is limited by side effects. Combination therapy with oophorectomy and either progesterone (10 mg/day) and/or tamoxifen (20 mg/day) is the only approach that has demonstrated reliable benefit and should be considered.[10] Chemical oophorectomy with analogs of luteinizing hormone–releasing hormone may eventually replace surgical oophorectomy as the primary treatment of this disorder.

To date, only lung transplantation offers any hope for cure and should be considered as definitive therapy for any failing patient. Approximately 50 percent of patients with lymphangioleiomyomatosis are alive at 3 years following transplant. Unfortunately, reports of recurrent disease in transplanted lungs also exist.

TUBEROUS SCLEROSIS

Tuberous sclerosis (Bourneville's disease) is a rare disorder that can be passed on in an autosomal dominant pattern or may occur (68 percent of the time) sporadically. It affects men and women equally. Mental retardation, seizures, and facial angiofibromas (adenoma sebacium) form the classic clinical triad. The features are variable, however, and some affected individuals can have normal intelligence. Skin lesions (hypopigmented spots on the trunk followed by adenoma sebaceum (wartlike lesions distributed in a butterfly pattern over the face and cheeks) are a prominent feature of tuberous sclerosis and are usually present in childhood.

In less than 1 percent of cases, tuberous sclerosis is associated with pulmonary manifestations that are indistinguishable from those of lymphangioleiomyomatosis. The onset is generally in the fourth decade of life and rarely before age 20 years. The complete triad of tuberous sclerosis is not commonly present in those who develop pulmonary involvement.[14] When pulmonary involvement is present, there is a marked female predominance. Most patients present with dyspnea. Pneumothorax (33 percent), hemoptysis, chest pain, and chylothorax can be seen. The radiographic appearance is similar to that of pulmonary lymphangioleiomyomatosis, described above. The primary histologic lesion is a hamartoma. Similar lesions occur in the brain and can calcify. A micronodular hyperplasia of type II pneumocytes has also been described. Renal lesions, angioleiomyomata, also occur with high frequency.

Pulmonary involvement in tuberous sclerosis carries a poor prognosis. Progressive disease with death due to respiratory insufficiency is common. Long-term survivors have been described and may be seen more frequently today because of improved management of the potential complications, especially cor pulmonale and pneumothorax. No effective treatment has been found. However, because of similarities to lymphangioleiomyomatosis, treatment with progesterone and/or oophorectomy in women is recommended.

REFERENCES

1. Banner AS, Carrington CB, Emory WB, et al: Efficacy of oophorectomy in lymphangioleiomyomatosis and benign metastasizing leiomyoma. *N Engl J Med* 305:204–209, 1981.
2. Bonetti F, Chiodera PL, Pea M, et al: Transbronchial biopsy in lymphangiomyomatosis of the lung. HMB45 for diagnosis. *Am J Surg Pathol* 17:1092–1102, 1993.
3. Burger CD, Hyatt RE, Staats BA: Pulmonary mechanics in lymphangioleiomyomatosis. *Am Rev Respir Dis* 143:1030–1033, 1991.
4. Corrin B, Liebow AA, Friedman PJ: Pulmonary lymphangioleiomyomatosis: A review. *Am J Pathol* 79:348–382, 1975.
5. Baldi S, Papotti M, Valente ML, et al: Pulmonary lymphangioleiomyomatosis in postmenopausal women: Report of two cases and review of the literature. *Eur Respir J* 7:1013–1016, 1994.

6. Berkman N, Bloom A, Cohen P, et al: Bilateral spontaneous pneumothorax as the presenting feature in lymphangioleiomyomatosis. *Respir Med* 89:381–383, 1995.

7. Bernstein SM, Newell JD, Adamczyk D, et al: How common are renal angiomyolipomas in patients with pulmonary lymphangioleiomyomatosis? *Am J Respir Crit Care Med* 152:2138–2143, 1995.

8. Carrington CB, Cugell DW, Gaensler EA, et al: Lymphangioleiomyomatosis. Physiologic-pathologic-radiologic correlations. *Am Rev Respir Dis* 116:977–995, 1977.

9. Crausman RS, Lynch DA, Mortenson RL, et al: Quantitative CT predicts the severity of physiologic dysfunction in patients with lymphangioleiomyomatosis. *Chest* 109:131–137, 1996.

10. Eliasson AH, Phillips YY, Tenholder MF: Treatment of lymphangioleiomyomatosis. A meta-analysis. *Chest* 96:1352–1355, 1989.

11. Kitaichi M, Nishimura K, Itoh H, Izumi T: Pulmonary lymphangioleiomyomatosis: A report of 46 patients including a clinicopathologic study of prognostic factors. *Am J Respir Crit Care Med* 151:527–533, 1995.

12. Taylor JR, Ryu J, Colby TV, Raffin TA: Lymphangioleiomyomatosis. Clinical course in 32 patients. *N Engl J Med* 323:1254–1260, 1990.

13. Muller NL, Chiles C, Kullnig P: Pulmonary lymphangiomyomatosis: Correlation of CT with radiographic and functional findings. *Radiology* 175:335–339, 1990.

14. Valensi QJ: Pulmonary lymphangiomyoma, a probable *forme fruste* of tuberous sclerosis. *Am Rev Respir Dis* 108:1411–1415, 1973.

36 | The Lungs in Patients with Inborn Errors of Metabolism*

Jack A. Elias

INTRODUCTION

A variety of diseases are collectively referred to as *inborn errors of metabolism*. In most of these disorders, "stored" material is deposited in the interalveolar septa or alveoli. The diverse manifestations of these diseases are poorly defined.

NIEMANN-PICK DISEASE

Niemann-Pick disease (NPD) is an autosomal recessive disorder characterized by the excessive accumulation of sphingomyelin (types A and B) and unesterified cholesterol (type C) in cells of reticuloendothelial and parenchymal tissues of viscera and/or the brain. Three types of NPD have been described, based on the nature of the primary molecular defect.

Type A NPD is an acute disorder that affects infants, almost half of whom are Jewish. The onset is insidious, and the children manifest difficulties in feeding, failure to thrive, progressive psychomotor deterioration, and hepatosplenomegaly. The chest radiograph shows diffuse reticular infiltration. These infants generally die within the second year of life. In type B NPD, most patients are in good health until late infancy. These infants manifest hepatosplenomegaly and lymphadenopathy and increased susceptibility to pneumonia. They die during their juvenile years. Type C NPD involves viscera and the central nervous system. The initial symptoms usually occur after the first or second year and occasionally after the sixth year of life. Psychomotor deterioration is progressive. Hepatosplenomegaly is less striking than in the other types of NPD. These patients often die between the fifth and fifteenth years of life.

The lungs, particularly in type A, are increased in weight and have a yellow, mottled surface. Microscopic examination reveals cells in the pulmonary septa and alveoli that are characteristic of this disease.

Types A and B NPD can be diagnosed with biochemical assays of sphingomyelinase in fresh blood samples and frozen tissue. The diagnosis of type C NPD requires analysis of cellular cholesterol esterification and the demonstration of filipin-cholesterol staining in cultured fibroblasts during LDL uptake. Enzyme analysis is not reliable for heterozygote studies; molecular genetic identification is required. The peripheral smear, bone marrow, and/or lymph nodes or liver should be examined for foamy cells using special histochemical preparations.[1]

---

*Edited from Chap. 78, "The Lungs in Patients with Inborn Errors of Metabolism," by Adachi M. In: *Fishman's Pulmonary Diseases and Disorders,* 3d ed., edited by Fishman AP, Elias JA, Fishman JA, Grippi MA, Kaiser LR, Senior RM. New York, McGraw-Hill, 1998, pp 1179–1192. For fuller discussion of topics dealt with in this chapter, the reader is referred to the original text, as noted above.

GAUCHER'S DISEASE

Gaucher's disease is an autosomal recessive disorder in which a deficiency of β-glucosidase is associated with the accumulation of glucosyl ceramide in a variety of organs. Type 1, the "adult form," is most common and usually occurs in Ashkenazi Jews. It is a chronic disorder that may start comparatively soon after birth, usually lasting into childhood. Patients with this form lack neurologic manifestations but do have hepatosplenomegaly, thrombocytopenia, anemia, bone pain, fractures, and Gaucher cells in their bone marrow. Pulmonary hypertension and severe pulmonary arteriosclerosis occur in some patients.[2] The reticular pattern of pulmonary infiltration that is characteristic of NPD is rare.

In type 2, the children develop normally until the age of 3 to 6 months. Thereafter, hepatosplenomegaly and lymphadenopathy become prominent, Gaucher cells are found in the bone marrow, high levels of serum acid phosphatase are noted, and progressive psychomotor deterioration is seen. The type 3 disorder presents with a more protracted course of neurologic alterations. Patients with the type 3 variant also show splenomegaly, slowly progressive hepatomegaly, and osteolytic lesions. Pulmonary infiltration is often noted on radiologic examination. However, the typical reticular pattern is rarely seen.

Gaucher cells are the histologic hallmark of this disease. They are round or polygonal in shape, 20 to 80 μm in diameter, contain cytoplasmic fibrils that give the appearance of striation and stain pink to red with the modified periodic acid–Schiff stain for cerebroside.[2] The pulmonary pathology of this disease has not been extensively described in the literature. In descriptions of fatal cases, investigators have reported heavy lungs with diffuse interstitial infiltrates, Gaucher cells infiltrating the alveolar septa and filling the alveoli, glomoid lesions in pulmonary arterioles, grade A3 hypertensive pulmonary vascular disease, and marrow emboli containing Gaucher cells. A variety of malignancies including multiple myeloma, Hodgkin's disease, leukemias, and carcinomas of the lung and other organs have also been associated with the disorder.

Bone marrow transplantation has been utilized in severe Gaucher's disease. It was successful in restoring β-glucosidase in mononuclear white blood cells and plasma with complete engraftment of the enzymatically normal donor cells. However, Gaucher cells persisted in the bone marrow.

For diagnosis, all suspected cases should have a careful radiologic survey of the lungs and bones, identification of Gaucher cells in smears from the bone marrow, and assays of β-glucosidase in leukocytes or cultured fibroblasts. If liver biopsy or splenectomy is undertaken, glucosyl ceramide and β-glucosidase activities should be quantitated in fresh-frozen tissue (1.0 g) and light and electron microscopy undertaken. For heterozygote studies, molecular genetic identification is required.

GM$_1$ GANGLIOSIDOSIS

Three types of GM$_1$ gangliosidosis have been recognized. Type 1 is an infantile form with generalized gangliosidosis, accompanied by bone involvement and psychomotor retardation. Early in the disease, the lungs are unremarkable. Later, bronchopneumonia is common, often causing patients to die before the age of 2 years. Chest x-ray abnormalities similar to those in Hurler's disease are observed, and foamy cells are demonstrable in smears of bone marrow. The type 2 disorder is a late infantile, juvenile form with milder bone abnormalities and progressive motor and mental deterioration. Visceral histiocytosis is less common, but neuronal lipidosis occurs more often than in type 1. Children with this variant live 3 to 10 years. The type 3 disorder is an adult, chronic form with juvenile onset of progressive cerebellar dysarthria and slow but progressive motor and intellectual impairment. Long-term survival is characteristic of this variant. The lungs of affected individuals have foamy histiocytes with membrane-bound inclusions and complex proteolipids in their alveoli and infiltrating their septa. The disease is due to a deficiency in GM_1 galactosidase and the accumulation of ganglioside GM_1. A diagnosis can be confirmed by analysis of β-galactosidase activity in leukocytes, urine, and skin. Ultrastructural studies of rectal mucosal biopsies can also be useful.[3] Since enzyme studies are unreliable for heterozygotes, gene analysis is required for carrier detection.

SULFATIDE LIPIDOSIS (METACHROMATIC LEUKODYSTROPHY)

Five categories of sulfatide lipidosis have been identified. It is classified as either congenital, late infantile, early juvenile, late juvenile, or adult, based on the age of onset of clinical manifestations. In addition, two other types have been identified: multiple sulfate deficiency (MSD) and cerebroside-4-6-sulfatase activator deficiency.[4] The clinical manifestations of these disorders largely reflect the striking changes in the white matter of the brain that occur during the course of the disease. MSD, however, begins with respiratory difficulty in early infancy followed by progressive psychomotor deterioration.[5]

Patients afflicted with this disease show a marked increase in the concentration of cerebroside sulfatides in their brain and viscera. This abnormality is secondary to the reduced activities of arylsulfatase A and to a lesser degree arylsulfatase B in this disorder. Arylsulfatase C is affected only in MSD. These abnormalities result in the widespread accumulation of metachromatic inclusion bodies in histiocytes in the alveolar septa of the lungs of these patients. These diagnoses are established by quantitating the arylsulfatase A activity in leukocytes or cultured skin fibroblasts from patients who are suspected to have the disorder. Analysis for sulfatase A in the urine is rapid and simpler but less reliable. Heterozygotes can be identified by leukocyte and fibroblast assays for arylsulfatase A and cerebroside sulfatase.[4]

GALACTOSYLCERAMIDE LIPIDOSIS (GLOBOID-CELL LEUKODYSTROPHY—KRABBE'S DISEASE)

Three clinical forms of galactosylceramide lipidosis (GL) have been described. In most, clinical symptoms are first noted in 3- to 6-month-old infants and progressive psychomotor deterioration culminates in death within 2 years. The late-infancy form is rare and manifests as mental deterioration, pyramidal signs, and visual impairment in children 2 to 6 years old. In the adult form, visual impairment is noted in 10- to 35-year-old individuals. Patients with this disease variant also exhibit slowly progressive motor deterioration and usually survive 2 to 10 years from presentation. The primary defect in these disorders involves the enzyme galactocerebroside β-galactosidase and is transmitted as an autosomal recessive.[6] This leads to a marked increase in the galactosylceramide concentrations in the white matter of the brain. In visceral organs, histiocyte-derived giant cells, similar to globoid cells, are seen. A diagnosis is established by quantitating the activity of galactocerebroside β-galactosidase in serum, leukocytes, or cultured fibroblasts.

GLYCOSPHINGOLIPID LIPIDOSIS (FABRY'S DISEASE)

Glycosphingolipid lipidosis (GSL) is transmitted by a gene on the X chromosome that controls the hydrolytic enzyme α-galactosidase A. Thus, it is seen most often in men but can be seen in isolated cases of heterozygous women. The clinical picture results from the progressive accumulation of globotriaosyl (ceramide) in most visceral organs as well as the brain. GSL presents in childhood or adolescence with severe burning pain and telangiectasis. The latter are symmetrical and most commonly involve the superficial layers of the skin, oral mucosa, and conjunctivae. Some patients with this disease develop pulmonary alterations ranging from obstructive disease of the airways to diffuse interstitial abnormalities.[7] Pulmonary function tests in older patients may reveal airflow obstruction, a reduced diffusing capacity, and a reduction in the $\dot{V}_{max_{25}}$ values.[8] Pathologically, lungs from these patients are congested and have vacuoles in alveolar epithelium, airway vascular smooth muscle cells, and endothelial cells. Toluidine blue–staining laminated inclusions are also seen in endothelium and type II cells. Affected patients can be identified by demonstrating an increase in globotriaosylceramide and by assaying hydrolase activity in serum, leukocytes, tears, and cultured skin fibroblasts.

MUCOPOLYSACCHARIDOSIS

The term *mucopolysaccharidosis* (MPS) refers to a group of autosomal recessive genetic diseases that are characterized by abnormal tissue deposition of acid mucopolysaccharide (glycosaminoglycans). Seven major forms of the disease have been recognized: Hurler syndrome (MPS I), Scheie syndrome (MPS I S, formerly V), Hunter syndrome (MPS II), Sanfilippo syndrome (MPS III), Morquio syndrome (MPS IV), Maroteaux-Lamy syndrome (MPS VI), and Sly syndrome (MPS VII). The most severely affected patients (except for those with type I S) commonly have respiratory involvement, particularly obstructive disease of the airways. Microscopic examination of these tissues reveals cells with abnormal deposits that are variously called clear cells, gargoyle cells, Hurler's cells, or balloon cells. Frozen sections exhibit metachromatic material that stains with toluidine blue and gives a positive reaction in alcian blue preparations.

The excretion of urinary mucopolysaccharides is markedly increased in many of these disorders. Although metachromatic material can be demonstrated in polymorphonuclear leukocytes and lymphocytes, the diagnosis can be established only by measuring urine mucopolysaccharides, with precise identification of the substance excreted. The characteristic enzyme defect of each disorder should also be studied in leukocytes, serum, or fibroblasts from the patient being evaluated.

GLYCOGEN STORAGE DISEASE

Patients with Pompe's disease [glycogen storage disorders (GSD) type II] manifest hypotonia by 2 months of age. Cardiomegaly and heart failure are also common. Most patients die within the first year of life. A rare few survive up to 15 years. The disease is transmitted as an autosomal recessive and is the result of an alteration in the gene for acid α-glucosidase. Histologically, GSD is characterized by the massive accumulation of glycogen granules in the cytoplasm of the parenchymal cells of most organs, including the lungs. Foamy alveolar macrophages are also noted. Glycogen is also present in smaller amounts in cartilage cells and mucosal and bronchial epithelial cells.[9] A diagnosis of GSD is based on the demonstration of increased tissue glycogen concentrations and a deficiency of α-glucosidase activity using urine, muscle tissue, and/or cultured fibroblasts.

DISORDERS OF AMINO ACID METABOLISM (MAPLE SYRUP URINE DISEASE)

Maple syrup urine disease (MSUD) (leucinosis, branched-chain ketonuria) is occasionally associated with bouts of respiratory embarrassment for which there is no infectious explanation. In this autosomal recessive disorder, affected infants often manifest respiratory distress, apneas, and a need for respiratory assistance within the first weeks of life. Severe psychomotor deterioration and seizures also occur and the children usually die from recurrent infections within the first year. With the help of a synthetic diet, some patients have survived for as long as 13 years.

MSUD results from abnormalities in the genes of the branched chain α-ketoacid dehydrogenase complex. These mutations increase levels of urinary leucine, isoleucine, valine, and plasma branched-chain ketoacids.[10] Patients with this disease have a maple syrup–like odor of their urine. The diagnosis should be verified by studies of the amino acids and ketoacids in blood and urine and enzymatic studies of leukocytes or cultured skin fibroblasts and lymphoblasts.

CYSTINE STORAGE DISEASE (LIGNAC-FANCONI DISEASE)

This disorder causes widespread pathologic changes in many organs. It is inherited as a simple Mendelian recessive and manifests in children as severe rickets or dwarfism with marked photophobia, amino aciduria, and death from infection or renal dysfunction. Tissue deposits are seen in a variety of organs including the lungs. In tissue sections treated with concentrated sulfuric acid and phosphotungstic acid, peribronchial birefringent crystals that form radiating clumps are noted. These deposits provoke no cellular reaction and do not alter pulmonary function.

REFERENCES

1. Adachi M, Volk BW: Methodology: Histochemistry, in Volk BW, Schneck L (eds): *The Gangliosidoses.* New York, Plenum Press, 1975, pp 249–264.
2. Schneider EL, Epstein CJ, Kaback MJ, Brandes D: Severe pulmonary involvement in Gaucher's disease. *Am J Med* 63:475–480, 1977.
3. Suzuki Y, Sakuraba H, Oshima A: β-galactosidase deficiency *(β-galactosidosis):* GM_1 gangliosidosis and Morquio B disease, in Scriber CR, Beaudet AL, Sly WS, Valle D (eds): *The Metabolic and Molecular Bases of Inherited Diseases,* 7th ed, vol 2. New York, McGraw-Hill, 1995, pp 2785–2823.
4. Kolodny EH, Fluharty AL: Metachromatic leukodystrophy and multiple sulfatase deficiency: Sulfatide lipidosis. In Scriver CR, Beaudet AL, Sly WS, Valle D (eds): *The Metabolic and Molecular Bases of Inherited Diseases,* 7th ed, vol 2. New York, McGraw-Hill, 1995, pp 2693–2739.
5. Murphy JV, Wolfe HJ, Balazs ER, Moser HW: A patient with deficiency of arylsulfatases A,B,C, and steroid sulfatase associated with storage of sulfatide,

cholesterol sulfate and glycosaminoglycans, in Bernsohn J, Grossman HJ (eds): *Lipid Storage Disease.* New York, Academic Press, 1971, pp 67–110.

6. Suzuki K, Suzuki Y: Globoid cells leukodystrophy (Krabbe's disease) deficiency of galactocerebroside β-galactosidase. *Proc Natl Acad Sci USA* 66:302–309, 1970.

7. Wise D, Wallace HJ, Jellinek EH: Angiokeratoma corporis diffusum: A clinical study of eight affected families. *Q J Med* 31:177–206, 1962.

8. Rosenberg DM, Ferrans VJ, Fulmer JD, et al: Chronic airflow obsruction in Fabry's disease. *Am J Med* 68:898–904, 1980.

9. Spencer H: *Pathology of the Lung.* Oxford, UK, Pergamon Press, 1985, pp 753–754.

10. Chaung DT, Shih VE: Disorders of branched chain amino acid and keto acid metabolism, in Scriver CR, Beaudet AL, Sly WS, Valle D (eds): *The Metabolic and Molecular Bases of Inherited Diseases,* 7th ed, vol 1. New York, McGraw-Hill, 1995, pp 1239–1277.

Part Six | ALVEOLAR DISEASES

37 | Alveolar Hemorrhage Syndromes*

Daniel B. Rosenbluth

Alveolar hemorrhage is a potentially catastrophic complication of many nonimmune and immune disorders. Hemoptysis, infiltrates on chest radiographs, hypoxemia, and progressive respiratory insufficiency are common. Nonimmune causes include endobronchial tumors, arteriovenous malformations or aneurysms, ulcerative tracheobronchitis, hemorrhagic pneumonia, bronchiectasis, congestive heart failure, uremia, thrombocytopenia or coagulopathy, pulmonary venoocclusive disease, and massive pulmonary embolism.

Immune alveolar hemorrhage results from diffuse injury to the pulmonary microvasculature (termed *capillaritis*). Causes are listed in Table 37-1.

DIAGNOSIS

A presumptive diagnosis of alveolar hemorrhage can often be made by a combination of clinical and serologic findings and bronchoalveolar lavage (BAL) fluid. Grossly bloody BAL fluid, large numbers of hemosiderin-laden macrophages, and the absence of purulent secretions strongly support alveolar hemorrhage as a cause of pulmonary infiltrates, and BAL is usually adequate to exclude infectious etiologies. Urinalysis for microscopic hematuria, red cell casts, and proteinuria as well as measurement of renal function should always be done in the diagnostic evaluation of alveolar hemorrhage.

The Role of Lung Biopsy

Pulmonary capillaritis can be diagnosed by transbronchial biopsy, but this diagnosis is made with greater confidence when a larger biopsy specimen is obtained by video-assisted thoracoscopy or limited thoracotomy. The role of open or thoracoscopic lung biopsy is controversial owing to the risks of the procedure in patients with severe alveolar hemorrhage and respiratory failure. The potential for postoperative infection and air leaks may be increased by the corticosteroid or immunosuppressive agents used to treat many of these syndromes. Histologic and serologic features of the autoimmune pulmonary hemorrhage syndromes are found in Table 37-2.

The Role of Percutaneous Kidney Biopsy

Necrotizing glomerulonephritis occurs in most immune-mediated alveolar hemorrhage syndromes. Percutaneous kidney biopsy should be performed in any patient with suspected alveolar hemorrhage who has abnormalities on urinalysis or renal function tests.

*Edited from Chap. 79, "Alveolar Hemorrhage Syndromes," by Lynch JP, Leatherman, JW. In: *Fishman's Pulmonary Diseases and Disorders,* edited by Fishman AP, Elias JA, Fishman JA, Grippi MA, Kaiser LR, Senior RM. New York, McGraw-Hill, 1998, pp 1193–1210. For fuller discussion of topics dealt with in this chapter, the reader is referred to the original text, as noted above.

TABLE 37-1   Etiology of Autoimmune Diffuse Alveolar Hemorrhage
Anti–basement membrane antibody disease (Goodpasture's syndrome)
Antineutrophil cytoplasmic antibody (ANCA) mediated vasculitis (e.g., Wegener's granulomatosis, microscopic polyangiitis, Churg-Strauss syndrome, pauci-immune glomerulonephritis)
Idiopathic rapidly progressive glomerulonephritis
Collagen vascular disease (e.g., systemic lupus erythematosus)
Immunocompromised status (e.g., bone marrow transplant, AIDS)
Exogenous agents or drugs (e.g., trimellitic anhydride, isocyanates, D-penicillamine, cocaine)
Idiopathic pulmonary hemosiderosis (pathogenesis unknown)

THERAPY OF IMMUNE-MEDIATED ALVEOLAR HEMORRHAGE

Because of the rarity of the immune-mediated pulmonary-renal syndromes, controlled, randomized trials evaluating therapy are lacking. Corticosteroids are part of standard therapy for all the immune-mediated alveolar hemorrhage syndromes. For systemic necrotizing vasculitis, cyclophosphamide (or occasionally other immunosuppressive agents) is combined with corticosteroids. For severe, fulminant autoimmune alveolar hemorrhage, high-dose intravenous ("pulse") methylprednisolone (1 g daily for 3 days) is advised (irrespective of underlying etiology), even while a diagnostic workup is pursued. Delaying pulse therapy in a critically ill patient for even a few hours may be catastrophic. Rapid resolution of bleeding can occur, often within 24 to 72 h of initiation of therapy. Following the 3-day pulse, corticosteroids (dose of methylprednisolone 60 to 120 mg per day or equivalent) should be continued for a few days, until control of the bleeding and extrapulmonary manifestations has been achieved. The subsequent dose and rate of corticosteroid taper must be individualized, based upon clinical, radiographic, and serologic response. Cyclophosphamide or other immunosuppressive agents should be withheld until a specific diagnosis mandating treatment with these agents has been substantiated. Plasmapheresis is a central component of therapy for anti-GBM disease but has no routine role for other disorders.

SPECIFIC SYNDROMES

Goodpasture's Syndrome

Anti–glomerular basement membrane (anti-GBM) disease (Goodpasture's syndrome) accounts for about one-quarter of the cases of immune-mediated alveolar hemorrhage. Typically, anti-GBM disease manifests as alveolar hemorrhage and rapidly progressive glomerulonephritis (RPGN). Most often it affects individuals between age 20 and 45 years of age, with a male predominance.

Most patients present with progressive dyspnea, widespread alveolar infiltrates, hypoxemia, and hemoptysis. A key feature is the presence of glomerulonephritis. Without therapy, progressive renal insufficiency ensues, often resulting in end-stage renal failure within days to weeks of the onset of symptoms. In up to one-third of patients with anti-GBM disease, glomerulonephritis occurs without alveolar hemorrhage. Alveolar hemorrhage without renal disease is exceptionally rare. Chest radiographs typically reveal dense bilateral alveolar infiltrates, often with air bronchograms. With cessation of

TABLE 37-2 Autoimmune Diffuse Alveolar Hemorrhage: Pathology and Serology

	Lung pathology		Renal pathology		Serology
	Histopathology	Immunofluorescence	Histopathology	Immunofluorescence	
ABMA disease (Goodpasture's syndrome)	±Capillaritis	Linear	Variable	Linear	ABMA (±p-ANCA)
Wegener's granulomatosis	Capillaritis (±granulomatous)	Negative	Segmental necrosis, crescents	Pauci-immune	ANCA (c-ANCA>>p-ANCA)
Microscopic polyangitis	Capillaritis	Negative	Segmental necrosis, crescents	Pauci-immune	ANCA (p-ANCA or c-ANCA)
Systemic lupus erythematosus	Capillaritis	Granular	Variable	Granular	ANA
Idiopathic pulmonary hemosiderosis	±Capillaritis	Negative	Normal	—	Negative

KEY: ABMA, anti–basement membrane antibody; ANA, antinuclear antibody; ANCA, antineutrophil cytoplasmic antibody; p-ANCA, perinuclear antineutrophil cytoplasmic antibody; c-ANCA, cytoplasmic antineutrophil cytoplasmic antibody.

bleeding, infiltrates may resolve within 24 to 36 h. Anemia is present in more than 90 percent of cases.

Serologic assays for anti-GBM antibody are invaluable in confirming the diagnosis and monitoring the adequacy of therapy. Radioimmunoassays or enzyme-linked immunosorbent assays (ELISA) for anti-GBM antibody are highly sensitive (>95 percent) and specific (>97 percent), but results are usually not available for several days. Although the height of serum anti-GBM antibody titer does not correlate with severity of disease, changes in titer over time may be a guide to efficacy of therapy.

Histopathology

Percutaneous kidney biopsy is the preferred invasive procedure to substantiate the diagnosis of anti-GBM disease. Light microscopy demonstrates a proliferative or necrotizing glomerulonephritis, often with cellular crescents. Although these microscopic features are nonspecific, bright linear deposits of immunoglobulin G (IgG) and complement (C3) along glomerular basement membranes are pathognomonic of anti-GBM disease. Lung biopsy is rarely necessary.

Pathogenesis

Antibodies are directed against the $\alpha3$ chain of type IV collagen, which is present in both alveolar and glomerular basement membranes. The stimulus for these antibodies is unknown. Exposure to cigarette smoke, hydrocarbon-containing solvents, hard metal dust, influenza A2 virus, chlorine gas, and D-penicillamine have been associated with anti-GBM disease.

Treatment

Plasmapheresis, corticosteroids, and cyclophosphamide have reduced mortality to <20 percent. Early treatment is critical, as the prognosis for recovery of renal function depends upon the initial extent of injury. Plasma exchange daily or every other day for 2 to 3 weeks, until the clinical course has improved and serum anti-GBM antibodies are nondetectable, is recommended. Immunosuppressive therapy is required to inhibit antibody production and rebound hypersynthesis which may occur following discontinuation of plasma exchange. Cyclophosphamide (2 mg/kg per day) or azathioprine (2 mg/kg per day) combined with prednisone (1 mg/kg per day) is used. For life-threatening alveolar hemorrhage, pulse methylprednisolone therapy is used, as in other autoimmune disorders. The dose of cyclophosphamide is maintained for the duration of therapy unless complications such as leukopenia necessitate dose reduction. The corticosteroid dose is gradually tapered over the next several weeks. Immunosuppressive or cytotoxic therapy may be discontinued within 3 to 6 months provided that a sustained remission has been achieved and anti-GBM antibodies have disappeared.

ANCA-Associated Vasculitides

Wegener's granulomatosis and microscopic polyangiitis are two ANCA-associated diseases that may result in alveolar hemorrhage.

Systemic Lupus Erythematosus

Alveolar hemorrhage is a potentially catastrophic complication of systemic lupus erythematosus (SLE), with mortality rates as high as 50 percent. It is rarely the sole or presenting feature of SLE. Glomerulonephritis is usually lacking. The diffuse pulmonary infiltrates must be differentiated from other pulmonary complications of SLE, including lupus pneumonitis, opportunistic infections, congestive heart failure, uremia, and pulmonary embolism. Provided that clinical features are consistent, the diagnosis of alveolar hemorrhage may be established by BAL and transbronchial lung biopsy.

Prospective, controlled trials evaluating therapy have not been performed. As with other causes of immune alveolar hemorrhage, high-dose intravenous pulse methylprednisolone (1 g daily for 3 days) is recommended for severe alveolar hemorrhage. The dose may be tapered to 60 to 120 mg of methylprednisolone or equivalent by the fourth day, with a gradual taper thereafter. For mild cases, high-dose prednisone (1 mg/kg per day) may be adequate initial therapy. Symptoms, serial chest radiographs, complete blood counts, and anti-DNA titers reflect the efficacy of therapy and guide the rate of taper of corticosteroid. Immunosuppressive or cytotoxic agents may be considered for alveolar hemorrhage refractory to corticosteroids, but data are limited. Plasmapheresis has been associated with anecdotal successes for acute flares of SLE or alveolar hemorrhage.

Alveolar Hemorrhage Complicating Bone Marrow Transplantation

Diffuse alveolar hemorrhage occurs in 3 to 31 percent of autologous or allogeneic bone marrow transplants (BMTs). Opportunistic infections or thrombocytopenia account for some of the cases, but a distinct syndrome of alveolar hemorrhage unrelated to infection is well accepted. Risk factors for alveolar hemorrhage include age >40 years, underlying solid tumors, severe oral mucositis, and renal failure. Diffuse alveolar hemorrhage usually develops 10 to 50 days after BMT. Chest radiographs typically demonstrate bilateral infiltrates. Serosanguinous or frankly bloody BAL fluid, with negative stains for infectious organisms, supports the diagnosis of alveolar hemorrhage. Mortality rates in patients requiring mechanical ventilatory support typically exceeds 50 percent. Secondary infections are serious and potentially lethal.

A retrospective analysis of alveolar hemorrhage in marrow transplant recipients noted improved survival in patients receiving high-dose corticosteroids (generally 125 to 250 mg of methylprednisolone every 6 h for the first 4 to 5 days) compared with low-dose corticosteroids (<30 mg per day methylprednisolone or equivalent) or supportive therapy. The incidence of infection was no higher in patients receiving corticosteroids. Alveolar hemorrhage or bloody BAL fluid may be seen in infectious causes of pneumonia (particularly due to CMV or *Aspergillus* spp). Because high-dose corticosteroids could be disastrous under these circumstances, infectious etiologies must be rigorously excluded.

Alveolar Hemorrhage Complicating HIV Infection

Diffuse alveolar hemorrhage can complicate human immunodeficiency virus (HIV) infection. The incidence and clinical significance of alveolar hemorrhage is not clear, as additional pulmonary processes (e.g., opportunistic infections, Kaposi's sarcoma) are usually present.

Alveolar Hemorrhage Due to Exogenous Agents

Trimellitic anhydride, isocyanates, D-penicillamine, lymphangiography dye, cocaine, warfarin, and prophylthiouracil are rare causes of alveolar hemorrhage. Glomerulonephritis has occurred in alveolar hemorrhage associated with D-penicillamine but not with the other agents. Smoking or snorting of cocaine or intravenous use of "crack" cocaine has been associated with hemoptysis and varying degrees of alveolar hemorrhage, including rare fatalities.

Immediate avoidance of the implicated agent or drug is essential. A brief course of high-dose corticosteroids is warranted. Plasmapheresis or cytotoxic agents may be considered for fulminant cases refractory to corticosteroids.

Idiopathic Pulmonary Hemosiderosis

Idiopathic pulmonary hemosiderosis (IPH) is a rare cause of alveolar hemorrhage that occurs primarily in infants and children. A history of milk or gluten sensitivity is common and a subset of adults with celiac sprue manifest IPH, which may respond to elimination of gluten from the diet. Extrapulmonary or renal involvement is lacking. Serum or tissue antibodies (including ANCA, immune complexes, anti-GBM antibody) are also absent. A diagnosis of IPH can be made *only* when other specific causes of DAH have been *reliably* excluded.

Recurrent episodes of alveolar hemorrhage over several years are characteristic. Hemoptysis may be absent, particularly in young children who may be unable to expectorate. Iron-deficiency anemia is characteristic and can be marked. Spontaneous remissions without long-term sequelae have been cited in up to 25 percent of cases. Recurrent episodes of alveolar hemorrhage can lead to pulmonary fibrosis, progressive respiratory failure, and cor pulmonale.

Although corticosteroids are considered the mainstay of therapy, an epidemiologic survey of 30 children with IPH concluded that corticosteroids did not alter the long-term course.

BIBLIOGRAPHY

Green RJ, Ruoss SJ, Kraft SA, et al. Pulmonary capillaritis and alveolar hemorrhage. Update on diagnosis and management [published erratum appears in *Chest* 1997 Jul;112(1):300]. *Chest* 110(5):1305–1316, 1996.

38 | Pulmonary Alveolar Proteinosis*

Daniel B. Rosenbluth

Primary pulmonary alveolar proteinosis (PAP) is a rare disorder of unknown etiology resulting from the accumulation in the alveoli of a proteinaceous material, rich in phospholipids. Congenital PAP affects neonates, a subset of whom are deficient in surfactant-associated protein B (SP-B).

Secondary PAP is observed in association with acute silicoproteinosis, exposure to aluminum dust, titanium dioxide, and other inorganic dusts; hematologic malignancies; myeloid disorders; and acquired immunodeficiency syndrome (AIDS).

PATHOGENESIS

Pulmonary alveolar proteinosis has been postulated to have a relationship to impaired macrophage maturation or function. Mice lacking a functional granulocyte-macrophage colony-stimulating factor (GM-CSF) gene develop lung pathology resembling PAP.

Deleterious effects of silica and other inorganic dusts on the alveolar macrophage are thought to play a role in the genesis of secondary PAP. Impaired macrophage function may account for the increased incidence of nocardial, fungal, and mycobacterial infections in PAP.

PATHOLOGY

On light microscopic examination, the alveoli are filled with a granular periodic acid–Schiff (PAS) base-reactive eosinophilic material without interstitial inflammation or fibrosis, but these may develop in the course of this disease. The large amount of sediment in lung lavage yields primarily phospholipids and surfactant-associated proteins.

CLINICAL FEATURES

PAP has a fourfold higher incidence in men and occurs predominantly between the ages of 20 and 50. Patients describe a gradual onset of a slowly progressive dyspnea commonly with a dry cough. Less frequently there is pleuritic chest pain, intermittent low-grade fevers, and weight loss.

On lung auscultation, there are fine end-inspiratory crackles. Clubbing is sometimes observed.

Chest radiographs show bilateral perihilar airspace disease in a "batwing" distribution simulating the pattern of acute pulmonary edema. On computed tomography (CT) of the chest, a patchy airspace consolidation is commonly seen.

*Edited from Chap. 81, "Pulmonary Alveolar Proteinosis," by Persson A. In: *Fishman's Pulmonary Diseases and Disorders,* edited by Fishman AP, Elias JA, Fishman JA, Grippi MA, Kaiser LR, Senior RM. New York, McGraw-Hill, 1998, pp 1225–1230. For fuller discussion of topics dealt with in this chapter, the reader is referred to the original text, as noted above.

Pulmonary function tests reveal a restrictive pattern with diminished diffusing capacity and arterial hypoxemia.

Fungal pathogens, *Nocardia,* and mycobacterial infections—most commonly due to *Mycobacterium avium intracellulare* complex—are present in increased frequency in lavage fluid and tissues in PAP. PAP-like material with *Pneumocystis carinii* in patients with AIDS suggests a causal relationship in rare instances.

DIAGNOSIS

Transbronchial biopsies of affected lung segments frequently yield sufficient tissue to establish the diagnosis of PAP; when coupled with the findings in the bronchoalveolar lavage, they permit a high degree of confidence in the diagnosis. Bronchoalveolar lavage yields a milky or grossly opaque lavagate containing few lipid-laden macrophages and large amounts of eosinophilic PAS-positive extracellular material. The increased incidence of infections in PAP necessitates that culture and careful examination of the biopsy and lavage for infectious agents be performed.

THERAPY

The only treatment recognized to be effective is mechanical removal of the proteins and lipids by alveolar lavage. Whole-lung lavage for the treatment of PAP is performed under general anesthesia with a double-lumen endotracheal tube to allow ventilation of one lung while the other is being lavaged. Patients frequently experience marked improvement in their symptoms soon after lavage.

PROGNOSIS

Some patients with primary PAP undergo spontaneous remission. The response to a single whole-lung lavage can be quite dramatic, but most patients require repeated lavages to maintain adequate gas exchange. A significant number have accompanying fibrosis, which worsens the prognosis. Therapy for the congenital PAP associated with SP-B deficiency is currently limited to lung transplantation.

The prognosis of secondary PAP is related to the cause. While whole-lung lavage may improve PAP from silica exposure, the long-term prognosis may be poor owing to pulmonary fibrosis. The prognosis of PAP associated with malignancy is coupled with the successful treatment of the underlying malignancy. PAP associated with immunosuppression may be secondary to an infectious agent, and the prognosis is linked to the successful treatment of the pathogen.

BIBLIOGRAPHY

Rosen SH, Castleman B, Liebow AA, et al: Pulmonary alveolar proteinosis. *N Engl J Med* 258:1123–1142, 1958.

Shah PL, Hansell D, Lawson PR, et al: Pulmonary alveolar proteinosis: Clinical aspects and current concepts on pathogenesis. *Thorax* 55:67–77, 2000.

Part Seven | **DISORDERS OF THE PULMONARY CIRCULATION**

39 Pulmonary Hypertension and Cor Pulmonale*

Alfred P. Fishman

Pulmonary hypertension invariably precedes cor pulmonale, or enlargement of the right ventricle by dilation and/or hypertrophy. In acute conditions, dilation predominates; in chronic cor pulmonale, right ventricular hypertrophy becomes a prominent feature. If pulmonary hypertension is severe and unrelieved, right ventricular failure will ensue—i.e., the diagnosis will be cor pulmonale and heart failure.

THE NORMAL PULMONARY CIRCULATION

The normal pulmonary circulation is a low-resistance, highly compliant vascular bed with low vascular tone. Because of these features, the normal cardiac output at rest is accommodated with low pulmonary arterial pressures, which only increase slightly during moderate exercise. Sample hemodynamic values are shown in Table 39-1.

Pulmonary vascular resistance is calculated as a ratio of the pressure drop across the pulmonary vascular bed divided by the cardiac output (pulmonary blood flow), as follows:

$$\text{Pulmonary vascular resistance} = \frac{\begin{array}{c}\text{mean pulmonary} \\ \text{arterial pressure} \\ \text{(mmHg)}\end{array} - \begin{array}{c}\text{pulmonary arterial} \\ \text{wedge pressure} \\ \text{(mmHg)}\end{array}}{\text{pulmonary blood flow (L/min)}}$$

Using the units indicated above, the normal pulmonary vascular resistance is 1.0 unit or less. Resistance may also be expressed in $\text{dyne} \cdot \text{s} \cdot \text{cm}^{-5}$ by multiplying the numerator of the above equation by 80; expressed in this way, normal pulmonary vascular resistance is approximately 50 to 100 $\text{dyne} \cdot \text{s} \cdot \text{cm}^{-5}$.

In practice, this resistance equation is more meaningful for the abnormal than the normal pulmonary circulation because the abnormal vessel walls correspond more closely to the hemodynamic conditions on which the formulation is based.

ETIOLOGIES OF PULMONARY HYPERTENSION AND COR PULMONALE

Pulmonary hypertension is usually secondary to an identifiable disease process rather than being primary ("unexplained" or "idiopathic"). The mechanisms by which these underlying conditions cause pulmonary hypertension vary considerably (Tables 39-2 and 39-3).

---

*Edited from Chaps. 82 and 83, "The Pulmonary Circulation" and "Pulmonary Hypertension in Cor Pulmonale," by Fishman AP. In: *Fishman's Pulmonary Diseases and Disorders,* 3d ed., edited by Fishman AP, Elias JA, Fishman JA, Grippi MA, Kaiser LR, Senior RM. New York, McGraw-Hill, 1998, pp 1233–1296. For fuller discussion of topics dealt with in this chapter, the reader is referred to the original text, as noted above.

TABLE 39-1 Representative Normal Hemodynamic Values at Sea Level

	While at Rest	During Moderate Exercise
Cardiac output (L/min)	5–6	16
Heart rate (beats/min)	80	130
Right atrial pressure (mmHg)	4–6	6–8
Pulmonary artery pressures (mmHg)		
Systolic	20–25	30–35
Diastolic	10–12	11–14
Mean	14–18	20–25
Pulmonary wedge pressure (mmHg)	6–10	10–14
Systemic arterial pressure (mmHg)	120/80	150/95
Mean	90–100	110–120
Pulmonary vascular resistance (units)	0.70–1.00	0.6–0.90

TABLE 39-2 Conditions Associated with Pulmonary Hypertension

Hyperkinetic
  Intracardiac shunt lesions
    Atrial septal defect, ventricular septal defect, anomalous venous return
    (total and partial)
  Pulmonary arteriovenous fistulas
Passive
  Elevated left ventricular end-diastolic pressure
    Coronary heart disease, cardiomyopathy, aortic valve disease, constrictive
    pericarditis
  Mitral valve stenosis or obstruction
  Left atrial obstruction
    Myxoma, neoplasm, thrombus
  Pulmonary venous obstruction
    Neoplasm, adenopathy, fibrosing mediastinitis
Obliterative
  Pulmonary parenchymal disease
    Obstructive physiology (bronchitis, emphysema, bronchiectasis, talcosis)
    Restrictive physiology (fibrosis of any causes, thoracic cage abnormalities)
  Pulmonary arteriopathy
    Scleroderma, systemic lupus erythematosus, other collagen vascular
    disease and vasculitis schistosomiasis
  Congenital stenosis
Obstructive
  Pulmonary embolism—acute and chronic
    Venous thromboemboli, tumor emboli
  Pulmonary arterial thrombosis
    Sickle cell disease, Eisenmenger's syndrome (e.g., tetralogy of Fallot)
Vasoconstrictive
  Hypoxemia
    Sleep apnea syndromes, neuromuscular disorders, high-altitude disease
Diet-related pulmonary hypertension (e.g., anorectic agents, toxic oil
syndrome, L-tryptophan, crack-cocaine)
HIV infection
Idiopathic
  Primary pulmonary hypertension, including pulmonary venoocclusive
    disease (small intrapulmonary veins)
  Coexistent portal and pulmonary hypertension
  Persistent fetal circulation

TABLE 39-3 Evaluation of Suspected Pulmonary Hypertension

Laboratory studies—complete blood count, coagulation profile, liver function tests, collagen vascular screen
Chest radiograph
Electrocardiogram
Pulmonary function tests—spirometry, lung volumes, diffusing capacity, arterial blood gas
Ventilation/perfusion lung scan—pulmonary angiogram (if lung scan or clinical history suggests proximal pulmonary embolism)
Echocardiogram
Exercise test
Right heart catheterization

PATHOGENESIS OF PULMONARY HYPERTENSION

The major factor responsible for pulmonary hypertension is an increase in pulmonary vascular resistance. This increase is localized primarily in the precapillary arteries and arterioles and may be anatomic or vasoconstrictive in origin; often both mechanisms are involved, although the anatomic changes invariably predominate.

RESTRICTED VASCULAR BED

Primary pulmonary hypertension (PPH) is a consequence of intrinsic pulmonary vascular disease, which progressively limits pulmonary arterial distensibility and increases pulmonary vascular resistance. Histologically, the disease is characterized by proliferative and obstructive changes in the small muscular arteries and arterioles—i.e., the "resistance vessels."

In the evolution of pulmonary hypertension, as the pulmonary vascular tree is progressively curtailed and becomes less distensible, lesser and lesser increments in pulmonary blood flow (cardiac output) suffice to cause large increments in pulmonary arterial pressures. Eventually, even the resting cardiac output is enough to sustain high pulmonary arterial pressures.

Oxygen Tensions

Alveolar hypoxia is a potent stimulus for pulmonary vasoconstriction acting on the small pulmonary arteries and arterioles; systemic arterial hypoxemia augments the local effects of alveolar hypoxia. In chronic hypoxic states, the effects of these pulmonary vasoconstrictive stimuli are often augmented by increased blood viscosity due to secondary polycythemia.

Acid-Base Status

Acidosis (pH <7.2) also elicits pulmonary vasoconstriction. Acidosis acts synergistically with hypoxia, whereas alkalosis diminishes the vasoconstrictive response to hypoxia.

Carbon Dioxide

Unlike the direct vasoconstrictive effects of acute hypoxia on the precapillary ("resistance") vessels, acute hypercapnia acts by way of the acidosis that it produces. Chronic hypoxia—as occurs in respiratory failure or is induced by metabolic alkalosis due to diuretics—depresses ventilation, thereby augmenting alveolar hypoxia and contributing to hypoxic pulmonary vasoconstriction.

DIAGNOSIS OF PULMONARY VASCULAR DISEASE

Extensive pulmonary vascular changes must be present before pulmonary hypertension develops. When symptoms do develop, they occur first during exertion, presenting as easy fatigability, dyspnea, chest pain, or presyncope/syncope. Right heart failure occurs subsequently and manifests itself as peripheral edema, early satiety, or right-upper-quadrant pain.

Symptoms

No symptom is specific for pulmonary hypertension. The most frequent initial symptom of pulmonary hypertension is exertional dyspnea. This dyspnea, as is the case with easy fatigability, is often blamed on anxiety or being "out of shape." Its mechanism is unclear.

Syncope or presyncope (light-headedness during exertion) is also commonly seen in pulmonary hypertension, usually during exertion. Most frequently, this symptom occurs later in the course of the disease in patients with high resting pulmonary arterial pressures. The cause of syncope is held to be the inability to increase cardiac output adequately during exertion (coupled with exercise-induced systemic vasodilation) or a bradyarrhythmia. It usually indicates a poor prognosis.

Chest pains occur in up to 50 percent of patients with severe pulmonary hypertension; these often resemble typical angina and are thought to be a consequence of right ventricular ischemia.

Hemoptysis may occur from different pulmonary vascular sites, depending on etiology of the underlying disease. In postcapillary pulmonary vascular disorders, the bleeding generally arises from dilated submucosal veins in the airways; in precapillary pulmonary hypertension, aneurysms of alveolar capillaries may be responsible. In instances of pulmonary hypertension in which parenchymal disease is involved, inflammation can cause bleeding by involving the pulmonary microvasculature.

Hoarseness occurs in long-standing, severe pulmonary hypertension. It is due to paralysis of the left vocal cord as the left recurrent laryngeal nerve is compressed between the aorta and the left pulmonary artery (Ortner's syndrome).

The advent of right heart failure and elevation of systemic venous pressure leads to early satiety or right-upper-quadrant epigastric pain due to hepatic congestion and distention of Glisson's capsule.

Signs

The physical signs of pulmonary hypertension are similar regardless of the underlying etiology or pathogenetic mechanism. Early on, the jugular venous pulse configuration is dominated by the *a* wave. As the pulmonary hypertension progresses and right heart failure and tricuspid insufficiency develop, the *a* wave becomes less prominent and the *v* wave becomes proportionally larger. A right ventricular S_4 may be present with the prominent *a* wave. The right ventricle becomes palpable at the lower left sternal border or in the subxiphoid region, and pulmonary arterial valve closure becomes palpable in the second intercostal space.

On auscultation, P_2 is accentuated and S_2 is initially narrowly split. Often a sharp systolic injection click is heard over the pulmonary artery in the second left intercostal space. A right atrial S_3 gallop is often present. A tricuspid insufficiency murmur is frequently heard at the left sternal border. Due to the relatively large pressure gradient present across the tricuspid valve in pulmonary hypertension, the murmur present is high-pitched and quite different from the low-pitched, blowing insufficiency murmur associated with organic tricuspid disease. This murmur may not evidence significant respiratory variation. A pulmonic insufficiency murmur may also be appreciated.

In addition to presenting with the signs and symptoms of right ventricular hypertrophy or right heart failure, attention to the possibility of pulmonary hypertension may be drawn by unexplained arterial hypoxemia. Frequently, the hypoxemia responds poorly to the administration of supplemental oxygen—i.e., it suggests a right-to-left shunting mechanism in the lungs. This shunt may reflect either congenital heart disease, increased flow through vessels in parts of the lungs that are poorly ventilated, or a reopened foramen ovale. An intravenous injection of technetium-99m microaggregated albumin (MAA) may be useful for distinguishing between the latter mechanisms: a patent foramen ovale shunts particles to the systemic circulation, where they will be trapped in the brain, liver, and kidneys; imaging with a gamma camera will reveal the radioactive particles in these organs. Pulmonary microvessels trap the imaging agent within the lungs, so that imaging studies over systemic organs will be negative.

Early Detection of Pulmonary Hypertension

The diagnosis of pulmonary hypertension in its early stages calls for awareness of certain associations. In some diseases, pulmonary hypertension may be part of the natural history. These diseases include widespread interstitial disease, the CREST variant of systemic sclerosis, chronic obstructive lung disease, lupus erythematosus, and thromboembolic disease. More easily overlooked are other associations, such as a family history of primary pulmonary hypertension; the ingestion of an appetite-suppressant drug (e.g., Phen/fen); cirrhosis of the liver; Raynaud's phenomenon; HIV infection; drug abuse (e.g., ingestion of L-tryptophan or the intravenous injection of cocaine); and hypothyroidism.

Diagnostic Studies

The unexpected finding of right ventricular hypertrophy on either an electrocardiogram or an echocardiogram, or of right heart enlargement or enlargement of the pulmonary arteries on a chest radiograph, should raise concern as to the presence of pulmonary hypertension and trigger further investigation. Except for cardiac catheterization (including measurements during exercise), currently available diagnostic techniques are more useful in following the course of documented pulmonary hypertension than for detecting early pulmonary hypertension.

Conventional laboratory tests sometimes shed light on the etiology of an unexplained pulmonary vascular disorder. For example, polycythemia raises the possibility of chronic hypoxia or hemoglobinopathy; hypercoagulable states suggest thrombosis; abnormal liver function studies raise the possibility of concurrent pulmonary hypertension and portal hypertension;

positive serologies can suggest the presence of a systemic connective tissue disorder.

Chest radiographs and pulmonary function tests (spirometry, lung volumes, and diffusing capacity) are useful in suggesting disorders of the airways, intrinsic pulmonary parenchymal disease, or abnormalities of the mediastinum. A ventilation/perfusion lung scan is necessary to distinguish between unresolved clot obstructing large vessels (which are surgically treatable) and other causes of unexplained pulmonary hypertension. Pulmonary angiography is generally reserved for patients with either a clinical history or a lung scan suggestive of large obstructing pulmonary emboli in the major pulmonary arteries. An echocardiogram can demonstrate structural cardiac abnormalities such as valvular disease, septal defects, or myxomas. Right heart catheterization remains necessary for determining the degree of the pulmonary hypertension, excluding certain cardiac lesions, and testing the effectiveness or vasodilator agents. (See Table 39-3 on page 455.)

Primary Pulmonary Hypertension (PPH)

Remarkable progress has been made in recent years in understanding the pathogenesis of pulmonary hypertension and in managing patients with primary and secondary pulmonary hypertension. Until two decades ago, the diagnosis of PPH was a death sentence, with a life span of about 2 to 3 years. Since then, a rapid succession of observations has improved prognosis and outcomes: after showing that chronic vasodilator therapy could cause a clinical remission in about 25 percent of patients with PPH—i.e., in those with a vasoconstrictive component to the disease—it was demonstrated that continuous intravenous prostacyclin improved quality of life and survival in most patients who apparently had no vasoconstrictor component to the pulmonary hypertension, possibly by "remodeling" of the pulmonary circulation. Fresh approaches to treatment were prompted in part by the demonstration of circulating mediators, such as endothelin and thromboxanes, along with upsets in the normal balance of vasoactive mediators in blood and urine. Currently, the search is on for new vasodilator agents and inhibitors and new methods of delivery of pulmonary vasodilator agents.

One by-product of the changes in management has been the advent of specialized centers for initiating therapy and providing instructions to personal physicians. It should also be noted that despite these advances in understanding, diagnosis, and treatment, the 5-year mortality of primary pulmonary hypertension is of the order of 50 percent, underscoring the need for new forms of management. An important recent insight is that pulmonary hypertension associated with known etiologies shares a histopathology with PPH. Among the known etiologies are scleroderma hypertension, anorexigen-induced pulmonary hypertension, HIV-associated pulmonary hypertension, and portal-pulmonary hypertension. The similarities in histopathology have encouraged trials of vasodilator agents in pulmonary hypertension of known cause (e.g., scleroderma).

A promising avenue with respect to the prevention of pulmonary hypertension is the discovery of the gene that causes familial primary pulmonary hypertension—i.e., protein receptor 2 (BMPR2). This mutated gene is a common feature of primary pulmonary hypertension and is believed to set the stage for a second mutation that culminates in the disease. It may serve as a marker for susceptibility to pulmonary hypertension.

TREATMENT OF PULMONARY HYPERTENSION

The treatment of pulmonary hypertension is directed toward reversing the underlying pathogenetic process while relieving hypoxemia, hypercapnia, or acidosis, which might be contributing to pulmonary vasoconstriction. In addition to specific measures, several general therapies apply to patients with pulmonary hypertension regardless of etiology.

Oxygen Supplementation

In patients who develop arterial hypoxemia—either at rest, during exertion, or while asleep—oxygen therapy is directed at relieving hypoxic pulmonary vasoconstriction and decreasing the threat of hypoxia-induced arrhythmias. Careful monitoring is required to avoid inordinate levels of oxygenation, which can decrease respiratory drive, thereby decreasing alveolar ventilation and worsening respiratory acidosis. Carefully adjusted oxygen therapy has been shown to reduce mortality in patients with cor pulmonale and right heart failure and to improve cognitive function and quality of life. Desirable levels of arterial oxygen tension are of the order of 60 mmHg (or an arterial oxygen saturation of about 90%).

Treatment of Heart Failure

Right heart failure in pulmonary hypertension and cor pulmonale is often reversible if the exacerbating factors can be controlled. The usual therapies for heart failure are used: a low-salt regimen, digitalis, and diuretics. Phlebotomy to decrease the circulating blood volume (and hematocrit) may be needed to maintain the benefit. Diuretics should be given with care, particularly in patients with abnormalities of ventilatory control, because metabolic alkalosis may complicate their use; alkalosis, in turn, can contribute to ventilatory insufficiency by depressing the ventilatory response to CO_2. Moreover, diuresis may increase blood viscosity by increasing the hematocrit. In critically ill patients, overdiuresis can result in inadequate filling of the right heart and may compromise cardiac output and arterial oxygenation.

Anticoagulation

Pulmonary hypertension predisposes to pulmonary vascular thrombosis, especially when right ventricular failure supervenes. Instead, thrombi in the small muscular arteries and arterioles are common findings at autopsy in pulmonary hypertensive patients. Moreover, anticoagulation has been shown to prolong life in patients with primary pulmonary hypertension.

Vasodilator Therapy: Prostacyclin (Epoprostenol)

Prostacyclin (epoprostenol) is the "gold standard" for the vasodilator therapy of pulmonary hypertension. The continuous infusion of prostacyclin delays the need for surgery, improves quality of life, decreases morbidity, and improves survival of those who do go to surgery. This conclusion is based on 30 years of experience with its use in primary pulmonary hypertension. The agent is administered intravenously: acutely for testing responsiveness of the hypertensive pulmonary circulation; by chronic intravenous infusion for continuous treatment. The latter has increased life expectancy from a median survival of 4.3 years to 12 years. Recent reports indicate that inhaled prostacyclin may be an effective substitute for the intravenous form. The mechanism by which prostacyclin lowers pulmonary arterial pressures appears largely to involve "remodeling" of the small pulmonary arteries and arterioles.

In Europe, iloprost, an analog of prostacyclin, also administered intravenously, is more readily available than prostacyclin. It appears to be the therapeutically equivalent and is more readily available and less expensive.

Vasodilator Therapy: Calcium-Channel Blockers

Up to 25 percent of patients with primary pulmonary hypertension have a vasodilator response to such agents as prostacyclin, nitric oxide, or adenosine. In the absence of right ventricular failure, these patients without heart failure may respond to long-term therapy with calcium-channel blockers; those with heart failure are treated with the long-term intravenous infusion of prostacyclin. Should prostacyclin fail to control symptoms or arrest progression of the pulmonary hypertension, transplant surgery is an option.

Vasodilator Therapies under Trial

Currently a variety of pharmacologies and gene therapies are being tested for their effectiveness in pulmonary hypertension, along with less demanding routes of administration. The new agents include antiendothelins and nitric oxide synthases; the new routes include subcutaneous injection (of prostacyclin analogs), inhalation (prostacyclin), and oral forms (prostaglandin derivatives).

Surgical Therapy

Bilateral lung transplantation offers the prospect of restoring normal levels of pulmonary blood flow. In selected patients, bilateral lung transplantation may provide dramatic relief of cardiorespiratory failure. Its use is limited by unavailability of donors and by the threat of chronic lung rejection. The rejection is manifested as a bronchiolitis obliterans, culminating in death within a few years.

Another surgical therapy for advanced pulmonary hypertension and cor pulmonale is atrial septostomy. The procedure unloads the right ventricle at the expense of aggravating systemic arterial hypoxemia. It can be done by thoracotomy or by balloon dilation. As yet, a randomized controlled clinical trial has not been done.

BIBLIOGRAPHY

Badesch DB, Tapson VF, McGoon MD, et al: Continuous intravenous epoprostenol for pulmonary hypertension due to the scleroderma spectrum of disease. *Ann Intern Med* 132:425–434, 2000.

Barst ST, Maislin G, Fishman AP: Vasodilator therapy for primary pulmonary hypertension in children. *Circulation* 99:1197–1208, 1999.

Rich S (ed): Primary Pulmonary Hypertension. Executive Summary from the World Health Symposium. Geneva, Switzerland, World Health Organization, 1998. On Internet: (http://www.who.int/ncd/cvd/pph.html)

Rubin LJ: Primary pulmonary hypertension. *N Engl J Med* 336:111–117, 1997.

40 | Pulmonary Thromboembolic Disease*

Alfred P. Fishman

DEFINITION

Pulmonary thromboembolism refers to a systemic venous clot that has lodged in the pulmonary arterial tree. It is a complication of deep venous thrombosis (DVT), which is a common occurrence after surgery, injury, childbirth, stroke, heart failure, and prolonged immobilization. Mortality in untreated pulmonary thromboembolism is of the order of 30 percent, but this can be reduced to 2 to 8 percent with adequate anticoagulant therapy.

Most emboli arise from thrombi in proximal deep veins. However, many proximal thrombi originate in the calf and progress into the proximal veins before embolizing. The risk of recurrence of pulmonary emboli (PE) depends on the residual clot or the clot that propagates proximally after the original clot has fragmented and moved to the lungs.

The three components of Virchow's triad—i.e., stasis, hypercoagulability, and injury to the vessel wall—predispose to the development of venous thrombosis (Table 40-1). Venous *stasis,* most often a consequence of prolonged immobility or bed rest, is a major factor in the development of venous thrombosis. *Hypercoagulability* occurs because of either a predisposition to venous thrombosis or a failure of the mechanisms that normally inhibit propagation of thrombus. *Vascular injury* that exposes collagen in the subendothelial basement membrane to blood causes platelet activation, the release of chemotactic substances, and initiation of the clotting cascades. These factors are particularly important with respect to thrombi that form after trauma and surgery.

CLINICAL MANIFESTATIONS

The clinical manifestations of pulmonary thromboemboli range from the absence of signs and symptoms ("submassive pulmonary emboli") to circulatory collapse and death produced by massive emboli (Table 40-2). To a large extent, the clinical consequences are determined by three major factors: (1) antecedent cardiac and pulmonary function; (2) the size of the embolus and the extent of the pulmonary vascular bed that has been obstructed; and (3) vasoactive substances, both vasoconstrictor and vasodilator, and neurohumoral reflexes.

Individual clinical signs and symptoms—such as dyspnea, pleuritic chest pain, and hemoptysis—are neither sensitive nor specific for thromboembolism. A search for the presence or absence of risk factors for thromboembolism is essential in evaluating a patient for the possibility of pulmonary thromboembolism.

*Edited from Chap. 84, "Pulmonary Thromboembolic Disease," by Palevsky HA, Kelley MA, Fishman AP. In: *Fishman's Pulmonary Diseases and Disorders,* 3d ed., edited by Fishman AP, Elias JA, Fishman JA, Grippi MA, Kaiser LR, Senior RM. New York, McGraw-Hill, 1998, pp 1297–1330. For fuller discussion of topics dealt with in this chapter, the reader is referred to the original text, as noted above.

TABLE 40-1 Vichrow's Triad: Clinical States Predisposing to Venous Thrombosis

Stasis	Immobility
	Bed rest
	Anesthesia
	Congestive heart failure/cor pulmonale
	Prior venous thrombosis
Hypercoagulability	Malignancy
	Anticardiolipin antibody
	Nephrotic syndrome
	Essential thrombocytosis
	Estrogen therapy
	Heparin-induced thrombocytopenia
	Inflammatory bowel disease
	Paroxysmal nocturnal hemoglobinuria
	Disseminated intravascular coagulation
	Protein C and S deficiencies
	Antithrombin III deficiency
Vessel wall injury	Trauma
	Surgery

DIAGNOSTIC TESTS

Chest Radiography

The major value of the chest radiograph is in excluding other causes of dyspnea or chest pain. Often the chest radiograph is abnormal with such lesions as a parenchymal infiltrate, atelectasis, or a pleural effusion. However, all of these manifestations are nonspecific. Whether parenchymal infiltrates that accompany pulmonary thromboembolism are due to pulmonary infarction or hemorrhagic

TABLE 40-2 Incidence of Signs and Symptoms of Pulmonary Embolism

	Massive PE,[a] %	Submassive PE,[a] %	PE without preexisting cardiac or pulmonary disease,[b] %
Dyspnea	85	82	73
Pleuritic chest pain	64	85	66
Cough	53	52	37
Hemoptysis	23	40	13
Tachypnea	95	87	70
	(>16 breaths/min)	(>16 breaths/min)	(>20 breaths/min)
Tachycardia (>100 beats/min)	48	38	30
Increased pulmonic component of second heart sound	58	45	23
Rales	57	60	51
Phlebitis	36	26	11

[a]Data from NIH-sponsored urokinase and streptokinase clinical trials. (*Am J Med* 62:355–360, 1977.)
[b]Data from NIH-sponsored PIOPED study. (*Chest* 100:598–603, 1991.)

edema is debatable. Hypovascularity of a zone of the lung may be suggestive of thromboembolism, especially when accompanied by an enlarged pulmonary artery. "Hampton's hump"—i.e., one or more wedge-shaped, pleural-based densities—represents pulmonary infarction(s) secondary to pulmonary embolism.

As indicated below, the chest radiograph plays an important role in evaluating ventilation/perfusion lung scans.

Electrocardiogram

Although the electrocardiogram (ECG) can be helpful in suggesting an alternative diagnosis, such as pericarditis or acute myocardial infarction, it can, per se, neither make the diagnosis nor rule out pulmonary embolism. As a rule, the ECG is nonspecific, manifesting only a sinus tachycardia or nonspecific changes in the ST-T segments. In about one-fourth of patients with submassive pulmonary embolism, the ECG is normal.

Acute cor pulmonale can occur as a consequence of pulmonary embolism. The ECG may then show a p-pulmonale pattern, right axis deviation, right bundle-branch block, or the classic $S_1Q_3T_3$ pattern. However, these findings are not only infrequent but can also occur in conditions other than acute pulmonary embolism.

Arterial Blood Gases

The distinctive abnormalities in the arterial blood gases are respiratory alkalosis and hypoxemia accompanied by a widened alveolar-arterial difference in P_{O_2} (A-a gradient). However, arterial pH, P_{O_2}, and the A-a gradient are often either normal or only minimally perturbed. Variability in the degree of arterial hypoxemia has two important clinical implications: (1) a normal arterial P_{O_2} or A-a gradient does not exclude the diagnosis of pulmonary embolism and (2) in a patient suspected of thromboembolism, the presence of hypoxemia without obvious cause should encourage further evaluation for pulmonary thromboembolism.

It is worthy of emphasis that although the diagnostic value of individual signs and symptoms and of common tests is poor, the combination can enable accurate diagnosis or even the use of a predictor rule.

Ventilation/Perfusion Lung Scans

Ventilation/perfusion scans play an essential role in the diagnosis of suspected pulmonary thromboembolism. The technique is noninvasive, very safe, and has been extensively validated in clinical trials. In most pulmonary diseases or disorders other than pulmonary emboli, a perfusion defect is accompanied by ventilation defect; in contrast, pulmonary emboli usually elicit perfusion defects that are unaccompanied by ventilation defects. Based on the presence, size, and correspondence of ventilation and perfusion defects, scans for pulmonary emboli are classified into four categories: *normal, high probability, intermediate (or indeterminate) probability,* or *low probability.* Intermediate and low-probability scans are often considered together (see below) as "non-high-probability" scans.

A *normal perfusion scan* excludes clinically significant pulmonary emboli.

High-Probability Lung Scans

Large perfusion defects, particularly when multiple and unmatched by ventilation defects, are most apt to represent substantial embolic events. Scans of this type are highly specific; they predict the presence of pulmonary emboli with a high degree of accuracy. However, although highly specific, the high-probability scan is relatively insensitive in detecting pulmonary emboli. For example, in the PIOPED study (see bibliography), only in 41 percent of patients in whom pulmonary emboli were demonstrated by angiography were scans interpreted as *high probability*.

Because of residual perfusion defects due to previous embolism, the predictive value of the high-probability lung scans decreases in patients with a prior history of pulmonary embolism. In the patient who is a candidate for recurrent pulmonary embolism, lung scans after the course of anticoagulation is finished may help to set a new baseline for detecting future emboli.

Non-High-Probability Lung Scans

Intermediate- and low-probability lung scans are often considered together in dealing with patients suspected of PE, because perfusion defects in both of these categories are smaller or fewer in number than in high-probability scans and the management of the intermediate- and low-probability patient is similar. In patients suspected of having PE, intermediate- and low-probability scans are not diagnostic.

The combination of lung scan and clinical assessment can fail to diagnose or exclude pulmonary emboli in up to two-thirds of patients suspected of pulmonary embolism. The next recourse is either pulmonary angiography to disclose pulmonary emboli or a diagnostic measure that can suggest pulmonary thromboembolism by demonstrating thrombus in the lower extremities—e.g., impedance plethysmography, B-mode ultrasonography, or venography.

Pulmonary Angiography

The sensitivity of pulmonary angiography is of the order of 98 percent and its specificity is between 95 and 98 percent. Continuing improvements have made this technique relatively safe. However, indications generally depend on inconclusive or unavailable noninvasive diagnostic tests, the clinical state of the patient, and the need for a conclusive diagnosis. Contraindications are few but include allergy to iodine-containing agents, impaired renal function, left bundle-branch block, severe heart failure, and severe thrombocytopenia. Pulmonary hypertension increases the risk of pulmonary angiography.

Spiral Computed Tomography (Spiral CT)

Spiral computed tomography (sCT) enables direct visualization of emboli in the pulmonary arterial tree. It entails the administration of contrast material, usually nonionic contrast media. The times required for acquiring the images and for scanning are significantly less than those for conventional CT. Pulmonary emboli are seen as filling defects within the vessel, surrounded by opacified blood, or as a complete filling defect, which leaves the distal vessel completely unopacified. Although this technique was originally heralded as approaching pulmonary angiography as the "gold standard," subsequent observations have reduced sensitivity and specificity considerably. Variability in estimates of accuracy are attributable to variations from institution to institution in study design, investigator experience, and the segments of the pulmonary arterial tree under investigation. Spiral CT is most valuable for detecting emboli in the larger pulmonary arteries—main, lobar, and segmental.

Noninvasive Diagnosis of Deep Venous Thrombosis

Contrast venography is the gold standard for the diagnosis of venous thrombosis in the lower extremities. But it is an invasive procedure that exposes the patient to radiation and to the risks that attend the injection of large amounts of contrast medium. Accordingly, clinicians have come to rely increasingly on noninvasive techniques such as impedance plethysmography (IPG) and real-time (B-mode) ultrasonography.

Impedance Plethysmography (IPG)

Of the noninvasive modalities available for the diagnosis of deep venous thrombosis (DVT) in the lower extremity, IPG is the oldest and best validated. It is simple to apply and low in cost. Although the technique is excellent for detecting proximal DVT—in the popliteal, femoral, or iliac veins—it is not useful for the detection of thrombus in calf veins. Serial IPG is also useful in detecting *proximal propagation* of thrombi that begin in the calf veins, even though it is not useful in diagnosing thrombosis in the calf veins per se.

Real-Time (B-Mode) Ultrasonography

B-mode imaging ultrasound is used to evaluate the deep venous system of the leg for patency, intraluminal thrombi, vein compressibility, evidence of blood flow, and response to hemodynamic maneuvers. This technique seems to be most useful for the diagnosis of femoral or popliteal DVT; it is neither accurate nor reliable for thrombi in the calf or iliac veins. Unfortunately, the diagnostic yield from this method is operator-dependent, so that it is unclear whether the favorable sensitivities and specificities reported from some medical centers are achievable in conventional practice. At present, real-time (B-mode) ultrasonography cannot be recommended as the sole study for the diagnosis of proximal DVT in the lower extremities.

TREATMENT OF THROMBOEMBOLIC DISEASE

Heparin

The well-established treatment for venous thromboembolic disease involves anticoagulation using unfractionated heparin given intravenously followed by oral anticoagulation therapy using warfarin. Mounting evidence indicates that low-molecular-weight heparin (LMWH) can be substituted for unfractionated heparin in treating stable patients with pulmonary emboli. Insufficient evidence is as yet available for LMWH in the treatment of massive pulmonary emboli.

The start of therapy with unfractionated heparin involves an intravenous bolus, usually of 5000 to 10,000 U, followed by continuous intravenous infusion. The infusion rate is guided by the activated partial thromboplastin time (aPTT) targeted at 1.5 to 2.5 control values.

The heparin infusion is continued until oral anticoagulation with warfarin can be substituted. When adequate anticoagulation with warfarin has been achieved (see below), heparin is discontinued.

Two cautions in the use of heparin therapy have to be kept in mind:

1. Bleeding during heparin therapy is uncommon unless the aPTT is excessively prolonged, an invasive procedure is performed, or the patient has either a local lesion or a hemostatic abnormality.

2. The platelet count should be monitored during heparin therapy because of the possibility of heparin-induced thrombocytopenia, a rare but life-threatening complication. This complication appears to be more common with unfractionated than with LMWH.

The increasing popularity of LMWH stems from reports of equal effectiveness coupled with lower cost, shortened hospital stay, and better quality of life than afforded by unfractionated heparin.

Warfarin

Patients who require long-term anticoagulation should be switched to warfarin. The initial and maintenance dosages are the same: 5 mg daily. Adjustment of dosages depends on monitoring the prothrombin time.

In order to standardize oral anticoagulant therapy, the International Normalized Ratio (INR) has been widely adopted. The INR is determined as the ratio of the patient's prothrombin time to the mean value for a group of normals. For thromboembolism, an INR value of 2 to 3 is maintained for the duration of therapy. It should be emphasized that any patient who takes oral therapy requires frequent monitoring of the prothrombin time.

Concomitant

Heparin therapy should be continued for 4 to 5 days or until a therapeutic range of INR is achieved on at least 2 consecutive days. Effective therapy is obtained with an INR value between 2.0 and 3.0. Higher values increase the risk of bleeding complications.

The most common complication of oral anticoagulation therapy is bleeding. The risk is related to the intensity of the anticoagulation—e.g., when INR exceeds 3.0. Correction of a bleeding episode can be accomplished either by withholding warfarin or administering vitamin K (by mouth or intravenously) or fresh-frozen plasma.

The duration of anticoagulation varies with the risk of recurrent thromboemboli. One usual sequence for the patient on warfarin therapy who has experienced a first episode of thromboembolism is to maintain the therapeutic level of prothrombin time for approximately 4 months, reserving longer periods of anticoagulation for those who, at the start of anticoagulant therapy, had extensive DVT or large pulmonary emboli or continue to be at risk for recurrent thrombosis—e.g., prolonged inactivity, a hypercoagulable state, or a concurrent cancer.

In some patients, long-term therapy using heparin administered subcutaneously may be preferable to warfarin therapy. In that event, continuous infusion of heparin intravenously should be maintained for 1 week before switching to a dose-adjusted regimen of heparin administered subcutaneously.

Vena Caval Filters

For patients with venous thromboembolism in whom anticoagulation is contraindicated or for those who are unlikely to survive a recurrent embolic event, percutaneous placement of a filtering device into the inferior vena cava has become standard practice. Clotting of the filter is now uncommon and the filters can safely be used in conjunction with anticoagulation or thrombolytic therapy.

TABLE 40-3 Thrombolytic Therapy for Venous Thromboembolism

Agent	Loading dose	Hourly dose	Recommended duration
Streptokinase	250,000 IU over 30 min	100,000 IU/h	PE:24 h DVT:48–72 h
Urokinase	4400 IU/kg over 10 min	4400 IU/kg/h	PE:12 h DVT:not approved
Tissue-type plasminogen activator	None	50 mg/h	PE:2 h DVT:not approved

KEY: PE, pulmonary embolism; DVT, deep venous thrombosis; IU, international units.

Thrombolytic Therapy

The role of thrombolytic therapy in the treatment of thromboembolic disease is highly controversial. Currently, three thrombolytic agents approved by the U.S. Food and Drug Administration are available for the treatment of pulmonary emboli—streptokinase, urokinase, and recombinant tissue-type plasminogen activator (Table 40-3). The major reason for thrombolytic therapy is to promote the rapid clearance of clot from pulmonary arteries or from deep veins of the legs.

With respect to pulmonary emboli, these agents are generally reserved for *massive* clots that evoke hemodynamic instability or respiratory compromise. With respect to proximal thrombi in the deep veins of the legs, thrombolytic therapy results in more rapid and complete clearance of clot and better preservation of venous valves; it seems to evoke fewer long-term complications (venous stasis and ulceration) than does heparin therapy.

However, several practical considerations temper enthusiasm for the use of thrombolytic therapy in venous thromboembolic disease: (1) Thrombolytic therapy carries a greater risk of bleeding than does heparin therapy. (2) Optimal dosages and regimens for thrombolytic therapy, both in pulmonary thromboembolism and in DVT, have not yet been established. (3) Only few long-term trials that compare thrombolytic and conventional heparin therapies are available. Finally, after a course of thrombolytic therapy, standard anticoagulation is still necessary to prevent recurrent thromboemboli.

APPROACH TO MANAGEMENT

The approach to treating venous thromboembolism in a patient whose circulation and respiration are stable is based on the pivotal role played by deep venous thrombosis and the availability of noninvasive diagnostic methods to assess the amount of clot in both the legs and the lungs. However, this approach applies to conventional anticoagulation but not to thrombolytic therapy. In order for thrombolytic therapy to be seriously considered, the diagnosis of thromboembolic disease should be unequivocal. This requirement usually calls for invasive diagnostic tests, which run the risk of complications and morbidity in a patient with massive clots.

Certain key observations underlie the approach to management of a patient with submassive emboli whose respiration and circulation are stable.

1. The vast majority (>90 percent) of pulmonary emboli originate as DVT in the lower extremities.

2. Recurrent pulmonary emboli are associated with proximal DVT; conversely, recurrent PE are rare in the absence of proximal DVT.
3. Noninvasive evaluation of the lower extremities (particularly IPG), especially when repeated, can reliably establish or exclude the diagnosis of proximal DVT.
4. A low index of clinical suspicion coupled with a normal perfusion scan or a low-probability ventilation/perfusion reliably excludes pulmonary emboli.
5. High-probability lung scans, especially when clinical suspicion of thromboembolism is high and the patient has no prior history of thromboembolic disease, are reliable tests for establishing the presence of PE.
6. The outcome for patients in whom lung scans are not of high probability and in whom noninvasive evaluation (IPG) of the lower extremities for DVT are negative, especially on successive testing, is likely to be favorable, even if such patients are not anticoagulated.

Practical Aspects to this Approach

The patient suspected of having experienced PE and who is clinically stable is screened using ventilation/perfusion lung scans and IPG. If both studies are negative, other etiologies for the patient's symptoms are likely. If the lung scan is interpreted as of high probability and this interpretation is in keeping with the clinical impression or if the IPG is positive, the patient should be treated for venous thromboembolic disease. If the lung scan is not of high probability (but not normal) and the patient is clinically stable, the decision to treat is often based on the results of IPG. If the IPG is negative, particularly if negative on repeated testing, then the risk of recurrent thromboembolism is small and treatment for thrombotic disease need not be instituted. Thus, most clinically stable patients can be evaluated noninvasively for thromboembolic disease.

Pulmonary angiography and venography are reserved for unstable patients or patients in whom the risks of anticoagulation or thrombolytic therapy are so high that an unequivocal diagnosis of PE is necessary. Whether newer, less invasive diagnostic modalities—e.g., real-time ultrasonography, monoclonal antibody imaging, or magnetic resonance imaging—can be substituted for invasive procedures or used in an approach such as is outlined above has not yet been established.

BIBLIOGRAPHY

Fedullo PF, Auger WR, Channick RN, et al: Chronic thromboembolic pulmonary hypertension. *Clin Chest Med* 16:353–374, 1995.

PIOPED Investigators, The: Value of the ventilation/perfusion scan in acute pulmonary embolism. *JAMA* 263:2753–2759, 1990.

Rathbun SW, Raskob GE, Whitsett TZ: Sensitivity and specificity of helical computed tomography in the diagnosis of pulmonary embolism: A systematic review. *Ann Intern Med* 132:227–232, 2000.

Task Force Report on Pulmonary Embolism, European Society of Cardiology: Guidelines on diagnosis and management of acute pulmonary embolism. *Eur Heart J* 21:1301–1336, 2000.

41 | Pulmonary Edema*

Murali Chakinala and Daniel P. Schuster

Pulmonary edema is a frequently encountered entity that is associated with a variety of disease states. Despite the heterogeneous conditions leading to pulmonary edema, the clinical presentation, pathophysiology, and therapeutic options are fairly consistent.

DEFINITION AND CLASSIFICATION

Pulmonary edema can be anatomically classified as either *interstitial* or *alveolar*. Normally, the interstitium of the lung has the reserve to accommodate about 500 mL of fluid before symptoms or physiologic dysfunction is encountered. As additional extravascular fluid accumulates, the interstitial reserve is overwhelmed and alveolar edema occurs.

A more practical classification system is to distinguish *hydrostatic* edema from edema due to *increased permeability*. Hydrostatic edema, as seen in heart failure, results from an increased pressure gradient across the capillary wall. Edema formation from increased permeability, on the other hand, results from lung injury, with adult respiratory distress syndrome (ARDS) being the quintessential example. Despite these prototypical examples, pulmonary edema often results from a combination of increased hydrostatic forces and increased vascular permeability.

FLUID AND PROTEIN HOMEOSTASIS IN THE LUNG

The lung architecture accommodates large volumes of blood over an immense surface area. The endothelial cells that make up the capillary wall permit not only the exchange of diffusible gases but also the necessary efflux of inflammatory cells and various plasma proteins. A by-product of this arrangement is the leakage of fluid from the vascular compartment into the interstitial space, through intercellular junctions and possibly via endothelial cell membrane proteins (i.e., aquaporins). This interstitial space is continuous with the space surrounding the more proximal lymphatic ducts that begin at the junction of the respiratory and terminal bronchioles. Normally, excess interstitial fluid is evacuated away from the alveolus into the lymphatic system, finally returning to the venous system. Normal, pulmonary lymph flow is 10 to 20 mL/h.

Proteins (e.g., albumin) also move from the vascular space into the interstitial space via two forms of migration: transcellular and paracellular. Transcellular migration involves the formation of either intracellular vesicles or transendothelial channels that transport membrane-bound proteins across the endothelial cell. Meanwhile, paracellular transport allows migration of proteins through

*Edited from Chap. 85, "Pulmonary Edema," by Schuster DP. In: *Fishman's Pulmonary Diseases and Disorders,* 3d ed., edited by Fishman AP, Elias JA, Fishman JA, Grippi MA, Kaiser LR, Senior RM. New York, McGraw-Hill, 1998, pp 1331–1356. For fuller discussion of topics dealt with in this chapter, the reader is referred to the original text, as noted above.

469

"tight junctions" between neighboring endothelial cells. These junctions are linked with the cell's cytoskeleton by way of actin filaments. Fluctuations in intracellular Ca^{2+} concentration can alter actin confirmation and cytoskeletal shape, affecting the integrity of these junctions and providing a route for protein migration out of the vascular space during various disease states.

PHYSIOLOGY OF FLUID AND SOLUTE MIGRATION

The amount of extravascular lung water (EVLW) is simply the *difference* between the forces responsible for producing pulmonary edema and the forces that clear it (Fig. 41-1). These individual forces are illustrated by a derivation of Starling's basic law for transcapillary fluid movement:

$$EVLW = (K_{fc})([P_c - P_i] - \sigma[\Pi_c - \Pi_i]) - \text{lymph flow}$$

where K_{fc} = filtration coefficient for the conductance of water (i.e., product of the lung's surface area participating in fluid exchange and the hydraulic conductivity for water)

P_c and P_i = hydrostatic pressures within the capillary and interstitial spaces, respectively

σ = reflection coefficient for protein (i.e., vascular "permeability" to protein)

Π_c and Π_i = oncotic pressures within the capillary and interstitial spaces, respectively

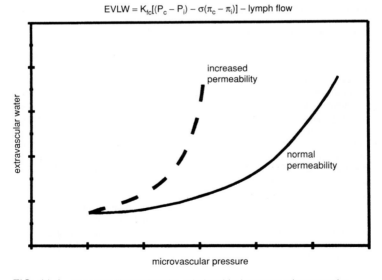

$$EVLW = K_{fc}[(P_c - P_i) - \sigma(\pi_c - \pi_i)] - \text{lymph flow}$$

FIG. 41-1   Diagram illustrating the relationship between microvascular pressure and the development of extravascular water in normal lungs and in those with increased vascular permeability to water and proteins. Note that extravascular water does not increase in the normal lung as microvascular pressure increases, a phenomenon attributed to several compensatory protective mechanisms (see text).

To summarize, fluid is driven out of the vascular space by the net hydrostatic gradient and is opposed by the net oncotic gradient; the difference, EVLW, is then minimized by further removal of fluid through lymphatics or other clearance mechanisms.

Because of gravity's effect and the architecture of the lung, P_c and P_i are not uniform throughout the lung. In regions of the lung below the left atrium, the increase in P_c is relatively greater than the increase in P_i. As a result, the difference in P_c and P_i is more pronounced in the dependent portions of the lung, favoring edema formation in these areas first.

While similar derivations can be used to explain *solute flux* across the capillary barrier, its measurement is further complicated by the semipermeable nature of the capillary membrane to larger solutes, depending on characteristics such as charge, size, and shape of the solute. *Ultimately, fluid and protein flux across the capillary membrane are separate but interdependent processes.*

DEVELOPMENT OF PULMONARY EDEMA

The pathogenesis of pulmonary edema can be divided into two sequential main events: the *escape of fluid from the vascular space into the interstitium* and the *leakage of fluid into the alveolar space*. The initial step towards edema formation is at least partially explained by alteration of the individual variables mentioned in Starling's equation, above. Clinical examples of these alterations are outlined in Table 41-1.

An important notion that highlights the interdependence of these variables is that as the forces that oppose fluid transudation (e.g., membrane conductivity for water and the capillary oncotic pressure) are minimized, the migration of fluid out of the vascular space becomes more sensitive to changes in *capillary hydrostatic pressure*. In terms of Starling's equation, as L_p increases, or σ or Π_c decreases, alterations in P_c have a greater impact on fluid migration out of the vascular space. But progressive changes in P_c do not necessarily cause proportional increases in EVLW, as numerous compensatory or "safety" mechanisms are built into the system. For instance, as protein-free fluid migrates into the interstitial space, P_i increases, Π_i decreases by dilutional effect, and lymph flow increases (as much as tenfold). Obviously, these protective forces are not 100 percent effective and can be overwhelmed.

TABLE 41-1 Disturbances in Variables of the Starling Equation Associated with Pulmonary Edema

Variable	Change	Clinical examples
L_P	↑	ARDS
σ	↓	ARDS
P_c	↑	CHF, volume overload, pulmonary venous hypertension (any cause) HAPE, NPE
P_i	↓	Upper airway obstruction, reexpansion pulmonary edema
π_c	↓	Severe hypoalbuminemia
π_i	↑	None known

KEY: ARDS, adult respiratory distress syndrome; CHF, congestive heart failure; HAPE, high-altitude pulmonary edema; L_p, hydraulic conductivity for water; NPE, neurogenic pulmonary edema.

Endothelial *membrane permeability* is also an important determinant of edema formation. Intracellular changes in calcium concentration, free oxygen radicals, and eicosanoids cause conformational changes in the endothelial cell cytoskeleton, which opens intercellular junctions and allows fluid to depart the vascular space. In this setting, relatively minor alterations in P_c would cause proportionally more leakage of fluid into the interstitial space, again exemplifying the interdependence of the individual variables.

The events transforming *interstitial edema* into *alveolar edema* begin when the rate of accumulating interstitial edema exceeds the normal capacity of the lung's various clearance mechanisms, such as lymph flow. With sufficient interstitial swelling, the epithelial barrier is disrupted and "alveolar flooding" occurs.

The mechanisms underlying disruption of the epithelial barrier are not entirely clear. Several routes may explain this final step in edema formation, including "upstream" breaches of the epithelial barrier near terminal bronchioles with subsequent filling of downstream alveolar units, as seen in congestive heart failure. Alternatively, direct epithelial cell injury and necrosis, as seen in acute lung injury, form breaches in the barrier at the alveolar level.

Damage to the epithelial cell barrier distinguishes the pulmonary edema created by increases in hydrostatic pressure (e.g., congestive heart failure) from increases in vascular permeability (e.g., ARDS). In ARDS, the same amount of EVLW will lead to a relatively greater amount of alveolar edema and worsened gas exchange than seen in congestive heart failure. Stated differently, it is not just the *amount* of EVLW but also its *location* (alveolar or interstitial) that affects the degree of respiratory impairment.

Additional contributions to edema formation are cellular damage from various *oxidant* compounds and *mechanical stress*. *Oxidants,* such as superoxide anions, hydrogen peroxide, and hydroxyl radicals, are directly or indirectly toxic to cell membranes. *Stretching and rupture* of capillaries can occur with extreme elevations of hydrostatic pressures secondary to pulmonary venous hypertension or increased capillary wall tension from alveolar hyperinflation during mechanical ventilation.

Less is known about the resolution of pulmonary edema. *Alveolar* edema probably resolves by multiple mechanisms, depending on degree and location of the epithelial injury. If the alveolar membrane is intact, resolution appears to be an active, energy-dependent process. Fluid is removed separately and more quickly than protein. Therefore, alveolar protein concentration increases as fluid is removed, making additional reabsorption take place against a rising oncotic gradient. While the exact routes for fluid reabsorption are not known, experimental evidence suggest roles for amiloride-sensitive Na^+ channels and separate water channels, such as aquaporins.

PATHOPHYSIOLOGY

Once pulmonary edema has accumulated, normal physiology is affected by disordered gas exchange, altered lung mechanics, increased work of breathing, and deranged pulmonary hemodynamics.

The main *gas exchange* disturbance is hypoxemia, due to increased right-to-left shunting from perfusion of atelectatic and fluid-filled alveoli. These units are unable to participate in normal gas exchange and cause ventilation/perfusion ($\dot{V}/\dot{Q}$) mismatching. A $\dot{V}/\dot{Q}$ of zero is equivalent to an intrapulmonary shunt, making hypoxemia refractory to supplemental oxygen and usually requiring positive-pressure ventilation for recruitment of atelectatic regions. In some cases, hypoxic vasoconstriction reduces the shunt fraction by limiting perfusion to poorly ventilated areas.

Altered *lung mechanics* in the form of worsened compliance is also encountered. Because edematous lungs are "stiffer," greater transpulmonary pressure is necessary to achieve a given increase in volume. The increased stiffness is not so much due to diminished elastic properties but is related to the reduced volume of aerated lung. Reduced or dysfunctional surfactant further reduces the volume of aeratable lung. In some patients, bronchial hyperreactivity increases airway resistance and accounts for the auscultory wheezes of "cardiac asthma."

The *work of breathing* can significantly increase in pulmonary edema and often signals the need for mechanical ventilation.

Last, mild to moderate pulmonary hypertension often develops with pulmonary edema. This *hemodynamic* abnormality mainly results from hypoxic vasoconstriction. Other likely contributors include nonhypoxic vasoconstrictive mediators, vascular compression by edema and alveolar collapse, in situ thrombosis, and vascular obliteration from associated inflammation.

CLINICAL FEATURES

In all cases of pulmonary edema, the hallmark manifestations are dyspnea, tachypnea, and increased work of breathing. Additional findings that offer clues to the etiology include angina (myocardial ischemia), orthopnea (left ventricular dysfunction), palpitations/dizziness (arrhythmia), pleural effusions (volume overloaded state), hypotension (acute myocardial infarction, acute mitral regurgitation, sepsis/ARDS), severe hypertension (hypertensive emergency), or fever (sepsis/ARDS).

The classic auscultory finding of pulmonary edema is inspiratory crackles (rales). These are produced by the sudden opening of small airways and alveolar units, which were closed from accumulation of edema and the bubbling of air through liquid in the airways. Rhonchi can also be detected in pulmonary edema secondary to congestive heart failure, suggesting that the site of escape of fluid is adjacent to larger airways—namely, terminal bronchioles (as mentioned above). Some patients have marked bronchial hypersensitivity to the extravascular fluid accumulation and present with diffuse wheezing, which can mislead the clinician to a diagnosis of "asthma."

Based on the degree and location of edema, presence of bronchospasm, effectiveness of hypoxic vasoconstriction in minimizing $\dot{V}/\dot{Q}$ mismatching, and severity of underlying lung disease, gas exchange abnormalities can vary. Typical findings are *hypoxemia* and *hypocapnia* (secondary to hyperventilation). *Hypercapnia* either suggests the presence of underlying lung disease (e.g., emphysema) or pending respiratory failure and the need for mechanical ventilation.

Early in the course of pulmonary edema, radiographic patterns can help to distinguish cardiogenic and noncardiogenic cases. In cardiogenic edema, notable features include cardiomegaly, prominent perihilar haze, peribronchial cuffing, peripheral septal lines or "Kerley's lines" (which represent engorged lymphatics traversing the interstitium from the level of the terminal bronchioles), pulmonary vascular redistribution, and pleural effusions. In contrast, plain radiographs of patients with noncardiogenic edema demonstrate diffuse and non-gravity-dependent opacities without the typical features of cardiac congestion.

Interestingly, computed tomography scans of ARDS patients reveal a propensity for infiltrates in the dorsal region of the lungs, even though lung injury, as measured by vascular permeability, is more evenly distributed. This heterogeneous appearance is at least partly due to atelectasis, as the infiltrates can be shown to improve by rescanning patients in the prone position. As pulmonary edema progresses to alveolar edema, the infiltrates of cardiogenic and noncardiogenic cases appear similar, with coalescence of infiltrates.

Measurement of cardiac and pulmonary indices with a pulmonary artery catheter (PAC) can be used to distinguish between cardiogenic edema (low cardiac output/index, high systemic vascular resistance, and elevated pulmonary artery occlusion pressure) and noncardiogenic edema (normal or supranormal cardiac function and normal occlusion pressure). The accuracy of these measurements are linked to numerous factors, including the location of the PAC, intravascular volume status, mechanical ventilation, use of positive end-expiratory pressure (PEEP), airway pressures, and degree of underlying cardiac disease. Despite frequent clinical and radiologic overlap of these disparate groups of patients, PAC can still be helpful in guiding therapy. While the measurement of EVLW and vascular permeability would be helpful, these parameters are not easily measurable in the clinical arena at the present time.

SPECIFIC CLINICAL SYNDROMES

Cardiogenic Pulmonary Edema

Elevations in capillary pressure may be secondary to depressed left ventricular contractility, severe elevation in afterload with reduced left ventricular compliance (i.e., diastolic dysfunction), brady- or tachyarrhythmias, acute myocardial ischemia/infarction, aortic or mitral valvular dysfunction (stenosis or regurgitation), or total-body volume overload in the setting of left ventricular dysfunction (usually due to dietary or medical noncompliance). Frequently, a combination of these factors is responsible for cardiogenic pulmonary edema.

Sympathetic nervous system activation can also contribute to the development of cardiogenic pulmonary edema. Venoconstriction and decreased systemic venous capacity redistribute blood from the periphery to the central venous system, leading to elevated pulmonary capillary pressures. This phenomenon helps to explain the effectiveness of venodilators and antianginals such as nitrates and opiates.

The staples of treatment include supplemental oxygen, diuretics, and venodilators (oral, topical, sublingual, or intravenous). Individualized therapies may include afterload reducers such as angiotensin converting enzyme inhibitors and nitroprusside (hypertensive emergencies), antiarrhythmic agents and cardioversion (atrial flutter/fibrillation or other supraventricular tachycardias), or dobutamine and dopamine (cardiogenic shock). Pulmonary edema in the setting of acute myocardial ischemia/infarction poses specific challenges; while antianginals, aspirin, and revascularization (i.e., systemic thrombolysis or primary angioplasty) are essential, beta blockers should be withheld in the setting of significant pulmonary congestion.

Adult Respiratory Distress Syndrome (ARDS)

While strict criteria defining ARDS are not uniformly established, certain key elements must be present: acute respiratory deterioration with severe hypoxemia, increased permeability of extravascular fluid secondary to diffuse epithelial injury, and bilateral radiographic infiltrates consistent with alveolar edema. In addition, the respiratory impairment of ARDS cannot be explained by left atrial or pulmonary capillary hypertension but may coexist with it.

ARDS can result from direct and/or indirect injuries to the lungs. Direct etiologies include inhalation of toxic gases (e.g., smoke, nitrogen dioxide, prolonged hyperoxia), aspiration of gastric contents, near-drowning, and pulmonary contusion. Indirect injury to the lung results from the systemic production of inflammatory mediators and activation of the host immune system. The most frequent clinical conditions that indirectly injure the lung and create ARDS include shock (especially septic shock), pancreatitis, severe trauma, and extensive burns.

While treatment of the underlying cause of ARDS is paramount, appropriate and *noninjurious* supportive measures for respiratory distress (i.e., mechanical ventilation) are also vital. The overall goal is to maintain basic cellular and physiologic function (e.g., gas exchange, organ perfusion, and aerobic metabolism) while minimizing iatrogenic complications (e.g., barotrauma/volutrauma, oxygen toxicity).

Because of increased susceptibility to pulmonary edema, careful fluid and hemodynamic management of patients with ARDS is essential and often necessitates the use of a PAC. The overall objective is to *keep the lungs "dry,"* allowing better gas exchange and lung compliance, *while maintaining adequate perfusion to the remaining organs.*

The adequacy and success of mechanical ventilation hinges on the recruitment of functional lung units and maintaining their patency throughout the respiratory cycle by the application of high positive end-expiratory pressure (PEEP), typically >13 cmH$_2$O. Low tidal volumes (5 to 7 mL/kg) will simultaneously reduce alveolar overdistention and the risk of volutrauma. This "protective ventilatory" strategy provides tolerable gas exchange (Pa$_{O_2}$ > 60, pH > 7.2), reasonable oxygen requirements (Fi$_{O_2}$ $< 60\%$), and acceptable airway pressures (peak airway pressures <45 cmH$_2$O and plateau pressures <35 cmH$_2$O) in the majority of cases. Adherence to these parameters reduces the incidence of barotrauma, volutrauma, oxygen toxicity, and overall complications of mechanical ventilation. In the minority of cases, additional measures such as pharmacologic muscle paralysis, pressure-control and inverse-ratio ventilation, prone positioning, inhaled nitric oxide, and tracheal gas insufflation may still be needed.

Miscellaneous

Some of the less frequently encountered etiologies of pulmonary edema include *high-altitude pulmonary edema (HAPE), neurogenic pulmonary edema, upper-airway obstruction, reperfusion edema, and aspiration or inhalation of foreign material.* The pathogenesis of these various entities also centers around derangements of the basic components of the Starling equation. Treatment is mainly supportive, often including positive pressure ventilation, and prognosis is usually determined by the underlying disease process and not by the pulmonary edema.

BIBLIOGRAPHY

Acute Respiratory Distress Syndrome Network, The: Ventilation with lower tidal volumes as compared with traditional tidal volumes for acute lung injury and the adult respiratory distress syndrome. *N Engl J Med* 342:1301–1308, 2000.

Gattinoni L, Pesenti A, Torresin A, et al: Adult respiratory distress syndrome profiles by computed tomography. *J Thorac Imaging* 1:25–30, 1986.

Gropper MA, Wiener-Kronish JP, Hashimoto S: Acute cardiogenic pulmonary edema. *Clin Chest Med* 15:501–515, 1994.

Jackson RM, Veal CF: Re-expansion, re-oxygenation, and rethinking. *Am J Med Sci* 298:44–50, 1989.

Matthay MA, Folkesson HG, Campagna A, Kheradmand F: Alveolar epithelial barrier and acute lung injury. *New Horizons* 1:613–622, 1993.

Mitchell JP, Schuller D, Calandrino FS, Schuster DP: Improved outcome based on fluid management in critically ill patients requiring pulmonary artery catheterization. *Am Rev Respir Dis* 145:990–998, 1992.

Schuster DP: The case for and against fluid restriction and occlusion pressure reduction in adult respiratory distress syndrome. *New Horizons* 1:478–488, 1993.

Schuster DP, Kollef MH: Acute respiratory distress syndrome. *Dis Mon* 42:265–328, 1996.

42 | Pulmonary Vasculitis*

Daniel B. Rosenbluth

Pulmonary vasculitis is the term applied to inflammation affecting the pulmonary circulation. It is usually part of a systemic process. The extrapulmonary manifestations may be more dramatic and consequential than those produced by the pulmonary involvement. Pulmonary vasculitis may be associated with a diffuse alveolar hemorrhage syndrome.

ANTINEUTROPHIL CYTOPLASMIC AUTOANTIBODY (ANCA)

Two patterns of ANCA-positive immunofluorescence are recognized when alcohol-fixed neutrophils are used as substrates. Cytoplasmic or cANCA displays a coarsely granular cytoplasmic pattern with central accentuation. In contrast, perinuclear or pANCA displays a tight rim of immunofluorescence around the nucleus, which bears resemblance to an antinuclear antibody. The chief target antigen for the cANCA pattern is proteinase 3, a serine proteinase in azurophil granules. Myeloperoxidase is the chief target antigen for the pANCA.

ANCA-ASSOCIATED VASCULITIDES

Comparative features of ANCA-associated vasculitidies are shown in Table 42-1.

Wegener's Granulomatosis

The following are the criteria (commonly known as "Wegener's triad") for this condition: (1) necrotizing granulomatous inflammation of the upper

TABLE 42-1 Comparative Features of Wegener's Granulomatosis (WG), Churg-Strauss Syndrome (CSS), and Microscopic Polyangiitis (MPA)

Feature	WG	CSS	MPA
Asthma	0	++++	0
Eosinophilia (blood, tissue)	+/−	++++	0
History of allergy	0	++++	0
Upper respiratory tract	+++	++	+
Lower respiratory tract	+++	+++	+
Glomerulonephritis	++	+	++++
Skin lesions	++	+++	++
Mononeuritis multiplex	++	+++	+
Eye lesions	++	0	+
Joint symptoms	++	++	++
Cardiac disease	+/−	++	+/−

*Edited from Chap. 86, "Pulmonary Vasculitis," by DeRemee, RA. In: *Fishman's Pulmonary Diseases and Disorders,* 3d ed., edited by Fishman AP, Elias JA, Fishman JA, Grippi MA, Kaiser LR, Senior RM. New York, McGraw-Hill, 1998, pp 1357–1374. For fuller discussion of topics dealt with in this chapter, the reader is referred to the original text, as noted above.

and/or lower respiratory tracts; (2) generalized focal necrotizing vasculitis involving both arteries and veins; and (3) focal necrotizing glomerulitis.

In so-called limited Wegener's granulomatosis, there is no kidney disease and no evidence of systemic vasculitis. In the ELK classification of the disease, E stands for the ears, nose, and throat or upper respiratory tract; L for the lung; and K for the kidney. Under the ELK system, any typical manifestation in E, L, or K supported by typical histopathology or a positive cANCA test qualifies for the diagnosis of Wegener's granulomatosis.

Clinical Manifestations

Ear nose, and throat (E)   In the Mayo Clinic series, the most common symptom was nasal obstruction with nasal crusting and a serosanguineous discharge. Patients often complained of deep, central facial pain. A "saddling" deformity of the nose was the result of dissolution of the nasal cartilage. Chronic otitis media was frequent. Less often was chronic mastoiditis and cholesteatoma formation. Subglottic stenosis is often associated with other upper airway involvement but can be an isolated finding associated with cANCA.

Lung (L)   The lung was involved in 72 percent of 323 patients seen at the Mayo Clinic. Lung involvement may be asymptomatic or may produce cough and occasionally hemoptysis. Patients having diffuse alveolar hemorrhage invariably have severe dyspnea and may develop respiratory failure. Inflammatory cicatricial lesions involving the bronchial tree may result in atelectasis or recurrent obstructive pneumonias. The classic radiographic finding is bilateral pulmonary nodules of varying size and definition, cavitated in about half of patients. Infiltrates may accompany the nodular lesions. Significant pleural lesions are rare.

Kidney (K)   In the Mayo Clinic series, the kidney was involved in 57 percent of cases. The lesion is disclosed by abnormal findings such as proteinuria and urinary red blood cell casts. Kidney involvement is asymptomatic. Creatinine clearance and the serum creatinine may or may not be altered in early disease.

Miscellaneous   Other systemic manifestations of Wegener's granulomatosis include mononeuritis multiplex, necrotizing skin lesions, and uveitis.

Pathology

Where the clinical findings are typical or consistent and there is a positive cANCA, tissue may not be necessary to establish the diagnosis. There are no absolutely diagnostic pathologic features of Wegener's granulomatosis. The necrotizing granuloma dominates the pathologic finding, but infection, particularly due to fungi or acid-fast bacilli, must be excluded. Biopsies of the nose and paranasal sinuses may show only nonspecific inflammation without granulomas or vasculitis. A transbronchial lung biopsy may occasionally support the diagnosis, but more tissue from a thoracoscopic or open lung biopsy may be required if evidence elsewhere is not supportive. The chief finding in the kidney is focal necrotizing glomerulitis that takes the pattern of rapidly progressive, crescentic glomerulonephritis, which is nonspecific.

Laboratory Studies

Anemia is common. The eosinophil count is usually normal. The rheumatoid factor may be elevated in half of the cases. The erythrocyte sedimentation rate may be normal or very elevated. If elevated, it is valuable in following the activity of the disease, particularly during treatment. Indicators of kidney disease are important, particularly the routine urinalysis, serum creatinine, and creatinine clearance. Classic findings on urinalysis are proteinuria with red blood cell casts.

The presence of cANCA is closely associated with the diagnosis of Wegener's granulomatosis. In a large study of patients, specificity of cANCA for Wegener's granulomatosis was found to exceed 90 percent. On occasion, pANCA has been reported, mainly in patients in whom the condition is limited to the upper airway or lungs. Although clearly valuable in diagnosis, the relation of the ANCA titer to disease activity remains unsettled.

Clinical Course, Treatment, and Prognosis

The treatment of choice for Wegener's granulomatosis is cyclophosphamide (1 to 2 mg/kg/day orally) and prednisone (60 mg/day). Once control has been established, the dosage of prednisone is gradually tapered and cyclophosphamide is maintained for 1 year after the last evidence of stability.

In severely ill patients with rapidly progressive glomerulonephritis and/or alveolar hemorrhage, glucocorticoids are administered intravenously (e.g., a bolus of methylprednisolone 0.5 to 1 g) for 3 consecutive days followed by prednisone given orally along with cyclophosphamide. The use of pulse intravenous cyclophosphamide is controversial. In patients who do not tolerate cyclophosphamide, other cytotoxic drugs such as azathioprine have been used. The antimicrobial agent trimethoprim-sulfamethoxazole may be useful in therapy of limited disease or as an adjunct to therapy. For residual fibrotic damage to the nose, subglottic areas, trachea, or bronchi, surgical intervention should be considered. Such interventions are best performed when the underlying disease has been arrested. In 151 patients treated at Mayo Clinic, survival was 90 percent at 1 year, 87 percent at 2 years, and 76 percent at 5 years.

Allergic Granulomatosis and Angiitis—The Churg-Strauss Syndrome

Clinical Manifestations

Allergic granulomatosis and angiitis is a syndrome of severe asthma, fever, and hypereosinophilia accompanied by systemic vasculitis.

Respiratory tract Episodic cough, wheezing, and dyspnea are the cardinal manifestations. Pulmonary function testing will show airway obstruction relieved by inhalation of bronchodilators. The chest radiograph may show fleeting, patchy infiltrates suggesting Löffler's syndrome, or there may be extensive alveolar infiltrates consistent with eosinophilic pneumonia. Multiple poorly circumscribed nodules may occur, but they are usually small and do not cavitate. Diffuse alveolar hemorrhage may occur accompanied by a diffuse bilateral alveolar filling pattern.

The nose and paranasal sinuses are frequently involved, producing nasal obstruction and rhinorrhea. Nasal polyps and/or crusting are common findings. Abnormal sinus radiographs are seen in approximately one-half of patients.

Nervous system Neurologic manifestations occur in about two-thirds of patients. Peripheral neuropathy, especially mononeuritis multiplex, is typical, but distal symmetrical polyneuropathy is also common.

Skin About two-thirds of patients have dermatologic findings, most frequently subcutaneous nodules on the extensor aspects of the arms, hands, and legs.

Cardiovascular Cardiac disease is generally attributed to coronary vasculitis or eosinophilic endocarditis with subsequent endomyocardial fibrosis. In one review, the cause of deaths was cardiac failure in 47 percent and pericarditis in 32 percent.

Musculoskeletal Migratory polyarthritis, which is not erosive or destructive, is common, chiefly affecting the ankles, wrists, and knees. The activity of the arthritis tends to reflect the overall activity of the underlying disease. Diffuse myalgias are common, probably due to myositis.

Gastrointestinal Small bowel perforations, peritonitis, appendicitis, or mucosal ulceration may be encountered due to eosinophilic infiltration and/or vasculitis.

Pathology

The chief histopathologic findings are necrotizing extravascular granuloma (called the *Churg-Strauss granuloma* or *allergic granuloma*); necrotizing vasculitis of small arteries and veins; eosinophilia of vessels and perivascular tissues with lymphocytes, plasma cells, and histiocytes; and fibrinoid necrosis of vessel walls.

Clinical Course, Treatment, and Prognosis

Survival has been reported to be 90 percent at 1 year, 76 percent at 3 years, and 62 percent at 5 years in patients treated primarily with glucocorticoids. A short interval between the onset of asthma and the first signs of vasculitis portends an aggressive process.

Glucocorticoids are the mainstay of therapy. Cytotoxic agents are less effective than in Wegener's granulomatosis. Glucocorticoid therapy may be needed for years and even lifelong. To lower the risk of side effects, efforts should be made to establish an alternate-day regimen. In fulminating cases, glucocorticoid therapy begins with intravenous administration, as described for Wegener's granulomatosis, followed by an oral maintenance dosage of 60 to 80 mg of prednisone daily. The eosinophil count and sedimentation rate are valuable laboratory parameters in the assessment of the efficacy of treatment. Neurologic deficits may persist even after the underlying inflammatory disease has been suppressed.

Microscopic Polyangiitis

Microscopic polyangiitis (MPA) is characterized by inflammation of small vessels—including venules, arterioles, and capillaries—that is not mediated by immune complex deposition. Microscopic polyangiitis shares histopathologic findings with Wegener's granulomatosis and Churg-Strauss syndrome and is ANCA-positive in many cases, usually with pANCA.

Clinical Manifestations

The chief pulmonary manifestation is alveolar hemorrhage. Pleuritic pain, effusion, and pulmonary edema occur occasionally. Although MPA has histologic features of Wegener's granulomatosis and Churg-Strauss syndrome, the upper airway is much less prominently affected. Abnormalities of rheumatoid factor, antinuclear antibodies, and immune complexes are common.

Clinical Course, Treatment, and Prognosis

With varying regimens of prednisone, azathioprine, cyclophosphamide, or plasma exchange, the survival rate has been 70 percent at 1 year and 65 percent at 5 years. Pulmonary hemorrhage, which developed in nearly one-third, was the most formidable complication.

PULMONARY VASCULITIDES NOT ASSOCIATED WITH ANCA

Collagen Vascular Diseases with Pulmonary Vasculitis

Systemic lupus erythematosus, rheumatoid arthritis, dermatomyositis, and polymyositis may have elements of pulmonary vasculitis along with interstitial inflammation and fibrosis. The clinical manifestation of pulmonary vasculitis in these diseases is diffuse alveolar hemorrhage, particularly associated with systemic lupus erythematosus. Behçet's disease involving the respiratory tract occurs in 1 to 5 percent of patients. The most significant lesion is aneurysm of the pulmonary arteries with potential erosion into the bronchial tree and consequent exsanguination. Resection of the aneurysms is indicated and can be lifesaving. Takayasu's arteritis affects large vessels, particularly the aorta and its main branches. The pulmonary artery is involved in up to 50 percent of cases. Pulmonary hypertension may result from the pulmonary vasculitis. It is exceedingly rare.

Necrotizing Sarcoid Granulomatosis

The histology of necrotizing sarcoid granulomatosis is similar to sarcoidosis except for prominent necrosis and destructive vasculitis. The granulomas may become confluent and are reflected in the appearance of multiple, bilateral nodular lesions on the chest radiograph. Hilar adenopathy, as seen in stage I sarcoidosis, does not occur, nor do other features of classic sarcoidosis, such as skin involvement or uveitis. The pathology appears to be confined to the thorax. Despite the extent of disease apparent on the chest radiograph and the nature of the pathology, most patients are asymptomatic, which is typical of sarcoidosis generally. Pathologically, veins and arteries are affected by a destructive process that involves the elastic muscular layers of arteries and veins, but neither thrombosis nor aneurysm formation are seen. The prognosis is good, with frequent spontaneous remissions and a good response to glucocorticoids.

BIBLIOGRAPHY

Sullivan EJ, Hoffman GS: Pulmonary vasculitis. *Clin Chest Med* 19:759–776, 1998.

43 | Pulmonary Arteriovenous Malformations*

Daniel B. Rosenbluth

STRUCTURE

Most pulmonary arteriovenous malformations (PAVMs) have a pulmonary arterial supply and pulmonary venous drainage. Approximately 80 percent have a single feeding and a single draining vessel; the remaining 20 percent are complex, with two or more of each. More than one-third of patients have two or more PAVMs. In general, multiple PAVMs correlate with hereditary hemorrhagic telangiectasia (HHT). In size, PAVMs range from those too small to be seen by radiography or angiography to those greater than 5 cm in diameter. Up to 65 percent of PAVMs are located in the lower lobes.

GENETICS

HHT is an autosomal dominant disease. Phenotypic variation ranges from asymptomatic to severely symptomatic and from cases with no or few mucocutaneous lesions to those with diffuse cutaneous telangiectasias. At least three chromosomal mutations may result in HHT. The gene products for two of these mutations are endoglin, the TGF-β receptor, and the TGF-β_2 receptor.

CLINICAL PRESENTATION

The mean age at detection is 38 to 39 years. PAVMs are uncommon in childhood. Pulmonary symptoms include dyspnea on exertion, orthodeoxia (desaturation in an upright position), and platypnea (dyspnea in an upright position), which occur in the presence of lower lobe PAVMs and hemoptysis in 10 to 15 percent of patients. Extrapulmonary symptoms include chest pain and epistaxis (largely seen in HHT). Headache is common in HHT patients. Transient ischemic attacks occur in 57 percent of patients with PAVM and symptomatic cerebrovascular accident in 18 percent.

Some 25 percent of patients may exhibit no findings at all. Hypoxemia is secondary to the right-to-left shunt, with resulting cyanosis and secondary polycythemia in advanced disease. The frequency of clubbing ranges from less than 10 to 20 percent and is nearly always associated with cyanosis. A pulmonary bruit may be heard in a minority of patients.

Telangiectasia has been reported in up to 66 percent of patients with PAVM. These small red vascular blemishes occur most frequently on the face, followed in descending order by the lips, nares, tongue, ears, hands, chest, and feet. They often increase in size and number with age. Cutaneous telangiectasias are seldom identifiable until the second or third decade.

*Edited from Chap. 87, "Pulmonary Arteriovenous Malformations," by Goodenberger DM. In: *Fishman's Pulmonary Diseases and Disorders,* 3d ed., edited by Fishman AP, Elias JA, Fishman JA, Grippi MA, Kaiser LR, Senior RM. New York, McGraw-Hill, 1998, pp 1375–1385. For fuller discussion of topics dealt with in this chapter, the reader is referred to the original text, as noted above.

A complete blood count may show polycythemia, although in patients with HHT, this tendency may be overcome by iron deficiency anemia. The severely affected person may have arterial hypoxemia at rest; those less severely affected may have orthodeoxia documented by supine and upright arterial blood gases. Blood gases on 100% oxygen may reveal a significant right-to-left shunt.

CLINICAL DIAGNOSIS

Diagnosis is approached differently in the two most common situations.

Evaluation of a Radiographic Abnormality

In evaluating an indeterminate pulmonary nodule, a computed tomography (CT) scan with contrast enhancement may show the typical lesion with feeding arteries and draining veins, but vascular tumors may cause false-positive results. A perfusion lung scan may detect a right-to-left shunt if technetium-labeled macroaggregated albumin passes through the lung and lodges in the brain and kidneys, resulting in radioactivity in those areas; but it does not differentiate intracardiac from intrapulmonary shunt.

Echocardiography, using agitated saline as contrast, is effective in the diagnosis of intrapulmonary shunt. With an intrapulmonary shunt there is a delay, averaging four to five cardiac cycles, of contrast appearance in the left heart. If contrast echocardiography is negative, no further workup for PAVM is indicated. If the contrast echocardiogram is positive, the definitive test is pulmonary angiography.

Screening of Probands or Relatives

The relatives of patients with PAVMs or HHT should be screened with contrast echocardiography to prevent central nervous system complications as the first manifestation of disease. Contrast echocardiography appears to be 100 percent sensitive and 100 percent specific. If it is positive, angiography should be performed.

COMPLICATIONS

Pulmonary Complications

Massive and life-threatening hemoptysis occurs in fewer than 10 percent of patients. Hemothorax occurs in approximately 9 percent of patients, presumably caused by rupture of large subpleural PAVMs into the pleural space. Pregnancy may cause PAVMs to enlarge.

Central Nervous System Complications

Neurologic complications secondary to PAVMs include abscess, paradoxical embolus, and hypoxemia. Brain abscess occurs in 3 to 5 percent of patients with PAVMs. Up to 1 percent of HHT patients have brain abscesses (1000 times the incidence in the general population). Paradoxical embolization to the brain or brain abscess may be the first manifestation of an occult PAVM.

TREATMENT

Early treatment of PAVMs consisted of thoracotomy and resection, but recently embolization of PAVMs has proved to be an excellent alternative with an apparent mortality of zero and few or no serious complications. The most common postembolization symptom is pleurisy sometimes accompanied by large pleural effusions, which resolve within several weeks.

For embolization the feeding vessel must be >2 to 3 mm in diameter. It is technically feasible to embolize most PAVMs. Approximately 6 percent of patients have diffuse, small PAVMs not amenable to embolization. Recanalization of the embolized vessel may occur. Successful embolization of most or all visible PAVMs results in abatement of hypoxemia and its complications. Occlusion of all large PAVMs appears to eliminate the risk of embolic stroke. Embolotherapy may reduce the risk of brain abscess, but abscess may recur even after successful therapy. Standard American Heart Association guidelines for antibiotic prophylaxis in endocarditis are advised before embolotherapy and for dental and other surgical procedures after successful embolotherapy.

BIBLIOGRAPHY

Gossage JR, Kanj G: Pulmonary arteriovenous malformations. A state of the art review. *Am J Respir Crit Care Med* 158:643–661, 1998.

Part Eight | **DISORDERS OF THE PLEURAL SPACE**

44 | Pleural Effusions: Nonmalignant and Malignant*

Daniel B. Rosenbluth

PLEURAL FLUID DYNAMICS AND EFFUSIONS

The pleural membranes line the space that separates the lungs from the mediastinum, diaphragm, and chest wall. The visceral pleura envelops the entire surface of the lungs, and the parietal pleura covers the inner surface of the chest wall, mediastinum, and diaphragm. The two pleural cavities are completely separate. Pain fibers are present in the connective tissue layer of the parietal pleura but not the visceral pleura. The parietal pleura is supplied by branches of systemic arteries, while the blood supply of the visceral pleura arises from the bronchial circulation. The capillaries of the visceral pleura drain into the pulmonary veins.

The parietal lymphatic system is the major route by which lymph leaves the pleural space. Its mesothelial surface is permeated by pores (stomas) that connect to a lymphatic network in the adjacent submesothelial layer. The visceral pleura is devoid of stomas and the underlying lymphatic vessels drain the pulmonary parenchyma.

Formation of Pleural Fluid

The composition of the thin layer of fluid between the parietal and visceral pleura is that of an ultrafiltrate of plasma (Table 44-1). The two linings act like semipermeable membranes, so the concentrations of small molecules, such as glucose, are similar in pleural fluid and plasma, whereas the concentrations of macromolecules (e.g., albumin) are considerably lower in pleural fluid than in plasma. Although the volume of fluid normally present in the pleural space is small (5 to 15 mL), the rate of turnover of pleural fluid is rapid and may be >1 L per day.

Because the hydrostatic pressure gradient in parietal pleural capillaries consistently exceeds the oncotic pressure gradient, fluid filters into the pleural cavity. In the visceral capillaries, the balance of hydrostatic and oncotic pressures promotes the reabsorption of fluid across the visceral pleural surfaces. Sodium and chloride are actively transported out of the pleural fluid. The balance of Starling forces across the pleural membranes and the solute-coupled fluid resorption by the mesothelium keep the volume of pleural at a minimum.

---

*Edited from Chaps. 88, 89, and 90, "Pleural Fluid Dynamics and Effusions," by Kinasewitz GT, "Nonmalignant Pleural Effusions," by Winterbauer RH, and "Malignant Pleural Effusions," by Sahn SA. In: *Fishman's Pulmonary Diseases and Disorders,* 3d ed., edited by Fishman AP, Elias JA, Fishman JA, Grippi MA, Kaiser LR, Senior RM. New York, McGraw-Hill, 1998, pp 1389–1410, 1411–1428, and 1429–1438. For fuller discussion of topics dealt with in this chapter, the reader is referred to the original text, as noted above.

TABLE 44-1 Normal Composition of Pleural Fluid[a]

Volume	0.1–0.2 mL/kg
Cells per mm^3	1000–5000
Mesothelial cells	3–70%
Monocytes	30–75%
Lymphocytes	2–30%
Granulocytes	10%
Protein	1–2 g/dL
Albumin	50–70%
Glucose	<Plasma level
LDH	<50% Plasma level
pH	≥Plasma

[a]Data from humans and animals.

The lymphatics in the parietal pleura provide both a safeguard against excess fluid and a mechanism for recovering proteins from the pleural space. Excess fluid in the pleural space increases lymph flow considerably.

Pleural effusions develop as a result of imbalances in the Starling forces, structural abnormalities in the vascular and mesothelial linings, impaired lymphatic drainage, or abnormal sites of entry—for instance, congenital defects in the diaphragm in a patient with ascites.

DIAGNOSTIC APPROACH

Clinical Appraisal

The hallmarks of pleural disease are pain, ipsilateral restriction of chest wall motion, breathlessness, fever, and an abnormal chest radiograph. A pleural effusion <300 mL of fluid is difficult to detect on physical examination. The percussion note over the fluid is flat, both tactile and vocal fremitus are absent, and breath sounds are diminished or inaudible. Above the effusion, compression of the lung produces the physical findings of consolidation. A pleural friction rub may be audible before the pleuritis has elicited an appreciable effusion. A massive effusion may push the trachea away from the diseased side.

Radiographic Evaluation

In the upright position, as little as 200 mL can be detected as blunting of the costophrenic angle on the lateral chest radiograph. Larger effusions (about 500 mL) are necessary to produce blunting of the costophrenic angle on the posteroanterior (PA) radiograph. Computed tomography (CT) may disclose an effusion that is undetectable by conventional radiography. It also permits a view of the underlying parenchyma, which may be obscured by the pleural disease. It is extremely sensitive in identifying the pleural thickening and calcifications due to asbestos exposure, and helpful in distinguishing between a peripheral lung abscess and a loculated empyema.

A subpulmonic effusion (accumulation of fluid between diaphragm and the inferior surface of the lung) is suspected when one or both hemidiaphragms appear elevated for no good reason. Clues to the presence of a subpulmonic effusion include blunting of the posterior costophrenic angle on the lateral radiograph, lateral displacement of the dome of the diaphragm on the PA radiograph, and widening of the distance between the top of the gastric bubble and the top of the left hemidiaphragm (>2 cm).

Occasionally, pleural effusions accumulate around a particular lobe, simulating lobar consolidation; in an interlobar fissure, simulating a nodule; or parallel to the heart border, simulating cardiomegaly. The explanation for these accumulations is localized obliteration of the pleural space, which forces fluid into unaffected parts of the pleural space.

Ultrasound is helpful in determining the presence and location of fluid in the pleural space and in guiding the aspiration of a loculated effusion.

Thoracentesis

Thoracentesis should not be performed in a patient with a bleeding tendency unless the underlying coagulopathy has been corrected. Some 50 to 100 mL of fluid provides sufficient material for diagnostic studies, whereas a larger quantity is removed during a therapeutic thoracentesis.

Thoracentesis is readily performed at the bedside with the patient sitting upright, with the arms and head supported by an adjustable table. The upper border of a moderate effusion is identified by the presence of a flat percussion note; the thoracentesis should be performed in the interspace below this level. The insertion site should be free of local disease so as to prevent contamination of the pleural space. Effusions <10 mm thick or loculated on decubitus radiographs should be localized by fluoroscopy or ultrasound before thoracentesis is attempted.

The skin is cleansed with iodophor or a similar antiseptic solution and the underlying tissues are infiltrated with local anesthetic. To minimize the risk of injury to intercostal vessels and nerves, the needle is introduced just above the upper edge of a rib and advanced with continuous gentle suction until fluid is obtained. If air is aspirated, the lung has been punctured and the needle should be withdrawn to minimize the risk of pneumothorax. To minimize the risk of lacerating the lung, a plastic catheter can be introduced through the needle and directed inferiorly into the dependent region of the pleural cavity, so that large quantities of fluid can then aspirated.

Complications of thoracentesis include pneumothorax, hemothorax, reexpansion pulmonary edema, and, rarely, air embolism. If a pneumothorax is large or causes breathlessness, aspiration or placement of a chest tube is indicated. Hemothorax usually follows trauma to the intercostal vessels.

Unilateral pulmonary edema occasionally follows *rapid* reexpansion of the lung. To avoid this complication, an effusion should be drained slowly and, as a rule, no more than 1 L of fluid should be removed at any one time.

Pleural Fluid Analysis

Normal pleural fluid resembles water in appearance and is odorless. Gross and microscopic examination of the fluid and determinations of the concentration of protein and lactic dehydrogenase (LDH) usually suffice to establish whether the effusion is a transudate; if so, additional studies are unlikely to yield useful information. If the effusion is an exudate, additional chemical assays and bacteriologic and cytologic studies should be obtained (Table 44-2).

Gross Features

Transudates are generally clear, with a slightly yellow tint. Exudates have a deeper color and more turbid appearance. Empyema fluid is opaque and viscous. Effusions rich in cholesterol have a characteristic satin-like sheen. Chylous effusions are milky.

TABLE 44-2 Useful Tests in the Evaluation of Pleural Effusion

Test	Abnormal value	Frequently associated condition
Red blood cells per mm^3	>100,000	Malignancy, trauma, pulmonary embolism
White blood cells per mm^3	>10,000	Pyogenic infection
Neutrophils	>50%	Acute pleuritis
Lymphocytes	>90%	Tuberculosis, malignancy
Eosinophils	>10%	Asbestos effusion, pneumothorax, resolving infection
Mesothelial cells	Absent	Tuberculosis
Protein, PF/S[a]	>0.5	Exudate
LDH, PF/S	>0.6	Exudate
LDH, IU[b]	>200	Exudate
Glucose, mg/dL	<60	Empyema, TB, malignancy, rheumatoid arthritis
pH	<7.20	Complicated parapneumonic effusion, empyema, esophageal rupture, TB, malignancy, rheumatoid arthritis
Amylase, PF/S	>1	Pancreatitis
Bacteriology	Positive	Cause of infection
Cytology	Positive	Diagnostic of malignancy

[a]Ratio of pleural fluid to serum.
[b]Concentration in international units.

Microscopic Appearance

The white blood cell count of most transudates is <1000/mm^3. Effusions with elevated white blood cell counts and a predominance of mature lymphocytes suggest neoplasm, lymphoma, or tuberculosis. Polymorphonuclear leukocytes predominate in effusions that accompany pneumonia and pancreatitis. Pleural fluid eosinophilia (>10 percent eosinophils) is often caused by air or blood in the pleural space.

Chemical Analyses

Protein and LDH measurements   Pleural fluid is classified as an exudate if it has any one of the following:

1. A ratio of concentration of total protein in pleural fluid to serum >0.5
2. An absolute value of LDH >200 IU
3. A ratio of LDH concentrations in pleural fluid to serum >0.6

If the effusion is an exudate, further analysis of the fluid may help determine its cause.

Glucose   Normally the concentration of glucose in pleural fluid equals that in serum; however, in bacterial infections of the pleura, rheumatoid disease, tuberculous pleurisy, and malignant effusions, the glucose concentration is usually less than that in serum.

pH   Pleural fluid pH < 7.2 can be expected in empyema, esophageal rupture, hemothorax, rheumatoid pleural disease, and systemic acidosis.

Amylase   The concentration of amylase in pleural fluid is high in effusions secondary to pancreatitis and esophageal rupture.

Complement and antibodies The ratio of complement in pleural fluid to serum complement levels is <0.4 in effusions due to rheumatoid disease and systemic lupus erythematosus (SLE).

Other chemical tests A high level of hyaluronic acid in a pleural exudate is suggestive of mesothelioma. High levels of adenosine deaminase and lysozyme may be helpful in distinguishing tuberculous pleural effusions from malignant pleural effusions.

Lipids In chylothorax and pseudochylothorax, the milky appearance is due to large quantities of lipids, chylomicrons in a chylothorax and lecithin-globulin complexes in pseudochylothorax. Triglyceride levels are high in chylothorax (>100 mg/dL) but low (<50 mg/dL) in pseudochylothorax. Lipoprotein electrophoresis will determine if the turbidity is due to chylomicrons.

Cholesterol Pleural Effusion

In tuberculosis or rheumatoid arthritis, the concentration of cholesterol is high, sometimes >1000 mg/dL. These levels greatly exceed those generally encountered in chylothorax. The cholesterol is produced by the inflammatory cells in the pleural effusion. Direct examination of the fluid discloses characteristic rhomboid-shaped crystals.

Bacteriologic Tests

In infectious pleuritis, Gram's stain and culture of the pleural fluid are of paramount importance. Recovery of an organism from culture (aerobic or anaerobic) clinches the cause of the infection. Acid-fast smears and cultures are routine in evaluating effusions of unknown origin.

Cytologic Tests

Malignant cells in the pleural fluid indicate tumor invasion of either the parietal or visceral pleura.

Pleural Biopsy

Closed-needle biopsy of the parietal pleura can be performed with thoracentesis to help diagnose malignancy or granulomatous pleuritis. A special needle, usually an Abrams or Cope needle, is used to obtain both fluid and the pleural specimen.

Pleural biopsy is complementary to cytologic examination of the pleural fluid; when the two tests are performed together, the results will be positive in two-thirds of patients who are ultimately shown to have malignant pleural disease. Pleural biopsy is diagnostic in 70 to 80 percent of patients with tuberculous pleuritis. In contrast, smear and culture of the fluid are positive in <25 percent.

When comprehensive evaluation fails to reveal the cause of the pleural effusion, thoracoscopy and visually directed pleural biopsy may be required.

TYPES OF PLEURAL EFFUSIONS

Pleural effusions occur in 25 to 50 percent of patients with congestive heart failure, pneumonia, malignancy, and pulmonary emboli. Together, these four disorders account for >90 percent of all pleural effusions. The initial step in establishing the cause of an effusion is to determine whether the fluid is a transudate or an exudate.

TABLE 44-3 Causes of Transudative Effusions

Congestive heart failure[a]
Nephrotic syndrome
Cirrhosis
Meigs's syndrome
Hydronephrosis
Peritoneal dialysis

[a]Responsible for >90 percent.

Transudates

Transudates are effusions containing low concentrations of protein or other large molecules. Although many disorders are associated with transudates (Table 44-3), the overwhelming majority are due to congestive heart failure. Hypoalbuminemia also leads to the development of transudative effusions in patients with the nephrotic syndrome and contributes to the pleural effusions that develop in patients with hepatic cirrhosis. The massive hydrothorax that sometimes complicates the ascites of hepatic cirrhosis occurs by passage of the ascitic fluid into the pleural space, either through defects in the diaphragm or via lymphatics. A similar mechanism is thought to be responsible for the pleural effusion that sometimes occurs in the course of hydronephrosis, as urine dissects from the retroperitoneal space to the pleural space. This effusion has a high creatinine level and is actually a urothorax. In Meigs's syndrome, hydrothorax is associated with ascites and a benign ovarian tumor (fibroma, thecoma, or granulosa cell tumor); in most instances, the effusion is on the right. Hydrothorax occasionally occurs during peritoneal dialysis; the chemical composition of the effusion is then similar to that of the dialysate.

Exudates

An exudate is fluid that contains higher concentrations of protein than do transudates. Pneumonia, pulmonary neoplasm, and pulmonary emboli account for over 80 percent of all exudates (Table 44-4).

NONMALIGNANT PLEURAL EFFUSIONS

Parapneumonic Effusions and/or Empyema

The most common cause of an exudative pleural effusion is pneumonia. Forty percent of patients with bacterial pneumonia will have a pleural effusion. Most parapneumonic effusions are small; if appropriate antibiotic therapy is initiated at this stage, the effusion usually does not progress and pleural drainage is frequently unnecessary. However, if the infection in the pulmonary parenchyma is unchecked and the infectious agent invades the pleural space, the effusion can rapidly expand, with an increase in the number of polymorphonuclear leukocytes and a fall in pleural fluid pH and glucose. Fibrin is frequently deposited in the pleural space, forming semipermeable barriers that envelop or loculate the infected spaces. Sampling of the infected space demonstrates pus and/or bacteria and establishes a diagnosis of empyema thoracis.

An uncomplicated parapneumonic effusion that enlarges in the face of antibiotic therapy, particularly if it causes respiratory discomfort, requires

TABLE 44-4 Causes of Exudative Effusions

Very common
 Parapneumonic
 Malignancy
 Pulmonary embolism
Common
 Abdominal disease
 Tuberculous
 Traumatic
 Collagen vascular
  (particularly rheumatoid and SLE[a])
Unusual
 Drug-induced
  (e.g., nitrofurantoin)
 Asbestos
 Dressler's syndrome
 Chylothorax
 Uremia
 Radiation therapy
 Sarcoidosis
 Yellow-nail syndrome
 Ovarian hyperstimulation syndrome

[a]Systemic lupus erythematosus.

drainage. In some instances, thoracentesis will suffice; however, many patients require a chest tube for adequate drainage. If the patient fails to improve clinically and radiographically within 48 h, ultrasonic or CT examination of the pleural space is performed to detect undrained loculated fluid.

The symptoms of empyema are nonspecific. Most patients complain of dyspnea, cough, and chest pain. In addition to fluid in the pleural space, most empyema patients also have a recognizable parenchymal infiltrate on chest x-ray.

Since the advent of beta-lactamase–resistant semisynthetic penicillins in the early 1960s, the organisms causing empyemas have shifted to anaerobic bacteria and aerobic gram-negative rods. Approximately 75 percent of patients with empyema have multiple infecting organisms. Anaerobic bacteria in the pleural space may originate in the mouth or from a subphrenic source via transdiaphragmatic spread. In children with empyema, the coagulase-positive *Staphylococcus* remains the predominant causative organism; anaerobic organisms are rare in patients younger than 18 years. Despite careful sampling, pleural fluids are culture-negative in up to 20 percent of patients with empyema.

The mortality from empyema ranges from 11 to 50 percent. A good outcome demands prompt recognition, appropriate antibiotic therapy, and adequate pleural drainage. The initial choice of antibiotics depends on the results of Gram's stain of pleural fluid and sputum. Antibiotics should be modified when the results of the cultures and sensitivities of the bacteria become available. For patients with empyema from community-acquired infection, the second-generation cephalosporins, cefotetan or cefoxitin, provide coverage against most aerobic Gram's-positive cocci, anaerobic bacteria including bacteroides species, and some gram-negative rods (*Haemophilus* species, *Klebsiella* species, *Escherichia coli,* and *Enterobacter* species). In the absence of a positive Gram's stain, erythromycin 2 g daily should be added to cover *Legionella* species and *Chlamydia pneumoniae*. For nosocomial infections, broader coverage is recommended, such as imipenem plus gentamicin. Initially, antibiotics are administered parenterally; however, should the infection prove to be caused by highly susceptible organisms, oral antibiotics are often substituted after the empyema is adequately drained and signs of sepsis have resolved. As a rule, antibiotics are continued until (1) the patient is afebrile and the white blood cell count is normal, (2) the tube thoracostomy drainage yields <50 mL of fluid daily, and (3) the radiograph shows considerable clearing. Typically, antibiotics are required for 3 to 6 weeks.

The criteria for drainage of a complicated parapneumonic effusion have been more difficult to establish. Pleural fluid of pH < 7.2, glucose <40 mg/dL, and LDH > 1000 IU/L indicates a patient with increased risk for needing pleural drainage; however, some patients meeting these criteria may be cured with antibiotics alone.

If the patient fails to show clinical and radiologic improvement in 48 h after placement of a chest tube, the drainage is either inadequate or, much less commonly, antibiotic selection is incorrect. In patients with inadequate drainage, the choices are (1) percutaneous insertion of additional chest tubes; (2) intrapleural injection of a fibrinolytic agent; or (3) thoracotomy with digital lysis of adhesions and operative placement of chest tubes with or without decortication.

Intrapleural streptokinase or urokinase can dissolve fibrin membranes and facilitate drainage of the pleural space. These agents are injected directly through a chest tube into the pleural space. The chest tube is then clamped for 4 h. This therapy can be repeated daily up to 14 days. Successful response is indicated by an increase in the amount of chest tube drainage, radiographic improvement, and decrease in the systemic signs of infection.

Criteria for tube removal are (1) control of fever and leukocytosis—usually after 7 to 10 days of therapy; (2) <50 mL of fluid draining per day; (3) expansion of the lung as fully as possible; and (4) sealing of a bronchopleural fistula if present.

Tuberculous Pleural Effusions

Tuberculous effusions are usually unilateral and moderate in size. In approximately one-third of patients, coexisting parenchymal disease is evident radiographically. If there is no radiographic evidence of parenchymal disease, the infection usually signifies primary tuberculosis. In 65 percent of patients with tuberculous pleuritis in whom the effusion resolves spontaneously, symptomatic parenchymal disease will occur within 12 months. Nonproductive cough, pleuritic chest pain, and fever occur in most patients; however, patients may be afebrile. Occasionally, the *initial* tuberculin skin test is negative; however, a repeat test within 8 weeks of the development of symptoms is invariably positive.

A tuberculous effusion is usually serous or serosanguineous but almost never frankly bloody. Mycobacteria are demonstrable on smear in less than 10 percent of patients, although 25 percent of tuberculous pleural fluids yield mycobacteria on culture. Typically, more than 50 percent of all white blood cells are mature lymphocytes. The eosinophil count rarely exceeds 10 percent, and mesothelial cells are rare. A pleural effusion adenosine deaminase (ADA) greater than 70 IU/L has shown a sensitivity of 98 percent and specificity of

96 percent for the diagnosis of pleural tuberculosis; however, histologic or bacteriologic confirmation of tuberculosis remains a necessity. The total protein content of the tuberculous effusion tends to be quite high. The concentration of glucose in pleural fluid is usually >60 mg/dL, and the pH varies.

Needle biopsy of the pleura demonstrates granuloma in approximately 80 percent of patients. Culture of the pleural biopsy is indicated, since *Mycobacterium tuberculosis* can be isolated from over 85 percent of biopsies.

With antituberculous therapy, the average patient becomes afebrile within 2 weeks, but fever may persist for 2 months. Radiographic clearing usually occurs in 6 to 12 weeks.

Fungal Pleural Effusions

Fungal diseases account for only 1 percent of pleural effusions. The most common cause is *Aspergillus* (usually *A. fumigatus*). The signs and symptoms mimic chronic bacterial infection of the pleura. In pleural fluid, clumps of hyphae appear as brown suspended particles. In patients with pleural aspergillosis, precipitating antibodies in the serum and the wheal-and-flare cutaneous reaction are almost always positive. Optimal therapy consists of surgical evacuation of the pleural cavity, closure or excision of any present bronchopleural fistula, and amphotericin B systemically.

Approximately 20 percent of patients with acute *Coccidioides immitis* infection show pleural disease on the chest radiograph, and most of these have pleuritic chest pain. Patients are almost always febrile; in about 50 percent of patients, parenchymal infiltrates accompany the pleural effusion. Pleural fluid examination reveals a predominance of lymphocytes, glucose concentration >60 mg/dL, and, rarely, eosinophilia. Pleural fluid cultures are positive for *C. immitis* in 20 percent of patients. Most patients with primary coccidioidomycosis and pleural effusion do not require systemic antifungal therapy.

Cryptococcosis is another rare cause of pleural effusion. More than half of the patients have serious underlying disease, most often either leukemia, lymphoma, or the acquired immunodeficiency syndrome. The pleural effusion is usually unilateral; cultures are positive for the organism in approximately 50 percent of patients. Cryptococcal pleural effusions have high titers of cryptococcal antigen. Patients with serious coexisting disease should receive amphotericin B and 5-fluorocytosine. Immunocompetent patients may recover without specific therapy.

Viral Pleural Effusions

Pleural effusions occur in approximately 10 percent of patients with adenovirus infections. On rare occasions, pleural effusions also occur with infections due to influenza virus, cytomegalovirus, herpes simplex virus, Epstein-Barr virus, and infectious hepatitis. Many self-limited effusions probably represent undiagnosed viral infections. A pleural fluid cell count usually reveals a predominance of mononuclear cells.

Parasitic Infections of the Pleural Space

Pleural pulmonary amebiasis is the most common complication of amebic liver abscess and is usually due to erosion of the abscess through the diaphragm. Empyema presents with sudden respiratory distress and pain and has a substantial mortality. The diagnosis is suggested by the discovery of "anchovy paste" or "chocolate sauce" pleural fluid. *Entamoeba histolytica* is usually demonstrable in the pleural collection. Treatment consists of metronidazole 750 mg PO tid for 5 to 10 days plus diloxanide furoate 500 mg three times a day for 10 days.

Infection by the fluke *Paragonimus westermani* is widely distributed in Africa, Asia, and South America. The cercariae are ingested orally, transit the intestinal wall, and migrate through the peritoneal cavity across the diaphragm into the pleural cavities and then into the lungs. The manifestations of paragonimiasis are eosinophilia and a cough productive of brown sputum with intermittent hemoptysis. Up to half of patients will have pleural effusions. The pleural fluid in paragonimiasis is unique in that the glucose is <10 mg/dL, the LDH level >1000 IU/L, the pH is <7.1, and the differential count reveals a high percentage of eosinophils. The diagnosis is established by finding operculated eggs in sputum or feces.

The hydatid cysts of *Entamoeba granulosus* form in the liver in 50 to 70 percent of patients and in the lung of 20 to 30 percent of patients. Pleural disease develops when either a hepatic or parenchymal lung cyst ruptures into the pleural space. The patient develops severe chest pain, dyspnea, and sometimes shock secondary to severe allergic reactions to parasitic antigens. The diagnosis is established by recognition of daughter cysts in the pleural fluid. Optimal treatment is surgical resection to drain the pleural space and removal of the original cyst.

Pulmonary Emboli

Pleural effusions occur in 30 to 50 percent of patients with pulmonary emboli. About 25 percent of the effusions are transudates and about 75 percent are exudates.

Pancreatitis

Some 20 percent of patients with acute pancreatitis develop pleural effusions. Most of the effusions are unilateral and left-sided. The effusion results from contact of the pleura with enzyme-rich peripancreatic fluid that gains access to the pleural space via transdiaphragmatic lymphatics or, less commonly, through a sinus tract between a pancreatic pseudocyst and the pleural space.

The diagnosis is established by demonstrating high levels of amylase in the pleural fluid. The concentration of glucose is normal. The white blood cell count may vary from 1000 to 50,000/mm^3 with a preponderance of polymorphonuclear leukocytes.

Pleural effusions secondary to pancreatitis usually resolve as the pancreatic inflammation subsides. If resolution has not occurred within 2 weeks, the possibility of a pancreatic pseudocyst or abscess is likely.

Esophageal Perforation

Approximately two-thirds of esophageal perforations occur as a complication of esophagoscopy. Other causes include esophageal carcinoma, gastric intubation, chest trauma, and rupture as a complication of vomiting (Boerhaave syndrome).

Perforation of the esophagus evokes an acute mediastinitis that often spreads through the mediastinal pleura to produce a pleural effusion, which is frequently complicated by a pneumothorax. The pleural effusion is usually left-sided. Radiographic findings include widening of the mediastinum and pneumomediastinum. Most of the morbidity is due to the infection of the mediastinum and the pleural space. Clinical symptoms are dominated by chest pain, usually severe. Hematemesis occurs in about half of the patients.

The pleural fluid is an exudate. The amylase level is high and the pH is very low (frequently <6.0). The amylase that has entered the pleural space through the esophageal defect is salivary. The treatment is exploration of the mediastinum, primary repair of the esophageal tear, and drainage of the pleural space and mediastinum.

Intraabdominal Abscess

A pleural effusion occurs in about 80 percent of patients with a subphrenic abscess. The pleural fluid is an exudate in which polymorphonuclear leukocytes predominate. The pleural fluid white blood count may be as high as 50,000/mm^3, but the pH > 7.2, and the glucose concentration exceeds 60 mg/dL. It is uncommon for the pleural fluid to become infected.

Collagen Vascular Diseases

Rheumatoid Arthritis

Pleural thickening and effusions are the most common pulmonary manifestations of rheumatoid arthritis. They occur in 8 percent of men and 2 percent of women with rheumatoid arthritis. The onset of rheumatoid pleural disease is usually rapid, i.e., over weeks to 3 months, when symptoms reach their peak. The incidence of pleural effusions increases in those patients who have high titers of rheumatoid factor and subcutaneous nodules. Pericardial effusion may occur concurrently. About one-third of patients with rheumatoid pleural effusions have no respiratory symptoms. The others notice some combination of pleuritic chest pain, cough, and dyspnea.

The pleural effusions are usually small. Most are unilateral. Intrapulmonary nodules and diffuse fibrosis sometimes accompany rheumatoid pleural disease. The pleural fluid in is usually an exudate. The predominant cell is either the polymorphonuclear leukocyte or, less often, the lymphocyte. In 80 percent of the patients, the concentration of glucose in the pleural fluid is <30 mg. The pH is usually <7.2, and the LDH concentration is >700 U. In many patients, the ratio of pleural fluid complement to serum complement is <0.4.

Most patients can be treated with a nonsteroidal anti-inflammatory/analgesic medication. Only one-third of patients require systemic corticosteroids for pleural disease. The response to steroids is good, with symptomatic relief and control of pleural fluid volume occurring in more than 75 percent of those treated. Fifty percent of patients (both treated and untreated) undergo resolution of the pleural disease within 4 months of onset.

About 20 percent of the patients develop a chronic, persistent pleural syndrome that tends to flare when therapy is stopped. The frequency of residual pleural fibrosis and restrictive ventilatory defects is higher in this group of patients.

Systemic Lupus Erythematosus (SLE)

Pleural effusions occur in up to 40 percent of patients with SLE. These are small in volume and bilateral in about 50 percent of the patients. Chest radiographs often show lesions other than the pleural effusions.

The pleural fluid is usually clear and yellow; the white cell count reveals a preponderance of polymorphonuclear leukocytes or lymphocytes. The concentration of complement in the pleural fluid is subnormal, and the ratio of pleural fluid to serum complement is <0.4. The pH of the SLE effusion is usually >7.2, the concentration of glucose is >60 mg/dL, and the LDH is <500 U. A pleural fluid antinuclear antibody (ANA) titer greater than or equal to 1:160 and a pleural fluid to serum ANA ratio greater than or equal to 1 is strongly suggestive of lupus pleuritis. The demonstration of lupus erythematosus (LE) cells in pleural fluid is diagnostic of lupus pleuritis. The pleural effusion associated with lupus usually responds well to corticosteroids.

Pleural Effusion from Drug Reactions

Few pleural effusions are induced by drugs. Most drug-induced pleural reactions are associated with a parenchymal abnormality. The symptoms sometimes are acute; i.e., chills, fever, cough, and dyspnea develop within hours to days after the offending drug is ingested. An acute reaction usually develops when prior use has sensitized the patient to the medication. Nitrofurantoin and procarbazine are identified with this pattern of acute illness. Acute pleuropulmonary reactions are often accompanied by eosinophilia in both blood and pleural fluid.

If the offending medication is continued, a chronic syndrome developing over weeks to months is apt to occur. Methysergide, dantrolene, and practolol tend to produce a chronic pleural syndrome with effusion and/or fibrosis. Pleural disease is occasionally not evident clinically until 2 to 3 years after the initial administration of the drug. The pleural changes are either unilateral or bilateral. After stopping of the medication, the pleural reaction improves in most patients over a period of 6 months; however, some are left with a fibrothorax.

Pleural Effusion Secondary to Asbestos Exposure

Three percent of asbestos workers develop pleural effusions. There is a direct relationship between the level of asbestos exposure and the development of the pleural effusion. The pleural effusion frequently develops within 10 years of the initial exposure, in contrast to the occurrence of pleural plaques and calcification, which usually do not occur until more than 10 years after the initial exposure.

Two-thirds of patients with asbestos-related pleural effusions are asymptomatic. Pleuritic chest pain and dyspnea are seen in the other third. The chest radiograph usually reveals a small or moderate unilateral pleural effusion. In 10 percent of patients, the effusions are bilateral. The pleural fluid is either serous or serosanguineous. The total white blood count in the pleural fluid may be as high as 20,000/mm^3, and either polymorphonuclear leukocytes or mononuclear cells predominate. Pleural fluid eosinophilia is common.

The diagnosis of asbestos pleural effusion is one of exclusion. Patients should be carefully evaluated for mesothelioma or bronchogenic carcinoma. In most patients, asbestos pleural effusion resolves in 1 to 2 years. Approximately 20 percent of patients will progress to massive pleural fibrosis; another 5 percent develop mesotheliomas. In 30 percent of patients the effusion waxes and wanes over a long period.

Chylothorax

More than 50 percent of chylothoraxes are related to tumor invading the thoracic lymph duct; and lymphoma is responsible for 75 percent of the malignancy-associated chylothoraxes. Trauma is the second leading cause, responsible for 25 percent of cases. Surgery is the most common cause of traumatic chylothorax, especially in operations that mobilize the left subclavian artery. Chylothorax may be a result of left subclavian lines complicated by clot which obstructs the thoracic duct ostium. Penetrating or nonpenetrating trauma to the chest can also produce the syndrome. Some 25 percent of chylothoraxes have no identifiable cause; they are presumed to be secondary to minor trauma. Pulmonary lymphangioleiomyomatosis has been associated with chylothorax.

The symptoms of chylothorax are related to the volume of fluid in the thoracic cavity. Fever and chest pain are absent. After trauma, the chylothorax usually develops in 2 to 10 days. A pleural fluid that is white, odorless, and milky in appearance suggests chylothorax. Pseudochylothorax accounts for approximately 10 percent of effusions rich in lipids; rheumatoid pleuritis and tuberculosis are the most common underlying diseases for pseudochylothorax.

Triglyceride concentrations greater than 110 mg/dL usually indicate a chylothorax. Levels below 50 mg/dL virtually exclude a chylothorax. In patients with the intermediate values (between 50 and 110 mg/dL), a lipoprotein analysis of the pleural fluid is performed; the demonstration of chylomicrons by lipoprotein analysis establishes the diagnosis of chylothorax. Not all chylous fluids have a classic milky appearance as almost half are either bloody or turbid in appearance. Therefore, determination of the triglyceride content of an exudative fluid of unknown etiology is a must.

The defect in the thoracic duct often closes spontaneously if caused by trauma. In the dyspneic patient, management begins with placement of either a pleuroperitoneal shunt or a chest tube. Efforts are then made to reduce chyle formation; these include placing the patient on constant gastric suction and keeping him or her at bed rest; fluid and nutrition are best supplied by parenteral hyperalimentation.

Malnutrition and lymphopenia are likely to occur in a patient with chylothorax if large amounts of lymph are drained. If lymph drainage has not stopped spontaneously within 7 days, surgical ligation of the thoracic duct is in order. At the time of surgery, an attempt is made to find the leak in the duct and to ligate on both sides of the leak. If the leak is not found, the thoracic duct is ligated both high and low in the thorax. Pleurodesis is a therapeutic alternative that is reserved for poor-risk patients who are not surgical candidates.

Lymphoma should be suspected in all cases of nontraumatic chylothorax. A CT study of the mediastinum should be done on all such patients; if there is evidence of intrathoracic tumor, the patient should undergo exploratory thoracotomy with appropriate biopsies. In a patient known to have lymphoma or metastatic carcinoma, chylothorax may simply be treated by mediastinal irradiation in anticipation that the leak will stop.

Hemothorax

The most common cause of hemothorax is penetrating and nonpenetrating chest trauma. Occasionally iatrogenic procedures, such as percutaneous placement of central venous catheters, produce a hemothorax.

Hemothorax should be considered to be present when the hematocrit of the pleural fluid is more than half that of the peripheral blood. Injuries that may result in hemothorax include pulmonary parenchymal laceration, intercostal vessel laceration, and rupture of pleural adhesions. Much less common is mediastinal injury causing damage of a major blood vessel. The vast majority of hemothoraxes are due to bleeding from the low-pressure pulmonary parenchymal vessels.

In most patients, an associated pneumothorax is found after both nonpenetrating and penetrating trauma. The treatment of choice is the immediate insertion of a chest tube. The chest tube is useful to (1) evacuate blood from the pleural space, thereby decreasing the incidence of empyema and/or fibrothorax; (2) stop bleeding from pulmonary parenchyma or pleural lacerations by apposing the pleural surfaces to create a tamponade; and (3) provide a quantitative measure of continued bleeding. Tube thoracostomy controls bleeding in about 85 percent of cases. Cardiac tamponade, continued bleeding, evidence of a major bronchial rupture, or sucking chest wounds require immediate thoracotomy. If bleeding is more than 200 mL/h and shows no signs of slowing over 4 to 6 h, thoracotomy should be seriously considered. Thoracotomy is not indicated for removal of retained blood in patients without active bleeding. Fewer than 1 percent of patients with hemothorax develop a fibrothorax.

Nontraumatic hemothorax is uncommon. When it does occur, it usually indicates pleural malignancy. It also occurs during anticoagulant therapy for pulmonary embolus. Other causes include bleeding disorders such as hemophilia or thrombocytopenia, complication of spontaneous pneumothorax, ruptured thoracic aorta, and pancreatic pseudocyst.

Postsurgical Pleural Effusions

Following an upper abdominal surgery, pleural effusions can be identified in up to 70 percent of patients. The effusions are usually small; they are greater in patients with postoperative atelectasis and in those with free abdominal fluid at the time of operation. Large effusions are particularly apt to occur after splenectomy. The effusions resolve spontaneously.

The incidence of pleural effusion following coronary artery bypass surgery is as high as 40 percent. The mechanism probably involves trauma to the pleura and pericardium during surgery. Effusions are frequently bilateral or unilateral on the left. Proper management is usually observation.

Post–Cardiac Injury (Dressler's) Syndrome

The post–cardiac injury syndrome consists of fever and pleuropericarditis developing after injury to the pericardium or myocardium. The syndrome has been described following myocardial infarction, cardiac surgery, and blunt chest trauma. Dressler's syndrome is thought to be an immunologic response to damage of the pericardium, and antibodies to cardiac antigens can be demonstrated in many patients.

Symptoms usually occur in the second or third week following myocardial injury. Almost all patients have a pericardial friction rub, and many have a pericardial effusion. Most patients have a peripheral leukocytosis and an elevated erythrocyte sedimentation rate. The pleural effusion may be either unilateral or bilateral and is usually small. Pericarditis is the dominant clinical feature. The pleural fluid is an exudate with a normal pH and a normal glucose level. Almost one-third of patients will have bloody pleural fluid. The pleural fluid cell population will vary from polymorphonuclear predominance to lymphocyte predominance. The diagnosis is one of exclusion.

Sarcoidosis

A pleural effusion can occur in up to 7 percent of patients with sarcoidosis. One-third of cases are bilateral. Pleural biopsy often reveals multiple non-caseating granuloma. Effusions are free-flowing; they rarely loculate and are generally small to moderate in size. The fluid is usually an exudate and invariably shows a predominance of lymphocytes. In some, the effusion may clear spontaneously or with corticosteroid therapy in 1 to 2 months; in others, the effusion can progress to chronic pleural thickening. Because of its rarity, the presence of a pleural effusion in association with pulmonary sarcoidosis should raise a possibility of other causes, including tuberculosis, pneumonia, or heart failure.

Uremic Pleuritis

The incidence of pleural effusions with uremia is approximately 3 percent; half of the patients are symptomatic with pleuritic chest pain and have pleural friction rubs on examination. The fluid is an exudate that is frequently serosanguinous or hemorrhagic. The glucose level is normal, and the differential white blood count reveals a predominance of lymphocytes in most patients. The diagnosis of uremic pleuritis is one of exclusion in the patient with chronic renal failure. Dialysis is the treatment of choice, and resolution occurs within 4 to 6 weeks in the majority of patients.

Yellow-Nail Syndrome

The *yellow-nail syndrome* involves thickening, yellowing, and curvature of all the nails in association with lymphedema, chronic pulmonary infections, and bronchiectasis. Pleural effusion occurs in approximately one-third of patients with the yellow-nail syndrome. The pleural effusions are bilateral half the time and vary in size from small to massive. The pleural fluid is a clear yellow exudate with normal glucose and predominantly lymphocytes in the pleural fluid differential. No specific treatment is available. If the effusion is large and produces dyspnea, pleurodesis should be considered.

MALIGNANT PLEURAL EFFUSIONS

A malignant pleural effusion is diagnosed by finding exfoliated malignant cells in pleural fluid or by demonstrating these cells in pleural tissue obtained by pleural biopsy. Effusions caused by malignancy in which neoplastic cells cannot be demonstrated in pleural fluid or pleural tissue are categorized as paramalignant effusions (Table 44-5). Lymphatic obstruction is the most common cause of a paramalignant effusion. Other causes of paramalignant effusions are bronchial obstruction with either pneumonia or atelectasis and trapped lung. Effusions can result from systemic effects of the tumor and from adverse effects of therapy.

Malignancies Associated with Pleural Effusions

Carcinoma of any organ can metastasize to the pleura. However, carcinoma of the lung is the most common malignancy to invade the pleura and produce malignant and paramalignant effusions, followed by carcinoma of the breast (Table 44-6). Lymphoma accounts for approximately 10 percent of all malignant pleural effusions and is the most common cause of chylothorax.

TABLE 44-5 Causes of Paramalignant Pleural Effusions

Cause	Comment
Local effects of tumor	
Lymphatic obstruction	Predominant mechanism for pleural fluid accumulation
Bronchial obstruction with pneumonia	Parapneumonic effusion; does not exclude operability in lung cancer
Bronchial obstruction with atelectasis	Transudate; does not exclude operability in lung cancer
Trapped lung	Transudate; due to extensive tumor involvement of visceral pleura
Chylothorax	Disruption of thoracic duct; lymphoma most common cause
Superior vena cava syndrome	Transudate; due to increased systemic venous pressure
Systemic effects of tumor	
Pulmonary embolism	Hypercoagulable state
Hypoalbuminemia	Serum albumin <1.5 g/dL; associated with anasarca
Complications of therapy	
Radiation therapy	
Early	Pleuritis 6 weeks to 6 months after radiation completed
Late	Fibrosis of mediastinum Constrictive pericarditis Vena caval obstruction
Chemotherapy	
Methotrexate	Pleuritis or effusion ± blood eosinophilia
Procarbazine	Blood eosinophilia; fever and chills
Cyclophosphamide	Pleuropericarditis
Mitomycin	In association with interstitial disease
Bleomycin	In association with interstitial disease

Pathogenesis

Impaired lymphatic drainage from the pleural space is the predominant mechanism for the accumulation of fluid associated with malignancy. Pleural fibrosis, usually observed in the more advanced stage of tumor involvement of the pleura, is at least partially responsible for the low concentrations of glucose and the low pH seen in some malignant pleural effusions and for the failure to achieve pleurodesis after instillation of chemical agents. A bloody, malignant pleural effusion usually results from either direct invasion of blood vessels, occlusion of venules, or tumor-induced angiogenesis.

TABLE 44-6 Causes of Malignant Pleural Effusions[a]

Tumor	n	Percent
Lung	641	36
Breast	449	25
Lymphoma	187	10
Ovary	188	5
Stomach	142	2
Unknown primary	129	7

[a]N = 1783. Combined data from nine series.

At diagnosis, pleural effusions are rare in Hodgkin's disease but not infrequent in non-Hodgkin's lymphoma. As Hodgkin's disease progresses, the incidence of pleural effusion increases and approaches 30 percent. Pleural effusion in Hodgkin's disease appears to result primarily from impaired lymphatic drainage. In non-Hodgkin's lymphoma, direct pleural infiltration is the predominant cause of effusion.

Clinical Presentation

Patients with carcinoma involving the pleura most often present with dyspnea on exertion and cough. Chest pain is often present because of the involvement of the parietal pleura, ribs, or chest wall. The respiratory symptoms of patients with pleural effusion due to lymphoma are indistinguishable in nature and frequency from symptoms due to carcinoma. About 20 percent of patients with lymphoma have no respiratory symptoms when the malignant pleural effusion is diagnosed.

Chest Radiography

A pleural effusion ipsilateral to the primary lesion is the rule in carcinoma of the lung. When the primary site of the cancer is elsewhere than the lung, with the possible exception of breast cancer, there seems to be no ipsilateral predilection and bilateral effusions are common.

Approximately 50 percent of patients who present with bilateral effusions and a normal heart size have a malignant effusion. If the mediastinum does not shift contralaterally in the face of a large pleural effusion (greater than 1500 mL), malignancy is almost always present and the prognosis is poor. The following diagnoses are then considered: (1) carcinoma of the ipsilateral main-stem bronchus resulting in atelectasis, (2) a fixed mediastinum due to malignant lymph nodes, (3) malignant mesothelioma (the radiodensity represents predominantly tumor with only a small effusion), and (4) extensive tumor infiltration of the ipsilateral lung radiographically mimicking a large effusion. Interstitial infiltrates with effusions (lymphangitic carcinomatosis) and multiple nodules with effusions also suggest a malignant disease.

Pleural Fluid Characteristics

Malignant pleural fluid may be serous, serosanguineous, or grossly bloody. The red cell count usually ranges from 30,000 to 50,000/μL. The number of nucleated cells in the pleural fluid is modest (1500 to 4000/μL) and consists of lymphocytes, macrophages, and mesothelial cells. In about one-half of malignant pleural effusions, lymphocytes predominate (50 to 70 percent of nucleated cells). Pleural fluid eosinophilia is rare (5 percent) in malignant effusions.

The pleural fluid in patients who have carcinoma of the pleura is usually an exudate; however, approximately 5 percent of malignant pleural effusions are transudates. These transudates are due either to concomitant congestive heart failure, atelectasis from bronchial obstruction, or the early stages of lymphatic obstruction.

In about one-third of patients with malignant pleural effusions at the time of diagnosis, the pleural fluid pH is low (less than 7.30), ranging from 6.95 to 7.29. In these low-pH effusions, the glucose concentration is also low.

About 10 percent of malignant pleural effusions have high amylase concentrations. The finding of a high level of salivary-like isoamylase in a patient without esophageal rupture essentially establishes the diagnosis of malignancy, most likely adenocarcinoma of the lung.

The effusion associated with malignant mesothelioma is an exudate with a modest number of nucleated cells (less than 5000/μL), predominantly mononuclear. In some instances of malignant mesothelioma, the viscosity of pleural fluid is greatly increased because of a high concentration of hyaluronic acid.

Diagnosis

Malignant pleural effusion can be diagnosed only by demonstrating malignant cells in pleural fluid or pleural tissue. Cytology is a more sensitive test for the diagnosis than percutaneous pleural biopsy. If the clinician suspects a malignant effusion, several hundred milliliters of fluid should be removed at the initial diagnostic thoracentesis. Percutaneous pleural biopsy should be reserved for the second thoracentesis if the initial pleural fluid cytologic examination is negative.

For the patient with suspected malignancy and negative pleural fluid and pleural tissue examination, options include observation for a few weeks with repeat studies, thoracoscopy, or open pleural biopsy. Bronchoscopy has a low diagnostic yield for an idiopathic pleural effusion without parenchymal lesions, ipsilateral mediastinal shift, or hemoptysis. The value of CT examination of the chest in an undiagnosed exudative effusion is unknown and probably not cost-effective. Under observation, a malignant pleural effusion would be expected to be stable or to progress and an effusion not due to malignancy to be stable or to regress over time. Failure to identify a malignant pleural effusion for several weeks is rarely a disservice to the patient who has incurable disease. Exceptions are those malignancies that tend to be responsive to therapy, such as breast cancer, prostate cancer, thyroid cancer, small cell lung carcinoma, germ cell neoplasms, and lymphomas.

Prognosis

The diagnosis of a malignant pleural effusion signals a poor prognosis. When pH and glucose concentrations in the malignant pleural effusion are low (7.30 and below 60 mg/dL, respectively), the patients' survival time is less (average 2 months) than in those with a normal pH and glucose (average 10 months).

A pleural effusion in the setting of lung cancer usually excludes operability; however, approximately 5 percent of these patients have a paramalignant effusion or effusion from another cause and may be operable and curable. Thus, it is essential to establish the cause of the pleural effusion before deciding that the patient is no longer a candidate for curative surgery.

Treatment

Asymptomatic patients need not be treated, but most will develop progressive pleural effusions that will require therapy. In the debilitated patient in whom a short survival is expected, periodic therapeutic thoracentesis on an outpatient basis is often preferable to hospitalization for tube thoracostomy and pleurodesis (Table 44-7).

Systemic chemotherapy is disappointing for the control of malignant pleural effusions. However, some patients with lymphoma, breast cancer, or small-cell carcinoma of the lung manifest a good response to chemotherapy. As a

TABLE 44-7 Management of Malignant and Paramalignant Pleural Effusions

Option	Comment
Observation	Asymptomatic; most will progress and require therapy
Therapeutic thoracentesis	Prompt relief of dyspnea; recurrence rate variable
Chemotherapy	May be effective in lymphoma, small cell lung cancer, breast cancer
Radiotherapy	Mediastinal radiation may be effective in lymphoma and with lymphomatous chylothorax
Chest tube drainage only	Usually not effective
Chest tube drainage with talc slurry	Control of effusion in >90 percent of cases
Thoracoscopy with talc poudrage	Control of effusion in >90 percent of cases
Pleuroperitoneal shunt	When other options have failed or not indicated; may be useful for chylothorax
Pleural abrasion and pleurectomy	Virtually 100% effective; requires thoracoscopy or thoracotomy

rule, radiation of the hemithorax is contraindicated in malignant pleural effusions from lung cancer. However, when involvement of mediastinal nodes predominates, radiotherapy may be helpful in patients with lymphoma and lymphomatous chylothorax.

The most cost-effective method of controlling a malignant pleural effusion is chest tube drainage and intrapleural instillation of a chemical agent. Currently, the most successful and widely used agents include talc by poudrage or slurry, the tetracyclines (minocycline and doxycycline), *Corynebacterium parvum* (available only in Europe), and bleomycin.

Before instituting chest tube drainage for intrapleural instillation of a chemical agent, it is necessary to demonstrate that thoracentesis with fluid removal improves dyspnea. The patient is a good candidate for pleurodesis if recurrence is rapid, if the expected survival is at least several months, if the patient is not debilitated, and if the pleural fluid pH is above 7.30.

The pleural space must be drained as completely as possible by tube thoracostomy. When the effusion is massive, the fluid should be drained slowly over the first several hours; the chest tube should be clamped intermittently to lessen the likelihood of unilateral pulmonary edema. It is useless to attempt to produce pleurodesis if the lung cannot be expanded fully. When the chest radiograph demonstrates that the effusion is absent or minimal and the lung is fully expanded, 5 g of talc in a slurry should be instilled into the pleural space. Following instillation, the tube should be clamped for 1 h. The chest tube can be removed when drainage is below 150 mL/day, usually within 24 to 48 h. If a large volume of drainage persists, a repeat dose of talc should be instilled. With the properly selected candidate and rigorously applied technique, the malignant effusion is controlled with talc poudrage or slurry in over 90 percent of cases. The degree of pain associated with talc has been variously reported from nonexistent to severe. Fever following talc poudrage or slurry is common. Other complications that have been reported with talc include empyema, arrhythmia, and respiratory failure, including adult respiratory distress syndrome (ARDS) and pneumonitis. The dose of talc used may play a role in the development of respiratory failure, as many reported patients had received 10 or more g of talc.

Pleural abrasion with or without pleurectomy is almost always effective in obliterating the pleural space and controlling a malignant pleural effusion. However, pleurectomy is a major surgical procedure associated with considerable morbidity and some mortality. Accordingly, this procedure is reserved for patients who are in good general condition and who have a reasonably long expected survival or who have failed a sclerosing agent procedure.

A further option available for the patient with intractable symptomatic malignant effusions who cannot undergo pleurodesis is a pleuroperitoneal shunt. The shunt may be particularly beneficial in refractory chylothorax, as it allows recirculation of chyle. Palliation is obtained in 80 to 90 percent of properly selected patients. The major problem has been shunt failure, which is most commonly due to clotting of the catheter.

BIBLIOGRAPHY

Antony VB, Loddenkemper R, Astoul P, et al: Management of malignant pleural effusions. *Am J Resp Crit Care Med* 162:1987–2001, 2000.
Light RW: *Pleural Diseases*. Philadelphia, Lea & Febiger, 1995.

45 | Pneumothorax*

Daniel B. Rosenbluth

A pneumothorax is the accumulation of air in the pleural space with secondary lung collapse. *Spontaneous pneumothorax* occurs without trauma or obvious cause, as opposed to *traumatic pneumothorax*. Primary spontaneous pneumothorax occurs in healthy persons and secondary spontaneous pneumothorax in persons with diseases that affect the lung.

PATHOPHYSIOLOGY

The pressure within the pleural space is negative with respect to the alveolar pressure during the entire respiratory cycle. Therefore air will move from the alveolus into the pleural space when a communication develops between the two, until there is equalization of pressure or the communication is sealed. The same happens with a communication between the chest wall and the pleural cavity. Pneumothorax results in decreases in the vital capacity and the Pa_{O_2}.

SYNDROMES

Primary Spontaneous Pneumothorax

Primary spontaneous pneumothorax occurs most commonly in men in the third and fourth decades of life; they tend to be taller and thinner than controls. Tobacco smoking increases the risk of spontaneous pneumothorax. The cause is most commonly the rupture of subpleural blebs or bullae on the apical portion of the upper lobes. The pathogenesis of these subpleural blebs or bullae is unknown.

Blebs are demonstrated on chest radiographs in only 20 percent of cases but are often found with computed tomography (CT); at thoracotomy, they are present in 85 to 100 percent of cases.

The rate of recurrence after a primary spontaneous pneumothorax is approximately 25 percent; this usually occurs within 2 years of the first episode and on the same side. The rate of recurrence may increase with each successive pneumothorax.

Secondary Pneumothorax

Chronic obstructive pulmonary disease (COPD) is the most common cause of secondary spontaneous pneumothorax. The incidence of spontaneous pneumothorax is high in patients with cystic fibrosis who are older and who have severe pulmonary disease. Other diseases associated with spontaneous secondary pneumothorax include asthma, sarcoidosis, tuberculosis, idiopathic pulmonary fibrosis, eosinophilic granuloma, lymphangioleiomyomatosis, and *Pneumocystis carinii* pneumonia (PCP).

*Edited from Chap. 91, "Pneumothorax," by Peters JI, Sako EY. In: *Fishman's Pulmonary Diseases and Disorders,* 3d ed., edited by Fishman AP, Elias JA, Fishman JA, Grippi MA, Kaiser LR, Senior RM. New York, McGraw-Hill, 1998, pp 1439–1451. For fuller discussion of topics dealt with in this chapter, the reader is referred to the original text, as noted above.

Traumatic Pneumothorax

Trauma is the most common cause of pneumothorax. The leading cause of iatrogenic pneumothorax is lung biopsy via transthoracic needle. The risk of pneumothorax with central venous catheterization is reported between 3 and 6 percent. Pneumothorax may also complicate thoracentesis, transbronchial biopsy, Wang needle aspiration, liver biopsy, intercostal nerve block, mediastinoscopy, and tracheostomy.

Mechanical ventilation is a frequent, potentially lethal cause of iatrogenic pneumothorax. The risk is increased if ventilated patients have chronic pulmonary disease, receive positive end-expiratory pressure, or have inadvertent right main-stem intubation. Clinically, patients become tachypneic and may fight the ventilator. Peak inspiratory pressure often rises suddenly from the fall in lung compliance. Any increased lucency in a supine chest radiograph should be evaluated by erect or decubitus views to detect the presence of a pneumothorax. If these films cannot be obtained, chest CT scan may be necessary.

Penetrating chest trauma produces a pneumothorax by allowing air to enter the pleural cavity directly through the chest wall; if the visceral pleural is penetrated, air may leak from the tracheobronchial tree. Any open chest wound must be occluded to assure adequate ventilation of the patient. Pneumothorax is also a frequent finding in patients with blunt trauma to the chest. Patients with traumatic pneumothorax may have coexisting injuries of the tracheobronchial tree or esophagus. Rupture of the esophagus usually produces a hydropneumothorax.

Catamenial Pneumothorax

Catamenial pneumothorax is a rare disorder in which pneumothorax, usually right-sided, occurs with menstruation and is usually recurrent. Its pathogenesis is unknown. It is usually treated with oral contraceptives to suppress ovulation. Since many patients are of childbearing age, thoracotomy with pleural abrasion or pleurectomy have been performed to prevent recurrent pneumothorax.

Pneumothorax in Acquired Immunodeficiency Syndrome (AIDS)

About 2 to 5 percent of patients with AIDS experience pneumothorax. Patients receiving inhaled pentamidine prophylaxis and those with a history of PCP are at greatest risk. The large number of pneumothoraces in patients with AIDS is thought to be secondary to the high incidence of subpleural cystic disease associated with PCP. Because of the necrotizing nature of PCP, spontaneous pneumothorax is notoriously difficult to treat. Persistent air leaks often require tube thoracostomy for 3 to 4 weeks, and up to one-quarter of patients require surgical intervention. Pneumothorax in patients with AIDS can also occur with pyogenic infections, Kaposi's sarcoma, cytomegalovirus, mycobacterial disease, and as a result of medical procedures.

CLINICAL FEATURES

The symptoms of pneumothorax are chest pain and dyspnea, which occur in 95 percent of patients. The pain is acute, localized to the side of the pneumothorax, and typically pleuritic. Cough, hemoptysis, orthopnea, and Horner's syndrome occur but are uncommon.

Small pneumothoraces (<20 percent) are usually not detectable on physical examination. In patients with obstructive lung disease, even larger pneumothoraces may be difficult to detect. Vital signs are usually normal with the exception of moderate tachycardia. Examination of the chest may reveal the affected side to be larger and to move less during breathing. Tactile fremitus is absent, the percussion note is hyperresonant, and breath sounds are absent or reduced on the side with the pneumothorax. A heart rate above 140 beats per minute, hypotension, cyanosis, or tracheal deviation suggests the possibility of a tension pneumothorax. Arterial blood gases show hypoxemia and perhaps hypocarbia from hyperventilation. In patients with secondary spontaneous pneumothorax, life-threatening hypoxemia and hypercarbia may be present.

RADIOGRAPHIC APPEARANCE

Pneumothorax is diagnosed by demonstrating the outer margin of the visceral pleura (and lung) separated from the parietal pleura (and chest wall) by a lucent gas space. The pleural line may be difficult to detect with a small pneumothorax. In erect patients, pleural gas collects over the apex, and the space between the lung and chest wall is most notable there. In the supine position, the juxtacardiac area, the lateral chest wall, and the subpulmonic region are the best areas to search for pneumothorax. When a suspected pneumothorax is not definitely seen on an inspiratory film, an expiratory film may help.

Avascular bullae or thin-walled cysts can be mistaken for a pneumothorax. A pneumothorax with a pleural adhesion may also simulate bullae or lung cysts. CT may be required to differentiate a loculated pneumothorax from a cyst or bulla.

Common radiographic manifestations of tension pneumothorax are mediastinal shift, diaphragmatic depression, and rib cage expansion.

THERAPY

The basic tenets of therapy for pneumothorax are to evacuate the free air, achieve closure of the leak, and either assess the risk of recurrence or ensure some means of reducing this risk.

Observation

Observation is generally reserved for asymptomatic patients with a small (<20 percent) unilateral pneumothorax. Serial chest radiographs should be performed over the initial 24 h to assess for further progression of the pneumothorax. Initial inpatient monitoring allows the use of adjunct measures such as supplemental oxygen, which increases the rate of absorption of pleural gas. Depending on the circumstances and level of patient compliance, follow-up may be done on an outpatient basis.

Aspiration

Aspiration of a pneumothorax involves insertion of a 16 or 18 Fr plastic catheter under local anesthesia using sterile technique in the second anterior intercostal space in the midclavicular line. Aspiration is performed until no further gas can be withdrawn and the catheter is removed. Follow-up chest radiographs are performed, with aspiration repeated once within 24 h if the first attempt is unsuccessful. If large volumes are aspirated without resolution or the second attempt is unsuccessful, a tube thoracostomy should be performed.

Long-Term Aspiration

Tube thoracostomy entails placement of an indwelling tube into the pleural space for continual removal of the interpleural gas. The tube is connected to a three-chamber system consisting of a fluid collection chamber attached to a water-seal chamber, to allow egress of gas from the pleural space in a one-way fashion, connected to a manometer bottle that regulates the degree of suction applied to the system. In most cases suction is applied for the initial 24 h. If an air leak exists, as evidenced by continual or intermittent egress of gas through the water-seal chamber, suction is maintained. When there is no active air leak, suction is discontinued and the tube may be placed to an underwater seal. After an additional 12 to 24 h, the chest tube may be removed if the pneumothorax does not recur. Persistence of an air leak for more than 72 h generally presages a leak that will not close by this regimen and should prompt consideration of more aggressive therapy.

A variation on the use of pleural drainage systems has been the substitution of a one-way valve to give the patient greater mobility. The most common is the Heimlich flutter valve, which may have some application in cases where long-term indwelling catheterization is required but surgical therapy is declined or not possible.

Pleurodesis

Chemical pleurodesis may be used in combination with tube thoracostomy or surgical therapy. A number of pleural irritants have been used, including quinacrine, silver nitrate, bleomycin, autologous blood, tetracycline, and talc. As an adjunct to tube thoracostomy, the chemical of choice is suspended in fluid and instilled through the tube. The tube is clamped for 6 to 8 h, then placed back to suction or water-seal. Periodically changing patient position during this period is believed to effect more even distribution of the irritant. Typical doses are 0.5 to 1.0 g of doxycycline in 50 to 100 mL normal saline, 600 mg of minocycline in 50 to 100 mL of normal saline, and 2 to 10 g of talc in 100 to 200 mL of normal saline. The most commonly described material is talc, which is insufflated during thoracoscopy or thoracotomy to coat the visceral pleural surface. General requirements for the performance of chemical pleurodesis via the tube are that pleural fluid output be less than 150 to 200 mL/day and that there be no air leak.

Mechanical pleurodesis may performed as part of a surgical procedure. It may consist of simple abrasion of the parietal pleural surface or stripping of the parietal pleura (pleurectomy). Pleurectomy has a greater potential for complications, including injury to an intercostal neurovascular bundle or excessive bleeding from the large raw surface area.

Operative Therapy

Operative therapy is indicated when the above-mentioned techniques fail, with a persistence or recurrence of the pneumothorax, or in patients with factors suggesting increased risk of later recurrence (Table 45-1). This risk of recurrence also includes an assessment of the potential morbidity to the patient should another pneumothorax occur.

TABLE 45-1 Indications for Surgery in Primary
Spontaneous Pneumothorax

First episode
  Prolonged air leak
  Incomplete reexpansion of lung
  Associated single large bulla
  Occupational hazard (flight personnel, divers)
  Absence of medical facility in isolated areas
  Tension pneumothorax[a]
  Hemopneumothorax[a]
  Bilateral pneumothorax[a]
Second episode
  Ipsilateral recurrence
  Contralateral recurrence after first pneumothorax[a]

[a]Relative indications.

Thoracoscopy

Thoracoscopy, or video-assisted thoracoscopic surgery (VATS), requires general anesthesia with double-lumen endotracheal ventilation. The entire lung can be inspected and a search for the air leak carried out. This area can then be closed with the use of a stapler, and the pleural surface abraded or talc-insufflated to achieve pleural adhesion following reexpansion of the lung. Long-term follow-up of recurrence rates has shown results similar to those for open thoracotomy.

Open Thoracotomy

Thoracotomy allows examination of the lung for the site of an air leak, enables lysis of previous adhesions that may lead to a loculated pneumothorax, and enables the release of a fibrotic peel that occasionally forms, leading to incomplete reexpansion of the lung. Drawbacks include the potential risks associated with general anesthesia, increased cost, and significant patient discomfort.

COMPLICATIONS

Tension Pneumothorax

A tension pneumothorax occurs when the visceral or parietal pleura is disrupted in such a manner that a one-way valve develops. During inspiration, the respiratory muscles contract and create negative intrapleural pressure, allowing for air movement into the pleural space. Then, during expiration, when the expiratory muscles relax, the pleural pressure becomes positive and the one-way valve prevents the egress of air from the pleural space.

    Tension pneumothorax is more common after a traumatic pneumothorax or with mechanical ventilation. A tension pneumothorax may develop because of improper connection of a one-way flutter valve to the chest tube. Patients appear acutely ill, with labored breathing, tachypnea, marked tachycardia, profuse diaphoresis, and cyanosis; they often exhibit distended neck veins, tracheal deviation to the side opposite the pneumothorax, subcutaneous emphysema, and hypotension. Patients receiving mechanical ventilation typically develop a sudden increase in peak and plateau pressures with a decrease in oxygen saturation.

Tension pneumothorax should be suspected in any patient with a pneumothorax whose condition deteriorates acutely, in any patient with cardiopulmonary collapse after a procedure known to cause a pneumothorax, and in any patient undergoing cardiopulmonary resuscitation who is difficult to ventilate or develops electromechanical dissociation. The decompensation of the cardiopulmonary status in patients with tension pneumothorax is usually attributed to diminished venous return and low cardiac output.

When the diagnosis of a tension pneumothorax is considered, confirmation by chest x-ray is desirable if time permits. The patient should be given a high concentration of oxygen, and a large-bore needle should be inserted into the second anterior intercostal space on the side with the pneumothorax. Optimally, the needle should be connected to a syringe partly filled with sterile saline. Air bubbling outward through the fluid confirms the diagnosis. The needle or its plastic outer sheath should be left in place and the patient prepared for immediate tube thoracostomy.

Bronchopleural Fistula

Most air leaks seal within 24 to 48 h. Patients with cystic fibrosis or COPD are at increased risk for the development of persistent bronchopleural fistula. For those who are not candidates for thoracotomy, the fistula may be localized by bronchoscopic balloon catheter occlusion and subsequently injected with a variety of substances to promote sealing of the air leak. However, most of these patients eventually undergo thoracoscopic surgery because these procedures usually fail and the air leak persists for more than 7 to 10 days.

Reexpansion Pulmonary Edema

Unilateral pulmonary edema may occur when the lung is rapidly reexpanded. It appears to be due to increased permeability of the pulmonary capillaries that are damaged by mechanical stress during reexpansion of the lung. Reperfusion injury due to free radicals may also be responsible for increased capillary permeability. The risk is increased with chronic pneumothorax and high suction pressures.

Typically, a persistent cough or tightness of the chest develops immediately after chest tube insertion; the patient develops hypoxemia and occasionally hypotension. Symptoms usually progress for 24 to 48 h. Up to 20 percent of cases have been fatal. If the patient survives the first 48 h, recovery is usually complete.

BIBLIOGRAPHY

Jenkinson SG: Pneumothorax. *Clin Chest Med* 6:153–161, 1985.
Sahn SA, Heffner JE: Spontaneous pneumothorax. *N Engl J Med* 342:868–874, 2000.

46 | Malignant Mesothelioma and Other Primary Pleural Tumors*

Daniel B. Rosenbluth

The most common tumors of the pleura are metastatic neoplasms. Tumors arising primarily from the pleura are rare and constitute a variety of malignant and benign lesions from several different cells of origin.

MALIGNANT MESOTHELIOMA

Epidemiology

The most common primary malignant tumor of the pleura is malignant mesothelioma. The incidence in the United States is estimated to be 2200 cases per year. The incidence is expected to drop in developed countries because of recent legislation aimed at reducing asbestos exposure, but it is predicted to escalate in the third world because of inadequate regulation of asbestos mining and widespread use of asbestos.

Etiology

The predominant cause of malignant mesothelioma is inhalational exposure to asbestos. The latency period from asbestos exposure to the development of mesothelioma is approximately 30 to 40 years. The exact mechanisms of asbestos carcinogenesis have not yet been fully elucidated. Although the lifetime risk of developing mesothelioma among asbestos workers is thought to be as high as 8 to 13 percent, there is no direct correlation of pleural disease incidence to the amount or duration of asbestos exposure. Peritoneal mesothelioma has been shown to occur more commonly in patients with heavy asbestos exposure.

Asbestos is the name for a group of hydrated magnesium silicate fibrous minerals divided into two major types: the serpentines and the amphiboles. Serpentine (chrysotile) fibers are curly and pliable, whereas the amphiboles (crocidolite, amosite, tremolite, anthophyllite, actinolite) are long and needle-like. Fibers with a high length-to-width ratio, such as crocidolite, are considered more carcinogenic. Amosite has an intermediate risk, chrysotile the lowest. Other fibrous materials, such as fiber glass, milled to the same size standards, may carry a similar cancer risk.

In rare cases malignant pleural mesothelioma has been associated with therapeutic irradiation, intrapleural thorium dioxide (Thorotrast), and inhalation of other fibrous silicates such as erionite.

*Edited from Chap. 92, "Malignant Mesothelioma and Other Primary Pleural Tumors," by Albelda SM, Sterman DH, Litsky LA. In: *Fishman's Pulmonary Diseases and Disorders,* 3d ed., edited by Fishman AP, Elias JA, Fishman JA, Grippi MA, Kaiser LR, Senior RM. New York, McGraw-Hill, 1998, pp 1453–1466. For fuller discussion of topics dealt with in this chapter, the reader is referred to the original text, as noted above.

Pathology

Grossly malignant mesothelioma is a firm, grayish tumor coalescing on the visceral and parietal pleural surfaces into discrete plaques and nodules. Adjacent structures are involved at an early stage, with invasion of the chest wall, pericardium, diaphragm, and interlobar fissures.

Malignant mesothelioma is classified into three histologic subtypes—epithelial, sarcomatoid, and biphasic. The epithelial subtype is the most common and differs from those with sarcomatoid histology in clinical course and presentation. It behaves much like metastatic carcinomas to the pleura, presenting with large pleural effusions and metastases to regional lymph nodes, while sarcomatoid tumors present with bulky tumor masses, minimal pleural fluid, and blood-borne metastases.

Clinical Presentation

Malignant pleural mesothelioma most commonly presents in the fifth to seventh decades of life. The most frequent presenting symptoms are nonpleuritic chest pain, dyspnea, and cough. Some patients are asymptomatic at diagnosis. Physical findings may include unilateral dullness to percussion throughout the hemithorax, palpable chest wall masses, and scoliosis toward the side of the malignancy.

Radiographic Presentation

The most common initial radiographic manifestation of pleural mesothelioma is a large unilateral pleural effusion with contralateral mediastinal shift. Occasionally, it presents as a pleural mass without pleural effusion. Only 20 percent of patients have radiographic signs of asbestosis, although many have evidence of pleural plaques and/or calcifications. In later stages of disease, ipsilateral mediastinal shift is seen secondary to encompassment of the lung by a thick rind of tumor and unilateral loss of lung volume. In advanced mesothelioma there may be mediastinal widening due to direct tumor invasion or lymph node involvement, enlargement of the cardiac margins secondary to pericardial invasion with effusion, and rib destruction or soft tissue masses extending from the chest wall. Chest computed tomography (CT) is important in detecting invasion of chest wall, ribs, and mediastinal structures. Magnetic resonance imaging (MRI) is helpful in discerning extension of pleural mesothelioma through the diaphragm into the peritoneal cavity.

Laboratory Studies

There are no specific serum biomarkers for malignant mesothelioma. Pleural effusions associated with mesothelioma are exudates, with elevated concentrations of protein and lactate dehydrogenase (LDH), and a lymphocytic predominance. With extensive involvement of visceral and parietal pleura, pleural fluid pH and glucose are commonly low. The effusion is characteristically highly viscous due to an elevated concentration of hyaluronic acid. An increased hyaluronidase level is suggestive but not diagnostic of mesothelioma. Pulmonary function testing typically demonstrates a restrictive pattern.

Diagnosis

Thoracentesis or closed pleural biopsy may not provide enough material to establish the presence of mesothelioma. Surgical intervention, via video-assisted thoracoscopic biopsy or open thoracotomy, is often necessary to make the diagnosis. Approximately 10 percent of patients who undergo a diagnostic procedure for mesothelioma will have seeding of the biopsy site with tumor cells, later developing chest wall recurrences. Prophylactic radiation therapy to the surgical incision or thoracentesis sites may prevent this complication.

Clinical Course and Complications

Mesothelioma exerts its morbidity and mortality via inexorable local invasion. Patients typically develop shortness of breath and chest pain as tumor obliterates the pleural space. Blood is shunted through the poorly ventilated trapped lung, leading to hypoxemia that is often refractory to supplemental oxygen. Dyspnea relates to abnormal lung and chest wall mechanics. Local invasion can result in dysphagia, hoarseness, cord compression, brachial plexopathy, Horner's syndrome, and superior vena cava syndrome. Distant metastatic disease, by hematogenous spread, is unusual in mesothelioma.

Mortality

Median survival of patients with mesothelioma is 6 to 18 months and is not significantly affected by current standard therapy. Patients die from local extension and respiratory failure; tumor extension below the diaphragm may result in death from small bowel obstruction.

Paraneoplastic Syndromes

Disseminated intravascular coagulation, migratory thrombophlebitis, thrombocytosis, Coombs-positive hemolytic anemia, hypoglycemia, and hypercalcemia associated with secretion of a parathyroid hormone–like peptide have been described in the setting of mesothelioma.

CURRENT APPROACHES TO TREATMENT OF MESOTHELIOMA

Response rates to single-agent chemotherapy have been dismal, ranging from 0 to 20 percent. Mesothelioma is more responsive to radiation than non–small cell lung cancer; however, "curative" radiotherapy involving therapy to the entire involved pleural surface is technically difficult and associated with a high risk of radiation pneumonitis, myelitis, hepatitis, and myocarditis. Most studies have shown no significant effect upon survival following high-dose external-beam irradiation. Radiation therapy may have a role in preventing chest wall recurrences after thoracoscopy/thoracotomy and in improving local control after pleurectomy or extrapleural pneumonectomy. Surgical intervention has been useful in palliating the major symptoms of the disease and may lead to some improvement in patient survival.

Palliation of disabling dyspnea may be achieved by drainage of the pleural effusion with pleurodesis. Unfortunately, chemical pleurodesis is often unsuccessful because the bulky tumor covering the pleural cavity prevents apposition of the pleural surfaces. Parietal pleurectomy—open surgical stripping of the pleura and pericardium from the apex of the lung to the diaphragm—is more successful than pleurodesis in reducing the recurrence of pleural effusion. The combination of parietal pleurectomy with postoperative intrapleural therapy and/or external beam irradiation has resulted in a median survival of 22.5 months and a 2-year survival rate of 41 percent in a select group of patients.

Pleuroperitoneal shunting is an alternative approach to relieving the rapid reaccumulation of pleural fluid in patients with mesothelioma. One potential risk of this procedure, borne out by anecdotal reports, is the rapid spread of mesothelioma to the abdomen, with subsequent development of bowel obstruction.

Extrapleural pneumonectomy (EPP) is a radical surgical procedure involving the complete removal of the ipsilateral lung along with the parietal and visceral pleura, pericardium with portions of the phrenic nerve, and the majority of the hemidiaphragm. EPP is associated with significant morbidity and an operative mortality of 5 to 35 percent. EPP alone has not been shown to prolong survival significantly, but EPP combined with sequential postoperative chemotherapy and adjuvant radiotherapy may improve survival.

Various forms of immunotherapy and gene therapy for mesothelioma are under investigation.

OTHER PRIMARY PLEURAL NEOPLASMS

Solitary, benign fibrous tumors of the pleura, previously referred to as "benign mesotheliomas," are approximately one-third as common as malignant mesothelioma and are thought to arise from a different cell of origin. The peak age range of affected patients is 40 to 70 years. There is no association of benign fibrous tumors of the pleura with asbestos exposure or other environmental agents.

Clinical Presentation

Solitary fibrous tumors of the pleura are usually diagnosed incidentally at routine chest radiography, but they can present with nonpleuritic chest pain, dyspnea, cough, or pleural effusion. Up to 40 percent of patients present with symptomatic hypoglycemia, thought to be secondary to elaboration of insulin-like growth factors. Clubbing of the digits is common, as are diffuse arthralgias.

Radiography

Benign fibrous tumors present radiographically as large, rounded, well-circumscribed pleura-based masses, but occasionally they can appear to be intraparenchymal. About 17 percent will present with an ipsilateral pleural effusion.

Pathology

Solitary fibrous tumors of the pleura typically arise from a pedicle on the visceral pleural surface, but they rarely invade the visceral pleura. They are well-circumscribed, firm, encapsulated, occasionally lobulated masses that vary in size. Histologic sections show interlacing spindle-like cells interspersed between areas of variably dense collagenous material. By electron microscopy the spindle cells lack the prominent microvilli and tonofilaments seen in malignant mesothelioma.

Treatment

Surgical resection of solitary, benign fibrous tumors of the pleura is curative.

Other Primary Pleural Tumors

A variety of benign and malignant neoplasms arising from multiple cell types of the pleural lining can occur, including soft tissue sarcomas, malignant and benign fibrous histiocytomas, fibromyxomas, and spindle-cell carcinoma. Each of these lesions has a characteristic immunohistochemical pattern.

BIBLIOGRAPHY

Testa JR, Pass HI, Carbone M: Benign and malignant mesothelioma, in DeVita VT Jr, Hellman S, Rosenberg SA (eds): *Cancer: Principles and Practice of Oncology,* 6th ed. Philadelphia, Lippincott, 2001, pp 1937–1969.

Part Nine | **DISEASES OF THE MEDIASTINUM**

47

The Mediastinum: Overview, Anatomy, and Diagnostic Approach*

Larry R. Kaiser and Joe B. Putnam, Jr.

The mediastinum lies centrally within the chest and spans the region vertically from the thoracic inlet to the diaphragmatic hiatus, transversely between the parietal pleura, and coronally between the sternum and vertebral column. Diseases of the mediastinum may affect any or all structures within the chest, with diverse effects both clinically and anatomically. Many patients, however, are asymptomatic, with the mediastinal mass found on routine screening chest radiograph. The location and mass effect on the heart or great vessels, the tracheobronchial tree, the esophagus, and nerves and other structures may produce specific clinical symptoms and may narrow the differential diagnosis. With the advent of the routine plain chest radiograph, computed tomography (CT) of the chest, magnetic resonance imaging (MRI), and various other diagnostic studies, the diagnosis of mediastinal lesions can be made more frequently and accurately.

The clinical presentation of the patient, the radiographic findings, and the location of the tumor all assist the clinician, who must consider the potential for neoplasia and infections as well as anatomic, congenital, or traumatic causes. Diagnosis of mediastinal masses may require histologic or other laboratory evaluation. Cytology (from fine-needle aspiration), core biopsy, or open (surgical) biopsy may be required for complete staging if neoplasia is suspected, as the treatment of mediastinal masses may be determined from histology and clinical staging.

ANATOMY

The mediastinum contains all soft tissue thoracic organs with the exception of the two lungs (Fig. 47-1). The mediastinal structures are separated from the thoracic cavity by the parietal pleura. The mediastinum is not fixed to the rigid thoracic structures and therefore can shift from its normal midline position by pressure (blood, air) or by compression from tumors. Acute displacement may impair venous return to the heart and can be fatal. Tumors that penetrate this pleura, by definition, invade the mediastinum. The paravertebral sulcus is a part of the hemithorax and not a true part of the mediastinum; however, the close juxtaposition of the mediastinal structures to the paravertebral sulcus and the radiographic appearances of tumors and abnormalities in this area typically allow these lesions to be grouped together with discussions of the mediastinum.

*Edited from Chap. 93, "The Mediastinum: Overview, Anatomy, and Diagnostic Approach," by Putnam JB Jr. In: *Fishman's Pulmonary Diseases and Disorders,* 3d ed., edited by Fishman AP, Elias JA, Fishman JA, Grippi MA, Kaiser LR, Senior RM. New York, McGraw-Hill, 1998, pp 1469–1484. For fuller discussion of topics dealt with in this chapter, the reader is referred to the original text, as noted above.

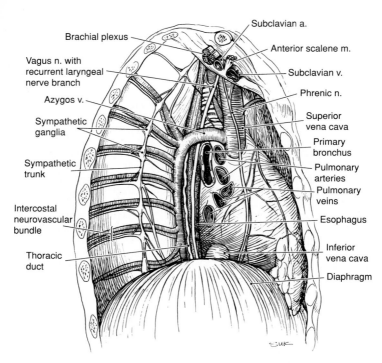

FIG. 47-1 The mediastinum as seen from the right thorax. The right lung has been removed. In adults, roughly 75 percent of mediastinal masses are benign and 25 percent malignant. In children, approximately 50 percent are benign and 50 percent malignant. The incidence of mediastinal tumors is often derived from large surgical series compiled over one or more decades. Series have been published from the early 1950s to the present. Diagnostic imaging, histologic diagnostic techniques, and surgical procedures have evolved considerably during the past 40 years, influencing the ability of the surgeon to improve selection of appropriate patients for treatment and to pathologically confirm the disease present within the mediastinum. Above is an approximation of incidence of mediastinal masses from various surgical series.

The thoracic inlet provides the superior limit of the mediastinum (Fig. 47-2A). Tumors in this area are further confined by the limited space within the thoracic inlet and may affect breathing by compression of the trachea. The diaphragm (Fig. 47-3) provides the inferior border to the mediastinum and separates the thorax from the abdomen. The structures within the mediastinum may be grouped together in various "compartments" and are listed in Table 47-1.

PNEUMOMEDIASTINUM

Pneumomediastinum (mediastinal emphysema) is an uncommon condition but is now being seen with increasing frequency due to the common use of mechanical ventilation—specifically certain modes of mechanical ventilation. Air (or gas) outside the normal confines of the respiratory and gastrointestinal tracts

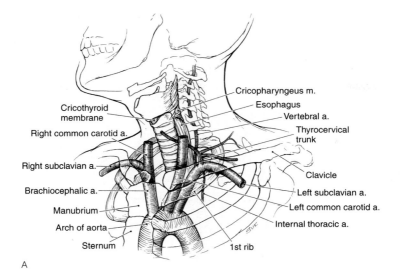

Cricopharyngeus m.
Esophagus
Vertebral a.
Thyrocervical trunk
Cricothyroid membrane
Right common carotid a.
Right subclavian a.
Clavicle
Brachiocephalic a.
Left subclavian a.
Manubrium
Left common carotid a.
Arch of aorta
Internal thoracic a.
Sternum
1st rib

A

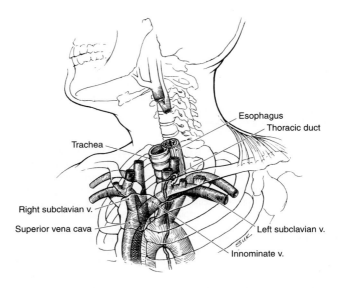

Esophagus
Thoracic duct
Trachea
Right subclavian v.
Superior vena cava
Left subclavian v.
Innominate v.

B

FIG. 47-2   The thoracic inlet. *A*. The superior border of the mediastinum is the thoracic inlet—a bony ring to protect the vessels, airway, and esophagus. *B*. The larynx is cut away to demonstrate the close apposition between the posterior membranous trachea and the esophagus. The great veins are shown overlying the aorta and great arteries. The thoracic duct enters the vasculature posteriorly at the level of the innominate and left subclavian veins.

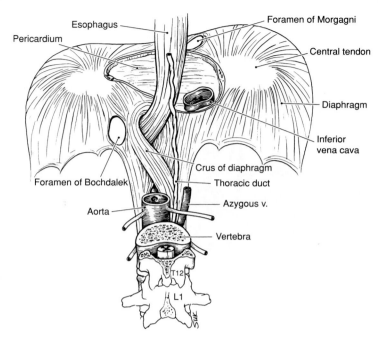

FIG. 47-3   Posterior view of the diaphragm. The anterior aspect of the vertebral bodies is identified. The hemiazygos and thoracic ducts are identified. The thoracic duct is formed by the cisterna chyli as it enters the chest through the anterior aspect of the aortic hiatus. Posteriorly the location of a Bochdalek hernia and anteriorly the location of a Morgagni hernia are shown. Note the relationship of the aortic hiatus and esophageal hiatus and the entrance of the inferior vena cava.

is always abnormal and always requires an explanation. Treatment is directed at the underlying abnormality if one can be identified. Pneumomediastinum, when present, is frequently associated with other forms of extraalveolar air, including pulmonary interstitial emphysema, pneumopericardium, pneumothorax, subcutaneous emphysema, pneumoretroperitoneum, and pneumoperitoneum. The key to understanding the distribution of extraalveolar air lies in the recognition of the common fascial planes that unite these areas. A pneumomediastinum that ruptures into the free pleural space results in a pneumothorax.

Idiopathic spontaneous pneumomediastinum is a rare, self-limited condition that most commonly affects young adult men. The majority of patients with spontaneous pneumomediastinum have predisposing factors that cause elevated airway pressure, which leads to alveolar rupture. Most commonly, this results from straining against a closed glottis, as during vomiting, coughing, or exercising. Spontaneous pneumomediastinum almost always presents with substernal pain, often pleuritic, which may radiate to the neck or back. Patients may experience either separately or in combination dyspnea, dysphagia, odynophagia, and dysphonia. Air in the subcutaneous tissues of the neck produces a characteristic change in voice quality—a higher-pitched

TABLE 47-1 Potential Mediastinal Diseases within the Mediastinal Compartments

Anterior compartment	Visceral compartment	Posterior compartment
Thymomas	Congenital cysts	Neurogenic tumors
Thymolipomas	Bronchogenic cyst	Arising from peripheral nerves
Carcinoid tumors	Enteric duplication cyst	Neurilemmoma (schwannoma)
Thymic cyst	Pericardial cyst	Malignant schwannoma
Thyroid (aberrant)	Miscellaneous (thoracic duct, neuroenteric cyst)	Neurofibroma
Germ cell tumors		Neurosarcoma
Teratomas	Primary cardiac/vascular tumors	Arising from sympathetic ganglia
Seminomas	Myxomas	Ganglioneuroma
Choriocarcinomas	Sarcomas	Ganglioneuroblastoma
Embryonal cell carcinoma	Miscellaneous cardiac sarcomas	Neuroblastoma
Malignant lymphomas	Lymphoma	Arising from paraganglia/receptors
Giant lymph node hyperplasia	Neural crest tumors	Pheochromocytomas
Teratomas	Pheochromocytoma	Paraganglioma (chemodectoma)
Parathyroid adenoma	Paraganglioma	Lymphoma
Parathyroid carcinoma		Mesenchymal tumors/soft-tissue sarcomas
Mesenchymal tumors and soft-tissue sarcomas		
Lipomas		
Liposarcomas		
Fibromas		
Fibrosarcomas		
Mesothelioma		
Lymphovascular tumors		
Lymphangiomas or cystic hygromas		
Hemangioma		
Angiosarcoma		
Primary carcinoma		

nasal tone—that the experienced clinician easily recognizes. Examination often reveals palpable subcutaneous emphysema in the neck. Auscultation of the chest may reveal a crunching or clicking sound heard over the pericardium, synchronous with the heartbeat (Hamman's sign). A chest radiograph usually demonstrates a thin radiolucent strip along a mediastinal fascial plane, most commonly along the left heart border. The aortic knob may be highlighted as well. Esophageal perforation is the condition most likely to be confused with spontaneous mediastinal emphysema. Worrisome features suggesting esophageal perforation include recent esophageal instrumentation, a history of esophageal problems, severe retching, the presence of a pleural effusion, or shock. A contrast esophagogram should be obtained immediately if there is any question of an esophageal perforation, since a delay in making this diagnosis often proves fatal. A high index of suspicion regarding esophageal perforation should always be present whenever a patient presents with mediastinal emphysema. Treatment of spontaneous mediastinal emphysema is supportive and is primarily directed at pain relief and reassurance. Prompt resolution is the rule.

Pneumomediastinum Associated with Mechanical Ventilation

Mechanical ventilation is commonly associated with pneumomediastinum and may often lead to life-threatening tension pneumothorax. Alveolar rupture results from high peak inspiratory pressures with subsequent elevated alveolar pressure associated with abnormal airways or parenchyma (decreased compliance). Classic predisposing factors include high tidal volumes, high levels of positive end-expiratory pressure, and "fighting" the ventilator. Air trapping with occult positive end-expiratory pressure (auto-PEEP) is probably an underrecognized cause of barotrauma. It is not clear if one mode of ventilation (pressure-controlled versus volume-limited) is associated with a decreased incidence of barotrauma.

Unlike spontaneous mediastinal emphysema, pneumomediastinum occurring in a patient on mechanical ventilation is potentially catastrophic because of its frequent association with tension pneumothorax. The chest radiograph should be closely examined to detect even a small pneumothorax; if such is present, tube thoracostomy should be promptly performed. Obviously, a sudden deterioration marked by hypotension and increased pulmonary pressures should prompt immediate attention with insertion of unilateral or bilateral chest tubes, depending on the clinical examination. The issue of prophylactic tube insertion is controversial and unresolved.

ACUTE MEDIASTINITIS

Acute mediastinitis is a life-threatening disorder that causes severe morbidity in the afflicted patient. All three mediastinal compartments can be affected; the anterior compartment most commonly after sternotomy for cardiac surgery, the middle compartment usually from esophageal perforation, and the posterior compartment from direct extension from the lung or spine. Instrumental perforation of the esophagus is the most common cause of acute mediastinitis in the United States.

Mediastinitis from Esophageal Perforation

Instrumental perforation of the esophagus now accounts for almost one-half of all esophageal perforation. Perforation is more common after rigid esophagoscopy, dilation of a stricture, and pneumatic dilation for achalasia, but it also occurs after variceal sclerosis, esophageal tube placement (nasogastric, Sengstaken-Blakemore, and salivary bypass tubes), and simple flexible esophagoscopy. Boerhaave's syndrome (postemetic rupture) was described in 1724 but still represents a diagnostic challenge and remains a major consideration in patients with otherwise unexplained mediastinitis. Patients usually present with the abrupt onset of severe substernal chest pain, which is pleuritic after forceful vomiting or retching. Dyspnea is common even in the absence of pneumothorax. Shock develops quickly and the patient usually appears gravely ill. A contrast esophagogram (usually with water-soluble contrast) should be performed immediately when the diagnosis is suspected, but one should be aware that this study has a false-negative rate of 10 percent. Flexible esophagoscopy is the definitive study in a patient in whom esophageal perforation is suspected but who has a negative esophagogram. Treatment should be instituted urgently and involves surgical debridement of necrotic tissue, secure closure of the perforation, correction of any distal obstruction, and wide drainage, usually performed through a left thoracotomy. Mortality is less than 10 percent if the perforation is recognized and repaired within 24 h, whereas mortality rises to 30 to 40 percent if more than 24 h has elapsed between perforation and repair.

Descending Necrotizing Mediastinitis

Mediastinitis occasionally develops after severe deep cervical infections that originate from the oropharynx. Most patients present with a mixed aerobic and anaerobic infection. Previously these infections had a fulminant, often lethal course with mortality as high as 40 percent. Extension of the cervical infection down the prevertebral or visceral space into the mediastinum leads to this syndrome of descending necrotizing mediastinitis. Computed tomography should be performed on all severe neck infections to identify signs of mediastinitis that may not be clinically apparent. Aggressive surgical drainage (cervical, substernal, and transthoracic) and antibiotics have reduced mortality, though prompt management is essential.

CHRONIC MEDIASTINITIS

Granulomatous mediastinitis is a disease of the mediastinal lymph nodes usually resulting from infection by *Histoplasma capsulatum* and occasionally from tuberculosis or other fungi. Coalescence of caseous mediastinal lymph nodes can result in a single large mass that incites a considerable fibrotic response, which can result in encapsulation and produce a mediastinal granuloma. Most authors suggest that there exists a spectrum of disease ranging from mediastinal granuloma to fibrosing mediastinitis. Mediastinal granulomas should be excised if symptomatic. Although complete excision is possible, the intense surrounding fibrosis places important structures at risk for operative injury. Evacuation of the granulomatous mass is usually a safer option.

Fibrosing Mediastinitis

Fibrosing mediastinitis may cause a variety of clinical syndromes due to the compression and/or erosion of vital mediastinal structures by the dense fibrous tissue reaction that is present. While the syndrome itself is rare, the commonly presumed causative agents—*Histoplasma* and (rarely) *Mycoplasma tuberculosis*—are relatively ubiquitous. Pathologic features include the presence of dense fibrotic tissue surrounding the trachea and hila of the lungs, often extending into contiguous structures. Compression of the airway, pulmonary arteries, or veins may occur because of this process. Histologic features include dense hyalinized collagenous tissue, aggregates of plasma cells and lymphocytes, and occasionally granulomas. Cultures are almost always negative, as are special stains for organisms. Symptoms are primarily caused by compression of vital mediastinal structures. Fibrosis around the right peritracheal area commonly causes superior vena cava syndrome. Subcarinal fibrosis can extend posteriorly to encase the esophagus or extend laterally to involve the pulmonary veins. Hilar fibrosis can obstruct either the tracheobronchial tree or pulmonary arteries. Rarely, constrictive pericarditis or obstruction of the trachea or proximal main bronchi can also occur. The signs and symptoms may progress over a period of time.

MEDIASTINAL COMPARTMENTS

No single concept covers all nuances of diseases within the mediastinum, as the boundaries of the mediastinal compartments are empiric. The simplest system divides the mediastinum into three compartments: anterosuperior, visceral (or middle), and paravertebral (or posterior).

Anterosuperior Compartment

Structures contained within it include the ascending aorta, the superior vena cava, the azygos vein, the thymus gland, lymph nodes, fat, connective tissue, transverse aorta, and great vessels. Common major lesions contained within the anterosuperior mediastinal compartment are thymomas, lymphomas, and germ cell tumors. Less common lesions are tumors of mesenchymal origin, vascular lesions, and displaced thyroid or parathyroid glands.

Middle Compartment (Visceral)

The superior pericardial reflection defines the superior border, while the diaphragm defines the inferior border. The posterior border extends to the spine. Contained within this compartment are the heart and pericardium, trachea and major bronchi, pulmonary vessels, lymph nodes, fat, and connective tissue. Lesions contained within the visceral compartment include cysts of the foregut, primary and secondary tumors of the lymph nodes, and, less commonly, pleural, pericardial, neuroenteric and gastroenteric cysts.

Posterior Compartment

The posterior compartment is also called the paravertebral compartment. It extends from the superior aspect of the first thoracic vertebral body to the diaphragm anteriorly and then posteriorly to the posteriormost curvature of the ribs. Contained within it are the sympathetic chain, vagus nerves, esophagus, thoracic duct, various lymph nodes, and the descending aorta. Lesions contained within it are primarily tumors of neurogenic origin.

Great differences exist between children and adults with respect to the location of mediastinal lesions. In adults, 65 percent of the lesions arise in the anterosuperior, 10 percent in the middle, and 25 percent in the posterior compartments; this distribution is reversed in children, in whom 28 percent of lesions arise in the anterosuperior, 10 percent in the middle, and 62 percent in the posterior compartments. In general, the incidence of posterior lesions is higher in children, whereas anterior lesions predominate in adults.

ANATOMIC STRUCTURES

Mediastinal structures may be conveniently placed into a particular mediastinal compartment that correlates to a varying degree with the radiographic appearance of the mass. Mediastinal masses commonly present on routine chest radiographs obtained for other purposes. Chest CT should be routine for all suspected or confirmed mediastinal masses. Although CT is poor with respect to distinguishing between cystic and solid structures, it provides excellent examination of the mediastinum. Indeed, the diagnosis of certain lesions—such as aortic aneurysms, mediastinal lipomatosis, and pericardial fat pads—is so straightforward with CT that further search or biopsy is not necessary. MRI is superior to CT imaging in three specific circumstances: when preoperative determination of a tumor's invasion of vascular or neural structures is crucial, when coronal or radial body sections are necessary, and when contrast material cannot be given intravenously because of renal disease or known allergy to contrast.

Invasive Biopsy Procedures

The decision to biopsy mediastinal masses is not straightforward. Biopsy before resection is not necessary in some cases and potentially harmful in others. The likelihood of a positive biopsy depends on several factors: (1) the presence, or absence, of local symptoms; (2) the location and extent of the lesion; (3) the presence or absence of various tumor markers; and (4) gallium uptake by the lesion. Locally asymptomatic lesions should not undergo biopsy before removal if they do not extend beyond the anterior compartment, show no increase in levels of tumor markers, and do not take up gallium. Surgical approaches to obtain tissue from mediastinal lesions include cervical mediastinoscopy, extended cervical mediastinoscopy, anterior mediastinotomy (Chamberlain procedure), subxyphoid mediastinoscopy, and videothoracoscopy. Cervical mediastinoscopy, performed through a small incision in the suprasternal notch, can sample masses in the superior mediastinum or lymph nodes in the subcarinal and paratracheal location (levels 1, 2, 3, 4, 7, and 10 in the American Thoracic Society staging system). Anterior mediastinotomy performed through a small incision over the second or third rib on either side can sample lymph nodes in the paraaortic position (levels 5 and 6) or anteriormediastinal masses.

Substernal Goiter

Two-thirds of patients with a substernal goiter complain of a neck mass, but most are asymptomatic. Twenty-five percent complain of dyspnea or dysphagia and they can occasionally present with acute airway obstruction . The reported incidence of malignancy has ranged from 2.5 to 21 percent. A case can be made for recommending operation even for the asymptomatic substernal goiter but many of these patients are elderly and not particularly good candidates for operation. What is important to realize, however, is that despite the location in the mediastinum even when there is no connection with thyroid in the neck, essentially all of these lesions, with rare exceptions, can be removed via a cervical incision. Rarely is median sternotomy necessary in the hands of an experienced surgeon.

ANTERIOR MEDIASTINAL NEOPLASMS

Lesions of the Thymus

Thymoma is the most common primary neoplasm of the mediastinum, comprising approximately 15 percent of all thymic lesions. These tumors occur with equal frequency in men and women 40 to 60 years of age. Seventy-five percent present in the anterior mediastinum; more than 90 percent are visible on the chest radiograph. Thymomas generally are classified as either encapsulated or invasive, and we tend not to refer to these lesions as benign or malignant.

Tumor stage at the time of treatment correlates with prognosis better than tumor grade. Stage I lesions are lesions that are completely encapsulated and do not invade adjacent structures. Stage II lesions demonstrate microscopic invasion of adjacent structures, while stage III lesions grossly involve adjacent structures. Stage IV thymomas present with disseminated disease. Tumor-node-metastasis (TNM) staging has not been widely adopted. A peculiar characteristic of the benign histologic appearance of many of these lesions is that invasion of adjacent structures, and thus the stage of the tumor, can usually be more easily determined by the surgeon at the time of operation than by the pathologist at the time of microscopy. Five- and 10-year survivals of 74 percent and 57 percent, respectively, can be expected following a treatment regimen of operation and postoperative radiotherapy for all patients and postoperative chemotherapy for some patients with high-grade lesions. All patients in whom an invasive thymoma has been resected should receive postoperative radiotherapy, which is strongly recommended for all but stage I patients. Surgery alone is associated with a recurrence rate of approximately 28 percent, whereas radiation and surgery together yield a recurrence rate of 3 percent.

Paraneoplastic Syndromes

Myasthenia gravis is the most common thymoma-associated systemic syndrome. Myasthenia gravis is present in approximately one-third of patients with thymomas. This disorder may either precede or follow the development of thymoma by many years. Any type of thymic tumor may occur in patients with myasthenia gravis. Many other syndromes may also be related to thymoma. Red cell aplasia occurs in 5 percent of patients with thymomas. It is a rare disorder that results in a severe normochromic normocytic anemia. Erythroid precursors in the bone marrow are decreased or absent, so reticulocytosis is markedly decreased. Hypogammaglobulinemia occurs in 5 to 10 percent of patients with thymomas. It is more common in patients with both thymoma and rheumatoid arthritis, ulcerative colitis, many cytopenias, and some extrathymic cancers. Thymectomy usually has not proved beneficial.

Thymic Carcinoma

These are epithelial neoplasms of thymic origin with considerably more cytologic and architectural features of malignancy than manifested by thymomas. Several subtypes exist, with significant differences in outcomes after surgical resection. Patients with low-grade lesions (squamous cell carcinoma, mucoepidermal carcinoma, and basaloid carcinoma) sustained a 95 percent cure rate. However, treatment of high-grade lesions (lymphoepithelioid lesions, small cell or neuroendocrine lesions, clear cell and sarcomatoid carcinomas, and anaplastic tumors) yielded only a 15 percent long-term survival.

Lymphoma

Lymphomas constitute 10 to 14 percent of mediastinal masses in adults. They make up 20 percent of anterosuperior mediastinal masses and 20 percent of middle mediastinal masses, ranking second in frequency in both compartments. Lymphomas are rare in the posterior mediastinum. The numerous classifications proposed for lymphoma are generally no better for determining prognosis or managing patients than is simple classification into either Hodgkin's or non-Hodgkin's lymphoma. Diagnosis requires significant tissue samples. Fine-needle aspiration biopsies are not adequate in most circumstances, although the yield improves with radiologic (ultrasound or CT) techniques that target specific areas of the mediastinal mass. Biopsies under local anesthesia of more accessible cervical nodes or of mediastinal nodes by mediastinoscopy or anterior mediastinotomy (under general anesthesia) have the greatest yield.

Mediastinal Hodgkin's Disease

The age distribution of patients with mediastinal Hodgkin's disease is bimodal—20 to 30 years of age or greater than 50 years of age. Among young adults, men and women are affected equally, although mediastinal lymphoma is more common in older men than in older women. The nodular sclerosing subtype of Hodgkin's disease accounts for almost 90 percent of patients who present with mediastinal invasion. Of these, half have only mediastinal disease and the other half have mediastinal disease with associated neck disease. Systemic symptoms of night sweats, fever, malaise, and weight loss are common. Mild local symptoms such as pain and cough are not uncommon. Severe local symptoms, such as superior vena cava syndrome, are very uncommon.

Non-Hodgkin's Lymphoma

Whereas about 75 percent of patients with Hodgkin's disease present with mediastinal disease, only 5 percent of patients with non-Hodgkin's lymphoma present with mediastinal involvement. Abdominal lymph nodes, cervical lymph nodes, and lymphoid tissue of Waldeyer's ring are more commonly affected than are mediastinal nodes. Large irregular anterior and superior mediastinal masses are common and are often associated with large pleural effusions, large pericardial effusions, and large pulmonary parenchymal changes. Because lymph nodes other than mediastinal nodes and body fluids are more accessible, mediastinoscopic biopsy is not usually necessary. These malignancies may consist of T cells, B cells, diffuse large cell lymphomas, or lymphoblastic lymphomas. The treatment of a localized lymphoma that appears histologically to be aggressive consists of combination chemotherapy, either with or without radiation therapy of the affected field. Stages I and II patients can expect 5-year disease-free survival rates of 80 to 100 percent.

Germ Cell Tumors

Both benign and malignant teratomas are classified as germ cell tumors. They are the fourth most common lesion in the adult mediastinum. Most lesions in the adult (60 to 80 percent) are benign; in children, a smaller proportion (about 57 percent) are benign.

Mediastinal germ cell tumors are of several types. *Benign teratomas* constitute 70 percent of the lesions in children and 60 percent of the lesions in adults. The predominant malignant lesions are *seminomas,* which constitute 50 percent of all malignant lesions. Nonseminomatous malignant lesions include a mix of tumors: malignant teratomas, malignant teratocarcinomas, yolk sac tumors, endodermal sinus tumors, choriocarcinomas, and embryonal cell carcinomas.

All types of germ cell tumors that have been found in the testes have been reported to occur in the mediastinum. Nonetheless, compared to testicular tumors, extragonadal germ cell tumors are uncommon. Three percent of all germ cell tumors in adults and 7 percent of germ cell tumors in children are extragonadal. An even smaller percentage (1 to 2 percent) of germ cell tumors originate in the mediastinum. Blood levels of alpha-fetoprotein and human chorionic gonadotropin should be determined for all patients in whom malignant germ cell tumors are suspected. Management of these tumors does not require surgery initially, since the lesions are generally unresectable at presentation. Treatment with chemotherapy and radiotherapy is the mainstay. More aggressive regimens, particularly the addition of cisplatin, improve the results of treatment of extragonadal nonseminomatous tumors. In such responders who are left with a residual mass, resection is appropriate. Testicular tumors are more chemosensitive than all extragonadal tumors, and retroperitoneal tumors are more sensitive than mediastinal tumors. Any mass that remains after chemotherapy should be resected if two conditions are met: The patient has had a good response to the chemotherapy, and levels of tumor markers in serum fall to normal. Any tumor left behind is usually a benign teratoma or necrotic tumor mass that can potentially degenerate and redevelop malignancy. If the tumor markers do not fall but the tumor shrinks, surgery is of no benefit.

Benign Germ Cell Tumors (Teratomas)

These tumors are of multiple tissues that are foreign to the part of the body in which they develop. They consist of a disorganized mixture of derivatives of the three germinal layers—ectoderm, mesoderm, and endoderm. Consequently, they may contain elements of skin and its appendages, bone, cartilage, intestinal and respiratory epithelium, and neurovascular tissue. About 80 percent of these lesions are benign. A dermoid cyst (benign cystic teratoma) is a variant that contains sebaceous material within a lining of squamous epithelium.

MIDDLE MEDIASTINAL MASSES

Bronchogenic Cysts

Mediastinal cysts constitute 20 percent of all mediastinal masses, and bronchogenic cysts make up 60 percent of all mediastinal cysts. Symptoms are present in two-thirds of patients, usually from compression of adjacent structures. If the diagnosis of a bronchogenic cyst is made preoperatively and patients are asymptomatic, observation is an appropriate course. If there is any question of malignancy—based on radiographic appearance, positive cytology, or evidence of enlargement or recurrence—the lesion should be resected. The presence of symptoms—especially pain, cough, or hemoptysis—suggests the advisability of resection. Video-assisted techniques offer the opportunity to resect less threatening lesions with low morbidity.

Esophageal Duplication Cysts

Esophageal cysts are periesophageal lesions that are smooth and possess some form of gastroesophageal epithelial lining. Diagnosis is possible with esophageal ultrasound, chest CT scan, or contrast studies of the upper gastrointestinal tract. Resection is the therapy of choice, whether by thoracoscopic or open technique.

Neuroenteric Cysts

Neuroenteric cysts make up 5 to 10 percent of foregut lesions and are associated with vertebral anomalies. They have not only endodermal but also ectodermal or neurogenic elements. They are usually connected by a stalk to the meninges and spinal cord. They present in infants before 1 year of age and are uncommon in adults. A CT scan showing a cystic mediastinal lesion with an associated vertebral abnormality—such as congenital scoliosis, hemivertebrae, and spina bifida—should prompt consideration of neuroenteric cysts.

Pericardial or Pleuropericardial Cysts

Pericardial cysts are commonly located in the cardiophrenic angles. They have fibrous walls and contain clear, watery fluid. Pericardial cysts are benign, and if the diagnosis is secure, resection is not necessary. If symptoms develop or if the lesions cannot be differentiated from hernias, bronchogenic cysts, or sequestration, resection is necessary.

Thoracic Duct Cysts

These cysts are rare. They may arise at any level of the thoracic duct but do not retain a communication with the thoracic duct. The lesion may distort the trachea or esophagus. Observation is appropriate if the diagnosis can be made preoperatively, since there is no malignant potential. Ligation of the thoracic duct may be necessary to resect a thoracic duct cyst.

POSTERIOR MEDIASTINAL MASSES

Neurogenic Tumors

Most patients with neurogenic tumors are asymptomatic, so the initial diagnosis is usually made on chest radiographs obtained for other reasons. A rare patient may present with a pheochromocytoma or a chemically active neuroblastoma. CT scanning is necessary to rule out intraspinal extension along the vertebral nerve roots (so-called dumbbell tumors). These patients often present with symptoms of spinal cord compression. About 10 percent of patients with mediastinal neurogenic tumors have extension through a vertebral foramen. Although the vast majority of these lesions are benign, approximately 1 to 2 percent are malignant. The CT scan typically shows a smoothly rounded homogeneous density abutting the vertebral column. For patients with dumbbell extensions through the intravertebral foramina or lesions abutting on the thoracic vessels, MRI may be useful in demonstrating involvement of the vertebral column and extension into the spinal cord. Nerve sheath tumors account for 65 percent of all mediastinal neurogenic tumors.

Tumors of Nerve Sheath Origin

Benign lesions are classified as either neurilemoma (schwannoma) or neurofibromas. Neurilemomas are more common than neurofibromas. Twenty-five to 40 percent of patients with nerve sheath tumors have multiple neurofibromatosis (von Recklinghausen's disease). Malignant tumors (neurogenic sarcomas or malignant schwannomas) are unusual. The incidence of malignancy is greater in tumors that are part of von Recklinghausen's disease (10 to 20 percent). Neurilemomas are well encapsulated, firm, and grayish tan.

SUPERIOR VENA CAVA (SVC) SYNDROME

Malignant tumors, such as lymphoma, bronchopulmonary cancers, thymic malignancies, and germ cell tumors of the mediastinum, account for more than 90 percent of all SVC obstructions. Lung cancer is most common, especially small cell cancer, although lymphoma is also common. Other malignancies are rare. Five to 10 percent of cases of SVC obstruction are due to benign causes. Most result from invasive monitoring techniques, such as the placement of central venous lines, Swan-Ganz catheters, and interventional techniques, such as the placement of pacemakers and central venous catheters for chemotherapy. Congestion of venous outflow from the head, neck, and upper extremities results in swelling of the face, neck, arms, and upper chest. Patients may have headaches, dizziness, tinnitus, and a bursting sensation. In addition, the face may appear cyanotic even though capillary refill is normal. Venous hypertension in SVC syndrome may lead to serious consequences (e.g., jugular venous and cerebrovascular thrombosis). It is important to obtain tissue from the mediastinal neoplasm causing the SVC syndrome in order to direct therapy. Once a diagnosis is established, treatment should begin as soon as possible.

REFERENCES

1. Mountain CF: A new international staging system for lung cancer. *Chest* 89(suppl):225S–233S, 1986.
2. Kern JA, Daniel TM, Tribble CG, et al: Thoracoscopic diagnosis and treatment of mediastinal masses. *Ann Thorac Surg* 56:92–96, 1993.
3. Mathisen DJ, Grillo HC: Clinical manifestation of mediastinal fibrosis and histoplasmosis. *Ann Thorac Surg* 54:1053–1058, 1992.
4. Shields TW: The mediastinum and its compartments, in Shields TW (ed): *Mediastinal Surgery.* Philadelphia, Lea & Febiger, 1991, p 4.
5. Cohen AJ, Thompson L, Edwards FH, Bellamy RF: Primary cysts and tumors of the mediastinum. *Ann Thorac Surg* 51:378–386, 1991.

Part Ten

DISORDERS OF THE CHEST WALL AND NEUROMUSCULAR DISEASES

48 | Disorders of the Chest Wall*

Robert M. Senior

The chest wall consists of the abdomen, the bony structure of the rib cage, the respiratory muscles, and the spine and its articulations. It is one of the components of the inspiratory pump, and its normal function is needed for effective ventilation. Kyphoscoliosis and previous thoracoplasty are the chest wall diseases that most profoundly embarrass ventilatory function. Flail chest may result in respiratory failure, especially when there is associated lung contusion. Diseases directly involving the respiratory muscles and obesity also affect chest wall function.

KYPHOSCOLIOSIS

Kyphoscoliosis is a common spinal deformity that characteristically consists of a lateral displacement or curvature (scoliosis), an anteroposterior angulation (kyphosis), or both. The abnormalities are readily appreciated on chest radiographs and their severity is determined by measurement of the acute angle formed by the two limbs of the convex primary curvature. This angle is called the *Cobb angle*. A Cobb angle greater than 100 degrees is considered a severe deformity. Most cases of kyphoscoliosis are idiopathic, often beginning in childhood. Secondary causes are disease of the vertebrae, vertebral connective tissue, neuromuscular diseases such as polio, and muscular dystrophy (Table 48-1). Severe kyphoscoliosis is easily recognizable on physical examination, but in children and adolescents the changes in spinal curvature may be subtle. The dorsal hump is due to the angulated ribs rather than to the spine. With severe kyphoscoliosis, signs of right-sided heart failure may be present.

Pathophysiology

Severe kyphoscoliosis has a profound impact on pulmonary function. Total lung capacity can be markedly reduced, with relative preservation of residual volume. Decreased thoracic compliance is the principal basis for the restriction, but inspiratory muscle weakness and decreased lung compliance from microatelectasis may also contribute to the restrictive process. Reductions in maximal inspiratory and expiratory strength may be due not to intrinsic muscle disease but to changes in geometry of the chest wall affecting the mechanical advantage of the inspiratory muscles. In idiopathic kyphoscoliosis, the severity of the restrictive process is proportional to the severity of spinal deformity, but secondary kyphoscoliosis does not exhibit as strong a

---

*Edited from Chap. 97, "Nonmuscular Diseases of the Chest Wall," by McCool FD, Rochester DF. In: *Fishman's Pulmonary Diseases and Disorders,* 3d ed., edited by Fishman AP, Elias JA, Fishman JA, Grippi MA, Kaiser LR, Senior RM. New York, McGraw-Hill, 1998, pp 1541–1560. For fuller discussion of topics dealt with in this chapter, the reader is referred to the original text, as noted above.

TABLE 48-1 Causes of Kyphoscoliosis

Idiopathic
Neuromuscular disease
  Muscular dystrophy
  Poliomyelitis
  Cerebral palsy
  Friedreich's ataxia
Vertebral disease
  Osteoporosis
  Osteomalacia
  Vitamin D–resistant rickets
  Tuberculous spondylitis
  Neurofibromatosis
Disorders of connective tissue
  Marfan's syndrome
  Ehlers-Danlos syndrome
  Morquio's syndrome
Thoracic cage abnormality
  Thoracoplasty
  Empyema

correlation between vital capacity and the degree of spinal deformity because other factors such as neuromuscular weakness may have more effect on vital capacity than the spinal deformity.

Kyphoscoliosis results in reduced lung and chest wall compliances that increase the elastic load on the respiratory muscles. The increased elastic load imposed with every breath may place these patients at risk of developing inspiratory muscle fatigue. To compensate for the increased load on the inspiratory muscles, these patients may adopt a rapid shallow breathing pattern. Low tidal volumes reduce the work per breath but increase dead-space ventilation and can lead to microatelectasis. Reductions in expiratory flow rates usually reflect the overall restrictive process rather than airway disease. Hypoxemia in severe kyphoscoliosis is due to ventilation/perfusion mismatch or to underlying atelectasis and shunt; hypoventilation worsens hypoxemia. With severe kyphoscoliosis, persistent hypoxemia leads to pulmonary hypertension, right ventricular hypertrophy, and cor pulmonale. Exercise capacity in patients with severe kyphoscoliosis is limited by reduced ventilatory capacity. Impairment of exercise performance in adolescents and adults with moderate scoliosis can be attributed to deconditioning and lack of regular aerobic exercise rather than to ventilatory limitation.

Disordered breathing during rapid-eye-movement (REM) sleep may contribute to the development of respiratory failure. While awake, patients may rely more on the intercostal and accessory muscles to assist the diaphragm in displacing the stiff chest wall. With REM sleep, the intercostal and accessory muscles may become hypotonic and hypoventilation may ensue. Oxyhemoglobin desaturation during sleep in these patients appears to be more severe than that seen during sleep in patients with chronic obstructive pulmonary disease (COPD). A second cause of nocturnal hypoventilation is recurrent episodes of obstructive sleep apnea from intermittent upper airway obstruction during REM-induced hypotonia of the pharyngeal muscles.

Clinical Course

Patients with idiopathic kyphoscoliosis <35 years of age tend to be asymptomatic even though they may have severe degrees of kyphoscoliosis. In contrast, middle-aged patients with severe idiopathic kyphoscoliosis tend to develop dyspnea, decreased exercise tolerance, and acute respiratory infections and are at risk for respiratory failure. The onset of respiratory failure is usually insidious. When respiratory failure occurs, it is often attributed to the spinal deformity alone; however, the cause is often multifactorial, involving factors such as inspiratory muscle weakness, advanced age, disordered ventilatory control, sleep-disordered breathing, intrinsic airway disease, and underlying cardiac disease. Impaired ventilatory drive is seldom a factor, as patients with kyphoscoliosis usually have normal or only slightly low ventilatory responses to CO_2.

Treatment

General Measures

Patients with mild to moderate kyphoscoliosis have little impairment of breathing or overall lifestyle and do not require treatment to prevent ventilatory failure. Pregnancy usually poses no added risk of respiratory complications. With kyphoscoliosis severe enough to lower the vital capacity to <1 L, however, the risk of respiratory complications may be high, and patients may be advised to avoid pregnancy. Immunizations against influenza and pneumococcal pneumonia, prompt treatment of respiratory infections, avoidance of sedatives, and carefully monitored supplemental O_2 are the mainstays of medical therapy. Physical training can improve exercise tolerance in the inactive scoliotic patient. If the patient develops hypercapnia and cor pulmonale, intermittent positive pressure breathing (IPPB) and chronic ventilatory support become necessary. Since sleep-related disorders represent a potentially treatable or reversible cause of respiratory failure, sleep should be evaluated in patients who are developing CO_2 retention. IPPB should be part of the conservative approach. It improves lung mechanics, resting Pa_{CO_2}, and oxygenation for up to 4 h following treatment. It probably decreases microatelectasis, thereby improving lung compliance and ventilation/perfusion matching and decreasing the work of breathing. For acute respiratory failure refractory to the IPPB and medical measures, ventilatory support is needed.

Noninvasive Ventilation

Long-term nocturnal ventilation has resulted in improvements in alveolar gas exchange, ventilation, cardiac function, activities of daily living, quality of life, and sleep quality and decreased hospitalizations for respiratory illnesses. Improvement may be related to reversing atelectasis, improving lung compliance, and resting the diaphragm. Nocturnal ventilation may be administered via either negative or positive pressure. Negative pressure is delivered by devices such as a cuirass and a body-wrap ventilator can be used to treat chronic respiratory failure, but these devices can induce upper airway obstruction during sleep and can present a problem in terms of custom fitting a cuirass to the deformed chest wall. In the past, positive pressure has been delivered via a tracheostomy; however, to avoid the complications of tracheostomy, positive pressure is now more commonly delivered via nasal or face mask.

Spinal Surgery

The long-term benefits of spinal surgery on pulmonary function remain controversial. It is generally accepted that surgical procedures are not useful in improving pulmonary function in adults. In children and adolescents, there may be a role for corrective surgery.

Thoracoplasty

Thoracoplasty was frequently used for treating cavitary pulmonary tuberculosis and empyema in the 1940s and 1950s. Thoracoplasty entails removal of a number of ribs and intercostal muscles. In recent years, thoracoplasty has been used to a limited extent to treat postpneumonic and postresectional empyema.

Of the disorders affecting the chest wall, thoracoplasty is second only to kyphoscoliosis in producing a severe restrictive pattern and increased work of breathing. The degree of restriction does not correlate with the extent of thoracoplasty (number of ribs removed or the number of surgical stages) as it is due primarily to a reduction in respiratory system compliance. Progressive lung fibrosis related to underlying granulomatous disease, fibrothorax, phrenic nerve damage, scoliosis, and previous lung resection may also contribute to the reduced lung volumes. The restriction may worsen with time because of progressive scoliosis or reduced respiratory system compliance associated with aging. Airflow obstruction—due to chronic bronchitis from cigarette smoking or chronic bronchitis from old tuberculous lung disease—is common. The obstructive component becomes more common with aging. Chronic airflow obstruction leads to hyperinflation, which reduces inspiratory muscle efficiency. Determining the presence and severity of airflow obstruction may help identify those at greater risk for developing respiratory failure. Although they may be asymptomatic for long periods after the surgery, respiratory failure occurs in many of these individuals, acutely over days or weeks or chronically over years.

ANKYLOSING SPONDYLITIS

Ankylosing spondylitis results in rigidity of the spine and limitation of rib cage mobility. Respiratory complaints such as dyspnea and chest wall pain are uncommon and may be related to chest wall restriction, kyphosis, or to upper lobe fibrobullous disease.

The reduction in respiratory system compliance is similar to that seen in kyphoscoliosis, but there is typically only mild restriction in total lung capacity (TLC) (80 percent predicted) and vital capacity (VC) (70 percent predicated). Since the rib cage is often fixed in an inspiratory position, both functional residual capacity (FRC) and residual volume (RV) may be increased above the predicted levels, which can be mistakenly interpreted as coincident obstructive disease. With the development of osteoporosis, kyphosis may also occur and contribute to the mild restrictive process. In elderly patients with osteoporosis and a moderate degree of kyphosis (Cobb angles of 46 to 80 degrees) posterior fusion of the ribs may play a greater role in limiting rib expansion and vital capacity than the degree of kyphosis. Inspiratory muscle weakness may also be involved in the mild restrictive deficit in these patients; exercise capacity may be mildly reduced, in part by impaired inspiratory muscle performance. Gas exchange is usually unimpaired. Upper airway obstruction is an infrequent complication of ankylosing spondylitis and is due to involvement of the cricoarytenoid cartilage. Patients may present with hoarseness or stridor.

Approximately 1 percent of patients will develop fibrobullous upper lobe lesions. This complication, seen especially seen in males, may progress to marked fibrosis, honeycombing, and cavity formation. Usually, these patients are asymptomatic, but they are at risk for pneumothorax and *Aspergillus* or atypical mycobacterial infection.

Treatment

Cardiorespiratory fitness and spinal mobility may be enhanced by institution of exercise and physiotherapy programs, but the effects of pulmonary rehabilitation on pulmonary function have been equivocal. Because thoracic surgery for fibrobullous disease is often complicated by bronchopleural fistula, it is recommended only for the treatment of massive hemoptysis. Corticosteroids do not prevent progression of the fibrobullous disease.

FLAIL CHEST

Flail chest denotes a condition in which a segment of the rib cage is disconnected from the rest of the chest and deforms markedly with quiet breathing. It is produced by double fractures of three or more contiguous ribs or combined sternal and rib fractures. The most common cause is blunt chest trauma following falls or automobile accidents. Pulmonary complications, which occur in approximately 60 percent of patients with flail chest, are pulmonary contusion, hemothorax, and pneumothorax. The harmful effects of blunt chest injuries on gas exchange are related primarily to pulmonary contusion and pain rather than to the flail segment per se. Typically, flail chest without pulmonary contusion causes short-term but not long-term pulmonary dysfunction.

With flail chest, the negative intrathoracic pressure during inspiration is unopposed and may displace the uncoupled part of the rib cage inward. Any reduction in lung compliance due to pulmonary contusion or microatelectasis or an increase in airway resistance further increases the degree of negative pleural pressure during inspiration and worsens paradoxical chest wall motion. Paradoxical motion of the chest wall increases the work of breathing because the inspiratory muscles must shorten more than normal for a given tidal volume. Also, regional reductions in lung compliance due to coincident pulmonary contusion increase the pleural pressure needed to inhale.

Treatment

Therapy includes measures to control pain, assistance with mechanical ventilation if necessary, and possibly stabilization of the flail segment. Adequate pain relief is imperative not only for patient comfort but also because it reduces splinting and improves tidal volume, vital capacity, and the clearance of respiratory secretions by cough. It can be accomplished by direct intercostal nerve blocks or by use of epidural anesthesia. The importance of stabilizing the flail segment has been controversial. Initially, tape, strappings, and external devices were used to stabilize the flail segment. "Pneumatic splinting" by positive pressure ventilation via tracheostomy for a 3- to 5-week period was the mainstay of therapy for many years. However, in a large study, mortality averaged 18 percent for continuous mechanical ventilation and 6 percent for intermittent mandatory ventilation (IMV), while patients who were not mechanically ventilated had no mortality and the morbidity was significantly lower than in either of the ventilated groups. Consequently, at present ventilator management is not recommended unless respiratory failure accompanies flail chest.

If ventilatory support is needed, use of a low-impedance system such as high-flow continuous positive airway pressure (CPAP) has been shown to produce less chest wall distortion than an IMV circuit. Such a mode may reduce the likelihood of developing inspiratory muscle fatigue. A randomized, controlled trial of CPAP versus mechanical ventilation in patients who had similar degrees of blunt thoracic trauma showed that patients treated with CPAP had significantly fewer days of treatment, intensive care, and total hospitalization.

PECTUS EXCAVATUM

Pectus excavatum is the most common chest wall deformity seen by pediatricians and primary care providers. Its incidence is approximately 8 per 1000, and it is three times more common in boys than in girls. Pectus carinatum, a disorder in which the sternum is protuberant, is less common than pectus excavatum. The most frequent complaint in patients with pectus deformity is an unattractive chest wall, but complaints of exercise intolerance are also very common. Exercise performance may be normal or only mildly diminished. Patients with pectus carinatum or excavatum have either normal pulmonary function or a mild reduction in TLC and VC. Using lateral chest radiographs, the ratio of the transthoracic diameter to the sternovertebral distances and the absolute distance between the posterior aspect of the lower sternum and the anterior face of the vertebral column have been used as indices of chest wall deformity.

Surgical repair can provide cosmetic benefits; subjective improvement in exercise tolerance and relief of dyspnea have also been noted following surgery. However, despite the marked improvements in the radiologic appearance of the pectus deformity and the subjective improvements in exercise tolerance, the physiologic benefits of corrective surgery are questionable.

OBESITY

Obesity is considered mild when body weight is 120 to 150 percent of ideal body weight and severe when body weight is greater than 150 percent of ideal. Patients are classified as exhibiting either simple obesity or the obesity hypoventilation syndrome (OHS). Patients with simple obesity are eucapnic. OHS is characterized by CO_2 retention and is frequently accompanied by obstructive sleep apnea. Both groups often complain of exercise intolerance and dyspnea on exertion. Obesity is strongly associated with obstructive sleep apnea. The prevalence is much higher in males than in females. For a given degree of upper body obesity, men have more severe obstructive sleep apnea.

With simple obesity there is generally no restrictive ventilatory defect unless the obesity is marked. Then, the VC may be reduced by 25 percent but the TLC and FRC can still be within the range of normal. When TLC is significantly reduced, other explanations for the restrictive process should be sought. Mildly obese men whose obesity is more centrally distributed have lower values of FVC, FEV_1, and TLC than those with more peripheral obesity.

In patients with OHS, lung volumes are smaller than in simple obesity. Expiratory reserve volume (ERV) is reduced to 60 percent of that predicted in simple obesity and to 35 percent of that predicted in OHS.

The adverse effects of obesity on pulmonary function cannot be entirely explained by the absolute load of adipose tissue in the chest wall, as similar degrees of obesity in simple obesity and OHS result in very different lung volume patterns. In simple obesity, chest wall and total respiratory system compliances are generally close to normal. In contrast, with OHS, the chest wall and total respiratory system compliance are generally quite reduced. The reduced respiratory system compliance is thought to be due to weight pressing on the thorax and abdomen, increased pulmonary blood volume, and closure of dependent airways. The increased elastic and resistive loads imposed by the lung and chest wall, along with the threshold load imposed by the fatty deposits around the abdomen, require a greater reduction of pleural pressure to achieve a given tidal volume. Accordingly, the work of breathing is increased in both simple obesity and OHS. Inspiratory and expiratory muscle strength is generally normal in simple obesity and the inspiratory muscles are strong enough to overcome the mild reduction in lung and chest wall compliance, so that total lung capacity is not reduced. In OHS, inspiratory muscle strength may be reduced by 40 percent.

Airway resistance is increased in patients with obesity, in part because of the reduction in lung volume. The FEV_1/FVC ratio is normal in simple obesity and in OHS. Thus, increased airway resistance appears to lie in small airways rather than in the large airways. Gas exchange is often impaired in obese persons; however, hypoxemia may be mild or absent in simple obesity. In contrast, the arterial P_{O_2} is lower than normal in OHS. In both simple obesity and OHS, hypoxemia becomes more pronounced in the supine position. Mechanisms of hypoxemia are ventilation-perfusion mismatching and shunting. In OHS, hypoventilation further aggravates hypoxemia. In general, with obesity the lung bases are well perfused but poorly ventilated, owing to airway closure and alveolar collapse. Respiratory drive is clearly depressed in OHS.

Obese patients may alter their breathing pattern to compensate for the increased load placed on the respiratory system. During quiet breathing, the respiratory rate of simple obesity subjects is approximately 40 percent higher than in normal subjects. Tidal volume is normal in simple obesity at rest and during maximal exercise. In the person with OHS, breathing frequency is 25 percent higher than in the person with simple obesity, but the tidal volume is 25 percent lower. The rapid shallow breathing pattern in OHS worsens gas exchange in these subjects. Obese subjects have a higher minute ventilation, respiratory rate, heart rate, and oxygen consumption during treadmill exercise than normals, but exercise capacity is near normal in simple obesity.

Treatment

The optimal treatment for obesity is weight loss, but it is difficult for patients to lose weight and even harder for them to remain at the lower weight. With weight loss in the range of 40 kg, in simple obesity there is minimal change in VC, TLC, or compliance, but ERV increases and the arterial P_{O_2} may be increased by 4 to 8 mmHg. The improvement in gas exchange is more pronounced in those whose body weight is reduced to less than 130 percent of ideal. In OHS, the effects of weight loss on ERV and FRC are even more pronounced. VC and gas exchange are also improved following weight loss, but respiratory control remains essentially unaltered. A further benefit of weight loss is the abatement of obstructive sleep apnea. The episodes of apnea are diminished, and there is an improvement in daytime arterial blood gases. With persistent hypercapnia, noninvasive nocturnal mechanical ventilation has been employed in an attempt to improve daytime function and sleep quality . Positive-pressure ventilation may be delivered as either CPAP or intermittent positive-pressure ventilation by nose mask.

BIBLIOGRAPHY

Bolliger CT, van Eeden SF: Treatment of multiple rib fractures: Randomized control trial comparing ventilatory and nonventilatory management. *Chest* 97:943–948, 1990.

Collins LC, Hoberty PD, Walker JF, et al: The effect of body fat distribution on pulmonary function tests. *Chest* 107:1298–1302, 1995.

Conti G, Rocco M, Antonelli M, et al: Respiratory system mechanics in the early phase of acute respiratory failure due to severe kyphoscoliosis. *Intens Care Med* 23:539–544, 1997.

Ferris G, Severa-Pieras E, Vergera P, et al: Kyphoscoliosis ventilatory insufficiency: Noninvasive management outcomes. *Am J Phys Med Rehab* 79:24–29, 2000.

Jackson M, Smith I, King M, Shneerson J: Long term non-invasive domiciliary assisted ventilation for respiratory failure following thoracoplasty. *Thorax* 49:915–919, 1994.

Kearon C, Viviani GR, Killian KJ: Factors influencing work capacity in adolescent idiopathic thoracic scoliosis. *Am Rev Respir Dis* 148:295–303, 1993.

Meecham-Jones DJ, Paul EA, Bell JH, Wedzicha JA: Ambulatory oxygen therapy in stable kyphoscoliosis. *Eur Respir J* 8:819–823, 1995.

Morshuis W, Folgering H, Barentsz J, et al: Pulmonary function before surgery for pectus excavatum and at long-term follow-up. *Chest* 105:1646–1652, 1994.

Vgontzas AN, Tan TL, Bixler EO, et al: Sleep apnea and sleep disruption in obese patients. *Arch Intern Med* 154:1705–1711, 1994.

49 | Neuromuscular Diseases*

Robert M. Senior

EFFECTS OF NEUROMUSCULAR DISEASES ON VENTILATION

Neuromuscular diseases may impair the respiratory system as a vital pump. Depending on the particular disease, the respiratory pump may be impaired at the level of the cerebral cortex, brainstem, spinal cord, peripheral nerve, neuromuscular junction, or respiratory muscle (Table 49-1). In individuals with these disorders, respiratory failure may be precipitated by an acute

TABLE 49-1 Levels of Respiratory System Dysfunction Induced by Neuromuscular Diseases and Conditions

Level	Disease or condition
Upper motoneuron	
Cerebral	Vascular accidents
	Cerebellar atrophy
	Trauma
Spinal cord	Trauma
	Tumor
	Syringomyelia
	Multiple sclerosis
Lower motoneuron	
Anterior horn cells	Poliomyelitis
	Spinal muscle atrophy
	Amyotrophic lateral sclerosis
Motor nerves	Cardiac surgery
	Charcot-Marie-Tooth disease
	Diabetes
	Polyneuropathy
	Toxins
	Guillain-Barré syndrome
	Neuralgia amyotrophy
	Critical illness polyneuropathy
Neuromuscular junction	Myasthenia gravis
	Eaton-Lambert syndrome
	Botulism
	Organophosphate poisoning
	Drugs
Muscle	Dystrophy
	Acid maltase deficiency
	Malnutrition
	Corticosteroids
	Polymyositis

*Edited from Chaps. 98 and 99, "Effects of Neuromuscular Diseases on Ventilation," by Criner GJ, Kelsen SG, and "Pulmonary Rehabilitation in Neuromuscular Diseases," by Bach JR. In: *Fishman's Pulmonary Diseases and Disorders,* 3d ed., edited by Fishman AP, Elias JA, Fishman JA, Grippi MA, Kaiser LR, Senior RM. New York, McGraw-Hill, 1998, pp 1587–1595. For fuller discussion of topics dealt with in this chapter, the reader is referred to the original text, as noted above.

respiratory infection, fatigue, bronchial secretions, pulmonary infiltrations, atelectasis, pleural disease, and pneumothorax.

Patients with advanced respiratory muscle insufficiency adopt a pattern of rapid, shallow inspirations coupled with the inability to take occasional deep breaths. This pattern can lead to microatelectasis and decreased chest wall elasticity. Respiratory muscle dysfunction combined with increased work of breathing can lead to alveolar hypoventilation. Hypercapnia is a consequence of rapid shallow breathing and usually occurs when the vital capacity decreases to less than about half of predicted. Hypercapnia itself can contribute to decreasing respiratory muscle strength. The risk of pulmonary morbidity and mortality correlate with increasing hypercapnia.

Patients with respiratory muscle dysfunction often have concomitant weakness of expiratory and oropharyngeal muscles, which decrease peak flows during a cough. If peak cough flows do not exceed 3 L/s, cough will be inadequate to eliminate airway secretions. Peak cough flows are significantly reduced in patients who cannot take or cannot receive and hold a breath greater than 1.5 L. Peak cough flow is also decreased in patients in whom airflow is decreased because of dysfunction of the expiratory muscles or irreversible airway obstruction caused by tracheal stenosis, laryngeal incompetence, postintubation vocal cord adhesions or paralysis, or chronic obstructive pulmonary disease.

With respiratory muscle dysfunction, arterial hypoxemia and hypercapnia occur initially during rapid-eye-movement (REM) sleep. In time, the blood gas abnormalities gradually extend throughout most of sleep and eventually throughout daytime hours. Nocturnal oxyhemoglobin saturation <85 percent often occurs in patients whose arterial Pa_{CO_2} is >50 mmHg while awake.

Most patients with progressive neuromuscular weakness develop alveolar hypoventilation insidiously. Most often, alveolar hypoventilation is first recognized largely because of bronchial mucous plugging during a respiratory infection. Calcium-channel blockers, aminoglycosides, steroids, and benzodiazepines can reduce the ventilatory response to hypercapnia and hypoxemia. Beta blockers may increase airway resistance. Malnutrition, acidosis, electrolyte disturbances, cachexia, and infection can all aggravate ventilatory insufficiency acute respiratory failure. Acute ventilatory failure can develop in patients with acute cervical myelopathies, Guillain-Barré syndrome, myasthenia gravis, poliomyelitis, or multiple sclerosis.

Respiratory Muscle Function

Patients with neuromuscular disease may demonstrate fatigue, dyspnea, impaired control of secretions, recurrent lower respiratory tract infections, acute or chronic presentations of respiratory failure, pulmonary hypertension, and cor pulmonale. Respiratory muscle weakness may be the only presentation, as in muscular dystrophy, and may occur only late in the disease course. Relentless, progressive dysfunction of the respiratory muscles may occur, as in amyotrophic lateral sclerosis, or it may occur in a pattern of exacerbations and relapses as in multiple sclerosis. Patients with severe respiratory muscle weakness due to chronic neuromuscular disease may not complain of dyspnea or have any respiratory complaints. Reductions in inspiratory and expiratory mouth pressures do not correlate with general muscle strength assessment; however, patients with proximal myopathy are more likely to have significant respiratory muscle weakness.

The rapid, shallow breathing pattern found in patients with respiratory muscle weakness may be due to decreased generation of respiratory muscle force, but it may also be due to changes in lung and chest wall elastic recoil. A decrease in inspiratory muscle tone may lead to unopposed lung elastic recoil, which reduces lung volume. Once inspiratory muscle strength decreases to ~30 percent of normal, abnormalities in gas exchange (manifest primarily by hypercapnia) commonly occur. Expiratory muscle weakness is also common and leads to ineffectual cough.

Sleep-Related Breathing Disturbances

Impaired sleep quality, hypopnea, and hypercapnia are frequent in patients with neuromuscular disease. Episodes of nocturnal desaturation occur mostly during REM sleep associated with hypoventilation rather than upper airway obstruction. A direct relation has been found between the oxygen desaturation during REM sleep and the fall in vital capacity (VC) measured between the erect and supine positions. Abnormalities in nocturnal gas exchange antedate problems in daytime gas exchange. Patients with the most impaired gas exchange during REM sleep have the greatest degree of daytime hypercapnia.

CLINICAL FEATURES

In the early stages of neuromuscular disease, the patient may be asymptomatic. As respiratory muscle weakness progresses, dyspnea on exertion occurs, followed by dyspnea at rest. Disturbed sleep and daytime hypersomnolence from nocturnal hypoventilation may occur. If the expiratory muscles are affected, there may be impaired cough and repeated lower respiratory tract infections. As respiratory muscle weakness becomes more severe, respiratory failure may ensue. Dyspnea, hypoventilation, and impaired cough with or without recurrent lower respiratory tract infections may be the first clinical clues that a neuromuscular disease is present. Impaired swallowing due to bulbar dysfunction and peripheral limb muscle weakness are indications of neuromuscular disease.

Although the physical examination may yield normal results with early or mild impairment of the respiratory system, with established disease tachypnea at rest is typical. Other findings may include nasal flaring, intercostal muscle retraction, and palpable contraction of the sternocleidomastoid and scalene muscles. Inward paradoxical motion of the rib cage or abdomen may indicate a respiratory workload greater than the patient's respiratory muscle strength, or severe weakness of the diaphragm. When the diaphragm is severely paretic or paralyzed, it cannot counterbalance the negative changes in pleural pressure generated by contraction of the inspiratory muscles of the neck and rib cage. Instead of moving normally in a caudad direction, movement is paradoxically cephalad into the thorax, causing a paradoxical inward motion of the upper abdomen. Increased dyspnea occurs when patients assume the recumbent position due to hypoxemia, hypercapnia, and placement of the accessory inspiratory muscles at a mechanical disadvantage.

Radiographic Assessment

Fluoroscopy is often used in the assessment of diaphragm paralysis, with the patient making a forceful sniff in the supine position. In unilateral diaphragm paralysis, a positive "sniff" test may demonstrate paradoxical upward movement of the affected hemidiaphragm. However, sniff tests have a false-positive rate as high as 6 percent in normal persons. The use of the sniff test to diagnose bilateral diaphragmatic paralysis is limited by compensatory abdominal muscle contraction.

Pulmonary Function and Arterial Blood Gases

Spirometry and Lung Volumes

A reduced VC is a hallmark of chronic neuromuscular disease. The reduction is due respiratory muscle weakness and parallels the progression of the underlying disease. Large reductions in maximum respiratory pressures have to occur before VC is significantly reduced. The magnitude of the reduction is greater than expected solely on the basis of the reduction in inspiratory muscle strength, because decreased lung and chest wall compliance occur for unknown reasons. A decrease in VC greater than 25 percent on moving from the upright to the supine posture is a sign of diaphragmatic weakness and a greater likelihood of sleep-related hypoventilation. Reductions in lung and chest wall compliance also probably contribute. FEV_1 and FEF_{25-75} are often greater than normal in patients with neuromuscular disease because maximum expiratory flow can be achieved over most of the vital capacity with low driving pressures. A restrictive ventilatory pattern is demonstrated with reduced total lung capacity (TLC) and a normal or reduced functional residual capacity (FRC) are common. The residual volume (RV) is usually elevated and is a sign of expiratory muscle weakness.

Flow-Volume Loops

A flow-volume loop with the following features has a high degree of specificity and sensitivity in predicting respiratory muscle weakness: a reduced peak expiratory flow, decreased slope of the ascending limb of the maximum expiratory curve, a dropoff of forced expiratory flow near residual volume, and a reduction in forced inspiratory flow at 50 percent of vital capacity. Changes in the configuration of the flow-volume loop may reflect respiratory muscle weakness or malfunction of upper airway muscles: "sawtoothing" is seen in extrapyramidal disorders affecting upper airway muscles; plateauing of the inspiratory flow wave indicates extrathoracic airway obstruction that occurs in vocal cord paralysis caused by extrapyramidal neuromuscular disorders.

Maximum Voluntary Ventilation

Maximum voluntary ventilation (MVV) is an index of respiratory muscle endurance in the presence of normal expiratory flow rates. In patients with neuromuscular disease, airway resistance and FRC are usually within the normal range, so that MVV values correlate with respiratory muscle strength and may be even more sensitive than VC in detecting respiratory muscle weakness.

Maximum Static Inspiratory and Expiratory Pressures

Maximum pressures measured at the airway opening during a voluntary contraction against an occluded airway are the simplest and most commonly performed tests of respiratory muscle strength. Significant respiratory muscle weakness may occur without pulmonary complaints, and no correlation exists between respiratory muscle strength and generalized nonrespiratory muscle weakness. When PI_{max} falls below 30 cmH_2O, ventilatory failure commonly ensues. While maximum static airway pressures are useful measures of global respiratory muscle strength, they fail to assess individual respiratory muscle function. Since the diaphragm is the primary muscle of inspiration, and may be susceptible to isolated disease (e.g., phrenic nerve paralysis after open heart surgery or idiopathic diaphragmatic paralysis), specific testing of diaphragm strength is desirable in some patients.

Arterial Blood Gases

Arterial blood gas abnormalities usually occur only with severe respiratory muscle weakness. Hypoxemia is usually mild and may occur as a result of microatelectasis and subsequent intrapulmonary shunting or ventilation/perfusion mismatching. Measurement of arterial oxyhemoglobin saturation by pulse is an insensitive indicator of hypoventilation. Hypercarbia is an insensitive measure of respiratory muscle strength, as the Pa_{CO_2} does not increase until maximum inspiratory and expiratory mouth pressures are <50 percent of predicted.

NEUROMUSCULAR DISEASES

Upper Motor Neuron Lesions

Stroke

Hemispheric ischemic strokes reduce chest wall and diaphragm movement on the side contralateral to the cerebral insult. Bilateral hemispheric strokes are associated with Cheyne-Stokes respiration. Up to 50 percent of patients with strokes may have pulmonary aspiration due to upper airway dysfunction.

Spinal Cord Injury

The degree of respiratory impairment depends on the level and extent of the spinal cord injury. High cervical cord lesions (C1 to C3) cause paralysis of the diaphragmatic, intercostal, scalene, and abdominal muscles and almost always require ventilatory assistance. In some patients, spontaneous breathing can be accomplished by glossopharyngeal breathing or diaphragmatic pacing, because the phrenic nerve motoneurons (C3 to C5) remain intact. Patients with more caudal lesions (i.e., C4 to C5 level) usually require ventilatory support only during the period immediately after the injury and rarely require long-term ventilation. In the months following spinal cord injury below the C5 level, pulmonary function typically improves.

Patients with spinal cord injuries also have alterations in thoracoabdominal motion during tidal breathing, which is accentuated by changing from the erect to the supine position. In quadriplegic patients with relatively intact diaphragmatic function, the distribution of respiratory muscle weakness results in paradoxical inward motion of the upper rib cage during inspiration owing to weakness of the parasternal and scalene muscles. This pattern of abnormal thoracoabdominal movement is more marked in the supine than in the upright position. Patients with high quadriplegia (above C3 to C5) may be able to sustain short periods of spontaneous respiration because of inspiratory activity of the sternocleidomastoid and trapezius muscles.

Parkinson's Disease

Respiratory abnormalities are common in Parkinson's disease, with pneumonia being the most common cause of death. A substantial problem with

Parkinson's disease is glottic muscle dysfunction. An abnormal flow-volume loop contour showing regular or irregular flow oscillations commonly occurs, which correspond to rhythmic involuntary movements of glottic and subglottic structures. Physiologic evidence of upper airway obstruction may be present. Impairment of the upper airway muscles is occasionally severe enough to cause such obstruction. Treatment (e.g., with apomorphine) significantly improves maximum expiratory pressures and peak inspiratory flow.

Multiple Sclerosis

The three most common respiratory manifestations of multiple sclerosis (MS) are respiratory muscle weakness, bulbar dysfunction, and abnormalities in respiratory control. Acute respiratory failure rarely occurs. Even with severe disability and impaired respiratory muscle strength, patients with MS seldom complain of dyspnea. Clinical signs helpful in predicting respiratory muscle impairment are weak cough and inability to clear secretions, limited ability to count on a single exhalation, and upper extremity involvement. Advanced MS is frequently complicated by aspiration, atelectasis, and pneumonia. Treatment includes adrenocorticotropic hormone (ACTH), high-dose corticosteroids, immunosuppressive agents such as cyclophosphamide and azathioprine, intravenous immunoglobulin therapy, and plasmapheresis. Methylprednisone, 1 g daily for 5 days with or without prednisone taper, may be helpful in MS patients with severe respiratory complications. Plasmapheresis resolves clinical symptoms in patients with severe acute exacerbation and relapsing/remitting types of MS in acute exacerbation.

Lower Motor Neuron Lesions

Poliomyelitis

Early in the twentieth century, poliomyelitis was the most common cause of acute lower motor neuron disease in the United States. This has changed dramatically with the use of polio vaccine. Some patients develop progressive muscle weakness, termed *postpolio syndrome,* 20 to 30 years after the initial infection. Symptoms vary from mild to moderate deterioration of function, with fatigue, joint pain, or weakness that may progress to muscle atrophy. The weakness tends to progress slowly, with an average decline in muscle strength of ~1 percent a year.

Amyotrophic Lateral Sclerosis

Amyotrophic lateral sclerosis (ALS) is manifest by spasticity and hyperreflexia, muscle wasting, weakness, and fasciculations. Respiratory muscle impairment is usually evident in the advanced stages. Progression of respiratory impairment is much faster in ALS than in other chronic neuromuscular disorders. ALS patients show progressive reductions in FVC and MVV. In those with severe expiratory muscle weakness, the flow-volume curve near RV shows a sharp drop in flow. ALS patients in this group usually show lower maximum expiratory pressures, smaller VC, reduced expiratory reserve volume, and a higher RV than do ALS patients with more normal-appearing flow-volume curves. Difficulty in swallowing food or even saliva places ALS patients at markedly high risk for pulmonary aspiration. Special swallowing precautions, earlier placement of enteral feeding tubes, or antisialagogues may be required.

Disorders of Peripheral Nerves

Diaphragmatic Paralysis

Unilateral or bilateral diaphragmatic paralysis following phrenic nerve injury can result from cardiac surgery, trauma, mediastinal tumors, infections of the pleural space, or forceful manipulation of the neck. Phrenic nerve injury during open heart surgery is now one of the most common causes of unilateral and bilateral diaphragmatic paralysis and is due to cold exposure during cardioplegia or mechanical stretching of the phrenic nerve during surgery. Diaphragmatic paralysis may also occur with a variety of motor neuron diseases, myelopathies, neuropathies, and myopathies.

Bilateral diaphragmatic paralysis is characterized by severe restrictive ventilatory impairment, with VC being frequently <50 percent of predicted in the upright position and reduced to 25 percent in the supine position. The TLC is also markedly decreased, as well as FRC. In most patients with nontraumatic bilateral diaphragmatic paralysis, the most important clinical feature is orthopnea out of proportion to the severity of the underlying cardiopulmonary disease.

In patients with nontraumatic bilateral diaphragmatic paralysis, the diagnosis usually goes unrecognized until they present with cor pulmonale or cardiorespiratory failure and a chest radiograph showing elevation of both hemidiaphragms with volume loss and/or atelectasis at the lung bases. The diagnosis of bilateral diaphragmatic paralysis should be considered when any of the following abnormalities is present: (1) a 40 percent or greater reduction in VC in the supine compared to upright position or (2) fluoroscopically observed paradoxical movements of both hemidiaphragms during a sniff test.

Hemidiaphragmatic paralysis is more common than bilateral paralysis and is usually diagnosed from unilateral elevation of the hemidiaphragm on the chest radiograph. Most disorders reported as causing bilateral diaphragmatic paralysis have also been reported as causes of unilateral paralysis (e.g., cervical spondylosis, spinal cord injury, poliomyelitis, and muscular dystrophy). Other causes are pneumonia, trauma from central vein cannulation, and viral infections of the cervical nerve roots. Patient complaints and abnormalities on physical examination in unilateral diaphragmatic paralysis are usually the same as with bilateral diaphragmatic paralysis but are less striking. Orthopnea is a frequent complaint, but it is less dramatic than in bilateral paralysis.

Guillain-Barré Syndrome

Guillain-Barré syndrome (GBS) precipitates respiratory failure more often than any other peripheral neuropathy. Respiratory muscle weakness and specifically severe diaphragmatic weakness may be found in patients with GBS. Oropharyngeal muscles may also be impaired. Peripheral muscle strength does not correlate with the presence or absence of respiratory muscle weakness; however, ventilatory failure correlates with diaphragmatic weakness. An FVC of <12 to 15 mL/kg is a sign of imminent respiratory failure in GBS. Hypercapnia is a late sign of respiratory failure.

Respiratory treatment of GBS patients is mainly supportive. With bulbar involvement, special precautions for feeding and control of upper airway secretions may be required. Intubation and assisted ventilation may be indicated to avoid complications that arise from progressive respiratory failure, overwhelming pulmonary infections, or both. Aggressive pulmonary toilet, including repeated bronchoscopy, may be needed to decrease atelectasis and the incidence of nosocomial pneumonia. Plasmapheresis has produced short-term benefits. Plasmapheresis should be started within 2 weeks of the onset of symptoms or earlier if possible. Intravenous immunogammoglobulin (IVIG), given within 2 weeks after the onset of GBS, may also be effective therapy.

Critical Illness Polyneuropathy

Polyneuropathy presenting as prolonged weakness of the distal extremities may occur in critically ill patients. Patients with this syndrome have no history of neuropathy but have a prolonged stay in an intensive care unit, documented sepsis, and multiple organ failure. The mechanism for axonal damage in this syndrome is unknown. Possible causes include nerve toxins released during episodes of multiple system organ failure, antibiotics impairing neuromuscular transmission, protracted use of neuromuscular blocking agents, and hyperglycemia causing nerve ischemia by endovascular shunting. The clinical course is usually benign; however, recovery of nerve function may take 6 to 12 months.

Disorders of the Neuromuscular Junction

Myasthenia Gravis

In patients with moderate, generalized myasthenia gravis, pulmonary function tests show a mild reduction in FVC and moderate reductions in maximum inspiratory and expiratory mouth pressures.

Acute respiratory failure usually occurs in the setting of a myasthenic crisis or cholinergic crisis or as the initial presentation of the disease. A myasthenic crisis involves worsening of the basic underlying disease, usually precipitated by decreased anticholinesterase medication, surgery, administration of neuromuscular blocking medication, or emotional upset. The most common complications of myasthenic crisis are respiratory failure and recurrent pneumonias due to aspiration from bulbar involvement and impaired cough. In addition to mechanical ventilation, treatment includes anticholinesterase agents, high-dose corticosteroids, thymectomy, and plasmapheresis in patients refractory to steroid or immunosuppressive therapy. Anticholinesterase agents are the first line of treatment. Most patients improve significantly with anticholinesterase agents, but only a few regain normal function. Remissions can be induced in up to 80 percent of patients with the use of corticosteroids; however, corticosteroids may cause temporary worsening of muscle weakness, usually on the sixth to tenth days of therapy. Thymectomy improves survival and relieves clinical symptoms, even in the absence of thymoma. Thymectomy is indicated for thymoma because the risk for malignant transformation is high in patients less than 55 years of age. Plasmapheresis produces a temporary reduction in acetylcholine receptor antibody level and may be helpful in patients with respiratory failure not responding to anticholinesterase and immunosuppressive agents.

Eaton-Lambert Syndrome

Eaton-Lambert syndrome is a rare myasthenia-like illness that develops in association with tumors (especially small cell lung carcinoma); respiratory failure is infrequent.

Botulism

In botulism, weakness of the respiratory muscles requiring mechanical ventilation is frequent, especially with botulinum type A toxins. Recovery may take months, requiring prolonged mechanical ventilation.

Muscular Dystrophies

Duchenne's Muscular Dystrophy

Pulmonary symptoms are often minimal early in Duchenne's muscular dystrophy, despite significant weakness of the respiratory muscles. Reductions in maximum inspiratory pressure occur early and may precede the reduction observed in VC. Maximum expiratory mouth pressures are substantially lower than maximum inspiratory pressures, possibly decreasing effectiveness of cough. During the first decade of life, the FVC increases with growth and may mask early respiratory muscle dysfunction before it plateaus and progressively decreases at about ~5 percent per year after about age 12. Kyphoscoliosis is common and contributes to a restrictive ventilatory deficit. Severe nocturnal hypoventilation may occur during REM sleep and may contribute to the development of cor pulmonale. Hypercapnia is uncommon until very late, presumably due to relative preservation of diaphragmatic function. Death often occurs around age 20 as a result of progressive respiratory failure and pneumonia.

Management is mainly supportive. Ambulation should be maintained and encouraged as long as possible. Surgical correction may attenuate the scoliotic contribution to the fall in VC and improve patient morale and quality of life overall, but the downward trend in VC continues despite spine stabilization. Physiotherapy may be help prevent contractures, and weight control is important. Chest infections are treated with physiotherapy, postural drainage, and appropriate antibiotics. Vaccinations against pneumococcal pneumonia and influenza are advised. Assisted ventilation is required once respiratory insufficiency or symptoms of sleep-related breathing disorders are present. Intermittent facial positive-pressure ventilation prolongs survival and may attenuate the decline in FVC and MVV. Prednisone therapy may improve muscle strength.

Myotonic Dystrophy

Respiratory muscle weakness is common in myotonic dystrophy and can be severe despite mild limb muscle weakness. A chaotic breathing pattern may explain the higher prevalence of chronic hypercapnia in patients with myotonic dystrophy than in those with other forms of muscular dystrophy. Sleep-related breathing disturbances are common and may include both central and obstructive forms of sleep apnea. These patients are particularly susceptible to respiratory failure with general anesthesia and sedatives. Postoperative respiratory monitoring is essential. Pharyngeal and laryngeal dysfunction increases the risk of aspiration.

Facioscapulohumeral Dystrophy (FSH)

The FVC is significantly reduced in patients with FSH, although facial weakness complicates spirometric assessment. In 20 percent of patients with FSH, the disease affects pelvic girdle and trunk muscles, sometimes impairing respiratory function.

Limb-Girdle Dystrophy

Most patients have moderate respiratory muscle weakness with normal gas exchange. A few have been reported with chronic hypercapnia from severe diaphragmatic weakness or paralysis.

Acid Maltase Deficiency

This disease presents in three clinical forms: infantile, childhood, and adult. In adult-onset disease, there is progressive proximal muscle weakness. Respiratory failure or sleep-related complaints secondary to respiratory deterioration during REM sleep may be the initial presentation.

Mitochondrial Myopathy

Mitochondrial myopathy represents a new, heterogeneous group of disorders that affect mitochondrial function and may present as complex multisystem disorders. The clinical manifestations may include myalgia, exercise intolerance, proximal muscle weakness, and external ophthalmoplegia with unexplained respiratory failure. Once identified, patients should be cautioned to avoid sedatives; special attention is required when sedation or surgery is planned.

Acquired Myopathies

Pulmonary complications are the major cause of morbidity and mortality in dermatomyositis and polymyositis. These include interstitial pneumonitis, pulmonary vasculitis, recurrent aspiration from oropharyngeal dysfunction, and, rarely, hypoventilatory failure from respiratory muscle weakness. Respiratory failure is uncommon and is usually due to interstitial lung disease. Some 10 to 30 percent of patients have dyspnea, nonproductive cough, and hypoxemia, with radiographic evidence of diffuse interstitial lung disease and impaired gas exchange. Corticosteroids may be successful in the treatment of interstitial pneumonitis and myositis, especially if started early.

Systemic Lupus Erythematosus

Diaphragmatic dysfunction and respiratory muscle weakness with small lung volumes occur without apparent involvement of the peripheral skeletal muscles in patients with systemic lupus erythematosus. This has been called "the shrinking lung syndrome." The finding is due a myopathic process affecting diaphragmatic strength. It occurs even in the absence of a generalized myopathy.

Steroid Myopathy

Although acute myopathy secondary to high-dose steroid use was first described almost 20 years ago, the development of severe respiratory muscle weakness and prolonged respiratory failure following the use of high-dose steroids has received renewed interest. Most patients have received neuromuscular blocking agents along with high-dose steroids before weakness becomes evident. Some patients require months of mechanical ventilation before eventual recovery. The serum CPKs are often normal, and electromyography data show nonspecific changes. Because an underlying severe illness is present—often along with undernutrition, multiple medications, and disuse atrophy—it is difficult to incriminate steroids as responsible for the myopathic changes.

TREATMENT

The principles of managing respiratory dysfunction in patients with neuromuscular disease are (1) institution of preventive therapies designed to minimize the impact of impaired secretion clearance and alveolar hypoventilation on gas exchange and lower respiratory tract infections and (2) stabilization of patients who develop acute or chronic presentations of respiratory failure.

Preventive Therapies

Unfortunately, most patients with ventilatory dysfunction caused by a combination of respiratory muscle weakness, paralysis, or mechanical dysfunction of the chest wall are not treated until they develop respiratory distress. Indicators of impending or actual respiratory failure should be sought, including patient evaluation for symptoms of alveolar hypoventilation, measurements of vital capacity (sitting and recumbent), peak cough flows zunassisted and assisted, and oxyhemoglobin saturation and end-tidal CO_2 sitting and recumbent. Symptoms of alveolar hypoventilation can include daytime drowsiness, morning headaches, fatigue, impaired concentration, frequent sleep arousals, anxiety, and nightmares. Oxygen saturation is monitored overnight when there are symptoms of daytime hypoxemia, the vital capacity is substantially less supine, or the patient is more short of breath supine than sitting. If there is significant oxygen desaturation and/or alveolar hypoventilation is suspected, an arterial blood gas is obtained.

Patients are at risk for acute respiratory failure during respiratory infections or other events that tax respiratory musculature if they have <50 percent of predicted vital capacity when sitting or supine or their peak cough flows are <5 L/s. Patients at risk are taught how to receive intermittent positive-pressure ventilation (IPPV) via mouthpieces or nasal interfaces. They are provided with a manual resuscitator and placed on a regimen of air-stacking exercises several times per day. They and their care providers are taught manually assisted coughing and mechanical insufflation-exsufflation. They receive an oximeter and are instructed to monitor their saturation during respiratory tract infections and events causing fatigue or shortness of breath. Properly managed patients often have a decrease in oxygen saturation <92% temporarily, particularly when they are febrile, but pneumonia and gross atelectasis are rare and hospitalization is seldom indicated.

In disorders causing bulbar dysfunction, swallowing precautions and airway control measures are required. With advanced bulbar symptoms, a cuffed tracheostomy tube may be needed to protect the airway and facilitate suction of lower respiratory tract secretions.

Although respiratory muscle training improves strength and ventilatory endurance in normal subjects and in patients with pulmonary diseases, the wisdom of training the respiratory muscles of patients with significant neuromuscular dysfunction has been questioned. Breathing through resistive loads may be harmful and perhaps further damage or tire already weakened respiratory muscles. Also, the training techniques do not apply to upper airway and pharyngeal musculature. Quadriplegic patients may be a more appropriate group for respiratory muscle training since their muscles are intrinsically normal.

TABLE 49-2 Indications for Mechanical Ventilation in Patients with Neuromuscular Diseases

Acute respiratory failure
  Severe dyspnea
  Marked accessory muscle use
  Copious secretions
  Unstable hemodynamic state
  Hypoxemia refractory to supplemental O_2
  Acute severe gas exchange disturbances (increased Pa_{CO_2} with pH ≤ 7.25)
Chronic respiratory failure
  Symptoms of nocturnal hypoventilation (e.g., morning headaches, decreased energy, nightmares, enuresis)
  Dyspnea at rest or increased work of breathing impairing sleep
  Cor pulmonale due to hypoventilation, Pa_{CO_2} >45, pH <7.32 after treating reversible conditions
Nocturnal desaturation (Sa_{O_2}<88%) despite supplemental O_2 therapy

Management of Respiratory Failure

In some patients, the onset of respiratory failure is insidious, manifest by the gradual onset of dyspnea, daytime hypersomnolence, morning headaches, nightmares, enuresis, and easy fatigability. In patients with these symptoms, arterial blood gas analysis is warranted, especially if the vital capacity falls below 1.5 L. Daytime measurements may be misleading, however, because impaired gas exchange may occur only during REM sleep. Nocturnal oximetry or a full polysomnogram should be considered to exclude the presence of nocturnal hypoventilation. In patients who have chronic hypoventilation, uncompensated respiratory acidosis, hypoxemia refractory to supplemental oxygen, or worsening symptoms such as easy fatigability and morning headaches, the need for nocturnal mechanical ventilation should be anticipated.

In patients with severe respiratory impairment, mechanical ventilation may be indicated to augment or supplant spontaneous breathing (Table 49-2). Mechanical ventilation may be invasive or noninvasive depending on the circumstances (Table 49-3). Patients who present with severe dyspnea, CO_2 retention, and moderate to severe hypoxemia require intubation and mechanical ventilation. In patients with acute respiratory failure who are awake, alert, able to control their airways and do not have copious secretions, noninvasive ventilation be adequate.

Noninvasive Assistance of Ventilation

Noninvasive intermittent positive-pressure ventilation (IPPV) methods are versatile, convenient, and effective in a number of neuromuscular disorders (Table 49-4). Noninvasive IPPV is the preferred method for 24-h ventilatory support. It can be delivered via oral, nasal, or oral-nasal interfaces.

Noninvasive IPPV only at night or intermittently throughout the 24-h period may produce significant improvements in daytime gas exchange as well as patients' symptoms and functional status. Several hypotheses have been proposed to explain these improvements: (1) respiratory muscle resting treats patients who suffer from chronic intermittent fatigue; (2) preventing nocturnal hypoventilation resets the central respiratory center's Pa_{CO_2} threshold; (3) there is improved ventilation/perfusion matching;

TABLE 49-3 Invasive versus Noninvasive Mechanical Ventilation in Patients with Neuromuscular Disease

Invasive Ventilation (endotracheal or tracheostomy tube and positive-pressure ventilation)	Noninvasive Ventilation (no airway cannulation)
Copious secretions	Awake, cooperative patient
Inability to control upper airway	Good airway control
Inability to tolerate or failure of noninvasive ventilation	Minimal secretions
Impaired cognition	Hemodynamic stability
Unstable hemodynamics	Reversible cause of respiratory failure

and (4) improved lung and chest wall compliance occurs and decreases the work of breathing.

Negative-Pressure Ventilators

For many years, negative pressure body ventilators (NPBVs) were the predominant noninvasive method of ventilatory support for patients with ventilatory impairment due to respiratory muscle weakness or paralysis or mechanical dysfunction of the chest wall. These ventilators function by intermittently applying subatmospheric pressure to the thorax and abdomen, thus increasing transpulmonary pressure and inflating the lung. Tank ventilators are the most efficient form of negative-pressure ventilators; cuirass negative-pressure ventilators are less so. They are particularly suitable for overnight ventilatory support. However, they are very large, cumbersome, claustrophobia-inducing; they interfere with nursing care and are usable only with the patient supine. All forms of negative-pressure ventilation tend to induce obstructive sleep apnea due to upper airway collapse during a mechanically delivered breath. This

TABLE 49-4 Neuromusculoskeletal Disorders for which Noninvasive Intermittent Positive-Pressure Ventilation Has Proved Effective for Total Ventilatory Support

Myopathies
 Dystrophinopathies (Duchenne and Becker dystrophies)
 Other muscular dystrophies (limb-girdle, Emery-Dreifuss, facioscapulo-humeral, congenital, childhood)
 Congenital and metabolic myopathies (e.g., acid maltase deficiency)
 Inflammatory myopathies (e.g., polymyositis)
Neurological disorders
 Motor neuron diseases and spinal muscular atrophy
 Poliomyelitis
 Hereditary sensorimotor neuropathies
 Phrenic neuropathies associated with cardiac hypothermia, surgery, or trauma
 Guillain-Barré syndrome
 Multiple sclerosis
 Myelopathies
 Myasthenia gravis
Sleep-disordered breathing
 Obesity hypoventilation
Skeletal pathology
 Kyphoscoliosis
 Osteogenesis imperfecta

problem is overcome by other, more practical approaches, including intermittent abdominal pressure ventilator, noninvasive IPPV, and glossopharyngeal breathing.

Rocking Beds

Rocking beds and pneumobelts—abdominal displacement ventilators—have been used as ventilatory assist devices in patients with mild to moderate ventilatory failure. Both devices augment diaphragmatic motion by cyclically displacing the abdominal viscera against gravity. The bed rocks between 12 and 24 times per minute and may be adjusted to optimize patient comfort and achieve minute ventilation targets. The pneumobelt (see IAPV, below) is an inflatable bladder that is worn over the anterior abdomen and connected to a positive-pressure ventilator that intermittently inflates it. Tidal volume can be augmented by increasing bladder inflation pressures to target goals. Both devices should be seen as methods to assist ventilation in impaired patients rather than as mechanical ventilators. Both devices are limited by their constraints on patient posture. The rocking bed is bulky and limited by the degree of ventilatory assistance that it provides. Similarly, the pneumobelt requires that the patient be in the upright position, the amount of ventilatory assistance provided is limited, and it can produce discomfort when high bladder inflation pressures are required to sufficiently augment ventilation.

Mouthpiece IPPV With mouthpiece IPPV, air is delivered via a mouthpiece held between the lips and teeth. Since high tidal volumes are delivered, even patients with little vital capacity need to take only a few deep insufflations per minute. Patients can vary their tidal volumes and stack them to deeply expand the lungs in order to increase voice volume and peak cough flows. The patient has to learn palatal movements to prevent leakage out of the nose during insufflation and to open the glottis during each assisted breath. Mouthpiece IPPV is the most convenient, reliable, and effective method of daytime assisted ventilation.

Lipseal IPPV Patients who are unable to hold a mouthpiece can use a lipseal that holds the mouthpiece firmly in the mouth and minimizes air leakage around the mouthpiece and out of the mouth. Orthodontic bite plates and custom-fabricated acrylic lipseals can increase comfort and efficacy and eliminate risk of orthodontic deformity. High insufflation volumes, 1200 mL or more, are used to compensate for nasal leakage. Aerophagia, allergy to the plastic lipseal, and abdominal distention occur sporadically.

Nasal IPPV Nasal IPPV has become the conventional approach to relieving nocturnal hypoventilation. A variety of continuous positive airway pressure (CPAP) masks are available. Each design applies pressure to the paranasal area differently. It is impossible to predict which model will be most effective and comfortable for a particular patient. Patients may use different styles on alternate nights to vary skin contact pressure. Custom-molded nasal interfaces can be obtained commercially or in specialized centers. Because patients generally prefer to use mouthpiece IPPV or the IAPV for daytime aid, nasal IPPV is practical only for nocturnal use.

Intermittent abdominal pressure ventilation (IAPV) As described above, IAPV involves intermittent inflation of an elastic air sac that is contained in a corset or belt worn beneath the patient's outer clothing. Inflation moves the diaphragm upward, causing a forced exsufflation. During bladder deflation, the abdominal contents and diaphragm return to the resting position, and inspiration occurs passively. IAPV augments tidal volumes ~300 mL. It is usually inadequate in the presence of scoliosis or obesity.

Expiratory Muscle Aids

Expiratory muscle assistance is applied to the body as manual thrusts or as pressure changes applied directly to the airway to increase peak cough flows. Peak cough flows can also be increased by mechanical insufflation-exsufflation (MI-E), which consists of a positive-pressure insufflation followed by a sudden decrease in pressure, usually from ~+40 cmH$_2$O to −40 cmH$_2$O. When MI-E is used through a translaryngeal or tracheostomy tube, the tube cuff is inflated and a concomitant abdominal thrust is unnecessary. Patients invariably prefer MI-E to tracheal suctioning, and suctioning can be discontinued for most patients. The technique does not work if the patient cannot keep the airway open, when there is a fixed upper airway obstruction, or when upper airway dilator muscles cannot maintain sufficient patency to allow for adequate expiratory flows.

Glossopharyngeal Breathing (GPB)

Glossopharyngeal breathing requires the patient to use the tongue and pharyngeal muscles to add to an inspiratory effort by projecting (gulping) boluses of air past the glottis. The glottis closes with each gulp. One breath usually consists of 6 to 9 gulps of 60 to 200 mL each. It is important to monitor the efficacy of GPB during the training period by spirometry, measuring the milliliters of air per gulp, gulps per breath, and breaths per minute. GPB is taught to patients with less than 1 L of vital capacity. GPB can provide individuals without respiratory muscle function with normal alveolar ventilation for hours and can ensure safety when a ventilator is not being used or in the event of ventilator failure. GPB is rarely useful in the presence of an indwelling tracheostomy tube. The safety and versatility afforded by effective GPB are key reasons to eliminate tracheostomy in favor of noninvasive aids.

BIBLIOGRAPHY

Neuromuscular Diseases: Clinical Features

Carter JL, Noseworthy JH: Ventilatory dysfunction in multiple sclerosis. *Clin Chest Med* 15:693–703, 1994.

Kaplan LM, Hollander D: Respiratory dysfunction in amyotrophic lateral sclerosis. *Clin Chest Med* 15:675–681, 1994.

Lynn DJ, Woda RP, Mendell JR: Respiratory dysfunction in muscular dystrophy and other myopathies. *Clin Chest Med* 15:661–674, 1994.

Rochester DF, Esau SA: Assessment of ventilatory function in patients with neuromuscular disease. *Clin Chest Med* 15:751–763, 1994.

Teitelbaum JS, Borel CO: Respiratory dysfunction in Guillain-Barré syndrome. *Clin Chest Med* 15:705–714, 1994.

Zulueta JJ, Fanburg BL: Respiratory dysfunction in myasthenia gravis. *Clin Chest Med* 15:683–691, 1994.

Neuromuscular Diseases: Therapy

Bach JR: A comparison of long-term ventilatory support alternatives from the perspective of the patient and care giver. *Chest* 104:1702–1706, 1993.

Bach JR: Amyotrophic lateral sclerosis: Predictors for prolongation of life by noninvasive respiratory aids. *Arch Phys Med Rehabil* 76:828–832, 1995.

Bach JR, Alba AS, Saporito LR: Intermittent positive pressure ventilation via the mouth as an alternative to tracheostomy for 257 ventilator users. *Chest* 103:174–182, 1993.

Chailleux E, Fauroux B, Binet F, et al: Predictors of survival in patients receiving domiciliary oxygen therapy or mechanical ventilation: A 10-year analysis of ANTADIR Observatory. *Chest* 109:741–749, 1996.

Ferris G, Severa-Pieras E, Vergara P, et al: Kyphoscoliosis ventilatory insufficiency: Noninvasive management outcomes. *Am J Phys Med Rehab* 79:24–29, 2000.

Jubelt B, Agre JG: Characteristics and management of postpolio syndrome. *JAMA* 284:412–414, 2000.

Part Eleven | **SLEEP AND SLEEP DISORDERS**

50 | Sleepiness, Control of Ventilation, and Sleep-Disordered Breathing*

Richard J. Schwab

A number of physiologic alterations in the control and mechanics of breathing characterize sleep. These sleep-induced changes may disrupt normal sleep and contribute to the pathogenesis of cardiopulmonary disease, including the development of hypoxemia, alveolar hypoventilation, pulmonary hypertension, and cor pulmonale. In addition, many disorders—including asthma, chronic obstructive pulmonary disease, restrictive lung diseases, and cardiovascular diseases—may become worse during the night secondary to changes in the control of ventilation during sleep. Patients who present with unexplained hypercapnia, cor pulmonale, pulmonary hypertension, or alveolar hypoventilation may have a primary sleep disorder precipitating these phenomena.

NORMAL SLEEP

Within sleep there are two distinct states: (1) *non–rapid-eye-movement (NREM)* sleep [slow-wave, in reference to the slow, large electroencephalographic (EEG) rhythms that characterize this stage] and (2) *rapid-eye-movement (REM)* sleep (paradoxical or active sleep). The onset of sleep is initiated through NREM sleep, which is divided into four stages (1 to 4) based on EEG criteria. Each successive stage in NREM sleep represents a deeper stage of sleep [the threshold for arousal is highest in stage 3/4 (delta sleep) and the lowest in stage 1 sleep]. Normal adults, upon falling asleep, cycle through stages 1 to 3, entering stage 4 approximately 35 min after the onset of sleep.

REM sleep is characterized by episodic rapid eye movements, muscle atonia, and EEG activity that is similar to that in wakefulness. Dreaming and increased metabolic activity of the central nervous system are hallmarks of REM sleep. REM sleep and NREM sleep alternate throughout the night in cyclic fashion. Cycles of REM sleep last approximately 10 to 30 min and occur every 90 to 110 min. The normal latency to REM sleep is 90 min. As the night progresses, the REM cycles lengthen. REM sleep usually occurs in four to six discrete episodes that account for 20 to 25 percent of sleep; NREM makes up 75 to 80 percent of sleep time. Age influences the pattern of sleep stages during the night; total sleep time and delta sleep decrease with aging.

*Edited from Chaps. 100 to 103, "Stages of Sleep," by Morrison AR; "Changes in the Cardiovascular System During Sleep," by Pack AI, Kubin L, Davies RO; "Sleep Apnea Syndromes," by Schwab RJ, Goldberg AN, Pack AI; "Differential Diagnosis and Evaluation of Sleepiness," by Kryger MH, George CFP. In: *Fishman's Pulmonary Diseases and Disorders,* 3d ed., edited by Fishman AP, Elias JA, Fishman JA, Grippi MA, Kaiser LR, Senior RM. New York, McGraw-Hill, 1998, pp 1599–1648. For fuller discussion of topics dealt with in this chapter, the reader is referred to the original text, as noted above.

CONTROL OF VENTILATION DURING NORMAL SLEEP

The breathing pattern of normal subjects is often periodic in stages 1 and 2 sleep, particularly in the elderly, but it becomes regular in stages 3 and 4 sleep. In REM sleep, the pattern of respiration is often irregular, with periods of central apnea. Minute ventilation decreases during sleep primarily due to a decrease in tidal volume. As a consequence of this decrease in ventilation during sleep, Pa_{CO_2} rises, typically from the normal value of 40 mmHg to 45 to 46 mmHg. Paralleling this increase in Pa_{CO_2} is a decrease in the Pa_{O_2}. Hypoxemia and hypercapnia are greater in REM than in NREM sleep. In normal persons, who are operating on the flat part of the oxyhemoglobin dissociation curve, Pa_{O_2} does not fall to a level of arterial hypoxemia. However, in persons with low Pa_{O_2} during wakefulness, in whom arterial oxygenation is closer to the "knee" of the oxygen oxyhemoglobin dissociation curve, the fall in Pa_{O_2} during sleep may lead to significant hypoxemia. For example, patients with chronic obstructive pulmonary disease (COPD) may require supplemental oxygen during sleep but not during wakefulness.

Another major change that occurs during sleep is a decrease in the ventilatory response to hypoxia and to hypercapnia; decrements are greater in REM than NREM sleep. During REM sleep, atonia causes a decrease in the functional residual capacity, which, in turn, results in ventilation/perfusion mismatching (worsening hypoxemia and widening of the A-a gradient). These state-dependent physiologic changes in ventilatory function, which do not have major clinical significance in normal subjects, may have deleterious consequences in patients with underlying pulmonary and cardiovascular disease.

DAYTIME SLEEPINESS

Some 4 to 5 percent of the population complain of excessive sleepiness. Moreover, sleepiness plays an important role in both industrial and motor vehicle accidents. Possibly the most important cause of daytime sleepiness is sleep deprivation (a rampant problem in our society and a major problem in the medical profession). The amount time spent in nocturnal sleep has a strong relationship to the degree of daytime sleepiness. Regardless of cultural or environmental factors, most adults sleep 7 to 8 h per day. However, the adage that we require 8 h of sleep each night does not apply to everyone: some require more than 8 h; others require less. The loss of as little as 1 h of sleep per night will accumulate over time and lead to daytime sleepiness. The differential diagnosis of persistent daytime sleepiness is indicated in Table 50-1.

Daytime sleepiness can be measured subjectively and objectively. The most widely studied subjective measure of sleepiness is the Epworth Sleepiness Scale (ESS) (Table 50-2). The ESS was designed to measure sleep propensity in a single, standardized way and is based on questions relating to eight commonplace situations. The questions are self-administered and subjects are asked to rate on a scale of 0 to 3 how likely they are to doze off in each situation based on their usual habits. A normal result on the ESS is <10.

More objective, reliable, and reproducible is the Multiple Sleep Latency Test (MSLT). The MSLT is a series of 20-min naps performed at 2-h intervals throughout the day. The MSLT measures the time to the onset of sleep as determined by the EEG. The normal latency to stage 1 sleep on a MSLT

TABLE 50-1 Differential Diagnosis of Persistent Daytime Sleepiness

---

Sleep deprivation—a significant problem for the hospitalized patient
Sleep-disordered breathing (i.e., obstructive sleep apnea and obesity-hypoventilation syndrome)
Depression
Narcolepsy (classic tetrad: severe daytime sleepiness, sleep paralysis, hypnagogic hallucinations, cataplexy)
Insomnia
Sleep-related movement disorders (e.g., periodic limb movement disorder, bruxism, etc.)
Metabolic, toxic, and medication-induced hypersomnolence
Idiopathic hypersomnolence (central nervous system hypersomnolence)
Head injury
Circadian-rhythm sleep disorders

---

is greater than 10 min. The MSLT is particularly useful in diagnosing narcolepsy [short latency to stage 1 sleep (usually <5 min) and 2 REM onsets (normally REM sleep is not achieved during a 20-min nap)].

SPECTRUM OF SLEEP-DISORDERED BREATHING

Sleep disordered breathing should be considered as a continuum of abnormalities, i.e., a span of diseases that ranges from snoring to the upper airway resistance syndrome (UARS)—snoring that consists of related arousals

---

TABLE 50-2 Epworth Sleepiness Scale

In contrast to just feeling tired, how likely are you to doze off or fall asleep in the following situations? (This refers to your usual life in recent times. Even if you have not done some these things recently, try to work out how they would have affected you.) Use the following scale to choose the most appropriate number for each situation:

0 = Would never doze
1 = Slight chance of dozing
2 = Moderate chance of dozing
3 = High chance of dozing

SITUATION	CHANCE OF DOZING
Sitting and reading	_____
Watching TV	_____
Sitting inactively in a public place (i.e., a theater or a meeting)	_____
Being a passenger in a car for an hour without break	_____
Lying down to rest in the afternoon when circumstances permit	_____
Sitting and talking to someone	_____
Sitting quietly after lunch without alcohol	_____
In a car, while stopping for a few minutes in traffic	_____

without reductions in airflow—to obstructive sleep apnea to obesity-hypoventilation syndrome (Pickwickian syndrome). The span may be pictured as follows:

Snoring $\leftrightarrow$ UARS $\leftrightarrow$ hypopneas $\leftrightarrow$ obstructive apneas $\leftrightarrow$ hypoventilation

Snoring should not be considered normal; it is often the first manifestation of sleep-disordered breathing. Appreciable weight gain or loss may move an individual along this continuum of sleep-disordered breathing; individuals may change position on the continuum relatively abruptly. For example, alcohol can worsen the degree of sleep-disordered breathing since it preferentially suppresses the activity of upper airway dilator muscles.

EPIDEMIOLOGY AND RISK FACTORS FOR OBSTRUCTIVE SLEEP APNEA

Sleep apnea is an extremely common disorder. It is twice as common in men as in women.

In adults, the major risk factor for obstructive sleep apnea is obesity. Not surprisingly, it is fat in the neck that plays the largest role. Indeed, neck (or collar) size is the best predictor of the occurrence of sleep apnea: approximately 30 percent of men who snore and whose collar size is greater than 17 in. have obstructive sleep apnea. Neck size in women has not been as well investigated, but >15 in. increases the risk for sleep apnea.

Obesity is not the only risk factor for obstructive sleep apnea. Upper airway anatomy (macroglossia; enlargement of the tonsils, soft palate, and lateral walls; and retrognathia), genetic factors, endocrine disorders (hypothyroidism, acromegaly), and substances that reduce upper airway muscle tone (alcohol, sedatives, or hypnotics) also play a role.

CLINICAL PRESENTATION OF OBSTRUCTIVE SLEEP APNEA

Obstructive sleep apnea should be considered in all overweight or retrognathic patients who complain of habitual snoring and/or daytime sleepiness.

Symptoms

The cardinal symptoms of sleep apnea are excessive daytime sleepiness, sleep fragmentation, and loud habitual snoring. Witnessed apneic episodes (nocturnal grunting/gasping) are often reported. Patients may fall asleep at inappropriate times, as while watching television or reading, in the middle of a conversation, or while operating a motor vehicle. Patients with sleep apnea have a three- to sevenfold greater rate of motor vehicle accidents than do subjects without sleep apnea. Other common symptoms include personality changes (especially irritability), nocturia, morning headaches (this suggests hypercapnia and concomitant obesity-hypoventilation syndrome), intellectual impairment, reduction in libido, palpitations, and memory loss.

Physical Examination

All patients with sleep apnea should have a careful head and neck examination, with particular attention to the size of the bony and soft tissue oropharyngeal structures. Neck size should be measured at the cricothyroid membrane (>17 in. in men and >15 in. in women increases the risk for sleep apnea). Craniofacial risk factors for sleep apnea include retrognathia (see below), micrognathia, a narrow hard palate, nasal obstruction, an overjet (greater than a 3-mm anteroposterior distance between the upper and lower incisors during occlusion), and overbite (greater than a 3-mm vertical distance between the upper and lower incisors during occlusion). The nares should be examined for nasal polyps and nasal septal deviation.

Retrognathia is defined as a >0.5-cm retroposition of the gnathion (the most inferior point in the contour of the chin) relative to the plane of the nasion (from the deepest point of the superior aspect of the nasal bone to the base of the nose). As a rule, the forehead, maxilla, and mandible are aligned. If the mandible is behind these structures, retrognathia should be considered.

Upper airway soft tissue risk factors for sleep apnea include macroglossia, tonsillar hypertrophy, and enlargement of the soft palate/uvula and lateral pharyngeal walls. The tongue is considered to be enlarged if it is above the level of the mandibular occlusal plane. Tonsillar enlargement is defined as the presence of lateral impingement of greater than 50 percent of the posterior pharyngeal airspace. The uvula is considered enlarged if it is >1.5 cm in length or >1.0 cm in width. Lateral peritonsillar narrowing is defined as impingement of greater than 25 percent of the pharyngeal space by the peritonsillar tissues excluding the tonsils. Recent data indicate that lateral peritonsillar narrowing may be the most important anatomic risk factor for sleep apnea.

DIAGNOSIS OF OBSTRUCTIVE SLEEP APNEA

The "gold standard" for making the diagnosis of obstructive sleep apnea is an overnight polysomnogram, which demonstrates recurrent episodes of cessation of respiration (apnea) or decrements in airflow (hypopneas) during sleep associated with arousals and arterial oxyhemoglobin desaturations. Patients with obstructive sleep apnea exert respiratory effort (i.e., chest wall and abdominal wall movement), unlike patients with central sleep apnea, who lack respiratory drive.

An apnea is defined as cessation of airflow for at least 10 s. An apnea can be obstructive (no airflow but continued respiratory effort), central (airflow and respiratory effort both absent), or mixed. A mixed apnea is one that starts as a central event but then becomes obstructive during the same episode. Most patients with obstructive sleep apnea have both obstructive and mixed apneas.

Hypopneas (a decrement in airflow of 50 percent or more associated with a 4 percent fall in oxygen saturation and/or an EEG arousal) can produce clinical consequences similar to apneas. Therefore the Respiratory Disturbance Index (RDI), also called the Apnea/Hypopnea Index (AHI), has become the standard method for defining and quantifying the severity of obstructive sleep apnea. This index is determined as the number of apneas plus hypopneas per hour of sleep. A RDI >15 events/h is indicative of obstructive sleep apnea. In the hospitalized patient, nocturnal oximetry demonstrating recurrent oxyhemoglobin desaturations has been used as a screening test for sleep apnea.

CONSEQUENCES OF OBSTRUCTIVE SLEEP APNEA

Consequences of obstructive sleep apnea can be broadly divided into those related to excessive sleepiness and those related to the cardiovascular system. Excessive daytime sleepiness produces a number of different problems for patients with sleep apnea, including the possibility of vehicular crashes. Studies in driving simulators indicate that sleep apnea impairs driving ability. Indeed, patients with sleep apnea can be as impaired in driving skills as those who have blood alcohol concentrations above the legal limits.

Cardiovascular risks associated with sleep apnea include hypertension, myocardial infarction, cardiac arrhythmias, and stroke. The sleep health heart study (6000 adults who underwent sleep studies were followed for cardiovascular morbidity) demonstrated that patients with sleep apnea are at special risk for hypertension. Obstructive sleep apnea has also been demonstrated to be a significant risk factor for myocardial infarction and cerebrovascular accidents. Nocturnal cardiac arrhythmias—including atrial and ventricular tachycardia, heart block, and sinus pauses—have been reported during apneic episodes (nocturnal arrhythmias are often a clue to the diagnosis). These arrhythmias often resolve after treatment of the obstructive sleep apnea, so that a pacemaker may not be indicated. Pulmonary hypertension and right heart failure develop in approximately 10 to 15 percent of patients with severe sleep apnea.

TREATMENT OF OBSTRUCTIVE SLEEP APNEA

The first line of treatment for sleep apnea syndrome is medical management.

General Measures

All patients with sleep apnea should avoid alcohol, sedatives, and hypnotics. Alcohol reduces the tone of upper airway dilator muscles and increases the severity of snoring and apneas. Weight loss has been shown to decrease the severity of obstructive sleep apnea; indeed, very moderate reductions in weight have been shown to improve upper airway function. Unfortunately weight loss has proved difficult to achieve and sustain in this patient population. However, for all obese patients with obstructive sleep apnea, weight-management programs should be recommended. Bariatric surgery, performed laproscopically, has been proposed for very obese patients with severe sleep apnea and may be a promising technique.

Position Therapy

In some patients, apneas may be totally position-dependent—i.e., apneas occur in the supine but not in the lateral decubitus position. Position-dependent sleep apnea can be easily diagnosed with polysomnography, which will demonstrate a high RDI in the supine position but not in the lateral decubitus position. Position therapy can be accomplished by sewing pockets for one or two tennis balls into the back of a patient's nightshirt in order to try to prevent him or her from lying in the supine position. The long-term efficacy of position therapy is unknown. In general, patients who have significant symptomatology or severe sleep apnea should not be treated by this approach.

CPAP and Its Modifications

The *treatment of choice* for patients with obstructive sleep apnea is nasal CPAP therapy. CPAP is the most effective noninvasive therapy for sleep apnea. It has been shown to reduce the number of apneic and hypoxic episodes during sleep as well as to reduce daytime sleepiness and improve neuropsychiatric function in patients with obstructive sleep apnea. CPAP provides a pneumatic splint for the airway, preventing collapse during sleep, when upper airway dilator muscle activity is reduced. In using CPAP, it is important to ensure that patients have a good interface with the CPAP machine, with no air leaks.

Although CPAP use is associated with few serious complications, it is associated with a number of bothersome complaints. These include nocturnal arousals, nasal irritation, rhinitis, nasal dryness, aerophagia, mask and mouth leaks, facial skin discomfort, difficulty with exhalation, claustrophobia, and chest/back pain (secondary to lung hyperinflation). Nasal irritation and rhinitis can be treated initially with humidification of the CPAP system and, if they persist, with nasal steroids. Claustrophobia may be improved by switching from a nasal mask to nasal pillows. Aerophagia can be treated with changes in body position or the type of mask. Serious side effects are uncommon. The major obstacle in the use of CPAP is not serious side effects; instead, it is adherence to the therapy. Several studies have shown the use of CPAP to be 4.5 to 5.0 h per night with a 60 percent compliance rate.

A newer technique for delivering positive airway pressure allows independent regulation of the inspiratory positive airway pressure (IPAP) and expiratory positive airway pressure (EPAP). These bilevel systems can decrease the need for high levels of expiratory pressure while maintaining higher levels of inspiratory pressure. Thus, they may be particularly useful in patients requiring high levels of CPAP pressure or in those who complain of difficulty exhaling on CPAP. However, bilevel systems are more expensive than conventional CPAP therapy and the algorithms to adjust the inspiratory and expiratory pressures are essentially empiric.

The newest modification in CPAP systems is auto-CPAP. These CPAP machines adjust the CPAP pressure throughout the night rather than delivering one fixed pressure. The auto-CPAP units adjust pressure on the basis of detecting apneas and/or snoring and/or inspiratory flow limitation. The concept of adjusting CPAP pressures throughout the night is valid, since position changes and sleep-stage changes affect apnea severity. Theoretically, auto-CPAP units might improve compliance by reducing pressure-related side effects, since the mean pressure is lower than that of conventional CPAP. Moreover, autoadjustment of CPAP avoids both the concern that patients may have been prescribed an inadequate level of CPAP, and the patient can adjust to longer-term needs—e.g. as a result of weight loss or gain. However, these devices are more expensive than conventional CPAP units and it is not clear that they improve adherence.

Intraoral Devices

Another treatment modality that is now being used more commonly comprises intraoral devices. Several studies have demonstrated that oral appliances are an effective noninvasive alternative to CPAP in patients with mild to moderate sleep apnea. The most common and best-studied appliances are the mandibular advancing devices. In general, these devices clasp on to the upper and lower teeth, pulling the mandible downward and forward. Although a number of different oral appliances to advance the mandible are available, the "best" oral appliance is unknown. For these devices to effectively treat sleep apnea, the mandible should be advanced to 50 to 75 percent of the maximal forward protrusion of the jaw. These devices may be particularly effective in patients with retrognathia and micrognathia. However, use of oral appliances is limited by the fact that they have not been shown to be effective in other cases of sleep apnea. The current trend is to consider use of this treatment modality in individuals with mild to moderate disease—that is, a respiratory disturbance index of 15 to 40 events per hour—and in patients who fail CPAP. Side effects caused by oral appliances include excessive salivation, dental misalignment, and pain in or damage to the temporomandibular joint. Data about long-term outcomes using this approach are limited.

Surgical Treatment

In general, surgical therapy for patients with obstructive sleep apnea should be reserved for those who fail medical therapy or patients with specific anatomic abnormalities. Nasal surgery can be helpful if there is a discrete nasal obstruction or a significant deviation of the nasal septum. Similarly, patients with obstructive sleep apnea who have significant tonsillar or adenoidal hypertrophy may improve with surgical removal of these tissues. In children and adolescents with enlarged tonsils and adenoids, adenotonsillectomy is very effective in treating sleep apnea.

Uvulopalatopharyngoplasty (UPPP) has been the most common surgical procedure for adult obstructive sleep apnea. UPPP warrants consideration for patients with retropalatial obstruction who fail or refuse CPAP therapy. The procedure consists of removal of the tonsils and adenoids, uvula, distal margin of the soft palate, and excessive pharyngeal tissue. The success rate in patients undergoing a UPPP appears to be partially related to the site of obstruction: patients with retropalatal obstruction having better outcomes than those with retroglossal obstruction. Many patients who undergo a UPPP may still require nasal CPAP therapy. UPPP has at least a 50 percent failure rate and has several significant complications, including oropharyngeal pain, infection, hemorrhage, nasopharyngeal reflux, and rhinolalia. UPPP is more effective for snoring than for sleep apnea—i.e., an 80 to 90 percent success rate for snoring. Polysomnography should be performed after upper airway surgery to determine if the patient's sleep-disordered breathing has been abolished.

The surgical procedures for patients with retroglossal obstruction include genioglossal, hyoid, or maxillomandibular advancement. The genioglossal and hyoid advancements are often performed in conjunction with a UPPP. The surgical treatments of choice in patients with retrognathia or micrognathia are maxillomandibular advancement or sliding genioplasty.

Although tracheostomy is almost invariably effective in treating obstructive sleep apnea, it should be considered only in patients with very severe disease that results in incapacitating hypersomnolence, malignant arrhythmias, and/or cardiac failure who have failed medical or surgical therapy

OBESITY-HYPOVENTILATION SYNDROME (PICKWICKIAN SYNDROME)

Obesity-hypoventilation syndrome (Pickwickian syndrome) is defined by obesity, hypoventilation, and daytime hypercapnia ($Pa_{CO_2} > 45$ torr). Patients with obesity-hypoventilation syndrome present with resting hypoxemia and hypercapnia, hypersomnolence, pulmonary hypertension, and chronic right heart failure. Pickwickian syndrome usually coexists with obstructive sleep apnea.

The diagnosis of obesity-hypoventilation syndrome can be confirmed by demonstrating an increase in Pa_{CO_2} greater than 10 mmHg (for diagnostic

TABLE 50-3 Diagnostic Features of Obesity-Hypoventilation Syndrome

Clinical presentation
  Daytime symptoms of hypercapnia
    Chronic fatigue
    Morning headache
  Right-sided congestive heart failure/cor pulmonale with lower extremity
  edema unresponsive to diuretics
Laboratory findings
  Hypercapnia during wakefulness ($Pa_{CO_2} > 45$ torr)
  Hypoxemia during wakefulness and sleep ($Sa_{O_2} < 90\%$)
  Greater than a 10-torr increase in Pa_{CO_2} during sleep
  Respiratory acidosis during sleep (pH < 7.3)
  Nocturnal oximetry demonstrating persistent oxyhemoglobin desaturation
  Polysomnography demonstrating concomitant obstructive sleep apnea or
  evidence of hypoventilation

features, see Table 50-3). Ideally, an arterial line should be placed to sample blood gases. But if this is not possible, arterial blood gases should be determined before sleep and upon waking in the morning.

The management of the obesity-hypoventilation syndrome requires adequate ventilatory support and treatment of coexisting medical conditions. Supplemental oxygen alone is hazardous, since it lengthens periods of apnea and exacerbates respiratory acidosis. Diuretics improve right-sided congestive heart failure.

The treatment of choice for the obesity-hypoventilation syndrome is nocturnal noninvasive ventilation administered via a nasal or oral face mask. Nocturnal noninvasive ventilation in patients with obesity-hypoventilation syndrome corrects daytime and nighttime hypoxemia and hypercapnia, ameliorates sleep fragmentation, produces respiratory muscle rest, reduces pulmonary artery pressures, and improves right ventricular function. Although either conventional volume- or pressure-cycled ventilators can be used for noninvasive ventilation in patients with the obesity-hypoventilation syndrome, volume-cycled nasal ventilation is the modality of choice in these patients. In obese patients, pressure-cycled ventilators may not provide sufficient inspiratory pressure to ensure an adequate tidal volume. Regardless of the mode of ventilation, the minute ventilation should be adjusted to maintain the P_{CO_2} in the range of 40 to 50 mmHg.

CENTRAL SLEEP APNEA

Central sleep apnea is a much less common disorder than obstructive sleep apnea and is usually associated with an underlying neurologic disorder. In central sleep apnea, repeated episodes of apnea occur during sleep in the absence of respiratory muscle effort. The pathogenesis of central sleep apnea involves transient abnormalities of central drive to the respiratory pump muscles. Patients with central sleep apnea have clinical features that range from daytime sleepiness to end-stage pulmonary hypertension and right heart failure. These patients complain of daytime sleepiness secondary to sleep fragmentation from the central apneas.

The diagnosis of central sleep apnea is made by overnight polysomnography, which demonstrates repeated episodes of apnea in the absence of motion of the chest wall and abdomen. These apneic episodes may result in hypoxia, hypercapnia, and acidemia. CPAP may not be effective for the treatment of central sleep apnea, since the airway is already patent even though it does narrow somewhat because of the loss of motor output to respiratory muscles. The treatment of choice for central sleep apnea is nocturnal nasal noninvasive ventilation, which ensures a respiratory rate that will abolish the central apneas. Pressure-cycled ventilation, with a bilevel system and a backup respiratory rate, is usually effective. Ventilatory stimulants, such as acetazolamide, are not useful for conventional central sleep apnea but may be effective in treating central apneas associated with residence at high altitude.

UPPER AIRWAY RESISTANCE SYNDROME

This syndrome is characterized by recurrent arousals secondary to increased upper airway resistance (or crescendo snoring). Repeated arousals occur due to snoring or increased upper airway resistance. The arousals may result in significant sleep fragmentation and daytime sleepiness. The upper airway resistance syndrome has been associated with systemic hypertension.

Accurate diagnosis of the upper airway resistance syndrome calls for a polysomnogram with an esophageal balloon. Since most sleep laboratories do not use esophageal balloons, a less invasive method of diagnosing the upper airway resistance syndrome is by counting arousals associated with episodes of snoring. It seems likely, although unproven, that using snoring-related arousals to diagnose the upper airway resistance syndrome underestimates the prevalence of this disorder. If the snoring-related arousal index is >5 to 10 per hour, treatment should be considered. The treatment of choice is nasal CPAP, although oral appliances and possibly upper airway surgery may be effective therapeutic interventions.

CARDIOPULMONARY DISORDERS AGGRAVATED DURING SLEEP

Sleep can exacerbate a wide variety of cardiovascular-pulmonary disorders, including asthma, chronic obstructive pulmonary disease (COPD) and other pulmonary diseases, coronary artery disease, and congestive heart failure (CHF).

Asthma

Asthma is known to worsen during sleep. Two-thirds of asthmatics develop nocturnal bronchoconstriction. These asthmatic patients have been labeled "morning dippers"; they manifest falls in FEV_1, and peak flow decreases by 50 percent during sleep. Nocturnal bronchoconstriction is most common in patients with unstable asthma or in those recovering from recent asthmatic attacks. The nocturnal asthmatic attacks are not related to a specific stage of sleep. Asthmatic patients admitted to the hospital should be expected to develop decrements in expiratory flow rates during sleep. Therefore weaning an asthmatic patient from the ventilator at night should be performed cautiously. Treatment modalities include long-acting bronchodilators given before sleep to help prevent nocturnal bronchoconstriction.

COPD AND OTHER PULMONARY DISEASES

Patients with COPD often deteriorate at night. Arterial oxyhemoglobin desaturation during sleep in patients with COPD may decrease by 10 to 35 percent. Hypoxemic episodes are especially severe during REM sleep.

Hypercapnia can also be exacerbated during sleep in patients with COPD; more severe hypercapnic episodes occur during REM sleep than during NREM sleep. Cardiac arrhythmias can pose a problem during sleep in COPD patients. Cardiac ischemia, manifest by ST-segment depression on electrocardiography, can also occur in hypoxic COPD patients. Oxygen administration reverses most of these cardiac abnormalities.

Patients with a wide variety of lung diseases—including interstitial lung disease, cystic fibrosis, restrictive lung disease, and chest wall disease (e.g., kyphoscoliosis)—develop hypoxemia during sleep. Therefore any patient with significant lung disease is at risk for the development of hypoxemia during sleep, and supplemental nocturnal oxygen should be considered.

Cardiovascular Disease—CVD/CHF

Relatively little is known about the effect of sleep on cardiovascular disease. As noted above, ischemic episodes and arrhythmias occur frequently during sleep. Nocturnal angina is common in both REM sleep and NREM sleep, although there is no predominance in a particular stage of sleep. Patients with nocturnal angina should be suspected of having obstructive sleep apnea. Patients with CHF have a high incidence of sleep-disordered breathing, including Cheyne-Stokes respiration. CPAP has been shown to be effective in relieving Cheyne-Stokes respiration in patients with CHF. Nasal CPAP and administration of supplemental O_2 may be helpful additions to the standard pharmacologic treatment of CHF.

BIBLIOGRAPHY

Davies RJ, Ali NJ, Stradling JR: Neck circumference and other clinical features in the diagnosis of the obstructive sleep apnea syndrome. *Thorax* 47:101–105, 1992.

Guilleminault C, Stoohs R, Clerk A, et al: A cause of excessive daytime sleepiness. The upper airway resistance syndrome. *Chest* 104:781–787, 1993.

Kribbs NB, Pack AI, Kline LR, et al: Objective measurement of patterns of nasal CPAP use by patients with obstructive sleep apnea. *Am Rev Respir Dis* 147:887–895, 1993.

Naughton MT, Liu PP, Bernard DC, et al: Treatment of congestive heart failure and Cheyne-Stokes respiration during sleep by continuous positive airway pressure. *Am J Respir Crit Care Med* 151:92–97, 1995.

Nieto FJ, Young TB, Lind BK, et al: Association of sleep-disordered breathing, sleep apnea, and hypertension in a large community-based study. *JAMA* 283:1829–1836.

Schellenberg J, Maislin G, Schwab RJ: Physical findings and the risk for obstructive sleep apnea: The importance of soft tissue structures. *Am J Respir Crit Care Med* 162:740–748, 2000.

Schwab RJ, Gupta KB, Gefter WB, et al: Upper airway soft tissue anatomy in normal subjects and patients with sleep-disordered breathing. Significance of the lateral pharyngeal walls. *Am J Respir Crit Care Med* 152:1673–1689, 1995.

Sher AE, Schechtman KB, Picirillo J: The efficacy of surgical modifications of the upper airway in adults with obstructive sleep apnea syndrome. *Sleep* 19:156–177, 1996.

Sleep apnea, sleepiness and driving risk. American Thoracic Society. *Am J Respir Crit Care Med* 150:1463–1473, 1994.

Strobel RJ, Rosen RC: Obesity and weight loss in obstructive sleep apnea: A critical review. *Sleep* 19:104–115, 1996.

Young T, Palta M, Dempsey J, et al: The occurrence of sleep-disordered breathing among middle-aged adults. *N Engl J Med* 328:1230–1235, 1993.

Part Twelve | **SURGICAL ASPECTS OF PULMONARY MEDICINE**

51 | Surgical Aspects of Pulmonary Medicine*

Larry R. Kaiser

Estimates of the overall surgical mortality for pulmonary resection range in large series from 2 to 4 percent. The estimated mortality increases with the size of the resection—from less than 1 percent for a wedge resection, to 2 to 3 percent for a lobectomy, and to 6 to 8 percent for a pneumonectomy.

As may be expected from the estimated surgical mortality for lung resection, the morbidity associated with these operations is also high: complications are estimated to occur in 36 to 75 percent of patients undergoing pneumonectomy and 41 to 50 percent after lobectomy. The major causes of complications and death after pulmonary procedures include respiratory failure and pneumonia, myocardial infarction and arrhythmias, bronchopleural fistula and empyema, and pulmonary embolus.

PREOPERATIVE ASSESSMENT AND OPTIMIZATION

Lung Function

Unfortunately, preoperative tests presage only a small percentage of postoperative complications, and most complications appear to be random events visited on the patient and surgeon. The surgeon's impression of surgical risk, a skill honed over time, remains the most useful tool for selecting patients for resectional surgery.

Patients with preoperative arterial hypercapnia are apt to have pulmonary hypertension and are poor candidates for pneumonectomy, but they may be able to tolerate a lobectomy. Pulmonary function tests, in particular the FEV_1, in combination with lobar perfusion scans, allow a reasonable estimate of postresectional FEV_1 to within approximately 100 mL. A postresectional FEV_1 less than 40 percent of predicted or less than 800 mL is cause for concern but does not necessarily contraindicate resection. A study of the $D_{L_{CO}}$ in 165 patients who underwent lung resection identified it as the most important indicator of postoperative pulmonary complications or death. Another study focused on the maximal oxygen consumption ($\dot{V}_{O_2max}$): a $\dot{V}_{O_2max}$ of 20 mL/kg/min was associated with fewest complications, whereas a $\dot{V}_{O_2max}$ under 15 mL/kg/min was associated with 75 percent of the postoperative morbidity.

Optimization of Preoperative Pulmonary Function

Optimization of pulmonary function begins with smoking cessation. Even a short period of abstinence from cigarettes can improve the effectiveness of

*Edited from Chap. 104, "Perioperative Care of the Patient Undergoing Lung Resection," by Downey RJ, and Chap. 116, "Extrapulmonary Syndromes Associated with Lung Tumors," by Johnson BE, Chute JP. In: *Fishman's Pulmonary Diseases and Disorders,* 3d. ed., edited by Fishman AP, Elias JA, Fishman JA, Grippi MA, Kaiser LR, Senior RM. New York, McGraw-Hill, 1998, pp 1649–1660, 1841–1850. For fuller discussion of topics dealt with in this chapter, the reader is referred to the original text, as noted above.

mucociliary transport. Heavy smokers also maintain levels of carboxyhemoglobin that interfere with oxygen transport and delivery to peripheral tissues. However, the optimal time after smoking cessation for repair of the airway to be undertaken is unclear. Studies of patients undergoing abdominal surgery and coronary artery bypass surgery suggest that 8 weeks of abstinence are necessary to achieve a significant decrease in pulmonary complications.

In patients with evidence of reversible airway obstruction on pulmonary function tests or with episodes of symptoms suggestive of airflow obstruction, nebulized albuterol appears to be of benefit. Mucostasis, if present, may warrant the addition of mucolytics such as N-acetylcysteine, with due regard to the possible side effect of bronchoconstriction. Methylxanthines are added only for refractory cases. Similarly, although the condition of patients with reversible airflow obstruction generally improves with steroids, prednisone or other corticosteroids should be added reluctantly because of their effects on wound healing and rate of infection. If steroids are deemed necessary, the dosage in the postoperative period should be as low as possible. Patients who produce purulent sputum should be treated with oral antibiotics directed at the organism identified.

PERIOPERATIVE FACTORS REDUCING LUNG FUNCTION

Bed Rest and Respiratory Function

In normal adults, mismatches between alveolar ventilation and blood flow are small. In bedridden postoperative patients, however, ventilation and perfusion are badly matched.

Placing a normal patient in a recumbent position leads to changes in all lung volumes except the tidal volume. In a normal person, a change from upright to supine position decreases the vital capacity by 2 percent, total lung capacity by 7 percent, closing volume by 10 percent, residual volume by 19 percent, expiratory reserve volume by 46 percent, and functional residual capacity (FRC) by 30 percent. The decrements in volume that accompany changes to other than the supine position are small. It is interesting that these changes might be *less* in patients with chronic pulmonary disease. Finally, although arterial oxygen saturation decreased significantly in supine normal subjects, it did not do so in patients with significant airflow obstruction.

Bed Rest and Cardiac Function

Upon standing, approximately 500 mL of blood shift from the upper to the lower body. Upon assumption of the supine position, central venous return increases, resulting in a decrease in heart rate, peripheral vasodilatation, increased renal blood flow, and diuresis. Within an average of 24 h, the diuresis causes a 5 percent decrease in plasma volume, which continues to fall by 10 percent in 6 days and 20 percent in 14 days.

Prolonged recumbency also blunts cardiac responsiveness to rapid changes in posture. Bed rest increases the resting heart rate by 4 to 15 beats a minute; after bed rest, the increase in heart rate during exercise is more pronounced. For example, normal volunteers experienced an increase in heart rate to approximately 129 beats a minute during submaximal exercise; after bed rest, the same exercise drove the heart rate to approximately 165 beats a minute.

Alterations in Lung Function Secondary to Surgery

Thoracotomy alone decreases chest wall compliance to about half of preoperative levels and significantly increases work of breathing. As a result, vital capacity and oxygen saturation fall significantly in the first few postoperative days. Pain, among other factors, leads to diminished cough and decreased respiratory effort.

ROUTINE POSTOPERATIVE CARE OF THE PATIENT UNDERGOING LUNG RESECTION

Extubation and Postoperative Supplemental Oxygen

Essentially every patient can be extubated at the completion of a thoracotomy and pulmonary resection. Reintubation in the immediate postoperative period is rare.

Supplemental oxygen is supplied in the postoperative period if the patient's arterial oxygen saturation, measured by pulse oximetry, is less than 92 percent, either at rest or during exercise. The routine administration of increased concentrations of oxygen may be counterproductive, since each appliance attached to the patient hinders incrementally the patient's mobility.

Pain Control

The patient with reduced pulmonary reserve can ill afford the additional burden of a painful chest wall, which limits ambulation and cough. Following thoracotomy, all patients should receive either epidural administration of a local anesthetic or a narcotic or patient-controlled intravenous analgesia using either morphine or meperidine (Demerol). The complications associated with epidural opiates are numerous and include pruritus, ileus, urinary retention, and respiratory depression. Epidural analgesia does improve pulmonary function in the postthoracotomy patient and, despite concerns about complications, should not be withheld from the patient in whom pulmonary function is markedly impaired. Most of patients appear to tolerate postthoracotomy pain well with the use of patient-controlled anesthesia alone, particularly if a short course of oral ketorolac is used as an adjunct. In the late postoperative period, oral medications, such as oxycodone with acetaminophen (Percocet), are usually sufficient.

Antibiotics

Wound infection following thoracotomy is rare. Currently, it is recommended that a broad-spectrum antibiotic, such as cefazolin, be administered within 1 h of the skin incision, and continued for 24 to 48 h. Subsequent antibiotic administration should be based on clinical factors such as fever, radiographic infiltrates, leukocytosis, and sputum Gram's stain and culture results. There is no need to provide antibiotic coverage simply because a chest tube is in place.

Fluids, Electrolytes, and Oral Intake

A routine pulmonary resection is not associated with large fluid losses intraoperatively or sequestration of volume in the third space postoperatively. Administration of intravenous fluids consisting of 5% dextrose and 0.45% normal saline at 50 to 75 mL/h until the patient begins to take oral fluids is usually adequate to maintain intravascular fluid volume. Oral intake should be resumed as soon as the patient is able to take fluids by mouth. Blood transfusion is not necessary unless the hematocrit is less than 24 percent or if bleeding should continue. Transfusion of 250 mL of packed red blood cells increases the intravascular volume by 750 to 1000 mL because of the movement of extravascular volume into the intravascular space due to plasma osmotic forces. The increase in intravascular volume may be more dangerous than a low hematocrit. Furthermore, the intraoperative administration of blood is probably immunosuppressive and may be associated with a decrease in frequency of 5-year disease-free intervals.

Chest Tube Management

Chest tube placement is routine after thoracotomy to enable drainage of blood, serum, and air from the pleural space. Chest tubes are connected to suction for the first night after surgery and then to water seal. Chest radiographs are performed to ensure that effective removal of air and fluid is being achieved, but it is not necessary to repeat chest radiographs on a daily basis only for clinical indications. If increased air in the pleural space is seen after a tube has been connected to water seal, suction drainage should be reestablished to reexpand the lung, since air leaks will cease sooner when the lung is fully expanded and there is total pleural apposition.

Postpneumonectomy space drainage is managed differently from postlobectomy drainage. After pneumonectomy, the position of the mediastinum is a major concern. Shift of the mediastinal structures either into the pneumonectomy cavity or toward the residual lung can lead to either hemodynamic or respiratory compromise. To allow "balancing" of the mediastinum after a pneumonectomy, most surgeons leave a single chest tube in the pleural cavity, usually connected to a "balanced" drainage system. Suction should never be applied to a tube in a postpneumonectomy space. The tube can be removed in the recovery room or on the nursing unit once it is clear that the patient is not bleeding.

For resections other than pneumonectomy, chest tubes are removed when there is no air leak and fluid output has decreased to less than 300 mL a day.

Excessive drainage that persists for several days after surgery suggests the possibility of injury to the thoracic duct. When such an injury has occurred, the drainage initially is clear, as the patient is either not taking anything by mouth or is only taking clear liquids. As the patient resumes a normal diet, however, the volume increases and the character of the liquid changes from serosanguineous to creamy. Often, the diagnosis is apparent from only an examination of the pleural drainage containers. Following chemical confirmation that the fluid is chyle (triglyceride level >150), initial management is to deny the patient food by mouth and to provide total parenteral nutrition. If the leak is coming from a small branch of the duct and the drainage decreases in response to this management, the patient should receive a high-fat meal before the chest tube is removed in order to confirm that the leak has closed. If drainage remains greater than 500 mL a day for more than several days, ligation of the thoracic duct is indicated.

COMPLICATIONS AFTER LUNG RESECTION

Atelectasis and Pneumonia

Atelectasis, with or without superimposed pneumonia, is the most common postoperative complication following thoracic surgery. As previously mentioned, risk factors for the development of atelectasis include advanced age, obesity, and the continued use of tobacco.

Routine measures directed toward the minimization of postoperative atelectasis should be initiated early in the preoperative period and include education, smoking cessation, and the use of incentive spirometry. Postoperatively, the most important measures are deep-breathing techniques, incentive spirometry, early ambulation, and bronchoscopy as needed to relieve retention of secretions.

The mainstays in the prevention of atelectasis are deep inspiratory respiratory maneuvers performed either with or without an incentive spirometer. Carefully supervised programs of these maneuvers have been shown to reduce the incidence of atelectasis after laparotomy.

Chest physical therapy, although widely practiced, is of unclear benefit, is often poorly administered, and imposes a considerable physiologic load on the already compromised patient. Its use should be reserved for the patient with obstructive atelectasis secondary to mucous impaction in a major airway. Chest physical therapy increases oxygen consumption and carbon dioxide production to approximately 40 percent above resting values. For many patients with major obstruction of the airway, bronchoscopy is a preferred alternative. The use of a minitracheostomy inserted by a percutaneous technique via the cricothyroid membrane allows for placement of a suction cannula and is indicated for patients with retained secretions.

Air Leaks and Subcutaneous Emphysema

Division of the lung parenchyma usually results in transient leakage of air. Usually, these leaks seal within a few days after surgery, either as the result of adherence of the lung to the parietal pleura or by deposition of proteinaceous fluid on the lung surface. Occasionally, air leaks persist. Different clinics define a "prolonged leak" differently but usually in terms of 7 to 10 days. It is important that the chest tube drainage system be examined daily to ensure that it is an actual air leak and not a loose connection that allows air to enter the system.

Large air leaks in the immediate postoperative period are most worrisome as a possible sign of inadequate closure or disruption of a bronchus. Bronchoscopy should be done urgently to clarify whether the bronchial stump is indeed intact. If disruption is found, surgical reexploration with closure of the stump, reinforcement with autologous material, and drainage of the pleural cavity should be performed in order to minimize the chances of ongoing pleural infection.

Occasionally, massive subcutaneous emphysema may occur if either the loss of air from the lung into the pleural cavity exceeds the drainage capacities of the chest tube or the tube is positioned away from the site of the air leak. Chest tubes should be examined for patency. If all methods fail to reestablish patency of a chest tube, the tube should be removed and a new one inserted. Massive subcutaneous emphysema may be decompressed with bilateral infraclavicular incisions into the subcutaneous tissue.

Supraventricular Tachycardias

Recent studies suggest that supraventricular tachycardias occur in 17 to 20 percent of all patients undergoing lobectomy or pneumonectomy. The development of supraventricular arrhythmias after pneumonectomy is a marker for perioperative morbidity and mortality. The cause of the dysrhythmias is almost certainly multifactorial; suggested factors include intrapericardial resection, hypoxemia, hyperadrenergic tone, and atrial distention. A full discussion of the management of atrial arrhythmias in the postoperative period is beyond the scope of this chapter. Currently, the preferred drug is amiodarone, but procainamide may also be used.

Postpneumonectomy Pulmonary Edema

Postpneumonectomy pulmonary edema is a rare but often lethal complication of pneumonectomy. The removal of one lung is well tolerated if the pulmonary vasculature is normal; however, if preexisting pulmonary vascular disease is present, the reduced pulmonary vascular bed may be unable to accommodate the cardiac output without an inordinate increase in pulmonary arterial pressure. Overzealous administration of fluid may contribute to the formation of edema in the remaining lung.

The clinical presentation of postpneumonectomy pulmonary edema is that of a relatively uneventful initial 24- to 48-h postoperative period, followed by an increasing oxygen requirement usually culminating in increased work of breathing and ultimately requiring reintubation and mechanical ventilation. The pulmonary edema progresses despite aggressive efforts to effect a diuresis and other supportive measures. The development of this complication carries at least a 50 percent mortality. Current therapy is directed at limiting the administration of fluids perioperatively and providing supportive measures if the complication should arise.

Empyema/Bronchopleural Fistulas

Empyema is a rare complication after pulmonary resection and usually can be managed with continued pleural drainage. If empyema occurs later in the postoperative period (3 to more than 6 weeks), surgical intervention may be required either to drain a fixed space or to decorticate the lung in order to allow it to fill the pleural space. Disruption of a bronchial closure after lung resection occurs in less than 5 percent of patients. Although dehiscence of a lobar bronchus occurs occasionally after lobectomy, it rarely presents a challenge in management. Usually, chest tube drainage and antibiotics suffice; rarely is further surgical intervention required, but the surgeon should always be involved in the management of these patients.

Infection in a postpneumonectomy space presents far greater challenges in management. Infections may occur with or without a bronchopleural fistula. The typical patient with an infected pneumonectomy space usually returns for the first postoperative visit complaining of poor appetite, fatigue, low-grade fevers, and continued weight loss. If there is no communication with the bronchus, the operated hemithorax may be filled as expected when seen on the chest radiograph. If a space infection is suspected the fluid in the space should be sampled under sterile conditions and sent for Gram's stain and culture. The patient with a bronchial stump dehiscence may complain of production of watery brown sputum, and the chest radiograph will demonstrate a decrease in the fluid level as compared with the level seen on the radiograph at the time of discharge from the hospital. Both situations require drainage of the pneumonectomy space by means of a chest tube initially, followed by an open-window thoracostomy that entails resection of segments of rib in the most dependent area of the space and sewing of the skin edges to the thickened pleural edges. The window must be large and correctly positioned in the most dependent portion of the space in order to effect unobstructed drainage.

Rarely is it necessary or advisable to attempt to close a disrupted bronchial stump unless a complication, indicating a technical problem, occurs in the early postoperative period (within the first 7 days). With an early stump breakdown, operation is indicated to reclose the bronchus and to buttress the closure with a muscle flap. Most bronchial stump disruptions occur late, as described above, and the leak itself is a secondary problem best dealt with by an open drainage procedure. Most of the bronchial leaks are small and can be assessed by bronchoscopy performed at the time of the open-window thoracostomy. These leaks usually close after the establishment of effective drainage of the infected space. Occasionally, complete bronchial stump dehiscence may occur, resulting in the loss of a considerable amount of expired air, so that speech is difficult.

Once the open-window thoracostomy is created, most patients begin to gain weight and regain strength. Over time, the open window begins to close as the space contracts. There is no hurry to close an open-window thoracostomy, and many patients adjust well to its presence. Minimal care is required; a dry dressing, changed once or twice daily, is worn over the opening. The wound is not packed. After several months, depending on the patient's overall status, the window may be closed, usually by the transposition of a muscle flap to obliterate the remaining space. Either the latissimus dorsi or serratus anterior muscle or both may be used, depending on which was divided at the initial thoracotomy. The pectoralis major muscle may also be used.

Postpneumonectomy Syndrome

Postpneumonectomy syndrome is a rare complication, manifest by cough and dyspnea on exertion, that usually follows right pneumonectomy. It is due to progressive mediastinal shift with compression of the left main-stem bronchus by the vertebral column. The underlying cause of this complication of pneumonectomy is herniation of the contralateral lung into the vacant pleural space, causing compression of the main-stem bronchus between the aorta, the pulmonary artery, or the vertebral column. Repair is directed toward repositioning and stabilizing the mediastinum in the midline by a combined procedure of cardiopexy and placement of pliable, variable-volume tissue expanders into the empty pleural space.

Pulmonary Torsion

The increased mobility of the remaining lobe or lobes following pulmonary resection may, on rare occasions, lead to torsion of all or part of the residual lung, causing venous outflow obstruction and possibly pulmonary gangrene. The middle lobe with complete fissures is at highest risk, although any portion of residual lung can be affected. In order to reduce the risk of middle-lobe torsion, the middle lobe is secured to the remaining lobe following right upper or lower lobectomy.

Pulmonary torsion may be suggested by the radiographic finding of consolidated lung in association with fever, leukocytosis, and purulent, occasionally bloody sputum. The treatment is immediate surgical exploration with derotation of the affected lung, followed by fixation to surrounding structures. If the lung is not viable, lobectomy or completion pneumonectomy may be required.

Recurrent Laryngeal Nerve Injury

The left recurrent laryngeal nerve is at greater risk than the right because of the course of the left vagus nerve across the aortic arch and the location of the left recurrent nerve in the aortopulmonary window adjacent to the ligamentum arteriosum, where it "recurs." If either nerve is affected, unilateral vocal cord dysfunction results in hoarseness, increased risk of aspiration, and marked decrease in the effectiveness of cough and in the ability to clear secretions. For the patient with limited pulmonary reserve who has undergone surgery, with its attendant postoperative transient decrease in pulmonary function, vocal cord paralysis can be a devastating problem and may mean the difference between recovery and respiratory failure. The problem of aspiration because of inability to protect the airway is particularly serious.

Surgical correction of unilateral vocal cord paralysis is becoming increasingly popular. Techniques include injection of Gelfoam for temporary medialization, Teflon for permanent medialization, or surgical placement of a hand-crafted silicone elastomer implant. The success rate, as measured by symptomatic improvement in dysphonia and aspiration as well as reduced incidence of pneumonia exceeds 90 percent.

Wound Disruption

Disruption of a posterolateral thoracotomy wound is a distinctly uncommon event, but separation of the rib closure, though extremely rare, may cause problems. Cough becomes ineffective, as expired air is forced out not through the vocal cords but into the extrapleural space as the lung herniates. Effective ventilation may also be impaired to the point of hypoxia and hypercarbia. Chest wall dehiscence in the early postoperative period requires reexploration, debridement, and reclosure of the wound.

BIBLIOGRAPHY

Bolton JW, Weiman DS: Physiology of lung resection. *Clin Chest Med* 14:293–303, 1993.

Deslauriers J, Ginsberg RJ, Dubois P, et al: Current operative mortality associated with elective surgical resection for lung cancer. *Can J Surg* 32:335–339, 1989.

Pairolero PC, Arnold PG, Trastek VF, et al: Postpneumonectomy empyema: The role of intrathoracic muscle transposition. *J Thorac Cardiovasc Surg* 99:958–968, 1990.

52 | Thoracic Trauma*

Larry R. Kaiser

Chest trauma can be classified as either blunt or penetrating. *Blunt injury* most commonly results from motor vehicle accidents but may also result from falls or beatings. *Penetrating injuries* are the result of stab or gunshot wounds and occasionally of impalement.

The approach to diagnosis and treatment of injuries to the chest depends greatly on the mechanism of injury, which influences the incidence and type of associated injuries. Most or all gunshot wounds of the chest require thoracotomy for management, whereas blunt injury usually is managed non-operatively. The possibility of associated injuries, especially to the abdomen, must also be kept in mind and thoroughly investigated prior to initiating a treatment plan.

Physicians managing patients with chest injuries must be prepared to make quick but accurate judgments and decisions and to act on them. With the development of trauma systems in most cities, more critically injured patients are surviving long enough to make it to the hospital, and the time spent prior to taking the patient to the operating room may make the difference between survival and mortality. The thoracic surgeon should be involved as soon as the patient arrives in the emergency room, although many chest injuries will not require operation.

INITIAL MANAGEMENT

Ensuring Airway Patency and Breathing

The initial goal in the resuscitation of any patient sustaining a traumatic injury is to establish adequate oxygenation and ventilation. Of primary importance is the establishment of a patent airway. Foreign objects as well as intrinsic laryngeal tissue, as in laryngeal fracture, can also obstruct the airway. As initial management, an oropharyngeal or nasopharyngeal airway can be inserted to maintain patency of the airway. Endotracheal intubation may be performed for apnea, to protect the airway from blood or secretions, or for hyperventilation in cases of severe head trauma. In cases of severe maxillofacial injury, a tracheostomy may need to be performed.

Once patency of the airway has been established, it must be verified that breathing is adequate. In the intubated patient, a carbon dioxide monitor can be connected to the endotracheal tube in order to establish that gas exchange is adequate and that the tube is properly situated. Mechanical ventilation may be instituted as necessary.

---

*Edited from Chap. 105, "Thoracic Trauma," by Kaiser LR, DiPierro FW. In: *Fishman's Pulmonary Diseases and Disorders,* 3d ed., edited by Fishman AP, Elias JA, Fishman JA, Grippi MA, Kaiser LR, Senior RM. New York, McGraw-Hill, 1998, pp 1661–1670. For fuller discussion of topics dealt with in this chapter, the reader is referred to the original text, as noted above.

Emergency Department Interventions

Once adequate oxygenation and ventilation have been established, the primary resuscitation effort must rule out other life-threatening chest injuries. Simple, open, and tension pneumothoraces, hemothoraces, and pericardial tamponade are injuries that require immediate attention.

Simple Pneumothorax

Simple pneumothorax is created when a tear in the pleura allows entry of air into the pleural space with resultant loss of negativity in intrathoracic pressure. If an injury to the lung parenchyma produces an air leak, the air accumulates in the pleural space, with each breath markedly increasing intrathoracic pressure, thereby shifting the mediastinum toward the opposite hemithorax. This so-called tension pneumothorax is immediately life-threatening because of the limitation of vena caval blood flow, which results in hypotension, tachycardia, and cardiac arrest.

Treatment of simple pneumothorax requires insertion of a chest tube into the pleural space under sterile conditions, usually through the fifth or sixth intercostal space in the anterior axillary line, and connection of the tube to suction.

Tension Pneumothorax

Especially following penetrating trauma, a high index of suspicion for tension pneumothorax should be maintained while remembering that insertion of a large-bore needle into the second intercostal space may result in injury to the lung if the diagnosis is incorrect.

Clinical findings that support the diagnosis of tension pneumothorax include hypotension, absent breath sounds on the involved side with tympany on percussion, tracheal deviation toward the opposite side, and difficulty in mechanically ventilating the patient because of high airway pressures. Once the diagnosis of tension pneumothorax is suspected, treatment should be initiated immediately without waiting for chest radiograph confirmation. A rush of air exiting via the needle confirms the diagnosis as treatment is initiated. Tube thoracostomy should be performed for definitive management. It should always be kept in mind that not every pneumothorax that results from trauma is a tension pneumothorax.

Pneumothorax and Open Chest Wound

When a pneumothorax is associated with an open chest wound after penetrating trauma, initial management is designed to restore a seal to the thoracic cavity. This is accomplished by applying a sterile occlusive dressing to the wound immediately followed by placement of a chest tube. The dressing allows some air to escape from the pleural space but does not allow air from the outside to enter.

Hemothorax

Both blunt and penetrating injuries of the chest may be associated with hemothorax, but this finding is far more common following penetrating trauma. Absence of breath sounds over the injured hemithorax and dullness to percussion are the characteristic physical findings. When the quantity of blood in the chest is small, the chest radiograph, which is usually taken as an anteroposterior film while the patient is supine, may show only haziness on the involved side.

Hemothoraxy is managed by insertion of a large-bore (36 Fr or greater) chest tube and blood volume replacement if necessary. Additional therapeutic maneuvers are based on the documentation of continued blood loss. Depending upon the extent of parenchymal injury, bleeding may have ceased by the time the chest tube is inserted. Thus, after the accumulated blood has drained, little if any further drainage will occur. If blood continues to drain and the patient is hypotensive and tachycardic in spite of volume replacement, exploration of the chest is indicated. An intraabdominal injury should be ruled out; if suspected, the appropriate procedures must be initiated. Even in the hemodynamically stable patient, if blood continues to drain from the chest tube at a rate of greater than 200 mL/h for 2 or 3 h, the patient should be surgically explored. Following chest tube insertion, if the decision is made to observe the patient, a chest radiograph should be repeated within several hours of the insertion to ensure that blood is not accumulating in the chest.

Cardiac Injury

Penetrating injury to the chest may involve not only the pulmonary parenchyma but also, not infrequently, the heart. Many patients with these injuries live long enough to make it to the hospital despite evidence of cardiac tamponade, which can be managed temporarily by massive replacement of the blood volume. Cardiac tamponade results when the intrapericardial pressure becomes high enough to impede the low-pressure venous return to the heart, resulting in circulatory collapse. Aspiration of as little as 10 to 20 mL of blood from the pericardial space often relieves intrapericardial pressure sufficiently to restore adequate circulation until the patient can be transported to the operating room for definitive repair of the inciting injury to the myocardium, usually the right atrium or ventricle. On rare occasion, blunt chest injury may cause cardiac tamponade. However, although myocardial rupture secondary to blunt trauma is usually fatal, an occasional patient with rupture of the atrium will survive to reach the emergency department (ED).

Emergency Department Thoracotomy

Occasionally, a patient with a penetrating injury to the chest who arrives at the ED loses vital signs soon after arrival. A thoracotomy performed in the ED allows immediate control of an exsanguinating thoracic injury and enables open cardiac massage while the patient is being transported to the operating room. The decision to perform an ED thoracotomy is a difficult one and requires consideration of the time required to transport the patient to the operating room in the particular hospital. Indications for ED thoracotomy vary from institution to institution.

The survival rates for patients undergoing emergency center thoracotomy is less than 10 percent.

BLUNT THORACIC TRAUMA

Tracheobronchial Injuries

Tracheal disruption may follow blunt injury to the neck and is usually identified by the presence of subcutaneous emphysema. The more common injury to the tracheobronchial tree that results from blunt trauma is disruption of a main-stem bronchus, usually resulting from sudden deceleration either as a result of a motor vehicle accident or fall. Since the left main-stem bronchus and carina are tethered by the aortic arch, sudden deceleration of this fixed structure may result in a tear or total disruption of either the right or left main bronchus. Blunt injuries causing tracheobronchial disruption are often associated with simultaneous injuries to adjacent structures, including the great vessels (especially the descending thoracic aorta), esophagus, manubrium, mandible, and cervical spine. Usually such coincident injuries are fatal. Those patients with a tracheobronchial injury who do survive long enough to reach the hospital usually have only the isolated injury, implying that individuals with other injuries have already died in the field. Findings associated with tracheobronchial injuries in addition to subcutaneous emphysema include hemoptysis, respiratory distress, change in voice, pneumothorax, or hemothorax. Pneumothorax is present only if the airway rupture communicates with the pleural space, a circumstance that does not always occur because of the dense, fibroconnective tissue around the carina and mainstem bronchi. In fact, more commonly, the only finding, even in the presence of complete bronchial disruption, is the presence of deep cervical or mediastinal air that is appreciated only on the chest radiograph. As noted above, pneumothorax may follow bronchial disruption, but the evidence of an airway injury is usually not apparent until after a chest tube is placed. When suction is applied to the chest tube, the patient may become significantly more dyspneic, a situation relieved only by discontinuing the suction. Also, as a consequence of the large air leak, the lung expands incompletely despite increasing suction. Although the combination of these findings almost ensures the diagnosis, bronchoscopy should always be done even if suspicion is low that the airway is injured. Bronchoscopy clearly delineates the injury and confirms the location—information crucial for planning the operative approach.

In patients with suspected injury to the cervical or mediastinal trachea, intubation of the trachea beyond the injury is performed under direct vision under bronchoscopic guidance. If airway injury is not suspected, blind endotracheal intubation may suffice but can result in further problems. Tracheostomy should be avoided if at all possible. In patients with unilateral bronchial injury, intubation of the opposite main bronchus is desirable. Most tracheobronchial ruptures occur within 2.5 cm of the carina, and the trachea or bronchi may be completely disrupted.

The principles of managing airway rupture include debridement of devitalized tissue and primary repair for tracheobronchial injuries. The bronchus is either repaired or reanastomosed with sutures so as to be airtight. Usually the airway is managed just as it is in elective carinal or main bronchial sleeve resections, scrupulously avoiding the use of extracorporeal oxygenation and systemic heparinization.

Pulmonary Contusion

Pulmonary contusion occurs during blunt thoracic trauma as the force of impact is transferred through the chest wall to the lung parenchyma. The anatomic manifestation of contusion is disruption of alveolar-capillary interfaces and resultant collection of blood and protein in the interstitium and alveoli. Both the physiologic derangements and the presentation of patients with this type of injury are variable and range from asymptomatic to severe hypoxia and the need for mechanical ventilation. In addition to associated injuries, preexisting medical conditions greatly influence the course of patients with pulmonary contusions. Patients with chronic obstructive pulmonary disease, heart failure, or renal failure are predisposed to shunting in the involved segment of lung parenchyma and should be mechanically ventilated at the first suggestion of systemic hypoxemia. Similarly, the degree of pulmonary vascular reactivity influences the severity of injury from pulmonary contusion and the subsequent clinical course. Pulmonary vasoconstriction occurs after pulmonary contusion, apparently serving to reduce that intrapulmonary shunt created by perfusing-injured, poorly ventilated parenchyma. Patients unable to vasoconstrict adequately experienced larger shunt fractions than do those with more reactive pulmonary vasoconstriction.

Pulmonary laceration often complicates pulmonary contusion. In the transfer of energy to the chest wall during blunt trauma, shear forces are often generated that are capable of tearing the lung. Although most lacerations resolve spontaneously, elastic recoil of the lung can extend the laceration and form a cavity or a pulmonary pseudocyst. Potential complications of these cysts include infection, abscess formation, hemoptysis, air leak, adult respiratory distress syndrome (ARDS), and death.

The findings on chest radiograph in pulmonary contusion range from small nodular patchy infiltrates to frank consolidation involving a significant portion of the pulmonary parenchyma. These findings become evident within a few hours of injury in the classic presentation of pulmonary contusion. The usefulness of the chest radiograph in the management of contused lung is limited by the time lag between the appearance of abnormalities in gas exchange and the appearance of the injury on chest radiograph. Chest computed tomography (CT) scans define the extent of injury more accurately than do chest radiographs and can allow rapid classification and quantification of pulmonary parenchymal damage.

The management of pulmonary contusion consists mainly of adequate analgesia and pulmonary toilet along with supplemental oxygen as needed. Endotracheal intubation and mechanical ventilation may be required, depending on the extent of the contusion and the presence of associated injuries.

Rib Fracture

The designation *simple rib fracture* usually refers to a nondisplaced fracture of a rib without injury to the lung or pleura. The most common mechanism for simple rib fractures is direct impact such as occurs in a fall or in a motor vehicle accident. Clinically, simple rib fractures may present with manifestations ranging from pain isolated to the involved rib to pneumonia secondary to splinting and hypoventilation caused by the pain. Point tenderness is present over the fracture site and a step-off may be palpated at the point where the fractured ends overlap. In patients with underlying lung disease, the anteroposterior chest radiograph is most useful in establishing the absence of associated injuries, such as pulmonary contusion and pneumothorax.

The management of rib fractures may sometimes be dictated in part by which ribs and how many are injured. Fracture of the first or second ribs requires significant force and can be associated with major vascular or nerve injury as a result of the proximity of these ribs to the subclavian vessels and the brachial plexus. Although fractures of these two ribs are not necessarily an indication for an arteriogram, certain associated injuries do require angiographic study. Abnormalities in pulse or in the neurologic examination of the upper extremities or a hematoma at the base of the neck should prompt an arteriogram. Other indications include palpable displacement of the first rib and a widened mediastinum on the chest radiograph. Fracture of the lower ribs may be associated with injury to the liver or spleen.

Regardless of etiology, all rib fractures caused by trauma require repeated chest radiographic examinations to screen for radiographic evidence of pulmonary contusion or other complication such as hemothorax. Pulmonary complications of rib fractures can result from pain and splinting and include retained secretions, atelectasis, ventilatory failure in patients with limited pulmonary reserve, and empyema.

The cornerstone of the management of rib fractures is the management of secretions. This can only be accomplished by adequate analgesia. Options for analgesia with rib fractures include narcotics, intercostal nerve blocks, and occasionally epidural infusion of narcotic.

Flail Chest

Flail chest is an even better indicator of extensive injury. It occurs when a section of the chest wall becomes unstable because of multiple rib fractures. This segment moves paradoxically with respiration, causing respiratory embarrassment. There has been a continuing debate regarding whether the segmental, paradoxical chest wall motion or the underlying lung contusion is responsible for the ventilatory abnormalities seen in these patients. The force of the injury required to cause a flail segment causes a significant contusion, and it is likely that the contused lung contributes most significantly to the derangement in gas exchange.

Because of the evolving views concerning the pathophysiologic mechanism, the treatment of flail chest has changed dramatically over the years. The early approach reflected the belief that the chest wall deformity was responsible for the ventilatory compromise and consisted of external stabilization of the chest wall with sandbags. Operations were also performed for internal fixation of the flail segment. Subsequently, internal pneumatic stabilization with positive-pressure ventilation was used in a further effort to prevent the paradoxical chest wall motion produced by spontaneous respiration.

In time, more attention was directed toward the underlying pulmonary contusion as the significant pathophysiologic mechanism. Current treatment for flail chest avoids mechanical ventilation until mandated by standard criteria. There is no physiologic reason to institute positive-pressure ventilation solely to prevent paradoxical chest wall motion. Management is directed toward the pulmonary contusion and control of pain. Continuous epidural analgesia has proven to be an excellent adjunct in the overall management of these patients, since the relief of pain lessens splinting, improves chest wall mechanics, and decreases the risk of atelectasis and pneumonia. Aggressive pulmonary toilet and secretion management are also important in the overall management of these patients.

If a segment of the chest wall is completely disrupted, operative fixation may provide a necessary adjunct. In this injury, the bellows mechanism of the chest is severely disordered by the major skeletal deformity consisting of complete separation of the ribs from each other, with maintenance only of the integrity of the overlying skin. In this injury, the flail is severe, and operative repair with wire stabilization of the flail segment and reconstruction of the chest wall is often necessary for restoration of the bellows.

Sternal Fracture

Sternal fracture most commonly occurs during motor vehicle accidents in which there is direct impact of the anterior chest on the steering wheel. Sternal fractures also are occasionally associated with single or multiple costochondral dislocations. The association of these two injuries can lead to flail chest with paradoxical motion of the sternum during spontaneous respiration. Other injuries associated with sternal fracture include flexion injuries of the vertebral column, tracheobronchial rupture, aortic disruption, and myocardial contusion or rupture. Isolated sternal injury is a relatively rare injury, since the force required to fracture the sternum usually results in other injury, which is often fatal.

Palpation of the sternum and the costochondral junctions may reveal point tenderness and a crepitance or step-off over the fracture. Sternal fractures are difficult to detect on anterior or oblique films. Patients suspected of having a sternal fracture should have lateral views with a specific request for sternal view. Simple undisplaced sternal fractures require no treatment. Displaced fractures with overlapping fragments may require operative reduction, debridement, and direct wire fixation. Claviculosternal dislocations may compress the structures traversing the thoracic inlet including the trachea, major vessels, and the brachial plexus. Treatment of the sternal fracture may need to be delayed depending on the presence of other associated injuries.

Diaphragmatic Injury

Injury to the diaphragm should be considered in any penetrating or blunt injury to the chest, abdomen, or lower back. When a diaphragmatic injury is noted, primary suture repair of the rent usually suffices, but occasionally repair with prosthetic mesh is required. Regardless of etiology, all diaphragmatic injuries should be repaired because there is a significant risk of incarceration and possible strangulation of abdominal viscera through the hernia as well as pulmonary compromise secondary to compression.

In those patients who do not undergo emergency laparotomy, the diagnosis can be delayed for several months or even years. Diaphragmatic injuries can occur with penetrating injuries as well as from blunt trauma, although the injuries incurred from a blunt mechanism tend to produce larger rents in the diaphragm. Patients with missed diaphragmatic injuries often complain of midepigastric pain or symptoms of bowel obstruction as abdominal viscera herniate into the chest. Examination may reveal a scaphoid abdomen without significant tenderness to palpation. Auscultation of the chest may reveal bowel sounds. The chest radiograph shows what appears to be an elevated hemidiaphragm, hydrothorax, hydropneumothorax, an air-fluid level, and evidence of abdominal viscera. These findings are most often seen on the left side because, after right-sided diaphragmatic injuries, the liver protects the abdominal viscera from herniating into the right chest. Occasionally, the liver itself may herniate after right-sided injuries. An easy diagnostic test is the introduction of a nasogastric tube. If the tube coils into the left chest, the diagnosis of gastric herniation through the diaphragmatic injury is made, and operation is indicated for repair of the diaphragm and restoration of the abdominal contents into the abdomen. Similarly, an upper gastrointestinal series or barium enema can be performed to evaluate the viscera with respect to herniation into the chest.

PENETRATING INJURY OF THE LUNG

Penetrating injuries of the lung occur from stab or gunshot wounds. An occasional impalement injury may also be seen. The degree of injury sustained by the lung ranges from small lacerations caused by knife injuries to massive destruction with shotgun blasts. In addition, the type of firearm used will define the amount of injury. Most civilian penetrating thoracic injuries can be managed with tube thoracostomy alone because of relatively minimal injury to lung parenchyma. Hilar injury or significant parenchymal injury requiring resection carries a high mortality.

The management of penetrating thoracic injury begins with placement of a chest tube. One indication for operation in such patients is an initial drainage of 2 L or more of blood. The patient who remains hypotensive following volume replacement requires operation. In those with less initial drainage, continuing drainage of 150 to 200 mL of blood every hour for 3 to 4 h is another indication for operation. Additional indications include hemoptysis, shock, and cardiac tamponade.

CONCLUSION

For purposes of classification, a distinction must be made between blunt and penetrating trauma to the chest, yet the management of many of these injuries, no matter what the cause, is similar. An injury confined to the chest most often results in a favorable outcome; the difficulty lies in the fact that most chest trauma is associated with other injuries. Many multiple-injury patients with chest trauma never make it to the hospital. Those who do must be managed by a team of individuals consisting of trauma and thoracic surgeons as well as physicians trained in critical care. The initial management of patients with thoracic trauma often requires quick and accurate decision making, as in the case of the patient who presents with a tension pneumothorax. It behooves all physicians who deal with critically ill patients to be familiar with the care of patients with chest trauma.

BIBLIOGRAPHY

Dee PM: The radiology of chest trauma. *Radiol Clin North Am* 30:291–306, 1992.
Robison PD, Harman PK, Trinkle JK, Grover FL: Management of penetrating lung injuries in civilian practice. *J Thorac Cardiovasc Surg* 95:184–190, 1988.
Symbas PN, Justicz AG, Ricketts RR: Rupture of the airways from blunt trauma: Treatment of complex injuries. *Ann Thorac Surg* 54:177–183, 1992.
Trinkle JK, Furman RW, Hinshaw MA, et al: Pulmonary contusion—Pathogenesis and effect of various resuscitative measures. *Ann Thorac Surg* 54:177–183, 1992.
Ziegler DW, Agarwal NN: The morbidity and mortality of rib fractures. *J Trauma* 37(6):975–979, 1994.

53 | Lung Transplantation*

Larry R. Kaiser and John C. Wain, Jr.

Lung transplantation has been used as a successful therapeutic intervention for a variety of end-stage pulmonary parenchymal and vascular diseases over the past 15 years. Advances in recipient and donor selection, surgical technique, and postoperative management have improved early survival. The criteria for the use of either isolated lung transplantation or heart-lung transplantation continue to be defined, with the role for heart-lung transplantation lessening over the past decade. A relative shortage of donor organs has been the major constraint on wider application of this treatment. In addition, chronic rejection in the pulmonary allograft, manifest as obliterative bronchiolitis, remains a major obstacle to long-term patient survival.

HISTORY

Clinical lung transplantation was undertaken first by Hardy in 1963. Between 1963 and 1978, however, at least 38 attempts were made at isolated lung transplantation, and only one patient survived to hospital discharge. The major cause of mortality beyond the first postoperative week in these patients was bronchial dehiscence. In addition, most of the patients were greatly debilitated at the time of the procedure, frequently ventilator-dependent or in a state of multisystem and multiorgan failure, hindering their ability to survive.

It has since been shown that despite initial concerns about the physiology of allograft ventilation, isolated single-lung transplantation is also appropriate for patients with end-stage chronic obstructive pulmonary disease (COPD). Isolated single- and double-lung transplantation has also been successfully applied to patients with primary pulmonary hypertension or Eisenmenger's syndrome (with correction of the congenital shunt), for whom combined heart-lung transplantation was initially devised. As the utility of isolated lung transplantation for these pulmonary diseases has been demonstrated, the need for heart-lung transplantation has diminished.

RECIPIENT SELECTION

General Considerations

The evaluation of a potential candidate for lung transplantation should include a complete assessment of cardiopulmonary function and of the patient's general health, in addition to a thorough evaluation of psychosocial status. Potential recipients should be patients with an end-stage pulmonary parenchymal or vascular disease who have a limited life expectancy and for whom no effective alternative therapy is available. However, since the average waiting time in the United States for donor lungs is more than 550 days, a *life*

---

*Edited from Chap. 106, "Lung Transplantation," by Wain JC Jr. In: *Fishman's Pulmonary Diseases and Disorders,* 3d ed., edited by Fishman AP, Elias JA, Fishman JA, Grippi MA, Kaiser LR, Senior RM. New York, McGraw-Hill, 1998, pp. 1671–1694. For fuller discussion of topics dealt with in this chapter, the reader is referred to the original text, as noted above.

expectancy of 2 years or less is considered a critical criterion for patients who deserve further evaluation as potential transplant recipients.

Absolute contraindications to lung transplantation include *bone marrow failure* and *hepatic cirrhosis,* the latter to be distinguished from reversible hepatic dysfunction due to right heart failure, which resolves following lung transplantation. An *active malignancy precluding long-term survival,* which in the case of most solid tumors implies a disease-free survival beyond 5 years, is also an absolute contraindication. A host of additional factors may be considered relative contraindications to lung transplantation. The age of the recipient may be a significant factor in view of the limited number of donor organs and the presumed subclinical organ dysfunction associated with the aging process that increases the potential for postoperative complications. Other contraindications are evidence of psychosocial instability that would preclude compliance with the necessary posttransplant regimens and active use of tobacco products during the wait for transplantation. Obesity or cachexia can increase the risk for perioperative morbidity. The same is true of the continued need for high doses of steroid therapy (e.g., more than 20 mg of prednisone per day).

Respiratory failure requiring mechanical ventilation before transplantation also increases the likelihood of complications. Prolonged mechanical ventilation results in colonization of the lower respiratory tract with significant microbiologic pathogens and a degree of deconditioning and protein wasting that significantly increases the perioperative risk of transplantation.

Chronic renal disease may affect eligibility for lung transplantation. All immunosuppressive regimens have some element of renal insufficiency as a complication of therapy, as do many of the antimicrobial regimens required for the management of these patients.

Severe peripheral vascular disease may be a limiting factor since vascular disease is also frequently associated with significant coronary or aortic disease. Infectious diseases have a profound effect on the morbidity and mortality of lung transplantation. Colonization of the respiratory tract with potential pathogens in patients with end-stage pulmonary disease requires careful assessment of anatomic changes in the airways and determination of antimicrobial susceptibility. Most bacterial flora in transplant candidates have a pattern of antibiotic sensitivity that can be identified preoperatively in order to define a perioperative antibiotic regimen. However, *Pseudomonas cepaciae,* a pathogen found in approximately 15 percent of patients with cystic fibrosis, is often highly resistant to antimicrobials and is a relative contraindication to transplantation unless a suitable pattern of antibiotic sensitivity can be identified before transplantation.

Viral diseases in a potential lung transplant recipient can also have a significant impact on the outcome of transplantation. Active hepatitis B or C in the lung transplant candidate increases both early and late mortality because of the effect of hepatic dysfunction on perioperative complications and the accelerated progression of these diseases in patients requiring chronic immunosuppression. Cytomegalovirus (CMV), a DNA-type virus that is incorporated into the host genome, can cause both a systemic illness and a pneumonitis in immunosuppressed patients. The serologic CMV status of the recipient is therefore an important determination to make before transplantation.

Immunologic study of potential transplant candidates includes assessment of ABO status and cross-matching for transfusion. All patients are currently matched to donors by ABO status, most commonly with ABO-identical donors; virtually all patients require some transfusion in the perioperative period. MHC status is also assessed preoperatively, primarily for use in studies of postoperative outcome, such as the effect of HLA-DR mismatching or donor-recipient microchimerism on chronic rejection.

Specific Disease States

The most common indication for lung transplantation is *obstructive lung disease,* with COPD accounting for 30 percent of all lung transplants and emphysema due to alpha$_1$-antitrypsin deficiency accounting for 15 percent of all lung transplants. *Restrictive lung diseases* are the indication for lung transplantation in 20 percent of patients who undergo lung transplantation. The most common cause is idiopathic pulmonary fibrosis (IPF), which accounts for 15 percent of lung transplant patients, whereas a variety of interstitial lung diseases with mixed physiologic characteristics account for the remainder (Table 53-1). Progression of the disease may be variable, but patients often deteriorate precipitously, developing progressive hypoxemia and pulmonary hypertension. As a result, the mortality of these patients while they await transplantation is more than 20 percent. Two other factors in patients with interstitial lung disease are also important: many of these diseases are systemic, and the effects of the disease on extrapulmonary organs may result in a sufficient number of relative contraindications to exclude the patient from consideration for transplantation; a number of these diseases, including sarcoidosis and lymphangioleiomyomatosis, have been shown to recur in the lung graft, underscoring the need for particularly cautious screening of such patients as potential candidates for transplantation.

TABLE 53-1 Disease-Specific Indications for Lung Transplantation

Obstructive lung disease—FEV_1 <25% predicted, postbronchodilator
  Chronic obstructive pulmonary disease
  α_1-Antitrypsin deficiency
Restrictive lung disease
  Idiopathic pulmonary fibrosis—FVC <50% predicted, Pa_{O_2} <50 mmHg, Pa_{CO_2} >45 mmHg
    Pulmonary artery hypertension
    No response to steroid therapy
Interstitial lung disease
  Sarcoidosis
  Desquamative interstitial pneumonitis
  Lymphangioleiomyomatosis
  Chemotherapy- or radiation therapy–related fibrosis
  Collagen vascular disorders with primarily pulmonary involvement
  Eosinophilic granuloma or histiocytosis X
  Alveolar microlithiasis
Septic lung disease
  Cystic fibrosis—FEV_1 <30% predicted, FVC ≤40% predicted, Pa_{O_2} <60 mmHg, room air
  Bilateral bronchiectasis
    Hypogammaglobulinemia
    Postinfectious (childhood measles, pertussis, postpneumonia, or tuberculosis)
    Immotile cilia syndrome—Kartagener's syndrome
    Allergic bronchopulmonary aspergillosis
Pulmonary vascular disease
  Primary pulmonary hypertension—symptomatic disease
  Eisenmenger's syndrome

Septic lung disease, including cystic fibrosis and other types of bronchiectasis, accounts for 15 to 20 percent of patients undergoing lung transplantation. Many of these patients demonstrate significant short-term improvements in response to aggressive medical therapy, which includes postural drainage, intravenous and inhaled antibiotics, and nutritional supplementation. Once medical therapy has been optimized, however, a pattern of more frequent hospitalizations for "cleanouts," continued weight loss, and progressive functional impairment is indicative of a patient who has a limited life span and should be given priority for transplantation. However, because of the shortage of donor organs and the variability in the progression of the disease, donation of a lobe from a related donor may warrant consideration for some patients. Initial results of this approach, using bilateral isolated lobar transplants from two donors, have been encouraging for patients with cystic fibrosis, without entailing donor mortality or significant morbidity.

Pulmonary vascular disease, either primary pulmonary hypertension (PPH) or secondary pulmonary hypertension due to Eisenmenger's syndrome, accounts for 10 to 15 percent of patients requiring isolated lung transplantation and for 45 to 50 percent of patients requiring heart-lung transplantation. The criteria for identifying patients who may require transplantation relate to the risks of death due to the underlying disease. From registry data, it is apparent that a New York Heart Association (NYHA) class III or IV functional status, an elevated central venous pressure, a decreased cardiac index, and an elevated *mean* pulmonary artery pressure correlate with a poor prognosis. Episodes of near syncope, syncope, or near death, which tend to occur later in the course of the disease, are also associated with mortality. It should be noted, however, that alleviation of symptoms or physiologic abnormalities by medical therapy using high-dose calcium-channel blockers or prostacyclin infusions in PPH patients may significantly modify the natural history of the disease. Therefore symptomatic patients with PPH who do not respond to medical therapy are the ones best considered for transplantation. Heart-lung transplantation is primarily limited to patients with either significant biventricular dysfunction (e.g., severe valvular cardiomyopathy) or incorrectable congenital heart defects.

TRANSPLANT PROCEDURE SELECTION

Except for patients with bilateral septic lung disease or severe pulmonary arterial hypertension, single-lung transplantation (SLT) is optimal for the majority of end-stage pulmonary diseases that require transplantation. The surgical mortality for SLT ranges from 3 to 10 percent, relating to the specific transplant indication, the presence or absence of pulmonary hypertension, and the intraoperative need for cardiopulmonary bypass.

Double-lung transplantation (DLT) is the procedure of choice for patients with bilateral septic lung disease, such as cystic fibrosis, or for patients with pulmonary arterial pressures that are at near-systemic levels from either primary or secondary causes. Typically, however, surgical mortality is higher for DLT than for SLT, ranging from 10 to 15 percent.

Combined heart-lung transplantation (HLT) has been used successfully for virtually all end-stage pulmonary diseases that require transplantation. However, with the perfection of the techniques of SLT and DLT and in light of the significant limitations in supply of donor organs, the use of HLT has focused on patients with significant refractory right ventricular *diastolic* dysfunction (e.g., RVEDP more than 15 mmHg), significant intrinsic left ventricular dysfunction, or Eisenmenger's syndrome and irreparable shunt defects.

DONOR SELECTION

The most significant factor limiting wider application of lung transplantation is the supply of donor organs. Nearly half of all comatose patients will develop pneumonia within 1 week of intubation, probably owing to a combination of these factors. Brain death itself may also lead to neurogenic pulmonary edema. In cases of trauma that lead to brain death, significant injury to the thorax may occur, or the volume replacement required for the resuscitation of these patients may limit the suitability of the lungs for subsequent transplantation. As a result, only about 25 percent of cadaveric organ donors are potential lung donors.

Criteria for lung donation are meant to identify donors with evidence of good gas exchange in the absence of infection of the airways or parenchyma (Table 53-2). Both increasing age and prolonged tobacco use are known to correlate directly with anatomic alterations in the pulmonary parenchyma—which, despite preservation of gas exchange function in the donor, may result in impaired graft function in the recipient. Chest radiographs should reveal a normal lung on the side of the proposed lung donation. Finally, the size of the donor lungs, based on direct measurement or correlated to body surface area as estimated by donor height, is a useful parameter for one to use when selecting lungs for a particular recipient.

Adequate gas exchange has been defined as a Pa_{O_2} greater than 300 mmHg on mechanical ventilation, with an Fi_{O_2} of 1.0 and positive end-expiratory pressure (PEEP) at least 5 cmH$_2$O. Minute ventilation should be adjusted to achieve normocarbia, with a tidal volume of 10 to 15 mL/kg and an appropriate respiratory rate.

Owing to the requisite endotracheal intubation, which bypasses the defense mechanisms of the upper airway, all lung donors will have some evidence of colonization of the lower respiratory tract by potential pathogens. A distal tracheitis is uniformly present after 72 h of intubation. For this reason, bronchoscopy is a critical step in the evaluation of any potential lung donor.

LUNG PRESERVATION

The ideal method of pulmonary preservation has not yet been identified. With current techniques, however, satisfactory graft function can be obtained after ischemic intervals as long as 6 to 8 h. As with other vascularized solid organs

---

TABLE 53-2 Characteristics of a Suitable Lung Donor

Age <60 years
Cigarette smoking <30 pack-years
No significant prior thoracic surgery on the side of the donor lung
Normal chest radiograph of the donor lung
Adequate gas exchange of the donor lung
  Pa_{O_2} >300 mmHg on Fi_{O_2} 1.0, PEEP ≥5 cm H$_2$O
  Pv_{O_2} >450 mmHg on Fi_{O_2} 1.0, PEEP ≥5 cm H$_2$O
Bronchoscopic evaluation demonstrating absence of mucosal inflammation
No significant pulmonary trauma or anatomic abnormalities

used for transplantation, the lung consists of a heterogeneous population of cells, of which the vascular endothelial cell appears to be the most sensitive to ischemia. Ischemic injury to the pulmonary vascular endothelium increases its permeability and results in pulmonary edema, the common end point for assessment of injury in models of pulmonary preservation techniques. Hypothermia is the major method used clinically to limit ischemic injury to these cells. *Hypothermic flush perfusion* is the method most commonly used for pulmonary preservation in clinical practice. This technique consists of flushing the pulmonary vasculature with a cold solution after systemic heparinization of the donor, followed by extraction and transport of the lungs inflated with 100% oxygen.

The administration of prostanoids, either prostaglandin E_1 (PgE$_1$) or prostacyclin, into the pulmonary circulation before flush perfusion has been shown to improve lung preservation. Most flush solutions are administered at a temperature of 4°C, while topical cooling is carried out by filling of the pleural cavity with iced crystalloid solution. After extraction, the lungs are immersed in crystalloid and packed in ice, resulting in a transport temperature of 1 to 4°C.

POSTOPERATIVE MANAGEMENT

Ventilation

In most cases, ventilatory management follows standard criteria. Significant barotrauma due to increased airway pressures is extremely uncommon after lung transplantation, and higher airway pressures may have a beneficial effect in minimizing postoperative pulmonary edema. Transition from volume ventilation to pressure ventilation before extubation may be useful to decrease the work of breathing and serves to minimize differences in compliance between the native lung and allograft following SLT.

Patients with emphysema who undergo SLT are an exception to the above guidelines. These patients require particular attention to airway pressures and to the compliance difference between the allograft and the native lung. Hyperinflation of the native lung may not only result in compromise of cardiac filling but also interferes progressively with ventilation of the allograft. Efforts to control hyperinflation of the native lung include use of slightly lower tidal volumes (9 to 12 mL/kg) accompanied by higher respiratory rates to preserve minute ventilation and lower levels of PEEP (1 to 3 cmH$_2$O).

In patients with significant pulmonary hypertension who undergo lung transplantation, the postoperative pulmonary hemodynamics are unique. In these patients, the right ventricle has been conditioned to generate peak systolic pressures against a markedly elevated pulmonary vascular resistance (PVR). Following lung transplantation, the PVR abruptly decreases to near-normal levels, accompanied by improved ventricular hemodynamics. Minimal catecholamine stimulation occurs when the patient awakes from anesthesia or is weaned from a ventilator, causing the right ventricle to respond by generating peak systolic pressures similar to those that existed preoperatively. The resultant abrupt increase in pulmonary artery pressure, in combination with increased capillary permeability due to ischemia and reperfusion injury and the absence of lymphatic continuity, causes fluid to accumulate rapidly in the donor lung. Preemptive treatment for this condition is necessary and requires maintenance of a high degree of sedation or even of muscle paralysis in the first 3 to 5 days after surgery. Following this period, patients can be awakened cautiously and weaned from the ventilator with standard methods while cardiac output, blood gases, and pulmonary artery pressures are closely monitored.

Antimicrobial Therapy

Bacterial prophylaxis entails the use of vancomycin for prophylaxis against gram-positive organisms in combination with a broad-spectrum antibiotic to provide appropriate coverage for organisms identified preoperatively from the sputum of the recipient. Postoperative antibacterial coverage should be modified if pathogens not already covered by the recipient-specific regimen are found in the sputum of the donor.

Routine prophylaxis for fungal organisms is useful when preoperative recipient sputum cultures have demonstrated the presence of *Aspergillus* species at any time before the transplant procedure, when there has been evidence of heavy overgrowth of yeast (e.g., *Candida*) in the donor sputum culture, or when cytolytic induction immunosuppression is used.

CMV infection remains a significant problem following lung transplantation. The incidence of CMV infection after lung transplantation is related to the preoperative CMV status of both the donor (D) and the recipient (R). The incidence of acute and chronic rejection and mortality are higher than among patients in whom CMV status is concordant. For this reason, many centers prefer to match D and R status. However, the use of ganciclovir prophylaxis has been shown to eliminate the incidence of primary disease and to improve the outcome of CMV-disparate lung transplants. *Pneumocystis carinii* infection in lung transplant patients has been eliminated by the routine use of trimethoprim-sulfamethoxazole beginning 1 week after surgery.

Immunosuppression

The induction of a state of relatively nonspecific immune suppression by pharmacologic means has been the key to successful clinical lung transplantation. The immunosuppressive regimens used for lung transplantation are based on the successful protocols that have evolved for renal and heart transplantation. Virtually all centers use a three-drug regimen for immunosuppression, with the hope of obtaining additive effects in terms of immune suppression while limiting drug toxicities. Although most centers use a combination of cyclosporine, azathioprine, and steroids for this purpose, tacrolimus is being more widely employed.

Rejection

Lung grafts contain a large population of immunocompetent cells, including lymphocytes and macrophages within the parenchyma, hilar and pulmonary lymph nodes, and bronchus-associated lymphoid tissue (BALT). Most of these cells are memory T cells. A prominent interaction occurs between donor and recipient immune cells during the early period after implantation. In view of these rapid and profound changes in immune cell populations, it is not surprising that rejection is common in lung allografts and that, in the case of heart-lung grafts, lung rejection may occur more frequently than, and independent of, rejection of the heart. A protocol of routine transbronchial biopsy of the lung for identification of histologic evidence of lung rejection is usually recommended for both heart-lung and isolated-lung transplants because of the likelihood of rejection that may occur with minimal clinical symptoms.

Typically, surveillance bronchoscopy is performed at 3 weeks, 6 weeks, 3 months, 6 months, 9 months, and 12 months after surgery. Bronchoscopy and biopsy are, of course, also performed for clinical symptoms or for changes in lung spirometry such as a decrease in FEV_1.

Because the incidence of acute rejection in the first 3 weeks after lung transplantation exceeds 90 percent at most centers, antirejection therapy is usually administered empirically for transplant recipients with the appropriate clinical syndrome, even in the absence of confirmatory biopsy findings, if no infectious cause is found by BAL. In most patients, symptomatic and radiographic improvement is seen within 48 h. Thereafter, the maintenance dose of steroids is usually increased for several weeks and then slowly reduced to prerejection levels.

Chronic rejection (CR) in the lung may affect either the pulmonary vasculature or the airway. Typically, CR is manifested by obstructive changes in the small airways. Clinically, progressive dyspnea occurs, although a gradual decline in FEV_1 or in expiratory flow rates often precedes symptoms. Histologically, this process is identified as bronchiolitis obliterans and consists of dense eosinophilic scarring of the membranous and respiratory bronchioles. Further progression of this process leads to worsening dyspnea and bronchiectasis with secondary infection. Although this form of CR is uncommon in the first 3 months after lung transplantation, up to 50 percent of patients develop it within 2 years, and the mortality at 3 years after diagnosis is 40 percent or higher. The term *bronchiolitis obliterans syndrome* (BOS) has been used to identify patients with CR of the lung involving the airways. The diagnosis of BOS is based on symptoms and objective changes in pulmonary function and does not require histologic evidence of bronchiolitis obliterans. Management of progressive BOS in its later stages is mostly palliative. At its most advanced stage, BOS is essentially an acquired form of septic lung disease, and management is similar to that required for other patients with septic lung disease awaiting lung transplantation. Retransplantation has been performed for some patients with BOS.

Complications

Surgical Complications

Major technical complications following lung transplantation have become increasingly rare with improvements in surgical technique and perioperative management. Some transplanted lungs demonstrate *acute graft dysfunction,* even without evidence of vascular anastomotic complications. As many as 20 percent of patients have severe early abnormalities of lung function, with rapidly progressive pulmonary edema, persistent pulmonary hypertension, and a markedly diminished pulmonary compliance that occurs rapidly after graft implantation. *Pleural effusions* are common after lung transplantation, particularly when a significant size disparity exists between the donor lungs and the thorax. Continued chest tube drainage following the primary procedure is not indicated as a preventive measure for these effusions and may actually lead to secondary infection and empyema.

Airway complications have been significantly less common in the recent experience with lung transplantation. Bronchial ischemia is the most common cause of postoperative airway complications. Most commonly, partial anastomotic dehiscence occurs, followed by formation of granulation tissue and eventually some degree of anastomotic stenosis. The overall incidence of airway complications in all lung transplant patients is 15 to 20 percent. Death due to extensive airway necrosis or secondary infectious complications occurs in 10 percent of patients who develop symptomatic airway complications.

Infectious Complications

Lung transplant patients have several unique attributes that account for a rate of infectious complications that is higher than the rate for other transplant recipients. An aggressive approach to the evaluation of all new pulmonary infiltrates, in either the lung graft or the native lung, is required in these patients. Flexible bronchoscopy with bronchoalveolar lavage (BAL) or protected brushing is needed for proper diagnosis of pulmonary infections after lung transplantation.

Bacterial pneumonia is the most commonly acquired infection after lung transplantation. Pneumonia occurs most frequently within 2 months of transplantation and is usually due to gram-negative bacilli. Diagnosis made with bronchoscopy and treatment with antibiotics administered intravenously lead to prompt resolution in most cases. Viral infections can be a major source of morbidity or mortality for lung transplant patients. *Cytomegalovirus,* a member of the human herpesvirus family, is the second most frequent cause of infection in the lung transplant patient and the most important opportunistic infection that occurs in these patients. Following infection with CMV, the virus remains in a latent state in the body; evidence of the infection can be identified from a positive serologic assay. Approximately 80 percent of adults are seropositive for CMV. The incidence of CMV infection in the lung transplant recipient is related to the serologic status of both donor and recipient. Primary CMV infection of an immunosuppressed host, such as the recipient of a lung transplant, is a potentially fatal systemic illness associated with viremia, pneumonitis, hepatitis, encephalitis, retinitis, and enterocolitis. Such patients require both ganciclovir (5 mg/kg intravenously twice a day) and CMV hyperimmune globulin (10 g intravenously every month) for prolonged courses of therapy until the disease is eradicated. Although ganciclovir is effective therapy for CMV in patients with pneumonitis or primary infection, the occurrence of CMV infection in these patients can lead to significant morbidity. CMV infection seems to elicit acute graft rejection in many instances, requiring a complicated treatment plan to balance the need for augmented immunosuppression against adequate treatment of the infection. In addition, CMV disease in some series appears to be a risk factor for the subsequent development of BOS, the most common cause of late mortality following lung transplantation.

Neoplastic Complications

Immunosuppression increases the risk of development of neoplasms after lung transplantation. The risk applies to a specific group of solid tumors, including squamous cell cancers of the lip and skin, Kaposi's sarcoma, soft tissue sarcomas, carcinomas of the vulva and perineum, and hepatobiliary tumors. The most common malignancy seen after lung transplantation is a type of B-cell lymphoid proliferation known as *posttransplant lymphoproliferative disorder* (PTLD). This represents a morphologically diverse group of polyclonal lymphoid proliferations. The pathogenesis of PTLD appears to be related to Epstein-Barr virus (EBV) infection of B lymphocytes that are stimulated to proliferate by the recipient's immunosuppression. Clinically, a distinction can be made between patients presenting with PTLD within 1 year after transplantation and those presenting with PTLD at later times. The early patients tend to have localized disease that responds to a temporary reduction in immunosuppression; their long-term prognosis is excellent. Patients who present after 1 year usually have disseminated disease that does not respond to reduced immunosuppression and requires cytotoxic chemotherapy for treatment. The mortality from lymphoma in these patients is 70 percent. Of interest is that the use of ganciclovir for prophylaxis against CMV disease in lung transplant patients may also help to control the incidence of PTLD, since ganciclovir also has significant activity against EBV.

RESULTS

Survival

Mortality following lung transplantation has decreased significantly over the past decade. The cause of this reduction is probably multifactorial—i.e., the result of technical improvements in the procedure, of improved recipient selection and preoperative management, and of increasing experience in perioperative management of these patients. In most recent series, surgical mortality following lung transplantation has been between 10 and 15 percent. The surgical mortality of DLT ranges from 15 to 20 percent as compared with that of SLT, which is usually 10 percent or less. This difference is attributable in large part to the increased likelihood of postoperative infectious complications in patients with septic lung disease who require DLT. Surgical mortality after HLT is usually slightly higher than for patients undergoing DLT, probably owing to the more advanced disease state of patients who require HLT.

Infection is the major cause of early mortality in lung transplant recipients, accounting for 30 to 45 percent of deaths. The likelihood of pulmonary infection is greatest in the first 100 days after transplantation, before recipient defense mechanisms (e.g., cough) are restored.

Long-term survival data indicate a cumulative survival rate of 70 to 80 percent at 1 year. Survival curves can vary significantly beyond 1 year, depending on the disease for which transplantation was performed. Patients with emphysema and those with pulmonary vascular disease appear to have a survival advantage over patients with restrictive lung disease or septic lung disease, in whom infectious complications or recurrence of native disease in the lung graft is more common. By 3 years, survival ranges from 75 percent in the former group to 55 percent in the latter group. At this interval, BOS begins to have a significant impact on survival as well, leading to an overall survival rate of less than 50 percent at 5 years. Causes of death in this period include infection, which has another peak of increased incidence throughout the second postoperative year, and BOS, which can be identified in half of the patients who survive to 3 years. Malignancy, usually PTLD, is the third most common cause of late mortality following lung transplantation.

Functional Results

Most patients surviving lung transplantation experience a highly significant improvement in their functional capability over their preoperative state. Improvements occur regardless of the native disease that led to transplantation. Unless BOS occurs, functional capacity based on the standards of reproducible exercise testing remains stable for at least 3 years. Controversy exists over the potential benefit of SLT as compared to DLT for younger patients with emphysema. Although the results of spirometry are obviously better in DLT recipients, exercise tolerance is initially similar in the two groups.

Retransplantation

Pulmonary retransplantation has been undertaken with increasing frequency in recent years. Retransplantation is used either as a method to correct an acute complication, such as graft failure or diffuse airway necrosis, or as a treatment for a chronic process in the graft, such as BOS or airway stenosis. These are technically challenging procedures, with a surgical mortality of nearly 50 percent. Factors contributing to a more favorable outcome include an ambulatory status before retransplantation, the use of ABO-identical grafts, and prior institutional experience with retransplantation; notably, retransplantation with a CMV-seronegative donor has also been associated with a favorable outcome. The long-term results of retransplantation are much worse than those of initial lung transplantation. One-year survival is about 45 percent, and 2-year survival is about 35 percent. BOS occurs with a frequency similar to that seen with primary lung transplantation and can be identified in one-third of patients 2 years after retransplantation.

SUMMARY

Significant progress has been made in the development of techniques of lung transplantation for all types of end-stage pulmonary diseases. Isolated lung transplantation has been applied with increasing success to the entire group of patients, including those with pulmonary vascular disease. A shortage of donor organs, however, remains the most significant obstacle to wider use of this method of treatment. Techniques of donor lung preservation and implantation allow ischemic intervals of 6 to 8 h for reasonable postoperative function. Surgical mortality is 10 to 15 percent, slightly lower for SLT and slightly higher for DLT and HLT. Functional results in survivors of the operation are excellent. Infection remains a significant source of morbidity and mortality in both the early and late postoperative periods. However, the most significant impediment to long-term survival is the development of chronic rejection in the lung allograft, manifest as BOS, in half of the patients by 3 years after transplantation. Further measures to prevent or treat this malady are critical to improving long-term survival rates following lung transplantation.

BIBLIOGRAPHY

Bando K, Paradis IL, Komatsu K, et al: Analysis of time-dependent risks for infection, rejection and death after pulmonary transplantation. *J Thorac Cardiovasc Surg* 109:49–57, 1995.

Bando K, Paradis IL, Similo S, et al: Obliterative bronchiolitis after lung and heart-lung transplantation: An analysis of risk factors and management. *J Thorac Cardiovasc Surg* 110:4–14, 1995.

Hardy JD: Lung homotransplantation in man. *JAMA* 186:1065–1066, 1963.

Mal H, Sleiman C, Jebrak G, et al: Functional results of single-lung transplantation for chronic obstructive lung disease. *Am J Respir Crit Care Med* 149:1476–1481, 1994.

Sundaresan S, Trulock EP, Mohanakumar T, et al: Prevalence and outcome of bronchiolitis obliterans syndrome after lung transplantation. *Ann Thorac Surg* 60:1341–1346, 1995.

Toronto Lung Transplant Group: Unilateral lung transplantation for pulmonary fibrosis. *N Engl J Med* 314:1140–1145, 1986.

Part Thirteen | NEOPLASMS OF THE LUNGS

54 | The Solitary Pulmonary Nodule: A Systemic Approach*

Larry R. Kaiser and Alan M. Fein

DEFINITION

A solitary pulmonary nodule is defined as a single discrete pulmonary opacity that is surrounded by normal lung tissue and is not associated with adenopathy or atelectasis. There is some difference of opinion on the upper size limit for a nodule. Some early series included lesions up to 6 cm. At present, most authors consider a nodule to be a lesion less than 3 cm in diameter. A lesion 3 cm or larger is more likely to be malignant and is called a mass.

INCIDENCE AND PREVALENCE

The frequency with which a solitary pulmonary nodule is identified on chest radiography is on the order of 1 to 2 per thousand chest radiographs. Most of these are clinically silent, and about 90 percent are noted as an incidental finding on radiographic examination. The prevalence of malignancy in nodules varies widely, depending on the patient population; thus, many case series may not be directly comparable. Surgical series in the era before computed tomography (CT), including both calcified and noncalcified nodules, reported an overall malignancy rate of 10 to 68 percent. Series that have used chest CT to screen out benign-appearing calcified nodules show much higher overall malignancy rates: 56 to 100 percent.

MALIGNANT SOLITARY PULMONARY NODULES

Risk factors for malignancy have been identified from studies of large series of solitary pulmonary nodules and include patient's age, smoking history, nodule size, and prior history of malignancy. Risk of malignancy increases with age. These findings correlate with those of previous studies, which also show that malignancy is very rarely found in patients under the age of 35.

Nodule size is closely correlated to risk of malignancy. Several series have demonstrated an increased incidence of malignancy with increasing nodule size. Nodules larger than 3 cm will be malignant 80 to 99 percent of the time, while those under 2 cm in size will be malignant in 20 to 66 percent of cases.

A history of current or prior extrapulmonary malignancy will greatly increase the probability that a nodule is malignant. Depending on the series, 33 to 95 percent of such nodules have proved to be malignant—most

*Edited from Chap. 110, "The Solitary Pulmonary Nodule: A Systemic Approach," by Fein AM, Feinsilver SH, Ares CA. In: *Fishman's Pulmonary Diseases and Disorders,* 3d ed., edited by Fishman AP, Elias JA, Fishman JA, Grippi MA, Kaiser LR, Senior RM. New York, McGraw-Hill, 1998, pp 1727–1738. For fuller discussion of topics dealt with in this chapter, the reader is referred to the original text, as noted above.

representing metastases but some second primaries. The most common histologic types of metastatic nodules are adenocarcinomas of colon, breast, or kidney; head and neck tumors; sarcoma; and melanoma.

Primary bronchogenic carcinoma is the most common malignant tumor that presents as a solitary pulmonary nodule. Histologically, adenocarcinoma and squamous cell carcinoma make up the majority; of the two, adenocarcinoma is slightly more common. Less frequent as a solitary pulmonary nodule is the bronchoalveolar cell carcinoma. Small cell carcinoma that presents as a solitary pulmonary nodule is rare. Other rare primary lung tumors that may present as solitary pulmonary nodules are bronchial carcinoids (1 to 5 percent), which are usually peripherally located; lymphomas; hemangioendotheliomas; and sarcomas.

Metastases may present as solitary pulmonary nodules in patients who have known primary malignancies or in whom the presence of primary malignancy is unknown. In up to 40 percent of such patients, who manifest only a single nodule on chest radiograph, CT scan may show other nodules that are not disclosed by plain chest radiograph. Even though the lesion is solitary, in patients with an established diagnosis of cancer, up to 95 percent of these nodules will be malignant upon resection. Because of this high likelihood of malignancy, a nodule in a patient with an established diagnosis of cancer should be treated differently from other solitary nodules. Assuming no other obvious metastatic spread, one should consider proceeding directly to biopsy. Even in the presence of a known malignancy, some of these nodules may represent a second primary pulmonary malignancy that is similar in histologic appearance. Immunohistologic and other confirmatory marker studies may be indicated to determine the nature of the nodule. A solitary pulmonary nodule in a patient with a history of malignant disease should be removed as long as there is no other evidence of recurrent or metastatic disease.

BENIGN SOLITARY PULMONARY NODULES

Benign solitary pulmonary nodules are more common in the young and in nonsmokers. They include both infectious and noninfectious granulomas, benign tumors such as hamartomas, vascular lesions, and rare miscellaneous conditions (Table 54-1).

Infectious granulomas make up more than 90 percent of all benign nodules. The offending agents will vary, depending on geographic location. Among the most common causes are histoplasmosis, coccidioidomycosis, and tuberculosis. Other, less common causes are dirofilariasis (dog heartworm), mycetoma, echinococcal cyst, and ascariasis. A history of exposure is important in establishing a possible infectious origin. Clues such as prior travel history, places of residence, occupation, and pets may be invaluable in some instances.

Noninfectious granulomas sometimes occur as solitary pulmonary nodules in systemic diseases such as sarcoidosis, in which nodules are not invariably accompanied by hilar adenopathy; rheumatoid arthritis, usually in patients with active disease who will often have subcutaneous nodules; and Wegener's granulomatosis.

Miscellaneous causes of solitary pulmonary nodules have been described. Some of the more common conditions are lung abscess; rounded or spherical pneumonia; pseudotumor, which represents fluid in an intralobar fissure; hematomas after thoracic trauma or surgery; and fibrosis or scars resulting

TABLE 54-1 Differential Diagnosis of Solitary Pulmonary Nodules

Malignant tumors
Bronchogenic carcinoma (adenocarcinoma, large cell, squamous, small cell)
Carcinoid
Pulmonary lymphoma
Pulmonary sarcoma
Plasmocytoma
Solitary metastases (colon, breast, kidney, head and neck, germ cell, sarcoma, thyroid, melanoma, others)

Benign tumors
Hamartoma
Adenoma
Lipoma

Infectious granulomas
Tuberculosis
Histoplasmosis
Coccidioidomycosis
Mycetoma
Ascaris
Echinococcal cyst
Dirofilariasis (dog heartworm)

Noninfectious granulomas
Rheumatoid arthritis
Wegener's granulomatosis
Sarcoidosis
Paraffinoma
Others

Miscellaneous
BOOP
Abscess
Silicosis
Fibrosis/scar
Hematoma
Pseudotumor
Spherical pneumonia
Pulmonary infarction
Arteriovenous malformation
Bronchogenic cyst
Amyloidoma

from the resolution of infectious or inflammatory process. Rarer conditions presenting as solitary pulmonary nodules include silicosis, bronchogenic cyst, amyloidosis, pulmonary infarct, and vascular anomalies. Arteriovenous malformations may present as solitary pulmonary nodules. They may grow slowly and have a characteristic appearance on contrast-enhanced CT scan.

RADIOLOGIC TECHNIQUES

Plain Chest Radiography

Most solitary pulmonary nodules are discovered on routine plain chest radiograph while asymptomatic. Malignant nodules are usually identifiable on chest radiograph by the time they are 0.8 to 1 cm in diameter, although nodules 0.5 to 0.6 cm can occasionally be seen. Most will be identified on posteroanterior (PA) projection, but some will be seen only on lateral projection, so standard PA and lateral chest radiography should be obtained whenever possible. Once it has been ascertained that a true nodule exists, the first step is to make every effort to obtain previous radiographs for comparison. A nodule that has remained stable, with no increase in size, for 2 years, is very probably benign and warrants no further investigation. Conversely, a nodule that was not present on a comparable radiograph within the past 2 months is likely, having grown so rapidly, to be a malignancy. On rare occasions, small cell carcinoma may present as a solitary pulmonary nodule with a doubling time of less than 30 days.

Standard and Computed Tomography

CT has replaced plain tomography as a more sensitive tool in the evaluation of solitary pulmonary nodules. CT is indicated when one is assessing indeterminate nodules less than 3 cm in diameter or in staging of larger lesions. It can pinpoint the exact location of the nodule and provide three-dimensional images of the lesion. Thin-section high-resolution CT (HRCT) can better define the borders and the nodule's relation to adjacent structures, such as vessels and the pleura. It is more sensitive than standard tomography in detecting calcification patterns, and it can detect fat within a nodule—which, when coupled with calcification, is highly suggestive of a benign hamartoma. In up to 40 percent of cases, previously unseen synchronous lesions can be seen. CT may be useful in looking for hilar or mediastinal adenopathy, and in evaluating accessibility of nodules for biopsy or resection.

HRCT can quantify calcification in nodules even when they are not readily visible to the naked eye. Nodules with higher radiographic density are more likely to be benign. This technique has been suggested for indeterminate nodules smaller than 3 cm in diameter. Nodules that are bigger than 3 cm or that have suspect characteristics in the right clinical setting (e.g., an older smoker, spiculated borders) should be considered for biopsy or resection.

Another CT technique that may be helpful is incremental dynamic CT, which uses serially increasing doses of iodinated intravenous contrast to look for enhancement of nodules. Although malignant nodules enhance more than benign ones, benign lesions, such as hamartomas and tuberculomas, may also enhance. Further experience with this method is needed to determine its role in the evaluation of solitary pulmonary nodules. Spiral or helical CT may be useful in the evaluation of small nodules and to look for synchronous lesions. It has the advantage of scanning a large area during a single breath-hold, thereby eliminating respiratory artifact. Its ability to reconstruct images at different intervals and thicknesses also permits better detection of smaller nodules.

Other Radiologic Techniques

Positron emission tomography (PET) is useful in differentiating noninvasively between malignant and benign nodules. PET takes advantage of the fact that tumor cells have an increased glucose uptake and metabolism with the glucose becoming trapped in the tumor cell longer than in benign cells. A D-glucose analog labeled with a positron-emitting fluorine-18 radioisotope (fluorodeoxyglucose, or FDG) is injected into the patient, and uptake by the nodule is then measured. Malignant nodules demonstrate a higher uptake of FDG, with a sensitivity of 95 percent and specificity of greater than 90 percent. This technique has become widely available and is covered by Medicare when bronchogenic carcinoma is the presumed diagnosis. Carcinoid tumors and bronchoalveolar carcinoma do not take up glucose much differently than normal cells and thus have a higher rate of false-negative readings. A nodule found to be negative on PET imaging should be followed by serial CT scans to assure that no growth is occurring.

NODULE GROWTH RATE

Determination of nodule growth is based on the assumption that nodules are more or less spherical. Growth of a sphere must be considered in three-dimensional volume, not in two-dimensional diameter. The formula for volume of a sphere is $4/3(Pi)r^3$, or $1/6(Pi)D^3$, where r = radius and D = diameter. A nodule originally 1 cm in diameter whose diameter is now 1.3 cm has actually more than doubled in volume. Similarly, a 2-cm nodule has doubled in volume by the time its diameter reaches 2.5 cm. A nodule that has doubled in diameter has undergone an eightfold increase in volume. When old radiographs are available, growth rate and nodule *doubling time* (i.e., the time for a nodule to double in volume) can be estimated. Accepting the assumption that a tumor arises from serial doublings of a single cancerous cell, we can estimate that it will take 27 doublings for it to reach 0.5 cm, the smallest lesion detectable on chest radiography. By the time a nodule is 1 cm in diameter, it represents 30 doubling times and about 1 billion tumor cells. Depending on the exact growth rate, this theoretical 1-cm nodule has probably existed for years before it is detected, as malignant bronchogenic tumors have doubling times estimated at between 20 and 400 days. The natural history of a tumor usually spans about 40 doublings, whereupon the tumor is 10 cm in diameter and the patient has usually died. Squamous and large cell tumors have an average doubling time of 60 to 80 days. Adenocarcinomas double at about 120 days, and the rare small cell carcinoma that presents as a solitary pulmonary nodule can have a doubling time of less than 30 days. A nodule that has doubled in weeks to months is probably malignant and should be removed when possible.

Benign nodules have doubling times of less than 20 days or more than 400 days. A nodule that doubles in size in less than 20 days is invariably the result of an acute infectious process, while those that grow very slowly are usually chronic granulomatous reactions or hamartomas. Such nodules can be observed with serial radiographs.

The question often arises whether observing a solitary pulmonary nodule (less than 3 cm that probably has been growing for years) for 3 to 6 months increases the likelihood of metastatic disease. There is no convincing evidence to support this hypothesis. In fact, early detection of lung cancer by screening has not been shown to improve overall survival significantly.

BIOPSY TECHNIQUES

The issues of whether it is at all useful to biopsy an indeterminate solitary pulmonary nodule and, if so, how to do it remain controversial. Most experts agree that in certain clinical circumstances, a biopsy procedure is warranted. For example, in a patient who is at high surgical risk, it may be useful in establishing a diagnosis and in guiding decision making. If the biopsy reveals malignancy, it may convince a patient who is wary of surgery to undergo thoracotomy or thoracoscopic resection of a potentially curable lesion. Another indication for biopsy may be anxiety to establish a specific diagnosis in a patient in whom the nodule seems to be benign. Some chest physicians argue that all indeterminate nodules should be resected if the results of history, physical examination, and laboratory and radiographic staging methods are negative for metastases. Others argue that this last approach exposes patients with benign nodules to the risks of needless surgery. In such cases, a biopsy procedure sometimes provides a specific diagnosis of a benign lesion and obviates surgery.

Once it has been decided to biopsy a solitary pulmonary nodule, the choice of procedure is a matter of debate but includes fiberoptic bronchoscopy, percutaneous needle aspiration, thoracoscopic biopsy (usually with video assistance), and open thoracotomy.

Bronchoscopy

Traditionally, bronchoscopy has been regarded as a procedure of limited usefulness in the evaluation of solitary pulmonary nodules. Various studies have shown variable success rates, with an overall diagnostic yield of 36 to 68 percent, in nodules greater than 2 cm with bronchoscopic biopsy, brushings, and washings. In general, the yield for specific benign diagnoses has ranged from 12 percent to 41 percent.

The issue of determining the optimal bronchoscopic procedural approach is a complicated one and depends largely on the skill and experience of the individual bronchoscopist. Fluoroscopic localization of the nodule improves diagnostic yield and should be used when possible. Most authorities agree that bronchoscopic forceps biopsy, brush cytology, and bronchial washings are complementary and are routinely performed by most bronchoscopists. Future techniques, such as endoscopically guided bronchoscopic biopsy, may prove to be of use. It should be mentioned that routine preoperative staging bronchoscopy is of no value in asymptomatic patients with a solitary pulmonary nodule smaller than 3 cm because it has not been shown to alter management decisions.

Percutaneous Needle Aspiration

Percutaneous needle aspiration can be performed under fluoroscopic or CT guidance, the choice often depending on the availability and the experience of the operator. It is most useful as the initial procedure in peripheral lesions, in the outer third of the lung, and in lesions under 2 cm in diameter. It can establish the diagnosis of malignancy in up to 95 percent of cases and can establish specific benign diagnosis (granuloma, hamartoma, infarct) in up to 68 percent of patients. The use of larger-bore biopsy needles—such as 19 gauge, which provides a core specimen in addition to cytology—improves the yield for both malignant and benign lesions. The major limitation of percutaneous needle aspiration is its high rate of pneumothorax (10 to 35 percent overall); pneumothorax is more likely when lung parenchyma lies in the path of the needle.

Thoracoscopy

With the aid of fiberoptic telescopes and miniaturized video cameras, thoracoscopy has reemerged in the form of video-assisted thoracic surgery. This approach still requires general anesthesia but does not require a full thoracotomy incision or spreading of the ribs. The thoracoscope can be invaluable in the diagnosis and treatment of pleural disease and in the management of solitary pulmonary nodules. Video-assisted thoracic surgery allows the experienced surgeon to identify and wedge out peripheral nodules in most cases with minimal morbidity and mortality. Video-assisted thoracic surgery can spare patients with benign nodules the risks of open thoracotomy and can be useful for wedging out nodules in patients who have limited pulmonary reserve and cannot otherwise tolerate a lobectomy. Lobectomy is preferable to wedge excision or segmental resection for definitive therapy. Therefore, if a diagnosis of malignancy is made on frozen section at the time of video-assisted thoracic surgery and no contraindication exists, the procedure is usually converted to a formal thoracotomy and an anatomic resection is carried out. Video-assisted thoracic surgery is not indicated for lesions greater than 3 cm, as they are likely to be malignant and should be removed by open thoracotomy if the pulmonary reserve permits. Nor is the surgical technique indicated for centrally located lesions. Video-assisted thoracic surgery may be the initial procedure of choice for lesions that are not amenable to bronchoscopic or percutaneous needle aspiration biopsy because of the location—i.e., small peripheral lesions (outer third of lung), lesions located under ribs or the scapula, or lesions near areas of emphysema or bullous disease.

DIAGNOSTIC ALGORITHM

As is often the case in medicine, it is unwise to presume that an infallible algorithm can be provided for the evaluation of the solitary pulmonary nodule. Since no consensus can be reached on the basis of available data, the best that can be done is to offer recommendations. The pathway to be taken and final decision will rest on the individual clinician and patient. A 30-year-old nonsmoker, who is the mother of two children, and has an indeterminate lesion may not be willing to "observe serial radiographs" and therefore demand a resection; in contrast, a 75-year-old smoker with mild COPD and a lesion that seems to be a malignancy may decide to leave well enough alone and ignore it. The following recommendations represent one possible approach to a complex clinical problem:

1. On discovering a solitary pulmonary nodule, the clinician should determine whether it is a true solitary nodule, whether it is spherical, and whether it is located within the lung fields. Standard PA and lateral radiographs often suffice. A lateral radiograph may show the lesion to be superficial or may show other lesions hidden behind the diaphragm or the mediastinum. If the existence of the lesion remains in question, CT is indicated. A thorough history and physical may provide clues about the nodule's possible cause (a history of tuberculosis in an asymptomatic patient will suggest granuloma, while weight loss and adenopathy will point toward malignancy). Most of the time, solitary pulmonary nodules are asymptomatic.
2. Once it has been established that the nodule is truly solitary and a benign pattern of calcification is present, the nodule is considered benign and no further workup is necessary. Follow-up by serial radiographs is recommended every 6 months for a period of 2 years.
3. If prior chest radiographs are available and the nodule remains unchanged for 2 years or longer, no further workup is necessary. Follow-up with serial radiographs is recommended every 6 months to a year for 2 years.

4. Noncalcified nodules greater than 3 cm and of indeterminate stability are likely to be malignant and should be resected if adequate pulmonary reserve is present and if staging CT shows resectability. Mediastinoscopy may be required for staging if CT is equivocal.
5. Noncalcified nodules less than 3 cm and of indeterminate stability should undergo HRCT in a search for occult calcification. If a benign pattern of calcification is identified, no further workup is necessary. Follow-up by serial radiographs is recommended.
6. If no visible calcification is identified, a biopsy procedure is recommended. The initial procedure will depend on local availability, but bronchoscopy, percutaneous needle aspiration, or both will yield good results in the right setting. If no definite diagnosis is obtained or if the lesion is inaccessible to either bronchoscopy or percutaneous needle aspiration, thoracoscopy is recommended. If the lesion is inaccessible to thoracoscopy, open thoracotomy is required.

BIBLIOGRAPHY

Buckley JA, Scott WW, Siegelman SS, et al: Pulmonary nodules: Effect of increased data sampling on detection with spiral CT and confidence in diagnosis. *Radiology* 196:395–400, 1995.

Cummings SR, Lillington GA, Richard RJ: Estimating the probability of malignancy in solitary pulmonary nodules. *Am Rev Respir Dis* 134:449–452, 1986.

Dewan NA, Gupta NC, Redepenning LS, et al: Diagnostic efficacy of PET-FDG imaging in solitary pulmonary nodules. *Chest* 104:997–1002, 1993.

Guerney JW, Swensen SJ: Solitary pulmonary nodules: Determining the likelihood of malignancy with neural network analysis. *Radiology* 196:823–829, 1995.

Libby DM, Henschke CI, Yankelevitz DF: The solitary pulmonary nodule: Update 1995. *Am J Med* 99:491–496, 1995.

Mack MJ, Hazelrigg SR, Landreneau RJ, et al: Thoracoscopy for the diagnosis of the indeterminate solitary pulmonary nodule. *Ann Thorac Surg* 56:825–832, 1993.

Rubins JB, Bloomfield-Rubins H: Temporal trends in the prevalence of malignancy in resected pulmonary lesions. *Chest* 109:100–103, 1996.

Zwirewich CV, Vedal S, Miller RR, et al: Solitary pulmonary nodule: High-resolution CT and radiologic-pathologic correlation. *Radiology* 179:469–476, 1991.

55 | Non–Small Cell Lung Cancer—Clinical Aspects, Diagnosis, Staging, and Treatment*

Larry R. Kaiser

CLINICAL ASPECTS

Clinical Assessment

History

The most common initial symptom of non–small cell lung cancer (NSCLC) is cough, which is noted in 35 to 75 percent of cases. Dyspnea has been reported in 26 to 60 percent of patients presenting with NSCLC and is often an ominous development, signifying intrathoracic extension or dissemination. Among the thoracic complications of NSCLC giving rise to dyspnea are pleural effusion, atelectasis, postobstructive pneumonia, lymphangitic carcinoma, tumor microembolism, upper airway obstruction, and pneumothorax. Occasionally patients with chest wall involvement or mediastinal extension report dyspnea from pain-induced restriction of respiration. Chest pain is reported at presentation in 20 to 45 percent of cases of non–small cell lung cancer and usually arises via direct invasion or metastatic involvement of pain-sensitive intrathoracic structures. Most commonly, a peripheral tumor invades the costal parietal pleura and chest wall, giving rise to sharp, intermittent pleuritic pain. Hemoptysis is the sole presenting complaint in 5 to 10 percent of cases of NSCLC but may be one of the initial symptoms in up to 50 percent of new cases. Typically hemoptysis consists only of blood-streaked sputum, which is sometimes erroneously attributed to chronic bronchitis. Hoarseness is an initial complaint in 5 to 18 percent of cases of NSCLC and is often accompanied by cough. It usually indicates direct mediastinal extension or adenopathy that involves the left recurrent laryngeal nerve, thereby causing unilateral left vocal cord paralysis. Up to one-third of patients with NSCLC present with symptoms due to metastatic disease. The most common symptom is bone pain, which usually signifies metastatic involvement of a specific skeletal site. Symptoms reflective of central nervous system (CNS) metastases are next most common, especially those resulting from increased intracranial pressure, such as headache, nausea, and vomiting. Significant weight loss in NSCLC is deemed to have occurred when the patient has lost more than 10 lb or 5 percent of body weight. Weight loss reflects a complex interplay

---

*Edited from Chap. 112, "Non–Small Cell Lung Cancer—Clinical Aspects, Diagnosis, Staging, and Natural History," by Margolis ML. In: *Fishman's Pulmonary Diseases and Disorders,* 3d ed., edited by Fishman AP, Elias JA, Fishman JA, Grippi MA, Kaiser LR, Senior RM. New York, McGraw-Hill, 1998, pp 1759–1781. For fuller discussion of topics dealt with in this chapter, the reader is referred to the original text, as noted above.

TABLE 55-1 The Karnofsky Performance Scale

Definition	Percent	Criteria
Able to carry on normal activity and to work; no special care is needed.	100	Normal; no complaints; no evidence of disease.
	90	Able to carry on normal activity; minor signs or symptoms of disease.
	80	Normal activity with effort; some signs or symptoms of disease.
Unable to work; able to live at home; care for most personal needs; a varying amount of assistance is needed.	70	Cares for self; unable to carry on normal activity or to do active work.
	60	Requires occasional assistance but is able to care for most of needs.
	50	Requires considerable assistance and frequent medical care.
Unable to care for self; requires equivalent of institutional or hospital care; disease may be progressing rapidly.	40	Disabled; requires special care and assistance.
	30	Severely disabled; hospitalization is indicated, although death may not be imminent.
	20	Very sick; hospitalization necessary; active supportive treatment necessary.
	10	Moribund; fatal processes progressing rapidly.

of factors that vary from patient to patient, including depression, anorexia, metabolic derangements, increased work of breathing, pain, and cough. Circulating tumor necrosis factor, interleukins, and other cellular mediators are likely involved; thus, weight loss can be considered in part a paraneoplastic syndrome. Nevertheless, it remains an important historical element and prognostic factor in NSCLC. Performance status—a clinical index that reflects the global effect of the patient's comorbid diseases, age, weight loss, and tumor burden—is a vital consideration. Whether scored by the 10-point Karnofsky scale (Table 55-1), the 5-point Eastern Cooperative Oncology Group scale, or a dichotomous ambulatory/nonambulatory system, performance status consistently ranks among the most important prognostic variables in NSCLC. It has been estimated that only about 5 to 15 percent of patients are completely asymptomatic at the time of diagnosis. In most of these cases a chest radiograph performed as a routine upon hospital admission or as part of a "checkup" discloses an abnormality that proves to be a NSCLC. An important issue relating to asymptomatic presentations of NSCLC is that of screening. The concept that lung cancer could be detected at an early, more curable stage is attractive; yet screening tends to disclose relatively indolent cancers that might have remained clinically inapparent. In 1984 the results of a prospective multicenter trial were published that employed both sputum cytologies and chest radiographs to screen for early NSCLC among male smokers over the age of 45. The study demonstrated that chest roentgenography was a sensitive technique for detecting early-stage peripheral tumors, while sputum cytology, though less sensitive, permitted early recognition of many radiographically occult, central squamous cell carcinomas. Although a large proportion of early-stage tumors were detected and resected, it was extremely disappointing to find no change overall in lung cancer mortality in the screened population compared to a control population. Recently spiral computed tomographic (CT) scanning has been used to screen for lung cancers with the finding that about 10 percent of nodules detected actually proved to be lung cancer at the time of definitive therapy. A large prospective randomized trial of this screening modality is underway.

Physical Examination

Examination of the thorax must be meticulous. Stridor, a distinctly unusual presenting sign, must be recognized at once, since upper airway obstruction may progress with surprising rapidity once a critical airway diameter is reached. A localized wheeze must be distinguished from the generalized wheezing of chronic airflow obstruction. A disparity between the intensity of normally transmitted voice sounds compared with diminished breath sounds suggests an endobronchial tumor causing partial occlusion of a lobar or main-stem bronchus. Dullness and the absence of breath sounds over one lung may be accompanied by ipsilateral tracheal deviation in the case of atelectasis and a contralateral shift in the case of massive pleural effusion. When present, physical findings suggesting metastatic disease are valuable for planning the diagnostic and staging workup of non–small cell lung cancer.

Chest Imaging

As a widely available, inexpensive, and safe test that can simultaneously suggest the diagnosis and localize NSCLC, the standard chest radiograph remains the primary means for radiographic assessment. However, several important limitations pertaining to chest radiographs must be mentioned. First, up to 12 to 30 percent of lung cancers are missed on chest radiography; indeed, missed lung tumors are a leading cause for malpractice claims against radiologists. The superior spatial resolution, enhanced ability to detect calcium, and cross-sectional detail provided by CT scans address many of the shortcomings of chest radiographs. Such scans provide a clearer image of the primary lesion and its anatomic relationship to nearby chest structures. They also allow an evaluation of extrabronchial tumor, which aids in planning surgical or laser resection. Magnetic resonance imaging (MRI) generally affords few advantages over CT in imaging primary NSCLC. It is helpful in imaging apical lung tumors (see below); also, the increased intensity of recurrent lung cancer on T2-weighted images occasionally can be distinguished from the decreased signal of fibrotic lung. Nevertheless, MRI is typically reserved for specific staging problems in NSCLC (see below).

Many other imaging techniques—including ultrasound, fluoroscopy, bronchography, superior venography, and lordotic, oblique, and lateral decubitus films—are occasionally of value in answering specific questions relating to NSCLC and its intrathoracic complications. Also, positron emission tomography with fluoro-2-deoxyglucose has recently emerged as a potentially useful means of exploiting the high metabolic activity of NSCLC to demonstrate primary tumor and metastatic lesions.

Pulmonary Function Tests

Pulmonary function tests are usually obtained as part of the initial clinical assessment of patients with NSCLC. The severity of associated chronic airflow obstruction and adequacy of pulmonary reserve are paramount in planning treatment. The measurement of pulmonary function enters into the risk/benefit analysis in the management of the patient being considered for resection, but recent evidence suggests that even patients who classically would be considered to have poor pulmonary function often are surgical candidates. Patients who in the past would not have been considered for operation because of their pulmonary function routinely are undergoing resection based on information learned from patients with severe emphysema undergoing lung volume reduction surgery.

Clinical Presentations

Mediastinal Involvement

In roughly 40 percent of cases of NSCLC, the mediastinum is involved either by the presence of lymph node metastases or by direct extension, posing a critical clinical dilemma. Patients with mediastinal spread from NSCLC may be completely asymptomatic, but many complain of cough or vague chest pain and may exhibit symptoms and signs that reflect involvement of contiguous mediastinal structures. These include the phrenic nerve, left recurrent laryngeal nerve, pericardium and heart, pulmonary veins and arteries, aorta, superior vena cava, and esophagus. Massive adenopathy may also produce lymphatic blockade, resulting in pleural effusions or diffuse lymphangitic dissemination. Ultimately an invasive procedure such as mediastinoscopy, mediastinotomy, or thoracotomy is necessary to reliably define the mediastinum in NSCLC.

Pneumonia, Obstructive Pneumonitis, and Atelectasis

Patients with alveolar infiltrates on the chest radiograph are frequently referred to the pulmonary clinician because of concern for underlying NSCLC. One obvious concern in this setting is that the chronic infiltrate itself represents the diffuse form of bronchoalveolar cell carcinoma. Alternatively, a hilar mass or radiographically occult endobronchial lesion may cause a true obstructive pneumonitis. Atelectasis is frequently the predominant feature of obstructing NSCLC, particularly in the absence of infection. Atelectasis may vary from subsegmental to collapse of an entire lung.

Chest Wall Involvement

In up to 5 percent of cases, NSCLC invades the parietal pleura and chest wall. The most common presenting symptom in such cases is chest pain, which is initially described as an intermittent dull ache.

Pleural Effusion

Pleural effusion can be detected in 7 to 24 percent of lung cancer cases at presentation and is a common cause of dyspnea in patients with NSCLC. Effusion may also be associated with chest pain and cough or give rise to no symptoms at all. Malignant cells can be demonstrated on a single large-volume thoracentesis in about 60 percent of cases, depending on histologic type, with closed pleural biopsy adding to the yield. The finding of malignant cells in the fluid confirms stage IIIb disease and a relatively poor prognosis. Occasionally fluid formation is only indirectly related to the tumor, via obstructive pneumonia or atelectasis.

Superior Vena Cava Syndrome

Though superior vena cava syndrome may result from small cell carcinoma, lymphoma, metastatic carcinoma, and a host of benign causes, it remains an important presentation of NSCLC. Patients characteristically complain of headache, swelling of the face, neck, and upper extremities, or a host of thoracic symptoms such as dyspnea, cough, chest pain, and dysphagia. Syncope or dizziness associated with bending is also mentioned frequently. Physical examination may show facial edema, neck vein distention, and striking collateral venous engorgement over the anterior chest wall and upper abdomen.

Phrenic Nerve Entrapment

Occasionally NSCLC may involve either the left or right phrenic nerve via mediastinal extension, resulting in a paralyzed hemidiaphragm. Affected patients may be asymptomatic or complain of dyspnea, related in part to the decrements in FEV_1 and FVC resulting from hemidiaphragmatic paralysis. Phrenic nerve involvement is staged as T3 disease (stage IIIa); if this is the only mediastinal structure invaded, it is not a contraindication to surgical resection. Involvement of other mediastinal structures often may only be evident at the time of operation; thus, patients with phrenic nerve involvement should not, as a matter of course, be denied the option of surgery.

Extrathoracic Metastases

NSCLC frequently metastasizes to distant organs. Though the metastatic potential of NSCLC is less than that of small cell carcinoma, distant spread is demonstrable at presentation in over one-third of cases, particularly with the large cell undifferentiated and adenocarcinoma subtypes. The usual sites of distant metastatic disease include the adrenals, brain, liver, lung, and bone, though virtually any organ can be affected. Metastases may present at the same time as the primary tumor or occur much later, and they may be single or multiple, clinically silent or demanding of emergent diagnosis and treatment.

Adrenal Metastases

Adrenal metastases are present in roughly 35 percent of patients dying of NSCLC and are the most common metastatic site in patients dying of lung cancer within 1 month of surgical resection with curative intent. Moreover, adrenal abnormalities represent the *only* site of metastatic involvement in up to 5 percent of cases. Adrenal metastases are usually silent clinically.

Central Nervous System Metastases

Brain metastases are seen more frequently with the adenocarcinoma histologic subtype as compared with squamous carcinoma and carry a poor prognosis. Lung cancer is by far the most common cause for brain metastases, which are usually multiple but occasionally occur as solitary lesions (i.e., no other metastases present). The most frequent symptom is headache, and neurologic features most often suggest increased intracranial pressure.

Liver Metastases

Liver metastases are found in 30 to 45 percent of cases of NSCLC coming to autopsy. Unfortunately, the history, physical examination, and routine biochemical tests of hepatic function are unreliable indicators of liver metastases, though a general correlation with organ-specific and non–organ-specific clinical abnormalities has been repeatedly demonstrated.

Skeletal Metastases

Bone metastases in NSCLC tend to develop in trabecular bone and are usually osteolytic, but osteoblastic metastases are occasionally associated with adenocarcinoma. Bone metastases may be asymptomatic or produce pain and tenderness. The favored sites are the ribs, vertebrae, and long bones of the legs and arms.

Lymphatic Metastases

The initial lymph node stations involved by metastatic non–small cell lung cancer are intrathoracic and include 13 intrapulmonary, hilar, and mediastinal sites designated in the American Joint Committee on Cancer (AJCC) system. However, further lymphatic spread may occur in up to 42 percent of cases at presentation, especially to supraclavicular nodes, which are considered an N3 (stage IIIb) site.

Skin and Subcutaneous Metastases

Cutaneous metastases are rarely the first clinical manifestation of NSCLC; usually other metastases are evident and the prognosis is extremely poor. The most common locations are the chest, back, abdomen, scalp, and neck. The lower extremities are rarely affected, despite their relatively large surface area.

DIAGNOSIS

Sputum Cytology

Sputum cytology, first used to diagnose lung cancer in 1887, remains the principal noninvasive means for diagnosing NSCLC, with a sensitivity ranging from 20 to 77 percent, depending on patient selection and numerous technical factors. The yield is significantly higher with central versus peripheral, lower lobe versus upper lobe, and large versus small tumors. Sometimes a sputum cytology specimen is diagnostic of NSCLC but no abnormality is apparent on the chest radiograph or upper airway examination. In such cases a meticulous bronchoscopy with segmental sampling may be required to identify an early peripheral lesion. Unfortunately, an advanced tumor is sometimes found in spite of the negative chest film.

Fiberoptic Bronchoscopy

Fiberoptic bronchoscopy is probably the most frequently utilized and important test for diagnosing NSCLC. Suspicious endobronchial areas are usually sampled with a series of techniques, including washings, brushings, and forceps biopsy. Many experts perform washings after the brushings and biopsies to increase cellular yield, while brush biopsy usually precedes forceps biopsy to prevent sheets of red cells from coating the brush. Each of these modalities has an average yield of 50 to 85 percent. Transbronchial needle aspiration is an additional technique of particular value when the tumor is infiltrating deeply beneath intact mucosa or causing bronchial compression. If no endobronchial lesion is apparent, brushings, transbronchial forceps biopsy, and transbronchial needle aspiration contribute to the diagnostic yield, particularly if C-arm or biplanar fluoroscopy is employed. However, it is agreed that bronchoscopic yield is highly dependent on the size of the tumor. In one series, the yield was only 25 percent for malignant lesions under 2 cm, 40 percent for lesions between 2.0 and 3.0 cm, and 56 percent for those between 3.0 and 4.0 cm. Location is also a prime determinant; for central endobronchial lesions, the overall yield approximates 90 percent, while peripheral lesions are diagnosed in 50 to 60 percent of cases.

Despite its attractive features, fiberoptic bronchoscopy should not be performed in every patient with suspected NSCLC. For patients with a small undiagnosed but growing lesion on the chest radiograph, fiberoptic bronchoscopy contributes little in terms of diagnostic yield or staging (see below); such patients can frequently be referred directly to the surgeon for definitive diagnosis and treatment via a single procedure (resection). In addition, patients with inoperable tumors and those with unmistakable clinical evidence of metastatic disease are often best diagnosed via sputum cytology, transthoracic needle biopsy, or other techniques.

Transthoracic Needle Aspiration Biopsy

Unlike fiberoptic bronchoscopy, transthoracic needle aspiration is better suited for peripheral cancers, for which the diagnostic yield is maximized and incidence of transthoracic needle aspiration–related pneumothorax is minimized. As with fiberoptic bronchoscopy, the yield is clearly dependent on the size of the tumor. Though an overall yield of up to 94 to 100 percent has been reported in selected series, it can be as low as 15 percent for lesions less than 2 cm and about 50 percent for lesions between 2.0 and 3.0 cm. Transthoracic needle aspiration is perhaps most useful for patients with suspected NSCLC who cannot tolerate or refuse fiberoptic bronchoscopy and for inoperable patients who require a tissue diagnosis prior to embarking on a course of radiotherapy. Transthoracic needle aspiration must not be employed indiscriminantly. For a small, peripheral growing lesion in a heavy smoker, it is often prudent to proceed directly to operation rather than attempting a needle biopsy. In such cases a negative biopsy is seldom fully reassuring and surgical excision is still warranted. A positive transthoracic needle aspiration for NSCLC also mandates surgery, assuming the patient meets the usual operative criteria. Thus, patient management is not altered by transthoracic needle aspiration and it can be omitted in this setting.

STAGING

General Considerations

The stage of NSCLC is not only among the most powerful predictors of prognosis (along with weight loss and performance status) but also allows for meaningful comparisons among subsets of patients in terms of clinical characteristics and responses to treatment. In 1986, the AJCC substantially revised the TNM system for non–small cell lung cancer to reflect newly appreciated differences in prognostic groups and recent progress in thoracic surgery that enabled curative resection for several localized tumors previously considered unresectable. The new system, reproduced in its entirety in Table 55-2, is the foundation upon which rests much of the current

TABLE 55-2 Staging of Lung Cancer: 1986 American Joint Committee on Cancer System

Primary tumor (T)
TX   Tumor proven by the presence of malignant cells in bronchopulmonary secretions but not visualized roentgenographically or bronchoscopically, or any tumor that cannot be assessed, as in a retreatment staging.
TO   No evidence of primary tumor.
TIS   Carcinoma in situ.
T1   A tumor that is 3.0 cm or less in greatest dimension surrounded by lung or visceral pleura, and without evidence of invasion proximal to a lobar bronchus at bronchoscopy.[a]
T2   A tumor more than 3.0 cm in greatest dimension; or a tumor of any size that either invades the visceral pleura or has associated atelectasis or obstructive pneumonitis extending to the hilar region. At bronchoscopy, the proximal extent of demonstrable tumor must be within a lobar bronchus or at least 2.0 cm distal to the carina. Any associated atelectasis or obstructive pneumonitis must involve less than an entire lung.
T3   A tumor of any size with direct extension into the chest wall (including superior sulcus tumors), diaphragm, or the mediastinal pleura or pericardium without involving the heart, great vessels, trachea, esophagus, or vertebral bodies; or a tumor in the main bronchus within 2 cm of the carina without involving the carina.
T4   A tumor of any size with invasion of the mediastinum or involving heart, great vessels, trachea, esophagus, vertebral bodies or carina; or with the presence of malignant pleural effusion.[b]

Nodal involvement (N)
N0   No demonstrable metastasis to regional lymph nodes.
N1   Metastasis to lymph nodes in the peribronchial or the ipsilateral hilar region, or both, including direct extension.
N2   Metastasis to ipsilateral mediastinal lymph nodes and subcarinal lymph nodes.
N3   Metastasis to contralateral mediastinal lymph nodes, contralateral hilar lymph nodes, ipsilateral or contralateral scalene or supraclavicular lymph nodes.

Distant metastasis (M)
M0   No (known) distant metastasis.
M1   Distant metastasis present; specify site(s).

Stage grouping			
Occult carcinoma	TX	N0	M0
Stage 0	TIS	Carcinoma in situ	
Stage I	T1	N0	M0
	T2	N0	M0
Stage II	T1	N1	M0
	T2	N1	M0
Stage IIIa	T3	N0	M0
	T3	N1	M0
	T1–3	N2	M0
Stage IIIb	Any T	N3	M0
	T4	Any N	M0
Stage IV	Any T	Any N	M1

[a]The uncommon superficial tumor of any size with its invasive component limited to the bronchial wall, which may extend proximal to the main bronchus, is classified as T1.
[b]Most pleural effusions associated with lung cancer are due to tumor. There are, however, some few patients in whom cytopathologic examination of pleural fluid (on more than one specimen) is negative for tumor, and the fluid is not bloody and is not an exudate. In such cases where these elements and clinical judgment dictate that the effusion is not related to the tumor, the patients should be staged T1, T2, or T3, excluding effusion as a staging element.

preoperative evaluation of patients with NSCLC. A long-standing controversy continues to rage over the proper utilization of noninvasive staging tests. Some authors advocate ordering complete metastatic workups for patients with organ-specific or non–organ-specific clinical factors while omitting all scans if these features are absent. Our current staging system makes no allowance for the vast intrinsic biologic variability among NSCLCs, as detailed elsewhere in this text. It seems likely that "biologic staging" of tumors via their genetic characteristics will assume great importance in the near future.

Thoracic Staging

Computed Tomography of the Chest

The CT scan provides important information regarding the size of the mediastinal lymph nodes, the presence of other parenchymal lesions, and the status of the pleural space, thereby greatly facilitating the clinical staging of a given patient. However, despite its safety and utility, a number of limitations pertain to the use of CT scanning as a staging test in NSCLC. The accuracy of CT scanning of the mediastinum depends on the site of the lymph node involvement, the extent of lymph node dissection at the time of thoracotomy, technical details such as the type of scanner and spacing interval between cuts, and the patient population being studied. The inability of the CT scan to detect micrometastases has already been alluded to; it is equally important to note that enlarged inflammatory nodes are erroneously categorized as "positive" in as many as 20 percent of cases. Thus, the specificity and sensitivity of CT scans in detecting metastatic involvement of mediastinal nodes are probably in the range of 70 to 80 percent. CT is unable to reliably identify chest wall invasion, or distinguish resectable from unresectable invasion of the mediastinum or vertebral body except in advanced cases.

Magnetic Resonance Imaging of the Chest

MRI is subject to many of the same limitations described for CT scans, especially the tendency to miss small tumor-bearing nodes, in addition to its poorer spatial resolution characteristics. In fact, several studies have shown that MRI and CT scans are roughly equivalent for detecting mediastinal nodal involvement. Therefore, MRI cannot be endorsed for routine use for thoracic staging of NSCLC. Most prospective studies comparing thoracic CT scans and MRI in terms of other staging applications have also failed to reveal a clear advantage for either study. However, MRI can sometimes provide useful staging data and is the imaging modality of choice for apical (superior sulcus) lung tumors. For these lesions, the coronal and sagittal planar images obtainable by MRI more clearly delineate invasion into chest wall, vertebral body, subclavian vessels, and brachial plexus. Vertebral body involvement and invasion of neural foramina is much more clearly delineated on MRI than on CT, and MRI should always be performed when a primary tumor is in close proximity to vertebral body on CT scan.

Surgical Staging

The role of invasive staging and the specific procedures utilized deserve mention. In discussing stage, distinction must be made between *clinical stage* and *pathologic stage.* The former is based solely on noninvasive imaging studies, whereas the latter depends on actual histologic material obtained either by invasive staging studies or at the time of the surgical resection. A clinical stage is no more or no less than an assumption which is only as good as the noninvasive studies employed. In general, invasive staging is reserved for cases in which definitive assessment of mediastinal lymph node involvement will affect management, specifically whether to proceed with thoracotomy. Thus, the decision to employ surgical staging usually implies that the patient is free of distant metastases and consents to thoracotomy if surgical staging procedures are negative. The definitive invasive procedure for staging the mediastinum remains mediastinoscopy. This procedure, though seemingly simple to perform, yields information regarding both ipsilateral and contralateral mediastinal lymph node involvement. The information obtained from mediastinoscopy is operator dependent and relies greatly on the experience of the surgeon. Mediastinoscopy is a difficult technique to master and the morbidity that may occur during the procedure often causes the less experienced surgeon to avoid the procedure. The close proximity of a number of major vascular structures makes the procedure daunting even to the experienced practitioner. The vessels include the inominate artery, the aortic arch, the superior vena cava, the azygos vein, and the right main pulmonary artery. Unfortunately none of these structures are easily seen, and success requires that the operator know where they are located to avoid injury.

The left recurrent laryngeal nerve and the esophagus are also subject to injury. The presence of involved mediastinal lymph nodes, if ipsilateral, usually prompts the use of induction therapy prior to operation or sometimes nonoperative treatment with curative intent.

There are nodal stations that cannot be accessed by standard cervical mediastinoscopy. These include the aortopulmonary window (level 5), a common site for lymph node involvement in left upper lobe tumors, and the posterior subcarinal space (level 7). However, the anterior subcarinal space, usually representative of the contents of the posterior subcarinal space, is accessible to mediastinoscopic biopsy, and involved lymph nodes in the aortopulmonary window in the absence of other lymph node disease carries a prognosis equivalent to N1 (hilar) disease. The aortopulmonary window, a common site of nodal spread from tumors of the left upper lobe, may be reached with a parasternal mediastinotomy, or so-called Chamberlain procedure. An incision is made over the left second costal cartilage, the cartilage is excised, and the pleural reflection is swept laterally to access the aortopulmonary window in an extrapleural plane. Similarly, video thoracoscopy aids in the staging of lung cancer, although not in lieu of mediastinoscopy, which offers an opportunity to sample nodes on the right and left through one incision, but as an adjunct. This technique also visualizes the pleural space, especially useful in the patient with a pleural effusion and negative fluid cytology, so as to rule out diffuse pleural involvement and prevent an unnecessary thoracotomy. Other nodules seen on CT scan which may have an impact on treatment planning also may be excised and defined histologically prior to formal thoracotomy. Video thoracoscopic examination has not proven particularly useful in assessing resectability of a tumor where there is a question because of presumed invasion of an adjacent mediastinal structure.

Mediastinoscopy is performed through a small (2 cm) incision made in the neck 1 cm above the sternal notch. The area explored by mediastinoscopy, the superior mediastinum, is palpated first by inserting a finger along the anterior aspect of the trachea which also serves to develop the space and facilitate insertion of the mediastinoscope.

Obviously involved lymph nodes often may be palpated, but palpation alone is insufficient, since intranodal disease may be present which can only be identified if representative biopsies of the important nodal stations are taken following insertion of the mediastinoscope. Nodal stations most frequently sampled include levels 2 (upper paratracheal) and 4 (lower paratracheal) on the right, level 3 (pretracheal), level 7 (subcarinal), and level 4 on the left. Because the left level 4 lymph nodes occur at a slightly higher location, identifying separate level 2 nodes on the left can be difficult. It is not necessary always to sample all nodal stations; if there are nodes obviously involved, these, along with contralateral nodes, are all that is necessary to adequately stage the patient.

Extrathoracic Staging

Adrenal Glands and Liver

Because of frequent occult metastases to the adrenal glands, thoracic CT scans, when ordered to stage NSCLC, are routinely extended caudally to include them. Since 2 to 9 percent of the general population harbors incidental adrenal adenomas, the appearance of a unilateral adrenal mass on a staging CT scan for NSCLC poses a common and thorny problem. In the final analysis, needle or open biopsy may be necessary to resolve difficult cases. Liver imaging is also a standard component of extrathoracic staging of NSCLC, and CT scans, ultrasonography, and MRI may be employed for this purpose. Computed tomography, currently the favored modality, suggests metastatic foci in liver in a highly variable percentage of patients, depending on the presence or absence of clinical indicators suggesting metastatic disease. Unfortunately, single or multiple liver defects on CT scans may also result from cysts, abscesses, hemangiomas, etc. Difficult cases usually may be resolved with an MRI that may be able to differentiate hemangioma from metastatic disease. Occasionally liver biopsy either by needle or laparoscopy may be necessary to resolve the issue.

Central Nervous System (Brain)

There are excellent data to suggest that MRI of the brain, especially when combined with gadolinium-based contrast infusion, is more sensitive than CT for the detection of metastatic disease, particularly in delineating small lesions. Despite this knowledge, CT scan often is used as the screening modality of choice usually because of easier availability and lower cost. A suspicious CT scan prompts the performance of an MRI.

Up to 10 percent of patients may harbor brain metastases in the absence of all clinical factors. This finding, coupled with the usual futility of attempting curative thoracic surgery in the presence of brain metastases (with few exceptions), has led some clinicians to obtain a brain CT scan in virtually all patients with NSCLC. The standard test is currently the technetium-99m radionuclide scan. Unfortunately, as alluded to previously, skeletal uptake of this isotope is quite nonspecific, and degenerative vertebral changes and old traumatic rib foci produce false-positive scans in up to 40 percent of cases. A second problem lies in correlating the bone scan with clinical features suggesting metastases. Depending on the clinical scenario, spot skeletal films, MRI, or an open biopsy may be appropriate. Alternatively, the case for metastatic disease may rest solely on the bone scan, especially in poor surgical candidates with multiple characteristic scan abnormalities.

SURGICAL TREATMENT OF LUNG CANCER

Recognizing that operation is the best treatment for early-stage disease, it is important that the appropriate procedure be performed. Lobectomy remains the definitive resection for most lung cancers, since it is an anatomic resection which removes the regional lymph nodes that are located along the lobar bronchus. Doing less than a lobectomy must be considered a compromise, although a nonanatomic wedge excision is tempting for small primary tumors. Not only does a wedge excision not include the lobar bronchus, precluding evaluation of lobar lymph nodes, but it provides only a minimal parenchymal margin. The Lung Cancer Study Group (LCSG) addressed the question of lobectomy versus limited resection for T1N0 lesions (tumor <3 cm, negative lymph nodes) in a prospective randomized trial. The early analysis of the data demonstrated an increased incidence of local recurrence in the limited resection group but no difference in survival. The final analysis revealed superior survival for patients in the lobectomy group. Other studies have looked retrospectively at patients undergoing limited resection, which includes segmental resection, and have demonstrated long-term survivors, but the LCSG study stands alone as the only randomized trial.

For patients in whom lobectomy is not feasible, a lesser resection offers the best alternative, although admittedly it is a compromise. Patients in this category are those with borderline pulmonary function or those who have had previous pulmonary resections. Whenever possible the lesser resection should be an anatomic segmental resection, which takes the segmental artery and vein as well as the segmental bronchus with its accompanying lymph nodes. A classic segmental resection is a relatively difficult operation, and many surgeons do not possess a significant amount of experience in performing this procedure. The prototype segmental resections include the lingular resection and resection of the superior segment of the lower lobe, but any lung segment may be removed anatomically. The key to segmental resection is the identification of the segmental artery which, once ligated and divided, reveals the location of the segmental bronchus which is taken next. The segmental vein is divided last, and the parenchyma is divided with a stapler or "stripped" as was originally described.

Depending mainly on the location of the tumor, more extensive and complex resections than lobectomy may be required. The determination as to when to perform pneumonectomy is made at the time of operation, rarely preoperatively. Recognizing that even today pneumonectomy carries a perioperative mortality of at least 5 percent, we do everything possible to avoid removing an entire lung. There are only a few absolute indications for performing pneumonectomy for the experienced surgeon. These include such proximal involvement of the main pulmonary artery that it is difficult to place a clamp on the artery, endobronchial tumor so extensive as to preclude sleeve resection, and involvement of the confluence of the pulmonary veins or of the left atrium. A "difficult" fissure, unless tumor involves the artery in the fissure, is not an indication for pneumonectomy, nor is tumor crossing a fissure an absolute indication. Pneumonectomy, technically, is an easier operation to perform than lobectomy, requiring very little dissection and only several applications of the stapler. Sleeve resections, or bronchoplastic procedures, are technically more demanding procedures which result in the same bronchial resection as a pneumonectomy, yet preserve lung tissue. The prototypical bronchoplastic procedure is the right upper lobe sleeve resection, where the main bronchus is divided just proximal to the right upper lobe takeoff and the bronchus intermedius is divided just distal to the upper lobe bronchus. The right upper lobe, with tumor present at the lobar orifice, is thus removed with a portion of the main-stem bronchus, and the bronchus intermedius is anastomosed to the main-stem bronchus. Thus the proximal bronchial division occurs essentially at the same site as if a pneumonectomy had been performed. Other sleeve resections are possible on both the right and left side, all result in lung conservation and are associated with long-term survival equivalent to pneumonectomy, depending on the indications.

A complete pulmonary resection requires more than simply excision of the tumor and the surrounding lung parenchyma be it lobe or entire lung. The operation is incomplete without excision of lymph nodes to complete the staging assessment. We perform a mediastinal lymph node dissection even if mediastinoscopy has been performed. This procedure, where, at least on the right side, the entire contents of the superior mediastinum are removed, is the only one that assures complete lymph nodes staging. The hilar and peribronchial lymph nodes are removed with the lobectomy or pneumonectomy specimen but must be specifically searched for by the pathologist. Any sampling procedure of mediastinal lymph nodes depends on how the nodes to be sampled are chosen. The failure to include mediastinal lymph nodes as part of a resection results in incomplete information. The mediastinal lymph nodes should not only be removed as part of the resection but should also be labeled according to their location in the mediastinum.

Having removed the mediastinal lymph nodes, it is not uncommon to find microscopic disease in a node that grossly appears normal. Finding tumor in mediastinal lymph nodes portends a significantly worse prognosis and at least prompts thought regarding postoperative treatment. Postoperative adjuvant therapy, usually radiation therapy, has not improved survival. Numerous studies have been conducted to assess whether postoperative adjuvant therapy might improve prognosis in these high-risk patients. Thus far there is no evidence that postoperative therapy, whether chemotherapy, radiation therapy, or a combination of the two, improves survival in completely resected patients. The results of a recently completed prospective, randomized trial (ECOG 3590) where all of the American cooperative oncology groups participated also showed no benefit for chemotherapy combined with radiation therapy when compared with radiation therapy alone for patients with positive lymph nodes identified at the time of thoracotomy. The designation *locally advanced* includes a wide variety of lesions which extend outside of the lung parenchyma whether by direct extension or nodal involvement to involve other structures within the hemithorax. Certain criteria need to be fulfilled before considering extending the indications for resection, since the intent is to maximize survival. The most obvious criterion is the exclusion of disseminated disease, and thus it is key to complete an extent of disease evaluation before embarking upon a complex resection where the indications for resection have been extended.

N2 Disease

Classically the involvement of mediastinal lymph nodes with tumor precluded any attempt at surgical resection, since most of these patients died within 2 years due to the development of disseminated disease. Utilizing mediastinoscopy, mediastinal lymph node involvement may be detected prior to thoracotomy, saving the patient a needless operation. Contralateral nodal disease, which carries a significantly worse prognosis than ipsilateral disease, may also be detected at mediastinoscopy and if found usually takes the patient out of the realm of operative intervention even if combined with neoadjuvant therapy. Ipsilateral mediastinal lymph node involvement usually is treated with a preoperative regimen combining chemotherapy with radiation therapy and followed by resection approximately 3 to 4 weeks after completion of the induction therapy. At least two randomized trials have shown an advantage for chemotherapy prior to operation in this group of patients. Multiple other nonrandomized phase II trials of preoperative therapy have been carried out in patients with N2 disease utilizing chemotherapy alone or chemotherapy combined with radiation therapy. Resections following preoperative therapy can be extremely difficult and hazardous because of the fibrosis that often results as a response to the therapy. This is especially significant when there has been a response in involved lymph nodes, since the nodes are intimately associated with the pulmonary artery and its branches, often making resection quite tricky. Despite the numerous studies addressing preoperative therapy, whether chemotherapy alone or combined with radiation therapy, the question as to what role surgical resection plays in the outcome of patients with N2 disease remains unanswered. To date no conclusive studies have proved that operation is superior to radiation therapy in controlling local disease in these patients. One reason for this is the difficulty in accruing patients on a study where the randomization chooses between a surgical and a nonsurgical arm.

Thus, although there is a suggestion that neoadjuvant therapy results in improved survival when compared to surgery alone, this has not been confirmed in a phase III randomized, large multi-institutional trial. There is evidence, however, that 60 to 75 percent of patients with lymph node disease as the only site of spread respond to the preoperative regimens, a significantly greater response than when the same regimens are used in patients with disseminated disease, and over half of these patients will go on to resection. Between 10 and 20 percent of patients resected have no evidence of disease found on histologic examination of the resected material. The activity of the neoadjuvant regimen in this patient population cannot be denied. Whether surgical excision is required or radiation is an acceptable modality for local control remains to be determined. Of great importance is the consideration of quality of life in patients undergoing these combined regimens, an area that has not been adequately addressed. The quality-of-life measurement tools are available to incorporate into future studies so that additional information should be forthcoming.

Chest Wall Resection

Approximately 5 percent of lung cancers involve the chest wall by direct extension. This involvement may be limited to the parietal pleura or may invade the endothoracic fascia, intercostal muscle, or ribs. Chest wall involvement by direct extension is *not* a contraindication to resection unless vertebral bodies are invaded, and even then, under some circumstances, resection may still be completed. Chest wall pain is the most sensitive predictor of chest wall involvement in a patient with a peripheral lung lesion where there is a question of chest wall invasion. Neither the CT scan nor the MRI can distinguish between abutment and invasion unless there is gross invasion of bone. The radionuclide bone scan may be negative with chest wall involvement, especially if only the parietal pleura and muscle are involved. Lesions involving parietal pleura or other chest wall structures are staged as T3 primary tumors, but often definitive staging cannot be accomplished until the time of operation. It is particularly important to assess the mediastinum in these patients, since mediastinal lymph node involvement is the single best prognostic indicator. Three-year survival approaches zero in patients with chest wall and mediastinal lymph node involvement, underscoring the importance of invasive mediastinal lymph node staging, usually with mediastinoscopy, prior to considering thoracotomy in this patient group. Conversely, greater than 50 percent 5-year survival can be expected in patients with chest wall involvement with negative mediastinal lymph nodes as long as the resection margins are negative.

The chest wall resection should include at least one rib and preferably two above and below the area of chest wall invaded. Margins of 3 to 5 cm should also be taken anteriorly and posteriorly. The intent is to achieve negative margins so the resection should be wide; there is little if any additional morbidity to taking a somewhat larger piece of chest wall. Once the chest wall block is totally mobilized, the lobectomy and mediastinal lymph node dissection are completed. A mediastinoscopy should have been performed earlier, but a lymph node dissection should be done for complete staging. A posterior chest wall defect is reconstructed with polypropylene mesh, and a defect in the anterior chest wall should be reconstructed with a sandwich of methylmethacrylate cement and polypropylene mesh. Posteriorly the defect is covered additionally by the scapula, but anteriorly the rigid fixation provided by the methyl methacrylate and mesh eliminates any paradoxical motion that might interfere with mechanics of breathing. Interference with the mechanics of breathing is much less likely to occur with posterior defects.

Tumors Involving the Mediastinum by Direct Extension

Some centrally located primary tumors may involve structures in the mediastinum by direct extension. The assessment of this involvement, whether there is true invasion or just abutment and adherence, cannot be determined until the findings are seen intraoperatively and then often only as the dissection proceeds. The distinction between a T3 tumor involving the mediastinum and a T4 tumor depends on the mediastinal structure invaded. Tumors invading structures such as the phrenic nerve, mediastinal pleura or fat, the pericardium, or the diaphragm that may be readily removed are classified as T3 primary tumors and as such are in the stage IIIa group which also includes mediastinal lymph node involvement and tumors involving chest wall. T4 primary tumors involve those structures which usually are not considered to be resectable such as aorta, left atrium, superior vena cava, trachea, esophagus, or vertebral bodies. There are occasions when tumors involving these structures are resected, most commonly with lesions involving the vena cava or left atrium. Rarely if ever is a portion of aorta resected for excision of a lung tumor, but a lesion may involve only the muscular coat of the esophagus and thus may be amenable to resection. What is important to recognize, however, is despite the seeming ability to remove some of these invasive lesions, the prognosis for long-term survival is dismal. For T4 lesions, fewer than 10 percent of patients are alive at 5 years. From the viewpoint of the surgeon, though certainly recognizing the poor long-term survival with these tumors, in the absence of mediastinal lymph node involvement it is difficult to simply back out and leave the tumor in place when it is possible to resect the lesion with minimal morbidity. Such would be the situation where a portion of vena cava or a piece of left atrium is all that is necessary to complete a resection. Extensive involvement of one of these structures is an absolute contraindication to resection.

Palliative Resections

The goal of treatment in patients with advanced malignancies is to preserve the quality of life. This may require intervention with a potentially morbid treatment in order to relieve the patient of an unpleasant complication of the disease. Palliative radiation therapy is most often used in situations where the patient's quality of life is, or could be, substantially compromised. Although response rates to chemotherapy have improved, radiotherapy remains the mainstay of palliative therapy for distressing local symptoms of lung cancer. The selection of patients for palliative radiotherapy is often more difficult than is the selection for adjuvant or definitive treatment, since the goals may be less well defined. The presence of a large lung cancer in and of itself is not an indication for palliative radiotherapy, particularly when a patient has been shown to have distant metastases with minimal, or no, local symptoms. Fairly clear situations which call for palliative thoracic radiotherapy include the superior vena caval syndrome, hemoptysis, and significant pain. Cough, often due to partial bronchial obstruction, is frequently palliated by radiotherapy. Atelectasis is rarely reversed by radiotherapy, although consideration should be given to irradiation in order to prevent refractory postobstructive atelectasis and pneumonia when impending obstruction of a main-stem or lobar bronchus is identified by bronchoscopy. Palliative radiotherapy generally involves lower total doses and smaller fields than does definitive radiotherapy. Larger daily fraction size is used (250 to 400 cGy per day) in the attempt to achieve relatively rapid palliation and to minimize the number of trips to the radiotherapy department. In addition, late radiotherapy complications (which are related to larger fraction size) are less relevant in this patient population. There is no standard palliation regimen, and treatments have ranged from 1000 cGy once to a full course of 6000 cGy in 200-cGy fractions. A typical compromise palliative radiotherapy schema is to deliver 300 cGy in 10 fractions, which may be followed by a second similar course of treatment, either after a 1- to 2-week break or later, at the time of local progression.

Finally, radiotherapy plays an important role in the palliation of metastatic sites, including brain and bone metastases. Whole-brain irradiation, to a dose of 3000 cGy in 10 fractions, is appropriate therapy for multiple brain metastases. In addition to palliating neurologic symptoms in many patients, it appears to improve survival marginally more than can be achieved by steroids alone. In addition, patients with solitary brain metastases appear to benefit from a combination of whole-brain irradiation and surgical resection. Patients with solitary brain metastases who are not candidates for craniotomy may similarly benefit from high-dose focal stereotactic irradiation of metastases. For bony metastases, most patients will achieve at least partial pain relief from 2000 to 3000 cGy in 5 to 10 fractions. The appearance caused by disfiguring skin and subcutaneous metastases can be improved by similar modest dosages of irradiation. Occasionally, pain from adrenal metastases can be palliated with radiotherapy in patients in whom the radiotherapy field would not include an excessive amount of liver, kidney, or bowel.

There is essentially no role for palliative resections in the modern management of NSCLC. Morbidity resulting from the primary tumor usually may be managed using modalities other than operation. There probably is no justification for operation if less than a complete resection is anticipated. At the present time there is no role for surgical "debulking" in the management of the patient with unresectable disease. With the newer treatment planning modalities available, radiation therapy can be given accurately and in high doses to patients who are inoperable or unresectable. Patients with hemoptysis or postobstructive pneumonia may benefit from laser excision of the endobronchial disease combined with external beam radiation therapy and endobronchial placement of radioactive sources. Laser excision may be combined with stent placement to maintain open an obstructed bronchus or trachea. Chest wall pain usually is readily controlled by a course of radiation therapy.

Postoperative Mortality

Recent analyses identify that modern 30-day operative mortality from pulmonary resections should be less than 4 percent. Lobectomies and lesser resections should have a mortality between 1 and 2 percent, and pneumonectomies still carry a mortality of 6 to 7 percent. The mortality rate is directly proportional to increased age, associated diseases, and the extent of resection. Respiratory complications, not surprisingly, are the most common cause of postoperative mortality in patients undergoing pulmonary resection. Cardiac complications also account for a significant percentage of mortality, and technical problems such as hemorrhage, bronchopleural fistula, and empyema account for a small but significant percentage of complications leading to death.

Postoperative Morbidity

Approximately 30 percent of patients undergoing pulmonary resection will sustain a postoperative complication of which approximately two-thirds are minor and the other one-third nonfatal major complications. The most common complication is supraventricular arrhythmia, which occurs in up to 20 percent of patients, depending on how closely patients are monitored. Other minor complications include postoperative air leaks lasting greater than 7 days and atelectasis. Major nonfatal events most commonly are respiratory related, with patients developing significant infiltrates and pneumonitis. A small percentage of patients require reintubation in the postoperative period for respiratory failure usually related to the development of an infiltrate. There are no definitive predictors for postoperative pulmonary complications, although significant risk factors for major complications include age <60 years,

FEV_1 <2 L, weight loss >10 percent, associated systemic disease, and extent of disease. Pulmonary complications can be minimized with meticulous attention to postoperative respiratory maneuvers including chest physiotherapy and preoperative teaching.

Other complications of pulmonary resection include wound infections and disturbances in mental status, especially in older patients. Postpneumonectomy complications, fortunately, are unusual, but the most common one is empyema with or without a bronchial stump leak.

Prognosis Following Resection

Prognosis following pulmonary resection, which has been well analyzed, depends mainly on TNM stage, a classification which was last revised in 1986 (see Table 55-2). Short of disseminated disease, prognosis mainly depends on the status of the regional lymph nodes.

Sites of Recurrence

Patients with lung cancer die of disseminated disease, and a distant site is most commonly the first site of recurrent disease. Over 30 percent of patients with adenocarcinomas will develop brain metastases, a percentage significantly higher than for patients with squamous carcinoma. Other common sites of metastatic disease include bone, lung, liver, and adrenals. Patients with higher-stage disease have a significantly greater likelihood of developing disseminated disease. This recognition has led to the neoadjuvant treatment regimens in patients with N2 disease. Local recurrence is most commonly seen in association with distant disease. Isolated local recurrence is a rare phenomenon but is sometimes amenable to resection. This underscores the importance of a complete resection at the time of the initial operative procedure. Sites of local recurrence that may cause problems include the chest wall (pain), superior vena cava (SVC syndrome), and involvement of the left recurrent laryngeal nerve (hoarseness and swallowing problems). Symptomatic local recurrence often is treated with radiation therapy, and chemotherapy is employed for some patients who develop disseminated disease, while recognizing that cure is usually not possible in patients who have developed distant disease.

Refinements in surgical techniques and perioperative management of patients with lung cancer have allowed greater numbers of patients with localized and locally advanced disease to benefit from operative intervention. Many patients with mediastinal lymph node disease previously thought not to be operative candidates now are able to be operated upon with improved survival after a course of neoadjuvant therapy. Other patients with pulmonary function so compromised that it precluded resection now are often considered for resection using the minimally invasive techniques developed within the previous few years aided by better pain management and postoperative chest physiotherapy. It's safe to say that surgery will continue to play a major role in the management of patients with non-small lung cancer.

Treatment of Non–Small Cell Lung Cancer: Chemotherapy

Approximately 60 percent of patients with NSCLC have evidence of disseminated disease when first seen by a physician. Such data have led to the assumption that NSCLC is generally a systemic disease and that relatively few patients have localized disease that is amenable to a surgical approach. Unfortunately, patients with disseminated disease are rarely cured despite our best efforts. Therefore, because even patients with localized disease are likely to develop disseminated disease, systemic therapy is an important component of therapy. Historically, single chemotherapeutic agents have achieved only minimal response rates in NSCLC, so regimens that entail combinations of drugs have evolved as standard therapy, if any therapy can be designated as "standard" in this disease. Definition of the role of chemotherapy in the treatment of this disease continues to evolve. For example, controversy exists over the role and benefit of systemic chemotherapy in advanced-stage NSCLC. On the other hand, clinical trials during the past few years have shown the value of chemotherapy in treating localized disease.

Once a new active drug or combination has been identified, a randomized trial is necessary to determine whether it offers advantages over a previously established regimen. Although response rates are still being reported, survival is the major end point in treating NSCLC by chemotherapy. Small improvements in survival (e.g., additional 10 weeks), although statistically significant, are of dubious biologic and clinical significance. In addition, quality-of-life indices that are standardized and reproducible are now available as part of the evaluation of clinical benefit. It seems likely that future clinical trials will include quality-of-life and cost analysis as measurable end points.

LOCALLY ADVANCED NSCLC

The term *locally advanced* includes several different presentations of primary lung cancer, but all have in common the absence of disease outside of the chest. Some of these lesions are eminently resectable, others marginally resectable, and others out of the realm of resectability. Included in this group of lesions (stage IIA) are those with mediastinal lymph node impairment (N2 disease), direct extension into certain mediastinal structures (T3), direct extension into the chest wall (T3), and certain endobronchial lesions.

Lesions that directly invade the mediastinum but affect structures that are not usually considered resectable (e.g., aorta, esophagus, and vertebral bodies) are classified as T4 and are considered to be stage IIIB. About 40,000 cases of stage IIIA and IIIB disease occur per year in the United States. The best treatment approach to locally advanced disease has not yet been determined. A wide array of combined modality approaches have been used in stage IIIA patients (particularly those with N2 nodes). These include chemotherapy with surgery, radiation with surgery, chemotherapy with radiation (both sequentially and simultaneously), and chemotherapy with radiation and surgery. Unfortunately, some T3 patients have been included in many of these trials, again complicating interpretation of the results.

RADIATION THERAPY ALONE

Most patients with lung cancer receive radiotherapy as part of their treatment, either as initial management or later in the course of their disease. This may include thoracic radiotherapy and/or irradiation of sites of metastatic disease.

Thoracic radiotherapy (RT) for NSCLC is usually categorized as follows:

Neoadjuvant = preoperative
Adjuvant = postoperative
Definitive = cure without surgery as treatment goal;
with or without chemotherapy
Palliative = directed at relief of thoracic symptoms

Utilization of thoracic radiotherapy as part of the therapeutic regimen and the therapeutic goal of the therapy depends not only on tumor-related factors such as stage but also on patient-related factors such as pulmonary reserve and performance status. All these factors need to be considered when deciding whether to irradiate. Until recently, radiation therapy alone was the standard therapy for patients with N2 disease. This practice resulted in a 5-year survival of about 5 percent. A number of studies have been conducted that underscore the lack of effect of radiation as a single modality as well as the lack of improvement when a single drug is added to radiation therapy. Since combination chemotherapy that included a cisplatin-based drug regimen provided longer survival than did any single agent, combination chemotherapy was utilized in addition to radiation therapy in an attempt to improve results.

ADVANCES IN RADIOTHERAPY

Biologic Advances

As the understanding of the relationship between radiation and cellular kinetics has grown, mathematical models have been developed that allow us to predict the responses of both normal tissue and tumor to radiation. This capability has led to many creative new fractionation schemes designed to maximize the destruction of tumor while minimizing damage to normal tissue. The difference in cellular kinetics between tumor cells and normal cells makes these new schemes possible and attractive. Both tumor cells and normal cells are injured by radiation; however, normal cells usually have a greater ability to repair this damage than do the tumor cells and can repopulate more between fractions.

Hyperfractionation utilizes multiple daily fractions in an effort to reduce the late effects in normal tissue without decreasing tumor control. The overall treatment time is the same as conventional schedules, but multiple smaller fractions are given each day, and total doses are increased. By giving multiple smaller fractions, the normal tissues are able to repair a greater percentage of the damage during the course of treatment.

Tumor cells, however, are less able to repair the damage and therefore do not benefit as much from the smaller fractions. In general, hyperfractionation works well in situations where there is a large discrepancy in repair capabilities between tumor cells and normal tissue.

Accelerated treatment administers multiple fractions per day but also decreases the overall treatment time. Total dose and dose per fraction are similar to conventional treatment. It is designed to reduce the amount of repopulation that occurs during treatment of rapidly dividing tumors and, therefore, to improve local control.

Technical Advances

Another method of increasing local control is through three-dimensional conformal radiation therapy. Utilizing three-dimensional planning of both the tumor and surrounding normal tissue, the radiation field can be *conformed* to the tumor as the field moves around the patient. The advantage of this approach is that the radiation can be delivered in a more precise fashion allowing the tumor dose to be raised and the normal tissue dose to be lowered. In a comparison of three-dimensional and two-dimensional planning in nine patients with NSCLC, three-dimensional planning decreased the radiation dose to the ipsilateral lung by 11 percent and by 51 percent to the contralateral lung. Thus, three-dimensional planning allowed the tumor dose to be increased by 20 to 30 percent. Dose escalation studies are currently under way to establish the maximum tolerable dose of radiation that can be delivered with conformal techniques to patients with NSCLC.

CONCURRENT CHEMOTHERAPY AND RADIATION THERAPY

The rationale for concurrent therapy (i.e., chemotherapy given during a course of radiation therapy) is based on the concept that some drugs or drug combinations (notably cisplatin) may act synergistically with radiation. The trade-off, however, may be an increase in toxicity and a regimen that is not well tolerated by all potentially eligible patients. When given on a weekly basis with radiation, the cisplatin did not confer any advantage over radiation alone. However, several other studies have failed to demonstrate an advantage for concurrent therapy in locally advanced disease (Table 55-3). The greatest advantage with combined chemotherapy and radiation therapy is seen at the 2- and 3-year marks. At present, concurrent therapy probably should be limited to clinical trials, since the benefit is modest and the toxicity is somewhat greater than that from sequential therapy or use of a single modality.

TABLE 55-3 Randomized Trials in Stage II Disease: Radiation Alone vs. Radiation and Chemotherapy

Number of patients	Therapy	Median survival	Survival, years		
			1	2	3
155	RT	9.6	40	13	11
	RT/CT	13.8	55	26	23
353	RT	10	41	14	4
	RT/CT	12	51	21	12
238	RT	10.2	41	17	
	RT/CT	10.9	42	19	
114	RT	10.3	45	16	7
	RT/CT	10.4	45	21	5
95	RT	11			
	RT/CT	16			
309	RT		46	13	2
	RT/CT		54	26	16
			44	19	13
183	RT	41		9	
	RT/CT	35		15	

CHEMOTHERAPY AND RADIATION FOLLOWED BY SURGERY

Various theoretical considerations have led to trials of chemotherapy and radiation followed by surgery: (1) tumor cell subpopulations in locally advanced NSCLC may respond differently to radiation and chemotherapy, and cells resistant to one treatment method may be sensitive to the other; (2) chemotherapy may promote the emergence of radiosensitive cells, thereby increasing the total number of cells killed by continued radiation treatments; and (3) induction of cell cycle synchronization by certain drugs may increase cell killing by radiation and induce recruitment of tumor cells in G_0. Neoadjuvant irradiation requires a moderate dose, i.e., approximately 4500 cGy in standard daily fractions (180 to 200 cGy). Higher doses increase complications, particularly if pneumonectomy is ultimately required. A slightly lower total dose using a larger daily fraction (3000 cGy in 10 fractions of 300 cGy) completes treatment more rapidly. Because of improvements in the current use of concurrent chemotherapy and the knowledge that the occurrence of late radiotherapy complications are strongly related to the use of large fractions, daily fractions greater than 200 cGy are not often used as preoperative or postoperative therapy. Preoperative radiotherapy carries with it the potential disadvantage of limiting the ability to give additional radiotherapy if tumor proves to be unresectable or if residual disease remains after resection. After 4000 to 5000 cGy preoperatively, only about 3000 cGy of additional irradiation can be safely administered postoperatively; this is unlikely to sterilize aggressive residual disease and should probably only be given if indicated for palliation of local symptoms.

ADJUVANT THERAPY

It is well recognized that despite complete resection, most patients with locally advanced NSCLC will, at some time, develop disseminated disease. Even with stage I disease, as many as 20 percent of patients will die of disseminated disease within 5 years. With stage II disease, less than 50 percent of patients will be alive at 5 years; with stage IIIa N2 disease, at best 30 percent of patients will be alive at 5 years. These numbers make clear the need for some additional therapy to improve on the overall survival achieved by surgery. Currently, there is no generally accepted postoperative therapy for patients who have undergone complete resection whose disease has been well staged. This does not mean that patients are not treated postoperatively. There is general belief, despite the lack of data for support, that patients with nodal disease found at the time of surgery should receive postoperative radiation therapy. This belief is so strongly held that it is currently impossible in the United States to mount a trial comparing postoperative treatment with no treatment. The results of a recently completed prospective, randomized trial (ECOG 3590) where all of the American cooperative oncology groups participated also showed no benefit for chemotherapy combined with radiation therapy when compared with radiation therapy alone for completely resected patients with positive lymph nodes identified at the time of thoracotomy. Patients whose tumors cannot be completely resected have a poor prognosis, although radiation is usually used in an attempt to maximize local control. What defines an incomplete resection varies from leaving gross disease behind to finding microscopic disease in the highest lymph node removed to tumor cells present in the peribronchial soft tissue of the resected specimen. There is almost no use for a so-called palliative resection when dealing with a primary lung cancer. If a tumor cannot be completely removed, there is no sense in removing part of it. Locally recurrent disease following a complete resection must be treated on an individual basis. Rarely does local disease recur as an isolated phenomenon; most commonly it is associated with disseminated disease. Radiation therapy is used to treat symptoms related to the locally recurrent disease, the regimen differing somewhat depending on the presence or absence of disseminated disease. An occasional patient with a local parenchymal or chest wall recurrence may be a candidate for further resection. Certain areas of locoregional recurrence engender more concern than others. Specifically recurrence in the region of the superior vena cava is noteworthy, since it is best to avoid obstruction of this vessel. A particularly concerning area of local recurrence is the aortopulmonary window in the left chest, where involvement of the left recurrent laryngeal nerve has a significant impact on the quality of life. Patients with a paralyzed left vocal cord are not only hoarse but have difficulty caused by aspiration.

Unfortunately, once the nerve is involved, function of the vocal cord does not return even if radiation therapy is employed for the recurrent disease. Over time the voice improves as the contralateral vocal cord moves across the midline to appose with the paralyzed cord. The avoidance of local recurrence in certain areas is far preferable to attempts to treat it.

ADVANCED-STAGE NSCLC

The goal of chemotherapy in advanced-stage disease is palliation, since, with few exceptions, disseminated lung cancer, like most other solid tumors, is essentially impossible to cure. Among the issues that have been raised with respect to the relative value of chemotherapy in patients with disseminated disease are the response rate, survival data, cost-effectiveness, and the quality of life. Prognostic criteria play an important role in analyzing and constructing clinical trials. For example, patients with a poor performance status (spending more than 50 percent of time in bed, significant weight loss) are much less likely to respond to chemotherapy than those with better performance status. In patients with poor prognosis, it is important to assess the effect of treatment-related toxicity on overall quality of life and the cost-effectiveness of therapy.

Several studies have randomized patients with disseminated disease to receive either best supportive care or systemic chemotherapy. In addition, four meta-analyses have reviewed studies that randomized patients to best supportive care or chemotherapy. These data can be used to make the case for or against systemic chemotherapy (i.e., that the patients did live longer when treated or that the three additional months of survival had little biologic significance). In general, meta-analyses have shown a 10 percent increase in survival at 1 year but an increase in median survival of only 2 months. Whether to treat a patient with disseminated disease using chemotherapy or to treat symptoms as they arise often comes down to the judgment of the medical oncologist balanced against the wishes of the patient. Patients with poor performance status can be expected to have a poorer response to chemotherapy than those with relatively good performance status; therefore, they would not usually be offered chemotherapy. Adding to this uncertainty is the fact that experimental drugs are often advocated as first-line therapy in advanced-stage

NSCLC based on the overall outcome from standard therapy—which, as noted above, is generally limited to those with relatively preserved performance status.

NEW DEVELOPMENTS

The past few years have been marked by the appearance of several new antineoplastic agents, several of which have novel mechanisms of action. These new agents have led to renewed enthusiasm for the role of chemotherapy in NSCLC. These agents include docetaxel, camptothecins such as topotecan and irinotecan, gemcitabine, and tirapazamine. It remains to be determined whether some of these agents will be associated with higher response rates either alone or in combination with more conventional agents in NSCLC patients with localized or disseminated disease.

SMALL CELL LUNG CANCER

Small cell lung cancer (SCLC) is a paradox among neoplastic diseases. Untreated, it is a highly virulent malignancy, killing its victims in a matter of weeks. On the other hand, it is one of the most chemotherapy-responsive of cancers in that, with proper treatment, partial or complete remissions occur in the vast majority of cases.

Unfortunately, although many patients can be rendered free of clinical evidence of disease, most eventually relapse and die from this malignancy. Like all other lung cancers, SCLC is linked to a variety of environmental risk factors. By far the strongest association is with the use of tobacco: up to 98 percent of patients with SCLC have a history of smoking. In most populations, the incidence of SCLC rises with increasing tobacco exposure in a dose-dependent fashion, making the overall risk for smokers approximately 15-fold higher than for nonsmokers. Occupational risks for small cell carcinoma include exposure to bischloromethyl ethers, nickel, vinyl chloride, asbestos, cadmium, and radon daughters (in uranium miners). Other types of radiation exposure also appear to be significant risk factors, with an increased incidence of small cell carcinoma being reported in atomic bomb survivors and a higher incidence of the disease being noted in those exposed to therapeutic irradiation (patients treated for Hodgkin's disease or breast cancer). Industrial nations in general have an increased incidence of small cell carcinoma, possibly from higher levels of air pollutants.

The natural history of untreated SCLC is early dissemination and death. Unlike NSCLC, it is always considered a systemic disease at diagnosis, even if it appears clinically confined to the chest. Postmortem examinations performed on patients who died of other causes shortly after the complete surgical resection of their SCLC have demonstrated identifiable metastases in up to 70 percent. Evidence of distant spread can be found in virtually any organ system. The most common sites of involvement, however, are the liver, bone and bone marrow, and central nervous system. The median survival for untreated patients is 4 to 6 months if they have disease that is apparently confined to the chest and 5 to 9 *weeks* if they present with distant disease. Chemotherapy with or without irradiation can extend median survival to an average of 14 to 20 months for those with thorax-confined disease and 7 to 10 months for those with more extensive spread. At 2 to 3 years, a consistent 10 to 25 percent of limited-stage patients will still be alive, although cure is not guaranteed even in these relatively long-term survivors. Recent trials indicate that 2-year survival rates may be as high as 40 percent for aggressively treated limited-stage patients. Two- to 3-year survival remains a dismal 1 to 2 percent for those with metastases.

The diagnosis of SCLC is usually not difficult. There usually is a central lesion arising from a major bronchus and extending into nearby pulmonary parenchyma. Necrosis and hemorrhage are often present. The classic oat cell form of SCLC consists of sheets of heavily staining cells with scant cytoplasm, hyperchromatic nuclei, and nonprominent nucleoli. Although a detailed description of available antibodies is beyond the scope of this text, immunocytochemistry can be helpful in ruling in or out the diagnosis of SCLCs. Antibodies reacting against the common leukocyte antigen would suggest the alternative identification of non-Hodgkin's lymphoma, while markers suggesting neural differentiation (e.g., chromogranin A) point toward the diagnosis of SCLC.

In staging, SCLC patients with disease that can be confined in a tolerable radiation portal are considered in the limited-stage category (30 percent of all patients with small cell cancer); *all others* are defined as extensive stage (70 percent).

No aspect of the clinical presentation of SCLC distinguishes it from NSCLC or even neoplasms metastatic to the lungs. However, the duration of symptoms of SCLC tends to be very short because of the rapid dissemination of the disease. Typically patients are middle-aged or elderly smokers with symptoms attributable to their pulmonary and mediastinal disease: cough, dyspnea, chest pain, hoarseness, and/or hemoptysis. A chest radiograph typically demonstrates a central mass (75 percent of patients) with or without hilar nodal involvement.

As previously stated, with extremely rare exceptions, the therapy for SCLC always includes chemotherapy. Chemotherapy can markedly prolong survival for patients with both stages of small cell carcinoma and can effect a cure in a significant number of those with limited disease. A popular combination consisting of cyclophosphamide, doxorubicin (Adriamycin), and vincristine (CAV) and similar regimens with only minor modifications became the standard therapy until the mid-1980s, demonstrating response rates of 55 to 65 percent in those with extensive-stage cancer and rates up to 85 percent in limited-stage disease. From the mid-1980s till now, platinum-based regimens—especially etoposide-cisplatin (EP)—with or without CAV have become the therapy of choice in North America. Though not clearly superior (in terms of higher response rates) to CAV alone in randomized trials, EP is less toxic than CAV in extensive-stage patients. It has advantages that become even more apparent when it is used to treat limited-stage disease, as it is much easier to give in conjunction with chest irradiation. A number of new drugs have been shown to be active in SCLC. These include the microtubule assembly–promoting taxanes paclitaxel and docetaxel, the topoisomerase-I–inhibiting camptothecin derivatives CPT-11 and topotecan, and the nucleoside analog–antimetabolite gemcitabine. Additional studies are needed to define more precisely the role of these agents in combination therapy or possibly as single agents in the salvage setting.

In summary, chemotherapy has profoundly changed the natural history of SCLC. Though the best regimen is still not defined, the most important lesson in chemotherapy for SCLC is that one must give full-course treatment on the originally selected schedule. Arbitrary dose reductions or delays may decrease the overall cure rate. Questions remain regarding how best to add irradiation to combination chemotherapy. None of the randomized trials or the meta-analyses established the best *sequence* of chemoradiotherapy. The preponderance of evidence suggests that close administration of the two methods is superior, albeit with more toxicity. Early administration of irradiation may eliminate clones of tumor cells that are resistant to chemotherapy and thus boost the cure rate. However, it is apparent that giving concurrent chemotherapy and irradiation increases side effects and makes it more difficult to administer full-course chemotherapy on time. There are still no trials comparing any schedule of concurrent chemoradiotherapy with sequential (radiation after completion of chemotherapy) or alternating cycles (radiation and chemotherapy administered on a nonoverlapping, alternating schedule). Chest irradiation for extensive disease may improve local control, but it does not alter overall response rate, median survival, or cure rate. Its use should be limited to patients with symptomatic chest disease that requires radiation for palliation. The need for prophylactic cranial irradiation (PCI) is one of the most controversial areas in the treatment of SCLC. The brain has long been considered a sanctuary site from chemotherapeutic agents, and it is also an area to which SCLC commonly metastasizes. The recommendation for PCI is generally limited to those whose disease has been put into a complete remission, since the vast majority of long-term survivors (those most likely to benefit from PCI) come from this group. No trial has demonstrated a significant survival advantage for prophylactic radiation therapy, although most have found a decrease in CNS metastasis and possibly improved duration of survival without CNS disease. Additional studies are needed before PCI can be routinely recommended when not part of a clinical trial, but at this point it is prudent to withhold PCI from any patient not achieving a complete remission with chemotherapy, and then to apply the technique only after the entire course of drug therapy is finished (since neurotoxicity may be worse with concomitant chemoradiotherapy).

SCLC is distinct from the other three major histologic varieties of pulmonary neoplasms, which tend to behave similarly and be lumped together in classification schemes under the generic rubric *non–small cell lung cancer.* It is biologically more active, secreting multiple hormones and neural markers and giving rise to a number of paraneoplastic syndromes. It is always thought of as a systemic disease, and therapy nearly always includes some form of drug treatment. Though it is highly responsive to chemotherapy, and survival is markedly prolonged with this kind of treatment, the complete eradication of small cell carcinoma in individual patients remains a relatively rare event. Long-term survivors are still subject to a host of morbid cardiopulmonary conditions as well as secondary malignancies and recurrence of their small cell cancer. A number of questions remain regarding optimal chemotherapy drugs and combinations, dose and timing of irradiation, and the role of PCI.

BIBLIOGRAPHY

Albain KS, Crowley JJ, LeBlanc M, et al: Determinants of improved outcome in small-cell lung cancer: An analysis of the 2,580-patient Southwest Oncology Group Data Base. *J Clin Oncol* 8:1563–1574, 1990.

Ginsberg RJ, Rubinstein LV: Randomized trial of lobectomy versus limited resection for T1 N0 non-small cell lung cancer. Lung Cancer Study Group. *Ann Thorac Surg* 60:615–622, 1995.

Marino P, Pampallona S, Preatoni A, et al: Chemotherapy vs supportive care in advanced non-small-cell lung cancer: Results of a meta-analysis of the literature. *Chest* 106:861–865, 1994.

Miller JD, Gorenstein LA, Patterson GA: Staging: The key to rational management of lung cancer. *Ann Thorac Surg* 53:170–178, 1992.

Sause W: Combination chemotherapy and radiation therapy in lung cancer. *Semin Oncol* 21:72–78, 1994.

Silvestri GA, Littenberg B, Colice GL: The clinical evaluation for detecting lung cancer—A meta-analysis. *Am J Respir Crit Care Med* 152:225–230, 1995.

Sugarbaker DJ, Strauss GM: Advances in surgical staging and therapy of non-small-cell lung cancer. *Semin Oncol* 20:163–172, 1993.

Vokes EE, Bitran JD: Non-small-cell lung cancer: Toward the next plateau. *Chest* 106:659–660, 1994.

56 | Lung Tumors Other Than Bronchogenic Carcinoma: Benign, Malignant, and Metastatic*

Larry R. Kaiser and Steven M. Keller

Although bronchogenic carcinoma represents the overwhelming majority of primary pulmonary neoplasms, a great variety of tumors either originate in the lung or metastasize to lung. Benign neoplasms of the lung (Table 56-1) represent fewer than 1 percent of all resected lung tumors, and nonbronchogenic primary pulmonary malignancies (Table 56-2) account for 3 to 5 percent of all lung tumors.

BENIGN TUMORS

Hamartoma

Hamartomas are the most common benign lung neoplasms and consist of cartilage, connective tissue, fat, smooth muscle, and respiratory epithelium. Most often, such a tumor presents as a solitary asymptomatic parenchymal lung nodule that may gradually increase in size. Approximately 10 percent of hamartomas are endobronchial and cause obstructive symptoms. The diagnostic radiographic finding of a popcorn pattern of calcification occurs in fewer than 30 percent of patients. Percutaneous transthoracic needle biopsy yields diagnostic information in as many as 85 percent of patients. The patient with a known peripheral hamartoma may be safely observed, as malignant transformation is rare. Excision is indicated if the diagnosis is in doubt or there are associated sequelae of obstruction. Minimal amounts of normal lung tissue should be removed. Recurrences after complete excision are unusual, although a second primary hamartoma may occur.

Chondroma

Chondromas of the lung may occur in the parenchyma or airways. The former are usually asymptomatic, and the latter are associated with obstructive symptoms. A lung-sparing resection should be performed whenever possible.

Intrapulmonary Fibroma/Fibrous Tumor

Intrapulmonary fibrous tumors are contiguous with the visceral pleura and are histologically identical to localized fibrous mesotheliomas. The lung is the most common location of these extrapleural fibrous tumors.

---

*Edited from Chap. 115, "Primary Tumors Other Than Bronchogenic Carcinoma: Benign and Malignant," by Keller SM, Katariya K. In: *Fishman's Pulmonary Diseases and Disorders*, 3d ed., edited by Fishman AP, Elias JA, Fishman JA, Grippi MA, Kaiser LR, Senior RM. New York, McGraw-Hill, 1998, pp 1833–1840. For fuller discussion of topics dealt with in this chapter, the reader is referred to the original text, as noted above.

TABLE 56-1 Benign Tumors of the Lung

Solitary tumors	Other solitary tumors	Multiple tumors
Epithelial tumors	Alveolar adenoma	Benign metastasizing leiomyoma
Clara cell adenoma	Pulmonary paraganglioma— chemodectoma Lymphangioleiomyomatosis	
Mucous gland adenoma	Glomus tumor	Cystic fibrohis- tiocytic tumors
Oncocytoma	Nodular amyloid	
Squamous papilloma	Pleomorphic adenoma— mixed tumor	
Soft tissue tumors	Pulmonary meningioma	
Cavernous hemangioma	Sclerosing hemangioma— pneumocytoma	
Chondroma	Sugar tumor—benign clear cell tumor	
Fibroma/fibrous polyp	Teratoma	
Fibromyxoma		
Inflammatory pseudotumor— fibrous histiocytoma, fibroxanthoma, plasma cell granuloma		
Granular cell myoblastoma		
Hamartoma		
Leiomyoma		
Lipoma		
Neurilemoma— schwannoma		
Neurofibroma		
Pulmonary hyalinizing granuloma		

Inflammatory Pseudotumor (Plasma Cell Granuloma)

These tumors occur most often in adults but represent the most common benign lung tumor in children. Serial radiologic examinations rarely demonstrate enlargement and may even reveal a decrease in size. The diagnosis is infrequently made prior to resection. Microscopic examination demonstrates a mixture of inflammatory cells, including plasma cells, lymphocytes, and macrophages.

Granular Cell Myoblastoma

Granular cell myoblastomas are thought to arise from Schwann cells and are most commonly found in the tongue, skin, and breast. The tumor occurs in the lung with equal frequency in men and women at a median age of 38 years. Although the majority are endobronchial, they are usually discovered on a routine chest radiograph.

TABLE 56-2 Rare Primary Malignant Neoplasms of the Lung

Blastoma
Carcinoid tumors
Carcinosarcoma
Epithelioid hemangioendothelioma (IVBAT)
Malignant lymphoreticular disorders
 Hodgkin's disease
 Non-Hodgkin's lymphoma
 Plasmacytoma
Malignant melanoma
Malignant germ cell tumors
 Malignant teratoma
 Choriocarcinoma
Salivary gland–type tumors
 Adenoid cystic carcinoma
 Mucoepidermoid carcinoma
 Acinic cell tumor
Sarcoma
 Chondrosarcoma
 Osteosarcoma
 Soft tissue sarcoma
Miscellaneous
 Ependymoma, malignant
 Ewing's sarcoma
 Lymphoepithelioma
Pseudomesotheliomatous carcinoma

Leiomyoma

Primary solitary leiomyoma accounts for approximately 2 percent of all benign lung tumors. The tumor occurs with almost equal incidence in the proximal bronchi and parenchyma. Symptoms of obstruction are associated with the former, whereas the latter are found on routine radiographs.

MALIGNANT TUMORS

Pulmonary Blastoma

This biphasic tumor is composed of both malignant mesenchymal and epithelial components that resemble the pseudoglandular stage of the 3-month fetal lung. These tumors may be separated into two categories based on histologic features: well-differentiated fetal adenocarcinoma (WDFA) and biphasic blastoma. WDFA is a pulmonary blastoma with a malignant epithelial component but without a malignant stroma. The biphasic blastoma is composed of malignant mesenchyme without the malignant epithelium.

Carcinoid

Neuroendocrine or Kultschitzsky cells are the precursors of these low-grade malignant neoplasms, which represent the second most common tumors arising in the tracheobronchial tree and 0.5 to 1.0 percent of all bronchial tumors. Carcinoid tumors may be divided into typical and atypical subtypes, with the latter accounting for 11 to 24 percent of all carcinoids and having more malignant histologic and clinical features.

Approximately half the patients with carcinoid tumors are asymptomatic at presentation, and as many as 9 percent of tumors may be incidental findings at surgery or autopsy. The most common clinical manifestations include hemoptysis, postobstructive pneumonitis, and dyspnea. Occasionally a case of atypical carcinoid may present with metastatic disease. Bronchial carcinoids are the most common malignant lung tumors of childhood. Almost 75 percent of all carcinoid tumors are visible bronchoscopically; a bronchoscopic biopsy is usually diagnostic.

Treatment of both typical and atypical carcinoids localized to the lung consists of excision of the primary lesion and mediastinal lymph node dissection. This usually entails a lobectomy.

Epithelioid Hemangioendothelioma

Originally named *intravascular bronchoalveolar tumor* (IVBAT), this neoplasm has since been demonstrated to be of vascular endothelial origin rather than alveolar cell. The tumor is categorized as a low-grade sarcoma and is usually multifocal. No specific therapy is known, although excision of the rare solitary tumor is recommended. The 5- and 10-year survival rates are 61 and 55 percent, respectively.

Lymphomas

All the various elements of the lymphoreticular system are present within the lung and may undergo malignant degeneration. Non-Hodgkin's lymphoma, Hodgkin's disease, and plasmacytoma of the lung together make up approximately 0.5 percent of all primary lung tumors. Secondary involvement of the lung by these processes is much more common.

The low-grade small lymphocyte lymphomas represent 50 to 90 percent of all primary pulmonary lymphomas. The majority are B-cell lymphomas arising in the bronchus-associated lymphoid tissue (BALT). Patients are typically in their sixth decade and approximately half are asymptomatic. Resection is the treatment of choice for localized tumors. Long-term survival is excellent, although relapse may occur in the lung or other lymphoid tissue. Rarely, these tumors evolve into an aggressive systemic lymphoma.

Angiocentric immunoproliferative lesions, or angiocentric lymphomas (AIL/LYG), are the second most common group of pulmonary lymphomas. The diagnostic microscopic findings are those of lymphoid cells forming nodules and infiltrates in proximity to lymphatics. Despite aggressive treatment with multiple chemotherapeutic agents, the disease may ultimately involve other organs.

Large cell lymphomas are the least common of the pulmonary lymphomas and may be difficult to distinguish from AIL/LYG. Patients generally present with a solitary nodule; the diagnosis is made following resection. Treatment consists of adjuvant radiochemotherapy.

In order to diagnose primary Hodgkin's disease of the lung, the typical histologic features must be present within the lung substance but absent from regional lymph nodes and other common extrathoracic sites. Most patients are female and present with systemic (type B) complaints such as weight loss, fever, malaise, and night sweats. The chest radiographs demonstrate either unilateral (more common) or bilateral abnormalities. The most frequent histologic subtype is the nodular sclerosing variety. Combination chemotherapy and radiotherapy appear to be associated with the best survival.

Plasmacytoma

Primary plasmacytomas of the lung may present as parenchymal, endo-bronchial, or endotracheal tumors. An extrathoracic primary site must be assiduously sought. Patients whose neoplasms are identified following resection require no further treatment, but those tumors identified prior to surgery may be treated with radiotherapy. Patients require careful monitoring as they may develop multiple myeloma.

Salivary Gland–Type Tumors

Adenoid cystic carcinoma is the most common salivary gland neoplasm found in the lung. These tumors most frequently occur in the trachea or main-stem bronchi and cause symptoms of obstruction. Complete resection is the most effective treatment, although radiotherapy may be utilized for inoperable cancers and may be of benefit to patients who have had incomplete resections. Metastases to intraparenchymal and mediastinal lymph nodes do not preclude long-term survival, which approximates 55 percent.

Mucoepidermoid carcinomas occur most frequently in the main-stem bronchi but can arise peripherally. The majority of tumors are low-grade, as demonstrated by few mitoses and little nuclear pleomorphism and necrosis. Patients with low-grade tumors that are completely resected may be considered to be cured. High-grade tumors are much more aggressive, with 100 percent mortality rates between 11 and 28 months.

Sarcomas

Primary pulmonary sarcomas arise from the mesenchymal cells found in the bronchial or vascular walls and interstices of the lung parenchyma. Chondrosarcomas of the lung are usually slow-growing tumors that metastasize infrequently. They may occur either in the main bronchi or lung parenchyma and cause symptoms of obstruction. Patients with primary osteosarcomas of the lung generally present with cough or hemoptysis. Tumors are solitary and frequently have a diameter greater than 4 cm.

The variety of primary soft tissue pulmonary sarcomas reflects the range of mesenchymal tissue found in the lung (Table 56-3). The overall 1-, 3-, and 5-year survival rates were 55, 31, and 25 percent respectively, with a median of 13 months.

TABLE 56-3 Primary Soft Tissue Sarcomas of the Lung

Leiomyosarcoma
Spindle cell sarcoma
Rhabdomyosarcoma
Malignant fibrous histiocytoma
Angiosarcoma
Fibrosarcoma
Malignant hemangiopericytoma
Neurogenic sarcoma
Synovial sarcoma
Kaposi's sarcoma
Liposarcoma

Tumors Metastatic to the Lung

It is well known that the lung is a common site of metastatic disease. Approximately 30 percent of patients with malignant disease will, at some point in the natural history of the disease, develop pulmonary metastases. Importantly, 20 percent of patients dying of pulmonary metastases will have no other detectable sites of disease. The treatment of patients with pulmonary metastases, particularly those who present with isolated pulmonary metastases, becomes extremely important in attempts to prolong survival. Most pulmonary metastases are discovered by routine chest radiograph either as a synchronous event with a primary tumor or as a metachronous event in a routine follow-up examination. Pulmonary metastases can present with a myriad of radiologic findings. They are most commonly bilateral, well-defined with smooth edges, and located primarily in the periphery of the lung. Pulmonary metastases to lung parenchyma may occasionally metastasize to hilar or mediastinal lymph nodes, but this is an infrequent event for most solid tumors. However, involvement of hilar or mediastinal nodes with pulmonary metastases from melanoma, seminoma, and breast carcinoma is more frequently reported than with other solid tumors. Endobronchial metastases occur but are extremely uncommon with the breast, pancreas, colon, and kidney, being the most common tumors to present in this fashion.

For the patient with a known primary tumor who subsequently presents with multiple pulmonary lesions, more than likely the patient has metastatic disease and not a benign process. The probability that a solitary pulmonary nodule in a patient with a peviously known cancer is a metastasis depends on the histology and site of the primary tumor (Table 56-4).

Computed tomography (CT) is currently accepted as the "gold standard" for the evaluation of pulmonary metastases, allowing both assessment for operative intervention and evaluation of response to chemotherapy. High-resolution scanners can now detect nodules as small as 2 to 3 mm with anywhere from 60 to 90 percent specificity.

In general, patients with pulmonary metastases from a solid tumor are considered for resection only if the lung is the sole site of metastasis. Therefore the primary goal of the preoperative evaluation of patients is to determine the extent of disease and to ensure that the lungs are the only site of metastases. Since the majority of solid tumors that have metastasized to the lung can also metastasize to brain, bone, and liver, the preoperative assessment of the patient being considered for surgical resection of metastatic disease should include a CT scan of the chest, a bone scan, and either CT or magnetic resonance imaging (MRI) of the brain. If indeed the lung is the only site of disease, the patient is potentially eligible for surgical resection. Two groups of

TABLE 56-4 Diagnostic Probability of a Solitary Lesion in Patients with Known Cancer

Primary cancer	New primary lung cancer	Metastasis
Sarcoma	1	10
Melanoma	1	10
Head and neck, breast	2	1
Genitourinary, gastrointestinal, gynecologic	1	1

SOURCE: Adapted from Cahan et al.

patients with pulmonary metastases are not considered for resection: (1) those with metastases to other organs and (2) those whose physiologic status would not allow them to tolerate the planned resection.

The following are the minimum criteria for resection of pulmonary metastatic disease:

1. The primary tumor has been controlled.
2. There are no extrathoracic metastases.
3. The radiologic features are consistent with pulmonary metastases.
4. The pulmonary metastases are deemed completely resectable.
5. There is adequate pulmonary reserve to allow for complete resection of all metastatic pulmonary disease.
6. The patient's general medical condition permits the planned operation.
7. Effective systemic therapy is not available.

In the past, pulmonary metastasectomy was reserved for those patients with solitary lesions; however, patients with bilateral and multiple lesions are now routinely accepted as surgical candidates. The number of metastases may or may not be a prognostic indicator. The CT scan should be utilized to help select those patients in whom it should be possible to resect all disease. In those patients who undergo complete resection of pulmonary metastases, the number of metastases does not predict survival; but the ability to completely resect the disease is the one prognostic factor that independently predicts survival, and the number of metastases may influence the ability to resect all disease. Data from the International Registry of Lung Metastases has shown that primary tumor type, disease-free interval, and number of metastases were significant prognostic indicators.

All operative approaches for patients with metastatic pulmonary disease must attempt to achieve complete resection of all disease with maximal conservation of pulmonary parenchyma. The majority of pulmonary metastases are located at the periphery of the lung, which in most cases allows excision by wedge resection with only a small amount of surrounding normal lung tissue. A 1- to 2-cm margin appears to be adequate for resection, and this can be carried out with mechanical stapling devices or the electrocautery. Occasionally, more extensive anatomic resections are required because of the central location of the metastasis, and segmentectomy and lobectomy are both acceptable procedures. It is extremely uncommon for a pneumonectomy to be required for a patient with a central metastases, but if this is a possibility, it is crucial to evaluate the contralateral lung for other metastases and, more important, to make sure that the patient can tolerate a pneumonectomy. Whether a posterolateral thoracotomy, sternotomy, or bilateral thoracosternotomy incision is used to resect bilateral pulmonary metastases, the operative morbidity and mortality following any of these procedures remains consistently quite low.

After a complete resection of either unilateral or bilateral pulmonary metastases, the most common cause of death is recurrent disease in lung. Recurrence following complete initial pulmonary metastasectomy for soft tissue sarcoma occurs in 67 to 86 percent of patients. Of those patients in whom disease recurs following an initial complete resection, 49 to 77 percent will have resectable disease again limited to the lungs. On subsequent recurrence, approximately 70 percent will have resectable disease limited to the lungs. The long-term survival of patients undergoing pulmonary resection for metastatic disease varies by the histology of the primary tumor. However, for most patients with completely resected pulmonary metastases, the 5-year survival approximates 25 to 30 percent.

SPECIFIC TUMOR TYPES

Soft Tissue Sarcoma

In patients with primary soft tissue sarcomas, the lungs are the most common site of distant disease, accounting for approximately 88 percent of all metastases in most series. Pulmonary metastases remain the major cause of death in these patients. Approximately 20 percent of patients with extremity soft tissue sarcomas will present with isolated pulmonary metastases at some point in the natural history of their disease. For patients who develop pulmonary metastases after treatment of the primary soft tissue sarcoma, 80 percent will do so within the first 2 years of treatment. Since systemic chemotherapy offers little chance of long-term survival, resection of pulmonary metastases remains the standard treatment for patients with metastatic soft tissue sarcoma to lung who are deemed resectable. The overall 5-year survival after resection of pulmonary metastases approximates 25 percent in several series. Although prognostic factors such as disease-free interval and tumor doubling time have been associated with a prolonged survival, the only factor that consistently predicts long-term survival is the ability to achieve a complete resection.

OSTEOGENIC SARCOMA

The treatment of osteogenic sarcoma has been constantly evolving. Currently, multimodality therapy—including adjuvant and neoadjuvant chemotherapy, limb-sparing surgery, and salvage therapy after relapse—has translated into improved survival. The development of multidrug chemotherapy has improved survival. It has frequently been noted that many patients who have died from pulmonary metastases had no evidence of extrathoracic disease. Currently, patients with pulmonary metastases who have been treated with a combination of systemic chemotherapy and resection have an overall survival at 5 years that approximates 40 percent.

COLORECTAL METASTASES

Approximately one-third of patients with colorectal carcinoma develop pulmonary metastases. However, in only 2 to 4 percent of these patients are the metastases confined to the lung; the majority have metastases to other sites, usually to the liver. In patients with isolated pulmonary metastases from colorectal carcinoma, pulmonary resection has been associated with an improved 5-year survival. Patients with a history of colorectal carcinoma who present with a solitary pulmonary nodule have an equal chance of the nodule being a primary lung cancer or a metastasis from their previous cancer.

URINARY TRACT CANCER

For patients with renal cell carcinoma, the lung is the most common site of distant metastases, and approximately 50 percent of patients with renal cell carcinoma will develop pulmonary metastases. In patients with unresected pulmonary metastases, the 5-year survival is less than 5 percent. Since chemotherapy and immunotherapy have not improved long-term survival, resection of pulmonary metastases has been utilized in selected patients.

TESTICULAR CARCINOMA

For patients with metastatic germ cell carcinoma, multimodality therapy has become the standard of care. Cisplatin-based chemotherapy has dramatically improved the survival of patients with disseminated germ cell tumors. At present approximately 80 percent of patients with disseminated germ cell carcinoma are cured of their disease. If residual mass is present after completion of chemotherapy, and if the tumor markers (alpha-fetoprotein and beta-human chorionic gonadotropin) are normal, the residual mass should be resected.

MELANOMA

Although most patients with metastatic malignant melanoma have diffuse metastases involving multiple organs, a small group of patients present with pulmonary metastases only, and resection occasionally has translated into long-term survival. Of all the solid tumors in which pulmonary metastases develop and where resection of metastases is part of the treatment plan, melanoma is consistently associated with the lowest 5-year survivals despite a complete resection.

HEAD AND NECK CANCER

Approximately 40 percent of patients with squamous cell carcinoma of the head and neck present with distant metastases at some point during their course. In the majority of these patients the metastases are to the lung. Resection of pulmonary metastatic disease has resulted in 5-year survival in the range of 29 to 43 percent. One should also keep in mind the markedly increased incidence of other aerodigestive malignancies in patients with head and neck cancers. Thus a solitary pulmonary nodule cannot simply be assumed to be a metastatic lesion but more likely is a new primary lung cancer and should be treated accordingly.

BREAST CARCINOMA

Approximately 20 percent of patients succumb to the disease with only isolated pulmonary metastases. Currently, with high-dose multidrug chemotherapy and bone marrow rescue, relatively few patients with metastatic breast cancer are referred to the thoracic surgeon for resection of pulmonary metastases. However, resection may play a role in selected patients who fail chemotherapy but have isolated pulmonary metastases.

GYNECOLOGIC MALIGNANCIES

Resection of pulmonary metastases from uterine or cervical carcinoma has been associated with 5-year survival rates ranging from 24 to 52 percent. For choriocarcinoma metastatic to lung, the standard treatment is multidrug chemotherapy. However, occasionally the metastases become resistant to chemotherapy, and resection should be considered.

CONCLUSION

For most solid tumors metastatic to lung, effective chemotherapy that translates into prolonged survival is lacking. Therefore, in the very select group of patients with pulmonary metastases as the only site of metastatic disease, surgical resection is currently the accepted and best treatment available. However, resection of metastatic disease does have its obvious limitations; in the majority of patients, disease will recur, usually within 2 years of the initial resection. As more effective chemotherapy is developed, a multimodality approach to pulmonary metastases from solid tumors, which includes resection in some cases, may result in further improvements in survival for these unfortunate individuals.

BIBLIOGRAPHY

Burt M, Zakowski M: Rare primary malignant neoplasms, in Pearson FG, Deslauriers J, Ginsberg RJ, et al (eds), *Thoracic Surgery,* sec 3, *Lung.* New York, Churchill Livingstone, 1995, pp 807–826.

Casson A, Putnam J, Natarajan G, et al: Five-year survival after pulmonary metastasectomy for adult soft tissue sarcoma. *Cancer* 69:662–669, 1992.

Cerfolio R, Allen M, Deschamps C, et al: Pulmonary resection of metastatic renal cell carcinoma. *Ann Thorac Surg* 57:339–344, 1994.

Colby TV, Koss MN, Travis WD: Tumors of the lower respiratory tract, in *Atlas of Tumor Pathology,* 3d series. Washington, DC, Armed Forces Institute of Pathology, 1995.

Harpole DH Jr, Feldman JM, Buchanan S, et al: Bronchial carcinoid tumours: A retrospective analysis of 126 patients. *Ann Thorac Surg* 54:50–55, 1992.

The International Registry of Lung Metastases: Long-term results of lung metastasectomy: Prognostic analysis based on 5206 cases. *J Thorac Cardiovasc Surg* 113:37–49, 1997.

Koss M: Pulmonary lymphoproliferative disorders, in Churg A, Katzenstein AL (eds), *The Lung.* Philadelphia, Williams & Wilkins, 1993.

Mark J: Surgical treatment of pulmonary metastases, where do we stand? *Ann Surg* 218:703–709, 1993.

Miller DL, Allen MS: Rare pulmonary neoplasms. *Mayo Clin Proc* 68:492–498, 1993.

Pogrebniak H, Roth J, Steinberg S, et al: Reoperative pulmonary resection in patients with metastatic soft tissue sarcoma. *Ann Thorac Surg* 52:197–203, 1991.

Suster S: Primary sarcomas of the lung. *Semin Diag Pathol* 12:140–157, 1995.

57 Extrapulmonary Syndromes Associated with Lung Tumors*

Larry R. Kaiser and Bruce E. Johnson

Lung cancers are the most common tumors associated with paraneoplastic syndromes, which can be classified into endocrine, hematologic, and neurologic types. Endocrine and hematologic syndromes associated with lung tumors are listed in Table 57-1.

The endocrine syndromes are characterized by the ectopic production of biologically active peptide hormones by tumor cells that bind to receptors in adjacent or distant organs, giving rise to a clinical syndrome. The ectopic adrenocorticotropic hormone (ACTH) syndrome, the hyponatremia of malignancy, and hypercalcemia of malignancy are examples of this model. In order to establish the diagnosis of an endocrine paraneoplastic syndrome, the following criteria should be met: (1) a decrease in the level of the hormone after treatment of the tumor, (2) demonstration of hormone synthesis and secretion by tumor cells in vitro, (3) high concentrations of the hormone in the tumor, and (4) an arteriovenous gradient in hormone levels across the tumor bed.

Lung cancers also produce extrapulmonary syndromes by other mechanisms. Hematologic syndromes develop in patients with lung cancer through the production of cytokines by tumor cells that activate progenitor cells in the bone marrow. Neurologic syndromes, such as encephalomyelitis and subacute sensory neuropathy, are caused by the induction of antibodies directed against proteins expressed by the lung cancer cells and against antigens present on cells in the nervous system.

Although lung cancers produce and express various hormones, many (e.g., the gastrin-releasing peptide) do not cause a clinically evident syndrome. Other peptide hormones, such as ACTH precursors, are translated into prohormones, which are not processed into mature peptides. As a result, levels of the immunoreactive proteins in plasma are increased without a clinical syndrome.

In general, definitive treatment of the underlying tumor by surgical resection, radiotherapy, or chemotherapy is the most effective form of therapy for the paraneoplastic syndrome.

HYPERCALCEMIA OF MALIGNANCY

Hypercalcemia is the most common paraneoplastic syndrome. Approximately 1 percent of patients with lung cancer have hypercalcemia when first seen, but 10 to 20 percent of patients develop hypercalcemia during the course of their disease. Lung cancer is the most common solid tumor associated with

*Edited from Chap. 116, "Extrapulmonary Syndromes Associated with Lung Tumors," by Johnson BE, Chute JP. In: *Fishman's Pulmonary Diseases and Disorders,* 3d ed., edited by Fishman AP, Elias JA, Fishman JA, Grippi MA, Kaiser LR, Senior RM. New York, McGraw-Hill, 1998, pp 1841–1850. For fuller discussion of topics dealt with in this chapter, the reader is referred to the original text, as noted above.

TABLE 57-1 Endocrine and Hematologic Syndromes Associated with Lung Tumors

Syndrome	Tumor	Proteins/Cytokines
Hypercalcemia of malignancy	Non–small cell	Parathyroid hormone–related peptide Parathormone
Hyponatremia of malignancy	Small cell Non–small cell	Arginine vasopressin Atrial natriuretic peptide
Ectopic ACTH syndrome	Small cell Carcinoid tumors	Adrenocorticotropic hormone Corticotropin-releasing hormone
Acromegaly	Carcinoid tumors Small cell	Growth hormone–releasing hormone Growth Hormone
Granulocytosis	Non–small cell	G-CSF GM-CSF IL-6
Thrombocytosis	Non–small cell Small cell	IL-6
Thromboembolism	Non–small cell Small cell	Unknown

hypercalcemia, accounting for 30 to 40 percent of all paraneoplastic cases. Hypercalcemia is commonly seen in patients with squamous cell carcinoma of the lung, uncommonly in patients with adenocarcinoma, and very rarely in patients with small cell lung cancer.

Hypercalcemia in patients with lung cancer is usually not caused by local osteolytic effects of bony metastases. Most cases of hypercalcemia in patients with lung cancer are caused by the ectopic production of parathyroid hormone–related peptide (PTHrP) by tumor cells (humoral hypercalcemia of malignancy).

Treatment

Patients in whom lung cancer cannot be eradicated can be treated with intravenous saline plus furosemide diuresis. Subcutaneous calcitonin has a rapid onset of action and is most useful in severe cases. Mithramycin and long-acting biphosphonates, such as pamidronate, are effective for long-term control of hypercalcemia. Corticosteroids exert their effect through inhibition of dihydroxyvitamin D_3 synthesis and therefore have less effect in patients with elevated PTHrP.

HYPONATREMIA OF MALIGNANCY

Hyponatremia is a frequent complication in patients with cancer. More than 90 percent of cases occur in patients with small cell lung cancer. Some 10 to 15 percent of patients with small cell lung cancer and 1 percent of those with non–small cell lung cancer present with hyponatremia. Most of these cases are caused by the ectopic production of arginine vasopressin (AVP). This subset of hyponatremia is recognized as the *syndrome of inappropriate antidiuretic hormone* (SIADH). Ectopic production of atrial natriuretic peptide (ANP) may also play a role in the hyponatremia of malignancy, but the exact contribution of this hormone remains to be defined.

Treatment

In many patients, despite an initial tumor response to chemotherapy, the syndrome of hyponatremia persists or recurs after the cancer regrows. In these patients, the short-term treatment for mild hyponatremia is fluid restriction of 500 mL per day. Many patients with cancer cannot tolerate this level of fluid restriction for extended periods, so other treatments are usually required. Demeclocycline is the medication of choice for chronic management of SIADH in patients with small cell lung cancer.

In patients who present with severe, symptomatic hyponatremia, the intravenous administration of 3 percent hypertonic saline as well as furosemide is recommended.

ECTOPIC ACTH SYNDROME

Lung cancers are the most common neoplasms that cause ectopic ACTH production and Cushing's syndrome, accounting for 50 percent of all cases. Small cell carcinoma accounts for 80 to 90 percent of cases associated with lung cancers, but carcinoid tumors (10 percent) and bronchial adenocarcinomas (5 percent) have also been reported to produce biologically active ACTH.

Diagnosis

The diagnosis of ectopic ACTH syndrome is established by the demonstration of increased 24-h excretion of urinary free cortisol (more than 400 nmol a day), increased plasma cortisol level (more than 600 nmol/L), and increased plasma ACTH level (over 22 pmol/L), which do not decrease in response to the administration of high-dose dexamethasone.

Treatment

The treatment for a patient with ectopic ACTH production is to remove the source of the ACTH. When removal of the ectopic source of ACTH is not possible, medical therapy directed at decreasing adrenal secretion may be successful. Ketoconazole is an imidazole derivative that inhibits steroidogenesis at both adrenal and gonadal sites.

ACROMEGALY

Carcinoid tumors of the lung and intestine are responsible for 70 percent of cases of ectopic acromegaly. Ectopic production of growth hormone–releasing hormone (GH-RH) by tumor cells can be demonstrated in most patients, whereas a minority of tumors produce growth hormone.

Diagnosis

The diagnosis is established by the presence of increased levels of GH-RH and insulin-like growth factor 1 (IGF-1) in the patient's plasma, the absence of a pituitary tumor, and the demonstration of GH-RH or GH in tumor tissue by immunohistochemistry or mRNA expression studies.

HEMATOLOGIC SYNDROMES

Most hematologic syndromes associated with lung tumors are not as well characterized as the endocrine syndromes, because the ectopic hormone responsible for the syndrome has not been identified in most tumor tissues. In many of the hematologic syndromes, such as granulocytosis and thrombocytosis, clinical sequelae are often absent. As with the endocrine paraneoplastic syndromes, the most appropriate therapy for the hematologic syndromes is treatment of the underlying neoplasm.

Granulocytosis

Non–small cell lung cancer is the most common cancer associated with granulocytosis. Twenty percent of patients with non–small cell lung cancer have granulocytosis, with absolute white blood cell counts ranging from 10,100 to 25,000 (normal range is 4000 to 10,000).

Although granulocyte colony-stimulating activity can be demonstrated in serum and/or urine in 80 percent of the patients, the specific peptide hormone causing the syndrome has not been identified.

Thrombocytosis

Thrombocytosis is common in patients with lung cancer, afflicting 40 percent of those with both non–small cell and small cell tumors.

The pathogenesis of thrombocytosis in patients with lung cancer has not been definitively elucidated. IL-6, which is a cytokine for megakaryocytes, has been demonstrated in cell lines from patients with lung cancer and thrombocytosis, and increased levels of IL-6 have been demonstrated in the plasma of such patients.

Thromboembolism

Twenty percent of patients with lung cancer develop venous thromboembolism during the course of their disease. Twenty percent of patients who present with recurrent idiopathic venous thrombosis are found to have an underlying diagnosis of cancer. The spectrum of causes of thrombosis in patients with lung cancer is broad, including disseminated intravascular coagulation (DIC), Trousseau's syndrome (recurrent migratory venous thrombophlebitis), nonbacterial thrombotic endocarditis, and obstruction of great vessels.

NEUROLOGIC SYNDROMES (TABLE 57-2)

Encephalomyelitis, cerebellar degeneration, retinopathy, opsoclonus/myoclonus, and the Lambert-Eaton syndrome have all been associated with lung tumors, most commonly small cell lung cancer. Most of these neurologic paraneoplastic syndromes appear to be caused by an autoimmune response directed at antigens that are shared by the cancer cells and normal neural

TABLE 57-2 Neurologic Syndromes Associated with Lung Cancer

Syndrome	Tumor	Antibody	Antigen
Encephalomyelitis/ subacute sensory neuropathy	Small cell	Anti-Hu	Hu-D antigen: 35–40-kDa neuronal nuclear protein
Cancer-associated retinopathy	Small cell	Antirecoverin	23-kDa protein specific to photoreceptor cells (recoverin)
Lambert-Eaton syndrome	Small cell	Anti-P/Q channel	P/Q-type calcium channel

tissue. Unlike that of the endocrine and hematologic syndromes associated with lung cancer, the clinical course of the neurologic syndromes is typically independent of the course of the underlying disease.

Encephalomyelitis/Subacute Sensory Neuropathy

Currently, more than 70 percent of cases of paraneoplastic encephalomyelitis are diagnosed in patients with small cell lung cancer. Anti-Hu, a specific antibody that reacts with the HuD antigen expressed by lung cancer cells and neuronal tissues, has been associated with the development of this syndrome.

Paraneoplastic Cerebellar Degeneration

A syndrome of cerebellar degeneration has also been noted in patients with small cell lung cancer. This is believed to be a variant of the paraneoplastic cerebellar degeneration (PCD) observed in patients with gynecologic and breast tumors.

Opsoclonus and Myoclonus

Opsoclonus is a disorder consisting of involuntary rapid conjugate eye movements in vertical and horizontal directions. It is often associated with myoclonus in patients with solid tumors. This syndrome of opsoclonus/myoclonus has been associated with both small cell and non–small cell lung cancer in numerous case reports, but less is known about this syndrome than about the syndrome of paraneoplastic encephalomyelitis/subacute sensory neuropathy.

CANCER-ASSOCIATED RETINOPATHY

Cancer-associated retinopathy is a rare paraneoplastic syndrome that occurs predominantly in patients with small-cell lung cancer. Many autoantibodies have been identified in patients with this disorder; they bind to a photoreceptor-specific protein called recoverin. The clinical triad of photosensitivity, ring-scotomata visual field loss, and attenuation of retinal arteriole caliber is considered highly suggestive of cancer-associated retinopathy.

LAMBERT-EATON SYNDROME

The Lambert-Eaton syndrome afflicts fewer than 2 percent of lung cancer patients but has been reported in up to 5 percent of patients with small cell lung cancer. Sixty percent of all patients who present with the Lambert-Eaton syndrome have small cell lung cancer.

Biology

In patients with Lambert-Eaton syndrome and small cell lung cancer, an IgG autoantibody has been identified that binds to calcium channels in motor and autonomic nerve terminals, thereby inhibiting acetylcholine release.

Diagnosis

Clinical features include weakness of the pelvic girdle and thigh, fatigue, dry mouth, dysarthria, dysphagia, blurred vision, and muscle pain. Unlike the situation with myasthenia gravis, muscle strength improves with exercise and does not improve significantly with the administration of anticholinesterases (e.g., edrophonium). Electromyography performed in these patients demonstrates increased muscle action potential with repeated nerve stimulation. In patients with the Lambert-Eaton syndrome, IgG autoantibodies should be demonstrable in serum.

CONCLUSION

The paraneoplastic syndromes have long fascinated and perplexed oncologists, and only in recent years have the molecular bases for these syndromes been appreciated. This new knowledge has not only led to more effective palliation of symptoms but may also offer new clues to the pathogenesis of malignancy. The presence of signs and symptoms that suggest a paraneoplastic syndrome should prompt a search for malignancy.

BIBLIOGRAPHY

Block JB: Paraneoplastic syndromes, in Haskell CM (ed), *Cancer Treatment,* 4th ed. Philadelphia, Saunders, 1995, pp 245–246.

Dalmau J, Graus F, Rosenblum MK, Posner JB: Anti-Hu–associated paraneoplastic encephalomyelitis/sensory neuropathy: A clinical study of 71 patients. *Medicine (Baltimore)* 71:59–72, 1992.

Ralson SH, Gallacher SJ, Patel U, et al: Cancer-associated hypercalcemia: Morbidity and mortality. Clinical experience in 126 treated patients. *Ann Intern Med* 112:499–504, 1990.

Part Fourteen | **INFECTIOUS DISEASES OF THE LUNGS**

58 | Approach to the Patient with Pulmonary Infection*

Jay A. Fishman

OVERVIEW: THE PATIENT WITH PNEUMONIA

The clinical syndrome of pneumonia may include fever; pulmonary symptoms such as cough, sputum production, dyspnea, and pleurisy; or pulmonary lesions observed on radiographic examination. This syndrome is one of the most common problems in clinical medicine. Pneumonia is defined as inflammation of the pulmonary parenchyma caused by an infectious agent. Pneumonitis may be due to many etiologies, both infectious and noninfectious, and reflects only inflammation. A variety of eponyms have been applied to various forms of pneumonia that *may* reflect the epidemiology of the process and the likely causative organisms: aspiration pneumonia, community-acquired pneumonia, nosocomial pneumonia, pneumonia in the immunocompromised host, and atypical pneumonia. However, these descriptions may be misleading, and definitive microbiological diagnosis remains helpful in optimizing clinical care. Physical findings are often unreliable—particularly as reliance on radiologic techniques has displaced the physical examination as an art form. "Crackles" and rales are "heard" much more often than the actual incidence of pulmonary consolidation. Commonly, radiographic appearances are also "confused" with etiologic diagnoses: consolidation, bronchopneumonia, miliary patterns, nodules, abscesses, fluid collections, pleural effusions, interstitial pneumonitis, lymphadenopathy. The goal of the clinician is to define the etiology of pulmonary processes as rapidly as possible so as to facilitate management.

The physician must answer a series of questions in regard to each patient, which will provide useful clues to management:

1. Is the process life-threatening?
2. What is the time course of the process? Is it rapidly progressive or gradual? Is there time to delay therapy or diagnostic procedures? Does the patient need supplemental oxygen, assisted ventilation, surgery, blood products, monitoring or isolation?
3. Is this process infectious? Are there clues to a noninfectious process? Is there more than one process involved?

*Edited from Chaps. 119 to 125, "Microbial Flora and Colonization of the Respiratory Tract," by Johanson WG Jr, Dever LL; "Pulmonary Clearance of Infectious Agents," by Toews GB; "Approach to the Patient with Pulmonary Infections," by Swartz MN; "Principles of Antibiotic Use and the Selection of Empiric Therapy for Pneumonia," by Niederman MS; "Local Therapy and Pharmacokinetics of Antibiotics in the Lungs," by Klastersky JA, Aoun M; "Vaccination for Pulmonary Infections," by Simberkoff MS; "Microbial Virulence Factors in Pulmonary Infections," by Michel JL, Pier GB. In: in *Fishman's Pulmonary Diseases and Disorders,* 3d ed., edited by Fishman AP, Elias JA, Fishman JA, Grippi MA, Kaiser LR, Senior RM. New York, McGraw-Hill, 1998, pp 1883–1972. For fuller discussion of topics dealt with in this chapter, the reader is referred to the original text, as noted above.

4. Is the patient (host) otherwise normal? Immunocompromised? Is pulmonary and thoracic anatomy normal?

5. How can a diagnosis be achieved most expeditiously? What invasive procedures are done well at my institution?

6. Does the patient have supports in the community? Can he or she manage medications, other therapies, and follow-up visits?

7. What are the gross pathologic and pathogenetic features of the pulmonary process: frank pneumonia, focal infiltrate, lung abscess, chronic cavitary lesion, bronchiectasis, miliary lesions? As a corollary, since pulmonary infections are occasionally generated by the hematogenous rather than by the bronchogenic route, possible initiating factors in the pathogenesis of the pulmonary infection should be weighed.

8. What are the most common infections in the community or hospital or institution where this "infection" was acquired? In this appraisal, it is helpful to resort to clinical groupings: community-acquired, nosocomial, and pneumonia in the immunocompromised host. Each group is considered either typical, in that direct sputum examination or culture provides the diagnosis and includes primarily the common pneumonias for that group (e.g., bacterial or fungal), or atypical, in that the sputum examination and culture fail to provide a diagnosis; this subset would consist primarily of "atypical" agents including viruses, *Chlamydia, Mycoplasma,* or *Legionella* species.

9. Establish clinical clues:
   a. Epidemiologic history (i.e., travel, contacts, exposures, vaccines, medications, prior infections, or hospitalizations).
   b. Symptoms: Rate of progression, other systemic signs. Prior mild respiratory illness ("the flu") with improvement and then rapid deterioration is suggestive of bacterial superinfection of viral pneumonitis consistent with *Staphylococcus aureus* or other bacterial infection. The abrupt onset of illness with recurrent (over several days) shaking chills, particularly if associated with mild diarrhea for 1 or 2 days, might suggest Legionnaires' disease. The presence of extrapulmonary signs or symptoms is often a better clue to the nature of infection than are pulmonary symptoms.
   c. Physical examination: Skin lesions (e.g., endocarditis or gram-negative sepsis), lymph nodes, retinal examination, ear examination (bullous myringitis with mycoplasmal infection), periodontal disease or absent gag reflexes (with aspiration pneumonia), and neurologic disease (pulmonary-brain syndromes) are commonly ignored but provide valuable clues.
   d. Laboratory examination: Many systemic processes are reflected in abnormalities of blood counts, urinalysis, and routine blood chemistries. For example, the presence of mild liver function abnormalities might suggest Q fever, tularemia, miliary tuberculosis, or Legionnaires' disease. A hemolytic anemia with a markedly elevated level of cold agglutinins would direct attention to the possibility of *mycoplasma pneumoniae* pneumonia; the presence of pigmented casts in the urine and markedly elevated serum levels of creatine phosphokinase might focus attention on the possibilities of influenza virus pneumonia, Legionnaires' disease, or a pulmonary infiltrate associated with intravenous drug abuse.

10. Radiology: No radiographic findings are specific enough to define the microbial origin of a given pneumonia or pulmonary infiltrate. The only

definitive way to reach a specific etiologic diagnosis is through demonstration of the infecting organism—i.e., by examination of stained smears of sputum and pleural fluid or other biologic materials, by culture of respiratory secretions and blood, by demonstration of nucleic acids from an infecting microorganism, or by demonstrating an increase in antibody titer against the infecting microorganism. Nonetheless, the radiographic picture, taken along with other clinical information, can favor one or several etiologic agents. The number of pulmonary lobes involved in the process and the presence of pulmonary effusions are poor prognostic features.

a. Define the radiographic pattern as lobar or segmental consolidation, patchy bronchopneumonia, nodules (large, small, or miliary), or an interstitial process. Many large round pulmonary densities in a renal transplant recipient suggest *Nocardia* infection rather than *Pneumocystis carinii* pneumonia, whereas in a heroin addict with cough, fever, and pleuritic chest pain, such densities suggest acute right-sided endocarditis rather than pneumococcal pneumonia.

b. Compare with prior radiographs: Is the process old or new? Are there multiple processes? Has the patient had surgery in the intervening period? Is the spleen enlarged or absent?
Confounding variables: Is it too early in the process to detect radiologic changes (first 18 to 24 h)? Is the patient neutropenic (early viral or fungal pneumonitis) or otherwise immunocompromised (*P. carinii* pneumonia often occurs with minimal or no radiologic findings)? Dehydration is commonly cited as a cause of false-negative radiographs, but in general this concept is probably incorrect.

11. Examination of clinical specimens (appropriately stained smear of sputum or pleural fluid, blood buffy coat, skin lesions, throat swabs) often provides a provisional diagnosis. Examination of an appropriately stained smear of sputum can provide a shortcut to diagnosis if the findings are reasonably definitive.

a. Gram-stained smears provide information regarding the morphology and the tinctorial properties of bacteria (and some fungi) but also about the presence of polymorphonuclear leukocytes and squamous epithelial cells, the latter indicating that the specimen originated in the upper rather than the lower respiratory tract.

b. Other special staining methods provide additional data, including Kinyoun and modified acid-fast stains for mycobacteria. Wright-Giemsa or a variant such as Diff-Quik or direct fluorescent antibody staining of induced sputum samples for *P. carinii* or *Legionella pneumophila* may provide a diagnosis.

c. Culture of sputum or blood or other bodily fluids may provide a specific etiologic diagnosis when evaluation of a sputum smear have not supplied a provisional diagnosis, either because the infecting agent cannot be distinguished from components of the normal flora of the upper respiratory tract incorporated in the specimen or because the particular microorganism is not visible on Gram-stained smear (e.g., *Aspergillus* species or *Mycoplasma pneumoniae*).

d. In some patients, an etiologic diagnosis cannot be made on the basis of initial smears or cultures. In such circumstances, a definitive diagnosis can sometimes be made by alternative means: e.g., urinary antigen tests for *Legionella* or *Histoplasma* infections, antigenemia or nucleic acid polymerase chain reactions for viral processes (cytomegalovirus), or, retrospectively, by serologic means, as in psittacosis, Q fever, or adenovirus pneumonia.

e. Invasive diagnostic procedures: If a patient is critically ill, rapidly deteriorating, or unlikely to tolerate invasive infection [immunocompromised host, recent major surgery, heart failure, chronic obstructive pulmonary disease (COPD)] it is reasonable to consider more invasive diagnostic procedures. In particular, some empiric therapies carry potential toxicities that may be intolerable to specific patients. In addition, empiric antimicrobial therapy carries the risk of obscuring a specific microbiologic diagnosis. In such patients, only specific etiologic diagnoses can direct appropriate therapy. Invasive diagnostic procedures are used to obtain uncontaminated lower respiratory tract secretions or pulmonary tissue for microbiologic and histologic analysis. The selection of such procedures should be based on the nature of the illness and the likelihood of success for each procedure at the institution. Among the invasive procedures that are available are (1) protected specimen brushing (PSB), (2) plugged telescoping catheter (PTC) sampling, (3) standard bronchoalveolar lavage (BAL), (4) protected bronchoalveolar lavage (P-BAL or PTC-BAL), (5) transtracheal aspiration (now uncommon), (6) fiberoptic bronchoscopy with transbronchial biopsy, (7) needle biopsy of the lung, and (8) open lung biopsy via limited or video-assisted thoracotomy. Important considerations include the type and location of the pulmonary lesion, the ability of the patient to cooperate with the required manipulations, the presence of coagulopathies, and experience at the particular hospital in performing each of the procedures.

12. Antimicrobial therapy: In practice, initial therapy is empiric and based primarily on available clinical clues. The selection of drug(s) for empiric therapy depends on the clinical setting and on the gravity of the pulmonary process. The selection of antimicrobial agents is considered in Chap. 59.

NONINFECTIOUS PROCESSES MIMICKING PULMONARY INFECTIONS

The list of noninfectious disorders that mimic pulmonary infections is extensive (Table 58-1). These should be considered in the course of taking the initial history. The likelihood of noninfectious etiologies of pulmonary disease increases if the Gram-stained smear and culture of sputum are unrevealing, if the initial response to empiric antimicrobial therapy proves unsatisfactory, or if radiographic findings are atypical. Given the limited spectrum of histopathologic appearances associated with pulmonary inflammation, it should be expected that similar histologic appearances result from both infectious and noninfectious etiologies. The presence of a maculopapular skin rash, generalized lymphadenopathy, joint or rheumatologic symptoms, and/or peripheral eosinophilia should suggest hypersensitivity. However, as noninfectious and infectious processes often coexist, it is essential to exclude infectious causes of pulmonary dysfunction before treating, for example, hypersensitivity reactions. Immunosuppressive agents, notably corticosteroids, will reduce inflammation due to both infectious and noninfectious causes.

TABLE 58-1 Noninfectious Causes of Febrile Pneumonitis Syndrome (Mimics of Pulmonary Infection)

Drug-induced pulmonary disease
Extrinsic allergic alveolitis
Injury due to inhaled toxic gases, dusts, chemicals
Acute eosinophilic pneumonia
Pulmonary infiltrate with eosinophilia (PIE syndrome)
Chronic eosinophilic pneumonia
Interstitial lung disease associated with autoimmune/connective tissue disorders
  Systemic lupus erythematosus
  Polymyositis-dermatomyositis
  Mixed connective tissue disease
Interstitial lung disease associated with pulmonary vasculitis
  Wegener's granulomatosis
  Lymphomatoid granulomatosis
  Churg-Strauss syndrome (allergic angiitis and granulomatosis)
  Polyangiitis overlap syndrome
Intersitial lung disease associated with pulmonary airway disease
  Allergic bronchopulmonary aspergillosis
  Bronchocentric granulomatosis
  Bronchiolitis obliterans and bronchiolitis obliterans with organizing pneumonia
Acute or subacute interstitial pulmonary fibrosis (IPF, Hamman-Rich syndrome)
Chronic interstitial pneumonias of unknown origin
  Usual interstitial pneumonia (UIP)
  Lymphocytic interstitial pneumonia (LIP)
  Desquamative interstitial pneumonia (DIP)
  Giant cell interstitial pneumonia (GIP)
Pulmonary neoplasms
  Carcinoma or lymphoma
  Kaposi's sarcoma in AIDS
Sarcoidosis
Pulmonary infarction
Acute chest syndrome in sickle cell crisis
Radiation pneumonitis
Lipoid pneumonia (exogenous or endogenous)
Adult respiratory distress syndrome (ARDS)
Associated with extrapulmonary sepsis
Associated with oxygen toxicity, chemical inhalation or aspiration, or aspiration of gastric contents
  Associated with pancreatitis
  Associated with fat embolization
  Associated with shock of various etiologies
  Associated with drug overdose
  Associated with chest trauma
Pulmonary leukoagglutinin transfusion reactions
Miscellaneous
  Pulmonary alveolar proteinosis
  Plasma cell granuloma
  Histiocytosis X
  Idiopathic pulmonary hemosiderosis
  Goodpasture's syndrome
  Rheumatic pneumonia (in acute rheumatic fever)

TABLE 58-2 Noncytotoxic Drugs Capable of Inducing
a Picture Resembling Pulmonary Infection

Antimicrobial agents
  Nitrofurantoin
  Penicillins, cephalosporins
  Sulfasalazine, other sulfonamides
  Minocycline, tetracycline
  Amphotericin B (acting with leukocyte transfusions)
  Para-aminosalicylic acid
Anticonvulsants
  Phenytoin
  Carbamazepine
Diuretics
  Hydrochlorothiazide
Antiarrhythmics
  Amiodarone
  Tocainide
Narcotics
  Heroin
  Methadone
  Propoxyphene
  Cocaine

Drug-Induced Pneumonitis

Noncytotoxic Drugs

Drugs producing pulmonary reactions may be considered in two categories, noncytotoxic and cytotoxic drugs. Noncytotoxic drugs producing hypersensitivity pneumonitis include antimicrobials, anticonvulsants, diuretics, antiarrhythmics, tranquilizers, and antirheumatic agents (Table 58-2). Among the most common pulmonary reactions are those to sulfa drugs, phenytoin, nitrofurantoin, and amiodarone. Sulfasalazine (and other sulfonamides) can produce hypersensitivity lung disease that includes cough, fever, dyspnea, and peripheral hazy acinar or diffuse reticular infiltrates. Phenytoin can produce hypersensitivity responses in the lung 3 to 6 weeks after initiation of therapy. Fever, cough, and dyspnea are accompanied by radiographic findings of bilateral acinar, nodular, or reticular infiltrates. Nitrofurantoin can produce two patterns of pulmonary reaction: (1) acute, which occurs within 2 weeks of starting therapy and consists of dyspnea, nonproductive cough, chills, fever, crackles, eosinophilia, and diffuse interstitial or patchy infiltrates (often with pleural effusion), and (2) chronic, which is less common and occurs after months to years of continuous treatment. The picture of the chronic form is one in which exertional dyspnea and nonproductive cough appear gradually and are unaccompanied by fever; the pattern is not that of an acute pulmonary infection but rather that of diffuse interstitial pneumonitis or pulmonary fibrosis. Amiodarone may be associated with pulmonary side effects, often after 5 to 6 months of therapy. Exertional dyspnea, nonproductive cough, malaise, and fever (in about half the patients) are gradual in onset, over weeks to several months. The radiographic findings include peripheral areas of consolidation that affect primarily the upper lobes. In some instances, coarse reticular interstitial infiltrates are present. Withdrawal of the medication, coupled with the administration of corticosteroids, usually leads to complete resolution. Other common forms of drug-induced hypersensitivity pneumonitis include those due to hydrochlorothiazide and gold salts. Hydralazine, procainamide, and isoniazid are capable of inducing a lupus-like syndrome, which may include pleuropulmonary involvement.

Cytotoxic Drugs

Three clinical and pathologic patterns characterize cytotoxic drug–induced pulmonary disease: chronic pneumonitis with pulmonary fibrosis, acute hypersensitivity lung disease, and noncardiogenic pulmonary edema. A variety of predisposing factors may contribute to the development of these reactions. The cumulative dose of certain drugs (e.g., bleomycin, busulfan, and carmustine) appears to be particularly important. Combined exposures [e.g., doxorubicin (Adriamycin) and bleomycin] with dual patterns (cardiac failure and pulmonary injury) are common.

Syndrome of Acute or Chronic Pneumonitis with Fibrosis Essentially all types of cytotoxic drugs capable of inducing pulmonary disease can produce pneumonitis with fibrosis. The clinical manifestations develop over weeks to months and include nonproductive cough, progressive dyspnea on exertion, fatigue, and malaise. End-inspiratory crackles are audible on examination. The radiographic findings are consistent with those of an interstitial inflammatory process and pulmonary fibrosis. Fever is not common in this process other than with cyclophosphamide; over 50 percent of patients with pulmonary fibrosis due to cyclophosphamide exhibit fever. Distinguishing between the effect of the drugs and the underlying disease process is often difficult.

Syndrome of Hypersensitivity Lung Disease Methotrexate, bleomycin, and procarbazine cause an acute syndrome of dyspnea, nonproductive cough, fever, and occasionally pleuritic chest pain. The presence of blood eosinophilia and a skin rash suggests a hypersensitivity reaction. The radiographic findings include a diffuse reticular pattern and, in some patients, bilateral acinar infiltrates.

Extrinsic Allergic Alveolitis (Hypersensitivity Pneumonitis)

Inhalation of organic dusts may produce chills, fever, nonproductive cough, dyspnea, and pulmonary crackles within hours of exposure to organic dusts or vapors. The chest radiograph usually shows bilateral patchy acinar infiltrates, suggestive of pulmonary infection. The history of a specific exposure provides the clue to diagnosis, particularly when such episodes have been recurrent. Farmer's lung occurs with hypersensitivity to moldy hay containing *Thermoactinomyces* species and *Micropolyspora faeni.* "Air-conditioner" or "humidifier" lung is associated with exposure to similar moldy antigens stemming from occult microbial growth on these air-exchanging systems in offices and homes. In other hypersensitivity pneumonitides, the offending antigens may be of avian origin (pigeon breeder's disease) or from other environmental fungi contaminating natural products in industry (e.g., maple bark stripper's lung; moldy sugar cane in bagassosis).

Injury Due to Inhaled Toxic Gases, Dusts, Chemicals

Silo-filler's disease, an acute syndrome mimicking acute bacterial or viral pneumonia clinically and radiologically, can following exposure to nitrogen dioxide. A degenerative interstitial pneumonitis–like picture may result from exposure to organic (e.g., wood, mycotoxin-containing) and inorganic (e.g., silicates, tungsten carbide) dusts. Severe interstitial disease and organizing pneumonia have occurred among workers exposed to aerosols of organic chemicals (designed to polymerize on mixing) used in textile dyeing.

Chronic and Acute Eosinophilic Pneumonia

Chronic eosinophilic pneumonia usually has a course of weeks to months, characterized by fever, night sweats, nonproductive cough, and dyspnea. Pulmonary crackles are variably present. Chest radiographs show a characteristic pattern of peripheral acinar infiltrates that usually involve the upper lobes, resembling the appearance of butterfly pulmonary edema. Peripheral blood eosinophilia is common. Occasionally, chronic eosinophilic pneumonia has an acute onset. Even though the onset in such cases is acute, the course, if untreated (corticosteroids), is prolonged, as in typical chronic eosinophilic pneumonia. Acute eosinophilic pneumonia was initially described as an acute febrile illness with severe hypoxemia, diffuse pulmonary infiltrates, increased numbers of eosinophils in bronchoalveolar lavage (BAL) fluid, and prompt response to corticosteroid therapy without relapse. Drug hypersensitivity may be the cause in some cases. A subset has been described with the same acute onset with high fever, a radiologic picture of micronodular and diffuse ground-glass infiltrates, and spontaneous improvement without relapse.

Pulmonary Infiltrate with Eosinophilia

The term *pulmonary infiltrates with eosinophilia* (PIE syndrome) is used to encompass a wide range of definable clinical entities such as acute eosinophilic pneumonia, chronic eosinophilic pneumonia, allergic pulmonary aspergillosis, and Churg-Strauss vasculitis (see below). However, *PIE syndrome* should be used to refer to a syndrome consisting of fleeting pulmonary infiltrates, dry cough and mild wheezing, low-grade fever, and blood and pulmonary eosinophilia. Loeffler's syndrome, a form of PIE, may be associated with parasitic infestation (migration or hypersensitivity) with *Ascaris lumbricoides, Strongyloides stercoralis, Ancylostoma duodenale, Toxocara canis,* and others or due to drug hypersensitivity. Tropical eosinophilia is a similar syndrome—endemic to India and southern Asia, Africa, and South America—and most likely due to filarial infection.

Interstitial Lung Disease Associated with Connective Tissue Disorders and Pulmonary Vasculitis

A variety of connective tissue disorders and vasculitides mimic pulmonary infections. Systemic lupus erythematosus may be associated with transitory infiltrates, interstitial disease, or frank consolidation of a noninfectious nature. Interstitial pneumonitis occurs in 5 to 10 percent of patients with polymyositis and may be mistaken for a pulmonary infection, since pulmonary manifestations and fever may precede muscle weakness.

Three types of vasculitis commonly mimic pulmonary infection. Wegener's granulomatosis involves the lung in approximately 95 percent of cases. Radiologically, the lesions appear as patchy infiltrates or as nodular lesions, which may progress to cavities or lung abscesses. Superinfection of Wegener's granulomatosis of the lungs is common. Allergic angiitis and granulomatosis (Churg-Strauss syndrome) occurs in the setting of asthma and peripheral eosinophilia. It characteristically involves the lung, producing pulmonary infiltrates associated with granulomatous and vasculitic lesions. The polyangiitis overlap syndrome combines some of the characteristic features of classic polyarteritis nodosa and of allergic angiitis and granulomatosis, including some instances of prominent pulmonary impairment.

Interstitial Lung Disease Associated with Airway Disease

Allergic bronchopulmonary aspergillosis, characterized by cough, bronchospasm, fever, and intermittent pulmonary infiltrates, can suggest pulmonary infection, although an accompanying eosinophilia provides a clue to the true nature of the process. Eosinophilia may be absent in patients receiving corticosteroid therapy. Bronchocentric granulomatosis, a necrotizing process of unknown cause affecting small bronchi, may be associated with fever in some patients. The pulmonary lesions vary from mucoid impaction to diffuse and nodular infiltrates.

Bronchiolitis obliterans is an occasional complication of pulmonary viral or bacterial infections, cocaine toxicity, drug hypersensitivity, connective tissue disease, or inhalation of chemical irritants; it can also occur without apparent cause. It is a common presentation of lung injury and chronic rejection of transplanted lungs. It may present with patchy areas of pneumonitis, necrosis of bronchiolar epithelium, and occlusion of terminal airways by granulation tissue. Bronchiolitis obliterans with organizing pneumonia (BOOP) refers to cases in which the presence of organizing inflammatory polypoid masses in distal bronchioles and alveolar ducts is accompanied by a chronic pneumonitis with lipid-laden macrophages. Although many patients with BOOP respond promptly to corticosteroids, occasional patients undergo a rapidly progressive downhill course even with intensive therapy.

Chronic Interstitial Pneumonias of Unknown Cause

A variety of interstitial pneumonias—known as usual interstitial pneumonia (UIP), lymphocytic interstitial pneumonia (LIP), desquamative interstitial pneumonia (DIP), and giant cell interstitial pneumonia (GIP)—are conditions of unknown origin that are defined on histologic grounds. Most often they present clinically as subacute or chronic processes characterized by progressive dyspnea, cyanosis, nonproductive cough, pulmonary crackles, and a radiographic picture of diffuse reticulonodular infiltrates (more prominent at the lung bases) or a "ground-glass" pattern without fever. Thus, the clinical picture may not suggest pulmonary infection. In some patients, the onset is rapid and accompanied by fever suggesting an acute respiratory infection.

Pulmonary Neoplasms

Bronchial obstruction by a bronchogenic carcinoma may produce obstructive pneumonia ("drowned lung") or atelectasis. Fever and signs of consolidation/atelectasis may fail to respond to antimicrobial therapy. Recurrent pneumonia in the same portion of the lung should suggest this possibility. Hodgkin's disease and non-Hodgkin's lymphoma may present with fever, cough, dyspnea, and pulmonary lesions suggesting infection. In Hodgkin's disease, a single mass lesion may be present and cavitate, suggesting a lung abscess.

Sarcoidosis

In the patient with sarcoidosis and interstitial lung disease, fever is uncommon unless hilar adenopathy or other features, such as erythema nodosum, are present as well. Thus, this process is usually not mistaken for a primary pulmonary infection.

Pulmonary Infarction

Fever, dyspnea, pleuritic chest pain, leukocytosis, and segmental pleural-based infiltrates (and possibly accompanying pleural effusion) of pulmonary infarction suggest the presence of pulmonary infarction due to pulmonary embolus or septic emboli. Similar features are observed with pneumococcal pneumonia. The presence of blood-streaked sputum in this syndrome might suggest the possibility of *Streptococcus pyogenes* pneumonia with hemorrhagic tracheobronchitis. Occasionally, multiple round radiographic infiltrates in the lungs of a febrile, dyspneic patient with pulmonary emboli might suggest lung abscesses due to aspiration or septic emboli.

Lipoid Pneumonia

Exogenous lipoid pneumonia results from inhaling or aspirating fatty materials (oily nose drops, mineral oil). Endogenous lipoid pneumonia (often called *cholesterol* pneumonia) consists of chronic inflammatory foci containing cholesterol and its esters, derived from destroyed alveolar walls located either behind a bronchial obstruction or in lung parenchyma at a site of chronic suppuration. Sputum, fine-needle aspirates, or BAL specimens may reveal macrophages containing lipoid vacuoles, as demonstrated by fat stains (Sudan, oil red O).

Radiation Pneumonitis

The acute phase of radiation pneumonitis usually develops within 3 or 4 months of initiation of radiation therapy. It is characterized by fever, dyspnea, cough, and radiographic changes (infiltrates or ground-glass density) sharply demarcated geometrically to the portal of irradiation rather than to natural pulmonary anatomic divisions. This reaction might be mistaken for a bacterial pneumonia. The late phase of radiation pneumonia, characterized by pulmonary fibrosis, occurs 9 months or more after radiation therapy and is not accompanied by fever.

Miscellaneous Mimics of Pulmonary Infection

Pulmonary alveolar proteinosis usually begins slowly, with dyspnea as the principal symptom. Radiographic features are those of a bilateral diffuse, predominantly perihilar airspace disease. The radiographic but not the clinical manifestations might suggest pulmonary infection. Fever is usually absent. However, pulmonary alveolar proteinosis may be associated with hematologic malignancies associated with fever including lymphoma or acute leukemia. In addition, pulmonary alveolar proteinosis is sometimes complicated by pulmonary infections—e.g., nocardiosis (most frequently), cryptococcosis, aspergillosis, tuberculosis, pneumocystosis, and histoplasmosis.

Plasma cell granuloma is a postinflammatory pseudotumor of the lung. The combination of cough, fever, and radiologic changes of atelectasis and consolidation suggests the diagnosis of pulmonary infection associated with bronchial obstruction. This process is very similar to the previously described cholesterol pneumonia.

Eosinophilic granuloma of the lung (pulmonary histiocytosis X) usually is manifest as a noninfectious interstitial pulmonary process with dyspnea and nonprogressive cough. In about 15 percent of patients, however, fever occurs, suggesting the possibility of pulmonary infection. The radiographic findings are those of small nodules and reticulation or honeycombing; these findings in the febrile patient might suggest the diagnosis of miliary tuberculosis, invasive mycotic infection, *Rhodococcus equi,* or viral disease (e.g., varicella zoster).

Adult Respiratory Distress Syndrome (ARDS)

Many unrelated conditions involving the lungs primarily or having their initial impact elsewhere have in common the capacity to cause diffuse damage to the alveolar-capillary membrane and produce noncardiogenic pulmonary edema. The process progresses rapidly, with inflammatory cell infiltration and pulmonary fibrosis. Extensive pulmonary infiltrates are evident on chest radiographs. Superinfection of lungs injured by ARDS, often by nosocomial pathogens, is common. Many of the underlying processes producing ARDS are associated with fever, including pancreatitis, peritonitis, endocarditis, severe thermal injuries, as well as fulminant bacterial or viral infections.

Pulmonary Leukoagglutinin Transfusion Reactions

An acute pulmonary reaction may follow receipt of a blood transfusion with which there has been passive transfer of leukoagglutinins and antibodies cytotoxic to recipient lymphocytes. The clinical picture of an abrupt onset of chills, fever, tachycardia, cough, and dyspnea, accompanied by numerous fluffy and nodular perihilar infiltrates on radiograph, might easily be mistaken for an acute pulmonary infection. Pulmonary hemorrhage may also affect such patients, particularly after hematopoietic transplantation.

PULMONARY INFECTIONS: PATHOLOGIC AND PATHOGENETIC FEATURES

Pulmonary infections can be categorized according to their distinctive pathologic aspects, anatomic and radiologic features, and pathogenetic characteristics.

Bacterial Pneumonia

Bacterial pneumonia commonly results from bronchogenic spread of infection following microaspiration of pharyngeal secretions. Such particles reach terminal airways and alveoli to initiate infection, which has the anatomic distribution and radiologic appearance of subsegmental, segmental, or lobar consolidation. Pneumonia may be patchy in distribution, with a peribronchial and multifocal distribution, in association with aspiration and bronchial plugging, superinfection of preexisting chronic bronchitis, diffuse acute tracheobronchial inflammation (e.g., influenza, parainfluenza), and with specific infecting microorganisms (e.g., oral anaerobic bacteria). The progression of a pulmonary infiltrate or lobar consolidation to parenchymal destruction (necrotizing pneumonia or lung abscess) is usually the consequence of one or more of three factors: the intrinsic virulence of the infecting organism(s), the presence of bronchial obstruction or other anatomic abnormality, or immune compromise in the host.

Pneumonia may develop via the bacteremic rather than the bronchogenic route. The clinical setting and the radiographic pattern usually suggest this form of pathogenesis. The intravenous drug abuser with *Staphylococcus aureus* bacteremia and acute right-sided endocarditis will present with fever, cough, purulent sputum, a murmur of tricuspid insufficiency, numerous irregular infiltrates, and rounded densities on chest radiograph. Similarly, burn patients with *Pseudomonas aeruginosa* bacteremia and multiple nodular pulmonary densities are likely to have bacteremic *Pseudomonas* pneumonia with pulmonary bacterial arteritis. Septic pulmonary emboli, arising from septic thrombosis of the jugular vein may cause a clinical and radiographic picture suggestive of multifocal bronchopneumonia. On the chest radiograph, however, the lesions are nodular; histologically, they represent septic pulmonary infarcts (following emboli) upon which are engrafted pyogenic infection and abscess formation.

Lung Abscess

A lung abscess is an area of pulmonary infection with parenchymal necrosis. Lung abscesses may be solitary or may occur as multiple discrete lesions. Most often such an abscess is secondary to aspiration of anaerobic or anaerobic and aerobic organisms that are colonizers of the upper respiratory tract and may be associated with periodontal disease. Superinfection of damaged or infarcted lung tissue (e.g., as in aspirational pneumonia with chemical injury and anaerobic superinfection or primary anaerobic infection) progresses to necrosis and microscopic foci of abscess formation. Confluence of small necrotic foci can create one or more lung abscesses or lead to a progressively fibrotic, shrunken, and destroyed lobe. *Pulmonary gangrene* is an unusual consequence of severe pulmonary infection characterized by sloughing of a pulmonary segment or lobe. This process affects an entire segment or lobe secondary to thrombosis of both bronchial and pulmonary arteries with pulmonary infarction. The organism most commonly implicated has been *Klebsiella pneumoniae,* but others have been *Streptococcus pneumoniae, Escherichia coli,* mixed anaerobes, *Haemophilus influenzae,* and *Staphylococcus aureus.* If there is some degree of ball-valve bronchial obstruction, air may enter while contained pus may fail to drain, producing the radiographic picture of an air-fluid level.

Other causes of lung abscess are (1) progression of a bronchogenic pneumonia due to a pathogen with necrotizing potential (e.g., *K. pneumoniae*), or *Nocardia asteroides* in an immunocompromised patient, (2) bacteremic spread of infection, and (3) septic pulmonary emboli. Lung abscesses complicating necrotizing pneumonia should be distinguished from pneumatoceles; the latter are thin-walled, air-filled structures that often develop early in the course of staphylococcal pneumonia, particularly in infants and young children, and usually disappear over the course of a few months.

Bronchitis and Bronchiectasis

Acute bronchitis is an inflammatory process, usually of viral origin, confined to the bronchi and bronchioles; it does not extend appreciably to surrounding pulmonary parenchyma and is not evident on radiographic examination. Purulent inflammatory secretions are common even though there may be no discernible bacterial infection. Such purulent secretions represent bacterial superinfection. The diagnosis of an acute exacerbation of chronic bronchitis is based solely on clinical grounds; the manifestations are increased cough, dyspnea, and enhanced production of purulent sputum, with or without fever, in a patient with chronic obstructive pulmonary disease. Bacteriologic examination generally reveals large numbers of pneumococci or nontypable *H. influenzae,* either as infecting organisms or as chronic colonizers of the bronchial tree. Patients with acute exacerbations of chronic bronchitis tend to improve with antimicrobial treatment, while those with chronic bronchitis are less likely to improve with therapy.

Bronchiectasis is characterized by destruction of epithelial, elastic, and muscular elements of bronchi, resulting in their irreversible dilatation. The major proximate cause is repeated for chronic bacterial infection. However, predisposition to such infections may be a consequence of a variety of factors, including certain types of prior infection (pertussis, adenovirus, or rubeola infections, necrotizing pneumonia), bronchial obstruction, immunodeficiencies, congenital anatomic lung disease (e.g., congenital tracheobronchomegaly), and other hereditable disorders, such as ciliary dysfunctional states and alpha$_1$-antitrypsin deficiency. Currently, cystic fibrosis is the most common predisposing factor for bronchiectasis. As a result of repeated infections, stasis of secretions, and peribronchial fibrosis, bronchi are grossly distorted or completely destroyed. Although pneumonia or lung abscess may accompany recurrent acute infections, exacerbations are usually confined to bronchial and peribronchial tissues.

Chronic Cavitary Disease

Chronic cavitary pulmonary disease is most often related to tuberculosis, but may be seen in alpha$_1$-antitrypsin deficiency, echinococcal disease, Wegener's granulomatosis, and other structural disorders. Tuberculosis commonly begins with a focus of pneumonitis, usually in the subapical posterior portion of an upper lobe. This patch of pneumonitis occurs at a latent site of earlier metastatic infection (Simon focus) produced by lymphohematogenous spread from primary pulmonary tuberculous lesions. Progressive caseation necrosis at this site, followed by drainage of caseous material through the bronchial tree, produces a cavity. The cavity is encased in a rigid wall of fibrous tissue.

In addition to pyogenic lung abscess and pulmonary tuberculosis, other pulmonary infections can produce chronic cavities. These include *Nocardia* infections, *Rhodococcus equi* infections, actinomycosis, and chronic primary pulmonary mycoses (particularly histoplasmosis, occasionally coccidioidomycosis, uncommonly blastomycosis). Sporotrichosis can affect the lung and produce thin-walled cavities. Parasitic infestation of the lung (paragonimiasis, echinococcosis) can also form cavities.

Pulmonary cavities may also occur in noninfectious disorders (e.g., Wegener's granulomatosis, lymphoma or bronchogenic carcinoma, bland pulmonary infarcts, and intrapulmonary nodules of rheumatoid lung disease). Such cavitary lesions, as well as the cystic lesions that occur in chronic pulmonary sarcoidosis and in the markedly dilated bronchi of saccular bronchiectasis, can be the sites of *fungus balls*. These represent tangled masses of fungal hyphae and debris lying freely within pulmonary cavities, generally as noninvasive saprophytic growths in the immunologically normal host. The mycotic agent responsible most commonly *Aspergillus* species (usually *A. fumigatus*), and the fungus ball are called aspergillomas. Hemoptysis originating from the cavity wall is common and may be severe.

Miliary Lesions

Hematogenous dissemination of tuberculosis can follow initial infection in children or adults. It also can result from breakdown of formerly quiescent sites of pulmonary or extrapulmonary infection. Clinically unexplained fever may be accompanied by miliary lesions (like millet seeds, very small and uniform in shape) on the chest radiograph; histologically, these lesions are foci of granulomatous reaction. Similar radiographic lesions also occur in the course of hematogenously disseminated bacterial and mycotic infections including cryptococcosis and histoplasmosis.

VIRAL INFECTIONS OF THE RESPIRATORY TRACT

The Common Cold

Respiratory viral infections are a major cause of morbidity worldwide. Patients present with cough, sore throat, bronchoconstriction, fever, rhinitis, and suffusion of mucous membranes. The majority of these infections are upper respiratory infections, which are of significance as causes of discomfort and as predisposing conditions for lower respiratory infections. Spread is via aerosolized droplets and hand contact. The most prominent of the viral pathogens include rhinovirus and coronavirus, for which no specific antimicrobial therapies are available. Commonly, adenovirus, parainfluenza virus, respiratory syncytial virus (RSV), and influenza virus may also cause this syndrome. Less commonly, reovirus, enteroviruses, and picornaviruses may cause the same symptoms. Of nonviral etiologies, treatable infections with *M. pneumoniae* and *Chlamydia pneumoniae* also cause significant upper as well as lower respiratory infections. The main differential for this infection includes allergic, vasomotor, or atrophic rhinitis or nasal polyposis. These syndromes should be considered in patients with atopic history and recurrent upper respiratory infections. While these infections are generally self-limited, common complications include sinusitis, otitis, and bronchitis, exacerbations of chronic pulmonary disease (chronic bronchitis), asthma, and bacterial superinfection with pneumonia.

Viral Infections of the Lower Respiratory Tract

Infections with respiratory viruses occur predominantly in the winter and early spring. Influenza virus is the one agent that may be associated with sizable outbreaks or major epidemics of upper respiratory infections. Primary influenza viral pneumonia usually occurs in the setting of an outbreak of influenza A infections. It occurs primarily in patients with underlying heart disease (mitral stenosis), chronic pulmonary disease, or pregnancy and in immunocompromised individuals. Unlike secondary bacterial pneumonia after influenza—a complication that occurs after a period (1 to 4 days) of improvement following a typical influenzal upper respiratory illness—primary influenza pneumonia immediately follows typical influenza. Rarely, in the course of systemic infection with viruses whose principal impact is not ordinarily on the respiratory tract, viral pneumonia develops in an otherwise healthy person. Pulmonary infiltrates occur in 16 percent of young adults with varicella, but only 2 to 4 percent have clinical manifestations suggestive of pneumonia. Some cases of mild pneumonitis have been observed in patients receiving live varicella vaccine. Pneumonia in children with varicella is more likely to represent bacterial superinfection than primary viral pneumonia. On rare occasions, pulmonary infiltrates develop in patients with clinical infectious mononucleosis; the infiltrates represent atypical pneumonia due to Epstein-Barr virus.

A novel Hantavirus, Sin Nombre virus, emerged acutely in 1993, in the Four Corners area of New Mexico, Arizona, Colorado, and Utah. Cases had been reported worldwide but primarily in the West and Southwestern United States. The Hantavirus pulmonary syndrome begins with a 3- to 6-day prodromal period consisting of myalgias and fever, sometimes accompanied by gastrointestinal symptoms. The prodrome is followed by progressive cough, dyspnea, tachycardia, and hypotension. Bleeding may occur. Laboratory findings include hemoconcentration, leukocytosis, and thrombocytopenia. The chest radiograph demonstrates interstitial edema, peribronchial cuffing, and bilateral airspace (bibasilar and perihilar) disease. The patient suffers from pulmonary edema (interstitial and alveolar), consistent with a diffuse pulmonary capillary leak syndrome. The case fatality rate for the Hantavirus pulmonary syndrome is 50 percent. The principal host for Sin Nombre virus is the deer mouse, and infection is acquired through exposure to this rodent, rodent excreta, or contaminated dust.

In the immunocompromised host, viral infection is most often due to cytomegalovirus, although RSV, varicella zoster, and herpes simplex viral pneumonias may be seen in addition to common community-acquired viral infections. In this population, the frequency and intensity of viral illness exceeds that of the general population. Cytomegalovirus pneumonia in the solid organ transplant recipient occurs most often in seronegative (naïve) recipients of donor organs from seropositive (latently infected) individuals. The syndrome of hypoxia with diffuse interstitial infiltrates may predispose to or coexist with a similar syndrome due to *P. carinii*. This is most severe in the lung transplant recipient. By contrast, CMV pneumonitis in the hematopoietic transplant recipient (BMT) occurs with the activation of CMV in the seropositive recipient of cells form a seronegative donor. With engraftment, the naïve immune system reacts against CMV antigens expressed in the lungs. Superinfection is common and graft-vs-host disease may complicate the differential diagnosis.

Fungal Pneumonia

Fungal pneumonia occurs most often in immunocompromised hosts. However, in the normal host, infection due to the endemic or geographic fungi (*Histoplasma capsulatum, Coccidioides immitis*) or to *Cryptococcus neoformans* may be asymptomatic or may present with systemic signs often confused with acute bronchitis, viral infection, mycobacterial infection, or aseptic meningitis. Otherwise, fungal infection of the lungs is most common with anatomic defects (aspergilloma) or aspiration (*Candida* species) but is otherwise rare in individuals without immune defects. A few syndromes merit consideration. *P. carinii* causes pneumonia with prominent hypoxia and often few physical or radiologic findings in immunocompromised individuals, particularly those on corticosteroids. As this infection is easily prevented, consideration should be given to prophylaxis in any individual receiving chronic immunosuppressive therapy or with HIV infection or AIDS unresponsive to antiretroviral therapy. Aspergilloma is traditionally considered to be a noninvasive colonization of pulmonary cavities. However, gross hemoptysis may complicate management and dissemination may occur at the time of surgical resection. Immune suppression may convert benign disease into invasive pneumonia. Mucormycosis (due to the *Mucoraciae*) causes rapidly progressive sinus and lung infection, which requires surgical resection for cure. This infection is most common in diabetics.

Parasitic Pneumonia

Parasitic pneumonia is uncommon without endemic exposures. Pneumonia generally occurs when the normal life cycle of the organism includes the lungs.

Infection by *Entamoeba histolytica* causes pleuropulmonary disease as a result of (1) *sympathetic* reaction to an unruptured abscess within the liver, (2) empyema, after rupture of the liver abscess into the pleural space, or (3) parenchymal involvement with abscess, consolidation, or hepatobronchial fistula after rupture of a liver abscess. Amebae that have broached the mucosal barrier are thought to gain entry to the liver via the portal vein. Subsequent liver abscesses can be either purely amebic or mixed bacterial and amebic. Other less common routes exist, including hematogenous spread, which can lead to metastatic abscesses of brain, lung, and other organs. *Acanthamoeba* species cause subacute meningoencephalitis or keratitis often secondary to hematogenous spread of dermal or pulmonary disease. Some form of pulmonary complication occurs in 3 to 10 percent of patients with falciparum malaria. Noncardiogenic pulmonary edema can develop suddenly, even after appropriate antimalarial therapy has been instituted and even after parasites are no longer detected on blood smears. Acute acquired infection due to *Toxoplama gondii* in the immunocompetent host is generally asymptomatic, with cervical lymphadenopathy as the hallmark of disease. It may be confused with mononucleosis caused by Epstein-Barr virus or cytomegalovirus. Fever, malaise, sore throat, and hepatosplenomegaly are also seen, and the peripheral blood may manifest atypical lymphocytosis. Rarely, acute acquired disease may present with severe dissemination, marked by pneumonitis, hepatitis, encephalitis, polymyositis, or myocarditis. In the immunocompromised host, acute toxoplasmosis is most often associated with necrotizing encephalitis as a result of brain cyst reactivation, although myocarditis, hepatosplenomegaly, fever, and interstitial pneumonitis are also common. Pulmonary infections due to migrating worms include Loeffler-like syndrome with *Ascaris lumbricoides,* postobstructive pneumonitis, and systemic sepsis due to *Strongyloides stercoralis,* cysts and nodules due to *Echinococcus granulosus, Paragonimus westermani, Schistosoma* species, and pulmonary eosinophilia in filariasis.

CLINICAL SYNDROMES IN PNEUMONIA

In the patient with pneumonia, it is helpful, while microbiologic data are being gathered, to consider the relative frequencies of various causes as an aid in selecting initial antimicrobial therapy. Categorization of pneumonia by the clinical setting is often useful (Table 58.3).

Community-Acquired Pneumonia

The largest category of pneumonia consists of community-acquired pneumonia (CAP), an infection acquired outside the hospital by an immunologically normal host. Worldwide, the incidence of various pathogens in community-acquired pneumonia is relatively constant. However, the increased numbers of immunocompromised individuals and of elderly or disabled individuals who may reside in chronic care facilities and changing patterns of antimicrobial susceptibility have changed the spectrum of infection that may be encountered in outpatient practice. Over 3.5 million cases of community-acquired pneumonia are diagnosed each year in the United States. The main variable is the regional incidence of endemic infections, including tuberculosis, and the episodic occurrence of epidemic infections such as outbreaks of influenza virus or Hantavirus.

For over half of the patients with CAP, no causative pathogen can be identified. Up to 15 percent of CAP are due to aspiration or mixed bacteria. In most series, 20 to 65 percent are due to *S. pneumoniae* (pneumococcus).

TABLE 58-3 Categorization of Pneumonia by Clinical Setting

Community-acquired pneumonia
  Typical (i.e., classic) pneumonia
  Atypical pneumonia
Aspiration pneumonia
Pneumonia in the elderly
  Community-acquired
  Nursing home residents
Nosocomial pneumonia
Pneumonia in immunocompromised hosts
  Pneumonia in patients with immunoglobulin and complement deficiencies
  Pneumonia in patients with granulocyte dysfunction or deficiency
  Pneumonia in patients with cellular and combined immune deficiencies
  Neoplastic disease
  Solid organ and hematopoietic transplant recipients
  Untreated AIDS
  Immune reconstitution syndromes (AIDS, neutropenia)
  Severe combined immunodeficiency and congenital deficiencies
  Autoimmune and connective tissue disorders
  Other immunocompromised patients

Approximately 15 percent of patients have definable nonbacterial etiologies such as *M. pneumoniae, Chlamydia psitacci,* or viruses. These atypical pathogens are difficult to diagnose (and therapy is often of less than certain value). The atypical pathogens, the pneumococcus and *Legionella* species, and aspirational events account for many of the undiagnosed cases of CAP. Certain uncommon causes may be endemic, in particular geographic niches, including *Coxiella burnetii* (in Nova Scotia, Canada) or *Francisella tularensis* in Little Rock, Arkansas.

CAP is a major cause of infectious morbidity and mortality. Depending on the causative organisms, the mortality of CAP ranges from 10 to 15 percent for pneumococcal infection to 60 percent for *Pseudomonas aeruginosa.* Adverse clinical prognostic factors included comorbid conditions (neurologic or neoplastic disease, cirrhosis, congestive heart failure, respiratory compromise, diabetes, hepatic and renal dysfuction, immune deficiency), bacteremia, and multilobar involvement. *S. pneumoniae* is the preeminent bacterial cause of community-acquired pneumonia. *H. influenzae,* usually unencapsulated strains, may produce pneumonia in patients with chronic bronchitis or in the chronic alcoholic. Apart from *S. pneumoniae,* however, the most important pathogen in this type of patient, by virtue of its virulence and special antimicrobial agent susceptibilities, is *K. pneumoniae.* During an outbreak of influenza viral infections, bacterial superinfections often occur, usually in the elderly or in patients with chronic cardiopulmonary disease. Patients with secondary bacterial pneumonia often have up to 4 days of clinical improvement after the initial influenzal illness before the onset of overt pulmonary infection. The superinfecting microorganisms are the pathogens that would ordinarily colonize the upper airways but opportunistically invade a tracheobronchial tree that has been recently damaged. These organisms include *S. pneumoniae, H. influenzae, S. aureus, S. pyogenes, M. catarrhalis,* and *K. pneumoniae.* The use of antimicrobial agents at the time of the initial respiratory infection not only is useless against viral influenza but also may selectively promote the emergence of a more resistant bacterial flora in the respiratory tract. *S. aureus* is a very uncommon cause of community-acquired pneumonia. Indeed, the occurrence of several cases of *S. aureus* pneumonia in the community during the winter months is usually a good indicator of the presence of an ambient influenza outbreak. Pneumonia due to *S. pyogenes* is quite uncommon. Usually it occurs as a superinfection in a patient with influenza or as a primary pneumonia in the course of a regional outbreak of group A streptococcal infections (as still occurs from time to time when a new M-antigenic type appears in a community).

Atypical Pneumonia Syndrome

In the evaluation of patients with community-acquired pneumonia, it is often helpful to consider separately a group of patients whose illness is characterized by minimal sputum that does not reveal a predominant microbial etiology on routine smears (Gram stain, Ziehl-Neelsen) and cultures (including those for mycobacteria and *Legionella*). The clinical onset of illness is generally subacute, with a radiologic picture consisting of patchy infiltrates or an interstitial pattern than a lobar consolidation. Fever and peripheral leukocytosis are less common or intense than in common bacterial pneumonias. For convenience, this grouping has been designated *atypical pneumonia*.

The entities in the category of atypical pneumonia are highly heterogeneous. The syndrome may account for up to 60 percent of cases of community-acquired pneumonia. *M. pneumoniae* is the causative agent in about 25 percent of the cases of atypical pneumonia. Respiratory viruses are responsible for about another 30 percent. However, the predominant etiologic agent varies considerably with the season and the prevalence of influenza viruses in the community. *Chlamydia pneumoniae* (formerly known as *Chlamydia* strain TWAR) is an infectious agent that causes pneumonia and can be spread from person to person, appears to be responsible for 12 to 21 percent of cases of atypical pneumonia. This form of pneumonia typically occurs in young adults as a sporadic mild pneumonia but may have enhanced severity when coinfecting individuals with pneumococcal infection.

The epidemiologic and clinical characteristics of certain types of atypical pneumonias may provide a basis for suspecting these causes before results of specific laboratory tests become available. In adults, *M. pneumoniae* pneumonia, in contrast to bacterial pneumonia, often begins insidiously with malaise, fever, and prominent headache. Sore throat is common, but coryza is minimal or absent. Nonproductive cough develops over the next few days and is the hallmark of this disease. Skin rash (erythema multiforme) and bullous myringitis, usually appearing late in the course of illness, are uncommon findings; when present, however, they do suggest the diagnosis. Minioutbreaks of *M. pneumoniae* infection in households, schools, and military camps may not be appreciated because of the long incubation period (3 weeks) and the varied forms that the illness can assume.

Q fever, due to *C. burnetii,* is suspected on the basis of epidemiologic clues. Transmission of this disease to humans occurs as a result of inhalation of aerosols from surroundings contaminated by placental and birth fluids of infected livestock (cattle, sheep, goats), wild rabbits, and domestic animals (cats). Veterinarians, ranchers, and medical investigators, such as those who use goats or sheep to produce antibodies, are at particular risk. Since the incubation period of Q fever is approximately 20 days, a source of exposure during travel may easily be overlooked. Although the clinical picture resembles that of *M. pneumoniae* pneumonia, the onset may be more abrupt, with chills and high fever. Liver function abnormalities or clinical hepatitis in a patient with atypical pneumonia is suggestive of Q fever. In some geographic areas (Australia, France), hepatitis has been the most frequent clinical presentation of *C. burnetii* infection; in others (Spain, Nova Scotia), pneumonia has been the major presenting sign.

Chlamydia trachomatis causes pneumonia in the newborn but has not been proved to be a cause of pneumonia in adults. *C. psittaci,* the causative agent of psittacosis, is spread to humans by avian species. Although psittacine birds (parakeets, parrots) are the major reservoir, human infection can be acquired from pigeons, sparrows, and turkeys. In a patient with atypical pneumonia, the clinical features that raise the possibility of this etiology are relative bradycardia, splenomegaly and hepatomegaly, and hepatic dysfunction. *C. pneumoniae* variant TWAR produces atypical pneumonia without the usual bird-to-human transmission of *C. psittaci* infection. The clinical picture of TWAR-strain infection is indistinguishable from that of *M. pneumoniae* pneumonia.

Legionella infections (due to *L. pneumophila* and other *Legionella* species) account for 2 to 4 percent of cases of atypical pneumonia. Although *Legionella* is an important nosocomial pathogen, it is also responsible for community-based sporadic cases and major outbreaks. The occurrence of summer outbreaks associated with the use of air conditioners and evaporative condensers should call attention to this possible cause of atypical pneumonia. Various extrapulmonary manifestations have been attributed to Legionnaires' disease; among them are a relative bradycardia, diarrhea for 24 h at the onset of illness, confusion and obtundation, mild renal dysfunction (azotemia, microscopic hematuria, proteinuria), acute rhabdomyolysis, and mild hepatic dysfunction. Although many of these manifestations also occur with other pneumonias, the coincidence of several of these features should raise the possibility of *Legionella* infection. This is particularly important in view of the fact that the antimicrobial therapy (erythromycin, tetracyclines, flouroquinolones) for Legionnaires' disease differs from that for the more common bacterial pneumonias, and that if the disease is inadequately treated, the mortality from Legionnaires' disease can be as high as 15 percent. Recurrent chills, which occur over several days in Legionnaires' disease, are rare in pneumococcal pneumonia unless septic complications (e.g., endocarditis and pericarditis) develop. Although the initial radiographic picture of *Legionella* pneumonia is often that of an interstitial, segmental, or bronchopneumonic pneumonia, it progresses to lobar or multilobar consolidation if the disease is untreated, a picture that mimics pneumococcal or *Klebsiella* pneumonia.

The other noteworthy bacterial types of atypical pneumonia are those due to *F. tularensis* (tularemic pneumonia), *Yersinia pestis* (plague pneumonia), and *Bacillus anthracis* (anthrax pneumonia). These are uncommon causes of pneumonia, and among epidemiologic considerations bioterrorism must be considered when these agents are recognized (see Appendix, "Agents Potentially Associated with Bioterrorism"). Exposure to *F. tularensis* comes through contact with tissues of an infected animal (rabbit), animal bites (coyote, cat), inhalation of infectious aerosols, tick or deerfly bites, or ingestion of contaminated water or poorly cooked meat from an infected animal. Ulceroglandular tularemia, or the typhoidal form of tularemia, may be complicated by patchy pulmonary infiltrates. Indeed, it is likely that typhoidal tularemia often represents infection initially acquired via the bronchogenic route. Plague is less common than tularemia in the United States and is strictly localized to the southwestern states, including California. The diagnosis should be considered in a person from an endemic area who has a septic illness (septicemic plague) or painful localized lymphadenopathy with fever (bubonic plague) and a history of bites by rodent fleas or of handling tissues of infected animals, such as prairie dogs or coyotes. Pneumonia occurs as a complication in 10 to 15 percent of patients with bubonic or septicemic plague. Primary (inhalation) pneumonic plague is extremely rare and occurs only as a result of exposure to aerosolized particles from an infected animal or following close contact with cases of plague pneumonia.

Anthrax pneumonia (inhalation anthrax) is also extremely rare in this country; it is a consequence of the inhalation of anthrax spores during the processing or use of goat hair or wool (usually imported from the Middle East, Asia, or Africa). However, anthrax has been associated with colonization, pneumonia, and cutaneous infection as a result of bioterrorism (see Appendix). Clinical clues include dyspnea, a widened mediastinum, and rapid clinical deterioration.

The principal clues to the presence of pulmonary mycoses are epidemiologic. For example, the principal endemic areas for histoplasmosis in this hemisphere are in the midwestern United States and Central America. The organism is present in high concentrations in soil sites where avian, chicken, or bat excrement has accumulated. Movement of soil in such endemic areas by cleaning chicken coops, knocking down old starling roosts, or cleaning out old attics or basements can expose people to high concentrations of airborne spores that, when inhaled, produce an acute pneumonia. Atypical pneumonia in a person with this type of geographic exposure or in a spelunker should automatically raise the possibility of histoplasmosis. Blastomycosis occurs in most states in this country, but the endemic area is principally in the southeastern and south central areas. Rural exposure to soil contaminated with animal excrement appears to be a risk factor. Skin lesions, either verrucous or ulcerative, are the most common extrapulmonary manifestations of blastomycosis and afford a clinical clue to diagnosis. Coccidioidomycosis is endemic in the southwestern United States (California, particularly the San Joaquin Valley, and Arizona) and in neighboring portions of Mexico. Infection is usually acquired in these areas by inhalation of highly infectious arthrospores. Occasionally, major dust storms carry the arthrospores considerable distances from their soil source and produce unexpected outbreaks of infection. Archeologic digs sometimes cause infection in those living elsewhere who receive an artifact uncovered in the explorations. Erythema nodosum may be associated with any of the primary pulmonary mycoses but most often with coccidioidomycosis. The coincidence of this hypersensitivity skin lesion and an atypical pneumonia syndrome in a person from an endemic area suggests the possibility of one of these pulmonary mycoses.

Paracoccidioidomycosis (South American blastomycosis) is endemic to Brazil (mainly), Colombia, Venezuela, and Argentina; this disease is caused by *Paracoccidioides brasiliensis*. In adults, the manifestations of this disease are mainly pulmonary; radiographs show patchy or confluent areas of consolidation, often bilateral. Cases have occurred in North America and Europe, but in those instances, the patients had previously resided in endemic areas where initial infection presumably had been acquired.

Aspiration Pneumonia

Aspiration pneumonia may occur after an overt episode of aspiration (e.g., of gastric contents) or of bronchial obstruction by a foreign body. More often the predisposing circumstances are clear-cut (e.g., alcoholism, nocturnal esophageal reflux, pyorrhea, a prolonged session in the dental chair, epilepsy, or chronic sinusitis in a patient with absent gag reflex). In these circumstances, since the pneumonia may develop more insidiously than after overt aspiration, the relationship of the developing pneumonia to the predisposing circumstances may not be appreciated at the time. For this reason, specific questioning regarding such possible pathogenetic factors and evaluation of the gag reflex should be part of the examination of any patient with pneumonia.

If untreated, aspiration pneumonia may progress rapidly to a necrotizing process that is usually due to anaerobic organisms. The process may involve a pulmonary segment, a lobe, or an entire lung, with ultimate extension to the pleura ("putrid empyema"); in some patients, the necrotizing pneumonia culminates in lung abscesses. In others, aspiration produces an illness of several weeks' duration that is characterized by malaise, productive cough, and low-grade fever. If a chest radiograph is first taken after several weeks of untreated illness, it may show little if any evidence of pneumonia but will clearly identify a well-formed lung abscess.

In community-acquired aspiration pneumonia, insight into the etiologic agents has been obtained primarily from bacteriologic studies after transtracheal aspiration; these studies have provided a statistical basis for selecting the initial antimicrobial therapy. Anaerobic bacteria are etiologically implicated in about 90 percent of community-acquired aspiration pneumonias and lung abscesses. In 40 to 65 percent of these patients, anaerobic organisms are the sole infecting agents; in 40 to 45 percent, the cause is a mixture of anaerobes and aerobes. The most common anaerobes are *Prevotella melaninogenica, Bacteroides* species, *Porphyromonas* species, *Fusobacterium* species, peptostreptococci, peptococci, and microaerophilic streptococci. Beta-lactamase–producing *Bacteroides* species, *P. melaninogenica,* and members of the *B. fragilis* group are present in about 15 percent of cases. *P. melaninogenica* may be the most important contributor in such mixed infections. The aerobic indigenous flora in mixed aerobic-anaerobic infections are *S. viridans, M. catarrhalis,* and *Eikenella corrodens.* A rare form of anaerobic aspiration pneumonia (actinomycosis) that is community acquired is that due to *Actinomyces israelii,* part of the normal flora in the gingival crevice. The direct extension of such a necrotizing pneumonia to the pleura and chest wall is a characteristic finding that strongly suggests the diagnosis of actinomycosis.

Although anaerobic members of the oropharyngeal flora have a preeminent role in community-acquired aspiration pneumonia and lung abscess, occasionally colonizing gram-negative enteric bacilli such as *K. pneumoniae, E. coli,* and *Proteus* species may be the cause. Persistence of a necrotizing pneumonia or lung abscess despite antimicrobial therapy that would be expected a priori to be effective raises the possibility of an underlying obstruction, often in the form of bronchogenic carcinoma, particularly if the patient is edentulous.

Pneumonia in the Elderly

Community-acquired pneumonia in the elderly (over 60 years) primarily affects two groups: one population that lives at home and another that resides in nursing homes. The latter, from the point of view of oropharyngeal flora and the extent of exposure to antimicrobial agents, might be regarded as midway between community residents and patients in hospital. The clinical features of pneumonia in the elderly may differ in presentation from those in younger people. Infection has a more gradual onset, with less fever and cough, often with a decline in mental status or confusion and generalized weakness, but with less readily elicited signs of consolidation on examination. Eliciting a deep breath from the patient may be helpful in demonstrating a localized wheeze or rales that might otherwise be undetectable. Among the bacterial causes of community-acquired pneumonia in the elderly, *S. pneumoniae* is the most frequent, accounting for 30 to 60 percent of cases. *H. influenzae,* primarily nontypable strains, is the second most common cause (about 20 percent). *M. catarrhalis* is another cause of pneumonia in this age group, primarily in patients with chronic bronchitis. Aspiration pneumonia due to mixed aerobic-anaerobic flora occurs in this age group, particularly because of the presence of a diminished gag reflex or impaired pharyngeal motor function.

In nursing home residents or persons with recent hospitalizations, increased oropharyngeal colonization with gram-negative bacilli occurs, probably secondary to individuals exposed to antimicrobial agents in such institutions. Subsequent microaspirational events would predispose to pneumonia due to species such as *K. pneumoniae, E. coli* and other Enterobacteriaceae, and *P. aeruginosa.* In several studies, such gram-negative bacilli have been implicated as the cause in 25 to 40 percent of elderly nursing home residents with pneumonia. *S. aureus* is responsible for 2 to 10 percent of cases of community-acquired pneumonia in the elderly overall, more commonly in nursing home residents and during community outbreaks of influenza. *M. pneumoniae* pneumonia occurs primarily in young adults, but it can occur in the elderly. Among 64 patients with *M. pneumoniae* pneumonia severe enough to require hospitalization, 9 percent were over 65 years of age. Even in this age group, the mortality was low.

Nosocomial Pneumonia and Antimicrobial Resistance

Nosocomial pneumonia is the second most common nosocomial infection in the United States and occurs at a rate of 5 to 10 cases per 1000 hospital admissions. The incidence increases 6- to 20-fold in patients receiving assisted ventilation. The causes of nosocomial pneumonia are often distinct from those of community-acquired pneumonia and should serve to direct the clinician's thinking about etiology and therapeutic approach before results of cultures become available. In particular, the organisms causing pneumonia in medical institutions are often resistant to commonly used antimicrobial agents.

The cause of hospital-acquired pneumonia depends on the time of onset of the pneumonia, the type of hospital (community or university tertiary care), and whether the patient is intubated or in the intensive care unit. Thus, the "early onset" (first 3 days) bacterial pneumonia is more often due to *S. pneumoniae, H. influenzae,* and *M. catarrhalis,* whereas "late onset" (after 4 days) is more commonly (45 to 75 percent) due to aerobic gram-negative bacilli *K. pneumonae,* other Enterobacteriaceae, *Acinetobacter* species, and *P. aeruginosa.* In respiratory intensive care units, *Burkholdaria* (formerly *Pseudomonas*) *cepacia, Stenotrophomonas* (formerly *Xanthomonas*) *maltophilia,* and *Acinetobacter baumannii* (formerly *Acinetobacter calcoaceticus* variant *anitratus*) have been implicated in localized outbreaks of nosocomial pneumonia. In a study by the National Nosocomial Infections Surveillance System of respiratory tract isolates from adults with nosocomial pneumonia, *P. aeruginosa* was the most common pathogen found, and *S. aureus* was the most common gram-positive organism, at a frequency about one-third that of *P. aeruginosa.* Gram-negative bacilli rapidly colonize the oropharynx of ill, hospitalized patients, and they are the most common cause of aspiration pneumonia that occurs subsequently.

Nosocomial outbreaks of *Legionella* pneumonia have occurred in hospitals secondary to environmental problems related to potable water, air-conditioning systems, or water-cooling towers. Although in these circumstances immunocompromised patients have been particularly at risk, patients with alcoholism and chronic obstructive airway disease have also been particularly vulnerable.

In previous years, attention focused on nosocomial pneumonias of bacterial origin. However, it is now appreciated that hospital-acquired viral pneumonias are also of considerable import. During major influenza outbreaks, the incidence of nosocomial pneumonias increases and is accompanied by considerable mortality. These pneumonias represent primary influenza viral pneumonia or, more often, bacterial pneumonia complicating influenza.

In dealing with the individual patient, useful information is provided by awareness of the bacterial species that is most often implicated in nosocomial pneumonia in the particular hospital and the antimicrobial susceptibilities of sputum isolates from patients in that institution. The hospital epidemiologist or the physicians working in an intensive care unit can often provide insights into the cause of outbreaks of nosocomial pneumonia either in the hospital or in their specific sector. With respect to treating a particular patient, examination of Gram-stained sputum (or an endotracheal or bronchoscopic aspirate) is essential as a guide to the selection of initial antimicrobial therapy and in following the response to therapy.

Pneumonia in the Immunocompromised Host

In assessing the likely cause of a febrile pneumonitis syndrome in a patient with an underlying disorder of host defenses, it is helpful to distinguish among several categories of abnormal defense mechanisms. (see Chap. 66).

Hypogammaglobulinemia

Patients who have congenital or acquired deficiencies of the immunoglobulins are particularly susceptible to recurrent pneumonias caused by encapsulated bacterial species, particularly *S. pneumoniae* and *H. influenzae* type b.

Granulocyte Deficiency

This category includes patients who have deficiencies both in granulocyte function and in granulocyte numbers.

Defects in Granulocyte Function   Patients with the hyperimmunoglobulin E syndrome, characterized by chronic eczema, "cold" cutaneous abscesses, and mucocutaneous candidiasis, have a chemotactic defect for polymorphonuclear leukocytes. As a result, they are subject to recurrent skin and sinopulmonary infections. The principal bacteria causing pneumonia in these patients are *S. aureus, H. influenzae,* and, to a lesser extent, *S. pneumoniae.*

Patients with chronic granulomatous disease of childhood suffer from an inherited disorder of oxidative microbicidal activity of polymorphonuclear leukocytes and monocytes. These patients are subject to suppurative lymphadenitis, soft tissue and hepatic abscesses, and sometimes pneumonia. Pathogens producing infections in these patients are primarily *S. aureus,* Enterobacteriaceae (*K. pneumoniae, Serratia*), *Pseudomonas* species or *B. cepacia, Nocardia, Candida* species, and *Aspergillus* species.

Granulocytopenia Granulocytopenia (fewer than 500 or 1000 granulocytes per microliter of blood) is an important risk factor for bacterial and fungal infections. Pulmonary infections in the neutropenic host are often due to endogenous or nosocomial flora including gram-negative bacilli, *S. aureus,* and fungi such as *Aspergillus*. The duration of granulocytopenia and the overall health of the patient are as important as the depth of the neutropenia. Pulmonary infections that occur in recipients of bone marrow transplants represent a special case because of the combination of profound granulocytopenia, combined B-, T-, macrophage, and neutrophilic immunodeficiency, and graft-vs-host disease produced by intense cytotoxic drug or radiation therapy that is used to ablate the bone marrow. These patients are also predisposed to many viral infections (e.g., CMV), to *P. carinii* and *Nocardia asteroides,* and to intracellular pathogens.

Pneumonia that affects granulocytopenic hospitalized patients occurs most often via the microaspiration route. Although mixed anaerobic oral commensals may be responsible, gram-negative bacilli colonizing the oropharynx (particularly *P. aeruginosa*) are among the most frequent causative agents. Bacteremic spread of infection to the lung can also occur from an initiating site of infection in the perineum, intestinal tract, or urinary tract. However, although bacteremia occurs in 30 to 40 percent of patients with gram-negative bacillary pneumonia, the pulmonary infection generally precedes the bacteremia. Radiologic findings are often subtle; CT scans will detect infiltrates missed by routine radiographs.

Cellular Immune Deficiency

The number of immunocompromised patients with primary T-cell defects (i.e., function or numbers) has increased markedly in recent years on several accounts: (1) the prolonged survival of patients with neoplastic disease, (2) the increasing number of organ transplants (and the attendant use of calcineurin inhibitors), (3) the increasing number of patients with collagen vascular disease (treated with both cytotoxic agents, corticosteroids, and calcineurin inhibitors), and (4) patients with the acquired immunodeficiency syndrome (AIDS).

Radiographic Features of Pneumonia The radiographic features of pneumonia are discussed in detail elsewhere. No radiologic pattern provides a specific etiologic diagnosis. However, the radiographic pattern, combined with clinical and epidemiologic information, can narrow the diagnostic considerations while microbiologic data are being assembled (Table 58-4). Several radiographic patterns can be helpful in categorizing infectious and noninfectious causes: (1) airspace or alveolar pneumonia, (2) broncho- or lobular pneumonia, (3) interstitial pneumonia, and (4) nodular infiltrates. Although the chest radiographs of a particular patient may not fit neatly into one or another of these categories, identification of a predominant pattern can be helpful in directing attention to certain causes.

Alveolar Pneumonia

This form of infiltrate occurs when certain organisms, notably *S. pneumoniae,* induce inflammatory edema in peripheral alveoli. When the extent of the consolidation involves an entire lobe, this is the classic *lobar pneumonia*. But more often the process is not that extensive, although the pathogenesis is the same. An air bronchogram is characteristic. Loss of volume is absent

TABLE 58-4 Radiographic Features and Differential Diagnosis of Pneumonia in Immunocompetent Host

Consolidation/focal opacity	*Streptococcus pneumoniae, Mycoplasma pneumoniae, Haemophilus influenzae, Chlamydia pneumoniae* (TWAR), *Legionella* species, *Staphylococcus aureus, Mycobacterium tuberculosis,* and *"atypical"* mycobacteria (*M. avium* complex)
Cavitation	*S. aureus,* anaerobic bacteria, *M. tuberculosis,* Gram-negative aerobic bacteria, *Aspergillus* species, geographic/endemic fungi (*Histoplasma capsulatum, Coccidioides immitis, Blastomyces dermatiditis*)
Interstitial infiltrates	Viruses, *M. pneumoniae, M. tuberculosis,* geographic/endemic fungi, *Chlamydia psittaci*
Miliary	*Mycobacterium tuberculosis,* geographic/endemic fungi, viruses, *M. pneumoniae*
Lymphadenopathy	*M. tuberculosis,* viral (EBV, CMV, rubella), geographic/endemic fungi, *C. psittaci*

KEY: EBV, Epstein-Barr virus; CMV, cytomegalovirus.

or minimal during the acute stage of consolidation, but some atelectasis may develop owing to obstruction of bronchi by exudate during resolution of the process.

K. pneumoniae is another common cause of community-acquired pneumonia, which, like pneumococcal pneumonia, shows homogeneous parenchymal consolidation containing air bronchograms. Although *K. pneumoniae* pneumonia classically affects the right upper lobe and produces a dense, homogeneous lobar consolidation with bulging of the fissure, these features are not pathognomonic and cannot be relied on for diagnosis without supportive bacteriologic data. The propensity for *K. pneumoniae* to produce tissue destruction and abscess formation may, in fact, result in a shrunken rather than an expanded, lobe. Pneumococcal pneumonia may also cause bulging of the fissure, albeit less commonly and less prominently. Extensive alveolar consolidation may occur with a variety of other bacterial causes of pneumonia, including mixed anaerobes of aspiration pneumonia and a variety of gram-negative bacilli implicated in nosocomial pneumonias. Occasionally, an unusual configuration of airspace consolidation, *spherical pneumonia,* occurs, particularly in children, with pneumococcal or *H. influenzae* pneumonia. It has also been reported with Q fever.

In the immunocompromised host, alveolar consolidation on the plain chest radiograph may be delayed and appreciated only by chest CT scan. Among the infectious causes, bacterial agents are a major consideration. Common pathogens such as *S. pneumoniae* will cause infection in this group of patients, often of greater severity than in the normal host and with less radiologic evidence for infection. Bacterial superinfection of viral processes (e.g., influenza, CMV) is also common. However, if the consolidation is lobar or multilobar, *L. pneumophila* is an important possibility to consider. Other likely infectious agents are fungi (e.g., *Aspergillus*), *Nocardia,* and *M. tuberculosis.* Less often, viruses alone (e.g., CMV) elicit a predominantly alveolar pattern. Bilateral diffuse involvement with an airspace pattern resembling pulmonary edema is not uncommonly a feature of *P. carinii* pneumonia, but may also reflect viral or noninfectious etiologies.

Bronchopneumonia

In bronchopneumonia, the focus of infection and the inflammatory response is in the bronchi and surrounding parenchyma. Consolidation is segmental in distribution, and involvement is patchy; segmental involvement may become confluent to produce a more homogeneous pattern. Bronchopneumonic patterns are commonly observed in pulmonary infections due to *S. aureus* or nonencapsulated *H. influenzae*. With *S. aureus* infections, macro- and microabscess formation may occur rapidly. Also, pneumatoceles occur during the first week of lung impairment in about half the children with *S. aureus* pneumonia.

A bronchopneumonic pattern of consolidation is commonly observed when pneumonia is superimposed on underlying bronchiectasis or chronic bronchitis. In such predisposing circumstances, *S. pneumoniae* infection may produce a bronchopneumonic pattern rather than its usual lobar consolidation. In the presence of underlying emphysema, the radiographic pattern of pneumococcal pneumonia may also be altered from its usual homogeneous pattern to one that contains multiple radiolucencies (representing unconsolidated emphysematous areas) that may be misinterpreted as abscesses.

Segmental bronchopneumonia is the radiographic picture in pneumonia due to *C. pneumoniae* or *M. pneumoniae* and in many viral pneumonias. Any of the bacterial species that cause nosocomial pneumonia can produce a radiographic pattern of bronchopneumonic consolidation.

Interstitial Pneumonia (Peribronchovascular Infiltrate)

A reticular or reticulonodular pattern of infiltration is the radiographic representation of interstitial inflammation—i.e., a peribronchovascular infiltrate. In otherwise healthy persons, *M. pneumoniae* is high on the list of community-acquired causes of a radiographic pattern of interstitial pneumonia. In some instances, interstitial infiltration progresses to produce patchy consolidation of airspaces, most often in the lower lobes. Pneumonias due to respiratory viruses sometimes have an interstitial pattern that progresses to patchy segmental consolidation or to diffuse airspace disease that resembles pulmonary edema. A variety of noninfectious causes of interstitial lung disease (e.g., hypersensitivity lung disease, collagen vascular disease, and sarcoidosis) may also produce a reticular pattern on the chest radiograph.

In immunocompromised patients, particularly in those with AIDS, the infectious causes of interstitial pneumonia are broadened to include early *P. carinii* pneumonia and additional opportunistic viral agents (CMV, varicella zoster, herpes simplex, and probably EBV and possibly HIV). Noninfectious causes of a reticular pattern on chest radiography in an immunocompromised host include drug-induced (bleomycin, methotrexate, etc.) pneumonitis, early radiation pneumonitis, and pulmonary edema.

Nodular Infiltrates

Nodular infiltrates are considered here as well-defined large (greater than 1 cm on the chest radiograph) round focal lesions. Such a lesion may represent small aspirational abscesses (without air-fluid levels), a fungal or tuberculous granuloma, or a lesion of pulmonary nocardiosis. Multiple nodular infiltrates may also represent the necrotic lesions that develop in the lung secondary to the septic vasculitis produced by *P. aeruginosa* bacteremia or the consequences of fungemic spread of candidal infection from an infected intravascular catheter. Infected nodular pulmonary lesions are sometimes caused by septic pulmonary infarcts produced by infected emboli that originate from right-sided bacterial endocarditis, septic thrombophlebitis of pelvic veins, or septic jugular vein phlebitis. On rare occasions, similar nodular lesions are produced by necrotic (but not infected) pulmonary infarctions; primary or metastatic neoplastic lesions may have a similar appearance. Nodular lesions that undergo rapid necrosis with cavity formation can be a feature of Wegener's granulomatosis.

In the immunocompromised patient, nodular infiltrates may be due to bacteremic or fungemic spread of infection, often as a result of nosocomial infection caused by an infected intravenous catheter. In this type of patient, nodular lesions should bring to mind the possibilities of pulmonary nocardial infection, aspergillosis, or other fungal infections. Tuberculous granulomas in the lungs may develop or enlarge in the immunosuppressed patient. Metastatic neoplasm or lymphoma sometimes presents a similar radiologic picture. Multiple small nodules, larger than miliary lesions but smaller than the gross nodular lesions described above, raise the possibility of varicella zoster or CMV infection of the lung.

Miliary Pulmonary Disease

Disseminated miliary lesions of infectious nature suggest miliary tuberculosis, histoplasmosis, or blastomycosis in either the normal or immunosuppressed host. In the immunosuppressed patient, a miliary pattern may also be seen in disseminated cryptococcal infection or bacteremic spread of bacterial or candidal infection.

Computed Tomography (CT)

CT scanning of the chest may be helpful in certain situations in patients with pulmonary infections: in determining whether a pneumonia is necrotizing, whether consolidation is secondary to bronchial obstruction (as by hilar lymphadenopathy or by endobronchial tumor), whether a pleural effusion or empyema or loculated fluid collections explains failure of infiltrates to resolve, whether bronchiectasis is present, whether a circumscribed pulmonary density represents a fungus ball within a cavitary lesion, etc. When small granulomatous lesions are present, CT scanning can provide information on the extent of the process. When a single nodule is present, CT scanning can assist in determining whether needle aspiration is feasible and, if so, to direct the biopsy needle. In particular, in immunocompromised individuals, infiltrates not appreciated on plain films (e.g., *P. carinii*) may be demonstrated by CT scanning. This information greatly facilitates invasive procedures such as needle biopsy, video-assisted thoracoscopy, or bronchoscopy.

NONINVASIVE DIAGNOSTIC STUDIES

Noninvasive studies can provide information indicating the specific microbial cause of a pulmonary infection or can narrow the field of likely etiologic agents.

Direct Examination of the Sputum

Cytologic Examination

Examination of Gram-stained sputum smears can be of major value in pin-pointing a bacterial cause of pneumonia and guiding initial therapy. The most valuable bacteriologic information from sputum examination is that in which the results from stained smears and cultures are mutually confirmatory. The quality of a sample of expectorated or induced sputum submitted for examination is the prime determinant of the results that can be expected. Culture of sputum that consists principally of saliva is valueless. What are sought are lower respiratory secretions produced by a cough, not nasopharyngeal secretions. Cytologic examination provides an evaluation of the quality of the sample and its suitability for culture and interpretation of a Gram-stained smear made from it. Scanning of Gram-stained smears or application of specific quantitative criteria is helpful in selecting meaningful specimens for bacteriologic evaluation on smear and in culture. Squamous epithelial cells (normally exfoliated from the oropharynx), when present in numbers of 10 or more per low-power ($\times 100$) magnification field, indicate that the specimen is unsatisfactory; culture of such a specimen correlates poorly with results from culture of a transtracheal aspirate. The presence of numerous poly-morphonuclear neutrophils on Gram-stained smear (10 to 25 or more per low-power microscopic field) in the absence of an excessive number of squamous cells (see above) is indicative of a good specimen for bacteriologic evaluation.

Examination of Gram-Stained Smears for Bacteria

The oil immersion fields examined, and the immediately adjacent fields, should not contain any squamous cells; each should also contain at least three or four neutrophils. The presence of squamous cells not only indicates that the specimen is derived from the upper respiratory tract but also may be confusing to the uninitiated because of the large number of bacteria, often gram-positive diplococci, which might be mistaken for *S. pneumoniae,* adherent to the surface of these cells.

A variety of bacterial respiratory tract pathogens have rather characteristic morphologies and strongly suggest an etiologic role when present in con-siderable numbers in a suitable specimen of sputum (or in a transtracheal aspirate) that contains the proper numbers of inflammatory cells. Such organisms include *S. pneumoniae* (gram-positive oval or lancet-shaped diplococci), *H. influenzae* (small, pleomorphic gram-negative bacilli), *M. catarrhalis* (gram-negative, biscuit-shaped diplococci), or the similar-appearing *Neisseria meningitis,* enteric gram-negative bacilli (not distin-guishable from one another with respect to species except for large encap-sulated rods that are suggestive of *Klebsiella*), and *S. aureus* (large gram-positive cocci in small groups or clusters. Since normal oral flora include a variety of streptococcal species that are morphologically some-what similar to *S. pneumoniae,* sputum smears may be misinterpreted. Thus, a definite predominance of gram-positive diplococci in multiple appropriate oil immersion fields needs to be observed to implicate *S. pneumoniae.* A quantitative aspect to the evaluation has been suggested: at least 10 gram-positive lancet-shaped diplococci per oil immersion field foretells the isola-tion of *S. pneumoniae* from sputum cultures. With use of the aforementioned criteria (numbers of polymorphonuclear leukocytes, absence of epithelial cells, and numbers of gram-positive lancet-shaped diplococci), the specificity of Gram's stain for identifying *S. pneumoniae* is 85 percent, with a sensitivity of 62 percent.

Gram-stained smears can be helpful not only in the etiologic diagnosis of community-acquired bacterial pneumonia due to the usual respiratory pathogens but also in supporting a diagnosis of atypical pneumonia when sputum examinations repeatedly show neither neutrophils nor bacteria. Uncommon bacterial species may be implicated in a pulmonary infection on the basis of unusual morphology on Gram-stained smear: irregularly staining, beaded, delicate gram-positive branching filaments suggest either *Nocardia* or *Actinomyces*.

Several organisms, uncommon causes of pulmonary infection, have morphologic characteristics that may mimic other, more common respiratory pathogens. *Pasteurella multocida* and *Acinetobacter* species, both small gram-negative coccobacilli, have each been mistaken in sputum of patients with pulmonary infections for either *H. influenzae* or *M. catarrhalis,* or for a mixture of the two.

Sputum or pleural fluid with foul odor provides evidence of activity of anaerobic organisms in infective processes such as lung abscess, aspiration pneumonia, empyema, and, occasionally, bronchiectasis. In these settings, the findings on Gram-stained smear may corroborate the preliminary diagnosis. Organisms of the *P. melaninogenicus-asaccharolyticus* group are small gram-negative coccobacilli. *Fusobacterium nucleatum* is a long, tapering, pale-staining gram-negative bacillus with irregularly staining gram-positive internal granules. Purulent secretions or pus from such anaerobic infections contain numerous neutrophils and usually a mixture of bacterial species, including anaerobic and microaerophilic streptococci on stained smear.

Examination of Ziehl-Neelsen or Fluorochrome-Stained Smears for Mycobacteria

The number of new cases of tuberculosis in the United States steadily declined over past decades, reaching a nadir in 1995. During the period 1985 to 1991, the rate of development of new cases (often due to multidrug-resistant strains of *M. tuberculosis*) increased, primarily associated with microepidemics among the urban poor, racial and ethnic minorities, drug abusers, hospital and correctional facility populations, and patients with HIV infection. TB is again decreasing in AIDS in association with highly active antiretroviral therapies (HAART), but not in individuals without access to such therapies. Pulmonary tuberculosis in the aforementioned settings may take the form of chronic cavitary tuberculosis or forms more likely to suggest pyogenic or atypical pneumonia—i.e., progressive primary tuberculosis and tuberculous pneumonia. Acid-fast smears of sputum can provide the very first evidence of this desease. Mycobacteria are seen on smears of about 50 percent of specimens that subsequently prove to contain *M. tuberculosis*. Most laboratories currently employ a fluorochrome stain with auramine-rhodamine (mycobacteria fluoresce orange-yellow) for initial examination of sputum or other body fluids. A typical mycobacteria may be demonstrated on sputum smears of patients, usually older people with slowly progressive pulmonary disease. In patients with AIDS, disseminated *Mycobacterium avium-intracellulare* infection is usually diagnosed by isolation of the organism from blood culture (lysis centrifugation method) or by histopathologic diagnosis on biopsy.

However, the organism can be demonstrated on acid-fast smears and culture of respiratory secretions even though there may be little radiographic evidence of pulmonary infection directly attributable to its presence. Modified Ziehl-Neelsen–stained smears are helpful in detecting *Nocardia*.

Fungal Wet Mounts (Potassium Hydroxide, KOH Preparations)

Fungal wet mounts, smears stained with Calcofluor white chemifluorescent agent or phase-contrast microscopy, are employed when epidemiologic considerations suggest community-acquired pulmonary mycoses (particularly coccidioidomycosis and blastomycosis). They should be a routine part of evaluation of respiratory secretions and lung biopsy materials from immunocompromised patients in whom additional fungal pathogens (e.g., *Aspergillus* and *Mucor*) may be active. In patients with allergic bronchopulmonary aspergillosis, or with the unexpected detection of *Aspergillus* in sputum, fungal hyphae must be considered in the clinical context of each patient.

Direct Immunofluorescent Microscopy

Direct fluorescent antibody (DFA) staining can be useful in rapid diagnosis of respiratory tract pathogens. DFA staining reagents for *L. pneumophila* are commercially available. Their use is not recommended in examination of sputum specimens because of the presence of cross-reacting species (*Bacteroides* species, *Pseudomonas* species, *Bordetella pertussis*) in the upper respiratory tract. However, biopsy specimens of lung (needle, bronchoscopic, or surgical), bronchoscopic aspirates, BAL washings, and pleural fluid samples are suitable for DFA staining for *L. pneumophila*. Although a variety of stains (toluidine blue O, methenamine silver, Wright-Giemsa, Diff-Quik, Calcofluor) are useful in identifying *P. carinii* in induced sputa or BAL specimens, or on imprint smears of tissue specimens, the most widely used diagnostic technique utilizes immunofluorescence with monoclonal antibodies against *P. carinii*. Rapid viral diagnosis (RSV, influenza, parainfluenza, adenovirus) by DFA can be applied to specimens from bronchial lavage or brushings or from nasopharyngeal swabs or washings. Anti–*B. pertussis* DFA may be used on nasopharyngeal aspirate smears in the presumptive diagnosis of pertussis.

Smears for Diagnosis of *Pneumocystis* Infection

Since *P. carinii* pneumonia is an alveolar process, examination of routinely collected expectorated sputae for *P. carinii* is generally not regarded as rewarding in immunosuppressed patients with neoplastic disease or transplant recipients. In these patients, fiberoptic bronchoscopy and transbronchial biopsy, combined with BAL, provide the highest diagnostic yield. In patients with AIDS, however, induced sputum examination for *P. carinii* may be helpful. Sputum induction employing aerosolized, hypertonic saline provides a diagnosis in up to 80 percent of cases, particularly if coupled with microscopy of antibody-stained cytocentrifuged specimens. Immunofluorescent assays, with monoclonal antibodies to *P. carinii*, of induced sputum have a sensitivity of 69 to 92 percent, compared with that of 28 to 80 percent for tinctorial stains. Toluidine blue O and methenamine silver stains stain only the cyst (<10 percent of the organism burden) and not the trophozoite forms of *P. carinii*. Giemsa and Diff-Quik stain trophozoites and intracystic sporozoites. If results of examination of induced sputum are negative and clinical circumstances warrant further attempts at diagnosis, follow-up bronchoscopy with transbronchial biopsy or BAL is performed. The sensitivity of each of these procedures for diagnosis of *P. carinii* pneumonia is more than 90 percent.

Special Microscopic Examinations

Occasionally, in the setting of apparent pulmonary inflammation with features atypical for infection, microscopic examinations using stains other than Gram's stain may be indicated. For example, Wright-stained smears may show the presence of eosinophils in allergic pulmonary aspergillosis or other causes of pulmonary infiltrates that are accompanied by eosinophilia. Cytologic examination of exfoliated sputum using Papanicolaou's stain may reveal a pulmonary neoplasm. Birefringent calcium oxalate crystals (needle-like in rosettes or arranged like sheaves of wheat) in sputum cytologic specimens have been reported as suggesting pulmonary infection with *Aspergillus* (aspergilloma and, occasionally, invasive aspergillosis), a fungus that excretes oxalic acid as a metabolic product.

In the intubated or tracheotomized patient, whose tracheobronchial secretions commonly contain neutrophils and often some bacteria on Gram-stained smears, it may be difficult at times to distinguish between colonization and nosocomial pneumonia. The presence on light microscopy ($\times 400$) of characteristic elastin fibers with split ends (in a drop of tracheal aspirate to which a drop of 40 percent KOH has been added), in the appropriate clinical setting, is a strong indicator of a necrotizing pulmonary infection.

Intense bacteremias sometimes accompany pulmonary infections, and the etiologic agent may be demonstrable on stained smears of the buffy coat of centrifuged blood: pneumococci have been identified in Gram-stained or Wright-Giemsa–stained smears of buffy coats from splenectomized patients; occasionally, *M. avium-intracellulare* has been found intracellularly in acid-fast stains of buffy coats from patients with AIDS.

Additional special microscopic examinations may be indicated for immunocompromised patients who have patchy pulmonary infiltrates on the chest radiograph. For example, the presence of the hyperinfection syndrome of strongyloidiasis (often accompanied by *E. coli* bacteremia) can be established by the finding of filariform larvae in the sputum and in the stool after the latter is suitably prepared by concentration techniques. Although eosinophilia is often present in patients with strongyloidiasis, it may be absent in the hyperinfection syndrome.

Sputum Cultures

In most patients with the common types of community-acquired and nosocomial bacterial pneumonia, the etiologic diagnosis can be made on the basis of the combined results of a Gram-stained smear of sputum and of proper culture of a suitable exudative portion of a freshly obtained sputum specimen. The criteria for a proper sample of sputum have been noted above. Culture entails streak dilution on blood agar and McConkey media. Expectorated sputum should not be cultured anaerobically, since contamination with oral anaerobes is inevitable. Because patients with Legionnaires' disease often raise little if any sputum suitable for culture, most attempts to isolate *Legionella* resort to specimens obtained either by transtracheal aspiration, fiberoptic bronchoscopy, or lung biopsy or at thoracentesis. Cultures of such materials are plated on buffered charcoal-yeast extract (BCYE) agar. Occasionally, *Legionella* species can be isolated from sputum with the use of a semiselective medium, either BCYE or BCYE-containing cefamandole, polymyxin B, and anisomycin. Culture is the most definitive method for diagnosis of *Legionella* infection. Unfortunately, it may take 5 or more days for colonies to appear.

Cultures for mycobacteria are undertaken when clinical circumstances raise the possibility of pulmonary infections due to *M. tuberculosis* or atypical mycobacteria. Similarly, cultures of sputum for primary invasive mycotic agents (e.g., *H. capsulatum, B. dermatitidis,* and *C. immitis*) are dictated by clinical and epidemiologic circumstances. In immunosuppressed patients, cultures of sputum are also directed toward a variety of opportunistic fungi, including *C. neoformans, Aspergillus* species, and Mucoraceae.

Most hospitals do not have facilities for isolating viruses by tissue culture. This lack poses little problem in dealing with most community-acquired viral pneumonias, for which viral isolation is not necessary and the cost is prohibitive. However, viral isolation from throat washings is warranted in certain circumstances (e.g., to prove the presence of an outbreak of influenza), to establish that an outbreak among young children is due to respiratory syncytial virus, and to identify a specific viral agent, such as an adenovirus, as the cause of a serious pneumonia that is not responding to antibacterial therapy. In immunosuppressed patients with pneumonia, a variety of opportunistic viral infections (CMV, respiratory syncytial virus, varicella zoster virus, herpes simplex) are diagnostic considerations. In vitro testing of CMV may provide data regarding susceptibility to antiviral agents.

Cultures are grown in cell lines susceptible to the viral infections under consideration in either standard "tube cultures" or "shell vial" cultures (rapid culture achieved by centrifugation of specimens against the cultured cells). Viral replication in the tissue culture can be confirmed within 48 h after inoculation with use of fluorescent monoclonal antibodies. Because CMV and herpes simplex are frequently present in the oral secretions of immunosuppressed patients, isolation of these viruses is apt to be meaningful only if the materials used for the isolation procedure were obtained either by bronchoscopy with protected specimen brush (PSB) or with BAL, lung biopsy, or transtracheal aspiration.

Blood Cultures

Blood cultures should always be performed in patients with suspected bacterial pneumonia. Bacteremia occurs in approximately 30 percent of patients with pneumococcal pneumonia. Demonstration of bacteremia in other patients with pneumonia may indicate that the pulmonary infection is secondary to bacteremia originating from a focus of infection elsewhere (e.g., acute right-sided *S. aureus* endocarditis or *P. aeruginosa* infection of thermal burns). In patients with AIDS and disseminated *M. avium-intracellulare* infection, mycobacterial blood cultures are almost always positive. The lysis centrifugation technique permits ready and rapid isolation of the mycobacterium and quantifies the intensity of the bacteremia. *L. pneumophila* has been isolated with some frequency from automated radiometric blood culture bottles, but blind subculture onto BCYE agar is necessary because growth in the liquid medium does not achieve detectable levels.

Bacterial Antigen Detection in Sputum and Urine

The quellung reaction was extensively used in the preantimicrobial agent era to identify *S. pneumoniae* in sputum. It entails the use of light microscopy to detect capsular swelling after pneumococcal antiserum has been added to a loopful of sputum. The occurrence of the quellung reaction was shown to correlate closely with the presence of *S. pneumoniae* in sputum culture—in about 90 percent of the patients.

Pneumococcal antigens may be detected in the sputum of patients with pneumococcal pneumonia by enzyme-linked immunosorbent assay (ELISA), latex particle agglutination, or counterimmunoelectrophoresis. The first two are more readily available. ELISA is the most sensitive method. Antigen detection in sputum may have as high a sensitivity as 70 to 90 percent; but specificity is a problem, with about 20 percent false positives, probably due in part to the difficulty in distinguishing oropharyngeal contamination and colonization (e.g., in patients with chronic bronchitis without pneumonia). Antigen detection in the urine has been less sensitive, and the sensitivity of antigen detection in the serum has been even lower.

A radioimmunoassay and an enzyme-linked immunoassay for *L. pneumophila* antigenuria are commercially available and provide a means of rapid (under 24 h) diagnosis of *Legionella* pneumonia, particularly in patients without sputum production. The sensitivity of the radioimmunoassay is 89 to 95 percent, and the specificity is very high (estimated at 99 percent). The test is positive despite antimicrobial agent administration, and antigenuria may persist for weeks or months after recovery from pneumonia. It must be remembered that the assay is available only for *L. pneumophila* serogroup 1, and this serogroup is responsible for only 80 percent of *L. pneumophila* infections.

Rapid Viral Diagnosis by Antigen Detection

The need for methods that can rapidly identify viruses stems from the recent introduction of effective chemotherapy for several viral agents that cause pulmonary infections and from the long time (3 to 10 days) required for viral isolation and identification by standard tube culture. As noted earlier (under "Direct Immunofluorescent Microscopy"), DFA can be used to detect viral antigens (adenovirus, influenza A and B, parainfluenza, and RSV, as well as CMV and HSV) in specimens of bronchial brushings, BAL, or nasopharyngeal washings. Enzyme immunoassay can also be used to detect viral antigens in respiratory secretions. The presence of CMV antigenemia can be detected with the use of peroxidase-labeled antibody staining of peripheral blood buffy coat. The demonstration (culture, antigen) of CMV in BAL fluids may be interpreted variously in different clinical settings. Strict criteria for CMV pneumonia include demonstration of the virus, typical cytologic changes, and absence of other evident pathogens. This would be applicable in patients with AIDS, in whom CMV is frequently isolated but in whom CMV rarely causes pneumonia. In contrast, isolation of CMV from BAL fluid in bone marrow transplant recipients with pneumonia is sufficient evidence to make the diagnosis and institute treatment, in view of the high frequency and mortality of CMV pneumonia in these patients.

Serologic Tests

Serologic tests are sometimes of considerable help in establishing the causes of a number of pulmonary infections when the causative agents are difficult to isolate. However, this approach, requiring the demonstration of a fourfold or greater rise in titer between acute and convalescent samples, neither enables rapid diagnosis nor provides assistance in initial selection of antimicrobial therapy. Microimmunofluorescence serologic tests are of value in the diagnosis of psittacosis (*C. psittaci*). A fourfold rise in IgG or the presence of IgM antibody indicates recent infection. The indirect immunofluorescent antibody test (fourfold titer rise to 1:128 or higher indicates recent infection) may provide a retrospective diagnosis of Legionnaires' disease, but the antibody rise occasionally may not be demonstrable for 4 to 6 weeks after the clinical onset. Antibodies may persist for months or up to a year or more. Thus, a single titer of 1:256 or higher may reflect a prior *Legionella* infection. Cold agglutinins develop in about half the patients with *M. pneumoniae* pneumonia, but such antibodies occur in other conditions; complement fixation testing is the preferred diagnostic procedure. The most sensitive and specific serologic test for infection with *C. pneumoniae* is the microimmunofluorescence test. A fourfold rise in IgG titer or an IgM titer of 1:16 or more reflects an acute infection. The complement fixation test is usually used to confirm a diagnosis of Q-fever pneumonia, but microimmunofluorescence, microagglutination, and enzyme-linked immunosorbent assays have been used to diagnose acute *C. burnetii* pulmonary infection. Tularemic pneumonia can be diagnosed serologically with an agglutination test for *F. tularensis*.

Serologic tests are also helpful in the diagnosis of invasive infection due to the primary pulmonary mycotic pathogens. Serum IgM precipitins (latex agglutination, immunodiffusion) appear with primary coccidioidomycosis. Abnormally high complement fixation titers (at least 1:32) are present in most patients who have disseminated infection due to *C. immitis*. A fourfold increase in complement fixation titer to yeast and to mycelial phases of *H. capsulatum* (or possibly a single titer of 1:64 or higher) and the presence of H and M precipitin bands strongly suggest histoplasmosis. Complement fixation tests for blastomycosis lack sensitivity and specificity: titers of at least 1:8 suggest recent or active disease, particularly if precipitins to the A antigen are also present. Cryptococcal antigenemia is detectable from latex particle agglutination in patients with cryptococcal pneumonia or disseminated cryptococcal infection. Sporotrichosis can be diagnosed with a serologic agglutination test when the titer is 1:80 or greater.

Serologic tests (paired acute and convalescent sera) may be helpful for the retrospective diagnosis of infections due to influenza A and B, respiratory syncytial virus, adenoviruses, and parainfluenza viruses.

Molecular Diagnostic Testing

A variety of nucleic acid target amplification tests known as polymerase chain reactions (PCR) or hybridization assays are available for direct detection of pulmonary pathogens. PCR tests approved by the U.S. Food and Drug Administration (FDA) can detect *M. tuberculosis* (as distinct from nontuberculosis mycobacteria) directly from sputum and BAL specimens. These tests have shown a sensitivity of 90 to 100 percent in specimens that are AFB smear positive but a sensitivity of only 65 to 85 percent for specimens that are smear-negative. Consequently, these PCR assays have been approved for use only on acid-fast bacillus (AFB) smear–positive specimens. PCR assays for detection of *C. pneumoniae* and *M. pneumoniae* on nasopharyngeal or throat swab specimens are available to markedly shorten (by 1 to 2 days) the time required to isolate these organisms by culture (up to 3 weeks).

Other PCR tests that appear to increase detection of respiratory pathogens (*P. carinii, L. pneumophila*) are still at the stage of research tools. Although PCR tests for herpes simplex virus, cytomegalovirus, and adenovirus are available, their detection in respiratory tract specimens is difficult to interpret, since they might represent only upper respiratory colonizers, benign reactivation of latent infection, and may be unrelated to the process causing pneumonia.

Skin Tests of Delayed Hypersensitivity

The tuberculin skin test is of great importance in the evaluation of a pulmonary infection of unknown origin. The intermediate (5-tuberculin-unit) purified protein derivative (IPPD) test should be used if no information is available about previous testing. A positive test does not distinguish between prior and current infection, but in persons who are either less than 35 years old or members of high-risk groups (immigrant, HIV-positive), a positive reaction carries considerable diagnostic weight.

A negative second-strength PPD skin test in a patient who is not anergic is strong evidence against a tuberculous origin of a pulmonary process. However, several caveats are noteworthy: since it may take 4 to 6 weeks for the skin test to become positive, the tuberculin skin test may be initially negative in progressive primary pulmonary tuberculosis, and in the patient who was infected long ago, cutaneous hypersensitivity may wane; in the elderly person, in whom waning has occurred, repeat testing several weeks later may show a positive result (booster effect) even if the original IPPD skin test was negative.

Fungal skin tests do not distinguish between current and past infection; indeed, active disease is often accompanied by a negative skin test. The coccidioidin skin test is the best of the available tests, but the diagnosis of coccidioidomycosis is not excluded by a negative test. Blastomycin and histoplasmin skin tests are of little value because of frequent false-negative results and cross reactions. Also, the performance of the histoplasmin skin test may falsely elevate antibody levels to the *H. capsulatum* mycelial antigen.

A negative skin test response to a specific antigen must be interpreted in the light of possible anergy related to underlying conditions such as malnutrition, immunosuppressive and corticosteroid therapy, and AIDS. A battery of control antigens (mumps, *Candida, Trichophyton,* streptokinase streptodornase) serves to detect such anergy.

INVASIVE DIAGNOSTIC PROCEDURES

In certain circumstances, a more aggressive approach is required to uncover the cause of a pneumonia or other pulmonary infection. This should be considered in any patient with immune deficiency or who is critically ill in whom rapid therapy is critical or in whom drug toxicity may be a major concern (e.g., renal transplant recipients). Such procedures are best done prior to the initiation of antimicrobial therapy. Such an approach may also be required if the patient's condition continues to deteriorate despite empiric antimicrobial therapy. In the immunocompromised patient, early invasive diagnostic approaches are mandated by the large number of etiologic agents that may be responsible, the frequent involvement of many infectious or noninfectious agents in the pulmonary process, the multiplicity of antimicrobial choices available against different organisms, and the rapidity with which clinical deterioration may preclude further diagnostic and therapeutic actions. Among such invasive diagnostic procedures are bronchoscopy, bronchoalveolar lavage (BAL), open lung biopsy, and transthoracic needle aspiration, and video-assisted thoracoscopy (VATS). A choice has to be made among one of several invasive procedures. The choice depends on the experience and skill with the different procedures at a given hospital. Also important in determining the proper procedure are location and radiographic appearance of the pulmonary lesions. Fiberoptic bronchoscopy using specialized devices to shield against oropharyngeal contamination (protected specimen brushing) is used at some institutions to obtain tracheobronchial secretions for culture in certain acute bacterial pneumonias. A peripheral nodule or cavity (more than 1 cm in diameter) that is readily visualized on conventional (posteroanterior and lateral) radiographs and fluoroscopy, and is in an accessible location, may be aspirated and biopsied by needle percutaneously. A nodule that is inaccessible to needle aspiration, or a process placed peripherally, where the need for histopathology is not apt to be met by needle aspiration and biopsy, is best approached by open lung biopsy.

Flexible Fiberoptic Bronchoscopy with Lung Biopsy

Fiberoptic bronchoscopy in conjunction with transbronchial lung biopsy provides an etiologic diagnosis in about 50 to 80 percent of immunosuppressed patients who do not have AIDS and in 60 to 90 percent of patients who do have AIDS, in whom *P. carinii,* CMV, and *M. avium-intracellulare* infections are common. Contraindications to transbronchial biopsy include inability of the patient to cooperate, marked hypoxemia, bleeding disorders (particularly those associated with hypoprothrombinemia, thrombocytopenia refractory to platelet transfusion, and uremia), and pulmonary hypertension. In such patients, correction of bleeding tendency and/or open procedures may be preferred. Fiberoptic bronchoscopy combined with transbronchial biopsy and segmental BAL is the usual initial invasive diagnostic procedure in the immunocompromised patient with an undefined diffuse pulmonary process. If this fails to provide a diagnosis, open lung biopsy is indicated.

Tissue specimens are processed for histopathologic examination (hematoxylin-and-eosin stain, tissue acid-fast stains, Gomori's methenamine-silver stain, periodic acid–Schiff stain, tissue Gram's stain, and Dieterle silver stain). Impression smears from tissues are made with sterile slides, which, after appropriate fixation, are stained with Giemsa, Gram, Ziehl-Neelsen, and methenamine silver (for *P. carinii*) stains, as previously described. As indicated, DFA staining for *Legionella* and monoclonal antibody staining for *P. carinii* are performed on separate impression smears. Appropriate cultures are made with tissue obtained either transbronchially or at open lung biopsy.

Bronchoalveolar Lavage

In patients with AIDS, fiberoptic bronchoscopy coupled with wedged, terminal, subsegmental BAL has proved particularly useful, providing a diagnosis in more than 95 percent of cases of *P. carinii* pneumonia. BAL alone, without transbronchial biopsy, is often substituted in patients who are thrombocytopenic, on mechanical ventilation, or severely hypoxemic. The material obtained by BAL is processed for smear and culture. As indicated earlier, a variety of stains are available for demonstrating the presence of *P. carinii* in the cytocentrifuged material. Stained cytocentrifuged BAL specimens can also be helpful in establishing other diagnoses: Papanicolaou's stain is useful in detecting neoplastic cells and in identifying viral cytopathic effects in epithelial cells.

In at least two-thirds of immunosuppressed patients with CMV pneumonia, the diagnosis can be made from the finding of inclusion bodies in cytocentrifuged BAL specimens and with immunofluorescent monoclonal antibody staining. CMV is isolated more often on culture in these patients, but culture alone is not sufficient to establish the diagnosis, since viral isolation may represent only viral shedding in the presence of pulmonary disease due to other causes.

Invasive Diagnostic Testing in Ventilator-Associated Pneumonia

PSB with quantitative culture and protected-catheter BAL, also with quantitative culture, have been employed to obtain bacteriologic information while minimizing opportunity for contamination from colonization of the upper airway in patients with ventilator-associated pneumonia (VAP). The role of quantitative diagnostic techniques in the evaluation of patients with HAP and VAP remains controversial because of questions of accuracy of the results and what the threshold concentration of bacteria should be. In one study, tracheal aspirate cultures correlated with PSB cultures in patients with VAP, suggesting no added value to use of such an invasive procedure to direct initial therapy. At present, such invasive diagnostic testing is not considered a standard for routine management of patients with suspected VAP.

Percutaneous Transthoracic Needle Lung Biopsy

Percutaneous needle biopsy is often the invasive diagnostic procedure of choice for a sizable (greater than 1.0 cm) pulmonary nodule or cavity that is located peripherally. The use of smaller-gauge needles has reduced the frequency of pneumothorax as a complication. Diagnostic yields of 60 to 80 percent have been obtained in immunocompromised patients with pneumonia. This procedure has also provided the diagnosis in 70 percent of patients in whom the underlying lesion was granulomatous. The small core of tissue and aspirated fluid is examined by stained smear and culture for various infectious agents described above. Cytologic examination should be done for neoplastic cells. Because of the nature of the specimen, however, histopathologic examination may be unrewarding. In patients in whom respiratory status is tenuous, or in whom lymph node biopsy or sampling of pleural fluid may be desired, VATS or open biopsy may be preferred.

Open Lung Biopsy

Open lung biopsy or and more recently VATS, provides the most definitive procedure for histopathologic diagnosis in the immunocompromised host. It provides sufficient lung tissue for diagnosis and also makes it possible to sample several different sites. It is particularly suitable for evaluating processes that may not be infectious (e.g., neoplasm such as Kaposi's sarcoma, antineoplastic drug toxicity, drug hypersensitivity, and lymphocytic interstitial pneumonia). Open lung biopsy has provided a specific diagnosis in 60 to 90 percent of immunocompromised patients in whom it has been employed. Its major advantages include the ability to control bleeding, air leaks, and the airway. Its disadvantages relate to the thoracotomy: the need for general anesthesia, the inherent delay in preparing the patients for the surgical procedure, the need for intubation, the usual placement of a chest tube, and postoperative splinting due to incisional pain. Some of these complications are decreased in VATS. The mortality from the procedure is about 1 percent. Bleeding is a complication in about 1 percent of patients and delayed pneumothorax in about 9 percent. For the patient in whom the pace of the illness does not allow this sequential approach, open lung biopsy may have to be the first choice. It is also preferred in the patient who is unable to cooperate with fiberoptic bronchoscopy or in whom thrombocytopenia or hypoxemia presents additional problems for transbronchial biopsy.

Processing of lung biopsy specimens should include special stained imprint smears for *P. carinii*, bacteria (including *Nocardia* and mycobacteria), fungi, and viral inclusion bodies; cultures for bacteria, viruses, fungi, and mycobacteria; and tissue sections stained for histology and for infectious agents.

BIBLIOGRAPHY

Bartlett JG, Finegold SM: Anaerobic infections of the lung and pleural space. *Am Rev Respir Dis* 110:56–77, 1974.

Bartlett JG, Gorbach SL, Finegold SM: The bacteriology of aspiration pneumonia. *Am J Med* 56:202–207, 1974.

Bartlett JG, Mundy LM: Guidelines for community acquired pneumonia in adults, *Clin Infect Dis* 26:811–838, 1998.

Baselski VS, Wunderink RG: Bronchoscopic diagnosis of pneumonia. *Clin Microbiol Rev* 7:533–558, 1994.

Bates JH, Campbell GD, Barron AL, et al: Microbial etiology of acute pneumonia in hospitalized patients. *Chest* 101:1005–1012, 1992.

Burack JH, Hahn JA, Saint-Maurice D, et al: Microbiology of community-acquired bacterial pneumonia in persons with and at risk for human immunodeficiency virus type 1 infection. Implications for rationale empiric antibiotic therapy. *Arch Intern Med* 154:2589–2596, 1994.

Cooper JAD, White DA, Matthay RA: Drug-induced pulmonary disease. Part 1: Cytotoxic drugs. *Am Rev Respir Dis* 133:321–340, 1986.

Cooper JAD, White DA, Matthay RA: Drug induced pulmonary disease. Part 2: Noncytotoxic drugs. *Am Rev Respir Dis* 133:488–505, 1986.

Johanson WG, Jr., Pierce AK, Sanford JP: Changing pharyngeal bacterial flora of hospitalized patients. *N Engl J Med* 281:1137–1140, 1969.

Marrie TJ: Pneumonia and carcinoma of the lung. *J Infect* 29:45–52, 1994.

Marrie TJ, Durant H, Yates L: Community-acquired pneumonia requiring hospitalization: 5 year prospective study. *Rev Infect Dis* 11:586–599, 1989.

Mundy LM, Auwaerter PG, Oldach D, et al: Community-acquired pneumonia: Impact of immune status. *Am J Respir Crit Care Med* 152:1309–1315, 1995.

Murray JF, Mills J: Pulmonary infectious complications of human immunodeficiency virus infection. *Am Rev Respir Dis* 141: 1356–1372, 1582–1598, 1990.

Neiderman MS, Bass JB, Campbell GD, et al: Guidelines for the initial empiric therapy of community-acquired pneumonia: Diagnosis, assessment of severity, and initial antimicrobial treatment. *Am Rev Respir Dis* 148:1418–1426, 1993.

Niederman MS, Torres A, Summer W: Invasive diagnostic testing is not needed routinely to manage suspected ventilator-associated pneumonia. *Am J Respir Crit Care Med* 150:565–569, 1994.

Penner C, Maycher B, Long R: Pulmonary gangrene: A complication of bacterial pneumonia. *Chest* 105:567–573, 1994.

Pollock HM, Hawkins EL, Bonner JR, et al: Diagnosis of bacterial pulmonary infections during quantitative protected catheter cultures obtained during bronchoscopy. *J Clin Microbiol* 17:255–259, 1983.

Redman LR, Lockey E: Colonization of the upper respiratory tract with gram-negative bacilli after operation, endotracheal intubation, and prophylactic antibiotic therapy. *Anesthesia* 22:220–227, 1967.

Rello J, Quintana E, Ausina V, et al: Incidence, etiology, and outcome of nosocomial pneumonia on mechanically ventilated patients. *Chest* 100:439–444, 1991.

Shelhamer JH, Ogniebene FP, Masur H, et al: Respiratory disease in immunosuppressed patients. *Ann Intern Med* 117:415–431, 1992.

Trucksis M, Swartz MN: Bronchiectasis: A current view, in Remington JS, Swartz MN (eds), *Current Clinical Topics in Infectious Diseases*. Boston, Blackwell Scientific, 1991, pp 170–205.

| # Antimicrobial Therapy of Common Pulmonary Infections

Jay A. Fishman

OVERVIEW

Optimal antimicrobial therapy provides rapid killing (bactericidal, fungicidal) of pathogenic organisms without disrupting the normal flora of the individual's mucosal surfaces. Further, therapy should be reserved for *documented infections* that are susceptible to therapy (i.e., not for symptoms that may be due to viral or noninfectious causes). In addition, the narrowest spectrum of antimicrobial therapy should be used in each case, thus reducing the likelihood of the emergence of antimicrobial resistance in the individual (e.g., nosocomial infections) or in the community. However, *initial therapies for infections, and in particular pneumonia and other potentially life-threatening infections, are generally empiric.* That is, therapy is directed at the likely pathogens until microbiologic data are available to adjust the selection of agents. Mortality in community-acquired pneumonia, for example, is determined to a large degree by the correct selection of initial, empiric, therapy. In addition, one of the strongest arguments in favor of the microbiologic evaluation of patients (i.e., sputum Gram's stains, special stains, cultures) with severe pneumonia is not only the optimization of initial therapy, but also the ability to adjust therapy for the *patient failing to respond to initial therapy.* Once antimicrobial therapy is started (within 2 to 4 h), the ability to obtain meaningful culture data is markedly reduced.

Initial therapy of pneumonia is based on the clues provided by clinical, epidemiologic, and radiologic information (Tables 59-1 and 59-2) and by evaluation of Gram-stained, fungal, and AFB-stained smears of sputum and other microbiologic data (e.g., nasal swabs for direct immunofluorescence for influenza or respiratory syncytial viruses). In the case of a presumed bacterial pneumonia in which an etiologic agent is identified on the sputum smear, initial treatment is aimed at this organism.

COMMUNITY-ACQUIRED PNEUMONIA (CAP)

The etiology of CAP is generally unknown. While many studies implicate *Streptococcus pneumoniae* as the most common pathogen *identified,* over 50 percent of cases have no pathogen isolated despite extensive efforts. Common pathogens also include *Haemophilus influenzae, Moraxella catarrhalis, Klebsiella pneumoniae,* and *Staphylococcus aureus.* Common atypical pathogens (little sputum, often "viral" symptoms) include *Mycoplasma pneumoniae, Chlamydia pneumoniae, Legionella pneumoniae,* and viruses [influenza, respiratory syncytial virus (RSV), and adenovirus]. Tuberculosis and *Pneumocystis carinii,* and the geographic or endemic fungi (*Histoplasma capsulatum, Coccidioides immitis, Blastomyces dermatitidis*) must be considered in persons from endemic regions or with immune compromise. Dual or

TABLE 59-1 Clues to the Etiology of Pneumonia from the History and Physical Examination

Feature	Common Organisms
Environmental	
Exposure to contaminated air-conditioning cooling towers, recent travel associated with a stay in a hotel, exposure to a grocery store mist machine, visit or recent stay in a hospital with contaminated (by *L. pneumophila*) potable water	*Legionella pneumophila*
Pneumonia after windstorm in an endemic area	*Coccidioides immitis*
Outbreak of pneumonia in homeless shelters, jails, military training camps	*Streptococcus pneumoniae* *Mycobacterium tuberculosis* *S. pneumoniae* *Chlamydia pneumoniae*
Exposure to contaminated bat caves, excavation in endemic areas	*Histoplasma capsulatum*
Animal contact	
Exposure to infected parturient cats, cattle, sheep, or goats	*Coxiella burnetii*
Exposure to turkeys, chickens, ducks, or psittacine birds	*C. psittaci*
Travel history	
Travel to Thailand or other countries in Southeast Asia	*Burkholderia (Pseudomonas) pseudomallei (melioidosis)*
Pneumonia in immigrants from Asia or India	*M. tuberculosis*
Occupational history	
Pneumonia in a large-city health care worker	*M. tuberculosis*
Host factors	
Diabetic ketoacidosis	*S. pneumoniae* *Staphylococcus aureus*
Alcoholism	*S. pneumoniae* *Klebsiella pneumoniae* *S. aureus*
Chronic obstructive lung disease	*S. pneumoniae* *Haemophilus influenzae* *Moraxella catarrhalis*
Solid organ transplant recipient (pneumonia occurring >2–3 months after transplant)	*S. pneumoniae* *H. influenzae* *Legionella* spp. *Pneumocystis carinii* *Cytomegalovirus* *Strongyloides stercoralis*
Sickle cell disease	*S. pneumoniae*
HIV infection (with CD4 cell count ≤200/μl)	*P. carinii* *S. pneumoniae* *H. influenzae* *Cryptococcus neoformans* *M. tuberculosis* *Rhodococcus equi*

TABLE 59-1 (continued)

Feature	Common organisms
Physical findings	
Periodontal disease with foul-smelling sputum	Anaerobes, may be mixed aerobic-anaerobic infection
Bullous myringitis	Mycoplasma pneumoniae
Absent gag reflex, altered level of consciousness, or a recent seizure	Polymicrobial (oral aerobic and anaerobic bacteria) can be macro- or microaspiration
Encephalitis	M. pneumoniae
	C. burnetii
	L. pneumophila
Cerebellar ataxia	M. pneumoniae
	L. pneumophila
Erythema multiforme	M. pneumoniae
Erythema nodosum	C. pneumoniae
	M. tuberculosis
Ecthyma gangrenosum	P. aeruginosa
	Serratia marcescens
Cutaneous nodules (abscesses) and CNS findings	Nocardia species

SOURCE: From Clin Infect Dis 18:501–515, 1994.

mixed infections are common, including postinfluenza bacterial pneumonia with *Staphylococcus,* aspiration pneumonia, or pneumococcus with *C. pneumoniae*. Most cases of community acquired pneumonia are treated with oral antimicrobial therapy aimed at these common pathogens.

The initial decision regarding the need to hospitalize a patient should be based on the presence of comorbid conditions and the severity of the pneumonia. Studies of CAP emphasize the stratification of patients based on the severity of the infection and comorbid conditions (Table 59-3). The decision to admit a patient to the hospital should be based on both clinical appearance and social factors. The Pneumonia Outcomes Research Teams (PORT) outcomes study assigns point scores to clinical findings (Table 59-3). Major factors at presentation include the following:

- Age
- Respiratory rate >30/min, temperature >40°C, pH <7.35 (Pa_{O_2} <60 mmHg, glucose >139, hematocrit <30%, pulse >125/min are lesser indicators)
- Serum sodium <130, BUN >30 mg/dL (11 mmol/L)
- Coexisting diseases, especially cancer, liver disease (congestive heart failure, renal disease, cerebrovascular disease are lesser indicators)
- Social conditions: Cannot maintain oral intake, lack of home care supports

The American Thoracic Society and the Infectious Disease Society of America have proposed guidelines for the care of patients with pneumonia. In general, patients sick enough to be admitted to the hospital for the care of CAP (20 percent of pneumonia) and all patients with nosocomially acquired infection merit attempts to define causative pathogens (sputum Gram's stain and culture, blood cultures). Reducing excessive drug use will ultimately reduce the cost of health care overall as well as toxicity. But initial therapy is

TABLE 59-2 Differential Diagnosis of Common Patterns on Chest
Radiography in a Patient with a Clinical Picture of Pneumonia[a]

Focal opacity
  Streptococcus pneumoniae
  Mycoplasma pneumoniae
  Legionella pneumophila
  Staphylococcus aureus
  Chlamydia pneumoniae
  Mycobacterium tuberculosis
  Blastomyces dermatitidis
Interstitial
  Viruses
  M. pneumoniae
  Pneumocystis carinii
  C. psittaci

Interstitial pneumonia with
  lymphadenopathy
  Epstein-Barr virus
  Francisella tularensis
  C. psittaci
  M. pneumoniae
Cavitation
  Mixed aerobic anaerobic (lung
  abscess)
  Aerobic gram-negative bacilli
  M. tuberculosis
  L. pneumophila
  Cryptococcus neoformans
  Nocardia asteroides
  Actinomyces israelii
  Coccidioides immitis
  P. carinii

Bulging fissure
  Klebsiella pneumoniae
  L. pneumophila

Multifocal opacities
  S. aureus
  Coxiella burnetii
  L. pneumophila
  S. pneumoniae

Miliary
  M. tuberculosis
  Histoplasma capsulatum
  C. immitis
  B. dermatitidis
  Varicella zoster

Segmental or lobar pneumonia
with lymphadenopathy
  M. tuberculosis (primary infection)
  Atypical rubeola
  Fungi
Pneumatoceles
  S. aureus
  S. pyogenes
  P. carinii

Round pneumonia
  C. burnetii
  S. pneumoniae
  L. pneumophila
  S. aureus

[a]Only the microbial causes of the various radiographic patterns are given.
Each also has an extensive noninfectious differential diagnosis.
SOURCE: From *Clin Infect Dis* 18:501–515, 1994.

almost always empiric. Therapy delayed more than 8 h has a significant impact on survival. Clinical history is generally a good indicator of severity and helpful with regard to possible etiologies.

Antimicrobial therapy is selected based on penetration into the lung parenchyma and the likely etiologies of infection (Tables 59-4 and 59-5). When initial clinical and laboratory evidence suggests *S. pneumoniae* as the cause, penicillin or amoxicillin may be the preferred treatment. In view of the current frequency of penicillin resistance among pneumococci (about 25 percent in some areas of the United States), uncomplicated pneumonia due to such strains requires treatment with high doses of parenteral penicillin, a third-generation cephalosporin, or a latter-generation fluoroquinolone. Otitis or central nervous system disease militates against use of a penicillin for suspected pneumococcal infection (vancomycin $+/-$ ceftriaxone or cefotaxime $+/-$ macrolide).

TABLE 59-3 Scoring System for Hospitalization for Community-Acquired Pneumonia

Demographic Factor	Points	Demographic Factor	Points
Age		Laboratory and radiographic	
Men	Age (yr)	findings	
Women	Age (yr)	Arterial pH <7.35	+*30*
	−*10*	Blood urea nitrogen ≥	+*20*
Nursing home resident	+10	30 mg/dL	
Coexisting illnesses		Sodium <130 mmol/L	+20
Neoplastic disease	+*30*	Glucose, ≥250 mg/dL	+10
Liver disease	+20	Hematocrit <30%	+10
Congestive heart failure	+10	Partial pressure of arterial	
Cerebrovascular disease	+10	oxygen <60 mmHg	+10
Renal disease	+10	Pleural effusion	+10
Physical examination			
Altered mental status	+20		
Respiratory rate, 30/min	+20		
Systolic blood pressure			
<90 mmHg	+20		
Temperature <35°C or 40°C	+15		
Pulse, 125/min	+10		

Stratification of Risk Score

Risk class	Based on	Mortality (%)	Hospitalize?
I	Algorithm	0.1	No
II	<70 total points	0.6	No
III	71–90 total points	2.8	Brief
IV	91–130 total points	8.2	Yes
V	>130 total points	29.2	Yes

SOURCE: From *Arch Intern Med* 157:36–44, 1997, and *N Engl J Med* 336:243–250, 1997.

TABLE 59-4 Antibiotic Choice Guidelines Empiric Parenteral Antimicrobial Therapy[a]

Clinical Condition	Admitted to Regular Floor	Admitted to ICU and/or Severely Ill
Most patients (sputum Gram's stain not available, nondiagnostic, or suggestive of *Haemophilus influenza* or *Moraxella catarrhalis*)	Cefuroxime 750 mg IV q 8h (Ceftriaxone 1g IV q24h if being discharged on home IV antibiotic)	Ceftriaxone 1 g IV q24h + macrolide.[c]
	+/− macrolide.[b]	If unable to receive ceftriaxone, a fluoroquinolone.[d]
	If unable to receive cephalosporin, substitute a fluoroquinolone.[d]	
Clinical picture suggestive of **aspiration** of oropharyngeal secretions in the community	Penicillin 2 mU IV q4h (+ metronidazole 500 mg IV or PO q8h if lung abscess, suspected empyema, or severely ill).	If penicillin allergic, clindamycin 600 mg IV q8h or 300 mg PO qid.

TABLE 59-4 *(continued)*

Clinical Condition	Admitted to Regular Floor	Admitted to ICU and/or Severely Ill
Clinical picture, sputum Gram's stain, and/or culture suggestive of **Streptococcus pneumoniae**	Penicillin 2 mU IV q4h.	If non-life-threatening penicillin allergy, cefuroxime 750 mg IV q8h or ceftriaxone 1g IV q24h. If severe penicillin or cephalosporin allergy, vancomycin 1g IV q12h.
Clinical picture, sputum Gram's stain, and/or culture results suggestive of **Staphylococcus aureus**	Nafcillin 1.5g IV q4h	If nonthreatening penicillin allergy, cefazolin 1g IV q8h. If severe penicillin or cephalosporin allergy, or methicillin-resistant *S. aureus* strongly suspected or documented, vancomycin 1g IV q12h.
Patient hospitalized or in a chronic care facility within preceding ten days (including suspected aspiration) or sputum Gram's stain or culture results suggestive of **enteric gram-negative bacilli**	Ceftriaxone 1g IV q24h +/− gentamicin for initial 48 h until susceptibilities known. Add metronidazole 500 mg IV or PO q8h if lung abscess, suspected empyema, or severely ill.	If unable to receive cephalosporin, substitute a flouroquinolone[d] +/− metronidazole. If *Pseudomonas* suspected, use ceftazidime.

[a]These regimens are meant as guidelines only and cannot substitute for clinical judgment in individual circumstances; approach to patients with the most severe pneumonias must be made on clinical grounds. Doses should be adjusted for patients' renal function and age. Therapy should always be adjusted based on results of cultures and/or clinical responses.
[b]Macrolide: Erythromycin 500 mg PO qid or 1g IV q6h, clarithromycin 500 mg PO bid, or azithromycin 250 mg PO qd.
[c]Erythromycin 1g IV q6h or azithromycin 500 mg IV q24h.
[d]Fluoroquinolones: Later generation agents have improved antipneumococcal activity and include levofloxacin, gatifloxacin, and moxifloxacin.
NOTE: Ceftriaxone has poor activity for *Pseudomonas aeruginosa*. Ceftazidime 1g IV q8h has excellent activity against *P. aeruginosa* but poor activity for gram-positive bacteria such as *S. aureus*. In selected patients, ceftazidime plus an antistaphylococcal antibiotic or fluoroquinolone[d] may be substituted. Gentamicin 5 mg/kg, initial dosing interval based on estimated creatinine clearance; a trough level and adjustment needed if therapy is to be continued beyond initial period.

Modification of initial therapy is made on the basis of the results of sputum and blood cultures, urinary *Legionella pneumophila* antigen tests, or, if available, polymerase chain reaction (PCR) for *M. pneumoniae, C. pneumoniae*, and *Mycobacterium tuberculosis*. But if the causative agent cannot be identified in the sputum smear, initial therapy is directed at the likely agents.

TABLE 59-5 Penetration of Antibiotics into Respiratory Secretions

Good Penetration: Lipid-Soluble, Concentration Not Inflammation-Dependent

Quinolones
New macrolides: azithromycin, clarithromycin
Tetracyclines
Clindamycin
Trimethoprim/sulfamethoxazole

Poor Penetration: Relatively Lipid-Insoluble, Inflammation-Dependent for Concentration in the Lung

Aminoglycosides
β-lactams
  Penicillins
  Cephalosporins
  Monobactams
  Carbapenems

A variety of approaches for empiric therapy have been proposed when initial diagnostic tests have failed to provide guidance. Pneumonia in young adults considered manageable as outpatients might reasonably be treated with an oral macrolide (erythromycin, clarithromycin, or azithromycin) active against *M. pneumoniae, C. pneumoniae,* and *L. pneumophila.* Oral amoxicillin or a second-generation cephalosporin is an alternative. If epidemiologic factors suggest Q fever or psittacosis, a tetracycline is indicated in initial therapy. Pneumonia in persons 60 years of age and older and in those with coexisting conditions (e.g., chronic obstructive lung disease, congestive heart failure, chronic alcoholism, asplenia) who can be treated as outpatients might be treated with an oral second-generation cephalosporin active against *H. influenzae* and susceptible strains of *S. pneumoniae* or amoxicillin. Alternatives for patients with penicillin allergy would include an oral macrolide, doxycycline, or fluoroquinolone.

For patients with severe community-acquired pneumonia requiring hospitalization, treatment should include a parenteral second-generation (cefuroxime) or third-generation (cefotaxime or ceftriaxone) cephalosporin, with erythromycin or other macrolide added if the clinical picture suggests atypical pneumonia. Alternatively, fluoroquinolone may be used. In the special setting of an influenza viral outbreak, the possibility of a severe pneumonia being due to *S. aureus* superinfection should be considered, and therapy might include use of nafcillin or oxacillin. However, sputum production is frequently a feature of *S. aureus* pneumonia, and the organisms can usually be identified on Gram's stain of the sputum. In the alcoholic patient with a dense lobar consolidation and large gram-negative bacilli on stained smear of the sputum, *K. pneumoniae* is a likely cause, and treatment should include a second- or third-generation cephalosporin plus an aminoglycoside.

Initial treatment of community-acquired aspiration pneumonia or lung abscess would be directed at the normal aerobic and anaerobic bacterial flora of the upper respiratory tract that are etiologic (Table 59-6). Clindamycin or a combination of penicillin (or ampicillin) with metronidazole is the pharmacotherapy

TABLE 59-6 Microorganisms That Colonize
the Normal Upper Respiratory Tract[a]

Viridans streptococci
Streptococcus pyogenes
Streptococcus pneumoniae
Staphylococci, including *S. aureus*
Micrococcus spp.
Neisseria spp.
Moraxella (Branhamella) catarrhalis
Haemophilus spp., including *H. influenzae*
Lactobacillus spp.
Corynebacterium spp.
Obligate anaerobes
Candida spp.

[a]Often involved in aspiration pneumonitis.

of choice for initial treatment unless gram-negative infection is suspected (recent hospitalization), in which coverage must be broadened.

HOSPITAL-ACQUIRED PNEUMONIA

Hospital-acquired pneumonia (HAP) is often due to organisms with resistance to common antimicrobial agents. These may include *K. pneumoniae, Enterobacter, Acinetobacter, Serratia, Pseudomonas aeruginosa,* or *S. aureus.* The best guide to therapy is the sputum gram-stained smear and knowledge of the common organisms in the clinical facility or in the patient in the past. Antimicrobial resistance may emerge during therapy. For HAP, consideration of time of onset, severity, and presence of specific risk factors can be used to suggest pathogens likely to be implicated and provide some initial guidance in the selection of antimicrobial therapy while culture results are awaited. In patients with mild to moderate HAP with onset anytime after hospitalization and without unusual risk factors, a core group of organisms (*H. influenzae, S. pneumoniae,* methicillin-susceptible *S. aureus,* and non-pseudomonal enteric gram-negative bacilli) are likely to be responsible. Monotherapy in this setting generally uses a second- or third-generation cephalosporin or a beta-lactam–beta-lactamase inhibitor combination (e.g., ticarcillin-clavulanate, ampicillin-sulbactam). If the pathogen is likely to be an *Enterobacter* species and a third-generation cephalosporin is used, addition of another agent (e.g., gentamicin or tobramycin) is indicated because of possible chromosomal beta-lactamase induction.

In patients with mild to moderate HAP associated with specific risk factors, additional antimicrobial agents should be included along with those already indicated for the core group of pathogens. Thus, for example, if aspiration were a consideration, clindamycin might be added; if high-dose corticosteroids had been employed invasive diagnosis must be considered. If the patient were granulocytopenic, antipseudomonal therapy should be included (see below). In patients with severe HAP and/or onset late in hospitalization, other organisms (*P. aeruginosa, Acinetobacter* species) in addition to core pathogens should be considered. Such circumstances require initial combination therapy with an antipseudomonal penicillin or cephalosporin (or carbapenem) or an antipseudomonal combination beta-lactam–beta-lactamase inhibitor plus an aminoglycoside (or fluoroquinolone). In some patients, methicillin-resistant

S. aureus (MRSA) is also a consideration, and vancomycin may be added to the aforementioned combination therapies. Cognizance should always be taken of local epidemiologic data (e.g., in a given intensive care unit, clusters of cases of pneumonia that are due to organisms that are less common and more difficult to treat), such as *Acinetobacter* species or *B. cepacia*, and their antimicrobial susceptibility patterns.

In the febrile granulocytopenic patient who has received broad-spectrum therapy for presumed sepsis of unknown origin, the development of a pulmonary infiltrates may raise the question of a fungal infection (e.g., *Aspergillus*) that warrants addition of empiric antifungal therapy and invasive diagnostic procedures.

Extrapulmonary findings sometimes suggest the cause of a pulmonary process and thereby direct initial therapy. Thus, antiviral therapy would be indicated in the immunocompetent or immunosuppressed adult who has varicella zoster (or cytomegalovirus infection) and a diffuse pulmonary infiltrates. The patient with untreated HIV infection whose chest radiograph shows a bilateral interstitial or airspace process compatible with *P. carinii* pneumonia is likely, on statistical grounds, to have *P. carinii* pneumonia. However, all patients are susceptible to community-acquired pathogens and appropriate coverage must be included. Initial therapy using trimethoprim-sulfamethoxazole is appropriate for the mildly ill AIDS patient after obtaining an induced sputum for examination. Invasive diagnostic procedures are undertaken if the process progresses. In the AIDS patient whose illness is severe when first seen, whose course has progressed rapidly, whose radiographic picture is complex, and whose pulmonary infiltrates may represent several causes, not only is initial therapy begun with trimethoprim-sulfamethoxazole but also an invasive procedure is performed immediately to obtain a microbiologic diagnosis.

CONSIDERATIONS WHEN PNEUMONIA FAILS TO RESOLVE OR WORSENS DURING THERAPY

The need for microbiologic data is emphasized by the patient who fails to respond to initial therapy. In this situation, the physician must consider that the original diagnosis (microbiologic or etiologic) was incorrect or that superinfection has occurred. Added considerations might include the diagnosis of pulmonary infarction, malignancy, pulmonary vasculitis, drug reaction, or eosinophilic pneumonia. Additional specimens for microbiologic analysis should be obtained (sputum, bronchoscopy) recalling that polymicrobial infections are common. In addition, unusual pathogens—including *Mycobacterium tuberculosis, Actinomyces,* and *Nocardia*—can mimic pyogenic pneumonia.

The anatomy of infection merits consideration. Anatomic alterations (malignancy, pulmonary sequestration) will result in postobstructive infection that is difficult to eradicate. Similarly, empyema or pus in the pleural space will cause fever and pulmonary compression. Patients with endovascular infection or loculated pus under pressure (e.g., endocarditis, meningitis, septic arthritis, or abscesses of the spleen or kidney) may have extrapulmonary sites of metastatic infection.

Nosocomial pneumonia is diagnosed in patients hospitalized over 72 h. This is increasingly common in patients who require endotracheal intubation and assisted ventilation. In such patients, antimicrobial resistance must be considered, including *S. pneumoniae* (often resistant to penicillin, erythromycin, macrolides, and trimethoprim-sulfamethoxazole), *Pseudomonas* species, and with the induction of resistance in *Enterobacter* and *Acinetobacter* species.

ACTINOMYCOSIS AND NOCARDIOSIS

Actinomycosis is an indolent, infectious disease characterized by a pyogenic response and necrosis, followed by intense fibrosis. Occasionally, the pus contains minute yellow granules consisting of clumps of *Actinomyces* filaments. Actinomycosis is usually caused by *Actinomyces israelii,* but other species of *Actinomyces* and *Propionibacterium propionicum* (formerly *Arachnia propionica*) are occasionally responsible. Thoracic actinomycosis often occurs in people with carious teeth and periodontal disease, in whom the numbers of these bacteria are increased. Aspiration of infective material is the probable inciting event. Spread to the mediastinum is usually from pulmonary or, less commonly, cervicofacial disease. In tissue, *Actinomyces* organisms tend to grow in dense microcolonies or granules that may reach 4 mm in size. These are often called sulfur granules because they are usually yellow, although they do not contain much sulfur. Cultures should be made from diseased tissue or normally sterile body secretions under strictly anaerobic conditions and inoculated promptly.

Penicillin is the drug of choice for actinomycosis. In most cases, the drug should be given orally in maximal tolerated doses. In severe or rapidly progressive cases, penicillin should initially be given intravenously in high doses 10 to 20 million units per day. Tetracycline and clindamycin have also been used with good results. In vitro tests of susceptibility of *Actinomyces* to antimicrobials are of uncertain clinical relevance. Penicillin, erythromycin, cephaloridine, minocycline, rifampin, and clindamycin are very active. Organisms are inhibited by achievable concentrations of cephalothin, ampicillin, tetracycline, doxycycline, and chloramphenicol. A few strains are susceptible to sulfamethoxazole. Metronidazole is ineffective. Surgery should be used to eradicate bulk disease or fistulas. Empyemas should be drained. Surgery is sometimes required to relieve obstruction of mediastinal structures. Actinomycosis has a marked tendency to relapse; therapy should therefore be continued for from 6 to 12 months. The exact duration should depend on the extent of the disease within and outside the chest and the response to treatment.

Pulmonary nocardiosis is a subacute or chronic pneumonia caused by aerobic actinomycetes of the genus *Nocardia. Nocardia asteroides* is the most common pathogen, but *N. brasiliensis, N. otitidis-caviarum* (formerly *N. caviae*), *N. farcinica, N. nova, N. transvalensis,* and *N. pseudobrasiliensis* have all been associated with pulmonary disease. *N. asteroides* frequently disseminates to other sites or is associated with mycetoma or skin and connective tissue infection after transcutaneous inoculation or keratitis. The risk is increased in people with impaired cell-mediated immunity, especially in those with lymphoma, transplanted organs, or AIDS. Nocardiosis has also been associated with pulmonary alveolar proteinosis, tuberculosis, and chronic granulomatous disease. Disseminated disease occurs in one-half of cases of pulmonary nocardiosis. The central nervous system is the most common location of disseminated disease, while other common locations are the skin and subcutaneous tissues, kidneys, bone, and muscle. Nocardiae are thin, crooked, branching filaments that are weakly to strongly gram-positive and appear beaded. Sulfonamides are the antimicrobials of choice; 6 to 8 g of sulfisoxazole or sulfadiazine should be given daily in four to six divided doses. Resistance to sulfonamide has been documented. Nocardiosis may occur despite sulfonamide prophylaxis in immunocompromised hosts. In difficult cases, sulfonamide levels should be measured and dosages adjusted to keep serum levels between 100 and 150 g/mL. Many patients have been treated with the combination of sulfamethoxazole and trimethoprim, but it is unclear whether the combination is superior to the use of sulfonamides alone. If the combination is selected, 5 to 20 mg of trimethoprim and 25 to 100 mg/kg per day of sulfamethoxazole should be given in two or three divided doses. After the disease is brought under control, doses can be reduced to approximately 4 g per day of sulfonamides alone or to 5 mg of trimethoprim and 25 mg/kg per day of sulfamethoxazole for the remainder of therapy. Therapy is for the duration of immune suppression. Other agents have been used with success, including minocycline, ceftriaxone, amikacin, meropenem, imipenem, amoxacillin-clavulanate, fluoroquinolones, and macrolides; *N. nova* infections can be treated with a variety of combinations based on susceptibility testing. Newer beta-lactam antibiotics including cefotaxime, ceftizoxime, ceftriaxone, and imipenem are usually effective except in cases with *N. farcinica.* In most cases, isolates of *Nocardia* should be sent to an experienced reference laboratory for speciation and for susceptibility tests. The various pathogenic species differ in their susceptibility to second-line drugs. Surgery is used as it is for other infectious diseases of the chest. Empyemas should be drained. Abscesses usually respond to antimicrobial therapy alone. Reduction in immune suppression is desirable, but patients can be treated successfully for nocardiosis even if immunosuppressive therapy is continued. For nonimmunosuppressed patients, treatment of pulmonary nocardiosis should be continued for 6 to 12 months. Central nervous system disease requires treatment for 1 year unless all apparent disease has been excised. Immunosuppressed patients with pulmonary nocardiosis should be treated for at least 1 year. In some patients, including a few with advanced AIDS, much longer treatment is necessary. Patients should be carefully followed during therapy and for at least 6 months after therapy is stopped for signs of relapse. With prompt diagnosis and appropriate treatment, most patients should be cured.

SYSTEMIC ANTIFUNGAL AGENTS

Infections of the lungs due to the fungi are usually associated with immune deficiency, or structural abnormality, or both. Prompt diagnosis is essential to successful therapy of these infections, many of which are caused by angioinvasive molds including *Zygomycetes, Fusarium, Aspergillus* spp., *Pseudallescheria,* and others (see Table 59-7). Consideration of the epidemiology and host risk factors for these pathogens may be useful in establishing a specific diagnosis. Neutropenia remains a major risk factor for infection, particularly with

TABLE 59-7 General Principles in Management of Fungal Infections

Antimicrobial agents alone are generally inadequate for the cure of invasive fungal infection (e.g., *Aspergillus*). Surgical intervention is essential.
Early and *specific* diagnosis (biopsy and cultures) are essential.
Reduce immune suppression whenever possible.
Compromises must often be made based on the inherent toxicities of many antimicrobial agents.
The use of second-line agents that allow the progression of infection is unacceptable.
Recognition of antimicrobial resistance.
Demonstration of response and cure.

TABLE 59-8 Antifungal Agents for Invasive Mycoses

Amphotericin B
Liposomal polyenes
ABLC, ABCD, AmBisome
Liposomal nystatin
Azoles
Fluconazole
Itraconazole (PO/IV)
Voriconazole
Posaconazole (SCH56592)
Ravuconazole (BMS-207147)
Echinocandins
Caspofungin (MK-0991; Cancidas)
FK463 (Micafungin), VER-002
Others
Pradimicins
Sordarins

Aspergillus, but increasing numbers of patients with other risk factors, including organ transplantation and AIDS, develop infection. Among patients with solid-organ transplants, those undergoing lung transplantation are at particular risk for *Aspergillus* infection, with a clinical presentation ranging from an ulcerative tracheobronchitis to disseminated infection. Zygomycosis may be associated with necrotic skin lesions and associated with wound dressings.

Surgical debridement is critical to successful antifungal therapy whenever possible. A broad array of antifungal agents is now available (Table 59-8). Amphotericin B remains the standard therapy for critically ill patients with invasive fungal disease, but carries significant toxicity (see Table 59-9), most

TABLE 59-9 Amphotericin B—Properties of the "Gold Standard"

Activity
Binds to ergosterol; cell wall disruption
Considered cidal antifungal
Broad spectrum of activity
Despite limitations, the gold standard for therapy of systemic and invasive fungal infection
Few resistant fungi; emerging resistance
Administration
IV formulation for systemic infection; no oral form
Significant toxicities:
Infusion associated acute and largely cytokine-mediated: Headache, chills, nausea and vomiting, fever, dyspnea, tachycardia, bradycardia, arrhythmia, back pain, hypothermia, hypertension, hypotension
Nephrotoxicity: acute and chronic
Glomerular: ↓GFR, ↓renal blood flow
Tubular: urinary casts, renal tubular acidosis, magnesium and potassium wasting, nephrocalcinosis
Exacerbated by sodium deprivation (tubuloglomerular feedback, chloride wasting)
Renal arteriolar vasospasm? Calcium depletion during ischemia? Direct toxicity? Cytokines? Vasospasm?
Normochromic normocytic anemia, leukopenia, thrombocytopenia
Neurotoxicity: confusion, depression, seizures, paresis, leukoencephalopathy

TABLE 59-10 Antifungal Therapy: Preventing Toxicity of Amphotericin B

Considerations: Efficacy associated with high plasma levels and total dose
Sodium loading (>1 L IV normal saline, bolus or continuous)
  Maintain urine output (not mannitol)
  Correction of serum magnesium, potassium
  Hypotension (especially renal ischemia)
Concomitant nephrotoxins: aminoglycosides, calcineurin inhibitors, high-dose sulfamethoxazole, diuretics, cisplatin
Possible antagonism with azoles (itraconazole)—some animal data, few in vivo data; possible synergy with echinocandins?
Cytokine storm—anti-inflammatory, antihistamines

of which are largely avoidable (Table 59-10). Toxicity is reduced in the lipid forms of amphotericin B, the newer azoles; new classes of antifungal agents such as the echinocandins have activity against a broad spectrum of pathogens (see Tables 59-11 and 59-12). Mortality from invasive aspergillosis in high-risk patients remains high even with standard amphotericin B. New therapies such as the lipid formulations of amphotericin B have resulted in improved outcome in some patients, but overall responses are still poor. Newer triazole antifungals with improved activity against resistant yeast and molds (such as voriconazole, ravuconazole, and posaconazole) are in advanced development. In addition, new classes of antifungal drugs such as the echinocandins (including caspofungin, micafungin, and VER-002) and new formulations of other compounds (such as intravenous itraconazole and liposomal nystatin)

TABLE 59-11 Azole Antifungals

Activity
  Inhibit cytochrome P450 α-14 demethylase
  Block formation of ergosterol; inhibit cell growth
  Slower killing—considered static drugs
  Interactions with P450 drug metabolism
Toxicity: keto >> itra ≥ vori > flu (in general; individual patients may vary)
  Nausea/vomiting, hepatotoxicity, adrenals
  Significant drug interactions
  Visual effects: voriconazole (~25%)
  Reversible/transient/dose-related

TABLE 59-12 Echinocandins

Caspofungin (MK-0991; cancidas)
Micafungin (FK463); VER-002 (LY303366)
Mechanism: Inhibit cell wall β-1,3-glucan synthase
Characteristics
  Rapidly fungicidal for yeast
  Intravenous administration only
  Minimal renal toxicity
  Interactions with cyclosporine (liver function tests)?
Activity
  Yeasts (*Candida albicans*; non-*albicans*)
  Molds (*Aspergillus*; not Zygomycetes)
  Others (endemic mycoses; **not** *Cryptococcus*)
  Synergy with amphotericin B? with voriconazole?

TABLE 59-13 Respiratory Viral Infections: Clinical Syndromes, Treatment, and Prevention

Virus Group	Clinical Syndromes[a]					Antiviral Agent Approved[b]		
	Common Cold	Pharyngitis	Croup	Bronchiolitis	Pneumonia	Prophylaxis	Treatment	Vaccine
Adenoviruses	−	+	−	+	+	N	N	Y
Coronaviruses	++	−	−	−	−	N	N	N
Herpesviruses								
CMV[c]	−	+	−	−	+	Y	Y	N
EBV[d]	−	++	−	−	+	N	Y	N
HSV[d]	−	++	−	−	+	Y	Y	N
VZV[d]	−	−	−	−	+	Y	Y	Y
Orthomyxoviruses								
Influenza A, B, C	+	++	+	+	++	Y	Y	Y
Paramyxoviruses								
Measles	−	−	−	−	+	Y	N	Y
Parainfluenza 1, 2, 3	+	++	+++	++	−	N	N	N
Respiratory syncytial virus	−	+	++	+++	++	N	?	N
Picornavirus								
Enterovirus	+	−	−	−	−	N	N	N
Rhinovirus	+++	++	+	+	−	Y	N	N

[a] +++, most commonly isolated with syndrome; ++, common isolates; +, uncommon isolates; −, rarely or not identified with clinical syndrome.
[b] +Approved for use or experimental studies—demonstrate clinical benefit: Y, yes; N, no.
[c] Ganciclovir, foscarnet, cidofovir—all have significant toxicities.
[d] Acyclovir, famciclovir, valacyclovir, ganciclovir.

promise to further increase the antifungal armamentarium. Recent data suggest that voriconazole is as good or better than amphotericin B for *Aspergillus*. Aggressive therapy with high doses of antifungal agents appears to improve the outcome of invasive fungal disease. Combinations of antifungal therapies along with immune reconstitution may further improve responses. Prompt recognition of fungal infection combined with intensive antifungal therapy is needed for successful therapy of patients with invasive fungal infections.

VIRAL INFECTIONS OF THE RESPIRATORY TRACT

Viral infections are associated with tremendous morbidity worldwide and significant mortality only in the elderly, patients with comorbid illnesses (e.g., influenza), and relatively few therapeutic options (see Table 59-13). Most of these infections do not merit antimicrobial therapy. Viral infections in the immunocompromised host—including cytomegalovirus, herpes simplex virus, and shingles (varicella zoster)—may be therapeutic emergencies when affecting the lungs, central nervous system, or an allograft. The agents currently available for the treatment of CMV infection (ganciclovir, foscarnet, cidofovir) are associated with significant toxicities for bone marrow and kidney as well as the central nervous system.

BIBLIOGRAPHY

Baiter MS, Hyland RH, Low DE: Recommendations on the management of chronic bronchitis. *Can Med Assoc J* 151:5–23, 1994.

Bartlett JG, Dowell SF, Mandell LA, et al: Practice guidelines for the management of community-acquired pneumonia in adults. *Clin Infect Dis* 31:347–382, 2000.

Doern GV. Antimicrobial resistance with *Streptococcus pneumoniae* in the United States. *Semin Respir Crit Care Med* 21:273–284, 2000.

Fine, MJ, Auble TE, Yealy DM, Kapoor, *N Engl J Med* 336:243–250, 1997.

Greenberg SB: Respiratory herpesvirus infections: An overview. *Chest* 106:1S–2S, 1994.

Greenberg SB: Viral pneumonia. *Infect Dis Clin North Am* 5:603–621, 1991.

Marrie, TJ, Lau CY, Wheeler SL, et al: A controlled trail of a critical pathway for treatment of community-acquired pneumonia. *JAMA* 283:749–755, 2000.

60 | Community-Acquired Pneumonia*

Jay A. Fishman

ACUTE BRONCHITIS

Acute bronchitis is an inflammation of the tracheobronchial tree, usually in association with a generalized respiratory infection. It occurs most commonly during the winter months and is associated with respiratory viruses, including rhinovirus, coronavirus, influenza viruses, and adenovirus. *Mycoplasma pneumoniae, Chlamydia pneumoniae,* and *Bordetella pertussis* may also cause bronchitis. Secondary invasion with bacteria such as *Haemophilus influenzae* and *Streptococcus pneumoniae* may also play a role in acute bronchitis.

Cough is the most prominent manifestation of acute bronchitis. Initially the cough is nonproductive, but later mucoid sputum is produced. Still later in the course of the illness, purulent sputum is present. Many patients with acute bronchitis also have tracheitis. Symptoms of tracheal impairment include burning substernal pain associated with respiration and a very painful substernal sensation with coughing. Rhonchi and coarse crackles may be heard on examination of the chest; however, there are no signs of consolidation and the chest radiograph shows no opacity.

Most cases of acute bronchitis require measures directed only at relieving cough. Most are of viral etiology. For patients with fever or a predominant tracheitis component and purulent sputum, the sputum should be Gram-stained and cultured. If there is a predominant microorganism seen in the presence of more than 25 polymorphonuclear neutrophils and under 10 squamous epithelial cells per low-power field, antibiotic therapy directed against *S. pneumoniae* and *H. influenzae* should be instituted. Most patients, however, do not require antibiotic therapy for acute bronchitis—it is a self-limited disease. Acute exacerbations of chronic bronchitis as a part of chronic obstructive pulmonary disease (COPD) appears to benefit from antimicrobial therapy, even though the majority of these infections appear to be polymicrobial in origin.

---

*Edited from Chaps. 126 to 133, 144, and 145, "Infections of the Upper Respiratory Tract," by Durand M, Merchant SN, Baker AS; "Acute Bronchitis and Community-Acquired Pneumonia," by Marrie TJ; "Pneumonia in Childhood," by Pasternack MS; "Aspiration Disease and Anaerobic Infection," by Bartlett JG; "Empyema and Lung Abscess," by Finegold SM, Fishman JA; "Mediastinitis," by Rupp ME; "Bronchiectasis," by Swartz MN; "Systemic Infection, The Sepsis Syndrome, and the Lungs," by Teplick R, Fishman JA; "Legionellosis," by Yu VL, Vergis EN; "Mycoplasma, Chlamydia, and 'Atypical Pneumonias'," by Mufson MA. In: *Fishman's Pulmonary Diseases and Disorders,* 3d ed., edited by Fishman AP, Elias JA, Fishman JA, Grippi MA, Kaiser LR, Senior RM. New York, McGraw-Hill, 1998, pp 1973–2094 and 2235–2256. For fuller discussion of topics dealt with in this chapter, the reader is referred to the original text, as noted above.

PNEUMONIA

Definition

Pneumonia is defined as inflammation and consolidation of lung tissue due to an infectious agent. Pneumonia that develops outside the hospital is considered community-acquired. Pneumonia developing 72 h or more after admission to hospital is nosocomial, or hospital-acquired. There is still some debate as to whether nursing home–acquired pneumonia should be considered community-acquired or nosocomial pneumonia. For this reason, it is perhaps best to divide pneumonia into community-acquired and institution-acquired. (The latter category includes hospitals, nursing homes, extended care facilities, psychiatric institutions, and rehabilitation facilities.)

Epidemiology

The overall attack rate is about 12 cases per 1000 persons per year. The attack rates are highest at the extremes of age. Pneumonia is the sixth leading cause of death in the United States.

   The epidemiology of pneumonia has changed in recent years. This is due in part to changes in the population at risk and in part to the discovery of new microbial agents that cause pneumonia and changes in antimicrobial susceptibility of old microbial agents, such as *S. pneumoniae, H. influenzae,* and *Staphylococcus aureus.* Population changes include a continued increase in the number and proportion of patients who are 65 years of age or older. The annual incidence of pneumonia requiring hospitalization among persons in the age group 75 years or older is 11.6 per 1000 persons, compared with a rate of 0.54 per 1000 among persons aged 35 to 44. Likewise, there has been a steady increase in the number of immunocompromised individuals in the general population. This has created a subset of patients with community-acquired pneumonia who may be infected not only with the traditional pathogens that cause pneumonia but also with opportunistic pathogens. These individuals will often have severe or atypical presentation of infections. Newer pathogens recognized as causing pneumonia include *Chlamydia pneumoniae* and Hantavirus. *Pneumocystis carinii,* previously a rare cause of pneumonia in intentionally immunocompromised patients, is a common cause of pneumonia in untreated HIV-infected patients who are not receiving appropriate antimicrobial prophylaxis.

Clinical Manifestations

Symptoms that are suggestive of pneumonia include fever, chills, pleuritic chest pain, and cough. The cough may be nonproductive (dry) or productive of mucoid or purulent sputum. Sputum may be rusty in color and frankly bloody; in patients with a lung abscess (anaerobic infection), it may have a foul odor. For some time it was held that typical pneumonia (due to pyogenic organisms such as *Pneumococcus, Staphylococcus,* or *H. influenzae*) could be distinguished from that due to *Mycoplasma, Legionella,* and *Chlamydia pneumoniae*—so-called atypical pneumonia. The latter is said to be characterized by a more indolent illness than that of typical pneumonia, with a cough that is nonproductive or productive of mucoid sputum only. Careful studies have shown that one cannot reliably distinguish between typical versus atypical pneumonia on clinical grounds. However, this is not to say that a careful history and physical examination are not helpful in suggesting a cause of the pneumonia. Nonrespiratory symptoms such as headache, nausea, vomiting, abdominal pain, diarrhea, myalgia, and arthralgia are common symptoms in patients with pneumonia. It is wise to remember that the elderly complain of fewer symptoms with pneumonia than do younger patients.

Physical Examination

Fever is usually present, but some patients may be hypothermic (a poor prognostic sign), and some (20 percent) are afebrile at the time of presentation with their pneumonia. Crackles are heard on auscultation over the affected area of lung, and physical findings of consolidation (dullness to percussion, increased tactile and vocal fremitus, whispering pectoriloquy, and bronchial breath sounds) are present in about 20 percent of patients with pneumonia. A pleural friction rub is heard in about 10 percent of cases.

Radiographic Diagnosis

Clinical suspicion of pneumonia usually prompts a chest radiograph. An opacity on the chest radiograph is considered the "gold standard" for the diagnosis of pneumonia. However, this opacity may be due to infection, infarction, hemorrhage, edema fluid, malignancy, or inflammation caused by a variety of processes, such as vasculitis or adverse drug reactions. Several studies have shown that radiologists cannot differentiate bacterial from nonbacterial pneumonia on the basis of the radiograph. Certain radiographic patterns (Table 60-1) are more commonly associated with some microbial agents than with others.

Etiologic Diagnosis

Pneumonia represents a difficult challenge for the clinician, since the cause cannot be determined from the clinical presentation and data from microbiologic studies are not available for at least 48 h. Even then, in the case of microorganisms isolated from the sputum, one cannot be sure that this is the organism causing the pneumonia. The etiology of community-acquired pneumonia (CAP) as determined in prospective studies is given in Tables 60-2, 60-3, 60-4, and 60-5. Table 60-4 shows data for patients with severe pneumonia requiring admission to intensive care units. Table 60-5 gives the etiologic data for bacterial pneumonia in patients with HIV infection. Early in the course of the HIV epidemic, *P. carinii* accounted for most cases of pneumonia. Now, with widespread use of prophylaxis to prevent *P. carinii* pneumonia, it is evident that bacterial pneumonia is common in HIV disease. Indeed, the rates of pneumococcal pneumonia and *H. influenzae* pneumonia [without highly active antiretroviral therapy (HAART)] are 20 times higher among HIV-infected persons than in those of an age- and sex-matched population without HIV infection.

Admission Decision and Diagnostic Workup

Once a diagnosis of pneumonia has been made, the next decision is whether or not to admit the patient to hospital. There is considerable pressure to treat as many patients as possible as outpatients. In order to do this, it is important to know the factors that are predictive of a complicated course in pneumonia (Table 60-6).

Patients well enough to be treated as outpatients need minimal diagnostic workup. This should include a chest radiograph, complete white blood cell

TABLE 60-1 Differential Diagnosis of Common Patterns on Chest
Radiography in a Patient with a Clinical Picture of Pneumonia[a]

Focal opacity	Multifocal opacities
Streptococcus pneumoniae	*S. aureus*
Mycoplasma pneumoniae	*Coxiella burnetii*
Legionella pneumophila	*L. pneumophila*
Staphylococcus aureus	*S. pneumoniae*
Chlamydia pneumoniae	
Mycobacterium tuberculosis	
Blastomyces dermatitidis	
Interstitial	Miliary
"Viruses"	*M. tuberculosis*
M. pneumoniae	*Histoplasma capsulatum*
Pneumocystis carinii	*Coccidioides immitis*
Chlamydia psittaci	*B. dermatitidis*
	Varicella zoster
Interstitial pneumonia with	Segmental or lobar pneumonia
lymphadenopathy	with lymphadenopathy
Epstein-Barr virus	*M. tuberculosis* (primary
Francisella tularensis	infection)
C. psittaci	Atypical rubeola
M. pneumoniae	Fungi
Cavitation	Pneumatoceles
Mixed aerobic/anaerobic (lung abscess)	*S. aureus*
Aerobic gram-negative bacilli	*S. pyogenes*
M. tuberculosis	*P. carinii*
L. pneumophila	
Cryptococcus neoformans	
Nocardia asteroides	
Actinomyces israelii	"Round" pneumonia
C. immitis	*C. burnetii*
P. carinii	*S. pneumoniae*
	L. pneumophila
	S. aureus
Bulging fissure	
Klebsiella pneumoniae	
L. pneumophila	

[a]Only the microbial causes of the various radiographic patterns are
given—each also has an extensive noninfectious differential diagnosis.
SOURCE: From *Clin Infect Dis* 18:501–515, 1994.

count, electrolytes, creatinine, and oxygen saturation if pulse oximetry is
available to the physician. Attempts should be made to obtain sputum for culture in patients with COPD. In patients who are ill enough to be admitted to
hospital, two sets of blood cultures should be performed. About 10 percent
of patients with pneumonia have positive blood cultures. *S. pneumoniae* is
the most common cause of bacteremic pneumonia, accounting for 60 percent
of all cases.

Sputum Gram's Stain and Culture

A sputum specimen should be cultured only if a Gram-stained smear of a
representative portion shows more than 25 polymorphonuclear neutrophils
and fewer than 10 squamous epithelial cells per low-power field. The

TABLE 60-2 Guidelines for Determining the Etiology of Community-Acquired Pneumonia

Definite
  Blood cultures positive for a pathogen
  Pleural fluid positive for a pathogen
  Presence of *Pneumocystis carinii* in induced sputum or in bronchoalveolar lavage fluid
  A fourfold or greater rise in antibody titer to *Mycoplasma pneumoniae, Chlamydia pneumoniae*
  Isolation of *Legionella pneumophila* or a fourfold rise in antibody titer or positive urinary antigen test for *Legionella*
  Positive direct fluorescence antibody test for *Legionella* plus an antibody titer of ≥1:256 for *Legionella*
  Serum or urine positive for *Streptococcus pneumoniae* antigen
  Isolation of *Mycobacterium tuberculosis* from sputum
Probable
  Heavy or moderate growth of a predominant bacterial pathogen on sputum culture and a compatible Gram's stain
  Light growth of a pathogen in which sputum Gram's stain reveals a bacterium compatible with the culture results
  Aspiration pneumonia is diagnosed on clinical grounds.

SOURCE: Modified from Fang et al.

Gram's stain on such a specimen is useful. If only one morphologic type of bacteria is seen in such a specimen, it is likely that this microorganism is causing the pneumonia. Indeed, in one study, when more than 10 positive lancet-shaped diplococci were seen, the sputum was considered positive for pneumococci. This criterion was met in 62 percent of specimens that were culture-positive for *S. pneumoniae.* In patients with HIV infection, sputum production may be induced by inhalation of hypertonic saline, which irritates the tracheobronchial tree and produces bronchorrhea. This results in a specimen that is useful for examination for *P. carinii,* thereby obviating bronchoscopy. However, patients receiving second-line prophylaxis for *P. carinii* (other than trimethoprim-sulfamethoxazole) may need bronchoscopy to elucidate infection.

Patients who are ill enough to require admission to an intensive care unit for the treatment of pneumonia should have an aggressive diagnostic workup. This will usually include at least a bronchoscopy, with use of a protected brush to sample respiratory secretions and brochoalveolar lavage. If this is carried out before the initiation of antibiotic therapy, the diagnostic yield is up to 80 percent. When this procedure is performed after 72 h or more of antibiotic therapy, however, the microbiologic yield is much lower—18 percent.

Transthoracic needle aspiration can be used when the basal segment(s) of the lungs is (are) consolidated. A 20-gauge 3.5-in. needle is used to inject 2 to 3 mL of nonbacteriostatic saline into the lung. This is then aspirated and placed into a blood culture bottle. The diagnostic yield from this procedure ranges from 33 to 85 percent. Occasionally, patients with CAP require an open lung biopsy. However, this is usually a last resort in a patient whose condition continues to deteriorate and where there is no etiologic diagnosis despite the usual workup, including bronchoscopy.

TABLE 60-3 Etiology of Community-Acquired Pneumonia Requiring Hospitalization—North America

No. of patients studied	359	719	151 (154 episodes)
No. (%) patients with sputum cultured	336 (94)	257 (36)	None[a]
Location	Pittsburgh, PA	Halifax, NS	Little Rock, AR
Time period of study	Jul 1/86–Jun 30/87	Nov 1/81–Mar 18/87	1985
No. (%) with pneumonia of:			
Unknown cause	118 (32.9)	340 (47)	75 (48.7)
More than one cause	10 (2.8)	74 (10.3)	10 (6.4)
Streptococcus pneumoniae	39 (10.9)	61 (8.5)	9 (5.8)
Aspiration	12 (3.3)	52 (7.2)	Not stated
Mycoplasma pneumoniae	7 (2)	40 (5.6)	5 (3.2)
Influenza A virus	Not tested	40 (5.6)	7 (4.5)
Staphylococcus aureus	12 (3.3)	29 (4.0)	9 (5.8)
Haemophilus influenzae	39 (10.9)	27 (3.7)	2 (1.3)
Coxiella burnetii	Not tested	22 (3.1)	0
Influenza B virus	Not tested	17 (2.4)	0
Pneumocystis carinii	9 (2.5)	14 (1.9)	0
Legionella spp.	24 (6.7)	16 (2.2)	14 (9)
Mycobacterium tuberculosis	4 (1.1)	10 (1.4)	3 (1.9)
Chlamydia pneumoniae	22 (6.1)	18/301 (6)[b]	12 (7.8)
Postobstructive	19 (5.3)	13 (1.8)	Excluded
S. epidermidis	0	0	4 (2.6)
Aspergillus spp.	0	0	1 (0.6)
Nocardia spp.	0	0`	1 (0.6)
Francisella tularensis	Not tested	Not tested	5 (3.2)
Streptococcus spp.	10 (2.8)	19 (2.6)	4 (2.6)
Anaerobic bacteria	0	4 (0.6)	2 (1.3)
Other aerobic gram-negative bacteria	21 (5.9)	22 (3.1)	8 (5.2)

[a]This study did not use information from sputum cultures in determining cause. Some patients had a variety of invasive diagnostic procedures.
[b]Only 301 patients had serum samples tested for antibodies to *Chlamydia pneumoniae*.

An acute-phase serum sample should be obtained from all patients who are admitted to hospital with CAP. If the patient responds promptly to antibiotic therapy, there is no need to obtain a convalescent sample. If the patient responds poorly to therapy, however, a convalescent sample should be obtained 3 to 6 weeks after the acute-phase sample. The diagnostic battery ordered will depend on local epidemiologic conditions. In general, *M. pneumoniae; C. pneumoniae; Coxiella burnetti; Legionella pneumophila;* adenovirus; influenza A and B viruses; parainfluenza viruses 1, 2, and 3; and respiratory syncytial virus antibodies can be measured in most laboratories. The latter viruses may also be detected by direct fluorescent antibody staining (DFA) of nasal swabs for rapid diagnosis. Antibody titers to *S. pneumoniae* pneumolysin and detection of immune complexes to this antigen may be a tool for diagnosis of pneumococcal pneumonia in those who do not have sputum available for culture. *L. pneumophila* serogroup 1 infection can be reliably diagnosed from detection of antigen in urine with a radioimmunoassay or an enzyme-linked imunosorbent assay.

TABLE 60-4 Etiology of Community-Acquired Pneumonia in Patients Requiring Admission to an Intensive Care Unit

No. studied	60	92	67	53
Mean age (years)	54	53	56.8	52
No. (%) died	29 (48)	18 (20)	14 (21)	13 (25)
No. (%) with pneumonia due to (six most common causes listed):				
Unknown	25 (42)	44 (48)	45 (67)	25 (47)
Streptococcus pneumoniae	11 (18)	13 (14)	12 (17)	15 (28)
Haemophilus influenzae	7 (12)			
Legionella pneumophila	7 (12)	13 (14)	7 (10)	
Mycoplasma pneumoniae	4 (7)	6 (7)		3 (5)
Influenza virus	3 (5)			2 (4)
Staphylococcus aureus	2 (3)	1		2 (4)
Streptococcus species		3 (3)		
Chlamydia psittaci				2 (4)
Other aerobic gram-negative bacilli	2 (3)	5 (5)	8 (12)	

TREATMENT

The initial therapeutic approach to pneumonia is empiric and discussed in the previous chapter. Once the decision is made as to the severity of the infection (mild, moderate, or severe) and where the patient will be treated—at home, in hospital, or in an intensive care unit—general guidelines can be established for treatment (see Table 60-7).

Once the etiologic diagnosis has been made, treatment should be changed to employ the cheapest, narrowest-spectrum agent effective against that microorganism. For example, if *S. pneumoniae* is determined to be the cause of the pneumonia, penicillin therapy is still appropriate in most instances unless there is evidence of central nervous system or ear involvement. The overall mortality for those admitted to hospital for treatment of pneumonia is 20 percent. In patients with nursing home–acquired pneumonia, it may approach 40 percent.

TABLE 60-5 Etiology of Bacterial Community-Acquired Pneumonia in Patients with HIV Infection

Location of study	San Francisco, CA
Period of study	May 1990–April 1991
No. of pneumonia episodes	216
Cause of pneumonia, no. (%)	
Haemophilus influenzae	4 (1.9)
Streptococcus pneumoniae	66 (30.6)
Moraxella catarrhalis	1 (0.5)
Other streptococci	15 (6.9)
Cause unknown	54 (25)
Mixed infections	13 (6)
Haemophilus spp.	42 (19.4)
Klebsiella pneumoniae	4 (1.9)
Staphylococcus aureus	10 (4.6)
Pseudomonas aeruginosa	5 (2.3)
Serratia marcescens	1 (0.5)
Neisseria meningitidis	1 (0.5)

TABLE 60-6 Risk Factors for a Complicated Course or Mortality in Patients with Community-Acquired Pneumonia

Age >65 years
Comorbid illnesses that are likely to be made worse by the pneumonia, especially chronic renal failure, ischemic heart disease, congestive heart failure, and severe COPD
Concurrent malignancy
Postsplenectomy state
Altered mental status
Alcoholism
Immunosuppressive therapy
Respiratory rate >30 breaths per minute
Diastolic blood pressure <60 mmHg; systolic blood pressure <90 mmHg
Hypothermia
Creatinine >150 mm/L or BUN >7 mm/L
Leukopenia <3000/μL or leukocytosis >30,000/μL
O_2 <60 mmHg or P_{CO_2} >48 mmHg while breathing room air
Albumin <30 g/L
Hemoglobin <9 g/L
Pseudomonas aeruginosa or *Staphylococcus aureus* as the cause of the pneumonia
Bacteremic pneumonia
Multilobe involvement on chest radiograph
Rapid radiographic progression of the pneumonia defined as increase in the size of the pulmonary opacity of ≥50% within 36 h

A recent concept in therapy of pneumonia requiring hospitalization is an early switch to oral antibiotics. Patients who are stable by hospital day 3 (as evidenced by temperature of 37.5°C or less for 16 h, white blood cell count returning toward normal, normal hemodynamics, no requirement for auxiliary oxygen, no complications of pneumonia such as empyema, and ability to take antibiotics by mouth) can be switched to antibiotics and discharged shortly thereafter. About one-third of patients qualify for this therapy.

Radiographic evidence of resolution of pneumonia lags behind clinical resolution and correlates with age and the presence of COPD. In general, those who are under 50 years of age and have no COPD show radiographic resolution of pneumonia within 4 weeks. In contrast, resolution requires 12 or more weeks for those with pneumonia who are older than 50 years and have coexistent COPD or alcoholism. In about 2 percent of patients, pneumonia will be the presenting manifestation of carcinoma of the lung (postobstructive pneumonia). It is important to demonstrate that the pneumonia has resolved radiographically for those who are at risk for carcinoma of the lung. In general, all tobacco smokers and those who are 50 years of age or older and have pneumonia should have a chest radiograph to determine whether the pneumonia has completely resolved.

PREVENTION

Influenza vaccination of the elderly results in reduction in the rate of hospitalization for pneumonia and influenza by 48 to 57 percent. The role of pneumococcal vaccine has not been as clearly defined as that of influenza vaccine; however, the Advisory Committee on Immunization Practice recommends pneumococcal vaccine for persons older than 65 years of age.

TABLE 60-7 Initial Empiric Antimicrobial Therapy for Community-Acquired Pneumonia

---

1. Clinical presentation: not severe; *oral therapy*
   a. Previously well and/or <60 years old—macrolide or tetracycline
   b. Comorbid illness and >60 years old—cephalosporin (second-generation) or trimethoprim-sulfamethoxazole or amoxicillin plus beta-lactamase inhibitor
   If *Legionella* is a concern, add a macrolide
2. Clinical presentation: severe; *intravenous therapy*
   a. Treatment site: hospital ward—cephalosporin (second- or third-generation) ± macrolide ± rifampin
   Penicillin-allergic patients: trimethoprim-sulfamethoxazole plus macrolide
   b. Treatment site: ICU—cephalosporin (third-generation) with anti-pseudomonas activity and a macrolide ± rifampin or imipenem-cilastatin or ciprofloxacin + macrolide ± rifampin
3. Treatment site: nursing home
   a. Clinical presentation: not severe—cephalosporin (second-generation) or trimethoprim-sulfamethoxazole or amoxicillin–clavulanic acid
   Add a macrolide if *Legionella* is a concern
   b. Clinical presentation: severe—penicillin plus ciprofloxacin (oral) or cephalosporin (second-generation)[a] or ceftriaxone (intramuscular)[a]
   Penicillin-allergic patients: ciprofloxacin + clindamycin (intramuscular)

---

[a]Add a macrolide if *Legionella* is a concern.

Specific Pathogens

Streptococcal Pneumonia

S. pneumoniae is still a common cause of pneumonia. Patients with bactere-mic pneumococcal pneumonia are more likely to have diabetes mellitus, COPD, or alcoholism than those who have other causes of CAP. Capsular polysaccharide types 14, 4, 1, 6A/6B, 3, 8, 7F, 23F, and 18C are the most frequent causes of pneumococcal disease. Currently, 10 to 15 percent of *S. pneumoniae* isolates in the United States are intermediately or highly resistant to penicillin. These isolates are usually also resistant to erythromycin, tetracycline, and trimethoprim-sulfamethoxazole. Types 19A, 6A, 23, 19, 11, 6, 16, 9, and 14 are most frequently associated with penicillin resistance. The minimal inhibitory concentration (MIC) of penicillin for susceptible strains is under 0.06 μg/mL; isolates with MICs of 0.1 to 1 μg/mL are of intermediate resistance, and those with MICs of at least 2 μg/mL are highly resistant. These levels were established for central nervous system (CNS) infections, for which trough concentrations of penicillin at 10 times MIC are necessary for cure. Generally, with intravenous antibiotics, high concentrations can be achieved in pulmonary tissue, so even resistant strains of *S. pneumoniae* will usually respond to treatment with high doses of penicillin or a third-generation cephalosporin. Atypical infections (meningitis, sepsis, endovascular infections) due to *S. pneumoniae* should be treated with vancomycin and ceftriaxone until susceptibility data are available. Penicillin resistance should be considered a possibility, particularly if the patient has had beta-lactam antibiotic therapy in the preceding 3 months or if the patient is debilitated with an immunosuppressive illness.

Staphylococcus aureus

Pneumonia due to this agent is usually of sudden onset, affects persons with comorbid illnesses (except during influenza outbreaks, when healthy young adults may be infected), and is frequently complicated by cavitation (20 percent), pneumothorax (10 percent), jaundice (8 percent), empyema (5 percent), acute renal failure (5 percent), and pericarditis (2 percent).

Methicillin-resistant *S. aureus* (MRSA) is a rare cause of CAP. It does occur, however, and once established in a region, it can be a major problem. Vancomycin is used to treat MRSA, whereas cloxacillin or nafcillin is used to treat methicillin-susceptible strains. Surgical drainage is necessary for treatment of empyema. If multiple rounded opacities are seen in a patient with *S. aureus* pneumonia, suspect right-sided endocarditis. Toxic shock syndrome may complicate *S. aureus* pneumonia.

Haemophilus influenzae

This cause of pneumonia is more common in older patients with COPD. Both type B and non-B strains can cause pneumonia. About 30 percent of all *H. influenzae* isolates now produce beta-lactamase and hence are resistant to ampicillin and amoxicillin. Between 7 and 14 percent of *H. influenzae* isolates are resistant to trimethoprim-sulfamethoxazole. More than 90 percent of *H. influenzae* isolates are resistant to erythromycin; 1 to 2 percent are resistant to tetracycline. Amoxicillin–clavulanic acid and a second- or third-generation cephalosporin will reliably treat *H. influenzae* pneumonia. Sir William Osler died of *H. influenzae* pneumonia.

Streptococcus pyogenes (Group A Streptococcus)

This agent is uncommon as a cause of pneumonia. One of its presentations is pneumonia accompanied by explosive pleuritis. Cases of group A streptococcal pneumonia may be accompanied by "toxic strep syndrome." Clindamycin, 600 mg given intravenously every 8 h is superior to penicillin for the treatment of serious group A streptococcal infections. Jim Henson, creator of the Muppets, died of group A streptococcal pneumonia.

Mycoplasma pneumoniae

This agent accounts for up to 30 percent of pneumonias treated on an outpatient basis. The extrapulmonary manifestations of *M. pneumoniae* are many and include cold agglutinin–induced hemolytic anemia, thrombocytopenia, encephalitis, cerebellar ataxia, Guillain-Barré syndrome, Stevens-Johnson syndrome, and myocarditis. This is primarily a disease of younger patients, but it accounts for 5 percent of all cases of pneumonia in persons 65 years of age or older. Macrolides (erythromycin, clarithromycin, azithromycin) or tetracyclines are the treatment of choice.

Legionellaceae

This family, which includes 29 species and more than 49 serogroups, causes two clinical syndromes—Legionnaires' disease and a self-limited flu-like illness (Pontiac fever). *L. pneumophila* serogroup 1, the microorganism responsible for the 1976 outbreak in Philadelphia that gave this disease its name, accounts for 70 to 90 percent of the cases of Legionnaires' disease. The disease can be community- or hospital-acquired, and it can occur in sporadic, endemic, and epidemic forms. Exposure to contaminated water (showers, cooling towers, or even ingestion of such water and subsequent microaspiration) is the prime mode of acquisition. Older age, male sex, immunosuppression (especially with corticosteroids), nosocomial acquisition, end-stage renal disease, and infection with *L. pneumophila* serogroup 5 are risk factors for death from this infection. Erythromycin, 1 g given intravenously every 6 h, along with rifampin, 300 mg twice a day, is used to treat seriously ill patients with Legionnaires' disease. The disease may continue to progress for up to 4 days despite optimal therapy. Other options are doxycycline, 100 mg given twice intravenously in 24 h and then 100 mg optimal dose (OD) intravenously, and ciprofloxacin, 400 mg every 12 h intravenously. Relapses have occurred with treatment courses of less than 21 days.

Hantavirus

In May 1993, reports of deaths due to severe pulmonary disease were received by the New Mexico Department of Health. Many of the affected persons were residents of the Navajo reservation located near the Four Corners area of New Mexico, Arizona, Colorado, and Utah. Within a few months a new Hantavirus, Sin Nombre ("no name") virus, had been isolated and shown to be responsible for this outbreak, which had affected 17 persons. Hantavirus pulmonary syndrome (HPS) is characterized by a flulike prodromal illness, followed by rapidly progressive noncardiogenic pulmonary edema. Fever, myalgia, cough or dyspnea, nausea or vomiting, and diarrhea are the most common symptoms. Hypotension, tachypnea, and tachycardia are the usual findings on physical examination. Leukocytosis (often with a severe left shift), thrombocytopenia (median lowest platelet count 64,500 per mm^3), prolonged prothrombin and partial thromboplastin times, and elevated serum lactate dehydrogenase concentration are the most common laboratory findings. The mortality was high (88 percent) in the Four Corners outbreak. The initial chest radiograph showed infiltrates in 65 percent and no abnormality in 24 percent. Subsequently, 16 (94 percent) had rapidly evolving bilateral diffuse infiltrates. In the few months after identification of this new Hantavirus, two more new Hantaviruses were identified in the United States and cases of HPS continue to be reported. The deer mouse, *Peromyscus maniculatus,* is the primary rodent reservoir for this virus.

Chlamydia pneumoniae

This intracellular pathogen of humans is spread by aerosols. It causes sinusitis, pharyngitis, bronchitis, otitis media, and pneumonia. The last can be as a result of primary infection or as reactivation of latent infection. Primary infection affects mainly young adults and may be followed by reactive airway disease. Two weeks' treatment with doxycycline is adequate. Clarithromycin is very active in vitro against *C. pneumoniae,* but whether it is superior to doxycycline is not known.

The reactivation type of infection occurs in older adults, often as part of a polymicrobial infection. The rate of *C. pneumoniae* in this setting is unknown.

Diagnosis is by isolation of the organism from respiratory secretions or by serology. A greater than fourfold rise in IgM or IgG by microimmunofluorescence test or a single IgM titer of at least 1:16 or an IgG titer of at least 1:512 is considered diagnostic.

Aspiration and Anaerobic Infections

Aspiration pneumonia and anaerobic pleuropulmonary infections are distinctive but overlapping syndromes. Anaerobic bacteria are relatively common

pulmonary pathogens. *Aspiration pneumonia* refers to the pulmonary consequences that follow abnormal entry of fluid, particulate substances, or endogenous secretions from the upper airways or gastric contents into the lower
airways. The usual predisposing conditions are twofold. First, there needs to
be a compromise of the usual defenses that protect the lower airways, including glottic closure, cough reflex, or other clearing mechanisms. The second requirement is an inoculum that must be deleterious to the lower airways
by direct toxic effect, a bacterial challenge sufficient to initiate an inflammatory process, or an adequate volume to cause obstruction. Aspiration pneumonia consequently comprises several syndromes based on the inoculum
(Table 60-8). Anaerobic bacteria are the most common pathogens in this
setting, reflecting both pathogenic potential and numeric dominance in the
normal flora of the upper airways. Other aspiration syndromes are common
and merit consideration.

Chemical Pneumonitis   This refers to the aspiration of an inoculum that is
inherently toxic to the lungs. Examples include acid, animal fats such as milk
and mineral oil, and volatile hydrocarbons. These substances are toxic to the
lower airways, and they initiate an inflammatory reaction. The prototypic example based on extensive study is gastric acid pneumonitis as classically described by Mendelson and often referred to as Mendelson's syndrome. Factors

TABLE 60-8   Classification of Aspiration Pneumonia

Inoculum	Pulmonary sequelae	Clinical features	Therapy
Acid	Chemical pneumonitis	Acute dyspnea, tachypnea; tachycardia; cyanosis, bronchospasm, fever Sputum: pink, frothy Radiographic: infiltrates in one or both lower lobes Hypoxemia	Positive-pressure breathing Intravenous fluids Tracheal suction
Oropharyngeal bacteria	Bacterial infection	Usually insidious onset Cough, fever, purulent sputum Radiographic: infiltrate in dependent pulmonary segment or lobe ± cavitation	Antibiotics
Inert fluids	Mechanical obstruction Reflex airway closure	Acute dyspnea, cyanosis ± apnea Pulmonary edema	Tracheal suction Intermittent positive-pressure breathing with O_2 and bronchodilators
Particulate matter	Mechanical obstruction	Related to degree of obstruction and presence of infection; may produce recurrent infections	Extraction of particulate matter; antibiotics for infection

that contribute to hypoxemia are pulmonary edema, reduced surfactant activity, reflex airway closure, hyaline membrane formation, and alveolar hemorrhage. These patients' pulmonary function tests show decreased compliance, abnormal ventilation/perfusion, and reduced diffusing capacity. Severe disease often progresses to the adult respiratory distress syndrome (ARDS). The second potential complication is a superimposed bacterial infection, which may occur later in the course of events.

Gastric acid pneumonitis requires a pH of 2.5 or less for the inflammatory process to be initiated. There must also be a relatively large inoculum, usually 1 to 4 mL/kg. It is possible for smaller volumes to initiate a less dramatic presentation or to go undetected. Atelectasis occurs within seconds and is extensive by 3 min. There is also peribronchial hemorrhage, pulmonary edema, and bronchial epithelial cell degeneration. The alveolar spaces are filled with neutrophils by 4 h and hyaline membranes are seen within 48 h. Resolution begins by the third day and may be complete or may result in residual scarring of the pulmonary parenchyma.

The treatment of gastric acid aspiration includes tracheal suction to clear fluids and particulate matter that may be aspirated concurrently. Supportive care consists primarily of intravenous fluids due to decreased intravascular volume with hypotension. Studies in animal models show benefit with positive-pressure ventilation, large-molecular-weight colloids given intravenously, and sodium nitroprusside. It has been difficult to establish the role of these therapeutic interventions in patients with appropriate controlled trials, in part because of the relative infrequency of gastric acid pneumonia. The role of antimicrobial agents is also controversial. There is no evidence that bacteria play a role in the acute events either in the animal model or in patients; indeed, bacteria cannot survive at the pH of the inoculum necessary to initiate this process. Antibiotic administration to aspiration-prone patients has not proved useful.

Mechanical Obstruction Aspiration pneumonia may involve fluid or particulate material. In this form of aspiration pneumonia, the inoculum is not toxic to the lung but may cause obstruction or reflux airway closure. In most cases there is only transient, self-limited hypoxemia due to rapid clearance. Some patients develop pulmonary edema, however, with hypoxemia and reduced compliance apparently due to an intrinsic pulmonary reflex closure. The most important therapeutic intervention is removal of the foreign body, usually with bronchoscopy.

Pathophysiology and Microbiology

The bacteria implicated in anaerobic lung infections represent the normal flora of the oral cavity—primarily the gingival crevice, where anaerobic bacteria are found in concentrations that approach the geometric limits with which bacteria occupy space: 10^{12}/g. Compromised consciousness or dysphagia predisposes most frequently to clinically significant aspiration. Common conditions associated with clinically significant aspiration include alcoholism, general anesthesia, seizure disorder, drug abuse, esophageal lesions, and neurologic deficits. Numerous studies indicate that virtually all healthy persons aspirate but that this is usually inconsequential. The decisive factor for the development of lung complications depends on the frequency, volume, and character of the material in the inoculum. The conditions cited above as causing clinically significant disease are associated with more frequent aspiration or aspiration of large volumes—factors that define the populations at greatest risk. Additional conditions that appear to predispose to anaerobic infections include pulmonary infarction, obstruction due to carcinoma or a foreign body, and bronchiectasis. These conditions are associated with stasis or necrosis of tissue, which presumably accounts for the association with anaerobic infections.

A somewhat unique feature of anaerobic lung infections is the tendency for necrosis of tissue, resulting in abscess formation or a bronchopleural fistula associated with empyema. Virulence factors of anaerobic bacteria presumed to account for this association include the capsular polysaccharide of anaerobic gram-negative bacilli. The most extensively studied is the polysaccharide of *Bacteroides fragilis,* but the same observations appear to apply to *P. melaninogenica* and probably other anaerobic gram-negative bacilli as well. Another virulence factor possessed by most anaerobic bacteria is the production of short-chain fatty acids that inhibit phagocytic killing at low pH levels. Short-chain volatile fatty acids are metabolic products of anaerobic bacteria that are used to classify these organisms taxonomically, and they appear to be responsible for the putrid odor that is often a characteristic feature of infections by these organisms.

The recovery of anaerobic bacteria in pulmonary infections requires specimens of respiratory secretions that are devoid of contamination from the upper airways. The usual procedures satisfying this criterion are transtracheal aspiration (TTA), transthoracic aspiration, open lung biopsy, thoracentesis, and, most recently, protected brush bronchoscopy with quantitative cultures. In addition, there must be appropriate laboratory expertise for cultivation of anaerobic bacteria. Most published reports deal with the role of anaerobic bacteria in aspiration pneumonia or lung abscess, and these show recovery rates ranging from 62 to 100 percent. One of the best studies is by Beerens and Tahon-Castel, who used TTA to characterize the flora in lung abscesses; this series showed recovery of anaerobic bacteria, usually in pure culture, in 22 of 26 cases (85 percent). A more recent report by Gudiol and colleagues employed similar techniques and showed anaerobic bacteria in 37 of 41 cases (90 percent). Anaerobic bacteria are actually relatively common pathogens among patients with community-acquired pneumonia and presumably account for a substantial proportion of cases that are now considered enigmatic.

In the preantibiotic era, *S. pneumoniae* accounted for 60 to 70 percent of cases of empyema; studies at that time indicated that empyema fluid was putrid (and thus implicated anaerobes) in about 5 to 7 percent of cases. More recent studies of empyema have shown a sharp decrease in the frequency of empyema and a marked shift in the bacteriology, so that the pneumococcus accounts for only 5 to 10 percent of cases while anaerobes are found in 25 to 40 percent. Bartlett reported the highest yield of anaerobes (76 percent) in a collaborative study at Cook County Hospital in Chicago and two VA hospitals in Los Angeles.

The bacteriologic findings in anaerobic lung infections involve multiple bacterial species (Table 60-9). The major bacterial isolates in patients with anaerobic lung infections are *Peptostreptococcus, F. nucleatum,* and *P. melaninogenica.* These are considered the "big three" anaerobic bacteria in oral and pulmonary infections involving the oral flora. Aerobic and microaerophilic streptococci are commonly present as well and may be contributing factors in the pathogenic events. At least 15 to 25 percent of anaerobic bacteria responsible for lung infections are resistant to penicillin, almost always because of penicillinase production. These sensitivity data are

TABLE 60-9 Bacteriology of Anaerobic Lung Infections

	Bartlett and Finegold	Marina et al.
Period reviewed	1968–75	1976–91
Patients	193	110
Total anaerobic isolates	461	404
Major isolates		
Gram-negative bacilli		
Bacteroides fragilis group	38[a]	18
Pigmented Prevotella[b]	76	63
Nonpigmented Prevotella	—	40
Bacteroides ureolyticus	—	23
Fusobacterium nucleatum	56	34
Bacteroides species (other)	37	138
Peptostreptococcus/Peptococcus[c]	126	39
Gram-positive bacilli		
Clostridium spp.	18	12
Eubacterium spp.	18	22
Actinomyces	5	19
Lactobacillus	8	22
Propionibacteria	10	9

[a]Numbers indicate the total number of isolates. Some of the differences are due to taxonomic changes.
[b]Pigmented Prevotella comprises organisms previously classified as B. melaninogenicus.
[c]Most peptococci have been reclassified as Peptostreptococcus.

rarely available in individual cases: most patients with anaerobic pulmonary infection never have cultivation of the putative agent, and those who do are usually not subjected to susceptibility testing.

Clinical Features

Common clinical features of anaerobic pulmonary infections are summarized in Table 60-10, which categorizes the patients with respect to pneumonitis,

TABLE 60-10 Clinical Features of Anaerobic Pulmonary Infections[a]

	Lung abscess (83 points)	Empyema (51 points)	Pneumonitis (only) (79 points)	Total (213 points)
Age (median)	52 years	49 years	60 years	51 years
Peak temperature (mean, °F)	102.1	102.4	102.6	102.4
Peripheral leukocyte count (median/mm^3)	15,000	21,600	13,700	15,000
History of				
weight loss	36 (43%)	28 (55%)	3 (4%)	57 (30%)
Putrid discharge	41 (49%)	32 (63%)	4 (5%)	62 (32%)
Lethal outcome	3 (4%)	3 (6%)	3 (4%)	8 (4%)

[a]Based on retrospective chart review of 213 cases established by recovery of anaerobes as dominant flora in TTA, pleural fluid, or blood culture.
SOURCE: From Bartlett, and Marina et al., with permission.

lung abscess, or empyema. Although these are distinctive clinical syndromes, there is no evidence of microbiologic distinctions in their etiology. Anaerobic lung infections may be acute, subacute, or chronic. The first stage in the infection is pneumonitis with clinical features similar to those of pneumococcal pneumonia. Significant differences with anaerobic infections are the lack of rigors, a somewhat longer duration of symptoms before presentation, and a more frequent association with predisposing conditions for aspiration. Patients seen in this early stage of infection rarely have the features that are commonly associated with anaerobic lung infections, such as putrid sputum, tissue necrosis with abscess formation, and a chronic course. These infections presumably account for some and possibly many of the cases of community-acquired pneumonia in which no etiologic diagnosis is established despite extensive study; such cases account for 40 to 50 percent of cases in most series.

The initial stage of pneumonitis is often more subtle or neglected, so that many patients do not seek medical attention until the infection has been present for weeks or even months. Many of these infections progress to suppurative complications, with presentation as lung abscess or empyema. The studies by David Smith show that 7 to 14 days is required for cavity formation. Occasionally, patients present with chronic pneumonitis.

Chest radiographs in patients with anaerobic lung infections show infiltrates, with or without cavitation, that most frequently involve dependent pulmonary segments. The favored locations are the superior segment of the lower lobes or posterior segments of the upper lobes; these are dependent in the recumbent position. The basilar segments of the lower lobes are favored in patients who aspirate in the upright position. The right lung is more frequently affected, owing to the more direct takeoff of the right main-stem bronchus.

Laboratory Diagnosis

Uncontaminated specimens that are considered valid for anaerobic culture include pleural fluid, transtracheal aspirates, transthoracic aspirates, and specimens obtained at thoracotomy. The most common technique used in the early 1970s was TTA. It was critical to obtain the specimen before administration of antibiotics, since this treatment rapidly alters the cultivable flora. TTA is now rarely used, and relatively few physicians are trained in the technique.

An alternative specimen source that is gaining popularity is quantitative cultures of specimens obtained at fiberoptic bronchoscopy, either by bronchoalveolar lavage (BAL) or with the protected brush. Anaerobic bacteriology, as conventionally done, should not be used for bronchoscopic aspirates. It should be noted that quantitative culture of lower airway secretions improves diagnostic accuracy with virtually any specimen that is subject to contamination, including expectorated sputum and tracheostomy aspirates. The second criterion for documenting anaerobic infections of the lower airways is proper attention to transport and processing of specimens. These specimens should be expeditiously transported to the laboratory for prompt microbiologic processing. Technical expertise for recovering and identifying anaerobic bacteria is highly variable. Most of these infections are polymicrobial, and many of the organisms grow slowly in vitro. There is also great variation in the quality of in vitro susceptibility tests. These factors contribute to the necessity for empiric decisions regarding antibiotic selection.

Most anaerobic gram-negative bacteria have unique morphologic features that make them relatively easy to identify or suspect on direct Gram's stain. Peptostreptococci appear like their aerobic counterparts. These are usually mixed infections involving multiple bacteria, and about half of the cases demonstrate mixtures of aerobic and anaerobic bacteria. Thus, the detection of polymicrobial flora or bacteria with the unique morphology of anaerobes on any specimen that is devoid of contamination by normal flora represents an important clue to the probable presence of anaerobic infection.

TREATMENT

The most important component of treatment is antibiotics—except in the case of empyemas, for which the mainstay of treatment is drainage. The standard drug historically for aspiration pneumonia and lung abscess involving anaerobic bacteria has been penicillin, usually given intravenously or with high-dose oral treatment. These recommendations have been confounded in recent years by the observations summarized above; penicillinase production has been noted in up to 40 to 60 percent of strains of fusobacteria and *P. melaninogenica* as well as in many other anaerobic gram-negative bacilli. Therapeutic trials in patients with lung abscess involving anaerobic bacteria compared clindamycin to intravenous penicillin; clindamycin proved superior in terms of response rates and time to defervescence. Alternative regimens in which the anecdotal experience is favorable include amoxicillin-clavulanate and penicillin combined with metronidazole. Metronidazole should not be used as a single agent in patients with anaerobic lung infections, since there is a poor response in about 50 percent. The presumed explanation is the contributing role of aerobic and microaerophilic streptococci, which are resistant to this drug. There are many other antibiotics that might be successful in anaerobic lung infections but have not been studied. These include any combination of a beta-lactam with a beta-lactamase inhibitor (ticarcillin-clavulanate, ampicillin-sulbactam, amoxicillin-clavulanate, piperacillin-tazobactam), chloramphenicol, imipenem, meropenem, and selected cephalosporins such as cefoxitin or cefotetan. All these drugs have established merit in treating anaerobic infections at several anatomic sites. Macrolides (erythromycin, clarithromycin, and azithromycin) have not been extensively studied for anaerobic pulmonary infections, but they show good in vitro activity against most strains except fusobacteria. Penicillin is not active against many strains; nevertheless, this drug may be adequate for most patients, especially those characterized by pneumonitis without suppurative complications. The same applies to other penicillins, especially when used in high doses, including ampicillin and antipseudomonad penicillins. Oxacillin and nafcillin are much less active. Tetracyclines show limited activity against many anaerobic bacteria in vitro; vancomycin is active only against gram-positive anaerobes. Drugs that have virtually no activity against anaerobes include aminoglycosides, early-generation quinolones (later generations have some anaerobic activity but are more expensive than other agents), aztreonam, and trimethoprim-sulfamethoxazole.

PREVENTION OF ASPIRATION

Methods to prevent aspiration have been most extensively studied in hospitalized patients, especially those who are aspiration-prone. Most important is use of the semirecumbent or upright position. Additional factors that have variable degrees of success are tracheostomies, reduction of the stomach volume with suction or metoclopramide, feeding via gastrostomy or nasogastric tube, and neutralization of gastric acid with H_2 blockers or antacids. Many of these procedures actually predispose to aspiration or invite other sequelae. An example is the neutralization of gastric acid, which may reduce the risk of chemical pneumonia but may increase the risk of bacterial infection following aspiration of gastric contents. Tracheostomy is useful in some patients with repeated aspiration, but inflation of the balloon may occlude the esophagus and promote aspiration of upper airway contents. Patients who require nasogastric feedings are aspiration-prone; percutaneous endoscopic gastroscopy is an attractive method to address this issue, but study results are quite variable. An alternative method sometimes favored is a feeding jejunostomy. The use of surgery with gastroesophageal reflux has given variable results.

BIBLIOGRAPHY

Amberson JB Jr: Aspiration bronchopneumonia. *Intern Clin* 3:126–138, 1937.

Bartlett JG: Anaerobic bacterial infections of the lung and pleural space. *Clin Infect Dis* 16(suppl 4):S248–S255, 1993.

Bartlett JG, Finegold SM: Anaerobic infections of the lung and pleural space. *Am Rev Respir Dis* 110:56–77, 1974.

Bartlett JG, Finegold SM: Bacteriology of expectorated sputum with quantitative culture and wash technique compared to transtracheal aspirates. *Am Rev Respir Dis* 117:1019–1027, 1978.

Bartlett JG, Gorbach SL, Thadepalli H, Finegold SM: Bacteriology of empyema. *Lancet* 1:338–340, 1974.

Bartlett JG, Mundy LM: Community-acquired pneumonia. *N Engl J Med* 333:1618–1624, 1995.

Bates JH, Campbell GD, Barren AL, et al: Microbial etiology of acute pneumonia in hospitalized patients. *Chest* 101:1005–1112, 1992.

Beerens H, Tahon-Castel M: *Infections Humaines à Bactéries Anaérobies Nontoxigènes*. Brussels, Presses Académiques Européenes, 1965, pp 91–114.

British Thoracic Society Research Committee and the Public Health Laboratory Service: The aetiology, management, and outcome of severe community-acquired pneumonia on the intensive care unit. *Respir Med* 86:7–13, 1992.

Burack JH, Hahn JA, Saint-Maurice D, et al: Microbiology of community-acquired bacterial pneumonia in persons with and at risk for human immunodeficiency virus type 1 infection: Implications for rationale empiric antibiotic therapy. *Arch Intern Med* 154:2589–2596, 1994.

Ehler AA: Non-tuberculous thoracic empyema: Collective review of literature from 1934 to 1939. *Int Abstr Surg* 72:17–38, 1941.

Fang GD, Fine M, Orloff J, et al: New and emerging etiologies for community-acquired pneumonia with implications for therapy: A prospective multicenter study of 359 cases. *Medicine* 69:307–316, 1990.

Gudiol F, Manresa F, Pallares R, et al: Clindamycin vs penicillin for anaerobic lung infections: High rate of penicillin failures associated with penicillin-resistant *Bacteroides melaninogenicus*. *Arch Intern Med* 150:2525–2529, 1990.

Lemmer J, Botham MJ, Orringer MB: Modern management of adult thoracic empyema. *J Thorac Cardiovasc Surg* 90:849–855, 1985.

Levison ME, Mangura CT, Lorber B, et al: Clindamycin compared with penicillin for the treatment of anaerobic lung abscess. *Ann Intern Med* 98:466–471, 1983.

Lorber B, Swenson RM: Bacteriology of aspiration pneumonia: A prospective study of community- and hospital-acquired cases. *Ann Intern Med* 81:329–331, 1974.

Marina M, Strong CA, Civen R, et al: Bacteriology of anaerobic pleuropulmonary infections: Preliminary report. *Clin Infect Dis* 16(suppl):S256–S262, 1993.

Marrie TJ, Durant H, Yates L: Community-acquired pneumonia requiring hospitalization: 5-year prospective study. *Rev Infect Dis* 11:586–599, 1989.

Neiderman MS, Bass JB, Campbell GD, et al: Guidelines for the initial empiric therapy of community-acquired pneumonia: Diagnosis, assessment of severity, and initial antimicrobial treatment. *Am Rev Respir Dis* 148:1418–1426, 1993.

Örtqvist Å, Sterner G, Nilsson JA: Severe community-acquired pneumonia: Factors influencing need of intensive care treatment and prognosis. *Scand J Infect Dis* 17:377–386, 1985.

Pachon J, Prados MD, Capote F, et al: Severe community-acquired pneumonia: Etiology, prognosis and treatment. *Am Rev Respir Dis* 142:369–373, 1990.

Smith DT: Experimental aspiratory abscess. *Arch Surg* 14:231–239, 1927.

Spray SB, Zuidema GD, Cameron JL: Aspiration pneumonia: Incidence of aspiration with endotracheal tubes. *Am J Surg* 131:701–703, 1976.

Torres A, Serra-Battles J, Ferrer A, et al: Severe community-acquired pneumonia: Epidemiology and prognostic factors. *Am Rev Respir Dis* 144:312–318, 1991.

61

Nosocomial Respiratory Tract Infections and Gram-Negative Pneumonia*

Jay A. Fishman, David J. Weber, William A. Rutala, and C. Glen Mayhall

Nosocomial pneumonia has been defined as an infection of the lung parenchyma that was neither present nor incubating at the time of hospital admission. Nosocomial pneumonia is the second leading cause of hospital-acquired infection and accounts for approximately 19 percent of all nosocomial infections in the United States. It has been estimated that there are 150,000 to 200,000 nosocomial respiratory tract infections per year in the United States. Nosocomial pneumonia results in an average of 5.9 extra hospital days at a cost of $5683 in 1992 dollars. Overall, nosocomial pneumonia results in an estimated 7087 deaths and contributes to 22,983 deaths per year in the United States.

PATHOGENESIS

Bacteria may invade the lower respiratory tract by three major routes: aspiration of oropharyngeal flora, inhalation of infected aerosols, and, less frequently, hematogenous spread from a remote focus of infection (Fig. 61-1). Investigators have proposed bacterial translocation from the gastrointestinal tract as an additional mechanism of infection. The major cause of nosocomial pneumonia is believed to be colonization of the oropharynx and gastrointestinal tract by pathogenic microorganisms followed by aspiration of these pathogens and the development of pneumonia in the setting of impaired host defenses (see Chap. 60). Aspiration of oropharyngeal secretions has been noted in approximately 45 percent of normal subjects during sleep. Several problems commonly affecting hospitalized patients are associated with an increased frequency or volume of aspiration: altered consciousness, abnormal swallowing, depressed gag reflexes, delayed gastric emptying, and decreased gastrointestinal motility. Oropharyngeal colonization with aerobic gram-negative bacilli is favored by coma, hypotension, acidosis, azotemia, alcoholism, diabetes mellitus, leukocytosis, leukopenia, pulmonary disease, use of nasogastric or endotracheal tubes, and antibiotic use. Thus, hospitalized patients, especially those in intensive care units (ICUs), have an increased frequency of oropharyngeal colonization by more pathogenic aerobic gram-negative bacilli and are often at increased risk for aspirating this more pathogenic flora.

*Edited from Chap. 143, "Nosocomial Respiratory Tract Infections and Gram-Negative Pneumonia," by Weber DJ, Rutala WA, and Mayhall CG. In: *Fishman's Pulmonary Diseases and Disorders,* 3d ed., edited by Fishman AP, Elias JA, Fishman JA, Grippi MA, Kaiser LR, Senior RM. New York, McGraw-Hill, 1998, pp 2213–2234. For fuller discussion of topics dealt with in this chapter, the reader is referred to the original text, as noted above.

734

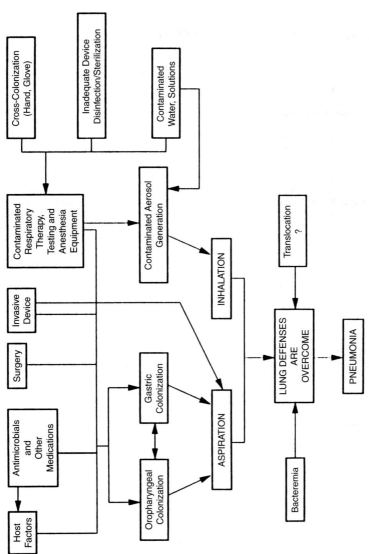

FIG. 61-1 Pathogenesis of nosocomial bacterial pneumonia. *(Based on data of Tablan et al., with permission.)*

The importance of oropharyngeal colonization in nosocomial pneumonia was demonstrated by Johanson and colleagues, who showed that pneumonia occurred in 23 percent of patients colonized with aerobic gram-negative bacilli but in only 3 percent of noncolonized patients. More recently, the stomach has been postulated as an important reservoir of organisms capable of causing nosocomial pneumonia. Normally, the stomach is rendered sterile by hydrochloric acid; however, elevations of gastric pH from normal levels to levels at or above 4 allow microorganisms to multiply to high concentrations. Elevated gastric pH may occur in patients with advanced age, achlorhydria, ileus, or upper gastrointestinal disease and in those receiving enteral feeding, antacids, or histamine$_2$ (H$_2$) antagonists.

Intubation for respiratory support is the most important risk factor for subsequent nosocomial pneumonia. Nasotracheal or orotracheal intubation predisposes patients to bacterial colonization and nosocomial pneumonia by a variety of pathophysiologic alterations: (1) sinusitis and trauma to the nasopharynx (nasotracheal tube), (2) impaired swallowing of secretion, (3) acting as a reservoir for bacterial proliferation, (4) increased bacterial adherence and colonization of airways, (5) ischemia secondary to cuff pressure, (6) impaired ciliary clearance and cough, (7) leakage of secretions around the cuff, and (8) suctioning often required to remove secretions. Contaminated respiratory care equipment may lead to nosocomial pneumonia by two routes. First, respiratory care equipment may serve as a reservoir for microorganisms, especially gram-negative bacilli. Fluid-containing devices such as nebulizers and humidifiers may become heavily contaminated by bacteria capable of multiplying in water. Pathogens may then be spread to the patient by hospital personnel or by aerosolization into room air. Second, contaminated equipment may lead to direct airway inoculation of microorganisms if it is directly linked to the ventilatory system or if contaminated medications are instilled by aerosolization. The role of contaminated respiratory equipment as a source or reservoir for nosocomial pneumonia has recently been reviewed.

Hospital personnel and the hospital environment also play important roles in nosocomial pneumonia. Cross-transmission between patients may occur when the hands of medical personnel become transiently colonized with pathogenic organisms. Such pathogens may be acquired from direct patient care or from contact with contaminated equipment or hospital surfaces. For this reason, it is crucial that health care providers carefully wash their hands before and after each patient contact. Patients may acquire respiratory infections—including influenza, respiratory syncytial virus, pertussis, group A streptococcus, diphtheria, and *Mycobacterium tuberculosis*—transmitted by the droplet or airborne routes from infected health care personnel, other patients, or visitors.

The hospital environment may also serve as a reservoir for *Aspergillus, Zygomycetes,* and *Legionella.* Nosocomial pneumonia may result when these pathogens are inhaled, especially if the patient is immunocompromised. The recovery of *Aspergillus* or *Zygomycetes* within hospitals has been variable, but commonly at least small numbers can be isolated from the air, accumulated dust, and environmental surfaces. More than 25 outbreaks of nosocomial fungal pneumonia have been reported. Sources of airborne fungi in hospitals have been reported to include (1) dust associated with hospital renovations; (2) outside construction, with an inadequate or malfunctioning hospital ventilation system; (3) contaminated cellulose fireproofing material; (4) contamination of the hospital air supply by pigeon droppings, helicopter flights from a roof helipad, or contaminated air filters and air-conditioning coils; and

(5) an inadequate filtration system, coupled with location of the outside air intake vent near a refuse container.

Nosocomial acquisition of *Legionella pneumophila* and *L. bozemanii* have been linked to contamination of hospital water supplies, and the association has been strengthened by use of molecular epidemiologic typing methods (e.g., DNA fingerprinting by pulsed-field gel electrophoresis) and clinical and environmental strains. *Legionella* can be isolated from more than 50 percent of the potable water supplies and more than 10 percent of the distilled water supplies in hospitals. The subjects of *Legionella* in hospitals and disinfection of water distribution systems for *Legionella* have been reviewed.

INCIDENCE

The incidence of nosocomial pneumonia varies among hospitals. The National Nosocomial Infections Surveillance (NNIS) system of the Centers for Disease Control and Prevention (CDC) noted that in 1984, the overall incidence of nosocomial pneumonia was 6.0 per 1000 discharged patients. The incidence varied by hospital type, being 4.2 in nonteaching hospitals, 5.4 in small teaching hospitals, and 7.7 in large teaching hospitals.

The incidence of ventilator-associated pneumonia has ranged from 11 to 54 cases per 100 patients, depending on the population studied. Intubation and mechanical ventilation represent the most important risk factor for nosocomial pneumonia, with a 6- to 21-fold increased risk. Rates among ICUs ranged from 6.0 in the pediatric ICU to 22.2 in the burn ICU. For this reason, the CDC and other investigators now report the incidence of nosocomial pneumonia as cases per 1000 days of mechanical ventilation. Several investigators have described the actuarial risk of pneumonia as a function of the duration of mechanical ventilation. Langer and associates showed that the rate of pneumonia was constant through the first 8 to 10 days of respiratory assistance and then decreased. By day 30 of mechanical ventilation, an episode of nosocomial pneumonia will have developed in more than 60 percent of patients. Fagon and coworkers reported the actuarial risk of pneumonia during mechanical ventilation as 6.5 percent at 10 days, 19 percent at 20 days, and 28 percent at 30 days. Ruiz-Santana and colleagues reported actuarial risks for pneumonia as 8.5 percent at day 3, as 21.1 percent at day 7, as 32.4 percent at day 14, and as 45.6 percent for ventilation after 14 days.

RISK FACTORS FOR NOSOCOMIAL PNEUMONIA

Many risk factors have been demonstrated to be associated with nosocomial pneumonia (Table 61-1). In general, these factors can be divided into several broad categories: (1) intrinsic host factors such as age, underlying medical disorders such as pulmonary disease, and nutritional status; (2) hospital factors such as abdominal or thoracic operations, antibiotic use, immunosuppression, and treatment in an ICU; (3) equipment and device use, especially intubation with mechanical ventilation; and (4) factors that increase the risk of aspiration such as depressed consciousness.

Intrinsic Factors

The incidence of nosocomial pneumonia is increased at the extremes of life. However, age is not an independent risk factor for nosocomial pneumonia. Rather, the increased incidence of pneumonia in the elderly was a function of an increased frequency of both intrinsic and hospital risk factors, such as

TABLE 61-1 Risk Factors for Nosocomial Pneumonia

Ventilator-associated pneumonia independent risk factors	Ventilated and nonventilated patients univariate risk factors for pneumonia
Age >60 years	Age >60 years
COPD/PEEP/pulmonary disease	Male sex
Coma/impaired consciousness	Smoking
Therapeutic interventions[a]	Underlying disease, rapidly fatal vs
Intracranial pressure monitoring	nonfatal/ultimately fatal
Organ failure	Simplified acute physiologic score >9
Large-volume gastric aspiration	ASA class IV
Prior antibiotics	Inspired O_2 >0.50
H_2 blocker +/− antacids	Prior care facility
Gastric colonization and pH	Alcohol intake
Season: fall, winter	Renal failure/dialysis
Ventilator circuit changes 24 vs 48 h	Intraaortic balloon pump
Reintubation	COPD
Mechanical ventilation ≥2 days	Chemical paralysis
Tracheostomy	Airway instrumentation
Supine head position	Aspiration before intubation
	Mechanical ventilation >2 days
	No prior surgery
Ventilated and nonventilated	H_2 blockers or antacids vs sucralfate
patients independent risk factors	Coma
Age >60 years	Head trauma
APACHE II >6	Cascade humidifier vs heat moisture
Trauma/head injury	exchanger
Impaired airway reflexes	Tracheostomy
Coma	Continuous enteral feeding
Bronchoscopy	Prior antibiotics
Nasogastric tube	Nosocomial maxillary sinusitis
Endotracheal intubation	Type of intensive care unit
Upper abdominal/thoracic surgery	Repeat intensive care unit admission
Low serum albumin	APACHE II score
Neuromuscular disease	Emergency surgery
	Nasotracheal tube
	Nasogastric tube
	Subglottic secretions

[a]Interventions were markers of severe underlying disease and included dopamine, dobutamine ≥5 μg/min, barbiturate therapy for increased intracranial pressure, and continuous intravenous antiarrhythmic or antihypertensive therapy.
KEY: APACHE, acute physiologic score and chronic health evaluation; ASA, American Society of Anesthesiology; COPD, chronic obstructive pulmonary disease; PEEP, positive end-expiratory pressure.
SOURCE: Adapted from Craven and Steger.

poor nutrition, neuromuscular disease, and endotracheal intubation. Intrinsic risk factors reported in the literature have included chronic lung disease, poor nutrition, and immunosuppression.

Hospital Factors

Management in an ICU has been reported as an important risk factor for the development of nosocomial pneumonia. Other important hospital factors are intracranial pressure monitoring, chest and abdominal surgery, large-volume gastric aspiration, reintubation, tracheostomy, prior antibiotic use, organ failure, and use of H_2-blocker therapy. Many studies have documented that the administration of antacids and H_2 blockers—used to prevent stress bleeding in critically ill ICU patients—has been associated with gastric bacterial overgrowth. Several studies and three metanalyses have demonstrated a lower rate of pneumonia in patients treated with sucralfate, a cytoprotective agent, than in those treated with antacids or H_2 blockers. In their review, Craven and Steger note that most current data using a clinical diagnosis of ventilator-associated pneumonia suggest that sucralfate provides similar protection against stress bleeding but poses a lower risk of nosocomial pneumonia. The use of a nasogastric tube is increasingly recognized as a risk factor for nosocomial pneumonia. Nasogastric tubes may increase the risk of nosocomial sinusitis, oropharyngeal colonization, reflux, and bacterial migration.

RISKS ASSOCIATED WITH RESPIRATORY DEVICES

Intubation with mechanical ventilation is the single most important risk factor for the development of nosocomial pneumonia. For this reason, intubation should be used only when medically necessary, and strict adherence to equipment maintenance is critical. Fluid-containing respiratory devices are the major environment-associated reservoirs for nosocomial pneumonia. However, most phases of respiratory support have been linked to nosocomial respiratory infections. These include mechanical ventilation bags, ventilators, aerosolized medications, bronchoscopy, suction catheters, and respiratory support personnel.

Flexible bronchoscopy has proved to be an invaluable diagnostic and therapeutic procedure. In general, the incidence of postprocedure fever or pneumonia has been reported to be less than 1 percent. However, the use of contaminated bronchoscopes has led to both pseudoepidemics and clinical infection. Pseudoepidemics with clusters of positive cultures of bronchoscopic washings have been linked to the use of contaminated bronchoscopes, contaminated tubing or suction devices, cocaine for topical use, and green dye added to the topical anesthetic. Microorganisms isolated in these cases included *Trichosporon cutaneum* and *Penicillium* species, *Pseudomonas aeruginosa, P. fluorescens-putida, Bacillus* species, *Mycobacterium* species, and *Rodotorula rubra.* Cross-transmission of respiratory pathogens has led to clinical infections with *M. tuberculosis, P. aeruginosa,* and *Serratia marcescens.* Factors leading to the use of contaminated bronchoscopes have included postdisinfection rinsing in tap water and disinfection with an iodophor, cetrimide-chlorhexidine, and 70% alcohol. Failure to sterilize damaged bronchoscopes or bronchoscope suction valves contaminated by *Mycobacteria* has been noted with both ethylene oxide and immersion in 2% glutaraldehyde for 30 min. Prevention of nosocomial infection related to contaminated bronchoscopes requires adherence to guidelines that delineate proper techniques of cleaning and disinfection of bronchoscopes.

MORTALITY

Nosocomial pneumonia is an important cause of mortality in hospitalized patients and contributes to 60 percent of all infection-related hospital deaths. ICU patients with nosocomial pneumonia have a 2- to 10-fold increased risk of mortality compared to patients without pneumonia. Independent risk

TABLE 61-2 Risk Factors for Mortality in Patients with Nosocomial Pneumonia

Aerobic gram-negative bacilli as pathogen(s), especially *P. aeruginosa*
Severity of underlying illness
Inappropriate antibiotic therapy
Advanced age
Shock
Bilateral infiltrates
Prior antibiotic therapy
Neoplastic disease
Duration of prior hospitalization
Supine head position in patients receiving mechanical ventilation

factors for mortality in nonventilated patients include infection with *P. aeruginosa,* bilateral infiltrates on chest radiography, and respiratory failure. The crude mortality for ventilator-associated nosocomial pneumonia has ranged from 13 to 70 percent, but most investigators have reported rates in the range of 20 to 40 percent. Many risk factors have been associated with mortality in ventilated patients (Table 61-2).

ETIOLOGIC AGENTS

The common etiologic agents of nosocomial pneumonia reported from the NNIS hospitals from 1990 to 1992 were *Staphylococcus aureus* (20 percent), *P. aeruginosa* (16 percent), *Enterobacter* species (11 percent), *Klebsiella pneumoniae* (7 percent), *Candida albicans* (5 percent), *Haemophilus influenzae* (4 percent), *Escherichia coli* (5 percent), *Acinetobacter* species (4 percent), and *S. marcescens* (3 percent) (Table 61-3). As a group, aerobic enteric gram-negative bacilli accounted for approximately one-third of all pathogens responsible for pneumonia. In ventilated patients, gram-negative bacilli have accounted for 58 to 83 percent of infections, gram-positive cocci for 14 to 38 percent, and anaerobes for only 1 to 3 percent. Polymicrobial infections were common. The importance of viral diseases—such as those due to cytomegalovirus, influenza, and respiratory syncytial virus—is unknown, but they have clearly been underreported.

The relevance of the NNIS data is called into question by reports that document the inability of clinical criteria to accurately identify cases of nosocomial pneumonia and the failure of expectorated sputum or tracheal aspirates to reliably identify pathogens in the distal areas of the lung (Table 61-4). Reports in which the diagnosis of pneumonia was made by an invasive procedure as well as more specific microbiologic criteria were used; the etiologic agents of pneumonia were *P. aeruginosa* (16 percent), *S. aureus* (20 percent), *Acinetobacter* species (14 percent), *H. influenzae* (10 percent), *S. pneumoniae* (4 percent), and other streptococci (4 percent). Enteric gram-negative bacilli (*E. coli, Enterobacter, Proteus, Serratia, Klebsiella,* and *Citrobacter*) accounted for only 13 percent of isolates. Thus, generalizing from NNIS data would overestimate the importance of enteric gram-negative bacilli and underestimate the importance of *Acinetobacter* species as causes of pneumonia in ventilated patients. The specific etiologic agents isolated in an individual institution will likely vary from these summary statistics depending

TABLE 61-3 Common Pathogens Currently Associated with Nosocomial Pneumonia

Pathogen	Frequency (%)[a]	Source of organism
Early-onset bacterial pneumonia		
S. pneumoniae	5–20	Endogenous; other patients
H. influenzae	<5–15	Respiratory droplet
Late-onset bacterial pneumonia		
Aerobic gram-negative bacilli	≥20–60	Endogenous; other patients, environment, enteral feeding; health care workers; equipment, devices
P. aeruginosa		
Enterobacter spp.		
Acinetobacter spp.		
K. pneumoniae		
S. marcescens		
E. coli		
Gram-positive cocci		
S. aureus	20–40	Endogenous; health-care workers; environment
Early- and late-onset pneumonia		
Anaerobic bacteria	0–35	Endogenous
Legionella spp.	0–10	Potable water; showers, faucets; cooling towers
M. tuberculosis	<1	Endogenous; other patients, staff
Viruses		
Influenza A and B	<1	Other patients, staff
Respiratory syncytial virus	<1	Other patients, staff; fomites
Fungi/protozoa		
Aspergillus spp.	<1	Air; construction
Candida spp.	<1	Endogenous; other patients, staff
P. carinii	<1	Endogenous; other patients (?)

[a]Crude rates of pneumonia may vary by hospital, patient population, and method of diagnosis.
SOURCE: Adapted from Craven and Steger.

on many factors, including patient demographics, patterns of antimicrobial use, environmental reservoirs for pathogens such as *Legionella* and *Aspergillus,* and the mix of host defects in the patient population.

DIAGNOSIS

Clinicians have traditionally relied on the presence of clinical findings (i.e., fever, cough, the development of purulent sputum, and evidence of consolidation on physical examination), radiographic evidence of new or progressing pulmonary infiltrate, and laboratory findings (Gram's stain of sputum and cultures of sputum, blood, tracheal aspirate, and pleural fluid). Many studies have demonstrated that clinical criteria with appropriate cultures of tracheal specimens may be sensitive for bacterial pathogens but are highly nonspecific, especially in intubated patients on mechanical

TABLE 61-4 Microorganisms Isolated from Respiratory Tract Specimens Obtained by Various Representative Methods from Adult Patients with a Diagnosis of Nosocomial Pneumonia

	Emori, 1993	Bartlett, 1991	Fagon, 1989	Torres, 1990
Hospital type	NNIS	Veterans	General	General
Patients studied				
Ventilated or nonventilated	Mixed	Mixed	Ventilated	Ventilated
Number	N/A	159	49	78
Number of episodes of pneumonia	N/A	159	52	78
Specimen culture	Sputum, tracheal aspirate	Transtracheal aspirate, blood, pleural fluid	Protected specimen brush	Protected specimen brush, lung aspirate, pleural fluid, blood
Culture results				
No organisms isolated	N/A	0	0	54%[a]
Polymicrobial	N/A	54%[a]	40%[a]	13%[a]
Number of isolates	8891	314	111	N/A
Aerobic bacteria				
Gram-negative bacilli	59%[b]	46%[c]	75%[c]	16%[d]
Pseudomonas aeruginosa	16%[b]	9%[c]	31%[c]	5%[d]
Enterobacter spp.	11%	4%	2%	0%
Klebsiella spp.	9	23	4	0
Escherichia coli	4	14	8	0
Serratia spp.	3	0	0	1
Proteus spp.	2	11	15	1
Citrobacter spp.	1	0	2	0
Acinetobacter calcoaceticus	4	0	15	9
Others	5	0	10	0
Haemophilus influenzae	5	17%[c]	10%[c]	0%[d]
Legionella spp.	N/A	N/A	2%[c]	2%[d]
Gram-positive cocci	26%[b]	56%[c]	52%[c]	4%[d]
Staphylococcus aureus	20%[b]	25%[c]	33%[c]	2%[d]
Streptococcus spp.	2	31	21	2
Others	4	0	8	0
Anaerobes	0	35%[c]	2%[c]	0
Peptostreptococcus	N/A	14%[c]	N/A	0
Fusobacterium spp.	N/A	10	N/A	0
Peptococcus spp.	N/A	11	N/A	0
Bacteroides melaninogenicus	N/A	9	N/A	0
B. fragilis	0	8	N/A	0
Fungi	7%[b]	N/A	0	1%[d]
Aspergillus spp.	N/A	N/A	0	1%[d]
Candida spp.	6%[b]	N/A	0	0
Viruses	1	N/A	N/A	N/A

[a]Percent episodes.
[b]Percent isolates.
[c]Percent episodes (percentages not additive owing to polymicrobial origin in some episodes).
[d]Percent patients with pure cultures.
KEY: NNIS, National Nosocomial Infection Surveillance System; N/A, not applicable: not tested or reported.
SOURCE: Adapted from Tablan et al.

ventilation. Blood cultures have been reported to yield the etiologic pathogen in approximately 10 to 20 percent of patients with nosocomial pneumonia. Among patients with severe nosocomial pneumonia, however, an additional source of infection has been present in up to 50 percent of those with positive blood cultures.

Several new techniques are now available for diagnosing nosocomial pneumonia or providing specimens for culture, including quantitative cultures of bronchoalveolar lavage (BAL) and quantitative culture of protected specimen brushing (PSB). The reported sensitivity and specificity of these methods have ranged from 70 to 100 percent and 60 to 100 percent, respectively. In the absence of a "gold standard," however, the sensitivity and specificity of these measures cannot be definitely determined. False-positive results using PSB have been attributed to prior antibiotic therapy or bacterial colonization of the lower airway. False-negative results may also occur in significant numbers. Invasive procedures used to diagnose pneumonia may lead to clinically important complications, including hypoxemia, bleeding, and arrhythmia.

A definitive algorithm cannot be provided for the diagnosis of nosocomial pneumonia. However, the following approach to nosocomial pneumonia is suggested (Table 61-5). Patients with suspected nosocomial pneumonia should undergo a careful history and physical examination to define the severity of pneumonia. An arterial blood gas or pulse oximetry should be performed both to aid in defining the severity of infection and to determine the need for supplemental oxygen. Mechanical ventilation should be considered for patients with hypoxia not correctable by supplemental oxygenation, hypercapnia, or inability to protect their airway. If the patient is suspected to have a communicable disease transmitted by the droplet or airborne route (e.g., respiratory syncytial virus, tuberculosis, influenza), appropriate respiratory precautions (droplet precautions or airborne precautions; see below) should be instituted. All patients should undergo chest radiography and have two sets of blood cultures done. The chest radiograph will aid in identifying the presence of pneumonia, the extent and location of infiltrates, and the presence of a pleural effusion. The radiographic appearance may provide clues to the cause of the respiratory failure. Other laboratory studies (complete blood count, electrolytes, liver function tests, tests of renal function, etc.) may be useful in patient management.

TABLE 61-5 Evaluation of Patients with Suspected Nosocomial Pneumonia

Routine Evaluation
 History
  Recent exposure to possible pulmonary infectious agents (e.g., influenza, tuberculosis)
  Travel
  Occupational exposures
  Animal exposure
  Immunocompromising conditions (e.g., steroids, risk factors for HIV)
 Physical evaluation
 Chest radiograph
  Measure of oxygen saturation (arterial blood gas or pulse oximetry)
 Obtain expectorated sputum in nonventilated patients and a tracheal aspirate in patients who have been intubated or have a tracheostomy. Send the specimen for Gram's stain and bacterial cultures. Consider additional diagnostic tests, depending on the clinical findings and epidemiologic

TABLE 61-5 (continued)

circumstances: viral culture, direct antigen testing for respiratory syncytial virus, *Legionella* DFA and culture, smear and culture for *Mycobacterium,* smear and culture for fungi, stain for *Pneumocystis carinii*

Evaluation to Exclude Extrapulmonary Sources of Infections
  Routine evaluation
    Blood cultures from two different sites
    Urine analysis and culture
    Examination of wounds if present
  Additional tests directed by history, physical examination, and laboratory findings

Consider removal of central and arterial vascular catheters, with semiquantitative culture of the subcutaneous portion and tip of the catheter in patients with positive blood cultures and/or evidence of sepsis

Consider lumbar puncture following head CT or MRI in patients at high risk (e.g., after neurosurgery) or with unexplained change in mental status

Consider radiographic imaging of the abdomen (CT or MRI) in patients with rigid abdomen, ileus, or localized or diffuse tenderness or at high risk for abdominal sepsis (i.e., after abdominal surgery, with pancreatitis, gastrointestinal bleeding, or carcinoma, or receiving high-dose corticosteroids)

Consider abdominal ultrasound in patients with right-upper-quadrant tenderness or abnormal liver function tests, or who are too unstable for transfer to CT

Obtain stools for *Clostridium difficile* toxin assay in patients with more than two watery stools per day. If fever persists without a discernible cause, consider CT scan of sinuses to exclude sinusitis, with aspiration of the maxillary sinus in patients with air–fluid levels or opacification, and/or consider nucleotide scan (gallium-67 scintigraphy, tagged white cell scan)

Additional Pulmonary Evaluation

If pleural effusion is suspected, obtain decubitus films, ultrasound, or CT. If pleural effusion is present, consider diagnostic thoracocentesis

Consider need to exclude thromboembolic disease: impedance plethysmography or Doppler ultrasound evaluation of the lower extremities; ventilation/perfusion scan of the lung; pulmonary arteriogram

Consider need for invasive diagnosis in patients with rapidly progressive pneumonia, severe pneumonia in intubated patients on mechanical ventilation, immunocompromised patients, and patients who have failed to respond to empiric therapy or have progressed on empiric therapy: bronchoscopy with protected specimen brush and bronchoalveolar lavage or protected bronchoalveolar lavage
  Evaluation to rule out atelectasis
    Inhalation of bronchodilators every 2 h for four treatments, then every 4 h
    Percussion or vibration over the area of the chest with new densities on chest radiography
    Repeat chest radiograph in 48 h

Consider Other Sources of Fever
  Incorrect antibiotic administration: incorrect dose, route, frequency
  Drug fever
  Noninfectious source of fever and pulmonary infiltrate (e.g., aspiration, hemorrhage)
  Foreign body
  Superinfection
  Overgrowth
  Development of drug-resistant pathogen

SOURCE: Adapted from Meduri.

When a pleural effusion is present, consideration should be given to obtaining a diagnostic thoracentesis, especially if the patient is toxic or a large effusion (greater than 10 mm on a lateral decubitus film) is present. The pleural fluid should be sent for complete blood cell count and differential, protein, glucose, LDH, pH, Gram's stain, and aerobic and anaerobic bacterial cultures. Consideration should also be given to fungal and mycobacterial stains and appropriate fungal and mycobacterial cultures.

In nonintubated patients, an expectorated sputum should be obtained for Gram's stain and bacterial culture. Epidemiologic or clinical findings should be reviewed, and consideration should be given to obtaining appropriate stains and cultures for viruses, fungi, mycobacteria, *Legionella,* and *P. carinii.* It is important, however, to remember that *expectorated sputum is neither sensitive nor specific for the diagnosis of nosocomial pneumonia.* Its major value is to identify the antibiotic susceptibilities of the organisms present and thereby aid in the proper choice of therapy.

In intubated patients, a tracheal aspirate should be obtained. The Gram's stain may reveal a predominant pathogen. The culture has been shown to have both poor sensitivity and specificity in identifying the etiologic agents of nosocomial pneumonia. Cultures obtained by tracheal aspiration may be of most use in excluding certain potential pathogens (e.g., methicillin-resistant *S. aureus*) and providing information about the antimicrobial susceptibility spectrum of isolated pathogens.

Consideration should be given to performing an invasive procedure to better assess the diagnosis of pneumonia and potential pathogens in the following circumstances: an immunocompromised patient with a broad range of potential pathogens (e.g., heart- or lung-transplant patient), a critically ill patient with severe hospital-acquired pneumonia (see below), and a patient whose condition does not improve with empiric antimicrobial therapy.

Clinicians should always consider other potential causes of fever and pulmonary infiltrate in the hospitalized patient—including atelectasis, acute radiation pneumonitis, large-volume gastric aspiration, pulmonary embolus with infarction, lung contusion (in trauma patients), pulmonary hemorrhage, and acute respiratory distress syndrome with diffuse alveolar damage.

THERAPY

General Considerations

Despite the development of broad-spectrum antibiotic agents, nosocomial pneumonia continues to carry an unacceptably high mortality. Initial empiric therapy of presumed nosocomial pneumonia may be guided by an assessment of disease severity, the presence of risk factors for specific organisms, and time of onset of nosocomial pneumonia (Fig. 61-2; Tables 61-6 to 61-8). The choice of a specific agent will depend on several factors. The first is the spectrum of antimicrobial susceptibility of respiratory pathogens causing nosocomial pneumonia at one's health care facility. It is important for all health care facilities to periodically review the pathogens causing nosocomial pneumonia and their susceptibility patterns and disseminate this information to clinicians. Second, a history of allergic reactions to antimicrobials should be obtained from all patients. Because of the possibility of cross-reactivity between beta-lactam antibiotics, the use of a cephalosporin in a penicillin-allergic patient should be considered only if the benefit exceeds the risk. Third, antimicrobial therapy should be chosen to minimize drug interactions. Fourth, in patients

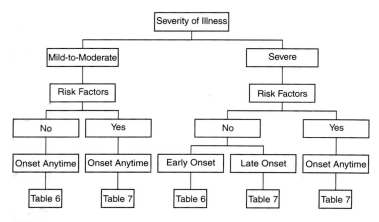

FIG. 61-2 Algorithm for classifying patients with nosocomial pneumonia. Specific drugs and doses, recommended in Tables 61-6, 61-7, and 61-8 are adapted from the American Thoracic Society Consensus Statement and represent the views of the authors. Doses provided are for an adult of average weight and normal renal and hepatic function. Doses may need to be adjusted depending on the patient's weight, age, renal function, hepatic function, use of interacting agents, and other factors. Physicians should be thoroughly familiar with the guidelines in individual drug manufacturers' inserts regarding dosing, drug interaction, contraindications, precautions, and administration.

with renal or hepatic dysfunction, specific drugs may be chosen to minimize the need for dose adjustment. Fifth, potential drug toxicities may provide relative contraindications to use in specific patients (e.g., avoidance of aminoglycosides in patients with neuromuscular disorders or avoidance of aminoglycosides in patients predisposed to renal dysfunction). Sixth, intrinsic patient factors—including age, pregnancy, and breast-feeding—may limit the choice

TABLE 61-6 Patients with Mild to Moderate Nosocomial Pneumonia, No Unusual Risk Factors, Onset Anytime, or Patients with Severe Nosocomial Pneumonia with Early Onset[a,b]

Core organisms	Core antibiotics
Enteric gram-negative bacilli (non-*Pseudomonas*) *Enterobacter* spp. *Escherichia coli* *Klebsiella* spp. *Proteus* spp. *Serratia marcescens* *Haemophilus influenzae* Methicillin-sensitive *S. aureus* *Streptococcus pneumoniae*	Piperacillin-tazobactam 3.375 g IV q 4 h *or* Piperacillin-tazobactam[c] 4.5 g IV q 6 h *or* Cefotaxime 1–2 g IV q 8 h *or* Ceftriaxone 1 g IV q 12 h *or* if allergic to penicillins/cephalosporins Clindamycin *or* vancomycin *plus* Ciprofloxacin IV *or* aztreonam

[a]Excludes patients with immunosuppression.
[b]Early-onset pneumonia, ≤4 days after hospitalization.
[c]Not an FDA-approved indication or dose.
SOURCE: Adapted from the American Thoracic Society.

TABLE 61-7 Patients with Mild to Moderate Nosocomial Pneumonia with Risk Factors, Onset Anytime[a]

Core organisms plus:	Core antibiotics plus:
Anaerobes (recent abdominal surgery, witnessed aspiration)	Clindamycin 600 mg IV q 8 h *or* Piperacillin-tazobactam 3.375 g IV q 4 h (alone)
Staphylococcus aureus (coma, head trauma, diabetes mellitus, renal failure)	+/− Vancomycin (until methicillin-resistant *S. aureus* excluded)
Legionella spp.	Erythromycin 1 g IV q 6 h +/− rifampin[b]
P. aeruginosa (prolonged ICU stay, steroids, antibiotics, structural lung disease)	Treat as severe nosocomial pneumonia (Table 61-4)

[a]Excludes patients with immunosuppression.
[b]Rifampin may be added if *Legionella* spp. are documented.
SOURCE: Adapted from the American Thoracic Society.

of antibiotics. Finally, if several equally efficacious and safe choices exist, the least costly regimen should be instituted.

The mechanism of bacterial action may be relevant in antibiotic selection and dosing. In general, bactericidal rather than bacteriostatic antibiotics are preferred. Beta-lactam antibiotics (penicillins, cephalosporins, carbapenems, monobactams) and vancomycin are bactericidal in a time-dependent fashion. Fluoroquinolones and aminoglycosides, which are bactericidal in a concentration-dependent fashion, exhibit killing more rapidly at high concentrations. In general, bactericidal antibiotics exhibit a prolonged postantibiotic effect in which bacterial replication is suppressed for a period after

TABLE 61-8 Patients with Severe Nosocomial Pneumonia with Risk Factors, Early Onset, or Patients with Severe Nosocomial Pneumonia, Late Onset[a,b]

Core organisms plus:	Therapy
P. aeruginosa	Aminoglycoside (gentamicin, tobramycin, amikacin)[c] *or*
Acinetobacter spp.	Ciprofloxacin 400 mg IV q 12 h *plus* one of the following:
Consider methicillin-resistant *S. aureus*	Piperacillin-tazobactam 3.375 g IV q 4 h *or* Piperacillin-tazobactam[d] 4.5 g IV q 6 h *or* Imipenem 500 mg IV q 6 h *or* Meropenem[d] 1.0 g IV q 8 h *or* Ceftazidime 2.0 g IV q 8 h *or* Cefepime 1–2 g IV q 12 h *or* Cefpirome[e] 2.0 g q 12 h +/− Vancomycin 1 g IV q 12 h

[a]Excludes patients with immunosuppression.
[b]Late-onset pneumonia, ≥5 days after hospitalization.
[c]Consider single daily dosing.
[d]Not an FDA-approved indication or dose.
[e]Not an FDA-approved drug.
SOURCE: Adapted from the American Thoracic Society.

antibiotic levels have fallen below inhibitory concentrations. These pharmacologic features may lead to specific dosing recommendations such as the use of single daily dosing of aminoglycosides.

A controversial area in the treatment of respiratory infections is the importance of antibiotic penetration into lung tissue. It remains unclear whether concentrations in bronchial secretions or in epithelial lining fluid are relevant for predicting efficacy in patients with pneumonia. Also controversial is the role, if any, of inhaled antibiotics in seriously ill patients with nosocomial pneumonia.

Specific Regimens

Initial empiric therapy for nosocomial pneumonia may be guided by severity, presence or absence of risk factors for specific pathogens, and length of hospital stay before the development of nosocomial pneumonia (Tables 61-6 to 61-8). In the absence of specific risk factors, the most common pathogens of early-onset nosocomial pneumonia are *S. pneumoniae, H. influenzae,* enteric gram-negative bacilli (*E. coli, Enterobacter* species, *Klebsiella* species, *Proteus* species, *S. marcescens*), and *S. aureus.* For these patients, a nonpseudomonal third-generation cephalosporin or beta-lactam–beta-lactamase inhibitor combination should be adequate.

In the presence of special risk factors, initiation of broader coverage may be warranted. Anaerobic bacteria are frequently isolated from the respiratory tracts of patients with witnessed gastric aspiration, recent thoracoabdominal surgery, or the presence of an obstructing foreign body in the airway. The significance of these anaerobes is unclear, however, since the aerobic bacteria are generally more pathogenic. Nevertheless, patients with witnessed gastric aspiration should be treated with a broad-spectrum agent with anaerobic coverage (e.g., piperacillin-tazobactam, imipenem, meropenem) or have a specific anaerobic agent added (e.g., clindamycin). Prolonged hospitalization, prior antibiotic therapy, and mechanical ventilation in an ICU increase the likelihood of infection with more resistant bacteria, including methicillin-resistant *S. aureus, P. aeruginosa, Enterobacter* species, and *Acinetobacter* species. In such patients, initial empiric therapy should include broad coverage.

The American Thoracic Society has provided a definition of severe hospital-acquired pneumonia (Table 61-9). Although few studies have evaluated severe

---

TABLE 61-9 Definitions of Severe Nosocomial Pneumonia

Admission to the intensive care unit
Respiratory failure, defined as the need for mechanical ventilation or the need for >35% oxygen to maintain an arterial saturation >90%
Rapid radiographic progression, multilobar pneumonia, or cavitation of a lung infiltrate
Evidence of severe sepsis with hypotension and/or end-organ dysfunction:
　Shock (systolic blood pressure <90 mmHg or diastolic blood pressure <60 mmHg)
　Requirement for vasopressors for more than 4 h
　Urine output <20 mL/h or total urine output <80 mL in 4 h (unless another explanation is available)
　Acute renal failure requiring dialysis

SOURCE: Adapted from the American Thoracic Society.

nosocomial pneumonia, it is reasonable to initiate very broad empiric antibiotic coverage in patients meeting this definition. As with mild to moderate nosocomial pneumonia, additional antibiotics will be necessary to treat methicillin-resistant *S. aureus* and *Legionella* species.

Immunocompromised Patients

The above guidelines were not designed to provide recommendations for the treatment of immunocompromised patients. The presentation and etiology of respiratory infection in immunocompromised patients depend on several factors: (1) the nature of specific host defense abnormalities, (2) the duration of immunosuppressing conditions, (3) the presence or absence of latent infections (e.g., cytomegalovirus), and (4) epidemiologic exposures. The patient's overall susceptibility to infection will reflect the net sum of all factors that alter host defenses, including underlying medical conditions, immunosuppressive therapy, and hospital-related interventions (e.g., indwelling lines).

PREVENTION

General Preventive Interventions

Prevention of nosocomial pneumonia begins with strict adherence to standard infection control guidelines (Table 61-10). Among the most important infection control guidelines are proper handwashing, institution of isolation precautions, and proper disinfection and sterilization of equipment. Patients with potentially communicable diseases should be rapidly evaluated and placed on

---

TABLE 61-10 General Methods to Reduce the Frequency of Nosocomial Pneumonia in Mechanically Ventilated Patients

General Methods
  Aggressive treatment of patient's underlying disease
  Review need and avoid antacids + histamine$_2$ blockers for stress ulcer prophylaxis
  Keep patient elevated at $\geq$30 degrees
  Review nutrition regimen and tube feeding procedures
  Extubate and remove nasogastric tube as clinically indicated
  Controlled use of antibiotics
Respiratory Care Equipment
  Discriminate between equipment with nebulizers and humidifiers
  $\geq$48-h circuit changes (tubing and humidifier) for mechanical ventilators with humidifiers; no changes for circuits with heat-moisture exchangers
  Proper removal of tubing condensate and education of staff to prevent washing contaminated condensate into the patient's trachea
  No transfer of equipment or devices between patients
  Review use and care of in-line medication nebulizers
Infection Control
  Surveillance in the ICU
  Education and awareness programs on nosocomial infection
  Handwashing and/or barrier precautions
  Review technique for suctioning patients; type of catheter used
  Review method of condensate disposal
  Use effective methods of disinfection of devices and equipment

SOURCE: Adapted from Craven and Steger.

appropriate isolation precautions. "Standard precautions" synthesize the major features of universal precautions (blood and body fluid precautions) and body substance isolation and apply them to all patients receiving care in hospitals, regardless of their diagnosis or presumed infection status. Standard precautions apply to blood; all body fluids, secretions, and excretions except sweat, regardless of whether or not they contain visible blood; nonintact skin; and mucous membranes. Standard precautions are designed to reduce the risk of transmission of microorganisms from both recognized and unrecognized sources of infection in hospitals.

Standard precautions include handwashing before and after patient contact, whether or not gloves are worn; wearing gloves when touching blood, body fluids, secretions or excretions, and contaminated items; wearing a mask and eye protection or a face shield during procedures and patient care activities that are likely to generate splashes or sprays of blood, body fluids, secretions, or excretions (e.g., bronchoscopy, arterial line placement); and wearing a gown during procedures and patient care activities that are likely to generate splashes or sprays of blood, body fluids, secretions, or excretions.

Airborne precautions are used for patients with a communicable disease transmitted by the airborne route, such as tuberculosis, varicella-zoster virus infections (with the exception of dermatomal zoster in the nonimmunocompromised host), and measles. Patients with these diseases should be placed in rooms with the following air-handling characteristics: private room, room at negative pressure with respect to the corridor, air directly exhausted to the outside or monitored high-efficiency filtration before the air is circulated to other areas of the hospital, and 6 to 12 air exchanges per hour. Personnel caring for patients with known or suspected tuberculosis should don an N-95 respirator before entering into the room. Droplet precautions are used for patients with diseases transmitted by the droplet route, such as pertussis, meningococcal pneumonia, pharyngeal diphtheria, rubella, measles, *H. influenzae* epiglottitis, mycoplasmal pneumonia, and group A streptococcal infections (in infants and young children). Droplet precautions consist of private room and limiting patient transport. Personnel should don surgical masks when working within 3 ft of the patient. Contact precautions are used for patients infected or colonized by direct contact, transient colonization of the hands of caregivers, or contamination of an inanimate object such as a medical instrument. Diseases requiring contact precautions include varicella-zoster infection, *C. difficile* infection, rotavirus, shigellosis, herpes simplex, methicillin-resistant *S. aureus,* and infection by multidrug–resistant pathogens.

Many reports attest to the ability of contaminated bronchoscopes to transmit pathogens leading to outbreaks or pseudo-outbreaks. For this reason, all endoscopic equipment should be rigorously cleaned immediately after use and then appropriately disinfected or sterilized.

Selective Decontamination with Antibiotics

In recent years, many studies have tried to determine whether selective decontamination of the digestive tract (SDD) is associated with a decreased incidence of nosocomial pneumonia. The SDD regimens have usually included a combination of nonabsorbable local antibiotics (e.g., an aminoglycoside, polymyxin B, and amphotericin) and intravenously administered drugs (e.g., cefotaxime, trimethoprim, or a quinolone). The local antibiotics have been applied as a paste in the oropharynx, and often also provided orally or through the nasogastric tube.

Craven and Steger recently summarized all trials employing SDD to prevent lower respiratory tract infection. They noted that despite several favorable reports, *two large double-blind, placebo-controlled trials did not demonstrate that SDD was beneficial.* Concerns have been expressed that the use of SDD may lead to the emergence of antibiotic-resistant pathogens and the lack of effect on the duration of mechanical ventilation or hospital stay and cost-effectiveness. For these reasons, many experts and the CDC do not support the routine use of SDD for all medical and surgical ICU patients.

Infection Control Guidelines to Prevent Nosocomial Pneumonia

Measures to prevent nosocomial pneumonia are based on an understanding of the risk factors associated with pneumonia (Table 61-11). Despite the use of these guidelines, however, the frequency of nosocomial pneumonia and subsequent morbidity is unacceptably high. Additional research to validate current preventive practices and innovative strategies to further reduce nosocomial pneumonia are sorely needed.

GRAM-NEGATIVE PNEUMONIA

Gram-negative pneumonias may be divided into several groups: community-acquired pathogens *(H. influenzae, Klebsiella, Bordetella pertussis),* hospital-acquired pathogens (enteric gram-negative rods, especially *E. coli, Enterobacter, Proteus,* and *Serratia*), and zoonotic pathogens *(Francisella tularensis, Yersinia pestis,* and *P. multocida).* The separation of gram-negative pathogens into community-acquired and hospital-acquired groups is only relative, as any of these pathogens may cause pneumonia in either setting. A large number of bacterial pathogens are gram-negative. Only the clinically most important species are discussed below.

Common Community-Acquired Pneumonias

Haemophilus influenzae

Microbiology and Epidemiology *H. influenzae* is a small, nonmotile, non–spore-forming bacillus that is often part of the normal flora of the human respiratory tree. Aerobic growth requires two supplements, called X and V factor. Because of these growth requirements *H. influenzae* must be cultured on chocolate agar or around a streak of *S. aureus* (a source of V factor) on a blood agar plate. In the latter method, *H. influenzae* will revolve around the *S. aureus* streak—a finding that allows presumptive identification.

H. influenzae is found only in humans; no animal or environmental reservoirs exist. At any given time, up to 80 percent of the population carries the organism. Most adults are colonized with nonencapsulated strains, but in 3 to 5 percent the isolates have a capsule (usually type b). Nonencapsulated strains are principally associated with chronic bronchitis, otitis media, sinusitis, and conjunctivitis. Encapsulated strains more commonly cause epiglottitis, meningitis, pneumonia and empyema, and bone and joint infections.

Transmission between people is via the large-droplet route or by direct contact. With the widespread use of *H. influenzae* vaccine, the incidence of invasive disease has dropped dramatically.

TABLE 61-11 Infection Control Measures for Prevention of Nosocomial Pneumonia Depending on the Presence of Specific Risk Factors

Risk factor	Infection control measures suggested to prevent nosocomial pneumonia
Bacterial pneumonia	
Host-related: age >65 years	
Underlying illness:	
Chronic obstructive pulmonary disease	Perform incentive spirometry, positive end-expiratory pressure, or continuous positive airway pressure by face mask.
Immunosuppression	Avoid exposure to potential nosocomial pathogens; decrease duration of immunosuppression, such as by granulocyte-macrophage colony–stimulating factor (GM-CSF).
Depressed consciousness	Administer CNS depressants cautiously.
Surgery (abdominal/thoracic)	Properly position patient; promote early ambulation; appropriately control pain.
Device-related	Properly clean, sterilize or disinfect, and handle devices; remove devices as soon as the indication for their use ceases.
Endotracheal intubation and mechanical ventilation	Gently suction secretions; place patient in semirecumbent position (30 to 45 degrees head elevation); use nonalkalinizing gastric cytoprotective agent on patients at risk for stress bleeding; do not routinely change ventilation circuits more often than every 48 h; drain and discard inspiratory tubing condensate, or use heat-moisture exchanger if indicated.
Nasogastric tube (NGT) placement and enteral feeding	Routinely verify appropriate tube placement; promptly remove NGT when no longer needed; drain residual; place patient in semirecumbent position as described above.
Personnel or procedure related	
Cross-contamination by hands	Educate and train personnel; wash hands adequately and wear gloves appropriately; conduct surveillance for cases of pneumonia, and give feedback to personnel.
Antibiotic administration	Use antibiotics prudently, especially on high-risk intensive care patients.
Legionnaires' disease	
Host-related	
Immunosuppression	Decrease duration of immunosuppression.
Device-related	
Contaminated aerosol from devices	Sterilize or disinfect aerosol-producing devices before use; use only sterile water for respiratory humidifying devices; do not use cool-mist room-air "humidifiers" without adequate sterilization or disinfection.
Environment-related	
Aerosols from contaminated water supply	Hyperchlorinate or superheat hospital water system; routinely maintain water supply; consider use of sterile water for drinking by immunocompromised patients.

TABLE 61-11 (continued)

Risk factor	Infection control measures suggested to prevent nosocomial pneumonia
Cooling-tower draft	Properly design, place, and maintain cooling towers.
Aspergillosis Host-related Severe granulocytopenia	Decrease duration of immunosuppression, such as by administration of GM-CSF; place patients with severe and prolonged granulocytopenia in protected environment.
Environment-related Construction activity	Remove granulocytopenic patients from vicinity of construction; if not already done, place severe granulocytopenic patients in protected environment; make severely granulocytopenic patients wear a mask when they leave their protected environment.
Other environmental sources of *Aspergillus*	Routinely maintain air-handling system and rooms of immunocompromised patients.
Respiratory Syncytial Virus Infection Host-related Age <2 years; congenital pulmonary/cardiac disease, immunosuppression	Consider routine readmission screening of patients at high risk for severe RSV infection, followed by cohorting of patients and nursing personnel during hospital outbreaks of RSV infection; consider prophylactic administration of RSV immunoglobulin (hyperimmune preparation).
Personnel or procedure related Cross-contamination by hands	Educate personnel; wash hands, wear gloves; wear a gown; during outbreaks, use private rooms or cohort patients and nursing personnel, and limit visitors.
Influenza Host-related Age >65 years; immunosuppression	Vaccinate high-risk patients before the influenza season each year; use amantadine or rimantadine for chemoprophylaxis during an outbreak.
Personnel-related Infected personnel	Before the influenza season each year, vaccinate personnel caring for high-risk patients; use amantadine or rimantadine for prophylaxis during an outbreak.

SOURCE: Adapted from Tablan.

Clinical Features and Diagnosis *H. influenzae* type b is an unusual cause of pneumonia in children between 4 months and 4 years of age. The clinical findings are similar to those of bacterial pneumonia due to *S. aureus* or *S. pneumoniae* except that the onset is more often insidious. Primary pneumonia in children is frequently associated with evidence of infection at other sites, including meningitis, epiglottitis, and bone and joint infection.

In adults, pneumonia may also be caused by nonencapsulated strains. Overall, *H. influenzae* is responsible for approximately 10 to 15 percent of adult pneumonias requiring hospital admission. Risk factors include alcoholism, underlying lung disease, and older age.

The onset of symptoms is generally abrupt. Common symptoms consist of fever, shaking chills, cough productive of purulent sputum, dyspnea, and pleuritic pain. Physical examination usually reveals acute illness with fever, tachypnea, lower lobe rales, and consolidation. Irrespective of age, the chest radiograph usually reveals a segmented, lobar, bronchopneumonic, or interstitial pattern. Pleural effusions are common, but empyema is rare.

Diagnosis is made from smear and culture on chocolate media. Sputum cultures are positive in about 70 percent of cases and blood cultures in 20 percent.

Treatment and Prevention *H. influenzae* strains increasingly produce beta-lactamase and therefore exhibit resistance to penicillin or ampicillin. The most active drugs include third-generation cephalosporins (cefotaxime, ceftriaxone) and combinations of penicillins with a beta-lactamase inhibitor (piperacillin-tazobactam, ampicillin-sulbactam, amoxicillin-clavulanate). Most strains are susceptible to trimethoprim-sulfamethoxazole, second-generation cephalosporins, and quinolones. The newer macrolides, azithromycin and clarithromycin, may also be used to provide oral therapy. Most patients respond to therapy within 24 h.

All children should be immunized according to current recommendations of the Advisory Committee on Immunization Practices and the American Academy of Pediatrics "Red Book" against *H. influenzae* type b.

Moraxella catarrhalis

Microbiology and Epidemiology *Moraxella catarrhalis* is a nonmotile, strictly aerobic, oxidase-positive gram-negative bacillus. The organism is part of the normal flora of the upper respiratory tract. *M. catarrhalis* may cause otitis media, sinusitis, bronchitis, and pneumonia.

Clinical Features and Diagnosis *M. catarrhalis* may cause pneumonia indistinguishable from that caused by *H. influenzae.* Sepsis is unusual.

Treatment and Prevention *M. catarrhalis* strains often produce beta-lactamases. The organism's susceptibility profile is similar to that of *H. influenzae.*

Bordetella pertussis

Microbiology and Epidemiology *Bordetella pertussis* is the causative agent of pertussis or whooping cough. The *Bordetella* organisms are tiny (0.2 to 0.5 by 0.5 to 2.0 μm) coccobacillary organisms that appear singly or in pairs and often have a bipolar appearance. The organism is a strict aerobe that exhibits optimal growth at 35°C. *B. pertussis* produces a number of biologically active substances that may play a role in disease, including filamentous hemagglutinin, adenylate cyclase toxin, dermonecrotic toxin, pertussis toxin, tracheal cytotoxin, and alpha-hemolysin. Occasionally, *B. parapertussis* and *B. bronchiseptica* may produce a clinical illness similar to that caused by *B. pertussis.*

More than 4500 cases of pertussis were reported to the CDC in 1994. However, CDC surveillance may detect as few as 10 percent of cases. Pertussis incidence is usually characterized by a cyclic pattern, with peaks occurring at 3- to 4-year intervals. The current levels of pertussis are considerably higher than levels reported between 1976 and 1980. Reasons for the resurgence of pertussis are unclear, but according to the CDC, the higher levels reported in recent years are not related to a decrease in vaccine coverage (about 70 percent for children aged 2) or to a substantive reduction in efficacy of diphtheria, pertussis, tetanus (DPT) vaccine.

Adolescents and young adults play an important role in transmitting pertussis to susceptible infants because immunization-induced immunity to pertussis wanes with increasing age. Furthermore, because booster immunizations are not given after the age of 6, immunity in adults is boosted only through inadvertent exposure to the organism. It has been estimated that approximately 50 million adults in the United States are susceptible to pertussis, and this number will continue to increase. Adults and adolescents are also an important vector in the transmission of pertussis to children because pertussis in adults is mild or "atypical" and frequently not diagnosed.

Humans are the only reservoir of *B. pertussis.* Transmission occurs by close contact via large aerosol droplets from the respiratory tract of symptomatic persons. Fomites play no role in transmission. The attack rate among immunized household contacts of children with pertussis may exceed 80 percent.

Clinical Features and Diagnosis The incubation period for pertussis ranges from less than 1 week to more than 3 weeks (average, 7 to 10 days). Classically, the early phase (catarrhal) is characterized by rhinorrhea, lacrimation, mild conjunctival injection, malaise, and low-grade fever. The later phase (paroxysmal) is characterized by cough paroxysms (the "whoop"), especially in children. Patients often exhibit leukolymphocytosis, and pulmonary consolidation may occur.

Pertussis in adults is characterized most commonly by upper respiratory tract symptoms or prolonged cough. Classic disease, including the whoop, can occur; however, 20 percent of infected adults may remain asymptomatic. Because the signs and symptoms in adults usually are nonspecific, pertussis is rarely considered in adults until a child contact develops classic disease.

Pertussis may be diagnosed with culture, direct fluorescent antibody (DFA) techniques performed on smears, serology, and polymerase chain reaction. Cultures must be obtained by the nasopharyngeal method and plated on either Bordet-Gengou or Regan-Lowe (preferred because of longer shelf life). Detection often requires 3 to 6 days of growth. Although culture is the "gold standard" method, newer serologic methods have demonstrated that culture is not a sensitive method of diagnosis. In addition, the ability to isolate *B. pertussis* in culture declines significantly when patients reach the paroxysmal phase of disease. Unfortunately, the currently available DFA lacks sensitivity and is subject to interobserver variability. Newer serologic tests are highly sensitive and specific, but are generally not clinically available.

Treatment and Prevention *B. pertussis* continues to be highly susceptible in vitro to erythromycin, although there have been several isolated reports of erythromycin-resistant strains. Chloramphenicol, ampicillin, and oxytetracycline have moderate activity. Most strains of *B. pertussis* are resistant to clindamycin, methicillin, and first- and second-generation cephalosporins. Erythromycin has been shown to decrease the duration of illness when administered early in the course of pertussis. Treatment of infected persons with erythromycin has been shown to eliminate pertussis organisms in a few days. For these reasons, erythromycin is the drug of choice for treatment and prophylaxis of pertussis. Some investigators prefer the use of the estolate preparation because it produces higher blood levels than the ethylsuccinate or stearate preparations. However, the use of a higher dose of erythromycin base (50 to 60 mg/kg a day) also has been reported to be effective. Treatment or prophylaxis requires a 14-day course of therapy. The newer macrolides, clarithromycin and azithromycin, are active in vitro against *B. pertussis.* Preliminary data from Japan suggest that they are clinically effective. However, they are not FDA approved for the prophylaxis or treatment of *B. pertussis.*

Immunization with DPT vaccine should be part of a routine childhood immunization program. Acellular pertussis vaccines are now FDA approved for use in children of all ages. As they demonstrate similar or improved efficacy and reduced toxicity, they should replace whole-cell pertussis vaccine.

Klebsiella

Microbiology and Epidemiology The family Enterobacteriaceae consists of a heterogeneous group of gram-negative bacteria, including *E. coli, Klebsiella, Shigella, Edwardsiella, Citrobacter, Enterobacter, Serratia, Hafnia, Proteus, Morganella, Providencia, Yersinia,* and *Erwinia.* Although many of these bacilli may cause pneumonia, *Klebsiella* is the most common enteric gram-negative rod that causes community-acquired pneumonia. However, it accounts for only about 1 to 5 percent of community-acquired pneumonias.

Although *Klebsiella* is a community-acquired pathogen, most patients who develop pneumonia have underlying medical ailments. Risk factors include alcoholism, chronic obstructive pulmonary disease, and diabetes mellitus.

Clinical Features and Diagnosis *K. pneumoniae* is an important cause of community-acquired lobar pneumonia. Classically, *Klebsiella* pneumonia has an acute onset and leads to a severe destructive lung infection. Symptoms include rigors (in about 60 percent of patients), high fever, productive cough, and pleuritic chest pain (in about 80 percent). The sputum has been described as "currant jelly" in quality. The classic radiographic picture is that of a swollen, infiltrated lobe. (This may produce the "bowed fissure" radiographic sign.) Complications are common and include abscess formation, cavitation, and empyema. Mortality is high because many patients have underlying illnesses and because of the destructive nature of the pneumonic process. *Klebsiella* may also cause less severe respiratory tract infections, such as bronchitis or bronchopneumonia.

A Gram's stain of the sputum may reveal short, plump, gram-negative bacilli. In many patients, however, the sputum is not revealing. Blood cultures are positive in up to 25 percent of patients. The mortality ranges from 20 to 50 percent in appropriately treated patients.

Treatment and Prevention *Klebsiella* strains are often sensitive to cephalosporins, the most active being the third- (ceftriaxone, cefotaxime) and fourth-generation cephalosporins (cefepime). Resistance due to expanded-spectrum beta-lactamases is an increasing problem, most notably in nosocomial cases. Therapy should be based on susceptibility testing. Other drugs with potential are piperacillin-tazobactam, carbapenems (imipenem, meropenem), and quinolones. No vaccine is currently available.

Unusual Community-Acquired Pneumonias (see also Appendix)

Tularemia

Microbiology and Epidemiology The etiologic agent of tularemia ("rabbit-skinner's disease") is *Francisella tularensis,* a small, gram-negative, nonmotile coccobacillus. Tularemia is a vector-borne disease. The tick vectors in the United States include *Amblyomma americanum* in the southeastern and south central states, *Dermacentor andersoni* in the West, and *D. variabilis,* which has the widest distribution of the three tick vectors. Tularemia may also be transmitted by the bite of the deerfly, *Chrysops discalis.* The reservoirs of *F. tularensis* include numerous small animals—especially rabbits, hares, muskrats, and beavers—and some domestic animals, as well as various hard ticks.

Approximately 100 cases of tularemia were reported to the CDC in 1994. The disease is widespread throughout the United States, but the greatest number of cases have been reported from Arkansas, Missouri, and Oklahoma. Cases occur in all months of the year; the incidence may be higher in adults in early winter during rabbit-hunting season and in children during summer, when ticks and deerflies are abundant.

In patients with pneumonia, tularemia may be transmitted from person to person. Patients with known or suspected tularemic pneumonia should be placed on droplet precautions.

Clinical Features and Diagnosis The incubation period of tularemia averages 3 to 5 days (range, 1 to 21 days). Tularemia usually starts abruptly, with onset of fevers, chills, headache, anorexia, malaise, and fatigue. Symptoms may also include myalgias, cough, vomiting, pharyngitis, abdominal pain, and diarrhea. Fever typically lasts for several days, remits for a brief period, and then recurs.

The clinical presentation largely depends on the route of inoculation. Clinical syndromes include ulceroglandular fever (in 21 to 87 percent of cases), which follows tick bites and animal contact; it is characterized by enlarged and tender local adenopathy and an ulcer at the inoculation site. Glandular tularemia (in 3 to 20 percent) occurs when patients present with tender regional adenopathy without evidence of a local cutaneous lesion. Oculoglandular tularemia (in up to 5 percent) is characterized by photophobia and lacrimation. Pharyngeal tularemia (in up to 12 percent) is acquired from contaminated foods or water and is characterized by exudative pharyngitis or tonsillitis. Typhoidal tularemia (5 to 30 percent) may result from any mode of transmission. Symptoms suggest multiorgan involvement and include fever, headache, chills, myalgias, nausea, vomiting, abdominal pain, and cough. Secondary pneumonitis may occur in up to 45 percent of patients.

Finally, tularemic pneumonia (in 7 to 20 percent of cases) may occur following inhalation of the organism. Symptoms include fever, cough, minimal or no sputum production, substernal chest tightness, and occasionally pleuritic chest pain. Physical examination is frequently nonspecific but may reveal rales, consolidation, or a pleural rub. Suggestive findings on physical exam include a cutaneous eschar, a tender enlarged lymph node, and pharyngeal exudate with tender cervical adenopathy.

The various clinical presentations of tularemia frequently lead to misdiagnosis. Pneumonic tularemia is in the differential diagnosis of a typical pneumonia, viruses, *Mycoplasma* and *Legionella* infections, plague, anthrax, Q fever, and psittacosis. The key to proper diagnosis is obtaining a history of potential exposure to *F. tularensis;* routine laboratory tests are nonspecific. *F. tularensis* may be recovered from the blood, lymph nodes, wounds, sputum, and pleural fluid when processed on special media. Tularemia presents a special hazard to laboratory personnel, and they should always be informed if tularemia is considered. The diagnosis is usually confirmed with serologic studies. Enzyme-linked immunosorbent assay (ELISA) is the preferred diagnostic test. Acute and convalescent sera are usually required.

Treatment and Prevention The drug of choice for treatment is streptomycin, administered at a dosage of 7.5 to 10 mg/kg intramuscularly every 12 h for 7 to 14 days. (The alternative is gentamicin.) The pediatric dose is 30 to 40 mg/kg per day intramuscularly in two divided doses for 7 days. Tetracycline and chloramphenicol have been used orally for therapy, but both are bacteriostatic and a high rate of relapse has been noted. Many other drugs (erythromycin, rifampin, cefoxitin, cefotaxime, ceftriaxone, quinolones) have demonstrated activity in vitro, but clinical studies of in vivo effectiveness are, in general, unavailable.

Prevention requires careful handling of animal skins and carcasses. Tick prevention includes the use of tick repellents, long pants, and high socks outdoors in the summer and a careful search for ticks at least twice per day with removal if any are found.

Pasteurellosis

Microbiology and Epidemiology Pasteurellosis is caused by *Pasteurella multocida,* a small, nonmotile, non–spore-forming gram-negative coccobacillus. On Gram's smear, the organisms generally appear as a single bacillus but may occur in pairs or chains. They frequently show bipolar staining. The organisms are aerobic and facultatively anaerobic and grow well at 37°C on blood, chocolate, and Mueller-Hinton agar but not on MacConkey's agar. Growth is facilitated by enriched media and increased carbon dioxide tension.

P. multocida has been isolated from the digestive system or respiratory tract of many animals, including domestic cats and dogs, large cats (e.g., lions), rodents, rabbits, cattle, swine, and horses. Carriage rates of *P. multocida* in oral or nasal secretions have been reported to be 70 to 90 percent in cats and 50 to 66 percent in dogs. Most human infections result from direct inoculation by bites or scratches. Infections following animal exposure in the absence of bites or scratches probably stem from contact with animal secretions. Human-to-human spread of infection has not been documented, and contaminated food and water have not been implicated as sources of infection.

Clinical Features and Diagnosis Infections with *P. multocida* may be divided into three categories: (1) soft tissue infections following animal bites or scratches, (2) oral and respiratory infections, and (3) serious invasive infection unrelated to animal bites, such as meningitis, intraabdominal infections, or ocular infection. The respiratory tract is second to animal bite wounds as a source of *P. multocida* isolates from humans. *P. multocida* may cause sinusitis, otitis media, tonsillitis, bronchitis, pneumonia, or empyema. Most patients who have *P. multocida* respiratory tract infections also have underlying pulmonary disorders such as bronchiectasis, carcinoma of the lung, obstructive pulmonary disease, or chronic sinusitis. In such patients, *P. multocida* may colonize the respiratory tree for long periods.

P. multocida may be diagnosed from culture of sputum with standard techniques.

Treatment and Prevention *P. multocida* is highly susceptible to many antibiotics, including penicillin G, ampicillin, piperacillin, second- and third-generation cephalosporins, chloramphenicol, and quinolones. Penicillin is the drug of choice. Less active agents include first-generation cephalosporins, aminoglycosides, vancomycin, erythromycin, and clindamycin.

Yersinia pestis

Microbiology and Epidemiology The genus *Yersinia* includes *Y. pestis, Y. enterocolitica,* and *Y. pseudotuberculosis. Y. pestis,* the cause of plague, is a gram-negative bipolar-staining bacillus. It grows aerobically on most culture media, including blood and MacConkey's agar, after 24-h incubation at 35°C.

Plague occurs worldwide, but most cases are reported from the less developed countries in Africa and Asia. In the United States, most cases are reported from the Southwest and occur between May and October. Man is an accidental host; the reservoir for *Y. pestis* includes rodents (especially rats), pigs, and birds. Plague is transmitted by flea bites, by ingestion of contaminated animal tissues, or by inhalation. In rare instances, pneumonic plague may be transmitted from person to person. Risk factors for acquisition include direct contact with rodents, the presence of shelter or food for wild rodents in the vicinity of the home, and inadequate protection against fleas for domestic cats and dogs.

Clinical Features and Diagnosis The major clinical syndromes of plague include bubonic plague, septicemic plague, and pneumonic plague. The incubation for bubonic plague is 2 to 8 days following the bite of an infected flea. Characteristically, patients suddenly develop fever, chills, weakness, headache, and then intense pain, with swelling of a regional lymph node (the "bubo"). Some patients develop septicemic plague, characterized by overwhelming sepsis. Secondary pneumonia may develop with hematogenous spread of bacteria during sepsis. Pneumonic plague is highly contagious and has a high mortality. Clinical findings, in addition to fever and lymphadenopathy, include cough, chest pain, and frequently hemoptysis. The chest radiograph most commonly reveals patchy bronchopneumonia, cavities, or consolidation.

As with other zoonotic disease, an epidemiologic exposure in the setting of an appropriate clinical syndrome should lead one to suspect plague. A bacteriologic diagnosis is easily made in most patients from smear and culture of a bubo aspirate. The smear should be processed for both Gram's and Wayson's stains. In pneumonic plague, the organism is readily isolated from sputum. Cultures may be sent to the CDC for identification, but all cultures should be handled with extreme caution, as they represent a significant risk to laboratory personnel. Serology can also be used to confirm the diagnosis.

Treatment and Prevention Streptomycin is the drug of choice for plague. It should be administered intramuscularly at a daily dose of 30 mg/kg in two divided doses for 10 days. In allergic patients, tetracycline is an acceptable alternative in a dose of 2 to 4 g a day in four divided doses for 10 days.

Prevention consists of avoidance of areas of the world with endemic or epidemic plague and extreme care when handling animal carcasses.

Nosocomial Pneumonias

Enterobacteriaceae

Microbiology and Epidemiology Enteric gram-negative bacilli are an important cause of nosocomial pneumonia. In certain patients—such as those in chronic care facilities, immunocompromised patients, or those with underlying lung disease—they are also an important cause of community-acquired pneumonia. Of the enteric pathogens, the most common agents in pneumonia are *Klebsiella, E. coli, Enterobacter, Proteus,* and *Serratia.* All these pathogens grow readily on blood or MacConkey's agar. These bacteria are normal flora of the gastrointestinal tract. As previously noted, hospitalization and other host factors (e.g., alcoholism) favor colonization of the oral cavity.

Clinical Features and Diagnosis The enteric bacteria are opportunistic pathogens that cause pneumonia in the setting of impaired host defenses. All may produce a destructive pneumonia. Characteristically, patients with pneumonia due to enteric pathogens have fever, chills, cough with production of sputum, shortness of breath, and pleuritic pain. The clinical features are not specific enough for one to be able to distinguish among the many enteric bacteria capable of causing pneumonia. In some patients—including immunosuppressed persons, the elderly, and patients with hematogenously spread pneumonia—the signs and symptoms of pneumonia may be reduced or absent. Blood cultures have been reported to be positive in 10 to 50 percent of patients, depending on the etiologic agent and the patient population. The radiographic findings do not allow microbiologic diagnosis, although they may be suggestive. As previously noted, the presence of a bulging fissure suggests pneumonia with *K. pneumoniae.* Gram-negative pneumonia is suggested by early necrosis and abscess formation, although it may also be seen with *S. pneumoniae, S. aureus,* and *Legionella.*

Treatment and Prevention The most active agents against gram-negative enteric pathogens are the third- and fourth-generation cephalosporins (cefotaxime, ceftriaxone, ceftazidime, cefepime), a penicillin combined with a beta-lactamase inhibitor (piperacillin-tazobactam), carbapenems (imipenem, meropenem), monobactams (aztreonam), and quinolones (ciprofloxacin). Aminoglycosides are also active but are rarely used as primary therapy. Some strains of *Klebsiella, Enterobacter,* and *Serratia* may be resistant to a number of antibiotics. Definitive therapy should be guided by in vitro susceptibility results and clinical response.

Pseudomonas aeruginosa

Microbiology and Epidemiology The family Pseudomonadaceae contains more than 150 species. However, the most important member of this family is *P. aeruginosa. P. aeruginosa* is an obligate, motile, rod-shaped (0.5 to 0.8 by 1.5 to 3.0 μm) gram-negative bacillus with a single flagellum. It may produce a variety of pigments, including pyocyanin (a pigment produced by approximately 50 percent of clinical strains), which causes colonies to appear blue or green. *P. aeruginosa* is capable of utilizing more than 30 organic compounds for growth. It grows optimally at 37°C.

P. aeruginosa can be isolated from soil, water, plants, and animals. Its minimal nutritional requirements allow it to reproduce in many ecologic niches in the hospital. Reservoirs discovered during outbreaks have included many moist devices and surfaces found in hospitals, including endoscopes, endoscope washers, disinfectants, food mixers, and enteral foods. *P. aeruginosa* may also be part of the normal flora of humans. *P. aeruginosa* is primarily a nosocomial pathogen and is the most common gram-negative bacillus causing hospital-acquired pneumonia. Within the hospital, *P. aeruginosa* acts as an opportunistic pathogen. Particularly vulnerable are patients with skin or mucous membrane disruption, intravenous catheters, urinary tract catheters, neutropenia, immunosuppressive medication, cystic fibrosis, and diabetes mellitus.

The pathogenesis of *P. aeruginosa* infections is very complex and includes many virulence factors. Key factors include the pili or fimbriae, which mediate adherence to respiratory epithelial cells; the mucoid capsule, which aids in anchoring the organism to its environment; cell-associated factors, which protect the organism from host phagocytes and complement; and extracellular enzymes and toxins, which promote penetration and impair host defenses.

Clinical Features and Diagnosis *P. aeruginosa* causes respiratory infection almost exclusively in patients with impaired respiratory host defenses. Only occasionally does *P. aeruginosa* cause community-acquired pneumonia, and then usually in patients cared for in extended care facilities or with chronic lung disease or other serious underlying illness. *P. aeruginosa* and *S. aureus* are the most important pathogens in patients with cystic fibrosis. Pneumonia due to *P. aeruginosa* is usually a fulminant infection and is characterized by fever, rigors, severe dyspnea, cough productive of sputum, cyanosis, and systemic shock. The chest radiograph commonly reveals a diffuse bilateral bronchopulmonary pneumonia with distinctive nodular infiltrates and small areas of radiolucency. Although pleural effusions are common, empyema is rare.

Bacteremic pneumonia may occur in severely neutropenic patients. Patients with bacteremic pneumonia characteristically have ill-defined hemorrhagic, nodular areas that are frequently subpleural. Central necrosis of these areas may occur.

Treatment and Prevention *P. aeruginosa* is typically treated with an aminoglycoside and an antipseudomonal penicillin (piperacillin), cephalosporin (ceftazidime, cefepime), carbapenem (imipenem, meropenem), or monobactam (aztreonam). The quinolones are also active, but only ciprofloxacin is currently available as an intravenous preparation. Despite therapy, the mortality from hospital-acquired pseudomonal pneumonia is approximately 70 percent. Unfortunately, no specific measures to prevent nosocomial pseudomonal infections are available at the present time.

BIBLIOGRAPHY

American Thoracic Society: Hospital-acquired pneumonia in adults: Diagnosis, assessment of severity, initial antimicrobial therapy, and preventive strategies. *Am J Respir Crit Care Med* 153:1711–1725, 1996.

Bartlett JC, O'Keefe P, Tally FP: Bacteriology of hospital-acquired pneumonia. *Arch Intern Med* 146:868–871, 1991.

Centers for Disease Control and Prevention: National Nosocomial Infections Surveillance (NNIS) Semiannual Report, May 1995. *Am J Infect Control* 23:377–385, 1995.

Chastre J, Fagon J-Y: Invasive diagnostic testing should be routinely used to manage ventilated patients with suspected pneumonia. *Am J Respir Crit Care Med* 150:570–574, 1994.

Chastre J, Trouillet J-L, Fagon J-Y: Diagnosis of pulmonary infections in mechanically ventilated patients. *Semin Respir Infect* 11:65–76, 1996.

Cook DJ, Laine LA, Guyatt GH: Nosocomial pneumonia and the role of gastric pH. *Chest* 100:7–13, 1996.

Craig CP, Connelly S: Effect of intensive care unit nosocomial pneumonia on duration of stay and mortality. *Am J Infect Control* 12:233–238, 1984.

Craven DE, Steger KA: Epidemiology of nosocomial pneumonia: New perspectives on an old disease. *Chest* 108(suppl):1S–16S, 1995.

Craven DE, Steger KA: Nosocomial pneumonia in mechanically ventilated adult patients: Epidemiology and prevention in 1996. *Semin Respir Infect* 11:32–53, 1996.

Daschner F, Kappstein I, Engels I, et al: Stress ulcer prophylaxis and ventilation pneumonia: Prevention by antibacterial cytoprotective agents? *Infect Control Hosp Epidemiol* 9:59–65, 1988.

Daschner F, Nadjem H, Langmaack H, Sandritter W: Surveillance, prevention and control of hospital-acquired infections: III. Nosocomial infections as cause of death: Retrospective analysis of 1000 autopsy reports. *Infection* 6:261–265, 1978.

Emori TG, Gaynes RP: An overview of nosocomial infections including the role of the microbiology laboratory. *Clin Microb Rev* 6:428–442, 1993.

Fagon J-Y Chastre J, Domart Y, et al: Nosocomial pneumonia in patients receiving continuous mechanical ventilation. *Am Rev Respir Dis* 139:877–884, 1989.

Fagon J-Y, Chastre J, Vuagnat A, et al: Nosocomial pneumonia and mortality among patients in intensive care units. *JAMA* 275:866–869, 1996.

Garner JS: Guideline for isolation precautions in hospitals. *Infect Control Hosp Epidemiol* 17:53–80, 1996.

Hanson LC, Weber DJ, Rutala WA: Risk factors for nosocomial pneumonia in the elderly. *Am J Med* 92:161–166, 1992.

Hart CA, Makin T: *Legionella* in hospitals: A review. *J Hosp Infect* 18(suppl A):481–489, 1991.

Jacobs S, Chang RWS, Lee B, Bartlett FW: Continuous enteral feeding: A major cause of pneumonia among ventilated intensive care unit patients. *J Parenter Enter Nutr* 14:353–356, 1990.

Johanson WG, Pierce AK, Sanford JP, Thomas GD: Nosocomial respiratory infections with gram-negative bacilli: The significance of colonization of the respiratory tract. *Ann Intern Med* 77:701–706, 1972.

Langer M, Mosconi P, Cigada M, et al: Long-term respiratory support and risk of pneumonia in critically ill patients. *Am Rev Respir Dis* 140:302–305, 1989.

Larson EL: APIC guidelines for handwashing and hand antisepsis in health care settings. *Am J Infect Control* 23:251–269, 1995.

Meduri GU: Diagnosis and differential diagnosis of ventilator-associated pneumonia. *Clin Chest Med* 16:61–91, 1995.

Rello J, Quintana E, Ausina V, et al: Incidence, etiology, and outcome of nosocomial pneumonia in mechanically ventilated patients. *Chest* 100:439–444, 1991.

Ruiz-Santana S, Garcia Jimenez A, Esteban A, et al; ICU pneumonias: A multi-institutional study. *Crit Care Med* 15:930–932, 1987.

Rutala WA: APIC guidelines for selection and use of disinfectants. *Am J Infect Control* 18:99–118, 1990.

Spach DH, Silverstein FE, Stamm WE: Transmission of infection by gastrointestinal endoscopy and bronchoscopy. *Ann Intern Med* 118:117–128, 1993.

Tablan OC, Anderson LJ, Arden NH, et al: Guideline for prevention of nosocomial pneumonia. *Infect Control Hosp Epidemiol* 15:587–627, 1994.

Torres A, Aznar R, Gatell JM, et al: Incidence, risk and prognosis factors of nosocomial pneumonia in mechanically ventilated patients. *Am Rev Respir Dis* 142:523–526, 1990.

Weber DJ, Rutala WA: Infection control in critical care units, in Moylan J (ed): *Surgical Critical Care.* St. Louis: Mosby, 1994.

Weber DJ, Rutala WA: Management of healthcare workers exposed to pertussis. *Infect Control Hosp Epidemiol* 15:411–415, 1994.

Weber DJ, Rutala WA: Nosocomial infections associated with respiratory therapy, in Mayhall CG (ed): *Hospital Epidemiology and Infection Control.* Baltimore: Williams & Wilkins, 1996, pp 748–758.

62 | Mycobacterial Infections*

Jay A. Fishman

HISTORY

Tuberculosis (TB) is a disease that has afflicted humankind throughout recorded history and before. Spinal lesions that are highly suggestive or classic for TB have been observed in a skeleton recovered from a grave near Heidelberg that dates from 5000 B.C., from a skeleton excavated from the Arene Candide Cave in Liguria, Italy, that dates from 4000 B.C., and from similar graves in Denmark and the Jordan Valley. *Mycobacterium tuberculosis* DNA has been recovered from a pre-Columbian mummy from Peru. The earliest records that are consistent with TB are Egyptian wall paintings that depict typical hunchback deformities and correlate with the findings of spinal TB in mummies. The first written description of TB is from India around 700 B.C. Hippocrates not only described the disease but also named it *phthisis,* which means to melt or to waste away. Aristotle noted its contagious nature. In Europe, tuberculosis rates peaked in the late eighteenth and early nineteenth centuries. With the introduction of industrialization and movement of people from the agrarian life of the countryside to the crowded cities, conditions were set for efficient person-to-person spread of the tubercle bacilli. It is estimated that as many as 10 percent of some populations died from tuberculosis, or consumption, as it was known at that time.

Presently, the number of deaths caused by tuberculosis worldwide exceed those caused by any other organism. It has been estimated that approximately one-third of the world's population is infected with the tubercle bacillus and that there are 8 million new cases and 3 million deaths annually from tuberculosis in the world. But it was not until Koch discovered the tuberculous bacillus in 1882 that the causative agent was discovered. Today TB describes an infection in humans that is caused by either *M. tuberculosis* or *M. bovis.* Infections caused by other mycobacteria should be referred to as disease caused by the specific mycobacterium.

PATHOPHYSIOLOGY OF TUBERCULOSIS

Overview

Initial infection with *M. tuberculosis* occurs by the airborne route. Since *M. tuberculosis* cannot penetrate mucus, the organism must bypass the mucous

*Edited from Chaps. 158 to 164, "The Epidemiology, Transmission, and Prevention of Tuberculosis in the United States," by Onorato IM, Ridzon R; "The Microbiology of the Mycobacteria," by van der Kuyp F; "Pathogenesis of Pulmonary Tuberculosis," by Dannenberg AM Jr, Tomashefski JF Jr; "Screening for Tuberculosis and Tuberculosis Infection in High-Risk Populations," by Bloch AB; "Clinical Presentation and Treatment of Tuberculosis," by Rossman MD, Oner-Eyuboglu AF; "Mycobacterial Infections and HIV Infection," by Chaisson RC; and "Diseases Due to Mycobacteria Other than Mycobacterium Tuberculosis," by Davidson PT. In: *Fishman's Pulmonary Diseases and Disorders,* 3d ed., edited by Fishman AP, Elias JA, Fishman JA, Grippi MA, Kaiser LR, Senior RM. New York, McGraw-Hill, 1998, pp 2431–2524. For fuller discussion of topics dealt with in this chapter, the reader is referred to the original text, as noted above.

barrier by staying suspended in the air until it arrives in the alveolar zone, where no mucus is present. Only organisms suspended in droplets between 1 and 10 μm are able to pass to the alveolar zone and avoid being safely eliminated. Although the minimal infecting dose for humans of *M. tuberculosis* is unknown, in rabbits and guinea pigs one to three live organisms may be sufficient. These organisms are initially ingested by alveolar macrophages. Since resident alveolar macrophages and nonactivated, recently arrived macrophages cannot kill intracellular *M. tuberculosis,* the organisms initially replicate within macrophages and rapidly increase in number. During this period, before the development of specific immunity, the organisms appear in draining lymph nodes and a bacteremia or hematogenous dissemination occurs.

This initial phase of uninhibited growth of *M. tuberculosis* ends with the development of an immune response. At the initial site of infection (primary infection), the organisms are usually completely eliminated. At the disseminated sites, however, the organism is not eliminated but only arrested. It is not known whether the organism is growing very slowly or is dormant during this period. Months to years later, for reasons that are not entirely known, the organism again begins to grow more rapidly, resulting in the development of symptomatic TB. Although these sites may be anywhere, they are most frequently in the apices of the lungs, bones, meninges, and kidneys. It is believed that the high tissue tensions of oxygen may be an important factor in the localization and continued growth of *M. tuberculosis* in these locations.

The Host Response

The *development of pulmonary tuberculosis* from its onset to clinical manifestations is dependent upon a series of interactions between the host and the bacillus. (1) An inhaled unit of one to three bacilli is ingested by an alveolar macrophage. Either the bacillus is destroyed before any lesion is produced or it multiplies within the alveolar macrophage, which dies and releases the amplified infectious agent. (2) Many of the bacilli are then ingested by and grow within phagocytes (monocytes, tissue macrophages, reticuloendothelial cells) that have emigrated from the bloodstream. These cells accumulate at the site, forming a microscopic lesion. (3) When the host becomes tuberculin-positive, a caseous center develops in this lesion. A lesion with a small caseous center (up to 2 mm in diameter) may enlarge or may heal (or stabilize) before it is detectable by radiography. (4) A larger caseous lesion may also heal or stabilize; or it may enlarge, shedding bacilli into the blood and lymph. (5) Alternatively, a caseous lesion may liquefy and form a cavity (from which the bacilli enter the bronchial tree). In the liquefied caseum, the bacilli will grow *extracellularly* (for the first time), and from the cavity they spread to other parts of the lung and to the environment. In general, at each step, the elimination of the bacilli is increasingly difficult and the interactions of the host with each separate tuberculous focus is often independent.

The host's activated macrophages can kill or inhibit ingested tubercle bacilli. The capacity of the host's alveolar macrophages to respond to infection and the intensity of this response is genetically determined; nonspecific activation of the macrophages determines whether an inhaled bacillary particle is able to establish a primary lesion. The degree of antigen-specific activation of macrophages from the bloodstream (via lymphocytes and their cytokines) is also genetically determined. Cytotoxic T lymphocytes can directly or indirectly kill nonactivated macrophages with replicating tubercle bacilli in their cytoplasm or activate such cells to avoid intracellular replication of bacilli. In addition, infected cells may undergo apoptosis (programmed cell death) to protect the host from dissemination of disease. The killing of such nonactivated macrophages eliminates the intracellular environment that is favorable to bacillary growth and replaces it with the extracellular environment of solid caseous (necrotic) tissue that is inhibitory to bacillary growth. The bacillus can multiply logarithmically within nonactivated macrophages (i.e., within monocytes that have recently migrated from the bloodstream into the local site of infection) and in liquefied caseous material. When the bacilli multiply extracellularly in the liquefied caseum, the resulting antigenic load causes more tissue necrosis, erosion of bronchial walls, and cavity formation, followed by spread of bacilli into the airways. The bacillus itself is nontoxic. It damages host tissue by means of the host's own immune response to tuberculin-like products.

In most people, tuberculosis is arrested as a single primary pulmonary lesion that is sufficient to produce a positive tuberculin reaction but is usually not large enough to be detected in a chest radiograph. In time, hosts with a primary lesion of any size develop both delayed-type hypersensitivity and cell-mediated immunity, which accelerate host responses to the bacillus. At secondary sites of bacillary lodgment, lymphocytes and macrophages then accumulate at an accelerated rate, causing an *exudative* or a *proliferative* response, depending on the tuberculin sensitivity of the host and on the number of tubercle bacilli, their rate of growth, and the quantity of their tuberculin-like products.

The various types of lesions and types of disease found in pulmonary tuberculosis sometimes change from one type to another or are a composite of several types. Multiple types of lesions often coexist in the lung. Furthermore, the disease as a whole may fluctuate between periods of exacerbation and remission.

Tuberculous pneumonia is an exudative response in the alveolar spaces, caused by the presence of numerous live and dead tubercle bacilli and their antigenic products. Small or extensive areas of pneumonia commonly occur when a liquefied caseous focus in the lung (or in a hilar lymph node) discharges its contents into the airways. Since the caseous material is impregnated with bacillary components, it causes a pneumonic exudate even if the number of intact bacilli is small. The initial exudate contains mononuclear cells, granulocytes, and a fibrinous coagulum of serum and cell proteins. In time, epithelioid cells, lymphocytes, plasma cells, fibroblasts, and, occasionally, giant cells appear. Caseous necrosis usually occurs. The confluence of progressing exudative lesions results in consolidation of small or large segments of the pulmonary lobe. At one end of the spectrum, such tuberculous pneumonia can result in death; at the other end, the pneumonia can undergo resolution with minimal scarring, especially if only small numbers of viable bacilli are present and the lung structure is preserved.

Pleurisy results when subpleural caseous lesions in the lung (or in the hilar lymph nodes) leak or rupture, discharging bacilli and their components into the pleural cavity. The spectrum of clinical disease includes mild, uncomplicated rougbenings of the pleural surface; large or small numbers of miliary tubercles on this pleural surface; serous effusions (from large or numerous surface lesions); or frank tuberculous empyema. The type of pleural disease is determined by (1) the number of live and dead bacilli, (2) the quantity of their tuberculin-like products in the caseous material, (3) the level of tuberculin sensitivity of the host, (4) the friction of the roughened visceral pleura against the parietal pleura, (5) the number and types of cells in the exudate, (6) the inherent ability of the host to localize and fibrose new sites of tuberculous infection, and (7) the presence or absence of superinfection with other bacteria. Tuberculous pleurisy may resolve completely or may heal with fibrosis, focal adhesions, and sometimes calcification. Depending on the amount of exudate in the pleural space, a large or small portion of the lung may collapse.

Childhood Tuberculosis: Lymphatic Spread and the Ghon Complex

Tuberculosis in children differs from tuberculosis in adults in several respects: (1) young children, especially infants, usually have lower native and acquired resistance to this disease; (2) their hilar lymph nodes more commonly become enlarged and caseous; (3) blood-borne dissemination occurs more readily but remains unusual; (4) calcification of caseous foci is more common; and (5) the primary pulmonary lesion in children is usually subpleural in well-ventilated regions of the lung, whereas such lesions in adults are usually subapical. Tubercle bacilli, either free or within immature macrophages (or granulocytes), spread via the lymphatics from the primary lesion to the hilar lymph nodes, where—in children (and in adults with low resistance)—the bacilli can cause large caseous lesions. The combination of one or more enlarged caseous hilar node(s) and a tuberculous focus in the lung periphery constitutes a Ghon complex.

A tuberculous hilar node may obstruct a bronchus by external compression or by extension of the disease process into the bronchial wall. The obstruction causes segmental or lobar collapse and pneumonitis, the so-called *right-middle-lobe syndrome.* Sometimes such a node ruptures into a bronchus, causing distally focal or diffuse pneumonic lesions.

Adult Tuberculosis: Endogenous and Exogenous Reinfection

As a rule, tuberculosis progresses more slowly in adults than it does in infants. Secondary endogenous tuberculous foci of lymphatic or hematogenous origin also occur less often in adults. However, the resistance of immunocompetent adults may be overwhelmed when a liquefied caseous focus ruptures and seeds large numbers of bacilli directly into a bronchus or into a blood or lymphatic vessel of appreciable size.

Reinfection- or adult-type tuberculosis may be caused by either exogenous or endogenous tubercle bacilli. This type of tuberculosis consists of a small to large pulmonary lesion that is most often in the subapical region and is unaccompanied by any marked enlargement of the hilar lymph nodes. Adult-type tuberculosis may occur as a primary infection in either adults or children with resistance high enough to restrict bacillary multiplication in the hilar nodes.

The active subapical lesion is frequently a localized area of bronchopneumonia containing macrophages, epithelioid cells, lymphocytes, giant cells, and fibroblasts. The lesion usually heals, and fibrosis results in a thickened pleura. Sometimes a cavity forms, either at the time of the initial subapical infection or, more commonly, years later if reactivation of a formerly dormant subapical lesion occurs. Then the disease may progress into one of the types described above. It is not known why the subapical region of the lungs is a favored site for the onset of adult-type tuberculosis.

Tuberculosis in the Immunocompromised Host

In immunocompromised patients, tuberculosis may be due either to reactivation disease or new primary exposures. In AIDS patients, the disease of reactivation often resembles childhood tuberculosis with hilar adenopathy, frequent lower lobe involvement, and absence of both cavitation and scar formation. In all immunosuppressed patients, the morphology of tuberculous lesions reflects poor host resistance. For example, in corticosteroid-treated patients, tuberculous lesions show abundant caseation with little or no encapsulation or granulomatous reaction. Large numbers of bacteria are usually present within the lesions. These changes are morphologically similar to those found experimentally in corticosteroid-treated tuberculous animals.

In patients with AIDS, the histologic pattern of tuberculosis generally correlates with the degree of immunosuppression. In premortem biopsy samples, the granulomas are more proliferative (and less exudative) than in necropsy-derived tissue. As the peripheral CD4 lymphocytes decrease, the type of necrosis changes from caseous to caseosuppurative (i.e., caseous necrosis containing neutrophils and more undigested nuclear debris). Also, the number of mycobacteria within lesions increases.

Infections with Nontuberculous Mycobacteria

The lung may be infected by inhalation of nontuberculous mycobacteria from the environment, or it may be infected by dissemination of nontuberculous mycobacteria from a primary site elsewhere, most often in the gastrointestinal tract. Since nontuberculous mycobacteria are organisms of relatively low pathogenicity, saprophytic colonization of the lung must be distinguished from overt pulmonary disease. The presence of granulomas in lung biopsy specimens, with or without demonstrable acid-fast bacilli (coupled with positive cultures from sputum or bronchial washings), establishes the diagnosis of nontuberculous mycobacteria lung disease in patients in whom the diagnosis could not be made by other criteria.

Chronic Progressive Pulmonary Disease

Nontuberculous mycobacteria typically infect persons with underlying chronic pulmonary conditions, such as pneumoconioses (especially silicosis), emphysematous bullae, chronic obstructive pulmonary disease, cystic fibrosis, prior tuberculosis, malignancies, esophageal disease with chronic aspiration (*M. fortuitum* and *M. chelonei*), and following gastrectomy (*M. xenopi*). In these patients, pulmonary infection with nontuberculous mycobacteria resembles reactivation infection with *M. tuberculosis,* both clinically and radiographically.

An increasing number of patients with pulmonary nontuberculous mycobacteria infection (usually due to *M. avium* complex) have no discernible predisposing lung disease. In this subgroup of patients, chest radiographs and computed tomography (CT) scans differ from those of classic tuberculosis. They have bilateral nodules associated with bronchiectasis, most frequently in the lower lungs.

Histopathologically, nontuberculous mycobacteria infections may show (1) many foamy histiocytes, (2) granulomatous endobronchitis and bronchiolitis, (3) epithelioid granulomas without caseation, (4) nonspecific organizing pneumonia, and (5) interstitial fibrosis without granulomas. Most patients with nonspecific organizing pneumonia or nongranulomatous interstitial fibrosis are immunocompromised. Lung disease caused by nontuberculous mycobacteria usually cannot, however, be differentiated histopathologically from that caused by *M. tuberculosis.* Both nontuberculous mycobacteria and *M. tuberculosis* usually produce caseating granulomas and similar types of cavitation, associated with variable degrees of fibrosis. No distinctive histopathologic differences are produced in lesions caused by different species of nontuberculous mycobacteria.

In general, chronic nontuberculous mycobacterial pulmonary disease tends to remain confined within the lung, with little tendency toward lymphatic or hematogenous spread to hilar lymph nodes or to extrathoracic viscera in the immunologically normal host. Exudative granulomatous pneumonia is present in about 10 percent of infections. Acid-fast bacilli are usually sparse within the caseum. When found, *M. kansasii* organisms often appear large and beaded.

Dimorphic mycobacterial granulomas are lesions with central suppuration (containing numerous neutrophils) surrounded by noncaseous granulation tissue (containing macrophages and epithelioid cells). Such granulomas are found in about 23 percent of pulmonary nontuberculous mycobacterial infections. Unfortunately, the incidence of dimorphic granulomas in *M. tuberculosis* infections is unknown because numerous neutrophils are often present during the early stages of caseous necrosis and when large numbers of tubercle bacilli occur during later stages of the disease.

Disseminated Disease

The lung is often affected in disseminated nontuberculous mycobacterial infection, a disorder that has become prevalent in patients with AIDS. Disseminated *M. avium* complex infection in AIDS patients usually occurs when the number of CD4 lymphocytes in the peripheral blood drops below 100 cells per cubic millimeter. Phagocytosis of mycobacteria by macrophages appears to be competent, but the killing of mycobacteria by such macrophages is impaired. Even before the outbreak of AIDS, nontuberculous mycobacteria were known as a cause of disseminated disease in immunocompromised hosts. The organisms producing disseminated disease in patients without AIDS were *M. avium* complex, *M. kansasii,* scotochromogens, and rapid growers, in order of decreasing frequency. In AIDS patients, the preponderant pathogen is *M. avium* complex, although most other species of nontuberculous mycobacteria can also sometimes cause disseminated infection. Disseminated *M. avium* complex disease is found at necropsy in approximately 15 to 24 percent of AIDS patients.

Among non-AIDS patients with disseminated *M. avium* complex infection, the lung was reported to be affected in 65 percent, followed by bone marrow, liver, lymph nodes (46 percent each), and spleen (22 percent). Histologically, disseminated *M. avium* complex disease in non-AIDS patients is usually characterized by poorly formed granulomas containing loose aggregates of mononuclear cells, abundant neutrophils, infrequent epithelioid cells, and focal necrosis. In bone and skin, however, there are often acute and chronic inflammatory areas and abscesses *without* granuloma formation. In most cases, acid-fast bacilli are scarce, but in 20 percent of one large series, tremendous numbers of acid-fast bacilli were seen within macrophages, just as in lepromatous leprosy.

Disseminated *M. avium* complex disease in AIDS patients predominantly affects the reticuloendothelial system, especially the spleen. The portals of entry of *M. avium* complex are thought to be the gastrointestinal and respiratory tracts. Histologically, the lesions at all sites consist of poorly formed granulomas or loose aggregates of striated macrophages, which usually contain numerous acid-fast bacilli. In the small bowel, periodic acid–Schiff–positive macrophages, laden with mycobacteria, histologically resemble those seen in Whipple's disease. In the lungs, however, granulomas or macrophage aggregates are not often seen.

M. avium complex has been cultured from the lung at necropsy in approximately 36 percent of AIDS patients with disseminated *M. avium* complex disease. But clinically significant pulmonary disease due to *M. avium* complex is uncommon and is usually overshadowed by coexistent opportunistic infections. Histologic evidence of *M. avium* complex pulmonary infection is usually minimal, even when lung cultures are positive for *M. avium* complex. However, a *minority* of AIDS patients develop clinically significant *M. avium* complex lung disease with necrotizing granulomas containing variable numbers of acid-fast bacilli. If the disease in their hilar lymph nodes extends into central bronchi, tumor-like masses of granulomatous tissue may obstruct the airways.

EPIDEMIOLOGY OF TUBERCULOSIS

Tuberculosis is a disease of overcrowding and poverty. The epidemiology of tuberculosis has changed drastically over the last half of the twentieth century—from a disease seen in older populations, with a steadily declining rate, to one of increasing incidence seen in younger, urban populations. In addition, the epidemiology has been changed by drug resistance, HIV, and immigration of foreign-born persons from areas with high rates of tuberculosis. Multidrug-resistant tuberculosis (MDR TB) has emerged as a significant public health threat and clinical challenge. Dramatic shifts have occurred in the epidemiology of tuberculosis. While 90 percent of disease in the United States was due to reactivation of latent infection in the past, more recent data suggest that up to 30 to 40 percent of new cases are now due to recent infection, with a higher incidence in cases of MDR disease.

Incidence in the United States

From 1953 to 1985, there was a steady decline in the number of tuberculosis cases reported in the United States; the average was between 5 and 6.1 percent per year (for case definition, see Table 62-1). In 1953, there were 84,304

TABLE 62-1 Centers for Disease Control and Prevention (CDC) Case Definition of Tuberculosis

---

Laboratory criteria for diagnosis:
Isolation of *M. tuberculosis* from a clinical specimen or, when a culture has not been or cannot be obtained, demonstration of acid-fast bacilli in a clinical specimen
For cases that lack laboratory confirmation, all elements of the clinical case definition must be met:
A positive tuberculin skin test (PPD[a])
Signs and symptoms compatible with tuberculosis, such as an abnormal, unstable (worsening or improving) chest radiograph or clinical evidence of disease
Treatment with two or more antituberculous medications
A completed diagnostic evaluation

---

[a]Purified protein derivative.

cases reported (53 cases per 100,000). This number steadily declined until 1985, when 22,201 cases were reported (9.3 cases per 100,000). From 1985 through 1992, annual rates rose, and in 1992 a total of 26,673 cases were reported (10.5 cases per 100,000). This represented a 20 percent increase over the 1985 case number. During this time, an estimated 51,700 excess cases were reported. Following public health efforts focused particularly on high-incidence areas, in both 1993 and 1994, total reported cases of tuberculosis declined compared to previous years. During 1995, the number of tuberculosis cases reported was 22,813 (incidence of 8.7 per 100,000).

Race/Ethnicity Distribution

Minority populations have been disproportionally burdened with tuberculosis. Socioeconomic status is probably the most important factor explaining the differences in white and nonwhite populations, and rates of tuberculosis are inversely related to income level. Even while tuberculosis rates in the United States were decreasing prior to 1985, the rate of decrease was less for the nonwhite than the white population. From 1985 through 1992, case numbers in whites continued to decrease, albeit not as sharply, and marked increases in case numbers were observed in minority populations. For example, between 1985 and 1992, cases among non-Hispanic blacks and Hispanics increased 26.8 and 74.5 percent, respectively. As the total number of cases declined between 1992 and 1995, so did numbers in minority populations. Except for Asian/Pacific Islanders and Native Americans, decreases were seen in all minority groups.

Age

In the elderly, most tuberculosis is not a result of newly acquired infection but rather of reactivation of latent infection acquired earlier in life; it reflects prevalence of the disease at the time that infection was transmitted. Tuberculosis in infants and children, on the other hand, serves as a sentinel event of recent infection. By virtue of the patients' young age, infection in children cannot be a remote event. Further, primary tuberculosis may develop within as many as 60 percent of untreated infected infants. As the incidence of tuberculosis declined in the United States, the median age of persons with tuberculosis increased; in 1985, the median age of persons with tuberculosis was 49 years. Nearly one-third of the total cases were in persons 65 years and older. With increasing cases, in 1985, the median age of tuberculosis fell to 43 years, and there were marked increases in cases of tuberculosis in younger groups, especially in medically underserved minority populations. In non-Hispanic blacks and Hispanics, cases in those 25 to 44 years old increased by 63 and 99 percent, respectively. Accordingly, case numbers in young children, who are the likely contacts of 25- to 44-year-old adults, also increased dramatically. For children from birth up to 14 years of age, cases increased 31 and 99 percent among non-Hispanic blacks and Hispanics, respectively. Despite the decline in cases in 1993 and 1994, cases in children under 15 years have not declined appreciably.

Place of Birth

Because tuberculosis is highly endemic in some countries of Central and South America, Africa, and Asia, persons who are born in these countries are more likely to have tuberculosis than U.S.–born persons. Place of birth for persons with tuberculosis has been included in reports to CDC since 1986. In 1994, some 32 percent of all cases occurred in foreign-born persons. For the years 1986 to 1993, the rate of tuberculosis in the foreign-born was 3.7 times higher than that in the U.S.–born population (30.6 per 100,000 versus 8.1 per 100,000, respectively). For those less than 15 years old, the rate in the foreign-born was 13.2 times higher than that in the U.S.–born (2.1 per 100,000 versus 27.7 per 100,000, respectively). Of 7627 cases of tuberculosis in foreign-born persons reported in 1994, the greatest number of cases were in persons born in Mexico (24 percent), the Philippines (14 percent), and Vietnam, (11 percent).

Clinical Site of Tuberculosis

Pulmonary tuberculosis accounts for approximately 80 percent of tuberculosis reported and has the greatest public health impact because of its infectiousness. Sites of extrapulmonary tuberculosis most commonly reported are disease of the pleura, the lymphatic system, and genitourinary tract as well as miliary disease. In children, meningeal and miliary tuberculosis are more common than in adults and account for approximately 20 percent of cases reported in newborns to 4-year-olds.

HIV and Tuberculosis

Infection with HIV is the strongest risk factor known for progression from latent infection with *M. tuberculosis* to active disease. Reactivation rates for those with *M. tuberculosis* and HIV infection have been estimated at 7 to 10 percent per year, making the *yearly* risk of reactivation equivalent to the *lifetime* risk of an immunocompetent host. In addition to the increased risk of reactivation of latent infection, persons with HIV infection who become newly infected with *M. tuberculosis* have an increased risk of developing primary disease, often with rapid progression. This has been illustrated in recent outbreaks of MDR TB. In persons with HIV infection, cavitary tuberculosis is less common than in the immunocompetent host. Extrapulmonary tuberculosis, on the other hand, is more common. In HIV infection, 40 to 60 percent of patients have extrapulmonary disease, usually accompanying pulmonary disease. An individual's HIV status does not appear to increase infectiousness for uninfected individuals.

The interaction between HIV and tuberculosis is reflected in the epidemiology of both of these diseases. The changing face of tuberculosis epidemiology in the United States was signaled, in 1985, by the reversal of the downward trend of cases and mirrored the epidemiology of reported AIDS cases. The number of individuals infected with either HIV or tuberculosis was similar with regard to age, racial/ethnic background, and geographic distribution. Tuberculosis case numbers decreased or remained stable in areas of low or intermediate cumulative AIDS incidence; in areas of high cumulative AIDS incidence, case numbers rose sharply. Racial/ethnic groups with the greatest burden of AIDS cases also experienced the sharpest increases in tuberculosis cases, and it has been estimated that HIV-infected individuals accounted for at least 50 percent of the excess cases seen in the United States. A serologic survey for HIV infection among patients attending tuberculosis clinics found a prevalence of 3.4 percent. However, the range of HIV seroprevalence varied from 0 to 46 percent, and coinfection between *M. tuberculosis* and HIV was most prevalent in the northeastern United States and in non-Hispanic blacks. Pulmonary tuberculosis was not classified as an AIDS-defining criterion until 1993.

Multidrug-Resistant Tuberculosis

Drug resistance in mycobacteria comes about through random spontaneous mutation. In a large population of bacilli, there will be a number of spontaneous mutations that confer resistance to a single antituberculous drug. Thus, upon exposure to a single drug, a small subpopulation of organisms resistant to that drug will be selected and eventually may make up the entire population of infecting organisms. This phenomenon is termed *acquired drug resistance.* Thus, in all treatment of tuberculosis disease, at least two drugs to which the organism is susceptible must be used. Each drug reduces the growth of organisms that are resistant to the other agent. Drug-resistant organisms can be transmitted to others directly. Persons with drug-resistant tuberculosis who have no history of prior tuberculosis treatment are said to have primary or initial drug resistance. Drug-resistant tuberculosis has been associated with increased treatment failure, defined as the failure of treatment to produce negative cultures and cure. In trials, treatment failure in patients with drug-resistant disease was 83 times higher than in patients with drug-susceptible tuberculosis (11.6 versus 0.15 percent, respectively).

MDR TB is generally taken to involve tuberculosis caused by an organism resistant to at least isoniazid *and* rifampin, the cornerstones of tuberculosis therapy. MDR TB poses problems from both a clinical and public health perspective. It is difficult to treat and generally requires a minimum of 18 to 24 months of therapy. Resection of affected tissues may be required. Patients with MDR TB remain smear- and culture-positive longer than patients with susceptible tuberculosis even when treated with two or more effective agents.

The greatest risk factor for the presence of MDR TB is a history of prior treatment for tuberculosis. Besides those with such a history, others who are at increased risk for drug resistance include persons from foreign countries and American communities where there are high rates of MDR TB. In a nationwide survey of drug resistance, 18 percent of *M. tuberculosis* isolates from foreign-born persons had resistance to at least one antituberculous medication. Resistance to isoniazid or streptomycin, which are the drugs used most commonly for the treatment of tuberculosis outside of the United States, is seen more often in foreign-born persons with tuberculosis. There have been eight nosocomial outbreaks of MDR TB investigated by the CDC, all of which involved patients who were HIV-infected. Common features to the outbreaks that contributed to the transmission included delay in diagnosis, delay in laboratory confirmation and susceptibility results, delay in therapy, and inadequate isolation of patients with infectious tuberculosis.

INTERPERSONAL SPREAD OF TUBERCULOSIS

In 1882, Robert Koch isolated the tubercle bacillus and demonstrated that it is the causative agent of tuberculosis. Tuberculosis is transmitted by airborne spread from person to person via infected respiratory secretions. Inhalation of droplet nuclei containing the tubercle bacillus may result in infection.

Respiratory droplets are produced when someone with pulmonary tuberculosis coughs, or, in the case of laryngeal tuberculosis, with speaking. While these respiratory droplets are airborne, water evaporates, leaving small 1- to 5-μm particles called *droplet nuclei*. Because of their small size, these droplet nuclei may remain suspended in air currents for hours and, when inhaled, may escape the host's upper airway defenses. When these droplet nuclei reach the alveoli, infection may result.

Infectiousness of a tuberculosis patient is dependent on the number of tubercle bacilli expelled into the air. The bacillary load is related to a number of factors, including presence of disease in the lungs, cavity formation, disease in the airways or larynx, presence or induction of cough, failure of the patient to cover the mouth while coughing, and presence of acid-fast bacilli (AFB) on microscopic examination of sputum specimens. *The period of infectiousness may be prolonged with inappropriate therapy of tuberculosis.*

Interpersonal spread of tuberculosis may be enhanced in areas of overcrowding, poor air circulation, or recirculated, unfiltered air. Rates of tuberculous infection in exposed contacts of individuals with active tuberculosis are also dependent on the duration of exposure. Children are less infectious than adults, because the tubercle bacilli are rare in their endobronchial secretions and they lack the tussive force of adults. Tuberculosis is not transmitted by fomites such as droplets on clothing or other inanimate objects. An increase of skin-test conversions in pulmonary fellows was attributed to time spent in contact with patients in intensive care units (ICUs) and performance of invasive procedures such as endotracheal intubation and fiberoptic bronchoscopy.

PREVENTION OF INFECTION

The CDC has issued guidelines for the prevention of transmission of tuberculosis in health care settings.

- Administrative controls are designed to reduce the number of persons exposed to a potentially infectious tuberculosis patient. This includes rapid identification, isolation, diagnostic evaluation, and treatment of patients likely to have tuberculosis. Hospitalized patients with confirmed or suspected tuberculosis should remain in AFB isolation until three consecutive sputums, obtained on separate days, are AFB smear–negative.
- Health care workers should be educated about tuberculosis to promote effective work practices such as correct use of respiratory protection.
- Engineering controls are used to prevent spread of potentially infectious droplet nuclei. Patients with known or suspected tuberculosis should be placed in a private room that has negative pressure with respect to the hallway and has at least six air changes per hour. Ultraviolet germicidal irradiation is also used in some institutions. Health care workers caring for tuberculosis patients should use personal respiratory protection.
- To assess nosocomial transmission of infection, health care workers should be screened periodically by tuberculin skin testing.

Preventive Therapy: Skin Testing and Therapy

Among immunocompetent hosts, tuberculosis infection acquired in childhood progresses to active disease at some time during life in approximately 10 percent. Risk is highest in the first several years after infection (half in

TABLE 62-2 Targeted Testing: Risk Factors for Tuberculosis

Increased Risk of Exposure	Increased Risk of Active Disease
Contacts of suspected cases	HIV-positive patients
Foreign-born patients	Recent infectious exposure
Group settings	Organ-transplant patients and other
Health care workers with	immunosuppressed hosts
high-risk clients	Silicosis
Medically underserved populations	Patients with head and neck cancer
High-risk racial or ethnic groups	Patients with hematologic
Infants and children exposed	malignancy
to high-risk adults	Patients with renal failure diabetes
Intravenous drug users	Gastrectomy patients
	Weight loss as a complaint
	Previously inadequately treated tuberculosis

the first 2 years). Certain medical conditions (see Tables 62-2 and 62-3) increase the risk of disease development. The most important of these is HIV infection. In a study of injecting drug users, the yearly risk of developing tuberculosis was 7 to 10 percent in those with *M. tuberculosis* and HIV infection.

A positive tuberculin skin test indicates latent infection. Preventive therapy is directed at eliminating the small number of tubercle bacilli residing in the body that may cause disease at a later date. While PPD is the best available diagnostic aid, clinical judgment remains critical. The CDC guidelines for screening and prophylactic treatment of latent tuberculosis infection (LTBI) were changed (2000) to reflect the changing epidemiology of disease.

- Screening is now "targeted" for groups with a high incidence of infection (household contacts, persons from endemic regions, contacts with high-risk individuals), or a higher than average risk for the progression of disease if

TABLE 62-3 Impairments of Pulmonary Defenses under Conditions of Poverty

	Mechanical	Phagocytic	T Cell	B Cell	Nonspecific
Cigarette use	+	+	+	+	+
Protein-energy malnutrition	+	+	+	+/−	+
Micronutrient deficiencies					
Vitamin A	+	−	−	−	−
Vitamin D	−	+	+	−	−
Iron	+	−	+	−	−
Zinc	+	−	+	−	−
Copper	−	−	−	+	−
Alcoholism	+	+	+	+	+
AIDS	+	+	+	+	+
Stress	−	+	+	+	+
Pollutants	+	+	+	+	+
Coinfection	+	+	+	+	+

SOURCE: Adapted from Bor and Epstein.

infected (HIV, recent infections, patients with MDR TB, children under 5 years of age, organ transplantation).

- Testing is focused on identifying and treating those individuals who may serve as a reservoir of disease in the community (see Table 62-2).
- Treatment is offered to *all* individuals with untreated latent infection *regardless of age.*
- Definitions for skin-test conversion have been revised (Table 62-4).
- Treatment regimens have also been revised, particularly those for immunocompromised hosts (Tables 62-4 and 62-5). The recommendation for preventive therapy depends not only on the extent of reaction to the tuberculin skin test (i.e., millimeters of induration) but also on the patient's risk factors for developing active tuberculosis (see Tables 62-2 to 62-4).

Intradermal purified protein derivative (PPD) [5 tuberculin units (TU),1 mL] injection will detect only 10 percent of those with primary tuberculosis initially and more with disseminated disease. For individuals with a history of a strong skin test, full-strength testing may cause skin necrosis and a 1-TU test is used if considered essential. A 250-TU test is not commonly used (booster more common) for individuals with low

TABLE 62-4 Recommended Guidelines for Preventive Therapy

Induration of PPD Skin Test	Indication for Preventive Therapy
≥5 mm	HIV infection (or with known risk factor for HIV and whose HIV status is unknown) Close contacts of an infectious case Chest radiograph consistent with old, healed tuberculosis with no or incomplete prior therapy Recent contact with infected individuals Immunosuppressed individuals (organ transplantation) Individuals from regions with low incidence of nontuberculous mycobacteria
≥10 mm	Diabetes mellitus Prolonged therapy with corticosteroids Hematologic/reticuloendothelial diseases associated with decreased cellular immunity (i.e., Hodgkin's disease, leukemia) Head and neck cancer Injecting drug user known HIV-negative Substantial weight loss or malnutrition From a country with high incidence of tuberculosis (<5 years) Medically underserved, low-income population Residents/employees of correctional, mental, or extended care facilities Children under 5 years of age Health care workers with clients with active infection Workers in mycobacterial microbiology laboratory
≥15 mm	All others without above risk factors Tuberculin skin-test conversions[a]

[a]Definition of a tuberculin skin-test conversion: an increase ≥10 mm within 2 years for any age group.

TABLE 62-5 Approved Therapies for the Treatment of Latent Tuberculosis Infection[a]

Drugs	Months of therapy	Interval of therapy	HIV-Negative	HIV-Positive or other high-risk persons[b]
INH 5 mg/kg/day to 300 mg + pyridoxine 25–50 mg/day	9	qd	A	A
INH 18 mg/kg/day +pyridoxine	9	biw DOT	B	B
INH	6	qd	B	C
INH	6	biw DOT	B	C
RIF (600 mg/day) + PZA (15–20 mg/kg/day)[a]	2	qd	B	B (?A)
RIF (600 mg/day) + PZA (50 mg/kg/day)[a]	2–3	biw DOT	C	C
RIF	4	qd	B	B

KEY: A, preferred; B, acceptable if necessary for compliance/directly observed therapy; C, use only when A and B not possible; DOT, directly observed therapy, used for compliance issues in twice-weekly (biw) regimens. Adult dosages only. Isoniazid (INH) used only with assumption of INH susceptibility. INH should not be given in first trimester of pregnancy if there is a likelihood of progression to active disease thought to be low; RIF/PZA, rifampin/pyrazinamide. For adverse effects of INH or INH-resistance (multidrug-resistant TB) likely. Rifampin (600 mg/day) plus pyrazinamide. Rifabutin may be considered as an alternative. Maximum recommended dose is 300 mg/day, but IDSA has recommended higher doses for use of single agent in high-risk individuals (600 mg/day). In some regimens ethambutol (15 to 25 mg/kg/day PO) or fluoroquinolone (levofloxacin 500 mg/day PO) have been substituted for rifampin with higher-dose PZA (25 to 30 mg/kg/day to a maximum of 2 g/day); however, the efficacy of these regimens is unproven [see *MMWR*, 49 (RR-6): 1–54, 2000]; HAART, highly active antiretroviral therapy.
[a] Severe hepatitis may occur with rifampin and pyrazinamide regimens [*MMWR* 50(34):733–735, 2001].
[b] HIV infection, new infection (skin-test conversion in past 2 years), old TB by chest x-ray; intravenous drug use, immunosuppression, lymphohematopoietic or head/neck cancer, renal failure, prior gastrectomy. Some prefer 12-month regimens for HIV-positive individuals. Role of HAART unclear, but those with decreased active disease still need therapy.

reactivity. PPD positivity to the standard 5-TU intradermal test is defined as follows:

- Induration of > 5 mm is positive for individuals considered at highest risk of progression from latent to active tuberculosis. These include HIV-positive, recent contacts of individuals with known tuberculosis, patients with chest radiographs suggestive of old tuberculosis, and immunosuppressed individuals. In areas with low incidence of atypical or nontuberculous mycobacteria, 5 mm of induration should suggest tuberculosis.
- Induration of >10 mm is considered positive for those individuals who do not meet the above criteria but have other risk factors for tuberculosis: those

from endemic regions (<5 years), high-risk groups, or group homes; intravenous drug users; and health care workers with infected clients.
• Induration of >15 mm is positive in persons without significant risk factors for tuberculosis.

All persons with positive PPD tests are candidates for therapy regardless of age.

False-Positive Reactions

A small percentage of tuberculin reactions may be caused by errors in administering the test or in reading results. However, false-positive results are commonly attributable to the presence in tuberculin of antigens shared with other mycobacteria. The potential sources of cross-reactions caused by these antigens are infection with nontuberculous mycobacteria and vaccination with bacille Calmette-Guérin (BCG). The larger the induration, however, the greater is the likelihood that the reaction represents infection with *M. tuberculosis.* The probability that a skin test reaction results from infection with *M. tuberculosis* rather than from BCG vaccination increases (1) as the size of the reaction increases, (2) when the patient is a contact of a person who has tuberculosis (especially if that person has infected others), (3) when a family history of tuberculosis exists or when the patient's country of origin has a high incidence or prevalence of tuberculosis, and (4) as the interval between vaccination and tuberculin testing increases (because vaccination-induced reactivity wanes over time and is unlikely to persist for more than 10 years). A history of BCG vaccination is not a contraindication to skin testing.

False-Negative Reactions

False-negative tuberculin skin test reactions have many potential causes. Nonresponsiveness to delayed-type hypersensitivity–inducing antigens like tuberculin is common among persons with impaired immunity (e.g., HIV-infected persons). Delayed-type hypersensitivity can be assessed with skin test antigens such as tetanus toxoid, mumps, and *Candida.* Most healthy persons are sensitized to these antigens. However, the scientific basis for anergy testing is tenuous and most skin test antigens used for anergy testing have no standardization. Thus, anergy testing is usually not part of screening for tuberculosis infection.

All HIV-infected persons should be tuberculin tested. Those who are tuberculin-positive (greater than or equal to 5 mm) should be evaluated for tuberculosis disease and placed on appropriate curative or preventive therapy. Preventive therapy should be administered to tuberculin-positive, HIV-infected persons regardless of age. If they are at high risk for tuberculosis, persons failing to react to tuberculin may be evaluated for anergy, although the lack of standardization of anergy testing practices should be considered.

Booster Phenomenon and Two-Step Tuberculin Skin Testing

Periodic use of the tuberculin skin test is valuable for the surveillance of tuberculin-negative persons at risk for exposure to *M. tuberculosis.* Repeated testing of uninfected persons does not sensitize them to tuberculin. However, delayed-type hypersensitivity resulting from mycobacterial infection or BCG vaccination will wane with years. Although subsequent initial skin test results may be negative, the stimulus of a first test may boost or increase the size of the reaction to a second test administered 1 week to 1 to 2 years later and thus may suggest an apparent—but false—tuberculin conversion.

Although the booster phenomenon may occur at any age, its frequency increases with age and is highest among persons more than 55 years of age and those who have had prior BCG vaccination. When tuberculin skin testing of adults is repeated periodically, as in employee health or institutional screening programs, an initial two-step approach can reduce the likelihood that a boosted reaction will be misinterpreted as the sign of a recent infection. If the first tuberculin test result is negative, a second 5-TU test should be administered 1 to 3 weeks later. A positive second result probably indicates boosting from a past infection or prior BCG vaccination. Persons having a boosted reaction should be classified as reactors, not converters. If the second result is negative, the person is probably uninfected, and a positive reaction to subsequent tests indicates a true tuberculin skin-test conversion (see "Definition of a Tuberculin Skin-Test Conversion," below).

Because of problems with continued cross-reactions with other mycobacteria, the specificity of the tuberculin test is less when serial skin testing is performed than when a single test is administered. Thus, serial skin-testing programs tend to overestimate the incidence of new tuberculosis infection in the tested population. Because of this potential for overestimation of incidence, serial skin-testing programs should be targeted to populations at high risk for continued exposure to infectious tuberculosis.

Definition of a Tuberculin Skin-Test Conversion

Recent tuberculin skin-test converters are considered at high risk. An increase in induration of greater than or equal to 10 mm within a 2-year period is classified as a conversion to a positive test among persons less than 35 years of age. An increase in induration of greater than or equal to 15 mm within a 2-year period is classified as a conversion for persons at least 35 years of age. Immunocompromised individuals should be considered PPD-positive for >5-mm induration regardless of prior status. Regardless of age, for employees in facilities where a person who has tuberculosis poses a hazard to many susceptible persons (e.g., health care facilities, schools, and child care facilities), an increase of greater than or equal to 10-mm induration should be considered positive.

Tuberculin Testing during Pregnancy

Studies in which the same patients were tested during and after pregnancy have demonstrated that pregnancy has no effect on cutaneous tuberculin hypersensitivity. Tuberculin skin testing is considered valid and safe throughout pregnancy. No teratogenic effects of testing during pregnancy have been documented.

Treatment of Latent Tuberculosis

A variety of regimens are now available for the treatment of latent tuberculous infection (LTBI) (see Table 62-5). Isoniazid (INH) is the single agent used most commonly in preventive therapy. The drug is given as a single daily dose of 5 to 10 mg/kg, not to exceed 300 mg/day. Hepatotoxicity and peripheral neuropathy are the most commonly seen adverse effects. Pyridoxine (25 to

50 mg/day) should be provided with any regimen containing INH. No more than 1 month of prescriptions should be given at one time (unless essential) to assure follow-up for signs of hepatitis. When considering the use of INH preventive therapy, the clinician must weigh the risk of INH toxicity during therapy against the lifetime risk of development of active tuberculosis. Because INH hepatotoxicity is age-related, INH preventive therapy was previously offered only to those younger than 35 years of age. However, in those who are at high risk of developing active tuberculosis, preventive therapy is now recommended regardless of age. Baseline liver function testing should be performed in anyone with liver disease, liver transplantation, or HIV; those who are pregnant or have recently given birth; users of other potentially hepatotoxic drugs or alcohol; or those over age 35. It is important to exclude active tuberculosis prior to initiating prophylaxis to avoid treatment of active disease with a single agent and potential emergence of resistance. General guidelines for the management of patients receiving INH include the following:

- Monitor for hepatitis and peripheral neuropathy.
- Pregnancy: await delivery in pregnant patients with LTBI except if there are significant risk factors for progression to active disease. Await end of first trimester in all patients if possible.
- Nursing is not a contraindication to INH.
- Screen household and other close contacts immediately and again after 3 months.

For those who have completed a full course of INH preventive therapy with good compliance, reduction in rates of tuberculosis may be as great as 70 percent. There is no evidence to suggest that preventive therapy with INH will lead to the development of INH resistance. If the infecting organism is thought likely to have primary INH resistance, INH preventive therapy will be of little benefit. For persons who are contacts of a source case with an isolate that is INH-resistant and rifampin-susceptible, rifampin is recommended as preventive therapy at a dose of 10 mg/kg per day, not to exceed 600 mg/day. There are few data on the use of this agent for preventive therapy in normal hosts; this use may be recommended based on experience in HIV-infected individuals with LTBI. Because of the difficulty of treatment of MDR TB, which carries higher morbidity and mortality, alternative preventive therapy for bacilli resistant to both INH and rifampin should be considered, especially in persons with a high risk of tuberculosis. Combinations of pyrazinamide, ethambutol, and a fluoroquinolone are usually used. There are no data on the efficacy of these alternative preventive therapy regimens. Before initiating one of these alternative regimens, physicians should seek advice from experts in the management of MDR TB. Severe liver injury has been associated with use of rifampin-pyrazinamide regimens for LTBI (CDC). The 2-month regimen should be used with caution, especially in those taking other medications or ethanol with potential hepatotoxicity. Close follow-up is needed.

BCG VACCINE

In 1908 Albert Calmette and Camille Guérin began to subculture a strain of *M. tuberculosis* from a cow with tuberculous mastitis. After 13 years and 230 serial subcultures, the strain was no longer virulent in animals, and in 1921 use of bacille Calmette-Guérin (BCG) in humans was begun. This is a live vaccine, and it is the most widely used vaccine in the world today. Due to genetic variation of strains and differences in production techniques, not all BCG vaccines are identical. *The vaccine does not protect against infection with the tubercle bacilli,* and the efficacy of BCG in preventing active disease has ranged from 20 to 80 percent in trials conducted. Explanations for this variability in vaccine efficacy may be related to differences in environmental mycobacteria, ethnic and race-based variations in immune responses, and different strains of BCG. Exposure to and infection with environmental mycobacteria may provide cross-protection against tuberculosis, and BCG may add little to that protection. In one meta-analysis of 26 trials, the estimated protective effect of BCG was 50 percent.

Vaccination with BCG usually produces a reaction to the tuberculin skin test, and there is no reliable way to distinguish tuberculin sensitivity caused by vaccination with BCG from natural infection with *M. tuberculosis.* Reactivity wanes over time and, in the absence of infection with *M. tuberculosis,* is not likely to persist over 10 years after vaccination. A diagnosis of *M. tuberculosis* infection should be considered for a BCG-vaccinated person with a positive skin test if any of the following conditions are met: (1) the size of the skin test induration is >10 mm, (2) there is history of contact with a person with tuberculosis, (3) there is a family history of tuberculosis, (4) the person's country of origin has a high prevalence of tuberculosis, or (5) several years have passed between vaccination and tuberculin skin testing. Administration of BCG is not a contraindication to tuberculin skin testing.

CLINICAL INFECTIONS WITH MYCOBACTERIA

Microbiology of Mycobacteria: Collection and Transportation of Specimens

The isolation of *M. tuberculosis* is the "gold standard" for the diagnosis of tuberculosis. A positive direct smear for acid-fast bacilli (AFB) in the proper setting may serve as presumptive evidence for tuberculosis but may also represent nontuberculous mycobacteria, known as mycobacteria other than tuberculosis (MOTT) (Table 62-6). These two groups of mycobacteria are indistinguishable on direct smear—with the exception of *M. kansasii,* which can be suspected from its larger size and banded appearance. In addition, 50 percent of patients whose cultures are positive will have a negative acid-fast smear. Thus, culture of *M. tuberculosis* is the only absolute way of confirming the diagnosis and to obtain antimicrobial susceptibility data.

Proper collection and transportation of specimens to be examined are critical. Early-morning sputum specimens, collected after awakening, have the highest yield in demonstrating AFB, since they represent secretions accumulated overnight. For ambulatory patients whose sputum specimens are collected in the clinic as well as for institutionalized patients with scant sputum production, sputum induction is desirable. Freshly expectorated sputum is the best sample to stain and culture for *M. tuberculosis.* Sputum samples more than 24 h old are frequently overgrown with mouth flora and are much less useful. If a patient is not spontaneously producing sputum, induced sputum is the next best specimen for study. It can be obtained by having the patient breathe an aerosol of isotonic or hypertonic saline for 5 to 15 min. If the patient cannot cooperate to give a spontaneous sputum sample, a gastric aspirate may be useful. Early-morning gastric lavage contains pulmonary secretions swallowed during sleep. Sterile water should be

TABLE 62-6 Genus *Mycobacterium*

Mycobacteria associated with human disease:
  Mycobacterium tuberculosis complex
    M. tuberculosis
    M. bovis
    M. africanum
  Mycobacterium avium complex
    M. avium
    M. intracellulare
  Mycobacterium scrofulaceum
  Mycobacterium kansasii
  Mycobacterium genavense
  Mycobacterium xenopi
  Mycobacterium szulgai
  Mycobacterium malmoense
  Mycobacterium haemophilum
  Mycobacterium marinum
  Mycobacterium ulcerans
  Mycobacterium leprae
  Mycobacterium fortuitum-chelonae complex
    M. fortuitum
    M. chelonae
Usually saprophytic mycobacteria:
  Mycobacterium gordonae
  Mycobacterium terrae complex
  Mycobacterium flavescens
  Mycobacterium smegmatis

used and Na_2CO_3 powder added to the bottle to neutralize gastric acid and protect the bacilli. This sample must be obtained in the morning, before the patient arises or eats.

Bronchoscopy to obtain specimens should be reserved until attempts to obtain proper spontaneously expectorated or induced specimens have failed and/or after proper initial specimens have been reported negative for AFB and confirmation or exclusion of mycobacterial disease remains essential. Sputum induction facilities and bronchoscopy suites should be equipped with negative airflow, and employees should wear appropriate respirators.

Other specimens submitted for mycobacterial examinations are urine, cerebrospinal fluid, joint and pleural fluid, and tissue biopsy specimens. Specimens should be transported for immediate processing but may be refrigerated to prevent overgrowth with contaminating organisms. A minimum number of three and preferably five sputum specimens should be obtained for staining and culture because of the fluctuation of the number of bacilli found. Once two initial direct smears are reported to yield AFB, additional pretreatment specimens may serve only to enhance the risk of infection to health care workers. To monitor the effectiveness of treatment for pulmonary tuberculosis, additional specimens need to be collected at weekly or biweekly intervals until at least two consecutive specimens are reported negative for AFB. A new series of specimens should be collected if there is clinical or radiologic suspicion of treatment failure or reactivation of the disease.

In most patients, the procedures mentioned above will be successful in providing positive material for culture. Smears of gastric contents for acid-fast bacilli are of limited value and are not recommended because of the presence of nontuberculous ingested AFB. However, gastric aspiration may be especially useful in the diagnosis of tuberculosis in infants, in whom the collection of spontaneous or induced sputum is almost impossible. In 75 percent of infants with pulmonary tuberculosis, the gastric aspirate can be positive. In a few cases, one may have to resort to bronchoscopy. The local anesthetics used during fiberoptic bronchoscopy may be lethal to *M. tuberculosis,* so specimens for culture should be obtained with a minimal amount of anesthesia. Irritation of the bronchial tree during the bronchoscopy procedure will frequently leave the patient with a productive cough. Thus, collection of the postbronchoscopy sputum can be another valuable source of diagnostic material.

Obtaining diagnostic culture material is not always possible. In 1994, only 80.2 percent of tuberculosis reported to the CDC had the diagnosis confirmed by positive cultures. In an additional 1.0 percent of the cases, only the smear was positive. In 11.5 percent of reported cases, both smears and cultures were reported as negative. Thus, in a significant number of cases, the diagnosis of tuberculosis was made in the absence of bacteriologic confirmation. In these cases, the diagnosis was made by a combination of a positive skin test, a compatible chest radiograph, and a therapeutic trial.

Direct Microscopic Examination

Direct examination of specimens by acid-fast stain is the first procedure performed on all specimens sent to the mycobacteriology laboratory. The presence of AFB provides supportive evidence of mycobacterial disease days or weeks before the culture report and final identification of the organism are available. In the proper setting, it may establish the need for isolation and prompt treatment of the patient. The standard acid-fast stain is the Ziehl-Neelsen procedure. The term *acid-fast* refers to the fact that dilute acids fail to remove basic dyes such as carbolfuchsin from the mycobacterial cell wall, owing to its lipid-rich complex structure. Review of acid-fast smears may require hours of time for proper examination by high-power, oil-immersion microscopy.

The fluorochrome acid-fast stain has replaced the standard Ziehl-Neelsen stain in many laboratories because it is more sensitive and allows the technician to review the slide at lower power, without oil. A larger number of fields can be examined in a much shorter time. A fluorescent microscope is required for the procedure, but most modern laboratories are equipped with this.

Microscopic examination is the most rapid diagnostic method available, but has relatively low sensitivity. More than 10,000 bacilli per milliliter are required for the average technician to demonstrate a positive result. This number may be as low as 1000 bacilli per milliliter using the fluorochrome stain with proper sputum concentration technique. The yield of microscopic examination also correlates with the extent of disease, the presence of cavitation, and the quality of the specimen. It is a good marker for the infectiousness and the response to treatment. A decrease in the number of organisms in sputum specimens during the first few weeks indicates response to treatment.

Direct smear-negative/culture-positive sputum specimens are frequently encountered in cases of pulmonary tuberculosis with minimal disease. This phenomenon may sometimes be found even in recent tuberculin converters with no radiologic abnormalities. The reverse may be seen in cases with advanced cavitary lesions with a significant amount of necrotic material. These patients may continue to excrete nonviable AFB for extended periods, sometimes for many months, with negative cultures. Occasionally, direct smear-positive/culture-negative reports may indicate bacilli with attenuated viability due to suboptimal chemotherapy.

For proper interpretations of the results of bacteriologic tests, it is crucial to consider the quality of the specimen submitted. The presence of elastic fibers in sputum wet mounts with potassium hydroxide indicates tissue necrosis and hence the fact that a proper specimen has been obtained.

CONVENTIONAL CULTURE TECHNIQUES

The traditional culture techniques followed by biochemical tests for the identification of mycobacteria require 4 to 8 weeks or more. Culturing of sputum and other specimens requires concentration of the material. Specimens from nonsterile sites need to be decontaminated. After such processing, specimens should be inoculated into both liquid and solid media. The solid medium may be the BACTEC 460 12B bottle or the Mycobacterium Growth Indicator Tube (MGIT)—both of which are manufactured by Becton Dickinson Laboratories, Cockeysville, MD—or one of the "automated" broth culture media. The latter are liquid media in bottles, whose contents are read out spectrophotometrically for the presence of one or more gases that indicate metabolism of mycobacterial organisms. Solid media can be any combination of egg based (Lowenstein-Jensen, for example) or non–egg based (Middlebrook). The broth and solid media will often be supplemented with antibiotics to further reduce the chance of contamination of the cultures. A biphasic medium, the Septi-check bottle (Becton Dickinson), is also available for isolation of mycobacteria. While it affords good overall recovery of mycobacterial isolates, it does not provide the timeliness that one derives from liquid media such as BACTEC or MGIT.

The broth culture medium provides for a turnaround time of about 10 to 12 days for *M. tuberculosis* and even less for many of the MOTT organisms. The agar medium requires about 3 to 4 weeks for colonies to be seen macroscopically. The use of a dissecting scope allows for the detection of "microcolonies" on solid media in 10 to 12 days—comparable to the time needed for liquid media. Once an isolate is recovered in broth or on solid media, identification should proceed as rapidly as possible. The *p*-nitroalpha-acetylamino-beta-hydroxy-propiophenone (NAP) test, a gene probe, or high-performance liquid chromatography (HPLC) should be employed. The conventional biochemical confirmation of *M. tuberculosis*—i.e., niacin positivity, nitrate positivity, and the presence of an unstable catalase—requires 3 to 4 weeks after isolation. The NAP test requires about 4 to 5 days, gene probes about 2 1/2 h, and HPLC about 5 to 8 h.

One of the most impressive recent developments has been the use of amplification of nucleic acids directly within the clinical specimen to avoid the delays of culturing. These amplification procedures require about 5 to 6 h of processing and are currently specific for *M. tuberculosis* complex only. A possible drawback is the fact that nonviable mycobacterial organisms may produce positive results. Moreover, many laboratories are unable to afford the high cost entailed. This is especially true in areas with a low incidence of tuberculosis. The sensitivity of these assays with smear-negative specimens has been only about 70 percent. Inconclusive tests are common with low levels of infection. DNA fingerprinting of mycobacterial DNA allows for the identification of individual strains of *M. tuberculosis*. DNA fingerprinting is based on analysis of the distribution of specific insertion sequences (e.g., IS6110) within the mycobacterial genome. Individual strains have their own banding pattern (restriction fragment length polymorphism, or RFLP). In addition to its diagnostic value, this procedure has proved to be extremely helpful in epidemiologic investigations to establish a link between cases in outbreaks of tuberculosis in various institutions and other congregate settings. Coupled with amplifications by the polymerase chain reaction (PCR), this link may alert the clinician to the presence of a specific drug-resistant isolate, allowing for the prompt selection of an effective drug regimen.

ANTIMICROBIAL SUSCEPTIBILITY TESTING

A poor therapeutic outcome is likely when chemotherapeutic agents are used to which more than 1 percent of bacilli in a given population demonstrate in vitro resistance. Drug susceptibility tests are performed by comparing the amount of growth in a medium containing various concentrations of the drugs with that in a control medium—i.e., one containing no drugs. The conventional method for susceptibility testing takes up to 4 weeks. This period may be significantly reduced by use of the BACTEC radiometric system. All *M. tuberculosis* clinical isolates should be tested.

SEROLOGIC DIAGNOSIS

Mycobacteria are rich in antigens that stimulate the production of antibodies and lymphokines. The development of a satisfactory serologic test should therefore be feasible. Attempts to develop such a test have been based on enzyme-linked immunosorbent assays (ELISA) and radioimmunoassays. To date, no test is available that meets criteria for its widespread use based on a high level of sensitivity, specificity, and relative simplicity.

CLINICAL IMPLICATIONS OF MYCOBACTERIA OTHER THAN *M. TUBERCULOSIS* (MOTT)

Historically, MOTT isolates from human material have been called paratuberculosis, opportunistic, pseudotubercle, unclassified, atypical, nontuberculous, and tuberculoid bacilli. Reported differences between MOTT and *M. tuberculosis* pulmonary disease are that MOTT tend to produce more thinwalled cavities with less pericavitary infiltrate and less frequently cause pleural effusions. The tuberculin skin test in MOTT disease may be entirely nonreactive or produce only small indurations. The clinical spectrum of disease caused by some MOTT has changed since their initial recognition. During the past quarter of a century, for instance, we observed a shift of pulmonary disease caused by *M. avium-intracellulare* complex (MAC) from afflicting predominantly middle-aged and elderly men with preexisting pulmonary disease to disease affecting increasing numbers of women with minor or no prior pulmonary pathology. During the past decade, the great majority of MAC encounters occurred as disseminated disease in patients with AIDS and other forms of immune compromise. In addition to MAC, the most frequent MOTT causes of human disease are *M. kansasii, M. marinum, M. fortuitum–M. chelonei complex,* and *M. scrofulaceum* (see Table 62-6).

M. tuberculosis is by far the most frequent cause of mycobacterial disease in the lungs. An organism that grows slowly, is nonpigmented, and is niacin-positive is likely to represent *M. tuberculosis.* Further confirmatory tests are necessary, the most recently developed being susceptibility to NAP.

M. bovis has been virtually eradicated in the United States and some other industrialized countries by destruction of tuberculin-positive cattle, which can spread the infection through milk. BCG, a low-virulence strain, is used for immunization against tuberculosis. This strain is occasionally the cause of disseminated disease in persons with certain cancers, to whom it has been administered therapeutically as a nonspecific potentiator of immunity or as local therapy for bladder cancer.

The third representative of *M. tuberculosis* complex, *M. africanum,* has characteristics intermediate between *M. tuberculosis* and *M. bovis.*

MAC, consisting of two organisms, *M. avium* and *M. intracellulare,* is by far the most frequent MOTT species associated with human disease. As mentioned earlier, MAC is a frequent cause of fatal disseminated disease in AIDS patients. The components can be separated by DNA probe technique and by seroagglutination. On the basis of glycolipid typing antigens, some 28 seroagglutination types are recognized. Unlike *M. tuberculosis,* all strains of MAC are naturally resistant to standard antituberculosis drugs. MAC is widely distributed in nature and may be found in soil and water and in various birds and mammals.

M. scrofulaceum is sometimes grouped with MAC because of shared genetic characteristics. The extended complex is then referred to as MAIS complex. *M. scrofulaceum* is a known cause of cervical adenitis in children and rarely causes pulmonary disease. It has been found in soil, water, and dairy products.

M. kansasii may be suspected in stained smears as large, cross-barred bacilli. Colonies are photochromogenic, developing pigment after exposure to light. Although it can be found in water, an *M. kansasii* isolate is more likely to represent a real pathogen than is the case with most other MOTT. It is the second most frequent cause of human disease among the MOTT; it usually causes pulmonary disease, although other organs may be affected. The disease responds very well to treatment with antituberculosis drugs in spite of some degree of resistance to isoniazid.

M. xenopi is peculiar for its geographic distribution and for the fact that its optimal growth temperature of 42 to 45°C is higher than that for other mycobacteria. Although it is rarely isolated in most parts of the world, its relative frequency is high in southeastern England, in Ontario, Canada, and in Scandinavian countries. It usually affects the lungs, and some outbreaks have been related to contamination of hot-water tanks. The response to drug treatment is variable.

M. marinum and *M. ulcerans* produce skin lesions. More benign lesions are caused by *M. marinum* from abrasions acquired in fish tanks, contaminated swimming pools (swimming pool or fish-tank granuloma), or in seal bites in aquarium workers ("seal finger"). The organism is photochromogenic and is generally susceptible to rifampin, ethambutol, and amikacin but resistant to isoniazid. *M. ulcerans* causes more severe necrotizing disease and is encountered in tropical areas, primarily in Africa, Australia, and Mexico. The disease is known as Bairndale ulcer in Australia and as Buruli ulcer in Uganda.

M. haemophilum almost exclusively affects immunosuppressed persons, in whom it causes painful subcutaneous nodules. The nodules may resolve spontaneously or develop suppuration and ulceration. This organism requires hemin or other iron sources for its growth in media.

M. fortuitum-chelonae complex is a group of rapidly growing mycobacteria. *M. chelonae* also known as *M. abscessus,* has been mostly associated with wound abscesses, although occasional reports of this organism as the cause of pulmonary disease have appeared in the literature. *M. fortuitum* is the occasional cause of pulmonary disease. Both organisms are found in the soil. *M. fortuitum* and *M. chelonae* are resistant to the first-line antituberculosis drugs. Isolates of *M. fortuitum* are usually susceptible to amikacin, ciprofloxacin, and sulfonamides, whereas isolates of *M. chelonae* are frequently susceptible to amikacin. Individual strains may be susceptible to other antimicrobial agents.

DISTINGUISHING MOTT FROM TUBERCULOSIS

The similarity of MOTT to *M. tuberculosis* is not restricted to the morphology by direct smear. Many organisms in the MOTT category cause disease that is clinically, radiologically, and histopathologically indistinguishable from tuberculosis. The main differences between the two groups are that the MOTT are ubiquitous environmental organisms and not transmitted from person to person. Disease caused by this group of organisms is therefore not infectious and does not require contact investigation. Most patients with progressive pulmonary disease caused by MOTT have preexisting chronic pulmonary disease such as bronchiectasis, pneumoconiosis, or healed tuberculosis or fungal disease. Isoniazid preventive therapy for tuberculosis is very effective; there is more limited experience in the prevention of MOTT disease in AIDS which suggests that improved survivals may be achieved with appropriate prophylaxis. Other differences are the sensitivity patterns to the usual antituberculosis drugs. There are also definite biochemical differences.

Some MOTT are not pathogenic; moreover, an isolation of even potentially pathogenic MOTT often represents contamination or the presence of a saprophytic relationship or colonization. An *M. tuberculosis* isolate, on the other hand, should be considered pathogenic. Rare exceptions include a single isolate from a usually nonsterile site such as sputum, especially when this includes a very low colony count. Such isolates may be the result of cross-contamination in the laboratory or during collection or transportation of the specimen.

Because MOTT organisms often appear as colonizers and because of their ubiquitous presence, it is clear that the mere isolation of a specific MOTT organism from a specimen does not necessarily establish the diagnosis of disease caused by that organism. There must be pathologic changes present that are consistent with disease caused by the MOTT under consideration. Other reasonable causes of the pathologic findings should be ruled out, and generally one expects evidence of progressive disease with multiple isolates. A single isolate is acceptable in the proper setting—for instance, when found in conjunction with histologic evidence of mycobacterial disease.

CLINICAL PRESENTATIONS OF PULMONARY TUBERCULOSIS

Signs and Symptoms

Because *M. tuberculosis* grows relatively slowly, pulmonary tuberculosis frequently develops insidiously without any striking clinical evidence of disease. Two major clinical syndromes are recognized. The first occurs with primary infection, and the second occurs with reactivation of latent or dormant foci.

The initial localized infection usually results in few or no clinical symptoms or signs. At the onset of tuberculin hypersensitivity (immune responses at 4 to 6 weeks), mild fever and malaise may develop, and occasionally other hypersensitivity manifestations (e.g., erythema nodosum) are noted. Thus, the initial infection with *M. tuberculosis* frequently is unrecognized. In general, only patients with some degree of immune suppression present with primary tuberculosis. This includes children under 1 year old, HIV-positive subjects, organ transplant recipients, and patients on chemotherapy. In most patients, the organism remains dormant either indefinitely or for many years, and when disease occurs, it may be secondary to a decrease in body immunity (Table 62-7).

Symptoms may be divided into two categories, systemic and pulmonary. Low-grade fever is the most frequently observed systemic symptom with more significant temperature elevations as disease progresses. The fever may develop in the late afternoon and may not be accompanied by pronounced symptoms. With defervescence, usually during sleep, sweating occurs ("night sweats"). Other systemic signs of toxemia—such as malaise, irritability, weakness, unusual fatigue, headache, and weight loss—may be present. In some reviews, cough, anorexia, and weight loss were the most common symptoms. With the development of caseation necrosis and concomitant liquefaction of the caseous area, the patient will usually notice cough and sputum, often associated with mild hemoptysis. Up to 10 percent of patients with a chronic productive cough may have active tuberculosis. Chest pain is often localized and pleuritic. Shortness of breath usually indicates extensive disease, with widespread involvement of the lung and parenchyma or some form of tracheobronchial obstruction, and therefore usually occurs late in the disease.

Physical examination of the chest is often completely normal early in the disease. The principal findings over areas of infiltration are posttussive rales (fine rales detected on deep inspiration, followed by full expiration and a hard cough). These are usually detected in the apexes of the lungs, where reactivation disease is most common. Percussion of the clavicles may reveal

---

TABLE 62-7 Populations with Increased Susceptibility to Tuberculosis

Nonspecific decrease in resistance
  Adolescence
  Senescence
  Malnutrition
Postgastrectomy state
  Uremia
  Diabetes mellitus
Decrease in resistance due to hormonal effects
  Pregnancy
  Therapy with adrenocortical steroids
Decrease in local resistance
  Silicosis
Decrease in specific immunity
  Lymphomas
  Immunosuppressive therapy
  Sarcoidosis
  Live virus vaccination
  HIV infection

dullness as the disease progresses. Other findings will also be present. Allergic manifestations may occur, usually developing at the time of onset of infection. These include erythema nodosum and phlyctenular conjunctivitis. The former is due to circulating immune complexes, with resultant localized vascular damage. Initially, erythema nodosum occurs in the dependent portion of the body and, if the reaction is severe, may be followed by a more disseminated process.

Laboratory Examination

Although routine laboratory examinations (Table 62-8) are rarely helpful in establishing the diagnosis, they may suggest the presence of a chronic inflammatory condition. A mild normochromic normocytic anemia may be present in chronic tuberculosis. The WBC count is often normal, and counts over 20,000/mL would suggest another infectious process; a leukemoid reaction may occasionally occur in miliary tuberculosis, but not in tuberculosis confined to the chest. Although a "left shift" in the differential WBC count can occur in advanced disease, WBC changes are neither specific nor useful. Other nonspecific tests may be elevated in active tuberculosis (sedimentation rate, alpha$_2$ globulins, and gamma globulin). Pyuria without bacteria on Gram's stain suggests renal involvement. Liver enzymes (transaminases and alkaline phosphatase) may occasionally be elevated before treatment. However, this finding is usually due to concomitant liver disease secondary to other problems, such as alcoholism, rather than to tuberculous involvement. On rare occasions, the serum sodium is low, owing to inappropriate secretion of antidiuretic hormone. This only occurs in advanced pulmonary tuberculosis.

A positive delayed hypersensitivity reaction to tuberculin (as discussed above) indicates the occurrence of a prior primary infection but not necessarily clinically active disease. However, very large reactions (greater than 25 mm of induration) are more frequently associated with active tuberculosis than smaller reactions. A negative reaction to tuberculin does not rule out the diagnosis, because the patient may be anergic or have specific anergy to tuberculin. Older persons with tuberculosis have a lower rate of tuberculin positivity than young adults.

TABLE 62-8 Biochemical Abnormalities in 265 Patients with Pulmonary Tuberculosis

Abnormality	Percent of patients with abnormality
Anemia	60
Leukocytosis with neutrophilia	40
Lymphopenia	17
Monocytopenia	50
Thrombocytosis	52
Sedimentation rate	80
Increased ferritin	94
Increased B$_{12}$	57
Abnormal RBC folic acid	17
Increased liver function tests	33
Hyponatremia	43
Hypoalbuminemia	72

SOURCE: Adapted from Morris et al., with permission.

Chest Radiography

Despite the introduction of new techniques for the radiographic evaluation of pulmonary lesions, the simple posteroanterior chest radiograph remains the primary laboratory test for suggesting the diagnosis of pulmonary tuberculosis.

Primary Tuberculosis

The most common radiographic appearance of primary tuberculosis is a normal radiograph. In primary tuberculosis, parenchymal involvement can occur in any segment of the lung. The airspace consolidation appears as a homogeneous density with ill-defined borders, and cavitation is rare except in malnourished or otherwise immunocompromised patients. Miliary involvement at the onset is seen in fewer than 3 percent of cases, most commonly in children under 2 years of age. An isolated pleural effusion of mild to moderate degree may be the only manifestation of primary tuberculosis.

Hilar or paratracheal lymph node enlargement with or without a parenchymal infiltrate is a characteristic finding in primary tuberculosis. In 15 percent of the cases, bilateral hilar adenopathy may be present and could be confused with sarcoidosis. Usually, the adenopathy is unilateral. Unilateral hilar adenopathy and unilateral hilar and paratracheal adenopathy are equally common. Massive hilar adenopathy may herald a complicated course. Atelectasis with an obstructive pneumonia may result from bronchial compression by inflamed lymph nodes or from a caseous lymph node that ruptures into a bronchus.

Reactivation Tuberculosis

In 95 percent of localized pulmonary tuberculosis, the lesions will be present in the apical or posterior segment of the upper lobes or the superior segment of the lower lobes, although reactivation tuberculosis may affect any lung segment. If only the anterior segment of the upper lobe is affected, tuberculosis is extremely unlikely. A person with lesions reported as inactive or stable by radiography can have sputum smears and cultures that are positive for *M. tuberculosis.*

The most common pattern of reactivation tuberculosis is of a focal airspace consolidation in a patchy or confluent nature. Frequently, linear densities connect to the ipsilateral hilum. Cavitation is common, but lymph node enlargement is rare. Because the lesions are usually chronic, destruction of tissue, fibrosis, calcification, and volume loss are usually present in the affected lung. The combination of patchy pneumonitis, fibrosis, and calcification should always suggest chronic granulomatous disease, usually tuberculosis.

Although the cavities that develop in tuberculosis usually have a moderately thick wall, a smooth inner surface, and no air-fluid level, thin- or thick-walled cavities, with or without air-fluid levels and little or extensive parenchymal infiltrate, can be observed in tuberculosis. Cavitation is frequently associated with endobronchial spread of disease. Radiographically, endobronchial spread appears as multiple small acinar shadows, usually in the superior segment of the lower lobes.

Besides the simple posteroanterior chest radiograph, lordotic films may be useful for demonstrating apical disease. Computed tomography may raise the suspicion of tuberculosis when cavitary lesions or multifocal lesions are observed that were not suspected on the plain film. In MDR disease, documentation of the extent of disease may be important if surgery is being considered. Currently, magnetic resonance imaging has little role in pulmonary tuberculosis.

Differential Diagnosis

Today, tuberculosis is a disease most frequently present in persons above 25 years of age. In adults, primary tuberculosis is becoming more common and may appear as a lower-lobe pneumonia. Young adults usually present with more symptoms (especially fever and night sweats) than the elderly. Common bacterial pneumonias are usually easily differentiated from tuberculosis. The localized alveolar infiltrate on the chest radiograph and the prompt response to antibiotic therapy usually differentiate bacterial pneumonia from tuberculosis. When in doubt, treatment for a bacterial pneumonia should be given first and tuberculosis therapy withheld until adequate sputums have been obtained and the response to antibiotics determined. Lung abscesses can usually be differentiated from tuberculous cavities by prominent air-fluid level, more common lower-lobe distribution, and clinical findings (associated with seizures, alcoholism, dental caries, etc.).

In the elderly, the major differential diagnosis is usually between tuberculosis and carcinoma of the lung. An important concept to remember is that carcinoma may cause a focus of tuberculosis to spread; thus, carcinoma of the lung and tuberculosis may be present simultaneously. In cases with the simultaneous presentation of carcinoma and tuberculosis, the diagnosis of tuberculosis frequently is made first, and the diagnosis of carcinoma is delayed for several months. Thus, if radiographic and clinical findings suggest carcinoma but the sputum has acid-fast bacilli, further procedures to diagnose carcinoma may still be indicated. Isolated involvement of the anterior segment of the upper lobe, isolated lower-lobe involvement, or the presence of irregular cavities would suggest carcinoma, and further diagnostic workup may be indicated despite acid-fast bacilli in the sputum smear.

Any type of infectious or granulomatous disease may be radiographically identical to tuberculosis. Three broad categories must be distinguished: fungi (histoplasmosis, coccidioidomycosis, and blastomycosis), bacteria (*Burkholderia pseudomallei*), and atypical mycobacteria (mainly *M. kansasii* and *M. avium* complex). Culture of the organism from the patient's sputum is the best way to differentiate these diseases, although serum antibody titers to fungi are also valuable.

COMPLICATIONS OF PULMONARY INVOLVEMENT

Pneumothorax

Although it is a relatively uncommon complication of tuberculous infection, the development of a pneumothorax requires rapid attention. After trauma, tuberculosis may be the second most common cause of bilateral pneumothorax in adults. Miliary tuberculosis can also rarely present as bilateral spontaneous pneumothorax. Unilateral pneumothorax has a broad differential, including *P. carinii* and other apical lung diseases.

Two postulated mechanisms can account for the development of a pneumothorax from tuberculosis. A bronchopleural fistula is created with the rupture of a cavity that connects the tracheobronchial tree with the pleural space.

Contamination of the pleural space results in spread of the infection to the pleura, with a tendency to produce pleural fibrosis, fibrothorax, and restrictive pulmonary dysfunction. Immediate therapy can prevent this complication. A second mechanism for the development of a pneumothorax from tuberculosis is the development of a subpleural bleb. This results from a submucosal bronchiolar lesion, with air trapping in an acinus or subsegment. When such a bleb ruptures into the pleural space, tuberculous infection of the pleural space does not necessarily follow. However, both occurrences should be treated with rapid expansion of the lungs by tube suction to avoid the possibility of further infection and fibrosis of the pleura with trapping of the lung. A bronchopleural fistula may persist after these episodes of pneumothorax and, especially if untreated, often results in mixed empyema because of complication of the tuberculous infection by secondary invaders.

Endobronchial Stenosis

Minor endobronchial disease is a common occurrence in tuberculosis, with exudative lesions and ulcerative lesions generally healing while lesions with scarring or bronchoglandular lesions often progressing to stenosis. Resected lung specimens will also frequently show either ulceration or stenosis of the draining bronchioles or bronchi. Stenosis of significance only rarely occurs in the major bronchi. At times, it results from involvement of the central lymph nodes draining into the lobar bronchi, with caseation, ulceration, and fibrosis. Since fibrosis due to tuberculosis tends to contract and aggravate the stenosis, resection of the affected lung segment may be required after chemotherapy has produced inactivity of the acute inflammatory reaction. Superinfection of the poststenotic segment is common.

Bronchiectasis

The endobronchial processes in tuberculosis may also result in bronchiectasis, which can be associated with active tuberculosis; sputum cultures should be sent to rule out an active process. In healed tuberculosis, the bronchiectasis is usually distal and frequently in the upper lobes. The so-called dry bronchiectasis (without sputum) is often the result of prior pulmonary tuberculosis and may manifest itself chiefly as low-grade hemoptysis. Bronchiectasis can result in life-threatening hemoptysis. Treatment for this complication is either bronchial artery embolization or surgery.

Empyema

Empyema rarely occurs from a primary infection with an associated tuberculous pleural effusion, since tuberculous pleural effusions usually clear with or without treatment. Empyema is more common later in the disease, occurring after a pneumothorax, and is often associated with debility and loss of resistance to infection. It is usually a part of a progressive, extensive parenchymal infection with caseation and cavitation, the presumed sources of pleural contamination. In many cases there is evidence of calcification of the pleura on the chest radiograph, and the process may have existed for many years. Because there is relatively poor penetration of antituberculous medication into the empyema cavity, chemotherapy alone is usually inadequate and may result in the development of drug resistance. Therefore, surgical removal of a calcified loculated empyema is necessary. For patients with mild symptoms, empyemectomy with lung resection is well tolerated. For chronic debilitated patients with severe symptoms, however, adequate drainage with a thoracostomy should be performed first; definitive surgery can be attempted later, when the patient is in better physical condition.

Late, Secondary Infections

If, after treatment of extensive tuberculosis, the patient is left with open, healed cavities as well as with areas of bronchiectasis, colonization of these areas can occur with a variety of infectious agents. Usually, colonization by aerobic and anaerobic upper respiratory bacteria results in a chronic productive cough, the syndrome of "wet" bronchiectasis. Other mycobacteria may be recovered during the development of inactivity and were at one time considered to be a sign of healing. However, the presence of other pathogenic mycobacteria does not rule out the possibility of active infection with *M. tuberculosis.*

Mycetoma

Aspergillus species are common in badly damaged lung areas, especially those that are cavitary. Patients with residual cavities develop precipitins to *Aspergillus* species and occasionally aspergillomas or "fungus balls." The finding of mycetoma does not rule out active tuberculosis, since 10 to 15 percent of patients may have active disease. Hemoptysis appears to be the major cause of death in these patients. Because systemic arteries may also feed the mycetoma cavity, bronchial artery embolization is not as effective for hemoptysis due to mycetoma as it is for hemoptysis due to bronchiectasis. Surgery is the best option for patients with significant hemoptysis. For patients who have little pulmonary reserve and may not tolerate surgery, a transthoracic catheter that is placed into the mycetoma cavity may be lifesaving.

Hemorrhage

Mild hemoptysis is very common in acute infection and not infrequently calls the attention of an otherwise unconcerned patient to the presence of serious disease. Young adults may have a higher incidence of hemoptysis than the elderly. Massive hemorrhage and death are dramatic events that occur in advanced cases of tuberculosis including rupture of a mycotic aneurysm of a branch of the pulmonary artery (Rasmussen's aneurysm) or aspergilloma or bronchiectasis.

Resection of the affected area had been the most widely used method of control in the past, and bleeding remains the main reason for surgery in patients today. The introduction of the technique of bronchial artery embolization has decreased the need for surgery and is 98 percent effective in the treatment of hemoptysis due to tuberculosis. Unfortunately, many patients die before this can be accomplished, and often (as in the case of aspergillomas) the areas are multiple and do not lend themselves to excisional therapy or bronchial artery embolization.

Hyponatremia

With extensive active disease, two interesting complications have been reported—the syndrome of inappropriate antidiuretic hormone (SIADH) and a reset osmostat. Both manifest themselves by abnormally low serum sodium.

However, the former is associated with the clinical and renal abnormalities associated with primary SIADH. A reset osmostat is characterized by decreased serum osmolality without clinical symptoms and the obligatory renal salt wasting found in SIADH. Both conditions disappear with control of the infection; they should be differentiated from each other, however, since SIADH requires metabolic control.

EXTRAPULMONARY MANIFESTATIONS OF TUBERCULOSIS

Extrapulmonary tuberculosis occurs as a result of exposure of superficial mucosal surfaces to infected respiratory secretions; contiguous spread of infection; and lymphohematogenous dissemination, commonly in immunocompromised hosts. Local progression of disseminated foci of infection may be the first sign of underlying immune compromise.

Local oral or gastrointestinal complications of tuberculosis, with oral or abdominal pain, are more common in patients with laryngeal involvement or those who come late to medical care. Among the observed lesions are nonhealing oral ulcers of the tongue or mouth, otitis media, gastric and duodenal ulcers, superinfection of preexisting gastrointestinal ulcers, perirectal abscess or obstructive lesions due to infection and scarring, hoarseness, and dysphagia with laryngeal infection. Localized symptoms (e.g., chest pain) may occur in association with extrapulmonary extension of infection by *M. tuberculosis*. Extension of infection or inflammation to the parietal pleura may be associated with pleurisy and fever. Pleural involvement may result in fusion of the visceral and parietal pleural surfaces (e.g., dry pleurisy when adjacent to an old cavity) or in serofibrinous effusion, often in association with primary infection or reactivation disease, and more often on the right side. Tuberculous empyema is uncommon. Granulomas are often seen on biopsy (60 percent), and cultures are generally positive despite negative acid-fast smears of pleural fluid.

Miliary tuberculosis may present with the initial manifestations in any organ system in proportion to blood flow: spleen, liver, lungs, bone marrow, kidneys, adrenal glands, or eyes. Symptoms may include splenomegaly or hepatomegaly with abscesses, primary hepatic disease with apparent cholangitis, leukopenia, anemia, thrombocytopenia, myelofibrosis, leukemoid reactions, Addison's disease, peritonitis, meningitis, choroidal tubercles, or pericarditis. Silent foci may serve as the source of miliary infection from the kidneys, prostate, bones, or deep lymph nodes. Renal infection is generally asymptomatic and temporally distant from the original infection. Patients present with "sterile" pyuria, hematuria, dysuria, and occasionally flank pain. Renal infection or miliary infection may cause epididymitis, orchitis, or prostatitis, and sexual transmission of infection may occur. Involvement of the fallopian tubes or uterus may cause dysfunctional bleeding, pain, or infertility.

Tuberculous meningitis generally occurs, in the normal host, several weeks into the illness via rupture of a subependymal tubercle (Rich focus) into the subarachnoid space rather than by direct seeding of the meninges or cerebrospinal fluid during bacteremia. The basal meninges are most commonly involved. Symptoms may reflect vasculitis (aneurysm, thrombosis, hemorrhage), hemiplegia, entrapment of cranial nerves (usually III, IV, VI, and occasionally VII), hydrocephalus, or uncommonly direct brain, meningeal, or spinal seeding with abscesses, transverse myelitis, radiculopathy, or spinal compression from paraspinous fibrosis.

Bone and joint involvement favors weight-bearing joints including the vertebral column, hip, and knee. Monoarticular disease favors joints with prior trauma. The presentation includes symptoms of arthritis and osteomyelitis with pain, often with fever and weight loss. Vertebral infections initially involve the anterior part of the vertebral body with spread to the intervertebral disk and the adjacent vertebrae. Sinus tracts may occur with presentations distant from the initial bony focus (e.g., with empyema from a lower thoracic infection). Neurologic complications (paraplegia or paresis) are not rare. Joint infections have high WBC counts (25,000 to 100,000), low glucose measurements, rice (fibrin) bodies, and negative smears with positive cultures in the majority. The yields of histologic and mycobacterial studies of synovial biopsies, as for the pleura, are high.

In AIDS, between 30 and 60 percent of patients with tuberculosis have extrapulmonary foci. Only half of those with extrapulmonary disease have identifiable concomitant pulmonary infection. Disseminated disease with multiple foci of involvement is common, including pneumonia, bilateral pleuritis, disseminated intravascular coagulation, omental and abdominal nodal involvement, and abscesses of multiple organs including prostate, liver, spleen, chest and abdominal wall, and pancreas.

Extrapulmonary foci in the immunologically normal host respond well to standard therapeutic regimens. Maximal, prolonged therapy is reserved for unique foci in the central nervous system or basal ganglia, in joints, or in bones, particularly in the spine.

HISTORY OF THE TREATMENT OF TUBERCULOSIS

Before chemotherapeutic agents were discovered, patients with tuberculosis were isolated in sanitariums for nutrition and rest. Lung collapse therapy was performed by pneumothorax or various surgical techniques that frequently left patients disfigured for life. In 1946, streptomycin was introduced as an effective antituberculosis drug and initially was used in tuberculosis patients by Feldman and Henshaw. However, it quickly became evident that streptomycin monotherapy resulted in relapse and the emergence of drug resistance. PAS, which was also used as monotherapy in 1944, could reduce the emergence of resistance to streptomycin as a two-drug combination. In 1953, isoniazid (INH) and pyrazinamide (PZA) were released for therapy. Following the development of ethambutol (EMB) in 1964, INH and EMB became the cornerstones of an 18-month treatment regimen. RMP was developed in 1965 and released for use in 1971. In the early 1980s, it was found that RMP and INH reduced the course of therapy to 9 months. Addition of PZA to this regimen shortened the duration of treatment to 6 months. Thus, in the 50 years since the introduction of the first effective drugs for the treatment of tuberculosis, the care of these patients has been transformed from long hospitalizations to a relatively short outpatient treatment regimen and cure. The challenge today is to ensure that patients receive proper treatment so as to avoid the development of drug-resistant strains and recrudescent infection.

Theoretical Basis For Effective Treatment Strategies

Effective chemotherapy is based on several considerations. The first is that only actively replicating organisms are killed by chemotherapy. In addition, differences in mycobacterial metabolic rate are associated with differences in mycobacterial susceptibility to antituberculosis drugs. Four major subpopulations of tuberculosis bacilli can be identified.

Group 1 The organisms living extracellularly in pulmonary cavities are metabolically very active and are rapidly and continuously growing in a hyperoxic and neutral-pH environment. These organisms are highly susceptible to streptomycin (SM), INH, and EMB.

Group 2 The organisms living extracellularly in closed caseous lesions are less or only intermittently metabolically active in a hypoxic and neutral-pH environment. This group of organisms is susceptible to rifampin (RMP) and INH.

Group 3 The intracellular organisms that live in the acid, hypoxic environment of macrophages have slow or intermittent growth; PZA and RMP are uniquely effective against these organisms, and INH is less effective.

Group 4 Some trapped organisms may become completely dormant and are unaffected by both antimicrobials and cellular immune mechanisms. Such persisting organisms can exist in tissues that healed with fibrosis and encapsulation.

Effective therapy for these bacterial subpopulations (Table 62-9) has to involve a bactericidal phase, during which most organisms (group 1) are rapidly killed, and a slower sterilizing phase, during which residual, susceptible, slowly or intermittently metabolizing organisms (groups 2 and 3) are inhibited or killed.

A second major consideration for effective chemotherapy is the presence of naturally occurring drug-resistant mutants. These mutants develop spontaneously at a rate of 1 in 10^7 to 10^{10} mutations per bacterium per generation. Their occurrence is less important in noncavitary pulmonary or extrapulmonary lesions, where bacillary populations are relatively small, whereas in a cavitary environment containing 10^8 to 10^9 bacilli, approximately 10 to 1000 organisms exist that are resistant to any single drug. In addition, the development of resistance to one drug is independent of the development of resistance to any other drug. Therefore, the probability of resistance to two drugs is the product of their individual rates (i.e., $10^{-7} \times 10^{-7}$ or only 1 out of 10^{14} organisms), a negligible number given an estimated population of

---

TABLE 62-9 Actions of First-Line Antituberculosis Agents

Drugs	Activity
Isoniazid (INH)	Bactericidal against both intracellular and extracellular bacilli
Rifampin (RMP)	Bactericidal against both intracellular and extracellular bacilli; a slower sterilizing phase against particularly slowly metabolizing organisms
Pyrazinamide (PZA)	Bactericidal against slowly metabolizing intracellular organisms; active at acid pH; good sterilizing activity synergistically with INH and other drugs
Streptomycin (SM)	Bactericidal against extracellular bacilli; active at neutral pH; effective against intracavitary bacilli
Ethambutol (EMB)	Bactericidal against both intracellular and extracellular organisms at 25 mg/kg; bacteriostatic at 15 mg/kg

10^9 bacilli. *Thus, antituberculosis therapy should always consist of at least two effective antituberculous drugs to prevent the emergence of drug-resistant mycobacteria.*

SPECIFIC ANTITUBERCULOSIS DRUGS

First-Line Drugs

Isoniazid

Because of its bactericidal effect and low cost, isoniazid (INH) is the most important drug used for the treatment of tuberculosis. INH should be included in all regimens except when a high proportion of INH-resistant organisms are present. INH is the hydrazide of isonicotinic acid, which most probably acts by inhibiting mycolic acid synthesis by mycobacteria. For INH to be effective, three things must occur. First, the drug has to be taken up by the organisms. Second, INH needs to be activated by a catalase-peroxidase enzyme within mycobacteria. The *katG* gene, encoding the catalase-peroxidase enzyme of *M. tuberculosis,* has been identified. In some highly INH-resistant isolates, either complete deletion or missense mutations are observed in the *katG* gene. Third, this activated form of INH interferes with mycolic acid synthesis. A second gene, *inhA,* encoding inhA protein active in mycolic acid synthesis, was cloned in 1994. The overexpression of this gene results in a phenotype of low-level INH resistance and cross-resistance to ethionamide. InhA protein also requires NAD or NADP as a cofactor, which is produced as a result of the interaction of INH with catalase-peroxidase enzyme. Because of these interactions of INH with mycobacteria, a single molecular test to identify INH-resistant organisms is unlikely.

INH has a bactericidal effect for both intra- and extracellular organisms and is well absorbed from the gastrointestinal tract, reaching serum levels equal to those following parenteral administration. The peak serum concentration of 3 to 5 μg/mL occurs 1 to 2 h after a dose of 5 mg/kg. The small molecular size of INH allows widespread distribution. The drug can be detected in serous membranes, caseous foci, cavities, and macrophages. INH is metabolized in the liver by both acetylation and oxidation via the cytochrome P450 system. The serum half-life is around 3 h in slow acetylators and 1 h in rapid acetylators. The inactive metabolites are excreted in the urine, accounting for 75 to 95 percent of a dose within 24 h. If the serum creatinine levels are higher than 12 mg/dL, these metabolites will accumulate in the body. In renal failure, INH should be administered after dialysis. The drug can be given by nasogastric tube, by intramuscular injection, or intravenously if the patient is unconscious.

When INH and phenytoin are administered together, an increase in serum concentrations of phenytoin will be observed, since INH is a noncompetitive inhibitor of diphenylhydantoin (DPH) metabolism. In such patients, the serum levels of phenytoin should be monitored and a dose reduction may be necessary. In cases of DPH intoxication, the drug should be discontinued for at least a week and then therapy restarted with low doses (100 to 200 mg/day). INH may also decrease the threshold for acetaminophen hepatotoxicity.

A major toxic manifestation of INH is peripheral neuritis. Susceptibility is highest in chronic alcoholics, persons with malnutrition, and slow acetylators. Major manifestations are sensory dysfunctions and numbness of the lower extremities. The syndrome is dose related (in 40 percent of patients at doses of 20 mg/kg/day, in 20 percent at 10 mg/kg/day, and in 1 to 2 percent at 5 mg/kg/day). Owing to its pyridoxinelike structure, INH competitively inhibits pyridoxine-requiring reactions. INH-induced depletion of pyridoxine stores can be prevented with pyridoxine 50 mg/day. Unless there is an obvious muscle weakness (i.e., atrophy or fasciculations), the symptoms of peripheral neuritis are reversible within a few weeks after withdrawal of INH and treatment with pyridoxine 100 to 200 mg/day. Autonomic dysfunctions, ataxia, muscle twitching, central nervous system (CNS) irritability, depression, acute psychosis, and encephalopathy are other neurologic symptoms that may also occur after INH therapy or overdose. Pyridoxine may terminate all these adverse effects.

The other major side effect of INH is toxic hepatitis. This is related to toxic drug metabolites. After acetylation, INH converts to hydrazine, which may be changed to a toxic agent, acetyl hydrazine. In addition, as RMP inducts the enzymatic conversion of INH to acetyl hydrazine, the hepatotoxic effect is potentiated when these drugs are used together. In the first months of therapy, a mild elevation of transaminase levels may occur in 10 to 20 percent of patients receiving INH. If the enzyme levels rise above three times normal values, the drug should be discontinued. Monthly monitoring of liver enzymes is recommended for all patients on INH therapy. The frequency of tests should be increased in patients who have elevated enzyme levels. INH causes a hepatocellular type of hypersensitivity reaction, and histology is indistinguishable from that of viral hepatitis. INH-induced hepatitis is age-dependent, occurring in 2 to 3 percent of patients over 50 years of age but seen in less than 1 percent of children. Fatal liver damage may occur in 1 to 2 percent of patients with INH hepatitis. This may be asymptomatic until jaundice develops. Before onset of jaundice, patients may suffer from weakness, fatigue, and generalized malaise. Therefore, patients may unknowingly continue taking INH after the onset of drug-induced hepatitis. Patients given INH should be warned about such symptoms and instructed to inform their physician promptly if such symptoms occur.

INH and RMP together produce hepatotoxicity more frequently than either drug alone. Risk factors for hepatitis are age greater than 35 years, slow acetylation, history of cholelithiasis, alcohol use, and preexisting liver disease. Liver transplantation has been successful in two patients who developed hepatic failure after either INH alone or INH and RMP therapy. Thus, liver transplantation may be a lifesaving therapy.

Rifampin

Rifampin (RMP) is bactericidal against intra- and extracellular bacterial populations. It is a semisynthetic antibiotic that inhibits RNA synthesis by inhibiting DNA-dependent RNA-polymerase enzyme, encoded by the *rpoB* gene. Most strains of *M. tuberculosis* are inhibited in vitro with 0.20 μg/mL RMP. RMP is considered to be a "sterilizing" agent. A standard oral dose of 600 mg/day in an adult may produce serum concentrations of 7 to 10 μg/mL in 1 to 2 h. RMP is metabolized in the liver and excreted in bile. As only 30 percent of the drug is excreted in the urine, dose reduction is not necessary in renal failure. RMP is able to penetrate into caseous foci, serous membranes, and macrophages. RMP does not pass the blood-brain barrier under normal conditions, but inflammation of the meninges causes an increase in penetration. RMP penetrates well into tissues and can be detected in urine, tears, sweat, and other body fluids, coloring them to red-orange. Patients should be advised of this harmless discoloration. RMP is a major antituberculosis drug; but because it is expensive, its use in therapeutic regimens in developing countries is limited. RMP can be given to unconscious patients either by nasogastric tube or by intravenous injection.

In nearly all isolates of *M. tuberculosis* resistant to RMP, a short region of 27 codons in the center of the *rpoB* gene was mutated. Most of these were missense mutations, although small in-frame insertions and deletions also occurred.

Major side effects of RMP are gastrointestinal upset, skin eruptions, and fever. Twenty percent of patients receiving high-dose intermittent RMP (600 to 1200 mg/day) develop an immunologically mediated influenza-like reaction, hemolytic anemia, acute renal failure, and thrombocytopenia. When these syndromes occur, RMP should be discontinued.

Another important adverse effect of RMP is its hepatic toxicity. An elevation in serum hepatic enzyme levels occurs in 5 to 10 percent of patients. Usually this resolves spontaneously, and therapy does not need to be altered or interrupted. The clinical presentation of hepatotoxicity varies from transaminase elevations to fatal hepatic necrosis. RMP is also a potent inducer of hepatic microsomal enzymes, resulting in an increased rate of metabolism of a number of drugs and, thus, a rapid elimination and diminished effect of these drugs, which include methadone, warfarin derivatives, glucocorticoids, estrogens, oral hypoglycemic agents, and antiarrhythmic agents.

Several studies have shown that the incidence of hepatitis in regimens containing both INH and RMP is approximately two to four times that of INH alone. Hepatic toxicity due to INH usually occurs after 2 months of therapy. In contrast, in INH and RMP combined therapies, jaundice may occur within the first 2 weeks of therapy and may be fulminant. The reason for this toxic effect was the accelerated production of toxic metabolites of INH due to the stimulation of hepatic microsomal P450 system by RMP.

There are several reports about renal toxicity due to RMP. The main histologic changes were tubulointerstitial nephritis, interstitial fibrosis, and tubular necrosis. Two patients developed crescentic glomerulonephritis with rapidly progressive renal failure. After discontinuation of RMP and addition of corticosteroids and other immunosuppressive agents, dramatic responses occurred. Further studies are necessary to document the incidence, mechanism, and treatment of RMP nephrotoxicity.

Pyrazinamide

Pyrazinamide (PZA) is a nicotinic acid derivative similar to INH, but cross-resistance with INH does not develop. PZA has bactericidal activity at acid pH which makes PZA particularly effective against slowly metabolizing intracellular bacilli. This "sterilizing" property has made PZA an essential component of short-course therapy. Regimens not including PZA require at least 9 months to succeed. This beneficial effect is limited to the first 2 to 3 months of treatment. PZA is absorbed from the gastrointestinal tract and distributed throughout the body, including the CNS. PZA is excreted from the kidneys. Serum levels of 30 to 50 μg/mL are achieved with doses of 20 to 25 mg/kg of PZA. It has a minimum inhibitory concentration (MIC) of 15 to 20 μg/mL.

Neither the mode of action nor the resistance mechanisms of PZA are clear. Konno and colleagues identified an enzyme, pyrazinamidase, that is toxic to pyrazinoic acid; they suggested that it may be absent in resistant strains. Studies done by Salfinger and colleagues in 1990 showed that pyrazinamidase was not present in all susceptible strains, but it was identified in some resistant strains.

The most adverse reaction of PZA is hepatotoxicity. After 2 months of therapy, 15 percent of patients who receive PZA at a dose of 3000 mg a day (40 to 50 mg/kg) develop liver dysfunction and 2 to 3 percent develop jaundice. Liver function should be monitored closely, and the treatment should be discontinued if elevations of SGOT levels occur. Another common side effect of PZA is hyperuricemia. Occasionally, mild nongouty polyarthralgias occur as a result of inhibition of urate excretion. This complication usually responds to nonsteroidal anti-inflammatory drugs. Clinical gout is rarely seen, and allopurinol therapy is usually indicated. Therapy is not necessary for patients who have only elevated urate levels without symptoms. Other side effects, such as skin rash and gastrointestinal intolerance, are rare.

Ethambutol

Ethambutol (EMB) is a bacteriostatic agent whose antibacterial effect is limited to *M. tuberculosis*. It has no activity on bacilli in the stationary growth phase. It is a unique butanol derivative that may block a step of cell wall synthesis. Following a 5-mg/kg oral dose, the peak serum level is approximately 4 μg/mL after 2 to 4 h. Serum half-life is approximately 4 h and is prolonged in renal failure. EMB may be bactericidal at 25-mg/kg doses, whereas it is bacteriostatic at 15-mg/kg doses. EMB is active against both intra- and extracellular bacilli. Most strains of *M. tuberculosis* are inhibited in vitro by 1 to 5 μg/mL of EMB. Cerebrospinal fluid concentrations are low (1 to 2 μg/mL) even in the presence of meningeal inflammation. It is often added to short-term therapy regimens when there is a concern about primary drug resistance.

The main toxicity of EMB is optic neuritis. This is manifest by central scotoma, decreased red-green color vision, decreased visual activity, and, rarely, concentric concentration of visual fields, leading to gun-barrel vision. This side effect is dose dependent and largely reversible. Optic neuritis occurs in 3 percent of patients taking 25 mg/kg but in less than 1 percent of patients taking 15 mg/kg. Patients should be questioned concerning visual symptoms, and tests of visual acuity and color vision should be performed. In cases of optic neuritis, the visual function returns after withdrawal of the drug. Like PZA, EMB may cause hyperuricemia and rarely gout. Skin rash, drug fever, and gastrointestinal disturbance are other rarely seen side effects.

Streptomycin

Streptomycin (SM) was the first major antituberculosis drug released. SM acts through inhibition of protein synthesis. It is effective only against extracellular bacterial populations in cavities, where the pH is neutral. SM must be administered parenterally, as it is not absorbed from the gut. Peak serum concentration of 40 μg/mL occurs approximately 1 h after a 15-mg/kg intramuscular dose. Most strains of *M. tuberculosis* are inhibited in vitro at a concentration of 8 μg/mL. SM's half-life is 5 h in blood.

Several mechanisms are responsible for resistance to SM. One of them is a mutation in the *rpsL* gene, encoding the S12 protein. Seventy percent of SM-resistant clinical isolates have modifications of the *rpsL* gene. An additional mechanism of resistance found by Kempsell's team in 1992 concerns the *rrs* gene, encoding 16S rRNA. Two conserved regions of this molecule are known to be engaged in SM resistance. Little is known about a third mechanism, a low-level resistance, which is found in about 30 percent of resistant clinical isolates that do not carry modifications of the genes mentioned above. In these strains, permeability or cell wall barrier modifications could be playing a role.

Although SM has good tissue penetration, it can enter the cerebrospinal fluid only in the presence of meningeal inflammation. Its major toxicity is irreversible eighth nerve damage, leading to vestibular dysfunction and, less frequently, deafness. It is a nephrotoxic drug like other aminoglycosides, and the frequency of renal toxicity is increased in patients with preexisting renal diseases or with simultaneous use of other nephrotoxic drugs. Renal and eighth nerve toxicity increases in patients above 50 years of age, in whom SM should be used very cautiously. Patients should be questioned regarding balance and asked to perform simple tests of vestibular function. In tuberculosis treatment, its use is usually limited to 2 months. Although SM itself is relatively inexpensive, the additional cost of needles and syringes increases the effective cost. Although it is routinely given intramuscularly, it can be given safely intravenously.

Second-Line Drugs

The second-line drugs include some older drugs that were used early in the treatment of tuberculosis; as less toxic regimens became available, however, their routine administration for tuberculosis was discontinued.

Para-amino Salicylic Acid

Para-amino salicylic acid (PAS) was the first oral antituberculosis drug that had strong bacteriostatic effect. This effect is potentiated when it is used in conjunction with SM or INH. As the drug is excreted rapidly, high doses are necessary to maintain bacteriostatic activity. The usual oral daily therapeutic dose is approximately 150 mg/kg; the total dose should not exceed 10 to 12 g/day. This total dose causes a high rate of adverse gastrointestinal effects, including nausea, vomiting, diarrhea, and epigastric pain. The half-life of PAS is about 1 h and is markedly prolonged in renal failure. PAS is well absorbed orally but does not cross the blood-brain barrier. In 5 to 10 percent of patients, PAS may also cause hypersensitivity reactions and, rarely, hepatitis, hypothyroidism, or hemolytic anemia. Adverse effects may be diminished by beginning therapy with a low dose and gradually increasing to a full dose over 7 to 10 days. To avoid gastrointestinal effects, PAS should be taken after eating. Antacids may also be helpful to reduce these side effects.

Ethionamide

Ethionamide has a structure similar to INH, but cross-resistance with INH is rare. Ethionamide is tuberculostatic at 0.6 to 2.5 μg/mL. Dosing is usually 1 g PO QD with peak serum levels of 20 μg/mL. It is well absorbed orally and hepatically metabolized. The optimum dosage is usually 1 g. It is almost completely and widely distributed in the body compartments. Nausea, vomiting, loss of appetite, and abdominal pain are the most common adverse effects. Serious neurologic reactions include headache, restlessness, diplopia, tremors, and convulsions. It is necessary to increase the dose to the full amount gradually. As it is very irritative for the gastrointestinal tract, a bedtime dose is recommended with an antiemetic and a hypnotic drug. Hepatitis may develop in 1 percent of patients. To monitor hepatotoxicity, monthly hepatic enzyme determination is necessary. In the presence of a fivefold elevation of liver enzyme levels, the drug should be stopped. If well tolerated, ethionamide can be a lifesaving agent in patients with drug-resistant tuberculosis.

Cycloserine

Cycloserine is a bacteriostatic drug. It is an analog of D-alanine and competes with it for incorporation into the cell wall. It is rapidly absorbed from the gut and is distributed to all compartments. Urinary excretion accounts for 70 percent of the active form of the drug, as only 30 percent is metabolized. Common side effects include neurologic and psychiatric disturbances ranging from headache, tremor, memory problems, and somnolence to psychosis (paranoid, depressive, or catatonic reactions) and seizure. Some patients with depression or anxiety have committed suicide. The usual dose is 15 to 20 mg/kg, with a maximal dosage of 1 g/day. Most of the adverse CNS effects are dose related and disappear when the medication is discontinued. To prevent serious psychiatric problems, periodic monitoring of mental status and serum drug levels is necessary. To diminish the potential for seizures and convulsions, pyridoxine at doses of 100 to 150 mg/day is helpful. Cycloserine may affect the elimination of phenytoin, especially when taken with INH. Dose reduction of phenytoin is necessary in these cases. In the presence of renal failure, the daily dose of the drug must be reduced.

Kanamycin

Kanamycin is an aminoglycoside antibiotic that acts on ribosomes, inhibiting protein synthesis. It is an agent that has limited activity against *M. tuberculosis*. The usual dosage is 15 to 30 mg/kg/day, 5 days a week, given intramuscularly with a maximum daily dose of 1 g. For the resistant strains of bacilli, serum concentrations of kanamycin should be in a range of 15 to 20 µg/mL. Ototoxicity is more common with kanamycin than with streptomycin or capreomycin. Hearing loss, tinnitus, and vestibular disturbances are the major symptoms of ototoxicity. Monthly audiometry monitoring is recommended following a baseline audiogram before therapy. Renal toxicity has greatly reduced the use of these aminoglycosides. Nephrotoxicity occurs at the same rate as for capreomycin. Regular monthly monitoring of serum creatinine and BUN levels is necessary. The frequency of monitoring should be increased in patients who have a history of renal disease. Kanamycin has a cross-resistance with streptomycin and amikacin.

Capreomycin

Capreomycin is chemically distinct from aminoglycosides, but it is likely to have cross-resistance with SM, amikacin, and kanamycin. It has the same therapeutic activity, pharmacology, and toxicity. Daily recommended dosage is 15 to 30 mg/kg by intramuscular injection. Maximum dosage should not exceed 1 g/day. After 2 to 4 months, the drug can be given three times or twice a week until the sputum cultures become negative. It is toxic to the eighth cranial nerve. In many patients (5 to 10 percent), hearing loss develops before vestibular dysfunction. Renal toxicity occurs more frequently than with SM. In elderly patients (over 60 years of age), in the presence of similar susceptibility to capreomycin and amikacin, capreomycin should be the first choice, since older patients seem to have more renal and eighth nerve toxicity with amikacin.

Amikacin

Amikacin is another aminoglycoside that is bactericidal against several species of mycobacteria in vitro. It has eighth nerve and renal toxicity, as do the other aminoglycosides. The usual dose is a single intramuscular injection of 15 mg/kg/day for 5 days a week. The same dose can be administered intravenously in 30 min. Average peak serum concentration is 21 μg/mL 1 h after administration of 7.5 mg/kg. The MIC for amikacin is 4 to 8 μg/mL. The major adverse effect is nephrotoxicity, and regular BUN and creatinine monitoring is necessary. If renal insufficiency occurs, the dose and frequency should be reduced. Other side effects are audiovestibular dysfunction and chemical imbalance (low levels of Ca, K, and Mg). Monthly audiogram monitoring is necessary, as for the other aminoglycosides. If a patient receives more than one injectable drug, the frequency of audiograms and kidney function tests should be increased. Monthly serum concentrations of the drugs should be monitored so that the dosage of aminoglycosides can be adjusted. There is cross-resistance to kanamycin and streptomycin.

Viomycin

Viomycin is chemically different from aminoglycosides but acts like them. In cases of SM-resistant tuberculosis, viomycin is used if other alternatives to aminoglycosides are not available. The dosage and duration of therapy are the same as for the other injectable drugs. Viomycin is less likely to show a cross-resistance with SM. To prevent side effects, kidney function should be monitored closely.

Thiacetazone

Thiacetazone is a thiosemicarbazole antibiotic that is not available in the United States because of its severe gastrointestinal, hepatic, bone marrow, and dermatologic toxicity. As it is very cost-effective, it is commonly used in many third-world countries. It is usually used with INH, as its bioactivity is related to INH. It has a bacteriostatic effect and is more toxic than INH. The recommended adult dosage is 150 mg/day or 450 mg twice a week. Commonly, INH 300 mg and thiacetazone 150 mg are combined in a single tablet. Thiacetazone may potentiate the vestibular toxicity of streptomycin. Cutaneous adverse effects may be very severe and may resemble exfoliative dermatitis or Stevens-Johnson syndrome. These reactions frequently occur in AIDS patients. For that reason, its usage is contraindicated in this patient group. There seems to be a better tolerance of this drug in African populations than in Asians.

POTENTIALLY EFFECTIVE DRUGS IN TUBERCULOSIS TREATMENT

Fluoroquinolones

Fluoroquinolones are broad-spectrum antibacterial agents that act by inhibiting DNA gyrase enzyme. They have activity in vitro against *M. tuberculosis.* There is no cross-resistance between fluoroquinolones and other antituberculosis drugs. The MIC for both ciprofloxacin and ofloxacin is between 0.25 and 2.0 μg/mL, and the predictable serum level for ofloxacin is 8.0 to 11.0 μg/mL. Unless there is evidence of higher activity of other quinolones, ofloxacin (one dose of 600 to 800 mg or two doses of 400 mg daily) or levofloxacin is recommended as the first choice among this family because of bioavailability. Newer agents of this class have not yet been studied in detail. The dose of ciprofloxacin is 750 mg twice a day or 750 to 1000 mg once a day. Both drugs have been used for MDR cases. Administration of quinolones with theophylline or calcineurin inhibitors increases serum levels and the risk of adverse effects from these agents. Ferrous sulfate and antacids with magnesium and aluminum may affect the absorption of quinolones.

Rifamycins

Several experimental rifamycins are active against *M. tuberculosis.* Rifabutin, a spiropiperidylrifamycin that is used against *M. avium* infections in AIDS, has 2- to 20-fold greater bactericidal effect against *M. tuberculosis* than rifampin. For that reason, some protocols use rifabutin as an antituberculosis drug, especially for MDR TB. As the two drugs have the same mechanism of action and a single-step mutation is responsible for RMP resistance, rifabutin should not be a treatment alternative for RMP-resistant tuberculosis. The serum concentration of rifabutin is 7 to 10 times lower than that of RMP. Rifabutin has a lower half-life (45 $\pm$ 6 h), and the C_{max}:MIC and MBC:MIC (C_{max} = maximum serum concentration MIC = minimal inhibitory concentration MBC = mean bactericidal concentration) ratios are similar to those of RMP. Important advantages of rifabutin are the extensive tissue distribution, higher intracellular penetration, lower enzyme-inducing activity, and no modification of activity when administered under fasting conditions or after a meal.

New Macrolides

These are semisynthetic derivatives of erythromycin. Currently, they are used against *M. avium–intracellulare.* Azithromycin, roxithromycin, and clarithromycin are thought to have significant activity against *M. tuberculosis.* Further studies are necessary to determine the role of these drugs for patients with tuberculosis.

Combination of Beta-Lactam Antibiotics and Beta-Lactamase Inhibitors

The beta-lactam antimicrobial agents have limited activity against mycobacteria, as these organisms produce beta-lactamases. In vitro, they have activity against *M. tuberculosis.* But even with the addition of beta-lactamase inhibitors, such as sulbactam and clavulanic acid, they do not appear to be clinically effective. At present, beta-lactam antimicrobials do not have a prominent role in the treatment of tuberculosis. However, they may be tried in patients with no other therapeutic option.

PRINCIPLES ON STARTING THERAPY

When a decision is made about initiating antituberculosis therapy, physicians should consider the following issues and try to avoid common mistakes (Table 62-10).

TABLE 62-10 Common Errors in the Management of Tuberculosis

Addition of a single drug to a failing regimen
Failure to identify preexisting or acquired drug resistance
Chest radiographic findings absent or misinterpreted
Inadequate primary regimen
Failure to identify and address noncompliance
Inappropriate isoniazid preventive therapy

---

1. Tuberculosis should be viewed as a disease with major public health implications.
2. Before starting therapy, at least three clinical specimens (generally, sputum samples) must be submitted for microbiologic evaluation for both AFB smears, culture and susceptibility testing.
3. In smear-negative cases, five or six sputum samples and, if necessary, bronchoalveolar lavage, gastric lavage, pleural biopsy, cerebrospinal fluid, or other samples should be sent for mycobacterial culture.
4. If no other cause can be found in a severely ill, smear-negative, presumed tuberculosis patient, antituberculosis therapy should be started immediately.
5. Initial therapy should be with four drugs when the incidence of primary drug resistance is greater than 4 percent, with the goal of at least two effective agents.
7. The emergence of drug resistance is usually due to noncompliance and failure to take all of the drugs. Directly observed therapy should be considered in all patients. When therapy is switched for reasons of resistance and nonresponse, at least two new agents should be added to replace the discontinued agents.
8. Therapy should never be stopped unless one is certain that the cultures are negative.

CURRENT ANTITUBERCULOUS THERAPY

The current therapeutic recommendations for new cases of tuberculosis are summarized in Tables 62-9, 62-11, and 62-12 on the basis of the ATS/CDC recommendations published in 1994. Specific recommendations for the care of HIV-infected individuals, the homeless, and populations of high endemicity for tuberculosis may be found at the CDC web site (www.cdc.gov/nchstp/tb) or through the American Thoracic Society (ATS) web site. The ATS and CDC currently recommend a 6-month regimen that is based on an initial 2-month "bactericidal phase," consisting of INH and RMP and PZA and either SM or EMB (if the INH resistance possibility is more than 4 percent), and a "continuation phase" of INH and RMP daily or twice weekly for 4 months as an alternative to 9 months of INH and RMP therapy.

The effectiveness of the therapy for tuberculosis was demonstrated in a U.S. Public Health Service study that compared a three-drug (INH, RMP, and PZA), 6-month regimen to the standard two-drug (INH and RMP), 9-month regimen. A rapid conversion of sputum in 16 weeks (94.6 versus 89.9 percent) and lower noncompliance rates (16.8 versus 29.2 percent) were observed without any change in relapse rates (3.5 versus 2.8 percent, respectively) 96 weeks after completion of therapy. Additional worldwide studies confirmed the efficacy of 6-month regimens in smear-positive patients. The initial addition of a fourth drug (SM) in smear-positive disease was superior to three drugs. Although PZA is the first choice as a third drug to add to INH and RMP for short-course therapy, there is no advantage in continuing PZA after the first 2 months of therapy. If the organism is resistant to INH or there is an intolerance to it, however, INH should be stopped and PZA maintained for the entire 6 months. Of interest is that when a good clinical and bacterial response to therapy is observed, whether the initial culture was resistant to either INH and SM did not change the results of 6-month therapy.

CHAPTER 62 MYCOBACTERIAL INFECTIONS **805**

TABLE 62-11 Current Recommendations for Therapy

Four-Month Therapy
Options 1, 2, and 3 (below, under 6-month therapy) can be administered for 4 months in patients who are not at high risk and have smear-negative, culture-negative pulmonary TB.

Six-Month Therapy
Option 1
Eight weeks of daily INH, RMP, and PZA, followed by 16 weeks of INH and RMP daily or two to three times per week.[a] In areas where the rate of primary INH resistance is not documented to be <4 percent, EMB and SM should be added to the initial regimen until susceptibility to INH, RMP, and PZA is demonstrated. Continue treatment for at least 6 months and 3 months beyond culture conversion. A TB medical expert should be consulted if the patient is symptomatic or smear culture–positive after 3 months.

Option 2
Two weeks of daily INH, RMP, PZA, and SM or EMB, followed by 6 weeks (by DOT) of the same drugs twice a week[a] and subsequently with twice-a-week administration of INH and RMP for 16 weeks (by DOT). A TB medical expert should be consulted if the patient is symptomatic or smear culture–positive after 3 months.

Option 3
Treat by DOT three times per week with INH, RMP, PZA, and EMB or SM for 6 months.[a] A TB medical expert should be consulted if the patient is symptomatic or smear culture–positive after 3 months.

Nine-Month Therapy
Nine months of daily INH and RMP or 1 to 2 months of daily INH and RMP, followed by 7 to 8 months of twice-weekly administration. EMB or SM should be added for the first 2 months if INH resistance rate is not documented to be <4 percent.

HIV-Related Tuberculosis
Option 1, 2, or 3 can be used for a total of 9 months and at least 6 months beyond culture conversion.[a] Patients should be followed much more closely, and in the presence of any problem with response to therapy, the evaluation should ensue.

KEY: INH, isoniazid; RMP, rifampin; PZA, pyrazinamide; SM, streptomycin; EMB, ethambutol; DOT, directly observed therapy.
[a]All regimens administered twice or three times per week should be monitored by DOT for the duration of therapy.

In cases in which both INH and PZA cannot be used, EMB and RMP have been recommended for 12 months, although there are not enough data about the efficacy of this approach. A third drug might be necessary to attain adequate success rates. If RMP cannot be used, INH, PZA, and SM may be used daily for 9 months or INH and EMB daily or twice weekly for 18 months.

If INH and RMP cannot be used together because of toxicity, it is wise to use at least three drugs to which the organism is sensitive and to continue therapy until culture conversion is documented, followed by at least 12 months of two-drug therapy. The standard 6-month regimen should be extended to 12 months in children with miliary, meningeal, or bone and joint disease.

A 9-month therapy regimen was shown to be very effective against most forms of tuberculosis. In the presence of INH resistance, addition of EMB to the regimen is recommended until culture sensitivity reports are available. If the incidence of primary INH resistance is documented to be greater than 4 percent, EMB at the beginning of therapy is recommended.

TABLE 62-12 Recommended Dosage for the Initial Treatment of Tuberculosis in Children[a] and Adults

	Dosage					
	Daily Dose		Twice-Weekly Dose		Thrice-Weekly Dose	
Drugs	Children	Adults	Children	Adults	Children	Adults
Isoniazid, mg/kg	10–20	5	20–40	15 max	20–40	15 max
	Max 300 mg	Max 300 mg	Max 900 mg	Max 900 mg	Max 900 mg	Max 900 mg
Rifampin, mg/kg	10–20	10	10–20	10	10–20	10
	Max 600 mg	Max 600 mg	Max 600 mg	Max 600 mg	Max 600 mg	Max 600 mg
Pyrazinamide, mg/kg	15–30	15–30	50–70	50–70	50–70	50–70
	Max 2 g	Max 2 g	Max 4 g	Max 4 g	Max 3 g	Max 3 g
Ethambutol, mg/kg[b]	15–25	15–25	50	50	25–30	25–30
Streptomycin, mg/kg	20–40	15	25–30	25–30	25–30	25–30
	Max 1.0 g	Max 1.0 g	Max 1.5 g	Max 1.5 g	Max 1.5 g	Max 1.5 g

[a]Children 12 years of age and younger.
[b]Ethambutol is generally not recommended for children whose visual acuity cannot be monitored (8 years of age). However, ethambutol should be considered for all children with organisms resistant to other drugs when susceptibility to ethambutol has been demonstrated or susceptibility is likely.

Dutt and colleagues observed a very good response in smear- and culture-negative pulmonary tuberculosis after 4 months of INH and RMP either daily or twice weekly. A study from Hong Kong showed that the smear- and culture-negative patients responded well to 4 months of either daily or thrice-weekly four-drug therapy. For this group of patients, a treatment period of 4 months is acceptable. The same regimen can be used for adults who are PPD-positive and seem to have an old healed lesion on their chest radiographs or as an alternative regimen to 12 months of preventive INH therapy for PPD-positive, sputum smear– and culture-negative adults.

MONITORING FOR ADVERSE REACTIONS

For evaluation of standard regimens, baseline measurements of a complete blood count, hepatic enzymes, serum bilirubin, and creatinine levels should be obtained. If PZA is used, serum uric acid levels should be monitored. Patients receiving EMB should have both visual acuity measurement and a red-green color perception testing. The baseline tests have two major goals— first, to detect abnormalities that would complicate the regimen and, if necessary, make rearrangements and, second, to monitor adverse reactions to drugs by comparing the baseline measurements with the follow-up results. The same tests should be repeated at monthly examinations. Patients with abnormalities detected on the baseline tests should be evaluated for the cause of this result. If symptoms suggesting drug toxicity occur, appropriate laboratory testing should be performed. Patients should always be informed about the common adverse effects of drugs (Table 62-13) before starting therapy.

DURATION OF OBSERVATION AND EVALUATION OF RESPONSE TO TREATMENT

Patients with Positive Pretreatment Sputum

To monitor conversion and detect the possible emergence of drug resistance, sputum smear and cultures should be obtained monthly or at least after 2, 4, and 6 months of therapy. With INH- and RMP-containing regimens, sputum should convert to negative within 2 months. If smear and culture results continue to be positive after 2 months of therapy, emerging drug resistance and noncompliance should be major concerns. A new drug susceptibility test should be performed immediately. Unless drug resistance is demonstrated, the regimen in use should be continued carefully under direct observation. If drug resistance occurs, at least two new drugs to which the organism is sensitive should be added to the therapy and administered under direct observation. Addition of a single drug to therapy should never be done, since it increases the risk of the rapid development of resistance to the new drug. Bacteriologic culture and susceptibility tests should be performed at monthly intervals until the cultures become negative. Relapse of drug-sensitive infections after adequate INH- and RMP-containing treatment is very infrequent. For patients who have completed a standard regimen and have had a satisfactory bacteriologic response, follow-up after completion of therapy is not necessary. In contrast, indications for prolonged follow-up include the patient with extensive disease, immunosuppressed patients, the persistence of radiographic findings after therapy, or suspicion of poor patient compliance.

TABLE 62-13 Side Effects of Antituberculosis Drugs			
Drugs	Most Common Side Effects	Tests to Detect	Remarks
Isoniazid	Peripheral neuritis, hepatotoxicity, hypersensitivity	SGOT, SGPT	Pyridoxine 25–50 mg as prophylaxis for neuritis; 100–200 mg as treatment
Rifampin	Hepatitis, GI upset (skin eruptions, fever[a])	SGOT, SGPT	Orange urine and other body secretions
Pyrazinamide	Hyperuricemia, hepatotoxicity (skin rash, GI irritation[a])	Serum uric acid level, SGOT, SGPT	NSAIDs for nongouty polyarthralgias; allopurinol for frank gout
Streptomycin	Eighth nerve damage, nephrotoxicity	Vestibular function, audiograms; BUN/creatinine	Use with caution in older patients or those with renal disease
Ethambutol	Optic neuritis (usually reversible), (hyperuricemia, gout, skin rash, drug fever, GI irritation[a])	Red-green color discrimination and visual acuity	Use with caution when eye test is not feasible
Ethionamide	GI intolerance, endocrine disturbances, hepatitis, hypersensitivity	SGOT, SGPT	Consider antiemetics or bedtime dosing
Cycloserine	Neurologic and psychiatric disturbances	Serum levels of drug, regular control of mental status	Pyridoxine needed
Capreomycin, kanamycin, amikacin, viomycin	Hearing loss, vestibular damage, renal toxicity, electrolyte disturbances	Audiogram, vestibular examination, BUN/ creatinine	Use with caution in older patients or those with renal disease, renal transplant
p-Amino-salicylic acid	GI intolerance, hepatitis, hypersensitivity	SGOT, SGPT	Consider antacids or dosing at mealtime
Ciprofloxacin, ofloxacin, levofloxacin,	GI intolerance, headache, restlessness, hypersensitivity, drug interactions	Monitoring for drug interactions	Avoid antacids, iron, zinc, and sucralfate, which decrease absorption
Clofazimine	Abdominal pain, skin discoloration (both dose related), photosensitivity		Consider dosing at mealtime; avoid sunlight; efficacy is unproven

[a]Less common side effects.

KEY: SGOT, serum glutamate oxaloacetate transaminase (aspartate aminotransferase); SGPT, serum glutamate pyruvate transaminase (alanine aminotransferase).

SOURCE: From Simone and Dooley, with permission.

A chest radiograph taken before the start of therapy is necessary to compare with one taken after the completion of therapy. Monthly chest radiographs during therapy are helpful but not as essential as sputum examinations. A chest radiograph taken at the end of therapy will also be useful in making comparisons with any future films.

Patients with Negative Sputum

In patients with radiographic abnormalities and clinical findings consistent with tuberculosis, diagnostic tests should be performed to isolate *M. tuberculosis*. If an alternative diagnosis cannot be established, treatment against tuberculosis should be started while culture results are awaited. For this group of patients, clinical evaluation and chest radiographs are the major indicators of response to therapy. If cultures are negative and radiographic changes have not occurred after 3 months of an INH- and RMP-containing regimen, the abnormality is probably due to another disease or a tuberculosis fibrotic scar.

Retreatment of Patients Who Have Relapsed

Patients whose sputum is persistently positive after 5 to 6 months of therapy are considered treatment failures. A current sputum specimen should be obtained for susceptibility testing. While susceptibility results are pending, the original therapy may be continued or at least three new drugs added to the therapy. Direct supervision of therapy should be implemented if that has not already been done. When the new susceptibility test results are received, a new regimen should be adopted in accordance with the results of the susceptibility tests. Patients who relapse after completing a regimen containing both INH and RMP and whose organisms were susceptible to the drugs at the outset of treatment may be restarted on their original therapy, since the organisms are still usually susceptible. In contrast, patients who relapsed after taking a regimen that did not contain both INH and RMP should be assumed to be infected with an organism that is resistant to all previous drugs and managed accordingly.

ADHERENCE AND DIRECTLY OBSERVED THERAPY

Nonadherence to therapy is a major reason for the failure of antituberculosis treatment. To overcome this problem, therapy should be given under direct observation if possible. A medical or other responsible person should observe as the patient ingests antituberculosis drugs. A health care worker may observe the patient in the "field" (patient's home, place of work, school, etc.) or in the clinic. Following the daily initial therapy, directly observed therapy (DOT) may be administered during the second phase. DOT is especially useful in alcoholic, drug-addicted, or homeless patients, as the risk of nonadherence is very high in these groups. Currently, only 10 to 12 percent of patients in the United States receive DOT.

The effectiveness of DOT was demonstrated in Baltimore by observation of a declining tuberculosis case rate, while similar cities that did not use DOT had unchanged or rising tuberculosis case rates. In Texas, after initiation of a DOT regimen, a fall in the frequency of primary drug resistance, acquired drug resistance, and relapses with MDR organisms was observed. This was in spite of the rising tuberculosis case rate and increasing rates of AIDS and homelessness. The cost of including supervision adds only $400 to the cost of unsupervised therapy. The cost of such therapy is insignificant compared to the cost of treatment for hospitalization for advanced tuberculosis or MDR tuberculosis.

TREATMENT OF DRUG-RESISTANT TUBERCULOSIS

Patients can become infected with mycobacteria resistant to drugs in two ways. The first is to become infected with resistant organisms. This is called primary resistance. The second is that the resistant organism develops in tuberculosis patients during therapy. This is called secondary resistance. In certain parts of the world, primary resistance rates to INH and SM may exceed 20 to 35 percent. In some Asian populations in the United States, the rate has been reported to be as high as 58 percent. In 1983, the CDC reported that primary resistance was most common for INH (4 percent), SM (3.8 percent), and ethionamide (1.1 percent). The rates for RMP, EMB, kanamycin, cycloserine, capreomycin, and PAS were less than 1 percent.

During the initial phase of treatment with a single drug, most of the susceptible bacilli are destroyed, but the small number of resistant mutants continue to grow and, after 2 weeks to several months, the resistant bacilli outgrow the susceptible bacilli; this is known as the "fall and rise" phenomenon. In a large population, additional mutations can occur, resulting in the doubling of resistant mutants. Basically, nonadherence to prescribed therapy and the use of inadequate therapy regimens cause the development of drug resistance. The best treatment for drug-resistant tuberculosis is to make sure the patient receives adequate treatment initially and prevent the emergence of drug resistance.

Current CDC recommendations are an initial regimen of four drugs when the primary INH-resistant rate in a community is greater than 4 percent. If resistance occurs, the basic principle of managing patients whose organisms are resistant to one or more drugs is the administration of at least two agents that have activity against *M. tuberculosis* strains. Isolated INH resistance is well documented. For patients infected with INH-resistant organisms, INH should be discontinued and PZA continued for the entire 6 months of therapy. When INH resistance is discovered during a 9-month regimen, INH should be discontinued. If EMB was given from the beginning of therapy, it should be continued with RMP for a minimum of 12 months. If EMB was not in the regimen, INH should be discontinued and two new drugs (EMB and PZA) added. The regimen can be adjusted when the results of the susceptibility test become available.

MDR is defined as the in vitro resistance of a strain of *M. tuberculosis* to two or more antituberculosis drugs. This is a very serious and difficult therapeutic problem. Clinically, the most important pattern of MDR is resistance to both INH and RMP. Goble and coworkers treated 171 INH-RMP–resistant patients under DOT. At least three new drugs not given previously (one parenteral, two oral) to which tuberculosis bacilli were fully susceptible were added to the regimen. In addition, drugs to which the organisms were at least partly susceptible or drugs previously given for a relatively short time were also added to the regimen. Of 171 patients in all, the sputum cultures of only 87 patients became negative within 1 to 8 months. Despite treatment, 47 percent remained sputum culture–positive and 12 percent of patients suffered relapses. Including those who had relapses,

44 percent had unfavorable outcomes. The ATS also recommends giving at least three new drugs to which the organism is susceptible. These regimens usually contain six or seven drugs. When both INH and RMP are ineffective, therapy should continue for 24 months after conversion of cultures to negative, as it may take several months for a patient with MDR TB to become culture-negative, the total duration of treatment may last well beyond 2 years, and adherence to therapy and drug toxicity become even greater problems during this period.

For patients who are infected with MDR organisms and in whom the preponderance of disease is in one lung or lobe, the therapeutic efficacy of surgery was studied by Iseman. Of 99 MDR patients, 27 had surgery and 25 remained sputum culture–negative for a mean duration of 36 months (combination of surgery and medical therapy).

SURGERY

Surgery is rarely used for the treatment of tuberculosis. Before the chemotherapeutic era, surgery was used as an adjunct to "resting" of the lungs. Operations such as artificial pneumothorax, artificial pneumoperitoneum, plombage, artificial phrenic nerve paralysis, thoracoplasty, pulmonary resection, cavity drainage, and decortication were performed as important adjunctive treatment for managing cavitary lesions, progressive local diseases, empyemas, and fibrothorax. Today, surgery has a role in curing treatment failures, such as MDR TB cases with localized disease (as mentioned above), chronic empyema, bronchopleural fistula, life-threatening hemoptysis unresponsive to arteriographic embolization, and closed pleural space evacuation.

ADJUNCTIVE CORTICOSTEROID THERAPY

Corticosteroids do not play a major role in the treatment of tuberculosis, but they are useful in some types of diseases. In fulminant miliary disease and obstructive lymphadenopathy, 20 to 30 mg of prednisone daily is very helpful to relieve symptoms, improve oxygenation, and abolish fever. Patients with tuberculous meningitis at stages 2 and 3 (uncomplicated cases) seem to benefit from corticosteroid therapy. Prednisone should be begun at 60 to 80 mg daily and gradually decreased after 1 to 2 weeks. Corticosteroid therapy has been recommended in the treatment of pericardial tuberculosis to prevent constriction.

TUBERCULOSIS IN HIV INFECTION

Mycobacterial infections are important complications of HIV disease. In the past decade, the emerging HIV pandemic has contributed to resurgent tuberculosis in developed countries, exacerbations of hyperendemic tuberculosis in developing countries, and unprecedented numbers of patients with disseminated *M. avium* complex (MAC) infections. Infections with other nontuberculous mycobacteria, such as *M. kansasii* and *M. haemophilum,* are also associated with HIV infection. With the advent of highly effective antiretroviral therapies, the incidence of tuberculosis as a manifestation of AIDS has been diminished somewhat in developed regions, but the absence of such therapies in developing regions has often allowed tuberculosis to progress unchecked. The World Health Organization estimates that at least 6 million adults are infected with both agents.

Pathogenesis

A number of immunologic defects have been noted in patients with HIV and *M. tuberculosis* infections, including reductions in CD4 cell levels, impaired T-cell proliferation, decreased cytolytic T-cell responses, deranged intracellular killing, and reduced cytokine elaboration in response to mycobacterial antigen challenge. Patients with latent tuberculosis infection and HIV have a 2 to 10 percent annual risk of developing active tuberculosis. The risk of reactivation rises as CD4 cell levels decline.

The early natural history of *M. tuberculosis* infection is also greatly affected by HIV disease. People with HIV infection who acquire new tuberculosis infections have an extraordinarily high rate of progressive, primary tuberculosis. The rapid progression of tuberculosis infection to tuberculosis disease in persons with HIV infection has resulted in epidemics of tuberculosis in institutions such as hospitals, nursing homes, and prisons as well as in community settings. While HIV has a major effect on the natural history of tuberculosis, there is also evidence that tuberculosis may affect the course of HIV disease. Activation of CD4 lymphocytes by tuberculosis enhances susceptibility to HIV infection in vitro, and HIV-infected CD4 cells stimulated by mycobacterial antigens have enhanced in vitro HIV replication. Cytokine elaboration by lymphocytes and macrophages in patients with tuberculosis and HIV—in particular, tumor necrosis factor and interleukin 1—may upregulate HIV expression.

Clinical Manifestations

The clinical features of tuberculosis in persons with HIV infection may differ considerably from those seen in patients without HIV infection. In patients with higher CD4 cell counts (more than 300/mm^3), tuberculosis may be more typical, involving the lungs predominantly with upper lobe infiltrates, with or without cavitation. As CD4 cell levels decline, tuberculosis in the HIV-infected patient is more likely to be disseminated, both within the lung and throughout the body. The pulmonary presentation of tuberculosis in these patients may mimic *Pneumocystis carinii* pneumonia, with diffuse interstitial infiltrates or alveolar infiltrates. Hilar adenopathy and lower-lobe infiltrates are found in patients with progressive, primary tuberculosis. In advanced HIV disease, extrapulmonary tuberculosis is more common. Sites of extrapulmonary invasion that are most prevalent are lymph nodes, urinary tract, meninges, and blood and bone marrow. Mycobacteremia is not unusual, particularly in patients with low CD4 cell counts.

The diagnosis of tuberculosis in the HIV-infected patient requires a high index of suspicion and the utilization of appropriate diagnostic tests. Acid-fast smears of respiratory secretions or tissue samples are useful in that positive smears are strongly suggestive of tuberculosis, even in populations where *M. avium* complex is more common. In addition, the sensitivity of acid-fast smears of respiratory secretions is not altered in advanced HIV disease. However, only two-thirds to three-quarters of HIV-infected patients with pulmonary tuberculosis will have a positive acid-fast smear. Rapid diagnostic methods—such as radiometric culture systems, nucleic acid amplification, and other novel techniques—are necessary to establish a timely diagnosis. Both bronchoalveolar lavage and transbronchial biopsy can be of value in diagnosing HIV-related pulmonary tuberculosis, as well as in determining the presence or absence of other pathogens, such as *P. carinii*. Biopsy is particularly useful for patients with pulmonary nodules or hilar or subcarinal lymphadenopathy; identification of granulomas or caseous necrosis is strongly suggestive of tuberculosis. Because of the moderate sensitivity of acid-fast smears, presumptive therapy for tuberculosis is often necessary after diagnostic studies have been performed and while cultures are pending.

As discussed above, the diagnosis of tuberculosis infection with the purified protein derivative (PPD) skin test is less sensitive in patients with HIV infection than in other populations. The sensitivity of the tuberculin skin test declines as CD4 cell levels fall in HIV-infected patients. The use of anergy testing in such patients is controversial. Even with advanced HIV disease, almost half of patients with active tuberculosis will have a positive PPD, giving the test important positive predictive value clinically.

Treatment and Prevention

Treatment of tuberculosis in patients with HIV infection is extremely effective when begun promptly. Early mortality from untreated or undertreated tuberculosis has ranged from 5 to 18 percent of patients in various series. When patients with HIV-related tuberculosis are treated with rifampin-based regimens, clinical responses are similar to those in tuberculosis patients without HIV infection. Several recent studies have indicated that short-course regimens (i.e., 6 months' treatment) are highly successful, with low relapse rates. Moreover, therapy given under direct supervision is associated with better outcomes and longer survival. Whereas earlier recommendations stated that HIV-infected tuberculosis patients should be treated for at least 6 months after conversion of cultures to negative, current guidelines recognize the high rate of success with conventional 6-month regimens. It should be emphasized, however, that even with appropriate therapy, between 2 and 5 percent of patients will relapse. For this reason, some clinicians still favor longer courses of treatment for patients with HIV-related tuberculosis. Use of thiacetazone in place of rifampin in developing countries has been associated with a high rate of serious cutaneous toxicities, and responses to thiacetazone-based regimens are poorer than those to rifampin-based regimens. Most tuberculosis experts agree that use of rifampin is both safer and more cost-effective than use of thiacetazone.

With the emergence of MDR TB, the CDC and ATS have recommended that the initial treatment of active tuberculosis consist of at least a four-drug regimen and that therapy be supervised unless adherence to treatment is assured. Treatment of MDR TB is frequently unsuccessful, even in immunocompetent patients, underscoring the importance of prevention of this complication. While recent reports emphasize longer survival of HIV-infected patients with MDR TB, cure rates are still low. The risk of developing rifampin resistance appears to be greatly increased in patients with HIV infection. The reasons for this phenomenon are not fully understood, but it has been suggested that malabsorption of medications may play a role.

MYCOBACTERIUM AVIUM COMPLEX

Mycobacterium avium complex infections are an increasingly common complication of HIV disease. Although *M. avium* complex is found widely in the environment, the incidence of disseminated *M. avium* complex in patients with HIV disease varies geographically. For example, although more than 15 percent of AIDS patients in the United States will develop *M. avium* complex disease, the disease is unusual in African AIDS patients. Within the United States, AIDS patients from some regions have a higher prevalence of *M. avium* complex than patients from other areas. The reason for these geographic differences in *M. avium* complex prevalence is not known. Intensive prospective studies of patients with HIV infection at risk for *M. avium* complex have failed to establish any connection between environmental exposures and subsequent disease.

The *M. avium* complex family comprises numerous organisms of varying serotypes from the species *M. avium* and *M. intracellulare.* While a large proportion of patients with pulmonary *M. avium* complex disease harbor *M. intracellulare,* most AIDS patients who get disease are infected with *M. avium.* Both monoclonal and polyclonal infections are known to exist, and the timing of the acquisition of initial infection is unclear. The most important predictor of disseminated *M. avium* complex is low CD4 lymphocyte count. Several prospective studies have shown that as CD4 counts fall to below $100/\text{mm}^3$, the annual incidence of *M. avium* complex bacteremia rises substantially. For patients with CD4 counts below $50/\text{mm}^3$, the risk of *M. avium* complex bacteremia is between 10 and 20 percent per year. Conversely, patients with CD4 counts of at least $100/\text{mm}^3$ are very unlikely to develop *M. avium* complex disease in the subsequent year. Patients found to have *M. avium* complex bacteremia, on the other hand, almost always have CD4 lymphocyte counts below $20/\text{mm}^3$. Other immunologic abnormalities that may contribute to the development of *M. avium* complex disease are impaired intracellular killing of organisms by macrophages, variations in cytokine production (especially interleukin-12), and derangements in antigen presentation to effector cells. Prior colonization of the respiratory and gastrointestinal tracts increases the risk of disseminated *M. avium* complex significantly, but most patients with *M. avium* complex bacteremia never show evidence of colonization. However, two-thirds of the patients who ultimately developed bacteremia never have evidence of colonization. Thus, screening of blood, stools, or sputum cannot be recommended routinely. Several recent studies suggest that bacteremia precedes dissemination and may be transient. Patients with transient bacteremia have less severe disease and longer survival than patients with sustained bacteremia. With sustained bacteremia there is ongoing seeding of organs and an increasing tissue burden.

Clinical Manifestations

Common symptoms of disseminated *M. avium* complex include fever, sweats, weight loss, diarrhea, and malaise. The onset of illness is usually insidious, and symptoms are often present for many weeks before the diagnosis is established. Accompanying clinical signs and laboratory abnormalities frequently include cachexia and weight loss, hepatosplenomegaly, anemia, neutropenia, and elevation of the alkaline phosphatase. In some patients, *M. avium* complex may be restricted to the lymph nodes, gastrointestinal tract, or lungs. *M. avium* complex infections of the lungs, including focal pneumonia and endobronchial lesions, may occur with or without bacteremia. Pulmonary impairment may be acute or chronic.

The diagnosis of disseminated *M. avium* complex disease is usually made from isolation of organisms from blood or bone marrow cultures. Patients in whom *M. avium* complex is identified in other tissues should have blood cultures performed to detect disseminated disease. Cultures should be performed with Bactec or another rapid culture assay so that results can be obtained expeditiously. Use of DNA-RNA hybridization probes allows speciation within 1 to 2 days after growth in liquid media. Isolating *M. avium* complex in stool or sputum does not necessarily indicate systemic disease, although patients with positive respiratory or gastrointestinal cultures, as noted above, are at increased risk of disseminated disease subsequently. In some circumstances, presumptive therapy for the disease may be initiated while cultures are pending, but long-term treatment should be based on isolation of the organism in culture. If blood cultures are unrevealing in a patient with suspected *M. avium* complex disease, a bone marrow aspirate and biopsy may confirm the diagnosis.

Treatment

Treatment of disseminated *M. avium* complex disease in patients with HIV infection has improved substantially since early in the AIDS epidemic. Early reports noted that standard antimycobacterial agents had minimal activity against this pathogen, although four- or five-drug combination regimens were shown to have moderate to good effect in some studies. Therapy against *M. avium* complex has been advanced considerably by the extended-spectrum macrolides clarithromycin and azithromycin (Table 62-14). These agents have been shown to have superior activity against *M. avium* complex disease. Clarithromycin given alone significantly reduces levels of bacteremia and is associated with clinical improvement. Lower doses of clarithromycin($\leq$1 g/day total) are better tolerated, with fewer gastrointestinal side effects than with high doses, and are associated with better survival, for unclear reasons. Treatment of *M. avium* complex bacteremia with clarithromycin alone is associated with emergence of drug-resistant organisms and recrudescence of

TABLE 62-14 Dosages of Drugs Used in Treating Adults with Atypical Tuberculosis

Rifampin	600–900 mg per day in a single dose
Isoniazid	300–600 mg per day in a single dose
Ethambutol	25 mg/kg daily in a single dose until cultures are negative for 6 months, then 15 mg/kg daily thereafter
Streptomycin, capreomycin, kanamycin, amikacin	15 mg/kg up to 1 g, once daily 5 days a week—when cultures are negative or significant toxicity occurs, dosages can be reduced and/or the drug given less frequently
Azithromycin	500–1000 mg per day in a single dose
Clarithromycin	500–750 mg twice daily
Ciprofloxacin	500–750 mg twice daily
Ofloxacin	800 mg per day in a single dose
Clofazimine	100–200 mg per day in a single dose
Rifabutin	300–600 mg per day in a single dose
Ethionamide	500–1000 mg per day usually in divided doses; give highest tolerated dose
Cycloserine	500–1000 mg per day usually in divided doses; give highest tolerated dose

symptoms. The mechanism for development of drug-resistant disease is selection of preexisting, innately macrolide-resistant *M. avium* clones during therapy. Azithromycin also reduces the level of bacteremia, and its use as monotherapy similarly results in emergence of drug-resistant disease. Resistant organisms usually begin to emerge after 2 to 3 months of treatment, and most patients will experience relapses with drug-resistant isolates after 4 or more months of monotherapy.

Combination therapy for disseminated *M. avium* complex is necessary to prevent the emergence of resistance. Regimens should consist of clarithromycin or azithromycin with at least one other antimycobacterial agent. Combination therapy with clarithromycin and ethambutol is clinically active and prevents relapses with drug-resistant organisms in a large proportion of patients. The addition of clofazimine to this regimen does not improve efficacy and is associated with greater mortality. The use of a three-drug regimen of clarithromycin, rifabutin, and ethambutol is also very effective. The use of clarithromycin and clofazimine results in high rates of relapse with drug-resistant organisms. The role of amikacin and ciprofloxacin remains unclear. In general, these agents are reserved for patients failing first-line therapy. The value of these agents in combination with clarithromycin has not been studied, however.

A major limitation to the treatment of *M. avium* complex disease is the occurrence of adverse reactions. Clarithromycin and azithromycin are associated with dose-related gastrointestinal toxicity, which affects up to one-half of patients. Common complaints include abdominal pain, nausea, vomiting, and diarrhea. Dose reduction or drug holiday may alleviate symptoms and permit further treatment. Taste and smell perversion occurs in 5 to 15 percent of patients treated with macrolides. Hepatotoxicity and rash are less common. Ethambutol is generally well tolerated, although gastrointestinal intolerance sometimes occurs. Optic neuritis is rare at doses of less than 20 mg/kg daily. Rifabutin, a semisynthetic rifamycin S derivative with activity against *M. avium* complex, may cause nausea, rash, and neutropenia. Discoloration of urine, tears, and sweat is a predictable complication in one-third to one-half of patients. Rifabutin-associated uveitis is common at high doses (450 to 600 mg daily) of the drug, particularly when clarithromycin and fluconazole are used concomitantly. Clearance of rifabutin by P450 cytochromes is inhibited by clarithromycin and fluconazole, resulting in higher serum concentrations of rifabutin.

Currently, routine testing of all *M. avium* complex isolates for drug susceptibility is not recommended. The value of susceptibility test results in predicting clinical outcomes is apparent only for clarithromycin. Making treatment decisions about patients who appear to be failing therapy is difficult. For a patient who develops symptoms of disseminated *M. avium* complex after an initial response, it is important to rule out other opportunistic diseases with similar signs and symptoms. Blood cultures should be obtained for mycobacteria and held for 4 to 6 weeks, as drug therapy may delay growth. If cultures are positive, testing for clarithromycin susceptibility is reasonable. For the patient known or thought to be failing treatment, at least two new agents should be added or substituted. Azithromycin should not be substituted for clarithromycin, as cross-resistance to these agents is the rule. Recently, interferon gamma has been shown to be active in controlling disseminated *M. avium* complex infections in patients without HIV. The efficacy of interferon gamma in patients with AIDS is not known.

TABLE 62-15 Guidelines for Prevention of *M. avium* Complex Disease in Patients with HIV Infection

1. Begin prophylaxis for patients with CD4 counts <75/mm^3.
2. Rule out active tuberculosis by clinical exam and appropriate laboratory studies.
3. Obtain mycobacterial blood culture to rule out subclinical bacteremia.
4. Regimens:Azithromycin, 1200 mg weekly
   or Clarithromycin, 500 mg twice daily
   or Rifabutin, 300 mg daily

Prevention

Because disseminated *M. avium* complex infection is a predictable late complication of HIV infection that occurs in a large proportion of patients, chemoprophylaxis to prevent disease is desirable in patients not responding to highly active antiretroviral therapy (HAART) or for whom HAART is not available. Guidelines for prevention of *M. avium* complex disease in patients with HIV infection are currently in flux. A summary of current guidelines for prevention of *M. avium* complex infections in patients with HIV is given in Table 62-15. It should be noted that therapy of the HIV infection should be initiated to attempt immunologic restoration and that drug interactions are common in the combination of HAART and antimycobacterial therapy. Because prophylaxis against *M. avium* complex reduces disease incidence and prolongs life, this therapy is generally considered standard for patients with CD4 counts under 50/mm^3. Clarithromycin 500 mg twice daily or azithromycin 1200 mg weekly is generally preferred as initial therapy; rifabutin 300 mg daily is an alternative.

OTHER MYCOBACTERIA

Patients with HIV infection are susceptible to a number of other mycobacterial infections, although these are less common than tuberculosis or *M. avium* complex. *M. kansasii* infections generally mimic tuberculosis, occurring in severely immunocompromised HIV-infected patients with cavitary or diffuse pulmonary infiltrates. Patients often have concomitant pulmonary infections, most often *P. carinii* pneumonia. Bacteremia, osteomyelitis, and soft tissue infections are also seen. Without therapy, the disease is generally progressive. Treatment with isoniazid, rifampin, and ethambutol for 12 to 18 months is recommended, and clarithromycin is also active against this organism.

M. genavense causes disseminated disease in advanced immunodeficiency, with bacteremia and other organ involvement. The organism grows poorly in liquid media and cannot be cultured on solid media. It is detectable with amplification of genomic sequences by the polymerase chain reaction, but this is not readily available in most settings. The diagnosis is suggested in HIV-infected patients with an *M. avium* complex–like illness who have weakly positive (low growth index) cultures that cannot be speciated or who have negative cultures but tissue samples showing acid-fast bacilli. Formal studies of treatment for *M. genavense* infections have not been conducted, but anecdotal information suggests that regimens active against *M. avium* complex are also effective for this organism. *M. haemophilum* may cause skin and soft tissue infections in AIDS patients, and case reports of infections with *M. fortuitum, M. chelonae,* and *M. xenopi* have appeared.

BIBLIOGRAPHY

American Thoracic Society: Treatment of tuberculosis and tuberculosis infection in adults and children. *Am J Respir Crit Care Med* 149:1359–1374, 1994.

Banerjee A, Dubnau E, Quemard A, et al: *InhA,* a gene encoding a target for isoniazid and ethionamide in *Mycobacterium tuberculosis. Science* 263:227–230, 1994.

Barnes PF, Bloch AB, Davidson PT, Snider DE: Tuberculosis in patients with human immunodeficiency virus infection. *N Engl J Med* 324:1644–1650, 1991.

Bor D, Epstein P: Pathogenesis or respiratory infection in the disadvantaged. *Semin Respir Infect* 6:194–203, 1991.

British Thoracic and Tuberculosis Association, Research Committee: Aspergilloma and residual tuberculous cavities—the results of a survey. *Tubercle* 51:227–245, 1970.

Burwen DR, Bloch AB, Griffin LD, Ciesielski CA. National trends in the concurrence of tuberculosis and acquired immunodeficiency syndrome. *Arch Intern Med* 155:1281–1286, 1995.

Cantwell MF, Snider DE, Cauthen GM, Onorato IM: Epidemiology of tuberculosis in the United States, 1985 through 1992. *JAMA* 272:535–539, 1994.

Centers for Disease Control: Guidelines for preventing the transmission of *Mycobacterium tuberculosis* in health-care facilities, 1994. *MMWR* 43(No. RR-13):57, 1994.

Centers for Disease Control: Prevention and treatment of tuberculosis among patients infected with human immunodeficiency virus: Principles of therapy and revised recommendations. *MMWR* 47(RR-20):1–51, 1998.

Centers for Disease Control: The use of preventive therapy for tuberculous infection in the United States. *MMWR* 39(RR-8):1–12, 1990.

Centers for Disease Control: Targeted tuberculin testing and treatment of latent tuberculosis. *MMWR* 49(49-RR):6, 2000.

Centers for Disease Control: USPHS/IDSA Guidelines for the prevention of opportunistic infections in persons infected with human immunodeficiency virus: A summary. *MMWR* 44(RR-8):9–10, 1995.

Centers for Disease Control: Update: Fatal and severe liver injuries associated with rifampin and pyrazinamide for LTBI; *MMWR* 50(34):733–736, 2001.

Chaisson RE, Benson CA, Dube MP, et al: Clarithromycin therapy for bacteremic *Mycobacterium avium* complex disease—A randomized, double-blind, dose-ranging study in patients with AIDS. *Ann Intern Med* 121:905–911, 1994.

Chaisson RE, Moore RD, Richman DD, et al: Incidence and natural history of *Mycobacterium avium*–complex infections in patients with advanced human immunodeficiency virus disease treated with zidovudine. *Am Rev Respir Dis* 146:285–289, 1992.

Colditz GA, Brewer T, Berkley C, et al: Efficacy of BCG in the prevention of tuberculosis: Meta-analysis of the published literature. *JAMA* 271:698–702, 1994.

Cremaschi P, Nascimbene C, Vitulo P, et al: Therapeutic embolization of bronchial artery: A successful treatment in 209 cases of relapse hemoptysis. *Angiology* 44:295–299, 1993.

Daley CL, Small PM, Schecter GF, et al: An outbreak of tuberculosis with accelerated progression among persons infected with human immunodeficiency virus: An analysis using restriction-fragment-length polymorphisms. *N Engl J Med* 326:231–235, 1992.

Dutt AK, Moers D, Stead WW: Smear- and culture-negative pulmonary tuberculosis: Four-month short-course chemotherapy. *Am Rev Respir Dis* 139:867–870, 1989.

Fine PEM: Variation in protection by BCG: Implications of and for heterologous immunity. *Lancet* 346:1339–1345, 1995.

Fischl MA, Uttamchandani RB, Daikos GL, et al: An outbreak of tuberculosis caused by multi-drug-resistant tubercle bacilli among patients with HIV infection. *Ann Intern Med* 117:177–183, 1992.

Garibaldi RA, Drusin RE, Ferebee SH, Gregg MB: Isoniazid-associated hepatitis. *Am Rev Respir Dis* 106:357–365, 1972.

Goble M, Iseman MD, Madsen LA, et al: Treatment of 171 patients with pulmonary tuberculosis resistant to isoniazid and rifampin. *N Engl J Med* 328:527–532, 1993.

Gonzalez-Montaner LJ, Natal S, Yongchaiyud P, Olliaro P, the Rifabutin Study Group: Rifabutin for the treatment of newly diagnosed pulmonary tuberculosis: A multinational, randomized, comparative study versus rifampicin. *Tubercle Lung Dis* 75:341–347, 1994.

Graham NMH, Nelson KE, Solomon L, et al: Prevalence of tuberculin positivity and skin test anergy in HIV-1–seropositive and –seronegative intravenous drug users. *JAMA* 267:369–373, 1992.

Hoover DR, Graham NMH, Bacellar H, et al: An epidemiologic analysis of *Mycobacterium avium* complex disease in homosexual men infected with human immunodeficiency virus type 1. *Clin Infect Dis* 20:1250–1258, 1995.

Iseman MD: Treatment of multidrug-resistant tuberculosis. *N Engl J Med* 329:784–791, 1993.

Jones BE, Young SM, Antoniskis D, et al: Relationship of the manifestations of tuberculosis to CD4 cell counts in patients with human immunodeficiency virus infection. *Am Rev Respir Dis* 148:1292–1297, 1994.

Kim YH, Kim HT, Lee KS, et al: Serial fiberoptic bronchoscopic observations of endobronchial tuberculosis before and early after antituberculosis chemotherapy. *Chest* 103:673–677, 1993.

Lecoeur HF, Truffot-Pernot C, Grosset JH: Experimental short-course preventive therapy of tuberculosis with rifampin and pyrazinamide. *Am Rev Respir Dis* 140:1189–1193, 1989.

Menzies D, Fanning A, Yuan L, Fitzgerald M: Tuberculosis among health care workers. *N Engl J Med* 332:92–98, 1995.

Morris CD, Bird AR, Nell H: The hematological and biochemical changes in severe tuberculosis. *Q J Med* 73:1151–1159, 1989.

Pape JW, Jean SS, Ho JL, et al: Effect of isoniazid prophylaxis on incidence of active tuberculosis and progression of HIV infection. *Lancet* 342:268–272, 1993.

Rossman MD, MacGregor RR (eds): *Tuberculosis.* New York, McGraw-Hill, 1995.

Simone PM, Dooley SW: The phenomenon of multidrug-resistant tuberculosis, in Rossman MD, MacGregor RR (eds): *Tuberculosis.* New York, McGraw-Hill, 1995, pp 219–311.

Stead WW, Senner JW, Reddick WT, Lofgren JP: Racial differences in susceptibility to infection by *Mycobacterium tuberculosis. N Engl J Med* 322:422–427, 1990.

Steele MA, Burk RF, Des Prez RM: Toxic hepatitis with isoniazid and rifampin. *Chest* 99:465–471, 1991.

Wallace JM, Deutsch AL, Harrell JH, Moser KM: Bronchoscopy and transbronchial biopsy in evaluation of patients with suspected active tuberculosis. *Am J Med* 70:1189–1194, 1981.

Wallis RS, Vjecha M, Amir-Tahmasseb M, et al: Influence of tuberculosis on human immunodeficiency virus (HIV-1): Enhanced cytokine expression and elevated β_2-microglobulin in HIV-1–associated tuberculosis. *J Infect Dis* 167:43–48, 1993.

63 | Fungal Infections of the Lungs*

Jay A. Fishman

OVERVIEW

Fungal pneumonia is rarely observed outside the broad group of immuno-compromised hosts. Diagnostic modalities for the fungi—e.g., blood tests, molecular assays—have lagged behind those for bacteria and viruses. As a result, the clinician is often confronted with the need for either empiric therapy or for invasive diagnosis via lung biopsy. The advent of newer antifungal agents with reduced toxicities compared with traditional amphotericin B deoxycholate (lipid-associated amphotericin, newer azoles, and echinocandin antimicrobials; see Table 63-1) has altered approaches to many fungal infections. This chapter will focus on some of the more common infections affecting the lungs. However, some general principles apply, which reflect the need for rapid and accurate diagnosis in the immunocompromised host (Table 63-2).

- Infections are a function of the nature of the immune defects of and the epidemiologic exposures of the host. Thus, neutropenic hosts are more often affected by *Aspergillus* species, line infections are most commonly *Candida* species, sinus infections in diabetics most often of the *Mucoraciae* group, patients with T-cell deficits (organ transplants, AIDS) with *Pneumocystis carinii, Cryptococcus neoformans, Histoplasma capsulatum* or *Coccidioides immitis*.

- Given the rapid progression of infection in the compromised host and the toxicities of antifungal therapies (including drug interactions), early invasive diagnosis is preferable to empiric therapy whenever possible.

- Inadequate therapy to avoid toxicity is unacceptable. Most toxicities can be managed with appropriate forethought (Tables 63-3 and 63-4).

- "Atypical" fungal infections are becoming more common. Thus, microbiologic data from biopsies of small nodules or skin lesions, unusual isolates form catheter infections, and surgical specimens should be believed and acted upon. These might include *Fusarium* species from blood cultures or pustules, *Paecilomyces* from nodular skin lesions, *Pseudoallescheria boydii (now Scedosporium species)* in sinusitis and endocarditis, pulmonary coin lesions due to *Penicillium* or *Cryptococcus or* pheohyphomycosis, and *P. carinii* pneumonia while on inadequate prophylaxis.

---

*Edited from Chaps. 146 to 150, "Actinomycosis and Nocardiosis," by Filice GA, Armstrong D; "Aspergillus Syndromes, Mucormycosis, and Pulmonary Candidiasis," by Sugar AM, Olek EA; "Endemic Mycoses of North America: Histoplasmosis, Coccidioidomycosis, and Blastomycosis," by Wheat LJ; Cryptococcal Infections," by Goldman MM; Wheat LJ; and "*Pneumocystis Carinii*," by Fishman JA. In: *Fishman's Pulmonary Diseases and Disorders,* 3d ed., edited by Fishman AP, Elias JA, Fishman JA, Grippi MA, Kaiser LR, Senior RM. New York, McGraw-Hill, 1998, pp 2257–2332. For fuller discussion of topics dealt with in this chapter, the reader is referred to the original text, as noted above.

TABLE 63-1 Antifungal Agents for Invasive Mycoses

Amphotericin B deoxycholate
Liposomal polyenes
  ABLC, ABCD, AmBisome
  Liposomal nystatin
Azoles
  Fluconazole
  Itraconazole (cyclodextrin/IV)
  Voriconazole
  Posaconazole (SCH56592)
  Ravuconazole (BMS-207147)
Echinocandins
  Caspofungin (MK-0991; Cancidas)
  Mycofungin (FK463); VER-002 (LY303366)
Others: pradimicins, sordarins

- The distinction between colonization and invasive disease (e.g., aspergilloma vs. aspergillosis) is often breached in the compromised host.

- The roles of newer antifungal agents remain to be clarified (Tables 63-5 and 63-6). The procurement costs for these agents are significant.

- Clinical trials of therapy for invasive fungal infections of the lungs, in particular those due to *Aspergillus* species, do not discriminate well between agents. In the most compromised individuals, mortality is at least 40 percent for every agent studied, and often higher.

PULMONARY ASPERGILLOSIS

Aspergillus species are ubiquitous molds that reproduce by formation of conidia; these are readily airborne and reach the airways by inhalation. Germination of conidia results in the production of hyphae, which are the forms associated with disease. *Pulmonary aspergillosis* is a general term for the lung disease caused by the genus *Aspergillus.* The three commonly described categories are allergic aspergillosis, colonizing aspergillosis, and invasive diseases. The spectrum of pulmonary aspergillosis is described in Table 63-7.

TABLE 63-2 General Principles in Management of Fungal Infections

Infections are often asymptomatic.
Invasive techniques to obtain specimens for histology and microbiological evaluation are critical.
Reversal of immune suppression is critical for successful management whenever possible.
Antimicrobial agents alone are inadequate for the cure of invasive fungal infection (e.g., *Aspergillus*). Surgical intervention is essential.
Compromises must often be made based on the inherent toxicities of many antimicrobial agents. However, the use of second line agents that allow the progression of infection is unacceptable.
Prior to cessation of therapy, there must be demonstration of response and "cure."

TABLE 63-3 Amphotericin B[a]

Activity
  Binds to ergosterol; cell wall disruption
  Considered a "cidal" antifungal
  Broad spectrum of activity
  Despite limitations, the "gold standard" for therapy of systemic and invasive fungal infection
  Few resistant fungi; emerging resistance
Administration
  IV formulation for systemic infection; no oral
  Dose-limiting toxicity
  Renal insufficiency
  Administration effects: chills, fever, anemia
  Electrolyte abnormalities (low K and Mg)
Significant toxicities:
  Infusion associated acute and largely cytokine-mediated: headache, chills, nausea and vomiting, fever, dyspnea, tachycardia, bradycardia, arrhythmia, back pain, hypothermia, hypertension, hypotension
  Nephrotoxicity—acute and chronic
  Glomerular: ↓GFR, ↓renal blood flow
  Tubular: urinary casts, renal tubular acidosis, Mg and K wasting, nephrocalcinosis
  Exacerbated by sodium deprivation (tubuloglomerular feedback, Cl wasting)
  Renal arteriolar vasospasm? Calcium depletion during ischemia? Direct toxicity? Cytokines? Vasospasm?
  Normochromic normocytic anemia, leukopenia, thrombocytopenia
  Neurotoxicity: confusion, depression, seizures, paresis, leukoencephalopathy

[a]Similar toxicities may be seen with lipid-associated forms of amphotericin B. While infusion-related side effects and nephrotoxocity are reduced in this class of agents, attention must be paid to hydration and electrolyte abnormalities.

There is overlap among these categories, and patients may exhibit characteristics of more than one process or progress from one category to another. Sputum from normal individuals may contain the fungus for many days after exposure in the absence of disease. Conversely, invasive pulmonary aspergillosis occurs in patients with prolonged and profound immune defects. Host immune status, in addition to the intensity of exposure, is the most important determinant of the disease process.

TABLE 63-4 Antifungal Therapy: Preventing Toxicity of Amphotericin B

Considerations: Efficacy associated with high plasma levels and total dose.
Sodium loading (>1 L normal saline IV, bolus or continuous)
  Maintain urine output (not mannitol)
  Correction of serum magnesium, potassium
  Hypotension (especially renal ischemia)
Concomitant nephrotoxins: aminoglycosides, calcineurin inhibitors, high-dose sulfamethoxazole, diuretics, cisplatin
  Possible antagonism with azoles (itraconazole)—some animal data, few in vivo data
  Cytokine storm—anti-inflammatory, antihistamines

TABLE 63-5 Azole Antifungals

Activity
  Inhibit cytochrome P450; α-14 demethylase
  Block formation of ergosterol; inhibit cell growth
  Slower killing—considered "static" drugs
  Interactions with P450 drug metabolism
Toxicity: ketoconazole $>>$ itraconazole $\geq$
voriconazole $>$ fluconazole (in general; individual
patients may vary)
  Nausea/vomiting, hepatotoxicity, adrenals
  Significant drug interactions
  Visual effects: voriconazole (~25%)
    Altered light perception
    Reversible/transient/dose-related

Epidemiology

Aspergillus species are ubiquitous and occur worldwide. The fungi grow well in many habitats and are commonly found on stored hay or grain, decaying vegetation, soil, dung, and organic debris. Inhalation of conidia probably occurs regularly, although disease is uncommon. A seasonal variation in the prevalence of outdoor spore levels may influence the development of extrinsic hypersensitivity disease, although no seasonal variation in the incidence of invasive pulmonary aspergillosis has been shown. Outbreaks of invasive pulmonary aspergillosis in oncology and transplant wards have been described in association with hospital construction, renovation, or suboptimal maintenance of ventilation systems. Pathogenic *Aspergillus* species have been isolated in the soil of indoor potted plants. Molecular epidemiologic methods utilizing DNA fingerprinting are useful for the investigation of the association between environmental sources of *Aspergillus* and infection.

Mycology and Host Defenses

Human infection has been caused by 19 species of the nearly 700 species described. The commonly isolated species include *A. fumigatus, A. flavus, A. niger,* and *A. terreus. A. fumigatus* is the most common cause of allergic

---

TABLE 63-6 Echinocandins

Caspofungin (MK-0991; Cancidas)
Micafungin (FK463); VER-002 (LY303366)
Mechanism: Inhibit cell wall β-1,3-glucan synthase
Characteristics
  Rapidly fungicidal for yeast
  Intravenous administration only
  Minimal renal toxicity
  Interactions with cyclosporine (liver function tests)?
Activity
  Yeasts (*C. albicans;* non-*albicans*)
  Molds (*Aspergillus;* not Zygomycetes)
  Others (endemic mycoses; **not** *Cryptococcus*)
  Synergy with amphotericin B? with voriconazole?

TABLE 63-7 Spectrum of Pulmonary Aspergillosis

Clinical Manifestation	Immune Status	Underlying Lung Architecture	Degree of Tissue Invasion
Simple colonization	Normal	Chronic obstructive airway disease	None
Hypersensitivity reactions			
Allergic bronchial asthma	↑	Normal	None
Allergic bronchopulmonary aspergillosis	↑	Excess airway mucus	None
Bronchocentric granulomatosis	↑	Excess airway mucus	None
Extrinsic allergic alveolitis	↑	Normal	None
Colonization			
Aspergilloma[a]	Normal	Preexisting cavity	None
Invasive disease			
Bronchial stump aspergillosis	Normal	Pneumonectomy	+
Chronic necrotizing pulmonary aspergillosis	↓	→	Normal +
Invasive pulmonary aspergillosis	↓↓↓	Normal	+++

KEY: ↑, hyperactive humoral response; ↓, suppressed immune response; ↓↓↓, severely depressed immune response, neutropenia.
[a]May have features of invasive disease surrounding the cavity.

pulmonary and invasive disease. *Aspergillus* species are rapidly growing, hardy molds, identified by the appearance of the colony and by microscopic examination of the spore-bearing structures. Microscopically, *Aspergillus* species are characterized by the production of narrow, uniform hyphae, 4- to 6-μm in width, with parallel walls and distinct septa. Dichotomous branching occurs at 45-degree angles. A wide range of microscopic appearances may be observed in clinical specimens. Other fungi such as *Fusarium* and *Scedosporium boydii* share the same microscopic appearance as *Aspergillus.*

Patient sputum specimens examined by direct mount or with KOH and ink may reveal the typical 45-degree branching hyphal fragments, often associated with eosinophils and Charcot-Leyden crystals in patients with allergic bronchopulmonary aspergillosis (ABPA). Stained tissue sections reveal regular hyaline septate hyphae best observed with periodic acid–Schiff (PAS) and Gomori's methenamine-silver (GMS) stains. Fungus ball specimens from cavities connected to open bronchi have hyphae that often appear lifeless and stain poorly, and, although seldom seen, the fruiting heads and conidia may appear well formed.

The conidia, or airborne spores, produced by *Aspergillus* species are small enough (2.5 to 3.0 μm) to reach the alveoli when inhaled. Pulmonary macrophages may kill the fungus under certain conditions in vitro, a function that is inhibited by corticosteroids. When first-line host defense mechanisms fail, germination of conidia results in production of hyphae. These hyphae may activate the complement cascade in serum, increase the generation of phagocytic chemotactic factors, and increase neutrophil degranulation. Once hyphae have formed, neutrophils can attach to and damage the fungal cells. Symptomatic pulmonary aspergillosis is reported among individuals with late-stage AIDS; because HIV-infected individuals have multiple immune defects, including defective neutrophil function, the role of T-cell immunity in host defense against *Aspergillus* remains unclear.

A. fumigatus produces several unique virulence factors, including a complement inhibitor and phagocytosis inhibitors including gliotoxin and aflatoxin. Gliotoxin impairs macrophage phagocytosis and the induction of cytotoxic T cells in vitro. The surface of resting conidia is coated by rodlike structures of a hydrophobic protein called *hydrophobin,* the significance of which is not clear. The production of different proteolytic enzymes (elastases, collagenases, trypsine) by *A. fumigatus* may play a role in breaching the mucosal–epithelial barrier and in degradation of host defense factors. Oxalic acid is produced by some species, especially *A. niger,* and presumably contributes to the inflammatory reaction around a fungus ball or *mycetoma* of the lung. Calcium oxalate forms in tissue and appears as birefringent crystals that may be seen in the microscopically examined sputum.

Clinical Manifestations

Hypersensitivity Reactions

Aspergillus species are important fungi that are involved in several distinct pulmonary syndromes. Clinical manifestations of *Aspergillus* infection are largely determined by the immunologic status of the individual and any underlying lung pathology. For example, atopic individuals represent a unique subset of patients in whom the fungal antigen can cause various responses, including allergic asthma, allergic bronchopulmonary aspergillosis (ABPA),

TABLE 63-8 Hypersensitivity Reactions to *Aspergillus*

	Asthma	Allergic Bronchopulmonary Aspergillosis	Extrinsic Allergic Alveolitis
Pathology	Hypertrophied mucous glands	Colonization of airways, viscid mucoid impaction, tissue eosinophilia	Lymphocytic infiltration of interstitium, noncaseating granuloma
Radiographic features			
Early	Normal hyperinflation	Migratory peripheral infiltrates, atelectasis, bronchiectasis	Diffuse alveolar-interstitial infiltrates
Late	Normal, hyperinflation	Fibrosis	Reticulonodular interstitial opacities
Skin test reactions to *Aspergillus* antigens			
Immediate	Positive	Positive	Positive
Delayed	Negative	Positive	Positive
Peripheral eosinophilia	Negative	Positive	Negative
IgG precipitins	Positive (up to 25%)	Positive	Positive
Serum IgE levels	Normal or mildly elevated	Marked elevation	Normal

or bronchocentric granulomatosis. In nonatopic individuals, airway colonization or extrinsic allergic alveolitis can occur as a result of massive or repeated inhalation of conidia. Early recognition of these syndromes is important so that appropriate treatment can be started early to prevent progression to permanent lung damage. Table 63-8 summarizes the hypersensitivity reactions to *Aspergillus*.

Simple Colonization

Aspergillus can exist on body surfaces and in bronchi without eliciting a pathologic response. Patients suffering from underlying chronic obstructive pulmonary disease (COPD) frequently require corticosteroids or antibiotic therapy for management of exacerbations and are consequently at increased risk for fungal colonization. Tissue invasion is not a feature of saprophytic colonization, although pulmonary aspergillosis may develop with the alteration of host defenses. Patients may show immunologic responses including increased IgE antibody, increased precipitins, and immediate or delayed skin reactivity to *Aspergillus* antigen. However, specific *Aspergillus* IgE or IgG antibody levels are not elevated.

Allergic Bronchial Asthma

Asthmatic patients may become sensitized to *Aspergillus* conidia as a consequence of thick bronchial secretions that trap fungal spores. The conidia seldom germinate in the bronchial airways. The syndrome develops in patients who are atopic and is perpetuated by inhalation of *Aspergillus* antigens, which typically cause acute bronchospasm. Transient infiltrates have been described during the immediate reaction but are not usual. As is typical in asthma of other etiologies, serum eosinophils and IgE antibody are increased. Immediate skin reactions to *Aspergillus* antigens are positive, but specific precipitating antibodies (IgG) are usually negative. Attenuation of spore exposure can diminish the frequency and severity of bronchospasm in this group of patients.

Allergic Bronchopulmonary Aspergillosis

Clinical Features Allergic bronchopulmonary aspergillosis (ABPA) occurs in atopic individuals with asthma or cystic fibrosis. The symptoms of ABPA include recurrent wheezing, malaise with low-grade fever, cough, sputum production (blood-streaked), chest pain, and pulmonary infiltrates. Patients may have a history of recurrent pneumonia and frequent antibiotic therapy. Chronic ABPA is characterized by cough and sputum production with superimposed acute exacerbations. Bronchiectasis becomes dominant with the development of clubbing and fixed radiographic abnormalities. Occasionally patients may present without symptoms or physical findings despite radiographic abnormalities.

The events involved in the development of ABPA occur when patients with asthma or cystic fibrosis develop bronchial allergic reactions to inhaled *Aspergillus* conidia. Mucous plugs form in the proximal bronchi and can progress to mucoid impaction resulting in atelectasis with transient pulmonary infiltrates. Mucous plugs often yield *Aspergillus* on culture. Repeated allergic reactions in the bronchi cause bronchiectasis in the proximal bronchi, where characteristic circular or oblong radiodensities are formed. These "ring signs" and "tram shadows" are observable on chest radiograph and represent small rims of chronic peribronchial inflammation around dilated bronchi.

Radiographic Findings Pulmonary infiltrates may be transient or permanent. Transient abnormalities may be the result of parenchymal infiltrates, mucoid impactions, or secretions in damaged bronchi. "Toothpaste" shadows result from mucoid impactions in damaged bronchi. "Gloved finger" shadows result from distally occluded bronchi filled with secretions. "Tramline" shadows are two parallel hairline shadows extending out from the hilum.

Permanent radiographic findings include proximal bronchiectasis, characterized by normal filling of bronchi distal to the sacular bronchial lesion. This finding is considered a strong diagnostic feature of ABPA, especially on computed tomography (CT) scans, which have greater sensitivity. Parallel-line or tramline shadows result from bronchiectasis with bronchial dilation; ring shadows are dilated bronchi *en face*. Late findings in ABPA include cavitation, local emphysema, contracted upper lobes, and honeycomb fibrosis. A normal chest radiograph does not rule out a diagnosis of ABPA, and bronchiectasis may be better demonstrated by narrow-section (3-mm) CT scans.

Diagnosis Patterson and coworkers have defined eight criteria for the diagnosis of ABPA. These are summarized in Table 63-9. Individuals meeting seven of eight criteria make the diagnosis of ABPA highly likely, and the presence of all eight criteria confirms the diagnosis. Brown mucous plugs containing eosinophils and hyphae may be present in expectorated sputum in

TABLE 63-9 Criteria for the Diagnosis of Allergic Bronchopulmonary Aspergillosis

Primary
  Episodic bronchial obstruction (asthma)
  Peripheral blood eosinophilia ($>1000/mm^3$)
  Immediate type skin reactivity to *Aspergillus* antigen
  Precipitating serum antibodies (precipitins) against *Aspergillus* antigen
  Elevated serum IgE concentrations (>1000 ng/mL)
  Elevated serum IgE and IgG antibodies specific to *Aspergillus fumigatus*
  History of pulmonary infiltrates (transient or fixed)
  Central bronchiectasis
Secondary
  Aspergillus fumigatus in sputum (by repeated culture or microscopic examination)
  History of expectoration of brown plugs or flecks
  Arthus reactivity (late skin reactivity) to *Aspergillus* antigen

SOURCE: Adapted with permission from Rosenberg et al.

up to 50 percent of patients with acute ABPA. Asthma, eosinophilia, and a history of unexplained pulmonary infiltrates should alert clinicians to the possibility of ABPA.

Patients with ABPA demonstrate a hypersensitivity reaction to *A. fumigatus* in the bronchial tree without tissue invasion. Type I and III reactions are involved in and around bronchial walls, where fungal antigens are released. Type I, IgE-mediated, immediate hypersensitivity reactions are thought to mediate the bronchospastic component of the syndrome, via the release of cytokines (chemokines) by mast cells, leading to eosinophilia and increased vascular permeability. The immediate type skin reaction is manifested by a wheal and flare (within 20 min) to skin-prick testing with *Aspergillus* antigens and is positive in nearly all ABPA patients. Immediate hypersensitivity to *A. fumigatus* is a useful screening test, since ABPA is very unlikely with a negative reaction. Difficulty with antigen standardization used in skin testing and serologic assays has been encountered and may explain the occasional failure to detect hypersensitivity. A recombinant antigen preparation has shown reproducible skin test results that correlate with serologic data and offers promise for standardization of antigen–allergen preparations.

Type III, Arthus, or immune complex–mediated reactions may account for the bronchial and peribronchial inflammation responsible for the radiographic pulmonary infiltrates. The IgG-precipitating antibodies form an antigen–antibody complex, leading to the delayed skin reaction (hemorrhagic cutaneous lesion at 4 to 10 h). These precipitating antibody complexes subsequently fix complement and liberate additional inflammatory factors that lead to chronic inflammation of bronchi resulting in bronchiectasis and pulmonary fibrosis. Granulomatous lesions and lymphocyte-mediated responses suggest that type IV immunopathogenic mechanisms may also have a role in ABPA.

Total IgE increases during acute flares of ABPA and is a good indicator of disease activity even in the absence of clinical exacerbation. However, elevated total IgE is not specific for ABPA and may be present in patients with other pulmonary diseases such as asthma. Approximately 5 percent of the total IgE is a specific component of IgE against *A. fumigatus* antigen and will also be elevated in ABPA. High titers of specific IgE antibodies reactive with *Aspergillus* may be more specific for ABPA. The level of IgE and IgG antibody in patients with ABPA to *A. fumigatus* is at least twice that of mold-sensitive asthmatic patients who demonstrate immediate skin reactivity to *A. fumigatus*. Specific IgG antibodies have been found to be elevated in most patients but do not correlate with disease activity.

Sputum cultures are positive for *Aspergillus* species in approximately two-thirds of all cases of ABPA. Because *Aspergillus* can colonize bronchi without producing disease, sputum cultures may be suggestive but are not diagnostic of this syndrome. Multiple positive cultures in a patient presenting with symptoms suggestive of ABPA support the diagnosis. Pulmonary function testing reveals reversible airway obstruction initially, followed by progressive fixed obstructive changes and hyperinflation. Restrictive airflow pattern and diminished carbon monoxide diffusing capacity become dominant in the chronic fibrotic stage of the disease. Patients studied chronically for ABPA demonstrated marked variability in pulmonary function measurements, and these measurements did not correlate with duration of ABPA or asthma.

No single clinical or immunologic feature is diagnostic of ABPA, and, although understanding and awareness has increased, ABPA remains an underdiagnosed disease. Asymptomatic pulmonary involvement occurs in ABPA and may lead to a delayed diagnosis and irreversible damage. Corticosteroid therapy for asthma may mask the signs of ABPA, allowing progressive decline in pulmonary function. Cystic fibrosis may also complicate the diagnosis of ABPA, since many of the clinical and laboratory features are similar.

Histopathology   Some of the histopathologic presentations associated with ABPA overlap with those of invasive disease. Thus, eosinophilic infiltrates may be present in invasive disease as well as in Loeffler's syndrome and in chronic eosinophilic pneumonia. These syndromes, as well as tropical eosinophilic pneumonia, may also be seen in the presence of parasitic infection with pulmonary migratory cycles, particularly filariasis and strongyloidiasis. Mucoid impaction associated with ABPA or other fungi may predispose to superinfection. Necrotizing granulomata in association with *Aspergillus* species in asthmatic patients may be observed and considered part of the ABPA syndrome. The distinction between ABPA, with fungal elements restricted to the airways, and invasive aspergillosis may be obscured by tissue necrosis or in immunocompromised individuals by poor granuloma formation.

Treatment   The five stages of disease activity proposed by Patterson and colleagues and Mendelson and coworkers are summarized in Table 63-10. No certain prognostic indicators for progression or regression of the disease have been identified. Aggressive treatment of the early stages may halt progression to the final debilitating stage.

Corticosteroid therapy is recognized as the treatment of choice. Prednisone is administered in a daily dose of 1 mg/kg or greater in order to see resolution of the chest radiographic changes. Prednisone 0.5 mg/kg per day is continued for 2 weeks and then decreased to an alternate-day dosage schedule. Maintenance corticosteroid therapy is continued for a minimum of 3 to 6 months and then gradually tapered no faster than 5 mg per month. Monthly IgE levels may be measured, and if there is a twofold increase in the total serum IgE, a chest radiograph should be obtained to rule out exacerbation of ABPA.

TABLE 63-10 Staging System For Allergic Bronchopulmonary Aspergillosis

Stage	Symptoms	Radiographic features	Laboratory features	Management
I. Acute	Fever, productive cough, wheezing	Pulmonary infiltrates, mucoid impaction	Blood eosinophilia, elevated serum IgE, positive skin test	Corticosteroids to achieve remission
II. Remission	Asymptomatic	Normal	Decrease in IgE and blood eosinophilia	Careful follow-up
III. Exacerbation	All or some of acute stage symptoms	All or some of acute-stage findings	At least a doubling of IgE in asymptomatic patients and an increase in IgE in symptomatic patients	Retreat with steroids to induce remission
IV. Corticosteroid-dependent	Symptomatic steroid requiring asthma	Variable	Usually continued elevation of IgE	Long-term steroids to control asthmatic symtoms and keep IgE levels at baseline
V. Fibrotic	Severe dyspnea, fibrotic lung disease as well as bronchospasm	Pulmonary fibrosis	Restrictive plus reversible and irreversible obstructive function tests; may have continued increased IgE	Long-term corticosteroids

SOURCE: Adapted with permission from Mendelson et al. and Patterson et al.

Itraconazole is an orally active triazole antifungal with low toxicity that often has activity against many *Aspergillus* isolates. Preliminary studies suggest that itraconazole may be a useful adjunctive therapy in ABPA to aid in clearing the airway of *Aspergillus* and to offer a steroid-sparing effect. Improvements in clinical, serologic, and pulmonary functional status were noted. Randomized comparative trials are needed to define the role of newer azoles, echinocandins, and itraconazole therapies in ABPA.

Inhaled corticosteroids may help to control the symptoms of asthma but do not prevent episodes of eosinophilic infiltration and mucous impaction and are generally not thought to have any influence on progressive lung damage. Parasitic infection should be excluded prior to starting steroid therapy. Inhaled antifungal agents such as nystatin or amphotericin B may offer temporary suppression of colonization, but penetration into plugged bronchi is limited, and recolonization occurs once therapy is ended. Meticulous bronchial toilet is important for clearance of *A. fumigatus* from the airway. Bronchodilators and physiotherapy with postural drainage are important adjunctive treatments. Increased oral fluids, use of expectorants, and, in selected patients, bronchial lavage may aid in the clearance of viscid mucus. Avoidance of environmental reservoirs of *Aspergillus* may help prevent exacerbations.

Bronchocentric Granulomatosis

Bronchocentric granulomatosis is characterized histologically by necrotizing granulomatous replacement of bronchial mucosa with eosinophilic infiltration of bronchioles. Blood vessels are not primarily affected. *Aspergillus* hyphae have been demonstrated within the lesions of approximately half of the patients described, but tissue invasion does not occur. First described in 1973 by Liebow, patients presented with chronic symptoms, malaise, cough, fever, dyspnea, chest pain, and hemoptysis associated with a focal lesion on chest radiograph, often in an upper lobe. The syndrome is associated with asthma in about half of the patients described and likely represents a severe manifestation of ABPA revealed as a localized pathologic reaction rather than the more generalized pulmonary pathology evident in ABPA. Diagnosis is made by biopsy or often retrospectively after removal of the lesion, which is curative, although some patients may require corticosteroid therapy for ABPA or if multiple lesions are present.

Extrinsic Allergic Alveolitis

Heavy or repeated exposure to *Aspergillus* conidia and mycelia may result in a hypersensitivity reaction affecting the alveoli in nonatopic individuals known as *extrinsic allergic alveolitis*. Malt workers, distillers, brewers, and others exposed to moldy straw or grain have suffered attacks producing cough, dyspnea, fever, chills, myalgias, and malaise 4 to 8 h after exposure to the antigen. Repeated exposure may lead to "malt worker's lung" or "farmer's lung" and to the development of granulomatous disease or interstitial fibrosis. The immunopathogenesis involves cell-mediated immunity (type IV response) and immune complex deposition (type III response) and likely involves an intricate interaction between these mechanisms.

Radiographic changes in the acute syndrome include diffuse alveolar-interstitial infiltrates that may resolve with removal of the inciting antigen. The chronic syndrome may reveal a fine reticulonodular interstitial infiltrate that may progress to pulmonary fibrosis with honeycombing. Serum IgG antibody (precipitins) against *Aspergillus* antigen are present; however, serum

IgE concentration is normal. Skin tests usually demonstrate an Arthus reaction at 4 to 8 h and occasionally may be preceded by an immediate wheal-and-flare reaction and followed by a delayed reaction (36 to 48 h later). The management of extrinsic allergic alveolitis involves removal or avoidance of the source of antigen exposure. Spontaneous recovery may occur once exposure has ended. Corticosteroids are helpful in aiding the resolution of acute symptoms and reduce the likelihood of structural damage. However, corticosteroids are not helpful once fibrosis has developed.

Aspergilloma

Saprophytic colonization of a parenchymal cavity by *Aspergillus* is referred to as *aspergilloma, mycetoma,* or *fungus ball.* A fungus ball consists of dead and living mycelial elements, fibrin, mucus, amorphous debris, inflammatory cells, and degenerating blood and epithelial elements. The mycelia mass may lie free within the cavity or be attached to the cavity wall by granulation tissue. Spontaneous lysis has been reported in 7 to 10 percent of cases, more often associated with bacterial superinfection. Bronchial epithelium or vascular granulation tissue may line the cavity, and surrounding lung may show pneumonitis. The usual species isolated is *A. fumigatus,* although others have been reported.

Pathophysiology The pathogenesis of aspergilloma usually involves the colonization and proliferation of the fungus in a preexisting pulmonary cavity (secondary aspergilloma). Many factors may act to predispose an individual to development of a fungus ball. Tuberculous cavitary disease is the most common, with other cavitary pulmonary disorders such as sarcoid, cavitary neoplasm, pulmonary fibrosis, lung abscess, bronchial cyst, asbestosis, histoplasmosis, blastomycosis, ankylosing spondylitis, brochiectasis, pneumonia, cyanotic heart disease, pulmonary infarction, ABPA, and invasive aspergillosis also associated. Up to 11 to 17 percent of patients with posttuberculous cavities have radiographic changes consistent with aspergilloma.

Primary aspergilloma, arising within the bronchial tree with a proliferation of *Aspergillus* and causing a pulmonary cavity to develop, is less common. The clinical conditions leading to the initiation of a cavitary process and fungus ball formation include (1) invasive pulmonary aspergillosis (IPA); (2) chronic necrotizing pulmonary aspergillosis (CNPA); and (3) ABPA. IPA may lead to primary aspergilloma during the period of bone marrow recovery, as the host is able to mount an inflammatory response and wall off the fungus. Pneumothorax may be a severe complication of pulmonary mycetoma that is reported as a rare occurrence in patients with hematologic malignancies. ABPA may cause bronchiectasis in the chronic phase of disease and result in aspergilloma secondary to growth of fungus distal to a plugged bronchus. Conversely, aspergilloma may provide a stimulus for the perpetuation of ABPA.

Clinical Features Many patients remain asymptomatic, although cough (productive if the lesion communicates with bronchial passages), dyspnea, malaise, and weight loss can be present. Hemoptysis is the most frequent symptom and can be fatal, occurring in 74 percent of patients according to the results of a review of nine separate series. Other associated symptoms include wheezing, chest pain, and, rarely, fever, more likely a consequence of underlying pulmonary pathology rather than due to the aspergilloma itself.

Chest radiograph reveals a solid round mass within a cavity (3 to 5 cm diameter) partially surrounded by a radiolucent cresent (Monod's sign). Movement of the fungus ball may be appreciated within the cavity when comparing upright and decubitus films. Upper lung fields more frequently demonstrate aspergillomas, most frequently in preexisting cavities secondary to tuberculosis and as a solitary lesion, but they can be bilateral and multiple. Chronic lung disease or local pneumonitis may obscure chest radiograph findings, and tomography may offer insight. CT scanning may easily demonstrate characteristic lesions and may be desirable in difficult cases. The only indicator of early disease may be thickening of a cavity wall or increased pleural thickening. Sputum cultures are often not helpful, since communication with the bronchus may not be present and specimen contamination with colonizing *Aspergillus* cannot be excluded. Multiple positive sputum cultures are more suggestive. Precipitating antibodies to *Aspergillus* antigens are present in the sera of most patients with aspergilloma. Eosinophilia, IgE, and skin-test reactivity may be seen in individuals who are allergic to the fungus, but are not consistent findings.

Treatment   Therapeutic options currently include systemic or local antifungal agents, surgical resection, or conservative management with careful follow-up, without specific medical or surgical intervention. Optimal management of patients with aspergilloma remains difficult and controversial. The major clinical concern is hemoptysis. The risk of severe recurrent events in patients with aspergilloma may not be as high as has been estimated. Often, the best management for asymptomatic patients is periodic chest radiographs without surgical intervention. Therapeutic considerations need to include the individual patient's health status with attention to the potential risks of treatment.

Surgical resection is indicated for patients with severe life-threatening hemoptysis, and some reviews have suggested surgical resection as a prophylactic therapeutic measure for all patients with aspergilloma, since resection is potentially curative. Patients in this category frequently have severe underlying pulmonary disease, leaving them poor surgical candidates and with a substantial postoperative complication rate. Patients suffering major hemoptysis and who are poor surgical candidates may alternatively undergo arterial embolization or cavernoscopic evacuation of aspergilloma as a palliative measure.

Systemic antifungals offer little benefit in treating aspergilloma, possibly because of inadequate penetration into the cavity. However, systemic antifungal therapy may help a subset of patients with systemic symptoms and locally invasive disease surrounding the aspergilloma (CNPA).

Direct intracavitary instillation of antifungal agents [amphotericin B, sodium iodide, natamycin, miconazole, ketoconazole, and 5-fluorocytosine (5-FC)] has shown promise in symptomatic patients with aspergilloma. Optimal dose and length of treatment remain to be determined. Complications can include mild hemoptysis, hypersensitivity to the antifungal agent, invasion of a hypervascular area resulting in hemorrhage, and recurrence of aspergilloma.

Oral suppressive antifungal therapy would be particularly useful in the inoperable group of patients with aspergilloma. Response rates to itraconazole have been variable. Long-term therapy is generally needed to prevent relapse.

Bronchial Stump Aspergillosis

Bronchial stump aspergillosis (BSA) is an unusual sequel to lung resection. Patients may present with a productive cough and hemoptysis, sputum that may be putrid, and, occasionally, expectoration of fungal material or suture thread.

The cause is secondary infection of silk suture material used to close the bronchus after pulmonary resection. A single line of suture penetrating the total layer of the bronchus from the mucosa to the serosa is most often used and is referred to as *Sweet's method.* Part of the suture thread protrudes into the bronchial lumen and may cause inflammation or infection. Incidence of BSA was found to be 1.5 percent when silk suture was used and was eliminated with the institution of nylon monofilament suture. Local inflammation, compromised tissue viability, and the high capillarity of silk thread favor *Aspergillus* infection.

The period from surgery to onset of disease usually ranges from 6 to 12 months, although one case was noted to occur after 3 years. One patient has been reported with mild hemoptysis and cough commencing 4 years after surgery, after an uneventful postoperative period. Fiberoptic bronchoscopy may reveal the silk thread and inflammatory changes such as hyperemia, swelling, granulation, and purulence. Biopsy of the bronchial mucosa shows necrotic areas and hyphae, and cultures are usually positive for *Aspergillus.* Simple removal of the suture during bronchoscopy with forceps is also curative. A related syndrome occurs at the site of bronchial anastomosis in lung transplantation recipients. At this relatively avascular site with mucosal and epithelial disruption, *Aspergillus* infection may become established. Such disease may present with persistent bronchial secretions, fever, or anastomotic leak. Eradication of such infection without surgical resection in these immunocompromised individuals is generally impossible. This infection may also progress to invasive aspergillosis.

Chronic Necrotizing Pulmonary Aspergillosis

Individuals with immune compromise as a result of corticosteroids, diabetes mellitus, alcoholism, or poor nutritional status or who have underlying pulmonary disease such as chronic obstructive pulmonary disease (COPD), sarcoidosis, inactive tuberculosis, pneumoconiosis, or radiation fibrosis may develop a slowly progressive form of aspergillosis. Patients are frequently chronically ill with complaints of fever, weight loss, productive cough, and hemoptysis. Chronic infiltrates may be evident on chest radiographs, which may progress to form an aspergilloma. A lesion may also begin as an aspergilloma and become locally invasive.

Sputum cultures and serum *Aspergillus* precipitins are often positive, and leukocytosis may be present. Tissue invasion of the cavity wall by *Aspergillus* hyphae, fibrosis, and a granulomatous reaction is evident by direct examination. Extent and progression of the disease appear to depend on the ability of a host to contain the fungus. Disseminated spread is uncommon.

Intravenous amphotericin B with or without oral 5-FC has resulted in occasional dramatic responses. Other agents merit study. Overall results with chemotherapy are, however, poor. Host defenses should be bolstered and immunosuppressive factors removed if possible. Surgical or percutaneous drainage may be necessary in patients with large necrotic cavities that do not drain via the tracheobronchial tree. Surgical resection should be reserved for patients who have failed antifungal therapy or who have clearly localized disease.

Invasive Aspergillosis

Invasive pulmonary aspergillosis occurs in the immunocompromised host most often following inhalation of *Aspergillus* conidia, although hematogenous dissemination from cutaneous or gastrointestinal source can occur.

Patients with acute lymphocytic and acute myelogenous leukemia with prolonged granulocytopenia during treatment are particularly prone to develop this form of disease. High-dose corticosteroids, especially when combined with other immunosuppressive agents in recipients of organ transplants, or chronic granulomatous disease, can cause immune dysfunction, predisposing such individuals to IPA. Patients usually die within 2 to 3 weeks unless immunosuppression is rapidly decreased. Invasive aspergillosis has been reported in apparently normal hosts, and heavy environmental exposure to *Aspergillus* spores has been linked to disease in both hospital epidemics and individual cases.

Once germination of conidia occurs, endobronchial proliferation of hyphae, occasionally with ulcerative tracheobronchitis (discussed below), leads to invasion of pulmonary arterioles and lung parenchyma and, finally, to ischemic necrosis. Hematogenous dissemination with thrombosis, hemorrhagic infarction, and invasion of distant organs may result from *Aspergillus* hyphae invading arterioles and occur in approximately one-third of cases. Thus, invasive aspergillosis can present with a similar clinical picture to other thrombotic and embolic diseases such as pulmonary embolism, cerebrovascular accidents, Budd-Chiari syndrome, and renal papillary necrosis. Invasive aspergillosis can spread to contiguous structures, across the diaphragm to the stomach, or from the lung to the heart or superior vena cava. The morphology of *Aspergillus* hyphae in tissue specimens is indistinguishable from that of several other fungi, such as *Scedosporium boydii* and *Fusarium* species, so that clinical correlation of the syndrome and culture identification are very important.

Clinical Features   Symptoms begin with fever, which may be followed by a mild, nonproductive cough suggestive of bronchitis. Pleuritic chest pain and progression to pneumonia occur within 1 to 2 days. The appearance of lesions by chest radiograph may be delayed in the leukopenic patient because of the impaired inflammatory response. The typical presenting finding may be one or more well-defined nodules or a patchy density. The lesions then progress to diffuse consolidation or cavitation. Cavitation tends to occur in patients if immunosuppression is decreased, as in leukemic patients during the period of recovering bone marrow function or when steroid therapy is reduced significantly; on occasion, this gives rise to massive hemoptysis.

Pleuritic pain and slight hemoptysis may suggest pulmonary infarction. Patients may expectorate necrotic tissue filled with hyphae. Cough, sputum production, and pleural effusion are either absent or minimal. Invasive aspergillosis must be strongly considered in susceptible patients who fail broad-spectrum antibiotics.

Extrapulmonary sites may be involved, including the highly vascular organs such as the kidney, liver, spleen, and central nervous system. Invasive disease of the nose and paranasal sinuses occurs in immunocompromised patients, and contiguous invasive spread into the orbit or into the cranial vault can result in a syndrome similar to rhinocerebral mucormycosis. Concomitant nasal ulceration and pulmonary infiltrate in the profoundly neutropenic host are suggestive of aspergillosis. *Aspergillus* is the most common fungal pathogen associated with sinusitis in the immunocompetent patient, but invasion into contiguous tissue rarely occurs.

Diagnosis   Tissue biopsy provides a definitive diagnosis. Histopathologic findings must demonstrate tissue or vascular invasion by hyphae that are morphologically consistent with *Aspergillus*. Early clinical, laboratory, and radiographic findings of invasive aspergillosis are often not present, making the diagnosis difficult. Invasive biopsy procedures in these patients are often precluded by severe illness and bleeding diathases, and unfortunately the diagnosis is often not made until postmortem examination. However, recognition of invasive fungal disease and early institution of therapy reduces the high mortality associated with IPA.

In the appropriate clinical setting, the CT "halo sign" of a zone of low attenuation surrounding a nonspecific pulmonary mass or infiltrate may prove to be helpful in the early diagnosis of IPA in patients with leukemia. However, this is nonspecific and may be seen in pulmonary infections due to *Nocardia asteroides* or Mucor infections. Magnetic resonance imaging may contribute to the early diagnosis of IPA by revealing the hemorrhagic content of pulmonary lesions typical in IPA. Positive blood cultures are rare, since fungemia is not sustained, although clumps of broken hyphae may sporadically embolize to end organs. In a highly susceptible patient, positive cultures of sputum, bronchoalveolar lavage fluid, or bronchial brushings are predictive of invasive aspergillosis, whereas negative cultures do not rule out disease.

Detection of *Aspergillus* antigens in sera or other body fluids or polymerase chain reaction for specific nucleic acids of *Aspergillus* may offer an early noninvasive method for the diagnosis of IPA. Antibody testing in IPA is usually not helpful, since patients with invasive aspergillosis often have greatly diminished or absent antibody production.

Treatment   The prognosis of patients with IPA is ultimately linked with the severity and outcome of the underlying disease. Although antifungal therapy may delay progression of IPA, bone marrow recovery in neutropenic patients is essential for cure. Even with restored immune function, progressive invasive aspergillosis may result in death.

Amphotericin B remains the drug of choice for invasive fungal infection. However, voriconazole and lipid-amphotericin have also proven useful. Empiric therapy with amphotericin or lipid-amphotericin should be started in patients with persistent fever and unexplained pulmonary infiltrates who cannot tolerate invasive procedures. Full-dose therapy should be given (0.7 to 1.5 mg/kg of amphotericin B). Nephrotoxicity, phlebitis, hypokalemia, hypomagnesemia, and anemia are adverse effects of amphotericin B that must be monitored (see Tables 63-3 and 63-4) . Therapy should be continued until demonstration of disease regression is documented. The duration of therapy is likely best individualized according to patient response, severity of disease, and immune status. The lipid-associated amphotericin agents (liposomal or lipid complex) have the advantage of reduced nephrotoxocity and reduced infusion-related side effects. In addition, higher doses (3 to 7 mg/kg/day) may be used with higher serum and tissue levels of drug. Studies do not yet clarify the benefits of such dosing or whether killing of fungus in tissue is improved as a result. Liposomal preparations provide an alternative to standard amphotericin B. The cost of these agents remains a limiting feature. They must be used with adequate prehydration with saline and attention to electrolyte abnormalities. Liposomal amphotericin has been associated with reduced infusion-related effects and approved for use in febrile neutropenia. Some strains of *Aspergillus* (e.g., *A. terreus*) are relatively resistant to amphotericin therapy.

Itraconazole is an oral and intravenous triazole antifungal that has been effective therapy for aspergillosis. Variable absorption and interpatient variation of serum levels have been problems. Oral absorption is dependent upon acid pH of the stomach. Itraconazole has been used in the treatment of IPA with reasonable success with adequate dosing (600 to 800 mg/day IV or PO if serum levels are obtained). The role for itraconazole in prophylaxis, primary treatment, and salvage therapy of invasive aspergillosis needs further study. However, some transplant patients have developed IPA while on prophylactic doses (200 to 400 mg per day) of itraconazole. Itraconazole may also be used to complete therapy for susceptible strains of *Aspergillus* following initial treatment and clinical response to amphotericin B. Concomitant use with amphotericin B has the potential for antagonism and adverse drug interactions. Itraconazole may be antagonistic for amphotericin B in animal models, but the in vivo correlate of this observation remains unclear. Ketoconazole has been shown in vitro and in animal models to be antagonistic of amphotericin. Preliminary trials with voriconazole suggest excellent anti-*Aspergillus* activity. The echinocandins have anti-*Aspergillus* activity, perhaps best used in combination with other active agents.

Combination antifungal therapy may be the future of care for IPA. Amphotericin B has been used in combination with flucytosine and rifampin in a variety of trials but no controlled trial data are available to prove the benefits of specific combinations. Preliminary data suggest that the echinocandins *may* have some synergistic activity when combined with amphotericin B.

Another modality of treatment is surgical resection alone or in combination with antifungal therapy in selected patients with localized lesions. Surgery may be indicated in patients with leukemia who develop pulmonary aspergillosis and require further chemotherapy or transplantation or when failure of medical therapy alone has occurred. Systemic therapy should be initiated *prior* to surgical manipulation of infected lung tissue to prevent systemic dissemination. In the nonimmunocompromised host sinusitis and BSA are the only two types of invasive aspergillosis that may be handled with surgery alone.

Mucosal colonization may be reduced by administration of antifungals either orally or locally. In a retrospective study of invasive aspergillosis, intranasal aerosolized amphotericin B was found effective in prophylaxis in neutropenic patients. Although positive nose cultures for *Aspergillus* have been shown to have predictive value for subsequent invasive disease, the observations in that study were uncontrolled. Itraconazole may also be useful for prophylaxis in neutropenic patients, and further controlled studies are needed. Success in reducing the rate of *Aspergillus* colonization and infection has also been attributed to effective mechanical air filtering systems.

Empiric treatment for aspergillosis with one or another form of amphotericin in neutropenic patients with fever and no response to antibacterial therapy is recommended. Early empiric therapy with amphotericin B appears to decrease morbidity and mortality among neutropenic patients at high risk for fungal infection. Four to seven days of fever while the patient is receiving broad-spectrum antibiotic therapy is a generally accepted course. Careful evaluation to exclude secondary bacterial infection not adequately treated by the antimicrobial regimen should occur prior to the commencement of antifungal therapy. Once fever resolves and bone marrow recovery is under way, antifungal therapy can be stopped provided that aspergillosis has been ruled out. Patients may suffer relapse if chemotherapy is resumed and neutropenia recurs.

Pulmonary Aspergillosis in AIDS

Pulmonary aspergillosis in patients with AIDS is relatively uncommon but increasing in frequency with prolonged survival of HIV-infected persons. Qualitative defects of neutrophils, alveolar macrophages, and corticosteroid use are generally present. All such patients have very low helper T-cell counts. Previously described cases have associated smoking of marijuana with invasive aspergillosis. Pneumonia due to other pathogens and the use of broad-spectrum antibiotics precede many cases of invasive aspergillosis. Cytomegalovirus disease is prevalent among the reported cases of invasive aspergillosis in AIDS and has been also associated with increased pulmonary infections in transplant patients. The association of CMV and *Aspergillus* infection in AIDS patients is unclear.

Symptoms of pulmonary aspergillosis in AIDS are nonspecific. AIDS patients may develop the whole spectrum of aspergillosis-related pulmonary disorders, including chronic cavitary, invasive, and bronchial forms of aspergillosis. Two patterns of aspergillosis that have been reported are possibly AIDS-specific. Termed *obstructing bronchial aspergillosis* and *pseudomembranous bronchial aspergillosis,* they resemble ABPA.

Another form of airway aspergillosis is ulcerative tracheobronchitis, which appears as inflammatory ulcers or nodules involving the main-stem and segmental bronchi on bronchoscopy. *Aspergillus* can be isolated on biopsy specimens, and the clinical and histologic features of the AIDS patients described were similar to those reviewed in patients without AIDS. Patients may present with fever, cough, dyspnea, or hemoptysis. Varying degrees of bronchial mucosal invasion occur, and subsequent disseminated aspergillosis occurred in two patients. *Aspergillus* ulcerative tracheobronchitis may therefore progress to IPA in the susceptible individual and warrants prompt investigation and treatment.

MUCORMYCOSIS

Mucormycosis refers to the acute and rapidly developing infection caused by fungi of the order Mucorales. Other names for this disease have been used in the past, such as, *phycomycosis* and *zygomycosis. Phycomycosis* is an outdated term derived from an earlier classification scheme, and *zygomycosis* is too vague, since all Zygomycetes do not cause the same clinical syndrome. The term *mucormycosis* is most useful to clinicians and will be used herein to describe this infection. Table 63-11 describes the taxonomic relationship of the pathogenic Zygomycetes.

Epidemiology

The Zygomycetes are ubiquitous fungi which are thermotolerant inhabitants of decaying organic matter. Species of Mucorales pathogenic to humans grow rapidly on any carbohydrate substrate and produce sporangiospores in large numbers. Spores become airborne, and inhalation of conidia occurs on a daily basis. Even though these fungi grow in many ecologic niches, the infrequency of disease due to these organisms attests to their low virulence potential in the human host. Patients with severe immune compromise, diabetes mellitus, or trauma are the most commonly affected, but mucormycosis is a rather rare development in any of these patient groups.

TABLE 63-11 Classification of the Agents of Mucormycosis and Related Diseases

I. Zygomycotina
  A. Zygomycetes
    a. Mucorales
      1. Mucoraceae
        iv. *Absidia*
          (a) *A. corymbifera*
          (b) *A. ramosa*
        ii. *Mucor*
          (a) *M. circinelloides*
        iii. *Rhizomucor*
          (a) *R. pusillus*
        iv. *Rhizopus*
          (a) *R. oryzae (R. arrhyziae)*[a]
          (b) *R. arrhizus*
          (c) *R. rhizopodiformis*
      2. *Cunninghamellaceae*
        i. *Cunninghalella*
          (a) *C. bertholletiae*
      3. Mortierellaceae
        i. *Mortierella*
          (a) *M. wolfii*
      4. Saksenaeaceae
        i. *Saksenaea*
          (a) *S. vasiformis*
      5. Syncephalastrum
        i. *Syncephalastrum*
      6. Apophysomyceae
        i. *Apophysomyces*
          (a) *A. elegans*
      7. Thamnidiaceae
        i. *Cokeromyces*
          (a) *C. recurvatus*
    b. Entomophthorales
      1. *Conidiobolus*
        i. *C. coronatus (Entomophthora coronata)*[a]
        ii. *C. incongruans*
      2. *Basidiobolus*
        i. *B. haptosporus (B. meristosporus; B. ranarum)*[a]

[a]Obsolete synonyms.

Rhinocerebral disease is most often associated with diabetic ketoacidosis, and the most commonly encountered genera is *Rhizopus*. Central nervous system mucormycosis is rare, occurring in severely debilitated patients usually as a result of the fungus spreading from the initial site of invasion through the nose and the paranasal sinuses or from intravenous drug use. Rhinocerebral infection may also occur in organ transplant patients or as a complication of severe cutaneous burn injury.

Pulmonary infection is associated with leukemia and lymphoma and other malignancies when patients are neutropenic, have decreased neutrophil function, and are diabetic, receiving corticosteroid therapy, and/or are receiving broad-spectrum antibiotics. It has also been observed in organ transplant recipients, particularly in diabetics. Increased risk for mucormycosis occurs in renal failure patients receiving the drug desferoximine, as an iron- or aluminum-chelating agent. Gastric involvement is encountered in children with kwashiorkor and immunosuppressed patients in concert with *H. pylori* or cytomegalovirus (CMV) infections.

Mycology and Pathogenesis

Zygomycetes are molds characterized by growth of wide, nonseptate hyphae in the environment and in tissue. They grow quickly, within 2 to 5 days on most media, as fluffy gray or brownish colonies. As the colony matures, the mycelium may darken and show a black pepper-like effect as large numbers of sporangia are formed. Cyclohexamide inhibits the growth of these fungi, and media that contain this compound, such as Mycosel and Mycobiotic agar, should not be used. All pathologic species grow at 37°C.

Microscopic examination for the presence and location of rhizoids, apophyses, and the morphology of the columellae differentiates the genera. Isolating and speciating the organism is important for treatment considerations. Issues of potential species-specific responses to antifungal drugs, determining the efficacy of therapy in eradicating the pathogen, or of whether a subsequent clinical isolate is the same, new, or contaminating are compelling reasons to identify the strain involved in an infection. The most commonly isolated genus is *Rhizopus,* followed by *Rhizomucor.*

The pathogenesis of mucormycosis begins with the inhalation of spores into the respiratory tract, where they are deposited in the nasal turbinates and may be inhaled into the pulmonary alveoli. Germination of spores into hyphae is followed by tissue invasion and progression toward blood vessels. Histopathologic characteristics include thrombosis and tissue necrosis after vascular penetration occurs.

Bronchoalveolar macrophages phagocytose *Rhizopus* spores and prevent their growth but do not kill them in the normal lung. Animals with diabetes mellitus or corticosteroid pretreatment experience a rapidly progressive pulmonary infection with hematogenous dissemination and death after inhalation of Mucorales spores. Macrophages recovered from the bronchial trees of the impaired animals reveal decreased ability to inhibit spore germination. Fungus-derived chemotactic factors, and the products of activation of the alternate complement pathway, recruit neutrophils into the site of infection.

Clinical Manifestations

Patient factors influence the particular mucormycotic syndrome exhibited. Assisted ventilation may promote the inhalation of spores or the aspiration of upper respiratory tract flora. Infection may remain localized in the lung or disseminate hematogenously. Some atypical presentations of pulmonary mucormycosis include disease in the absence of underlying systemic disease or predisposing factors, solitary nodules in a diabetic, multiple mycotic pulmonary artery aneurysms and pseudoaneurysms, or bronchial obstruction. A less fulminant, subacute clinical course is occasionally described in patients with diabetes mellitus, suggesting the need for aggressive diagnostic and therapeutic measures in patients who are at risk for this infection. Allergic *Rhizomucor* sinusitis affects immunocompetent individuals with or without nasal polyposis and is similar to the syndrome associated with *Aspergillus* sinusitis.

Patients with pulmonary mucormycosis often present with fever and may have other symptoms similar to a bacterial infection such as cough, dyspnea, or pleuritic chest pain. Hemoptysis may develop secondary to continued tissue necrosis and blood vessel invasion, and bronchopleural fistula and fatal pulmonary hemorrhage may result. Spread to contiguous areas of the lung and to the mediastinum occurs. Radiographic findings include infiltrate or a mass and, less commonly, pulmonary consolidation, cavitation, or an effusion. Radiographic pulmonary lesions due to Mucorales may expand very rapidly, particularly in the immunocompromised host. There is no specific lobar predilection.

Diagnosis

Mucormycosis, although a rarely encountered pathogen, is increasing in incidence and is potentially treatable. Aggressive diagnostic procedures including biopsy with histologic confirmation and culture may lead to earlier diagnosis and institution of treatment. The diagnosis of mucormycosis depends on demonstrating the organism in tissue. Routine laboratory studies are likely to be of low yield, and many specimens—including blood, sputum, gastric fluid, and nose swabs—are difficult to culture and often offer no diagnostic value. Sputum cultures are not reliable indicators of infection, since some species of Mucorales may occasionally be found in the sputum of individuals without clinical disease, and Gram's stain is not likely to be helpful. Invasive procedures are essential to provide histopathologic evidence of invasive disease, including bronchoscopy with transbronchial biopsy, percutaneous needle biopsy of the lung, or open lung biopsy must be employed. Touch slides prepared from the biopsy specimen with potassium hydroxide may reveal fungal hyphae. Tissue sections stained with hematoxylin-and-eosin will show the typical hyphae in infected tissue. These fungi stain poorly with the PAS and Gram's stains but very well by the Grocott's rapid silver stain. The use of lectin-binding stains on histologic preparations has been reported for the confirmation of the diagnosis of mucormycosis, but these are not widely available.

The fungi appear as broad (10 to 20 μm in diameter), nonseptate hyphae with branches occurring at a right angle. Rarely, occasional septa can be visualized. During the handling of tissues hyphae may collapse and fold, giving the characteristic ribbon appearance. It is recommended not to grind tissue for culturing. The differentiation of *Aspergillus* or *Fusarium* and *Scedosporium* subspecies from Mucorales hyphae in tissue involves visualizing thinner, more regularly shaped fungal elements with more frequent acute angle branching and the presence of septa in the former group. Culture and identification of the fungi will provide the specific genus and species. Agents of mucormycosis are rarely recovered from blood cultures.

Tissue histology of Mucorales infection reveals a neutrophil infiltrate (in the nonneutropenic host), necrosis, and invasion of blood vessels with thrombosis. An inflammatory vasculitis involves arteries and veins; in chronic cases, mononuclear cell infiltration is observed with occasional giant cells. Serologic diagnosis by fungal antigen detection remains investigational, and no assay of sufficient sensitivity or specificity has been identified.

Treatment

Mucormycosis is first and foremost a surgical disease. Without tissue resection, therapeutic failure is universal. Aggressive surgical debridement of necrotic tissue is an important intervention in the treatment of pulmonary mucormycosis. Removal of as much of the infected or devitalized tissue as possible while the infection is localized is of most benefit. Lobectomy is often required, and pneumonectomy may be necessary for proximal or extensive involvement. Repeated procedures may be needed. Rapid tapering of immunosuppressive drugs and corticosteroids should be carried out. Hyperglycemia and acidosis should be corrected, and neutropenia reversed if possible.

High-dose amphotericin B (1.0 to 2.0 mg/kg IV per day) is the standard therapy for mucormycosis. Liposomal formulations allow higher doses of amphotericin to be given, and reports indicate that successful outcomes were obtained in several patients with rhinocerebral mucormycosis treated with liposomal amphotericin B preparations. Further work to determine the efficacy of liposomal amphotericin B formulations in comparison to the standard preparation of amphotericin B needs to be completed. Mucorales subspecies are generally resistant to the azole class of antifungals. Voriconazole has been somewhat less effective for this indication. The addition of other agents such as rifampin to amphotericin B in an attempt to obtain synergistic antifungal activity is controversial and cannot be recommended as standard therapy. The application of in vitro susceptibility data for molds to in vivo conditions of infection is uncertain at best.

PULMONARY CANDIDIASIS

There are over 150 species of *Candida,* but only 9 are considered human pathogens. Of these, *Candida albicans*—a common skin, oral, and gastrointestinal saprophyte—causes significant morbidity in the forms of gastrointestinal disease (e.g., esophagitis, thrush), renal infection, and "line sepsis"; infrequently it also causes bronchopneumonia in the compromised host. More often, *Candida* seeds the lungs as a result of fungemia. Individuals with chronic mucocutaneous candidiasis have combined immune deficiencies of both the humoral and cellular limbs. *Candida krusei* and *Candida glabrata,* formerly *Torulopsis glabrata,* are opportunistic yeasts, infections with which have many characteristics in common with *C. albicans* infection in the compromised host, but they are less susceptible to azole antifungal agents. *C. glabrata* pneumonia may accompany fungemia in disseminated disease and is a common secondary invader. *C. tropicalis* is associated with disseminated infection in neutropenic patients and may be more pathogenic than other *Candida* species. *C. parapsilosis* seems to be the least pathogenic of the common types of *Candida* that cause fungemia. The virulence factors involved in the pathogenesis of *Candida* infections remain unclear. Histopathologic findings from biopsy or autopsy material provide a definitive diagnosis.

Epidemiology

Candida is widespread in the environment and a human commensal. The fungus is found in the human gastrointestinal tract, in the female genital tract, and on the skin. Alterations of the usual distribution and low colony counts of yeasts occur when the normal microbial flora is diminished by antibiotic therapy or when host defenses are impaired. Intravenous catheters and indwelling bladder catheters are common portals of entry. Indwelling intravenous catheters in place for total parenteral nutrition are particularly associated with the hematogenous spread of *Candida*.

Pathogenesis

Defense against *Candida* requires an intact immune system, particularly polymorphonuclear leukocytes (PMNs). PMNs play the initial role in the host response, followed by macrophages and granuloma formation. The addition of corticosteroids results in the proliferation of *Candida,* with the production of greater numbers of pseudohyphae and diminished cellular responses with increased tissue necrosis. *Candida* pulmonary infection occurs in chemotherapy-induced neutropenia, chronic granulomatous disease with myeloperoxidase deficiency, corticosteroid therapy, and diabetes mellitus. Maintenance of bacterial flora is an important defense that is frequently affected by antibiotic therapy as well as by other host factors such as nutrition and systemic illness. An immunocompromised state may be produced by the disruption of normal barriers, such as a surgical wound site or by gastrointestinal tract disuse or blind loops (Roux en Y), allowing fungi to penetrate the mucosa. Drugs for induction of immunosuppression for organ or bone marrow transplantation specifically diminish lymphocyte function and have been associated with *Candida* pulmonary infection. Table 63-12 lists some of the predisposing factors for *Candida* infection.

Clinical Manifestations

Persistent, often cryptic, fever is the most common clinical feature of *Candida* pulmonary disease. Patients may present without symptoms but subsequently develop symptoms of pneumonia (cough, sputum production, chest pain, and dyspnea). Physical exam and routine laboratory studies are often unremarkable. Chest radiographs may demonstrate a local or diffuse infiltrate involving one or both lungs, more often associated with infection acquired by the endobronchial route. A miliary–nodular pattern is more often associated with hematogenous seeding of the lung in disseminated candidiasis and often appears late in the clinical course of disease. Hepatic and splenic involvement may be the first signs of disseminated disease. Extrapulmonary manifestations such as skin lesions, myositis, or endophthalmitis may be the first signs of *Candida* fungemia. Multiple organ involvement prior to or concurrent with pulmonary findings, particularly kidney and myocardial failure, may indicate hematogenous seeding. Lung transplant patients may manifest an early (within 2 weeks) and fulminant *Candida* pneumonia. The association is probably due to occult aspiration in the donor followed by invasive pulmonary *Candida* infection after transplantation when immunosuppression is most intense. Infection of tracheal anatamoses is common without prophylaxis.

TABLE 63-12 Predisposing Factors for *Candida* Pneumonia

Abdominal surgery, trauma, mucosal erosion, or peptic
ulceration with perforation of the gastrointestinal tract
Indwelling catheters for intravenous alimentation, peritoneal
dialysis, urinary tract drainage
Intravenous drug use
High-dose, prolonged corticosteroid administration
Broad-spectrum antibiotic therapy
Neutropenia or hematologic malignancy
Diabetes mellitus
Colonization of multiple sites with *Candida*

A number of other forms of pulmonary disease have been described, including acute or chronic bronchitis and allergic asthma. Allergic bronchopulmonary candidiasis is a syndrome with a course and immunologic findings consistent with APBA, presenting with asthma, positive sputum culture for *C. albicans,* fleeting pulmonary infiltrates, immediate skin reactivity to *C. albicans* antigen, precipitating antibody against *C. albicans* antigen, elevated serum IgE concentration, and elevated serum IgE and IgG antibody against *C. albicans.* A significant decrease was observed in serum IgE levels and IgE antibody against *C. albicans* after corticosteroid treatment for 3 months. Allergic bronchopulmonary candidiasis should be considered in patients with this syndrome and negative serologic and skin tests to *Aspergillus.* Early diagnosis and treatment may prevent late fibrosis.

Diagnosis

The diagnosis of pulmonary candidiasis depends on convincing evidence that tissue invasion is present. The isolation of yeast from sputum is generally a reflection of colonization of the oropharynx and is common in the absence of deep infection in the respiratory tract. *Candida* is present in the oropharynx of approximately 20 percent of all patients with chronic lung disease. In the case of hematogenous spread of *Candida,* the sputum Gram's stain often does not contain yeast. Chest radiograph findings are nonspecific and often normal. Isolation of *Candida* from the blood may be helpful in disseminated disease. Lysis centrifugation blood cultures are the most sensitive and rapid way to recover *Candida* from blood. Serology to detect *Candida* antigen or metabolites of *Candida* in serum or other body fluids is currently not helpful, but polymerase chain reaction for *Candida* or panfungal nucleic acids are in use in many centers. CT scans of the abdomen may suggest invasive hepatosplenic candidiasis in compromised hosts with an unrevealing microbiologic evaluation.

Tissue invasion by *Candida* demonstrated on open lung biopsy histopathology is definitive, although such biopsy is difficult to perform in neutropenic patients with pneumonia. Gram's stain, KOH smear, and culture of lung tissue are only supportive of the diagnosis. Transbronchial biopsy revealing tissue invasion by *Candida* is an indication for treatment. Percutaneous needle biopsy and aspirate can be used to provide direct microscopic evidence for infection, although sampling for culture is often negative.

Treatment

The mainstay of treatment has been amphotericin B, and as in the case of other opportunistic infections, reversal of the factors affecting the immune status of the individual is crucial. In the setting of hematogenous spread, removal of indwelling intravenous lines or urinary catheters is also very important.

Amphotericin B in doses from 0.5 to 0.7 mg/kg per day may be given. The total dosage and duration of therapy are unclear. However, 1.5 to 3.0 g over 2 to 4 weeks is a general guideline. In our experience, patients with candidemia, of whom some had pneumonia, benefited by the addition of flucytosine to amphotericin B. The known adverse affects of flucytosine may limit its use in critically ill immunosuppressed patients and this agent must be used only with monitoring of serum 5-FC levels. The combination of rifampin with amphotericin B has shown synergy in vitro, but has been of little benefit in vivo.

Fluconazole has been shown effective for cryptococcal meningitis in AIDS patients, oropharyngeal candidiasis in patients with malignancy, hepatosplenic candidiasis, and candidemia. Fluconazole offers many advantages, and studies in fungemic patients are ongoing to evaluate its efficacy. Initiation of therapy with amphotericin B rather than fluconazole may be appropriate in the debilitated or critically ill patient with disseminated infection due to *Candida* subspecies with the completion of therapy or prolonged prophylaxis with fluconazole in the persistently immunocompromised host.

Extensive studies are underway with various preparations of amphotericin B. These preparations (liposomal amphotericin, amphotericin B lipid complex, amphotericin B colloidal dispersion) are better tolerated than conventional amphotericin B, even in much higher daily doses (up to 7 mg/kg per day). Randomized, controlled studies of efficacy and pharmacokinetics of these agents in systemic candidiasis are needed.

Prophylaxis of *Candida* pulmonary infection is not well studied. Ketoconazole and fluconazole have been efficacious in preventing oral *Candida* infections in cancer patients and AIDS patients and have reduced the incidence of deep fungal infections in patients undergoing bone marrow transplants. Routine use of these agents have enhanced the emergence of azole-resistant *Candida* species in some centers. Prophylaxis of pulmonary candidiasis is best achieved by eliminating or limiting those factors that predispose patients to *Candida* colonization and aspiration.

ENDEMIC MYCOSES

The endemic mycoses are restricted geographically, based on environmental and other factors that favor the growth of these organisms in the soil. *Histoplasma capsulatum* infects individuals in the Mississippi and Ohio River valleys of the midwestern United States, but is present on all continents except Antarctica including the tropical regions of Central and South America and areas in which bats, chickens, and starlings and other birds are present. *Histoplasma capsulatum var. duboisii* causes disease primarily in Africa. Coccidioidomycosis occurs primarily in the desert of the southwestern United States and in regions of Central and South America. Blastomycosis is present in the southeastern, Appalachian and midwestern regions of the United States but has been reported in Africa and in Europe. These mycoses are increasing in importance as causes for opportunistic disease in immunocompromised patients, including those with AIDS. Advances in diagnosis and treatment provide opportunities to improve the outcome of these patients.

HISTOPLASMOSIS

Histoplasmosis is the most common of the endemic mycoses and a major cause of morbidity in patients who live in endemic areas. It has emerged as a common presentation and complication of untreated AIDS. Understanding the clinical syndromes and untreated course of the infections is essential in the diagnosis of histoplasmosis and the management of patients with the disease. Improved laboratory tests have made it possible to diagnose severe cases more rapidly. Expanded treatment options are available with triazole antifungal agents and liposomal formulation of amphotericin B.

Mycology and Epidemiology

Histoplasma capsulatum grows as a mold in the soil and is found primarily in microfoci containing large amount of rotted bird or bat guano. Microconidia measuring 2 to 5 μm in diameter are the infectious particles in the mold phase of the organism. At temperatures above 35°C, *H. capsulatum* grows as a yeast, which is the pathogenic for that infects tissues. *H. capsulatum* is endemic in areas of North and Latin America but is found throughout the world. Factors accounting for its geographic distribution include humid environmental conditions and acidic, permeable soil characteristics. Bird and bat excrement enhance growth of the organism in soil by accelerating sporulation. Reactivation of latent infection may account for some cases in persons with previous histoplasmosis who become immunocompromised.

Pathogenesis

Infection develops when conidia are inhaled and germinate into yeasts or when old foci of infection reactivate. Cellular immunity plays the key role in defense against *H. capsulatum*. With development of specific T-cell–mediated immunity, cytokines, including gamma interferon and interleukin-12, activate macrophages to kill the fungus and halt progression of the disease. These defense mechanisms are sufficient to control the infection in immunocompetent subjects, explaining the subclinical or self-limited course characteristic of acute histoplasmosis.

Clinical Manifestations

Most clinically recognized infections are self-limited. The common self-limited presentations include acute pulmonary histoplasmosis, pericarditis, and rheumatologic syndromes.

Acute Pulmonary Histoplasmosis

Most patients present with symptoms of fever, cough, and retrosternal or pleuritic chest pain. Chest radiographs show mediastinal lymphadenopathy with patchy infiltrates. In rare instances, cavitation occurs in acute pulmonary histoplasmosis. Patients recover in a few weeks but may experience fatigue for months. Following heavy exposure, patients present with diffuse pulmonary impairment, which often causes respiratory insufficiency. Patients may present with obstructive symptoms resulting from enlarged mediastinal lymph nodes.

Rheumatologic Syndromes

Patients with acute histoplasmosis may experience arthritis or arthralgia accompanied by erythema nodosum. Chest radiographs usually show findings typical of acute pulmonary histoplasmosis, but they may be normal. Symptoms are best managed by treatment with anti-inflammatory agents but may recur when treatment is stopped.

Pericarditis

Pericarditis is another inflammatory complication of acute self-limited histoplasmosis, occurring in less than 10 percent of cases. Chest radiographs usually show mediastinal lymphadenopathy and an increase in the cardiac silhouette. Patients typically respond to anti-inflammatory treatment, but up to one-fourth of them exhibit pericardial tamponade. Late constriction is rare.

Chronic Pulmonary Histoplasmosis

Chronic pulmonary histoplasmosis occurs in patients with underlying lung disease and is characterized by recurrent symptoms, progressive lung infiltrates, fibrosis, and cavitation. Upper lobe infiltrates are present in nearly all cases, and cavities are found in most. Progression is manifested by cavity enlargement, formation of new cavities, spread to new areas of the lungs, and bronchopleural fistulas. Aspergilloma, bacterial infection, and malignancy must also be considered in evaluation of new masses or infiltrates in patients with chronic pulmonary histoplasmosis.

Disseminated Histoplasmosis

Progressive disseminated histoplasmosis occurs in about one in 2000 acute infections, usually in patients who are immunosuppressed or at the extremes of age. Fever and weight loss are the most common symptoms. Examination reveals hepatomegaly or splenomegaly in about half of the cases and lymphadenopathy in one-third. A sepsis presentation with shock; respiratory, hepatic, and renal failure; and coagulopathy may complicate severe cases. Meningitis or focal brain lesions occur in 10 to 20 percent of cases. Other common sites of dissemination are the oral mucosa, skin, and adrenal glands, seen in 5 to 10 percent of cases. Chest radiographs are abnormal in 70 percent of patients, usually showing diffuse interstitial or reticulonodular infiltrates.

Broncholithiasis

Lymph nodes and pulmonary granulomas calcify and may erode into adjacent bronchi, causing hemoptysis or obstruction. Patients may expectorate rock-like particles of tissue and experience recurrent and severe hemoptysis, bronchial obstruction, or tracheoesophageal fistula.

Mediastinal Fibrosis

Mediastinal fibrosis represents an exuberant scarring reaction to prior histoplasmosis. Mediastinal structures commonly affected are the superior vena cava, airways, pulmonary arteries or veins, and esophagus. Fibrosis may invade the thoracic duct, recurrent laryngeal nerve, or, in rare cases, the atrium. Chest radiographs show subcarinal or superior mediastinal widening, while CT scans reveal fibrotic restriction and invasion of mediastinal structures and calcification of the lymph nodes. Recurrent and often serious hemoptysis results from lung or airway damage and vascular compromise. Respiratory failure ensues in one-third of cases.

Pulmonary Histoplasmoma

Patients may develop a slowly enlarging pulmonary nodule, which has been called "enlarging histoplasmoma." These range in diameter from 8 to 35 mm and enlarge an average of 2 mm per year. Although these lesions are not associated with clinical symptoms, they may lead to concern about malignancy. Calcification occurs in the necrotic central and surrounding fibrous tissue. Histologically, they are characterized by a necrotic center surrounded by a fibrous-like capsule. Organisms may be seen in the necrotic center. These lesions are thought to represent an excessive fibrosis response to antigenic materials released from the central core into the surrounding tissue rather than progressive infection, a similar mechanism to that postulated for fibrosing mediastinitis. Results of serologic tests or cultures were not presented, but they probably would be negative in most cases on the basis of experience in patients with fibrosing mediastinitis or solitary coin lesions. Antifungal treatment would not be expected to alter the course of enlarging histoplasmomas and probably is not indicated.

Diagnosis

Diagnostic modalities include cultures, fungal stains of tissue or body fluids, and tests for antibodies and antigens. The role of each test varies with the severity of the infection. Serologic tests for antibodies form the basis for diagnosis in most patients with mild infections, whereas use of a battery of tests is needed in patients with more severe disease. Diagnosis can be established from culture or serologic testing for antibodies in most patients with chronic pulmonary histoplasmosis.

Antigen Detection

Detection of antigen in the body fluids offers a valuable approach to diagnosis in severe cases, including those with disseminated and extensive pulmonary histoplasmosis, providing results within 24 to 48 h. Antigen is found in the blood, urine, and bronchoalveolar lavage (BAL) fluid of most patients with disseminated histoplasmosis and in up to 75 percent of those with diffuse lung invasion during acute pulmonary histoplasmosis. Antigen may be found CSF of 25 to 50 percent of patients with chronic meningitis caused by histoplasmosis. Positive results caused by cross-reacting antigens occur in patients with African histoplasmosis, blastomycosis, paracoccidioidomycosis, and *Penicillium marneffii* infection. Cross reactions have not been recognized in patients with more common fungal infections, such as candidiasis, cryptococcosis, aspergillosis, or coccidioidomycosis. Antigen levels decline during the first year after treatment or spontaneously in patients with self-limited histoplasmosis and increase with relapse, providing a tool for monitoring therapy. Antigen testing is available only at the Histoplasmosis Reference Laboratory.

Fungal Stain

Fungal staining permits rapid diagnosis but with a lower sensitivity than culture or antigen detection. The highest yield is from bone marrow. *H. capsulatum* may be seen in peripheral blood smears in patients with severe disease. *Pneumocystis carinii, Candida glabrata, Blastomyces dermatitidis, Toxoplasma gondii,* and *P. marneffii* may be misidentified as *H. capsulatum.* Less experienced pathologists also may mistake staining artifacts for *H. capsulatum.*

Fungal Cultures

Cultures provide the strongest proof for histoplasmosis but are limited by low sensitivity (10 to 15 percent) in self-limited infections and delayed growth (2 to 4 weeks). In disseminated histoplasmosis, the highest yield is from bone marrow or blood—positive in more than 75 percent of cases. Several specimens must be cultured to achieve the highest yield. Cultures usually are negative in patients with mild acute pulmonary, pericardial, or rheumatogic manifestations and need not be performed.

Serologic Tests

Serologic tests are very useful but require familiarity with their limitations. Antibodies to *H. capsulatum* measured by immunodiffusion or complement

TABLE 63-13 Indications for Treatment in Patients with Histoplasmosis

Treatment indicated	Treatment not indicated
Acute pulmonary with hypoxia	Acute self-limited syndromes
Acute pulmonary >1 month	Acute pulmonary, mildly ill
Disseminated	Rheumatologic
Chronic pulmonary	Pericarditis
Mediastinal granuloma with obstruction or invasion of adjacent tissue	Fibrosing mediastinitis?
	Histoplasmoma
	Broncholithiasis
	Presumed ocular

fixation develop in most patients. Limitations of tests for antibodies include a 4- to 8-week delay in diagnosis while antibodies are being produced after acute infection, false-negative results in immunocompromised patients, and false-positive results in patients with blastomycosis, coccidioidomycosis, and paracoccidioidomycosis. Also, antibodies that persist after an earlier episode of histoplasmosis may cause confusion in patients with other diseases, such as malignancy, aspergilloma, or mycobacterial lung disease.

Histoplasmin Skin Test

Skin tests are not useful diagnostically because of high background rates of skin test positivity (50 to 80 percent) in endemic areas, false-positive results in patients with other fungal diseases, and false-negative results in patients with disseminated disease. Furthermore, skin tests boost antibody levels, compromising interpretation of serologic tests.

Treatment

Acute Syndromes

Diffuse Pulmonary Histoplasmosis Patients with acute pulmonary histoplasmosis causing hypoxia benefit from antifungal therapy and adjunctive corticosteroid therapy (Tables 63-13 to 63-15). Other patients with acute

TABLE 63-14 Drug Interactions of Azole and Triazole Antifungal Agents That Increase Concentrations of Other Drugs Metabolized by the Hepatic Cytochrome P450 System

Drug	Effect
Terfenadine	
Astemizole	Ventricular tachycardia
Cisapride	
Oral hypoglycemic	Hypoglycemia
Digitalis	Digitalis toxicity
Dihydropyridine, calcium-channel blockers	Edema, hyponatremia
Phenytoin	Phenytoin toxicity
Cyclosporine, tacrolimus	Renal failure
Rifabutin, rifampicin	Uveitis
Triazolam	Sedation
Midazolam	Sedation
Quinidine	Tinnitus
Warfarin	Bleeding

TABLE 63-15 Guidelines for Selection of Therapy for Endemic Mycoses

Infection	Moderately or Severely Ill	Mildly Ill	Maintenance
Histoplasmosis	Amphotericin B	Itraconazole	Itraconazole
Blastomycosis	Amphotericin B	Itraconazole	Itraconazole
Coccidioidomycosis	Amphotericin B	Fluconazole or itraconazole	Fluconazole or itraconazole

pulmonary histoplasmosis who remain moderate symptomatic for at least a month also may benefit from therapy, but controlled trials have not been conducted establishing efficacy in this situation. Amphotericin B is fungicidal and may induce a more rapid response in severely ill patients. Amphotericin B is preferred as initial therapy in patients who are more severely ill. Azoles or triazoles are fungistatic but are highly effective in patients with milder illnesses.

Mediastinal Granuloma Patients with obstructive symptoms or fistulas caused by mediastinal granuloma may benefit from antifungal therapy or surgery if the problem is sufficiently bothersome. Antifungal treatment or resection of enlarged mediastinal lymph nodes to prevent progression to fibrosing mediastinitis is not indicated, since progression of granulomatous mediastinitis to fibrosing mediastinitis has not been documented and must be rare. Rheumatologic syndromes and pericarditis are noninfectious inflammatory manifestations and respond to anti-inflammatory therapy. Antifungal therapy is not indicated unless the bone, joint, or pericardium is the site of disseminated infection.

Chronic Pulmonary Histoplasmosis Treatment improves survival, reduces symptoms, promotes radiographic healing, and eradicates *H. capsulatum* from the sputum. Most patients with chronic pulmonary histoplasmosis can be managed without hospitalization and respond well to treatment with itraconazole. Amphotericin B may be needed in patients with more severe respiratory insufficiency to achieve a more rapid response to therapy.

Disseminated Histoplasmosis Treatment is indicated in all patients with disseminated disease. The mortality for untreated disseminated histoplasmosis is 80 percent, but it can be reduced to less than 25 percent with therapy. Amphotericin B and itraconazole are highly effective therapy even in immunocompromised hosts, inducing a remission in 85 to 90 percent of patients.

Broncholithiasis Surgical therapy is required for patients with significant hemoptysis or recurrent pneumonia and for repair of bronchoesophageal fistulas. Antifungal therapy would not be expected to reduce the symptoms, since active infection is uncommon in such cases.

Mediastinal Fibrosis Antifungal treatment is not believed to improve the outcome of mediastinal fibrosis, but a few patients treated with ketoconazole showed some improvement. Antifungal therapy may be tried in patients with positive serologic tests and elevated sedimentation rates. Although most authorities discourage surgical therapy, improvement after resection of the scar tissue has been reported. Operative mortality is high.

Selection of Antifungal Agents

Amphotericin B   Amphotericin B may act more rapidly than other antifungal agents. Abatement of fever occurs within 1 week in more than 80 percent of patients with disseminated infection. Tolerability, however, is poor. Liposomal amphotericin B may overcome this limitation and permit more aggressive therapy of patients with severe illnesses. If the drug is used exclusively for treatment of disseminated or chronic pulmonary histoplasmosis, at least 30 mg/kg should be given over 2 to 4 months to adult patients. More commonly, however, treatment is changed to itraconazole after clinical improvement has occurred.

Itraconazole   Itraconazole was successful in 85 to 100 percent of cases with disseminated or chronic pulmonary histoplasmosis compared to 56 to 70 percent for ketoconazole. Itraconazole was effective in 85 percent of cases of disseminated histoplasmosis in patients with AIDS. Itraconazole requires an acidic gastric environment for solubilization and should be given with food or cola. Medications that reduce gastric acidity (H_2 antagonists are discouraged, and omeprazole is disallowed) should be avoided (Table 63-14). Blood concentrations should be measured during the second week of therapy 2 to 4 h after a dose in an effort to reach a concentration above 1 μ/mL and preferably higher (4 to 10 μ/mL).

Itraconazole is eliminated by hepatic metabolism. Hepatic enzyme inducers (rifampin, rifabutin, phenytoin, phenobarbital) reduce itraconazole concentrations. Treatment failures have occurred in patients receiving rifampin, the most potent of the cytochrome p450 inducers. Rifampin should not be given to patients receiving itraconazole for serious fungal infections. Rifabutin reduces itraconazole concentrations by about 75 percent and should be avoided if possible. If treatment with cytochrome P450 enzyme inducers is essential, itraconazole concentration should be monitored.

Itraconazole impairs hepatic metabolism of many drugs by inhibition of cytochrome P450 enzymes. This interaction causes an increase in blood concentrations of terfenadine, astemizole, and cisapride, potentially causing serious ventricular arrhythmias and even death. Such combinations should be strictly avoided. Interactions increasing the blood concentrations and toxicities of phenytoin, warfarin, oral hypoglycemics, digitalis, cyclosporine, and calcium-channel blockers also must be recognized so that these treatments can be monitored appropriately.

Ketoconazole   Ketoconazole is effective for treatment of histoplasmosis but appears to be less active than itraconazole. More gastrointestinal upset occurs with ketoconazole than with itraconazole. The pharmacokinetic and drug interaction profiles of ketoconazole and itraconazole are similar. While ketoconazole is only one-third as expensive as itraconazole, it remains a second choice for oral therapy because of its reduced efficacy and poorer tolerability.

Fluconazole   Fluconazole is less active in vitro than itraconazole for *H. capsulatum* and also appears to be less effective for treatment of histoplasmosis. Fluconazole 200 to 400 mg induced responses in 40 and 75 percent of cases in chronic pulmonary and disseminated histoplasmosis, respectively. Treatment with 800 mg daily may induce remission in AIDS patients with mild to moderately severe manifestations of disseminated histoplasmosis, but many relapse during maintenance treatment with 400 mg daily unless control of HIV infection is achieved.

Prevention

In two reports, fluconazole did not appear to reduce the occurrence of histoplasmosis in AIDS patients with low CD4+ lymphocyte counts, perhaps because of its relative weak activity against *H. capsulatum*. Itraconazole may be more effective if used in the suspension form that has better bioavailability. In general, prophylaxis cannot be supported in view of the lack of beneficial effect on mortality, the potential for drug interactions, toxicity, and the likely pressure for emergence of infection with triazole-resistant fungi, particularly candidiasis.

COCCIDIOIDOMYCOSIS

Coccidioidomycosis is the most serious of the endemic mycoses, often defying aggressive antifungal therapy. Recent outbreaks in southern California have placed large numbers of persons at risk for coccidioidomycosis. Whereas most cases are recognized within the endemic areas of the southwestern United States, increasingly cases are identified in travelers who have visited those areas.

Mycology and Epidemiology

Coccidioidomycosis is caused by the pathogenic fungus *Coccidioides immitis*. *C. immitis* is the most virulent of the pathogenic fungi, causing infection upon exposure to only a few conidia and severe disease with larger inocula. *C. immitis* grows as a mold with septate hyphae in the soil and on culture media and as an endosporulation spherule in the tissues of patients. Its arrow shaped arthroconidia are 2.5 to 4 by 3 to 6 μm in size and are the infectious particles found in soil. *C. immitis* converts to an endosporulating spherule at 37 to 40°C. Spherules measure 30 to 60 μm in diameter and contain multiple 2- to 5-μm endospores. Growth on fungal media occurs rapidly (in less than 5 days), and identification may be possible by the tenth day.

Coccidioidomycosis occurs in a spotty distribution in the southwestern United States, northern Mexico, and Central America. Growth is enhanced by bat and rodent droppings. Climates in the endemic areas are characterized by hot summers, mild winters, and arid conditions. Exposure is heaviest in the late summer and fall, when the soil is dry and conditions are windy—especially after rainy winters.

Workers exposed to soil are at increased risk for coccidioidomycosis. Cases most often are identified in construction or agricultural workers and archaeologists or students doing projects in the desert. However, large windborn outbreaks have exposed people many miles from the desert who had no direct exposure to contaminated soil. Coccidioidomycosis also is a threat to laboratory workers experimenting with live arthroconidia.

Coccidioidomycosis has become a serious opportunistic infection in patients with untreated AIDS in Texas, Arizona, and southern California. In Tucson, coccidioidomycosis was the third most frequently reported opportunistic infection in persons with AIDS, occurring in one-fourth of patients. Cases often are identified outside the endemic area in travelers who have visited the Southwest, emphasizing the importance of travel history in patients with compatible clinical syndrome. Disease also may develop outside the endemic region in persons who lived in those areas earlier, presumably through reactivation of clinically dormant foci of infection.

Pathogenesis and Pathology

Infection occurs following inhalation of arthroconidia of the mycelial phase of the fungus or reactivation of latent infection. Person-to-person transmission or exposure by direct inoculation is rare. Arthroconidia enlarge and form thick-walled spherules, which contain multiple endospores. Spherules rupture releasing endospores, which spread locally and disseminate hematogenously.

Cellular immunity and neutrophils both are engaged in host defense in coccidioidomycosis. Patients with deficient cellular immunity experience severe progressive forms of coccidioidomycosis. Pathologically, coccidioidomycosis is characterized by a pyogranulomatous reaction. In contrast to *H. capsulatum, C. immitis* is not an intracellular pathogen. The neutrophil response and caseous necrosis may lead to development of large abscesses, which often require surgical drainage. Abscesses also may spontaneously rupture or produce fistulas. Fibrosis may be prominent in the lungs or meninges. As with histoplasmosis, healed lesions frequently calcify. Tissue and blood eosinophilia may be pronounced in coccidioidomycosis.

Clinical Manifestations

About 40 percent of nonimmune persons experience symptoms 1 to 4 weeks after exposure to *C. immitis,* while the others have subclinical infection. Pulmonary illness is most common. More than 90 percent of symptomatic patients recover without treatment, while the rest develop chronic pulmonary or extrapulmonary complications. The illness is more severe in immunosuppressed persons, African Americans, and Filipinos.

Primary Pulmonary Coccidioidomycosis

Symptoms develop within a few weeks after exposure, depending on the intensity of the inoculum and the immunity of the patient. Flu-like symptoms include pleuritic or dull chest pain, nonproductive cough, fever, and malaise. Patients with more extensive pulmonary infection may experience dyspnea or respiratory failure.

Chest radiograms show patchy infiltrates, often with mediastinal adenopathy. Nodular coin lesions (coccidioidomas) and thin-walled cavities may follow in 5 percent of patients. Pleural invasion is uncommon (in less than 10 percent) and is characterized by pleuric pain, friction rub, and effusion. Pneumothorax, bronchopleural fistulas, or empyema may complicate such cases. Pericardial effusions are commonly seen less.

Rheumatologic Coccidioidomycosis

Women often exhibit erythema nodosum or multiforme as a manifestation of primary coccidioidomycosis. This manifestation is similar to that seen in histoplasmosis. Arthralgias or arthritis commonly accompanies the skin lesions. These manifestations resolve without antifungal treatment.

Chronic Pulmonary Coccidioidomycosis

Chronic fibrocavitary infection with progressive fibrosis and retraction similar to that seen with histoplasmosis and tuberculosis also may be seen in coccidioidomycosis. This manifestation is seen in patients with underlying lung disease and tends to progress without treatment.

Disseminated Coccidioidomycosis

Extrapulmonary dissemination occurs in less than 1 percent of persons with coccidioidomycosis and typically is diagnosed during the year after exposure. Sites most commonly affected are skin, bone, joints, and meninges. Skin manifestations include papules, pustules, plaques, nodules, ulcers, abscesses, and proliferative lesions. Organisms are readily demonstrated in skin lesions. A septic shock syndrome associated with respiratory failure has been described in patients presenting with focal or diffuse pulmonary coccidioidomycosis who later are found to have disseminated disease.

Meningitis is a particularly important complication because of its frequency and poor prognosis. Meningitis occurs in up to half of patients with disseminated coccidioidomycosis, often as the sole clinical manifestation of the disease. Patients with meningitis manifest headache, nausea, vomiting, and confusion. Cerebrospinal fluid shows lymphocytic pleocytosis.

Other sites of infection are lymph nodes, liver, peritoneum, kidneys, epididymis, prostate, testes, retina, ears, larynx, heart, thyroid, adrenal, pituitary, esophagus, and pancreas. Abscesses rarely occur in the brain or spinal cord. Brain abscesses may occur in the absence of meningitis or obvious sites of dissemination in other tissues; they are believed to develop as a consequence of hematogenous spread rather than direct extension from the meninges.

Pulmonary impairment is common in patients with disseminated coccidioidomycosis. Chest radiographs show diffuse reticulonodular infiltrates in most cases, but focal pulmonary lesions, nodules, cavities, adenopathy, and pleural effusions also may be seen. Miliary infiltrates represent hematogenous impairment of the lungs. Diffuse infiltrates appear to be more common in patients with AIDS than in other patient groups, and the prognosis is poor (70 percent mortality).

Diagnosis

Diagnosis of chronic pulmonary or disseminated coccidioidomycosis is made from fungal stain and culture. Examination of sputum is appropriate in patients with pulmonary manifestations. If the sputum examination yields negative results, bronchoscopy, which improves the yield, should be considered. Spherules may be seen in respiratory secretions or tissues. Cultures are usually positive from the above sites, with growth in 3 to 5 days in most patients. Blood cultures are seldom positive. Organisms isolated from cultures can be rapidly identified as *C. immitis* with DNA probe technology.

Serologic tests, positive in more than 80 percent of cases, is most valuable for diagnosis of coccidioidomycosis and has been reviewed in detail. Demonstration of elevated levels of antibodies to *C. immitis* often is the sole basis for diagnosis in patients with primary pulmonary coccidioidomycosis. The IgM antibody response to coccidioidin is first detected from tube precipitation. The IgG response measured by complement fixation follows the IgM response and persists longer. High titers of complement-fixing antibodies at a dilution of 1:16 or greater suggest severe infection and support the need to exclude dissemination. Detection of antibody in cerebrospinal fluid is invaluable for diagnosis of meningitis. Serial testing in patients with primary pulmonary coccidioidomycosis is helpful in monitoring recovery, as rising antibody titers suggest dissemination.

Skin Test

Skin testing is very useful for diagnosis of primary pulmonary coccidioido-mycosis. Development of positive skin tests precedes development of anti-bodies by several weeks. Additionally, antibodies remain undetectable in up to 20 percent of patients with self-limited illnesses and in 95 percent of asymp-tomatic skin test converters. Cross reactions with other mycoses are uncom-mon, and skin tests do not induce production of antibodies to coccidioidal antigens. The standard reagent should be diluted for use in patients with erythema nodosum, however, as severe reactions may occur.

Treatment

Treatment is less effective in coccidioidomycosis than in other systemic mycoses. Up to one-fourth of patients with disseminated coccidioidomy-cosis fail therapy, and a similar proportion of responders subsequently relapse. Outcome is worse in patients who have meningitis or chronic pulmonary infection than in those with primary pulmonary or other forms of disseminated disease. Outcome also is worse in persons with serious underlying immunosuppression.

Indications For Treatment

Acute pulmonary or rheumatologic manifestations of coccidioidomycosis usually resolve without treatment, but most other syndromes are progressive and eventually fatal. Therapy is appropriate in patients with disseminated or chronic pulmonary coccidioidomycosis and in those with symptomatic acute pulmonary infection who experience hypoxia or protracted morbidity (longer than 1 to 2 months) or are immunosuppressed. Persons who are seropositive or who previously experienced symptomatic coccidioidomycosis perhaps should receive therapy if they are to undergo intensive immunosuppression such as that required for organ or bone marrow transplantation.

Selection of Antifungal Agents

Amphotericin B is effective treatment in most cases. Amphotericin B is rec-ommended for initial therapy for patients who are severely ill or have diffuse interstitial infiltrates because of its fungicidal action and more rapid effect (Table 63-15). If it is used as the sole therapy, a total of at least 35 mg/kg is needed to achieve satisfactory and durable responses. Increasingly, however, amphotericin B therapy is being replaced by fluconazole or itraconazole after patients improve clinically. Ketoconazole was poorly effective and also moderately toxic at doses of 400 mg daily or higher used to treat coccid-ioidomycosis. Intravenous fluconazole (400 to 800 mg per day) and itra-conazole (and voriconazole in clinical trials) have been used for initial therapy of coccidioidomycosis. Fluconazole induced a clinical response in 79 percent of patients with meningitis, 76 percent with cutaneous and 86 percent with skeletal manifestations of disseminated infection. Response was poorer in patients with chronic pulmonary infection (55 percent). Itraconazole also has been used for treatment of coccidioidomycosis. Outcome was better in those with skeletal or cutaneous lesions than in those with chronic pulmonary coccidioidomycosis.

Chronic maintenance therapy is essential for all patients with meningitis, or-gan transplant recipients, chronically immune suppressed or with untreated AIDS, and perhaps in others who have relapsed after appropriate therapy or who have persistent foci of chronic infection that cannot be removed surgically. Recurrence or demonstration of active infection at autopsy following treatment supports this approach. Relapse appears to occur more commonly with fluconazole and ketoconazole than with itraconazole. Fluconazole or itraconazole 400 mg or more daily or amphotericin B 50 mg administered weekly are options, but have not been prospectively studied for this purpose. Fluconazole is preferred in patients with meningitis because of its cerebrospinal fluid penetration.

Coccidioidal Meningitis

Treatment of coccidioidal meningitis offers a special challenge. Amphotericin B, given intravenously and intrathecally, has been the treatment of choice for meningitis despite its toxicity and incomplete efficacy. The relatively poor response to amphotericin B is partly explained by its poor penetration into the cerebrospinal fluid. Aggressive treatment with high individual doses (1.0 to 1.5 mg) and overall courses (more than 40 mg total) of amphotericin B given intrathecally may improve responses.

Fluconazole is an attractive alternative to amphotericin B for treatment of coccidioidal meningitis because of its excellent penetration into the cerebrospinal fluid. Lifelong therapy to prevent recurrence is mandatory for patients with coccidioidal meningitis. Ketoconazole and itraconazole play a lesser role in treatment of meningitis.

Adjunctive Surgical Therapy

Surgical debridement or resection of infected tissue is often necessary as an adjunct to antifungal therapy in coccidioidomycosis. Chronic foci of pulmonary necrosis or cavitation may require resection to prevent progression during therapy or recurrence following therapy. Soft tissue, joint, or bone abscesses may require drainage or debridement.

BLASTOMYCOSIS

Blastomycosis is the least common of the endemic mycoses. The lack of good serologic or skin-testing reagents has prevented thorough investigation of the epidemiologic and clinical aspects of blastomycosis. Although its geographic distribution overlaps that of histoplasmosis, its environmental niche is poorly understood.

Mycology and Epidemiology

Blastomyces dermatitidis is a thermally dimorphic fungus producing mycelia with 2- to 10-μm dumbbell-shaped conidia at 25°C and doubly refractile broad-based budding yeasts varying in size from 8 to 30 μm at 37°C. Isolation of *B. dermatitidis* in the mycelial form from cultures may occur rapidly or require several weeks of incubation for slow-growing strains.

The organism may be found in microfoci enriched with animal excreta. Although the epidemiology of blastomycosis is incompletely understood, cases most often occur in the southeastern United States in a distribution overlapping that of *H. capsulatum*. Rare isolations from soil have occurred in samples from areas inhabited by farm animals and from beaver lodges or dams. Decaying organic matter enhances its growth in the environment. Several common source outbreaks have been reported, often in association with outdoor activities such as hunting, camping, or canoeing in wooded or swampy environments.

Pathogenesis and Pathology

Pulmonary disease follows inhalation of conidia and is often accompanied by hematogenous dissemination. Neutrophils are first recruited to sites of infection, but lymphocytes arrive later and lead to pyogranuloma formation. Cellular immunity plays a role in defense against *B. dermatitidis*, but perhaps less than against other endemic mycoses. Infection is more extensive and outcome is worse in immunosuppressed subjects.

Pathologically, blastomycosis is characterized by granuloma formation with central microabscesses, so-called pyogranuloma, but not by caseation as seen in histoplasmosis or tuberculosis. Histologic changes in the skin may resemble those of squamous cell carcinoma or keratoacanthoma.

Clinical Manifestations

Pulmonary Blastomycosis

Patients present with localized pulmonary impairment or with disseminated disease, each occurring in about half of patients. Presenting symptoms in patients with pulmonary blastomycosis include fever, cough, dyspnea, chest pain, and weight loss of an insidious onset. The course may be self-limited or chronic and progressive. Tracheal and endobronchial invasion also has been seen in patients with pulmonary blastomycosis.

Chest radiographs usually show focal alveolar infiltrates in the upper lobes, often nodular in character. Cavities occur in one-third of cases. A minority of patients present with miliary or diffuse infiltrates associated with respiratory failure. In contrast to the presentation of histoplasmosis, mediastinal adenopathy and calcification are uncommon (20 percent). Mass lesions may resemble those seen with lung cancer, occurring in about 15 percent of cases. Pleural involvement occurs in 20 percent of cases and may invade adjacent bone or soft tissues.

Disseminated Blastomycosis

Skin and bone lesions are the most common manifestations of disseminated disease, but many organs may be affected. Cutaneous lesions occur in half of patients with disseminated blastomycosis and may be acquired by hematogenous dissemination or direct inoculation. Typical lesions are painless erythematous nodules, which develop verrucous or ulcerative surfaces; they may be mistaken for skin cancer. Bone and joint lesions occur in less than half of patients with disseminated blastomycosis and are characterized by osteolysis.

Central nervous system (CNS) infection is manifested as meningitis, brain lesions, or epidural abscesses and are relatively common (at least 15%). CNS impairment is more common in immunocompromised patients, occurring in nearly 20 percent of cases. Chronic meningitis may be accompanied by intracranial or epidural abscesses. Isolated intracranial or epidural abscesses occur in 20 to 30 percent of these. Pulmonary affliction or dissemination to skin, bone, or other tissues commonly is found in patients with neurologic manifestations, assisting in diagnosis. Laryngeal impairment also has been reported frequently and may be mistaken for cancer visually and histologically. The larynx may be infected directly from the respiratory route or following hematogenous dissemination. The paranasal sinuses and ears also may be affected. Genitourinary tract impairment of the kidneys, testes, prostate, or epididymis also is relatively common in blastomycosis. Other sites of dissemination are the spleen, liver, pericardium, eyes, adrenal glands, and thyroid. Patients have presented with clinical findings of septicemia.

Diagnosis

Mycologic Diagnosis

Diagnosis is based on demonstration of organisms in culture or fungal stain. Cultures are positive in more than 90 percent of patients. *B. dermatitidis* has been isolated most frequently from bronchoscopy specimens, cerebrospinal fluid, or brain, skin, and blood. Of note is that fungal stains have been positive in most cases, providing a more rapid diagnosis.

Serologic Diagnosis

Tests for antibodies may be falsely negative or falsely positive and are not useful for diagnosis of blastomycosis.

Antigen Detection

Diagnosis by antigen detection can be useful in patients with extensive pulmonary or disseminated disease. A cross-reacting antigen may be detected in the *H. capsulatum* antigen assay in most patients with disseminated disease. Specimens of urine or blood may be submitted to the Histoplasmosis Reference Laboratory in Indianapolis for antigen testing.

Treatment

Indications for Treatment

First, a decision to treat must be made. Some patients with acute pulmonary blastomycosis after a point source exposure recover without treatment. Spontaneous recovery may be followed by symptomatic recurrence or extrapulmonary dissemination, however, making long-term follow-up important. Patients with persistent or recurrent symptoms after acute infection, chronic pulmonary disease, pleural involvement, or dissemination should be treated.

Selection of Antifungal Agents

Selection of antifungal agents should be individualized on the basis of illness severity. Amphotericin B is highly effective and is the treatment of choice for patients with severe manifestations or who are immunosuppressed (Table 63-15). In immunocompromised subjects, the response has been better to amphotericin B than to azoles or triazoles. Itraconazole (200 to 400 mg daily) is also highly effective in treatment of blastomycosis. Ketoconazole at doses of 400 to 800 mg daily for at least 6 months is reasonably effective, producing responses in more than 80 percent of patients. Relapse occurrs in some ketoconazole-treated patients, particularly those with immune compromise. Fluconazole is less effective in treatment of blastomycosis but can be used at doses of 400 to 800 mg daily if itraconazole is contraindicated.

Treatment should be continued until clinical and laboratory findings have normalized and radiographs stabilized to represent chronic residual manifestations of healed infection. Prolonged therapy often is needed in view of the slow response to therapy and significant risk of relapse after treatment is stopped. Lifelong maintenance therapy is essential in all patients with AIDS and may also be appropriate in those who require chronic immunosuppressive therapy or have relapsed after appropriate courses of therapy.

CRYPTOCOCCUS NEOFORMANS

Cryptococcosis is an illness caused by infection with the encapsulated fungus *Cryptococcus neoformans,* an organism with a worldwide distribution. Inhalation of *C. neoformans* initiates the infection in the lung, with hematogenous dissemination most often into the meninges. Although pulmonary infection may be discovered in the presence of disseminated infection, meningoencephalitis remains the most commonly diagnosed form of cryptococcal infection. In recent years, the incidence of cryptococcosis has risen because of AIDS and the increased use of immunosuppressive medications for other medical conditions.

Microbiology and Epidemiology

C. neoformans is a yeast that is characterized by its thick polysaccharide capsule. The yeast measures 4 to 6 mm in diameter, but the capsule thickness varies from 1 to more than 30 μm. Organisms are smaller and less well encapsulated in the environment, explaining their ability to reach the terminal airways after inhalation. *C. neoformans* grows readily in fungal media, allowing isolation in less than 48 h and identification with biochemical tests or DNA probes.

The fungus *C. neoformans* demonstrates no endemic pattern of distribution. Four serotypes of *C. neoformans* have been described. Serotypes A and D predominate in North America and Europe and grow best in composted bird droppings or rotted vegetation. Serotypes B and C are classified as *C. neoformans* var *gattii* and are more common in tropical and subtropical regions in association with eucalyptus trees rather than avian excreta. Outbreaks or clusters of cryptococcosis cases are rare. In most cases, a history of exposure to birds or dust is lacking. Person-to-person transmission does not occur, although cryptococcal infection has occurred via tissue transplantation and cutaneous infection has occurred after direct inoculation.

Cryptococcal infection can affect people with intact immune systems, although it is diagnosed most often in persons with underlying immune defects. Among those without immunosuppressive disease or therapy, the infection is rare, with an estimated incidence at 0.2 cases per million persons per year. Major risk factors include AIDS, patients with lymphoreticular malignancy (particularly Hodgkin's disease), patients requiring chronic corticosteroid therapy, recipients of solid organ transplants, and with sarcoidosis. The disease also appears to be more frequent in diabetics. There appears to be no race-related predilection for cryptococcosis, while the infection has been diagnosed in two to three times as many males as females—an observation that may be explained by inhibition of fungal growth due to estrogens or differential exposure to the organism in the environment.

Pathogenesis

Cryptococcosis is acquired by inhaling aerosols containing the yeast; it rarely occurs as a consequence of direct inoculation. Progressive disease often follows exposure in patients with impaired cellular immunity. In tissue, a mixed macrophage, lymphocyte, and plasma cell response is seen, but inflammation is often minimal in immunodeficient subjects. Granulomas are uncommonly found in the nervous system but may be seen in other tissues. Macrophages, natural killer cells, and T lymphocytes play the key roles in cellular defense against *C. neoformans*. Inflammatory cytokines (IL-2, IL-12, interferon gamma) and macrophage colony-stimulating factor enhance the antifungal activity of these cellular mechanisms. Humoral immunity complements cellular mechanisms in defense against *C. neoformans*.

Clinical Manifestations

Cryptococcal infection results in self-limited pulmonary disease in most healthy persons. Occasionally, isolated pulmonary cryptococcosis is diagnosed, but meningoencephalitis is the most commonly recognized manifestation of cryptococcosis and the most common cause of death from cryptococcal infection. Hematogenous dissemination to almost any tissue occurs in fewer than 25 percent of cases.

Pulmonary Infection

Isolated pulmonary infection may be identified in nonimmunosuppressed subjects, and saprophytic colonization has been observed in patients with underlying lung disease. There is no distinguishing constellation of signs or symptoms of pulmonary cryptococcosis. Normal hosts with pulmonary cryptococcal infection develop symptoms in up to one-half of cases, while have cryptococcosis diagnosed only after evaluation chest radiographic abnormality. In those who are symptomatic, the infection is often indolent, with some combination of dry cough, dull chest discomfort, and low-grade fever reported. Less commonly, night sweats, fatigue, weight loss, or hemoptysis may occur. The majority of isolated pulmonary infections in patients without immunosuppression have been shown to resolve over time without antifungal therapy. Occasionally, a chronic, slowly progressive pulmonary infection develops or disseminated infection manifested by meningoencephalitis or other organ involvement may present after apparent abatement or resolution of the pulmonary process.

Immunocompromised patients with pulmonary cryptococcosis have symptoms of fever and cough. Immunosuppressed patients with pulmonary cryptococcosis commonly develop meningoencephalitis, supporting the need for therapy in these patients. Since most immunocompromised patients receiving a diagnosis of pulmonary cryptococcosis have concurrent meningoencephalitis, it is critical to perform a lumbar puncture in immunocompromised patients with cryptococcal pneumonia even in the absence of clinical findings of meningitis.

The radiographic pattern can be correlated with the host's immune status. Well-defined nodular (single or multiple) infiltrates or well-defined patchy infiltrates are commonly seen in the normal host and may or may not be associated with symptoms. Diffuse pulmonary disease associated with diffuse interstitial infiltrates or widespread alveolar consolidation along with respiratory failure is more commonly seen in those who are severely immunodeficient. Diffuse infiltrates in a patient with AIDS may be mistakenly attributed to *Pneumocystis carinii* pneumonia, leading to inappropriate treatment with corticosteroids. The radiographic appearance in patients with less profound cell-mediated immune defects—such as those receiving corticosteroid therapy, transplant recipients, or patients with lymphoreticular malignancy—can vary widely, although most commonly nodular or patchy alveolar infiltrates are seen. Mass lesions may resemble malignancy. Cavitation is uncommon, and mediastinal adenopathy, pleural effusion, and calcification are rare. Empyema, pneumothorax, and pleural involvement suggesting Pancoast's tumor have been reported.

Meningoencephalitis

Meningoencephalitis is the most common manifestation of cryptococcosis. Typically, diffuse involvement of the cerebral cortex, cerebellum, and brain stem occur concurrently. A gradual onset of symptoms over a few months is typical, but a more rapid onset of symptoms occurs in patients with immunodeficiency. Presenting symptoms include fever, headache, nausea, and vomiting. Less than one-third of patients exhibit meningismus, altered mentation, or focal neurologic abnormalities. Elevated intracranial pressure is common and may cause serious problems, including death from brain-stem herniation. Focal brain lesions (cryptococcomas) are seen in about 10 percent of cases, either as isolated manifestations or in combination with meningoencephalitis. Imaging procedures more often show meningeal enhancement, hydrocephalus, cerebral edema, or cerebral atrophy.

Other Sites of Dissemination

Extraneural involvement occurs in up to half of patients who have cryptococcal meningitis. Hepatosplenomegaly and bone marrow suppression causing pancytopenia are seen commonly, in addition to occasional lesions in the skin, eyes, bones, or joints. Involvement of the prostate has been described in both AIDS and transplant patients. Other sites of dissemination are the heart, pericardium, muscle, gastrointestinal tract, peritoneum, thyroid, larynx, breast, placenta, urinary tract, and organ of Corti.

Diagnosis

Pneumonia

Diagnosis of cryptococcal pneumonia requires isolation of the organism from pulmonary secretions or tissues or visualization in histopathologic specimens. Sputum cultures reveal *C. neoformans* in up to 50 percent of cases. Growth of *C. neoformans* from sputum, while suggestive, does not establish a definitive diagnosis, as the organism can be recovered from the sputum of patients with lung disease due to other causes. If nodular or mass lesions are present, a fine-needle aspirate of the lesion should be considered for diagnosis. Cytologic examination as well as culture of the biopsied material should be performed. Bronchoalveolar lavage (BAL) may be the procedure of choice for those with interstitial or alveolar infiltrates. Cultures of BAL fluid or lung tissue yield the organism in 50 to 90 percent of cases, while fungal stains are positive less often. When present, pleural effusions may be positive for growth of *C. neoformans* in about 40 percent of cases.

In tissue, *C. neoformans* can be recognized as a globose or oval to lemon-shaped yeast with a polysaccharide capsule. Cryptococci may be difficult to visualize on routine hematoxylin-and-eosin–stained sections, although identification of the organism can be enhanced by the use of appropriate special stains. Cryptococci are uniformly positive with the Gomori methenamine silver and periodic acid–Schiff stains, as are other fungal organisms. More specific stains for *C. neoformans* include the Mayers mucicarmine stain, which stains the fungal capsule, and the Masson-Fontana melanin stain, which may detect capsule-deficient cryptococci in tissue.

Direct microscopic examination of BAL fluid sediment stained with India ink can help to identify the organism. Cryptococci may also be identified in sputum or pus after treatment with 10 percent sodium hydroxide.

In patients with cryptococcal pneumonia, the serum cryptococcal antigen is often detected and suggests dissemination beyond the lung. A negative serum cryptococcal test should not be used to exclude *C. neoformans* lung infection. Among immunocompromised patients with pulmonary cryptococcosis, the serum cryptococcal antigen may be positive in more than 95 percent of cases. Cryptococcal antigen testing may also be detected in lavage fluid and in pleural fluid, although antigen detection from these fluids has not been used routinely for diagnosis of pneumonia. Blood cultures may be positive for *C. neoformans* in severely immunocompromised hosts. It should be emphasized that once a diagnosis of pulmonary cryptococcosis is made, an *evaluation for extrapulmonary dissemination* should be initiated. A serum cryptococcal antigen test should be performed along with fungal blood culture and cerebrospinal fluid (CSF) examination; in men, a urine fungal culture after prostatic massage should be obtained.

Meningoencephalitis

The diagnosis of meningitis can be made initially on detection of cryptococcal polysaccharide antigen in CSF and confirmed by isolation of the organism from fungal cultures. Antigen also can be detected in serum in most patients with cryptococcal meningitis, often providing a clue to the diagnosis before lumbar puncture is performed. Encapsulated organisms may be seen with India ink staining. *C. neoformans* may be isolated from blood, skin lesions, bone marrow, urine, or other sites in up to two-thirds of patients.

Treatment

Treatment is indicated in patients with symptomatic pulmonary infections, especially if they are immunocompromised, and in all patients with meningoencephalitis or disseminated infection. Patients with a diagnosis of cryptococcosis at any site should be provided close follow-up for at least 1 year.

Pulmonary Cryptococcosis

For asymptomatic patients with isolated pulmonary cryptococcal infection and *no identifiable underlying immune deficits,* antifungal therapy may be withheld for 2 to 3 months as long as close observation is provided and any pulmonary lesions are stable or decreasing in size. Among nonimmunosuppressed symptomatic patients, asymptomatic patients whose disease progresses during observation, or patients with milder degrees of immunosuppression, amphotericin B is the treatment of choice for those who are more severely ill, while oral therapy with fluconazole is appropriate in milder cases or after a clinical and microbiologic response to amphotericin B. Intravenous amphotericin B at a dose of 0.3 to 0.6 mg/kg a day combined with oral 5-flucytosine at a dose of 75 to 100 mg/kg a day (divided into four daily doses) for 3 to 6 weeks can be used to treat cryptococcal pneumonia. The 5-flucytosine dose should be adjusted to keep serum levels less than 100 μg/mL and should not be used in the absence of monitoring of serum levels. Alternatively, amphotericin B alone at a dose of 0.5 mg/kg a day or higher or liposomal amphotericin (3 to 5 mg/kg/d) can be used for severe infections. After initial improvement is seen with a regimen containing amphotericin B, completion of therapy with oral fluconazole 400 mg daily is reasonable, with a suggested total duration of therapy of at least 3 months. The echinocandin agents do not appear to be effective for cryptococcosis.

Initiating treatment with oral fluconazole at a dose of 400 mg daily can be considered, particularly for normal patients and those with reversible forms of immunosuppression with mild infections, with a suggested duration of at least 3 to 6 months. As experience with oral therapy for these conditions is limited, consideration for treatment durations longer than 3 months should be given. In patients with immune deficits, disseminated infection and relapse are common, supporting the need for lifelong maintenance therapy after an initial induction therapy once cryptococcal infection is diagnosed.

Cryptococcal Meningitis and Disseminated Cryptococcosis in the Compromised Host

Induction Therapy In immunocompromised patients with cryptococcal meningitis, amphotericin B at doses of about 0.7 mg/kg a day, should be used for induction of remission. This may be coupled with 5-flucytosine. This is then followed by itraconazole or fluconazole, each 400 mg daily, to complete 10 weeks of induction treatment. Itraconazole seems to work as well as fluconazole during the consolidation phase of therapy, despite poor penetration into CSF. Cultures remain positive at the completion of therapy in some patients demonstrating the need for repeat lumbar puncture to prove sterilization of CSF. Aggressive management of elevated intracranial pressure is also important. Initial therapy with high dose fluconazole (800 mg daily) has also been used successfully. 5-Flucytosine and fluconazole interact synergistically for *C. neoformans.*

Liposomal preparations of amphotericin B are less toxic than the standard formulation and may be used at higher dosage but has been less well studied than traditional amphotericin B. The response to Ambisome was somewhat better than that to Abelcet for this indication in separate trials. Randomized trials are needed. If used, levels of 5-flucytosine should be monitored and maintained between 50 and 100 μg/mL to reduce toxicity.

Chronic Maintenance Therapy Chronic treatment is required to prevent recurrence in immunocompromised patients. Fluconazole 200 mg daily is more effective than amphotericin B 100 mg weekly for prevention of recurrence.

Development of Resistance Relative resistance of strains of *Cryptococcus* have been demonstrated in organ transplantation, AIDS, and other hosts with in vitro MICs to fluconazole over 64 μg/mL. Treatment failure caused by an amphotericin B–resistant strain also has been described. Higher doses of fluconazole and demonstration of microbiological cures will generally overcome problems with resistance.

PNEUMOCYSTIS CARINII

Since the original association of this organism with epidemics of "interstitial plasma cell pneumonitis" of young, malnourished children, *P. carinii* has been identified as a cause of pneumonia in a broad range of immunocompromised hosts (Table 63-16). The apparent incidence of *P. carinii* pneumonia has increased with the prolonged survival of immunocompromised patients and with improvements in diagnostic techniques for this pathogen. Particular susceptibility has been noted in patients receiving corticosteroid therapy and in those with AIDS.

TABLE 63-16 Conditions Associated with
Pneumocystis carinii Pneumonia

Acquired immunodeficiency syndrome (AIDS)
Chemotherapy (especially corticosteroids)
Radiation therapy
Organ transplantation
Neutropenia, CD4+ lymphopenia
Prematurity
Malnutrition (protein and calorie)
Malignancies (especially hematopoietic)
Congenital immune deficiency diseases
(cellular, humoral, combined)
Collagen vascular disease
Hematologic disorders
Cushing's syndrome
Nephrotic syndrome

Structure and Life Cycle

In humans and animals, three forms of the organism have been identified: trophozoite, cyst, and sporozoite (or "intracystic bodies"). The trophozoite, 2 to 5 μm in diameter, is either round or sickle-shaped and contains a nucleus, mitochondria, and vacuoles; it also includes pseudopodia and filopodia, used in limited motility. The cyst is 3 to 6 μm in diameter. Its cell wall consists of three layers, and its cytoplasm contains eight small pleomorphic intracystic (oval) bodies (sporozoites). Two other cystic forms have been described, but these are probably intermediates including empty or developing cysts (Fig. 63-1).

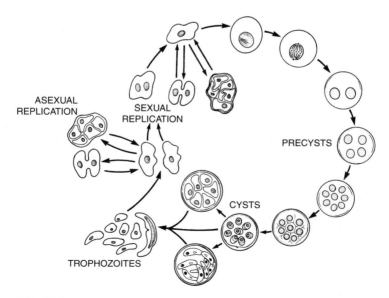

FIG. 63-1 The life cycle of *Pneumocystis carinii*.

Many small surface projections ("tubular expansions") form a branching network over the surfaces of the cysts and the trophozoites.

In the alveolus, *P. carinii* organisms are covered with a variety of glycoproteins derived from both the organism and the environment. Specific and nonspecific immunoglobulins, albumin, surfactant proteins, laminin, fibronectin, and other serum and lung proteins coat the surface. The organism itself produces a relatively limited array of surface glycoproteins that share antigenic epitopes. Most adult patients with *P. carinii* pneumonia carry antibodies to the major epitopes of the organism. The cell wall contains cholesterol but no ergosterol and does not appear to synthesize sterols de novo; this accounts for the lack of susceptibility to many of the antifungal antibiotics. The presence of chitin in the cell wall is controversial. The surface of *P. carinii* is carbohydrate rich with glucose, mannose, and β-1,3-glucan, which may play a role in phagocytosis of the organism by macrophages. The surface also contains carbohydrate-binding moieties, which may play a role in attachment to epithelial or surfactant layers.

Studies of the life cycle have used organisms derived from infected animals and passaged on a "feeder cell" layer of epithelial or fibroblastoid cells in tissue culture (Fig. 63-1). Both sexual and asexual intermediate stages have been postulated. Some differences exist in *P. carinii* grown in different hosts.

Research on *P. carinii* has been hampered by the difficulties encountered in propagating the organism in vitro. Studies have been performed on organisms derived from immunosuppressed rodents, which "spontaneously" develop *P. carinii* pneumonia. Hughes and coworkers have used this model to demonstrate the aerosol transmission of *P. carinii*. Cell culture techniques have not yet become useful diagnostically because of the difficulty in culturing the organism from infected human tissues.

Taxonomy and Molecular Biology

Phylogenetic data support the identification of *P. carinii* with the fungi (*Rhizopoda, Myxomycetes, Zygomycota, Schizosaccharomyces, Neurospora, Candida,* and the red yeasts in various studies), based on conserved mRNA sequences. The presence of separate genes encoding the thymidylate synthase and dihydrofolate reductase of *P. carinii,* the presence of a cyst wall rich in betaglucan that stains with periodic acid–Schiff and silver stains, the poorly developed mitochondria, the absence of typical protozoan intracellular organelles, and the airborne spread of infection all support this taxonomic position. The neutral lipid fraction of *P. carinii* includes a variety of phytosterols shared by plants and fungi, including *Physarum* species. However, the appearance of the organism with a thick-walled cyst with internal "sporozoites" and ameboid trophozoites, the absence of ergosterol, susceptibility to antibiotics used in the treatment of protozoan infections (pentamidine, atovaquone, sulfamethoxazole), and the existence of "antigenic variation" in the major surface glycoprotein (gp120, gpA, MSG) lend credence to identification with the protozoa.

It is likely that a new phylogenetic category may be needed for *P. carinii.* Unique cell wall components (glucans, phytosterols) and synthetic pathways (e.g., topoisomerases) may participate in the pathogenesis of infection due to *P. carinii* and may provide targets for the development of new antibiotics. Difficulty in ascribing *P. carinii* to one or another family may be further complicated by the apparent exchange of membrane lipids and perhaps glycoproteins between *P. carinii* and host cells. This may allow the adaptation of *P. carinii* to the host environment, decrease the effectiveness of the immune response, and enhance survival by decreasing the membrane synthetic demands of the organism.

The existence of different "strains" of *P. carinii* have been demonstrated using pulsed-field gel electrophoresis to establish chromosomal patterns. It appears that infections are often clonal, although many strains may coexist in the infected person. Characteristic chromosome patterns have not yet been associated with specific virulence or host characteristics. Characteristic shifts in the telomeric ends of the chromosomes suggest that genetic exchange is ongoing between chromosomes, as occurs in the mechanism of antigenic variation by movement of genetic cassettes noted in the subtelomeric region of the trypanosomes.

P. carinii expresses both unique and some common antigens in different host species. Surface antigens have been characterized at the glycoprotein and molecular levels. The major surface glycoprotein (MSG) represents the main humoral immunogen in the rat model, though other antigens (gp45 to 55) may have importance in human infection. Several MSG types (up to three) have been observed simultaneously in single infected humans and animals with monoclonal antibody staining and with genetic characterization. Because some antigens are shared between glycoproteins of differing sizes and between species, it is unclear whether a single organism can express more than one MSG or switch MSG expression during the life cycle. The MSG appears to represent a large family of related genes (more than 30), many of which are located in tandem repeated arrays in the subtelomeric regions and may contribute to the generation of the variety of antigenic types.

Epidemiology of Infection Due to *Pneumocystis*

The natural reservoir of infection remains unknown. Aerosol transmission of infection has been demonstrated animal models, and clusters of infections have developed in clinical settings—for instance, between HIV-infected persons and renal transplant recipients. *P. carinii* DNA has been detected by the polymerase chain reaction (PCR) in the air of hospital rooms, bronchoscopy suites, and clinics used by infected subjects. The frequency of infection varies both by institution and by geography. For example, it appears that the incidence of *P. carinii* in AIDS patients is much lower in Africa than in the United States. However, this may reflect limited diagnostic capabilities and the morbidity associated with the endemic level of tuberculosis and diarrheal pathogens in Africa, rather than a reduced epidemiologic exposure. The use of PCR technology suggests that carriage of *P. carinii* in African AIDS patients is, in fact, common.

Serologic testing has reinforced the view that subclinical infection is common and that a reactivation of latent infection is often a factor in the pathogenesis of *P. carinii* pneumonia. Most people have serologic evidence of exposure by age 4. The rate of identification of organisms in autopsy studies is less than 8 percent. An autopsy series from patients with malignant lymphoma or leukemia demonstrated a 5 percent incidence of identification of pulmonary *P. carinii,* compared with a less than 0.5 percent incidence in immunologically normal subjects. Molecular studies have suggested that *both reinfection and the reactivation of latent infection are significant factors in the incidence of disease.*

P. carinii pneumonia affects four categories of immunocompromised host: (1) *congenital,* caused by inborn immune defects in antibody-synthesizing capacity and/or in the cellular mechanisms responsible for delayed hypersensitivity; (2) *induced,* by immunosuppressive therapy, especially corticosteroids in the treatment of hematopoietic malignancies; (3) *acquired,* occurring as part of AIDS, often as the identifying opportunistic pathogen in HIV infection; and (4) *nutritionally deficient with epidemic infection,* seen primarily in neonates and infants.

P. carinii causes pneumonia in persons with a wide variety of underlying immune deficiencies (Table 63-16). T-cell immune defects are generally needed to initiate *P. carinii* infection although disease occurs in individuals with hypogammaglobulinemia. Passive transfer of immune T lymphocytes is protective against *P. carinii* pneumonia mice, whereas transfer of immune globulin alone is only partly protective. The risk of *P. carinii* pneumonia is greatest in the first 6 months after transplantation, after 3 to 6 months of oral corticosteroid therapy, and during periods of intensified immune suppression (for example, during the use of bolus corticosteroids or antilymphocyte therapies for graft rejection). In patients receiving lung transplants, the rate of asymptomatic isolation of *P. carinii* approaches two-thirds of the total in some series. Of these, up to half are expected to develop symptomatic disease without treatment. In AIDS, the risk increases with the progressive fall of the CD4-positive lymphocyte counts to below 200/cm^3 or to less than 20 percent of the total lymphocyte pool. The occurrence of *P. carinii* infection in persons not in these categories should suggest exposure to infected persons, other immunosuppressive effects (e.g., coinfection with cytomegalovirus, lymphoma, neutropenia), or, in the HIV-infected person, a rapid progression of viral infection with the accompanying decline in systemic immune function. Active infection due to cytomegalovirus (CMV) may also enhance the growth of *P. carinii* in any affected population. Whether CMV directly stimulates the proliferation of *P. carinii,* acts systemically as an immunosuppresive agent, or is simply a fellow traveler in the immunocompromised host remains to be settled. The clinical association of CMV with *P. carinii* may reflect similarities in the susceptible hosts or subtle shifts in the alveolar microenvironment. The incidence of infection varies between institutions and with the prophylactic regimens employed.

Corticosteroid use, neutropenia, and lung transplantation are also major predisposing factors in the development of infection. However, in most non-AIDS patients, the risk of disease is around 5 to 15 percent, depending on the nature and duration of the immune suppression. Clinically inapparent infection may develop during the weaning immunosuppressive agents. This is consistent with the limited inflammatory response generated by the organism in the susceptible host. Patients with *P. carinii* pneumonia generally have both antibodies and T lymphocytes directed at the organism at the time of presentation. Thus, the assumption has been made that such immunities are not protective, that the correlates of protection (the target antigens) have not yet been identified, that antigenic variation has "switched" the antigens expressed on the surface of the organisms, or that protection rests with the cellular immune control of alveolar macrophage function. In the presence of *P. carinii,* cytokine production and phagocytosis by alveolar macrophages are abnormal.

Clinical Presentation

The hallmark of infection due to *P. carinii* is the presence of marked hypoxemia, dyspnea, and cough out of proportion to physical or radiologic findings. In the transplant recipient or the person undergoing corticosteroid therapy, *P. carinii* pneumonia is generally acute to subacute in development and often masked by other processes, including allograft rejection or infection. In the AIDS patient with first episode of infection (i.e., untreated HIV infection), the evolution is more gradual (often 2 to 5 weeks) and constitutional symptoms and weight loss are prominent. Subsequent infections may evolve more rapidly. In the cancer patient receiving chemotherapy or in the organ or bone marrow transplant recipient, the use of corticosteroids, prior lung infection, abnormal pulmonary lymphatics (after heart, lung, or liver transplantation), and neutropenia may contribute to the absence of radiologically apparent disease. The rate of development of clinical infection is exacerbated by the presence of preexisting lung disease or other infections.

The presentation of *P. carinii* pneumonia is often complicated by a variety of factors. Prophylaxis with aerosolized pentamidine or with other second line prophylactic agents may delay or alter the presentation of disease. Coinfection may accelerate the progression of disease or alter the radiographic pattern; in particular, CMV, *Histoplasma capsulatum, Legionella* species, and mycobacterial species may contribute to the constitutional symptoms, to hypoxemia, and to the locality of pulmonary lesions. *Coinfection with CMV and other pathogens will be detected in more than half of the patients infected with P. carinii.* The expected mortality due to *P. carinii* pneumonia is increased in patients taking cyclosporine when compared with other imunocompromised hosts.

Extrapulmonary Pneumocystosis

P. carinii was known to cause extrapulmonary disease in the pre-AIDS era, but metastatic infection to significant degrees has been observed only in patients with advanced AIDS. Few cases of systemic infection due to *P. carinii* have been observed in patients receiving systemic prophylaxis with trimethoprim-sulfamethoxazole (TMP-SMX). Up to half of the patients with *P. carinii* pneumonia have PCR evidence of circulating DNA from this organism. In addition to the liver and spleen, sites of extrapulmonary disease have included eye, ear, lymph nodes, thymus, skin, mastoids, ascites, GI tract and omentum, pleura, kidney, bone marrow, pancreas, and adrenal glands, and it has been reported as a cause of thromboembolic disease. Vasculitis has been reported due to *P. carinii* as a cause of ischemic necrosis of digits.

Radiography

The Chest Radiograph

The chest radiograph plays a central role in the dignosis of *P. carinii* pneumonia, although no radiographic pattern is pathognomonic for *P. carinii* infection. The radiographic pattern depends on the patient's underlying or accompanying disease, the state of immunosuppression, and the duration of infection. Sometimes the chest radiograph is normal despite overt pulmonary disease. More often, the early stage of *P. carinii* pneumonia is manifest by fine, bilateral, perihilar, diffuse infiltrates that progress to an interstitial alveolar butterfly pattern; from the hilar region, the infiltrates spread to the apices or bases. Despite therapy, this pattern is often succeeded in 3 to 5 days by progressive consolidation, the appearance of air bronchograms, and complete opacification of the lung fields.

As in many of the "atypical pneumonias," unusual courses and patterns are seen: nodules, unilateral infiltrates, or even lobar consolidations. Small pleural effusions also occur. Distortions in pattern are commonly produced by prior radiation, drug-induced pulmonary injury, or concurrent infection with other organisms. The patient with recurrent disease may develop chronic interstitial markings, small cysts, or "honeycombing" on the chest radiograph. The distribution of cysts in pneumocystosis, when present at all, is more often diffuse, while peripheral or apical bullae are often seen without infection in intravenous drug abusers. Rarely, cavitary disease is seen in the absence of other pathogens; however, *P. carinii* can superinfect fungal or mycobacterial cavities.

The use of aerosolized pentamidine for the therapy and prophylaxis of *P. carinii* pneumonia has created problems in the diagnosis and treatment of pneumocystosis. The disease may present largely or solely in the upper lobes on chest radiograph. Similar disease may be seen without pentamidine use, suggesting a predilection of infection for the upper lobes. Cystic changes are more common in patients undergoing prophylaxis who develop *P. carinii* pneumonia. The development of spontaneous pneumothoraces may indicate the recurrence of *P. carinii* in the upper lobes despite ongoing prophylactic therapy. Pneumothorax may also complicate the management of intubated patients with *P. carinii* pneumonia; active pneumonia or fibrosis in the upper lobes is usually implicated. Undiagnosed, this complication is responsible for 50 percent mortality. Dense consolidation of tissues may suggest dual infection, often with a bacterial agent.

In lung transplant patients, rejection and infection often produce abnormal chest radiographs. In the first month, rejection of the transplanted lung will cause radiographic changes in up to 75 percent of patients. These changes include nodular and interstitial infiltrates in the perihilar area and the lower lobes, which may progress to consolidation. These changes may also occur with infection, of which CMV is the most common. CMV or *P. carinii* may be indistinguishable from organ rejection without biopsy. After the first month, rejection less often yields radiographic changes (about 25 percent), and the radiographic findings of infection are similar to those of other immunocompromised hosts.

Inflammation Imaging

Nuclear medicine scans are generally nonspecific and add little to the diagnosis of pulmonary pneumocystosis. However, a normal scan will generally exclude diffuse pulmonary infection due to *P. carinii*. The pattern of lymphoid interstitial pneumonitis (LIP) in children with AIDS is indistinguishable from that of *P. carinii* pneumonia. Some centers make a presumptive diagnosis of *P. carinii* pneumonia in the patient with AIDS when a decrease in the diffusing capacity of carbon dioxide ($D_{L_{CO}}$) is coupled with an abnormal chest radiograph and gallium scan. The clearance of radiolabeled inhaled diethylene triaminepentaacetic acid (DTPA) is also increased in *P. carinii* pneumonia (as in other pulmonary infections). Although these tests are usually abnormal in *P. carinii* pneumonia, they lack specificity.

Other Diagnostic Techniques

The chest CT scan will detect interstitial and micronodular disease not visible on routine chest radiographs. Further, the CT and magnetic resonance imaging (MRI) scans and ultrasound imaging are better suited to the definition of pneumocystomas occurring outside the lung. The sensitivity of CT scanning is essential for atypical presentations of *P. carinii* pneumonia and to guide the invasive collection of specimens.

Laboratory Findings

A number of nonspecific indicators of pulmonary processes have been used in the presumptive diagnosis of *P. carinii* pneumonia. In general, the patient will have a P_{O_2} less than 60 mmHg and a respiratory alkalosis. The serum lactic dehydrogenase (LDH) enzyme will be elevated in most cases of *P. carinii* pneumonia (over 300 IU/mL), with high levels (over 600 to 700 IU/mL) carrying a poor prognosis in the setting of histologically confirmed infection. Lymphoma, other diffuse pneumonias, and lymphocytic interstitial pneumonitis (LIP) may also raise the LDH level. Respiratory distress and respiratory failure requiring intubation carry a poor prognosis. The marked hypoxemia of *P. carinii* pneumonia is accompanied by a $P_{A_{O_2}}$-Pa_{O_2} gradient rise; gradients over 30 mmHg at the start of therapy are associated with a high mortality (and are an indication for the use of adjunctive corticosteroid therapy). Both LDH and the arterial oxygenation gradient will return to normal with successful therapy. Another nonspecific indicator of lung injury in *P. carinii* pneumonia is the angiotensin converting enzyme (ACE) level (also elevated by smoking and by sarcoidosis, among other causes). While pulmonary function testing may reveal abnormalities in oxygen exchange and compliance in *P. carinii* pneumonia, they are not useful diagnostically. Arterial blood-gas measurements are helpful in the management of patients with regard to decisions about intubation and the use of corticosteroids as an adjunct to initial antibiotic therapy. Corticosteroids are of greatest use in nonintubated patients with Pa_{O_2} of less than 75 mmHg and greater than 35 mmHg on room air, or a "hypoxemia ratio" (Pa_{O_2}/P_{O_2}) of less than 350 and greater than 75.

Sputum Examination and Histologic Diagnosis

The diagnosis of *P. carinii* pneumonia depends on the identification of characteristic organisms on examination of pulmonary specimens (Table 63-17). The methods used in making the diagnosis have been changed by the use of the induced sputum examination and bronchoscopic alveolar lavage (BAL) without biopsy and by immunofluorescent staining using monoclonal antibodies to *P. carinii*. As a result, the morbidity associated with diagnostic procedures has been reduced and the diagnosis of simultaneous pathogens by these methods is decreased.

The initial step in the diagnosis of *P. carinii* pneumonia should be a routine sputum examination for bacterial, mycobacterial, and fungal stains and cultures. Subsequently, the choice of diagnostic test depends on the status of the patient (ability to cooperate with sputum induction), the distribution of pulmonary disease, and the urgency of diagnosis. Given a single procedure, a more invasive test may be preferred. The diagnostic test of choice is the induced sputum examination, coupled with direct immunofluorescent staining for *P. carinii* and for mycobacterial smears and cultures. Some bacteria and fungi may not survive the hypertonic saline used for induction, and the yields for these pathogens do not exceed those of routine sputum samples. Induced sputum may be collected after 20 to 30 min of exposure to aerosolized hypertonic saline or water, or after oral hydration.

TABLE 63-17 Diagnostic Techniques for *P. carinii*

Technique	Yield	Complications	Comments[a]
Routine sputum	Poor	Rare	Cultures needed
Induced sputum	30–75%	Rare	First choice; excellent in AIDS
Transtracheal aspiration	Fair (with experience)	Common: bleeding, subcutaneous air	Rarely worthwhile
Gallium scan	Nonspecific	Injection site of infected patients	Positive in >95%
Bronchoalveolar lavage (BAL)	>50% (>95% in AIDS)	fever, bronchospasm	Bleeding, aspiration Wedged terminal BAL with immuno-fluorescence
BAL/brushing	As for BAL alone	As for BAL	Not useful for *P. carinii*
BAL/transbronchial biopsy	>90% (all patients)	See BAL; pneumothorax	Impression smears; cultures/pathology
Open lung biopsy	>95% (all patients)	Anesthesia, air leakage, altered respiration, wound infection	"Gold standard" for noninfectious/infectious processes; large sample
Needle aspirate	≤60%	Pneumothorax, bleeding	Best in localized disease

[a]All samples should be cultured and stained for bacteria (including mycobacteria), fungi, and viruses and examined for protozoa. Optimal procedures will depend on the locally available expertise.

Before the availability of immunofluorescent antibody staining techniques, smears were prepared from the mucoid, nonpurulent portion of the specimen and stained with Giemsa or Diff-Quik stain (for intracystic bodies of sporozoites and trophozoites) or with toluidine blue O or silver, which stains the cyst wall. Because cysts represent only 5 to 10 percent of the organism burden, many laboratories prefer the Giemsa to the more complex silver stain, but Giemsa-stained smears are more difficult to read. When a silver stain is used, a counter stain such as Gram's, Wright, Giemsa, hematoxylin, or trichrome may be required to identify intracystic bodies and to distinguish cysts from red blood cells and yeasts. In experienced hands, these stains should detect *P. carinii* in up to 85 percent of AIDS patients and in 60 to 75 percent of other immunocompromised patients. Proper induction and smearing techniques are critical to success.

The staining method of choice for sputum as BAL specimens is direct immunofluorescent staining with monoclonal antibodies. This method is costly, but significant cost savings may be achieved in terms of specimen preparation and examination time. Rapid staining with immunofluorescent monoclonal antibodies directed against surface antigens of *P. carinii* has a high degree of specificity and a sensitivity for screening of sputum smears.

This technique may detect 10 to 15 percent of *P. carinii* infections beyond the standard histologic stains. Some of the commercially available antibodies produce high backgrounds and some nonspecific staining; each laboratory must optimize the fluorescent staining technique. Smears may be improved through use of mucolytic agent (Mucomyst, dithiothreitol) just before preparation.

As with PCR testing, the heightened sensitivity of immunofluorescent staining, coupled with the use of either induced sputum or bronchoscopic lavage samples, may detect "infections" that are not of clinical significance. The meaning of a few organisms on smear in a patient with fever and cough may not be clear. Due to the broad antibacterial spectrum of TMP-SMX, response to therapy is only a partial confirmation of the existence of *P. carinii* pneumonia. AIDS patients will often have residual (dead) organisms in their sputum for many weeks after successful treatment. However, organisms found in the non–AIDS-immunosuppressed patient should suggest disease meriting therapy. Insignificant "colonization" of the respiratory tract before therapy has not been demonstrated; significant numbers of organisms have not been found by BAL in asymptomatic AIDS patients. Of note is that a negative smear does not indicate the absence of *P. carinii*. With use of ribosomal sequence–derived primers on pulmonary specimens, the PCR has more than 98 percent specificity and sensitivity, compared with a 78 percent sensitivity for immunofluorescence on the same samples. Serologic tests are useful only for epidemiologic studies.

The *histopathology* of *P. carinii*–infected lung is usually distinctive enough to be diagnostic even when organisms cannot be identified. In the adult, the disease appears to be predominantly alveolar. The airspaces are filled with a foamy eosinophilic exudate and appear honeycombed. The intraalveolar exudate consists of organisms, large amounts of surface glycoprotein, proteinaceous exudate from the lungs, and debris of macrophages and inflammatory cells. At the same time, the alveolar interstitium is infiltrated by polymorphonuclear leukocytes and lymphocytes. Patchiness in the distribution of disease within the lungs is common. In contrast to the adult disease, *P. carinii* pneumonia in malnourished infants has a major interstitial component: the interstitium is filled with fluid, plasma cells, and lymphocytes; these formed elements seem to overflow into the airspaces, which are also filled with a frothy eosinophilic exudate. In both forms, the organisms usually appear intermingled with alveolar macrophages in the alveolar exudate. By light microscopy, trophozoites predominate numerically (in more than 90 percent of the organisms), but cysts are more readily identified.

In AIDS, the interstitial inflammation is less marked than in other adult forms of *P. carinii* pneumonia, and greater numbers of both cysts and trophozoites are seen in the alveoli. While HIV-infected alveolar macrophages appear to bind organisms normally, internalization of *P. carinii* may be impaired and clearance of organisms delayed. Many dead macrophages are found in BAL samples from HIV- and *P. carinii*–infected lungs. In children with AIDS, the appearance is similar to that of adult AIDS, with the addition of some degree of plasma cell infiltration of the interstitium. Although hyaline membranes may line alveoli, they are not diagnostic of infection with *P. carinii*, since oxygen toxicity, alveolar proteinosis, or ARDS can evoke similar changes. These may coexist with *P. carinii* infection. In pediatric AIDS, lymphocytic interstitial pneumonitis, without evidence of an infectious origin, and bacterial pneumonia may mimic or coexist with *P. carinii* pneumonia.

Even when chest radiography indicates that *P. carinii* pneumonia has cleared, interstitial fibrosis is likely to be found at rebiopsy or autopsy. Unfortunately, the contribution of *P. carinii* to the residual fibrosis is often obscured by the tendency of superimposed infection, therapeutic agents, or intervening radiation therapy to elicit inflammatory responses in the interstitium. Subsequent infections are likely to present with more rapid progression to hypoxemia due to persistent restrictive lung disease. The demonstration of CMV by culture is not helpful in regard to the presence of CMV *disease.* Coinfection due to CMV and *P. carinii* is common, however, and may necessitate treatment for both entities.

Invasive Diagnosis of Pneumocystosis

In the immunocompromised patient with significant pulmonary disease, the inability to make a diagnosis of infection on examination of the induced sputum, or the failure to respond to appropriate therapy, should lead to a more invasive diagnostic procedure: BAL (with biopsies if possible), radiologically guided needle aspiration (for accessible cystic or mass lesions), or open lung biopsy. The choice of the specific test depends on the clinical condition of the patient and on the expertise available at the institution (Table 63-17). Pulmonary specimens obtained by invasive approaches should be processed for bacterial (including mycobacteria, *Nocardia, Actinomyces,* and *Legionella*), fungal, and viral evaluation in addition to making slides for rapid staining with fluorescent antibodies, toluidine blue O, silver, Diff-Quik, Giemsa, or Wright stain. Early diagnosis can be made and therapy initiated on the basis of such smears, especially in AIDS.

Often, accurate diagnosis in the non-AIDS patient may require invasive procedures despite the excellent yields of sputum induction and immunofluorescence. One element in the choice of procedure depends on the clinical state of the patient: patients who have an uncorrectable coagulopathy are poor candidates for either bronchoscopy with biopsy or open lung biopsy. Patients with atypical presentations or unique epidemiologic exposures have a higher incidence of dual processes or non–*P. carinii* infections. Institutions unfamiliar with the proper technique for sampling or handling specimens for the diagnosis of *P. carinii* infection should probably use lung biopsies, which are likely to be more rewarding. Because disease caused by *P. carinii* pneumonia may progress rapidly, the likelihood of success in treatment is greatest at the outset. Therefore, invasive procedures to disclose the organism and any secondary infections should be undertaken early in the course of the disease.

The demonstration of *P. carinii* organisms is necessary for diagnosis in the transplant recipient. No more than 15 to 25 percent of pulmonary infiltrates are caused by *P. carinii* in the non-AIDS patient, although regional and underlying disease-specific variations exist. Empiric therapy is more reasonable in the AIDS patient not receiving prophylaxis, as *P. carinii* pneumonia occurs in up to 90 percent of such persons; however, dual infections remain common. Empiric therapy in the transplant recipient may delay specific treatment for other opportunistic pathogens and subject the patient to avoidable toxicities of TMP-SMX or pentamidine. Demonstration of infection due to *P. carinii* should lead to successful treatment barring superinfection or ARDS.

Prophylaxis and Prophylactic Strategies

The spectrum of patients requiring anti–*P. carinii* prophylaxis has changed with evolving immunosuppressive regimens for organ transplantation, graft-vs-host disease and connective tissue diseases, intensive chemotherapeutic regimens for malignancy, and conversely, the decreasing incidence of opportunistic infections in AIDS. In most non-AIDS, immunocompromised patients, the risk of disease is of the order of 5 to 15 percent, depending on the nature and duration of the immune suppression. Routine anti–*P. carinii* prophylaxis has been reserved, in general, for centers or patient groups that are known to have a fixed high incidence of disease (i.e., on the order of 3 to 5 percent of susceptible hosts), or for individuals with recurrent *P. carinii* disease. At our center, 14 percent of nonprophylaxed renal transplant recipients develop *P. carinii* pneumonia. In solid organ transplant recipients, bolus corticosteroids and the calcineurin inhibitors contribute to the risk of *P. carinii* pneumonia. While mycophenylate mofetil may have some intrinsic anti–*P. carinii* activity, this does not appear to be protective in vivo. Patients who have undergone transplantation during or shortly after a course of corticosteroids (e.g., for COPD or autoimmune hepatitis) are at increased risk of *P. carinii* pneumonia *in the first weeks after transplantation* rather than 1 to 6 months after surgery. These individuals should receive prophylaxis prior to or immediately after transplantation. In single lung transplant recipients, prophylactic failure have been observed in the residual (native) lung despite successful protection of the allograft.

   The use of appropriate prophylaxis should prevent *P. carinii* pneumonia. In AIDS patients and in transplant recipients, the failure to utilize appropriate prophylaxis is generally a reflection of the toxicities associated with the necessary medications or a failure in compliance due to the large number of medications these patients may be expected to consume. Prophylaxis should be maintained in the stable transplant patient for at least 6 months after surgery. In liver and bone marrow transplant recipients with significant graft-versus-host disease or overall poor recovery, prophylaxis is extended to a full year. It should be noted that in transplant centers without a fixed, high incidence of *P. carinii* pneumonia, prophylaxis may be reserved for patients in whom chronic, high-level immune suppression, especially with corticosteroids, is needed to maintain graft function. If immune suppression cannot be reduced after a course of treatment for *P. carinii* pneumonia, prophylaxis should be maintained indefinitely. In Europe, where immunosuppressive regimens are often less intense, such reductions may not be feasible. Prophylaxis should be reinstituted with increases in immune suppression, including those resulting from pulse steroids or antilymphocyte therapies in transplantation, CMV infection in AIDS or transplantation, treatment of graft-versus-host disease following bone marrow transplantation, new-onset neutropenia, or similar conditions.

   In HIV infection, adults and adolescents with CD4 counts of fewer than 200 cells per cubic millimeter (or 15 to 20 percent of the total lymphocyte number), unexplained fever for more than 2 weeks, a history of oropharyngeal candidiasis, or rapid progression of disease, as measured by rising viral titers or falling CD4 counts, should receive prophylaxis. Prophylaxis in

HIV-infected children is recommended for CD4 cell counts of less than 1500/mm^3 for less than 11 months, fewer than 1000/mm^3 between 1 and 5 years, or fewer than 500/mm^3 after age 5, and in any child in whom the CD4 percentage falls to less than 24 percent. The greatest risk for children may be at 3 to 6 months of age, making the identification of the HIV-infected infant critical to survival.

Even with these observations, there are few clear rules regarding patients who "should" be on prophylaxis. However, experience dictates that these might include the following:

- AIDS patients with CD4+ lymphocyte counts below 200/mm^3 blood or less than 20 percent total CD4+ lymphocytes, rising HIV viral loads, persistent CMV infection, or recurrent opportunistic infections suggestive of persistent T-cell defects despite highly active anti-retroviral therapy (HAART) therapy. Transplant patients with CD4+ lymphopenia are expected to be at increased risk.

- Individuals receiving anti–T-cell therapies or corticosteroids over 20 mg per day of prednisone for a period of over 2 to 3 weeks (an arbitrary duration consistent with the life cycle of the organism and clinical observations).

- Solid organ transplant recipients depending on the incidence of infection in the institution ($>$ 5 to 10 percent without prophylaxis), but up to lifelong for heart, liver, and lung recipients and 6 months to a year posttransplant for kidney recipients. These recommendations are based on the periods of greatest risk due to intensity of immune suppression. Any transplant recipient with a history of *P. carinii* pneumonia or frequent opportunistic infections, who is receiving prophylaxis or therapy for CMV infection, or is treated for acute allograft rejection, merits consideration of *P. carinii* prophylaxis. Individuals with chronic graft dysfunction and who receive higher than usual levels of immune suppression merit prophylaxis. In transplant centers without a high incidence of *P. carinii* infection, prophylaxis may be reserved for the highest-risk individuals. If immune suppression cannot be reduced after a course of treatment for *P. carinii* pneumonia, prophylaxis should be maintained indefinitely.

- Use in neutropenic cancer patients is beneficial but challenging given the marrow suppression that may result from TMP-SMZ. Failure of marrow reconstitution may mitigate to prophylaxis with alternative agents.

Breakthrough Infection

The use of appropriate prophylaxis will generally prevent *P. carinii* pneumonia. Breakthrough infection rarely occurs in patients taking TMP-SMX routinely with adequate systemic absorption. Breakthrough *P. carinii* infections in patients on *non–TMP-SMX regimens* are often atypical in appearance. In these patients, bronchoalveolar lavage samples are *often negative* for *P. carinii,* and lung biopsy is often required for diagnosis. The occurrence of infection while receiving prophylaxis reflects (1) inadequate treatment prior to initiating secondary prophylaxis; (2) noncompliance; (3) inadequate dosing due to malabsorption, infection occurring before adequate tissue levels are achieved (e.g., pneumonia before the third dose of pentamidine for primary prophylaxis), or rapid metabolism; (4) acute immune suppression (antilymphocyte therapy) with use of a second-line prophylactic agent;

(5) high-level exposure in the community, a theoretical concern suggested by the clustering of cases; and/or (6) antimicrobial agent resistance that has not been fully documented. One example of "inadequate dosing" reflects the pharmacokinetics of a specific agent (e.g., extrapulmonary pneumocystosis in a patient receiving aerosolized pentamidine). Inadequate blood levels of active (unconjugated) sulfa drugs may reflect rapid hepatic metabolism (acetylation) in some individuals. The amount of unconjugated sulfa drug in serum varies between individuals from 15 to 70 percent.

Specific Agents for Prophylaxis

Trimethoprim-sulfamethoxazole (TMP-SMX, cotrimoxazole) This is the agent of choice for the prevention of *P. carinii* infection in patients who tolerate this agent. At a dose of one single-strength (80 mg TMP/160 mg SMZ) or one double-strength tablet per day, a wide variety of opportunistic infections are generally prevented, including *P. carinii,* most *Toxoplasma gondii,* and many community-acquired respiratory, gastrointestinal, and urinary tract pathogens. In addition, TMP-SMX will suppress *Isospora belli* (based on experience in AIDS) and most *Nocardia asteroides* (based on susceptibility data). However, infections due to *Nocardia* species (including *N. nova*) have been observed in both bone marrow and solid organ transplant recipients receiving TMP-SMX. While protection against *T. gondii* is incomplete in AIDS (80 to 90 percent effective), breakthrough toxoplasmosis is rare in extracardiac transplant recipients.

Studies of low- and high-dose regimens (single- or double-strength TMP-SMX) for prophylaxis in AIDS suggest no mortality advantage to the higher dose and earlier occurrence of toxicity in the high-dose group. For prevention of *P. carinii* infection, it is equally effective to administer the antimicrobial agents (single- or double-strength) 3 days per week.

Drug toxicity is common even with low-dose regimens, especially as mild hematopoietic suppression. Such toxicity is no table in combination with other marrow-suppressive agents (e.g., azathioprine, ganciclovir, cytoxan, allopurinol), malnutrition, or infection (CMV, hepatitis C virus). Significant toxicities generally evolve within the first month of therapy unless masked by immune suppression. Anemia, neutropenia, and azotemia have been related to trimethoprim levels in AIDS. Rash and hepatotoxicity have been related to serum sulfa levels. Some patients will not tolerate any dose of sulfa drugs due to significant rash, Stevens-Johnson syndrome, hepatitis (particularly in liver allograft patients), eosinophilic nephritis, or neutropenia. Hyperkalemia may be observed in the setting of baseline renal function as a result of interference by trimethoprim with the secretion of potassium at the renal distal tubule. This is reversible and more common during full-dose (intravenous) therapy than with prophylaxis. Treatment of TMP-SMX-induced neutropenia with folinic acid has been associated with treatment failure in some individuals. AIDS patients with mild intolerance of TMP-SMX will often tolerate the reintroduction of the drugs at reduced dose after resolution of acute toxicities (generally rash). In contrast, while marrow suppression may be tolerable, interstitial nephritis, hepatitis, and severe skin reactions *will generally recur* in solid organ and hematopoietic transplant recipients. Toxicity to transplanted organs may occur at *any level of drug* and, once established, rarely resolves without discontinuation of the agent. Thus, while oral and intravenous desensitization regimens allow the use of TMP-SMX in many AIDS patients otherwise intolerant of TMP-SMX, alternative agents should be used for prophylaxis in bone marrow and organ transplant recipients with similar, mild, drug-related toxicities (marrow suppression, nephritis, nausea, hepatitis) at least until graft function and immunosuppressive regimens are stable.

Alternative prophylactic regimens are available for the patient intolerant of TMP-SMX. Unfortunately all other prophylactic agents should be considered "second-line," in part because of diminished activities of most alternative regimens against pathogens other than *P. carinii*.

Pentamidine   **Aerosolized pentamidine (AP) isethionate** (300 mg every 3 to 4 weeks) was pioneered for primary and secondary prophylaxis in AIDS patients and is also well tolerated in solid organ and hematopoietic transplant recipients. Pentamidine aerosol prophylaxis is most effective when administered by experienced personnel with a nebulizer producing droplets in the 1 to 3 micron range. Up to 600 mg per month, accumulation of pentamidine in plasma does not occur. However, pulmonary pentamidine concentrations continue to rise for the first 6 months of aerosolized therapy. The benefit of adjusting patient positioning during inhalation is unclear. Breakthrough infection is seen in 10 to 23 percent of AIDS patients compliant with aerosolized pentamidine regimens for 1 year, with disease occurring in the most heavily suppressed patients. Breakthrough infection is often seen in the upper lobes either because the aerosolized drug may not reach the upper lobes or the growth of *P. carinii* may be favored in this region. Pneumothorax is a complication of *P. carinii* infection of the upper lobes, but a unique relationship with aerosolized pentamidine therapy has not been demonstrated. Chest radiographs are often unrevealing, while chest CT scans reveal diffuse interstitial disease. Either intravenous or aerosolized pentamidine (300 mg every 3 to 4 weeks) has been successful in prophylaxis of small series of transplant patients. However, in our experience, breakthrough infection exceeds 10 percent with pentamidine (intravenous or aerosol) in solid organ recipients, making this a less than optimal agent. Breakthroughs are generally seen in patients who have not yet received two or more doses of pentamidine (i.e., in the first 8 weeks of prophylaxis), in individuals with tissue-invasive CMV infection, in secondary prophylaxis after incomplete clearance of infections, during chemotherapy for hepatoma or post/transplantation lymphoproliferative disorder (PTLD), and in those who are receiving antilymphocyte globulins or high dose steroids for graft rejection.

Cough and bronchospasm are the common side effects of aerosolized pentamidine therapy and are generally reversible with bronchodilator therapy. Hypoglycemia or hyperglycemia has been observed and is particularly worrisome in pancreatic transplant recipients. Transient, mild hypoglycemia and nausea are more common following intravenous administration. The use of pentamidine prophylaxis requires the simultaneous administration of a second antimicrobial agent (e.g., quinolone) for antibacterial prophylaxis, which is not generally required in patients receiving TMP-SMX.

Dapsone   Dapsone (diaminodiphenylsulfone) with or without trimethoprim or pyrimethamine is widely used for prophylaxis in a variety of combinations. While low serum levels of sulfone are attained *in vivo*, therapeutic levels are maintained in alveolar fluids. Dapsone has equivalent activity to sulfamethoxazole and sulfadiazine *in vitro* assays of activity against the enzyme dihydropteroate synthetase at equivalent concentrations. Because of a long serum half-life, dapsone may be administered in doses from 50 to 100 mg/day to 100 mg/week. Breakthrough infection has been observed in transplant patients at doses up to 50 mg/day; toxicity begins to be limiting at 100 mg/day, limiting the utility of the drug as a single agent for prophylaxis or therapy. Therefore, pyrimethamine may be administered weekly (25 or 50 mg) to supplement dapsone (50 to 100 mg/day). TMP-SMX and dapsone have equal anti-*Toxoplasma* efficacy. Trials of dapsone at doses of 100 mg two or three times per week show equivalence to pentamidine therapy; doses of 50 to 100 mg/day are equivalent to TMP-SMX therapy. Trimethoprim may replace pyrimethamine in this regimen (100 to 200 mg/day) in patients with creatinine clearances over 15 mL/min.

Intolerance of dapsone (i.e., from mild side effects including anemia or rash to anaphylaxis) is roughly equivalent to that of TMP-SMX. In the transplant recipient, intolerance of TMP-SMX generally predicts intolerance of dapsone. Based on experience in AIDS, up to 40 percent of patients who discontinue prophylactic therapy with either of these agents due to toxicity will not be able to tolerate the other drug. Switching from TMP-SMX to dapsone cannot be recommended for individuals with severe side effects from either agent—including desquamation, neutropenia, severe nephritis, or hepatitis—or in documented G6PD deficiency. Toxicities observed with dapsone are long lived and may limit utility, especially in liver transplantation recipients. Dapsone is metabolized via the hepatic P450 system (CYP3A). This predicts interference with cyclosporine and tacrolimus metabolism, and increased serum dapsone levels in the presence of azole antifungal agents.

Atovaquone   Atovaquone has been FDA-approved for the treatment of mild to moderate *P. carinii* infections but may be most useful for prophylaxis. Atovaquone is a hydroxynapthoquinone and inhibitor of mitochondrial electron transport. Failure of atovaquone prophylaxis for *P. carinii* has been attributed to mutations in a ubiquinone-binding site on cytochrome *b*. Atovaquone undergoes enterohepatic circulation without metabolism and has a long serum half-life ($\geq$ 70 h). Atovaquone also has the potential unique advantage of activity against the bradyzooites (intracystic bodies) of *T. gondii*, a cause of encephalitis in AIDS and carditis in cardiac transplant recipients. Absorption is enhanced by fatty foods and decreased by diarrhea, malabsorption, and in AIDS patients. Bioavailability has been improved via reformulation as a liquid suspension. Rash, nausea, and elevated liver transaminases are occasionally documented. The incidence of rash correlates with the serum concentration. Experience suggests that bioavailability in AIDS patients is half to one-third that of other compromised hosts. Thus, in transplant or cancer patients, serum levels achieved with prophylactic doses in the range of 1000 to 1500 mg/day of liquid drug exceeds the MIC of atovaquone for rodent-derived *P. carinii*. Some patients complain about the flavor and color of atovaquone liquid (which stains clothes) but most find it preferable to aerosolized pentamidine. Atovaquone (1500 mg/day po) is effective as an alternative agent in TMP-SMX–intolerant solid organ transplant recipients.

Clindamycin and pyrimethamine   The combination of clindamycin and pryimethamine is effective as an alternative to TMP-SMX for both treatment and prophylaxis. However, while small prospective trials have indicated some efficacy for prophylaxis, clinical trials of the combination of clindamycin and primaquine for the prevention of pneumocystosis have been complicated by a high incidence of *C. difficile* colitis and of anemia (especially in G6PD-deficient hosts).

TABLE 63-18 Treatment of *P. carinii*[a]

Agent(s)(route)	Dose	Options
Trimethoprim and sulfamethoxazole (TMP-SMX) (IV/PO)	15 mg/kg/day TMP (to 20) 75 mg/kg/day SMX (to 100)	First choice; May treat through rash (reduce TMP or SMX by half); desensitize
Pentamidine isethionate (IV)	4 mg/kg/day 300 mg/day maximum 100 mg/day	Lower dose (2–3 mg/kg) after loading; IM not advised
Dapsone (PO) with TMP (PO/IV)	15–20 mg/kg/day (900 mg)	Methemoglobinemia, G6PD; *may* be tolerated in sulfadiazine allergy
Clindamycin (IV/PO) and primaquine	450–600 mg q6h 15–30 mg base qd	Methemoglobinemia, diarrhea (pyrimethamine for primaquine)
Atovaquone (PO) suspension	750 mg (PO) tid	Variable absorbance (better with fatty food); rash, occasional liver function abnormalities; few side effects
Trimetrexate (IV) with folinic acid (leucovorin)	30–45 mg/m²/day 80–100 mg/m²day	Leukopenia, anemia, thrombocytopenia; relapse common
Pyrimethamine (PO) with sulfadiazine (PO)	load 50 mg bid × 2days then 25–50 mg qd load 75 mg/kg, then 100 mg/kg/day	Not studied fully Maximum. 4 g in two doses; up to 8 g Like trimetrexate
Piritrexim (IV) with folinic acid	Under study	

[a]*Adjunctive therapies* (see text): Corticosteroids (high dose with rapid tapering), possibly gamma interferon, granulocyte-macrophage colony-stimulating factor.

Treatment of *P. carinii* Pneumonia

The incidence of *P. carinii* infection in AIDS patients has led to the development of a number of newer options for the treatment of this infection in all susceptible hosts (Table 63-18). Treatment should be initiated as soon as the suspicion of *P. carinii* infection is entertained. The short-term use of treatment (48 h) will not impair the diagnosis of infection if, for example, bronchoscopic or laboratory support services are unavailable. It is likely to be more useful clinically to obtain specimens for *P. carinii,* mycobacteria, *Legionella,* fungi, and routine cultures when these can be properly handled by the clinical laboratory. Further, because the pneumonia can be rapidly progressive, early therapy is essential. Treatment of *P. carinii* pneumonia should be successful if a 14- to 21-day course of therapy is tolerated.

The incidence of adverse reactions to antibiotics, necessitating switching of agents, is increased in the organ and marrow transplant recipient, as it is in AIDS patients. In general, side effects in transplantation are related to synergistic drug toxicities. For example, the bone marrow suppression seen in infection with CMV and treatment of this infection with ganciclovir may be further exacerbated with TMP-SMX. Generally, elevations in liver function tests in the liver transplant recipient or depression in the leukocyte count in the marrow recipient due to therapy with TMP-SMX is of concern in the transplant recipient but may be tolerable in other hosts. Nephrotoxicity is common in transplant recipients receiving calcineurin inhibitors receiving therapy with TMP-SMX, even with adjustment of dosing for renal dysfunction. Thus, while the incidence of intolerance by transplant recipients to one or another agent is somewhat less than the 50 percent seen in AIDS patients, significant toxicity remains a common feature of therapy. As was noted, resistance to antibiotics has not yet been demonstrated by *P. carinii.* Thus, changing antibiotics *other than for toxicity* does not appear to be indicated. While there are patients who appear to "do better" on one agent than another, it is much more common to recognize a second process (infection, tumor, allergy, ARDS) as complicating *P. carinii* pneumonia than a "resistant" infection. The chest radiograph is a less reliable indicator of failure than is oxygenation. Adding pentamidine to TMP-SMX offers no advantage over simply switching agents. Indeed, animal experiments suggest the possibility of antagonism between these agents when used in combination. As a rule, patients who need to be switched from co-trimoxazole to pentamide, or vice versa, do not fare as well as those who can be treated for 14 to 21 days with either agent alone. The success rate with either pentamidine or TMP-SMX for initial treatment is around 60 to 80 percent. Adjunctive therapies (see below) may also be more useful than switching agents.

The proper duration of therapy has not been studied but is generally 14 to 21 days in all patients. Residual organisms persist after treatment for a number of months (up to 3), but the role of these organisms in recrudescent or persistent infection is not clear. Following treatment with TMP-SMX, most residual organisms are dead; relapse in the non–AIDS-immunocompromised patient should not be expected *as long as immunosuppression can be reduced* (notably, with steroid therapy).

TMP-SMX is the agent of choice for the treatment of *P. carinii* pneumonia and extrapulmonary disease in all hosts. This combination antibiotic has the advantage of excellent tissue penetration, the most rapid clinical response of anti–*P. carinii* agents (3 to 4 days), and bioavailability from oral therapy comparable with that of parenteral administration. Survival without intubation and mechanical ventilation appears to be greater with TMP-SMX than with pentamidine (by up to 20 percent). The incidence of some of the side effects is related to serum concentrations and is also greater than with other agents. In part, this is a reflection of the use of dosage schedules derived for children in adults and in the setting of abnormal renal function. The proper dosing in adults has not been completely studied. Therapy is initiated at 15 to 20 mg/kg per day of the TMP component (100 to 150 mg/kg per day of SMX), divided into three or four doses. Therapy should be initiated intravenously if there is uncertainty about GI function or marked hypoxemia. Peak levels are obtained about 2 h after oral dosing and should approach the range of 100 to 150 µg/mL of SMX (5 to 15 µg/mL TMP). Levels of over 200 µg/mL of SMX are associated with a higher incidence of side effects, especially bone marrow suppression. After a clinical response is observed, the dosing can be reduced to 10 to 15 mg/kg per day in divided doses.

Therapy can be continued (with adjustments) despite mild side effects (rash, transaminase elevations, neutropenia) tolerable to the patient and physician. Dose reduction will often eliminate toxicity in AIDS patients. Desensitization to TMP-SMX may be used in the patient with mild intolerance. With renal dysfunction, dosing must be reduced; daily dosing is sufficient (3 to 5 mg/kg per day) for a glomerular filtration rate of 10 to 50 mL/min. Renal impairment developing in a patient taking TMP-SMX should prompt a search for urinary eosinophils and an assessment of the need for further therapy with this agent. Nephrotoxicity occurs frequently in the renal transplant recipient on full-dose therapy; this toxicity is both idiosyncratic and dose related. Nephrotoxicity often occurs without demonstrable urinary eosinophils, perhaps as a reflection of the use of corticosteroids for immune suppression. In these patients, interstitial eosinophils may be found on renal biopsy. The transplanted liver is particularly susceptible to TMP-SMX toxicity (eosinophilic infiltrates, hepatocyte necrosis, bilirubinemia) and may be confused with, or complicate treatment for, early rejection or systemic infection. The side effects of TMP-SMX are generally those of sulfa allergy: rash (including Stevens-Johnson syndrome), transaminase elevation, neutropenia, thrombocytopenia, erythema multiforme exudativum, and nephrotoxicity. The bone marrow suppression is marked in patients with underlying hematologic disorders; folinic acid supplementation is rarely useful and should be avoided in patients with acute leukemia.

Dapsone (100 mg orally per day), in place of SMX and in combination with oral TMP (15 mg/kg per day), is also effective alternative therapeutic regimen. Many AIDS patients intolerant of sulfamethoxazole will tolerate dapsone, which is metabolized by the liver (half-life at least 30 h). However, the long half-life and side-effect profile in the non-AIDS patient (hemolysis in G6PD deficiency, rash, hepatitis) may be particularly disadvantageous in the transplant recipient. Manifestations of sulfa and TMP toxicity may be masked by corticosteroids. Similarly, side effects of azathioprine (hepatitis, macrocytic anemia, neutropenia, hepatic venoocclusive disease) may be accentuated by TMP-SMX. In AIDS, the toxic side effects of TMP-SMX are generally those of the sulfonamide; however, trimethoprim allergy is not uncommon, and allergies to the "carriers" in the various preparations of TMP-SMX (dyes, coatings, filler) have also been reported. Both components of TMP-SMX interfere with folate metabolism. Leukopenia, thrombocytopenia, and anemia caused by co-trimoxazole are generally relieved by folinic acid, whereas drug rash, fever, azotemia, and increased blood levels of transaminases will reverse only when therapy is stopped. Folinic acid should not be used in patients with acute leukemia.

Pentamidine isethionate is the first alternative agent for the treatment of *P. carinii* pneumonia. Intravenous pentamidine isethionate is given by slow (1- to 2-h) infusion in 5 percent glucose solution as a single dose of 4 mg/kg per day. Evidence exists that lower doses (3 mg/kg per day) are equally effective. Pentamidine achieves therapeutic levels in the lungs slowly (in 5 to 7 days), owing to high levels of extrapulmonary tissue binding. Slow accumulation of pentamidine in pulmonary tissue may account for the delayed onset of activity when compared with TMP-SMX. However, increased serum levels and a long serum half-life and gradual accumulation in the lungs may play a role in the continued therapeutic effect after the cessation of therapy. Because this agent has a long serum half-life (6.4 h) and delayed excretion due to extensive tissue binding (more than 240 h), pentamidine tends to accumulate during therapy. The reduction of symptoms by pentamidine may be due in part to suppression of the secretion of tumor necrosis factor by alveolar macrophages as well as to treatment of infection. Pentamidine has largely been supplanted by TMP-SMX for therapy of *P. carinii* infection in the non-AIDS patient. But pentamidine continues to be used for infection in patients with adverse reactions to trimethoprim or the sulfonamides.

Idiosyncratic side effects include transient hypoglycemia, pancreatitis, diabetes (after prolonged therapy, with or without prior pancreatitis), pancytopenia, hypotension, and renal dysfunction—all of which are of greater significance in the recent organ transplant recipient than in most other hosts. These side effects are exacerbated by intravenous administration and in the presence of decreased renal function. Pentamidine should be avoided in pancreas transplant recipients, owing to the potential for islet cell necrosis. New diamidine compounds under development may have significantly superior therapeutic and side-effect profiles when compared to the parent molecule.

Alternative regimens have been developed as a reflection of toxicities observed in AIDS patients treated with either TMP-SMX or pentamidine. Atovaquone (750 mg orally three times a day) has been approved by the U.S. Food and Drug Administration (FDA) for the treatment of mild to moderately severe *P. carinii* pneumonia. Comparative trials between atovaquone (tablets) and TMP-SMX suggest that TMP-SMX is the preferred agent in patients who tolerate this therapy. Up to 7 percent of HIV-infected patients develop limiting toxicity on atovaquone (compared to 20 percent for TMP-SMX); however, significantly more patients failed therapy owing to lack of response in the atovaquone group than in the TMP-SMX group. Like TMP-SMX, atovaquone may *clear P. carinii* from the lungs in patients who complete a course of therapy better than other alternative agents, reducing the rate of relapsed infection.

Trimetrexate (45 mg/mL per day) *with* folinic acid (80 mg/mL per day) has been approved for use in moderately severe pneumonia. Trimetrexate is a dihydrofolate reductase inhibitor and is lipid-soluble, with a serum half-life up to 34 h. It will produce severe neutropenia in the absence of folinic acid supplementation (which should be continued for 3 to 5 days after cessation of trimetrexate), in some patients with simultaneous infections due to HIV or CMV, or during therapy with antiviral antibiotics. Side effects include fever, rash, leukopenia, and transaminase elevation. Infection relapse in AIDS patients has been somewhat more frequent than with other therapies. Piritrexim is pharmacologically similar to trimetrexate but has been most useful in combination with a sulfonamide.

The combination of clindamycin (600 to 900 mg intravenously every 6 to 8 h) and primaquine (15 to 30 mg base per day orally) is effective in mild to moderate infection, with the main side effect being *Clostridium difficile* colitis. Pyrimethamine (50 to 100 mg a day by mouth after 100- to 200-mg load) and sulfadiazine or trisulfapyrimidines (4 to 8 g a day) are also effective, but require folinic acid (10 mg a day) supplementation. Pyrimethamine will decrease the renal clearance of creatinine without attaining the glomerular filtration rate. The newer macrolides (azithromycin, clarithromycin) have little efficacy alone but appear to enhance the efficacy of sulfamethoxazole. However, this combination provides little benefit over TMP-SMX. The utility of DFMO (α-difluoromethylornithine) has not been established. Newer agents include the echinocandins (glucan synthase inhibitors), which block formation of cysts, the 8-aminoquinolines, the dicationic substituted bis-benzimidazoles (pentamidine derivatives), isoprinosine, bilobalide (a sesquiterpene from *Gingko biloba* leaves), quinghaosu albendazole, proguanil, terbinafine, guanylhydrazones, and some nonquinolone topoisomerase inhibitors.

Adjunctive therapies to the treatment of *P. carinii* pneumonia include corticosteroids and, potentially, colony-stimulating factors. The use of adjunctive corticosteroids was developed to prevent the early deterioration of AIDS patients with documented *P. carinii* pneumonia, but has now achieved acceptance for all patients with this infection. The use of corticosteroids (prednisone, 40 to 60 mg three or four times a day, orally or intravenously) in the first 72 h after admission may reduce pulmonary inflammation to a degree sufficient to avoid intubation. When studied in AIDS patients, the use of corticosteroids in patients with a $P_{A_{O_2}}$ of 35 to 72 mmHg or with a hypoxemia ratio of 75 to 350 was of significant benefit in terms of preventing deterioration in oxygenation in the first 7 days of therapy, mortality, and the avoidance of intubation (50 percent reduction). After such therapy the exercise tolerance and survival of patients were also improved. Slow steroid tapering is necessary to avert relapse of pulmonary inflammation. Patients experience an increase in oral thrush and herpes simplex after 2 to 3 weeks of therapy and tapering.

The response to therapy is generally excellent in patients who receive a diagnosis before respiratory failure. The ability to reduce immune suppression or to supplement the immune response (see above) also improves the rapidity of clearance of infection. The failure to observe clinical improvement by days 4 to 5 (TMP-SMX) or 5 to 7 (pentamidine) should suggest the presence of another process: fibrosis, adult respiratory distress syndrome (ARDS), dual infection (especially cytomegalovirus (CMV)), abscess, bronchial obstruction, drug allergy, carcinoma. Bronchoscopic lavage and biopsy for microbiology and pathology, or chest tomography (CT scan), may be revealing in these patients.

BIBLIOGRAPHY

Aisner J, Murillo J, Schimpff SC, et al: Invasive aspergillosis in acute leukemia: Correlation with nose cultures and antibiotic use. *Ann Intern Med* 90:4–9, 1979.

Albelda SM, Talbot GH, Gerson SL, et al: Pulmonary cavitation and massive hemoptysis in invasive pulmonary aspergillosis. *Am Rev Respir Dis* 131:115–120, 1985.

Ampel NM, Dols CL, Galgiani JN: Coccidioidomycosis during human immunodeficiency virus infection: Result of a prospective study in a coccidioidal endemic area. *Am J Med* 94:235–240, 1993.

Angus RM, Davies M-L, Cowan MD, et al: Computed tomographic scanning of the lung in patients with allergic bronchopulmonary aspergillosis and in asthmatic patients with a positive skin test to *Aspergillus fumigatus*. *Thorax* 49:586–589, 1994.

Baughman RP, Dohn MN, Frame PT: The continuing utility of bronchoalveolar lavage to diagnose opportunistic infection in AIDS patients. *Am J Med* 97:515–522, 1994.

Bennett JE, Dismukes WE, Duma RJ, et al: A comparison of amphotericin B alone and combined with flucytosin in the treatment of cryptococcal meningitis. *N Engl J Med* 301:126–131, 1979.

Bigby PD, Margolskee D, Curtis J, et al: Usefulness of induced sputum in diagnosis of pneumonia in patients with acquired immunodeficiency syndrome. *Am Rev Respir Dis* 133:515–518, 1986.

Bozzette SA, Finkelstein DM, Spector SA, et al, and NIAID AIDS Clinical Trials Group: A randomized trial of three antipneumocystis agents in patients with advanced human immunodeficiency virus infection. *N Engl J Med* 332:693–699, 1995.

Bradsher RW: Blastomycosis. *Clin Infect Dis* 14(suppl):S82–S90, 1992.

Broaddus C, Dake MD, Stulbarg MS, et al: Bronchoalveolar lavage and transbronchial biopsy for the diagnosis of pulmonary infections in the acquired immunodeficiency syndrome. *Ann Intern Med* 102:747–752, 1985.

Cameron M, Bartlett JA, Gallis H, Waskin HA: Manifestations of pulmonary cryptococcosis in patients with acquired immunodeficiency syndrome. *Rev Infect Dis* 13:64–67, 1991.

Chave J, David S, Wauters J, Francioli P: Transmission of *Pneumocystis carinii* from AIDS patients to other immunosuppressed patients: A cluster of *Pneumocystis carinii* pneumonia in renal transplant recipients. *AIDS* 5:927–932, 1991.

Clark RA, Greer D, Atkinson W, et al: Spectrum of *Cryptococcus neoformans* infection in 68 patients infected with human immunodeficiency virus. *Rev Infect Dis* 12:768–776, 1990.

Coffey MJ, Fantone J, Stirling MC, Lynch JP: Pseudoaneurysm of pulmonary artery in mucormycosis. Radiographic characteristics and management. *Am Rev Respir Dis* 145:1487–1490, 1992.

Coker RJ, Viviani M, Gazzard BG, et al: Treatment of cryptococcosis with liposomal amphotericin B (AmBisome) in 23 patients with AIDS. *AIDS* 7:829–835, 1993.

Coleman DL, Dodek PM, Luce JM, et al: Diagnostic utility of fiberoptic bronchoscopy in patients with *Pneumocystis carinii* pneumonia and the acquired immune deficiency syndrome. *Am Rev Respir Dis* 128:795–799, 1983.

De Lalla F, Pellizzer G, Vaglia A, et al: Amphotericin B as primary therapy for cryptococcosis in patients with AIDS: Reliability of relatively high doses administered over a relatively short period. *Clin Infect Dis* 20:263–266, 1995.

Denning DW, Stevens DA: Antifungal and surgical treatment of invasive aspergillosis: Review of 2,121 published cases. *Rev Infect Dis* 12:1147–1201, 1990.

Dismukes WE, Bradsher RW Jr, Cloud GC, et al: Itraconazole therapy for blastomycosis and histoplasmosis. *Am J Med* 93:489–497, 1992.

Drutz D, Catanzaro A: Coccidioidomycosis. Parts 1 and 2. *Am Rev Respir Dis* 117:559–585, 727–771, 1978.

Edman JC, Kovacs JA, Masur H, et al: Ribosomal RNA sequence shows *Pneumocystis carinii* to be a member of the Fungi (letter). *Nature* 334:519–522, 1988.

Edwards LB, Acquaviva FA, Livesay VT, et al: An atlas of sensitivity to tuberculin, PPD-B, and histoplasmin in the United States. *Am Rev Respir Dis* 99 (suppl):1–132, 1969.

Fishman JA: *Pneumocystis carinii* and parasitic infections in transplantation. *Infect Dis Clin North Am* 9:1005–1044, 1995.

Fishman JA: Case records of the Massachusetts General Hospital. *N Engl J Med* 332:249–257, 1995.

Gagnon S, Boota AM, Fischl MA, et al: Corticosteroids as adjunctive therapy for severe *Pneumocytis carinii* pneumonia in the acquired immunodeficiency syndrome: A double-blind, placebo-controlled trial. *N Engl J Med* 323:1444–1450, 1990.

Gerson SE, Talbot GH, Hurwitz S, et al: Prolonged granulocytopenia: The major risk factor for invasive pulmonary aspergillosis in patients with acute leukemia. *Ann Intern Med* 100:345–351, 1984.

Girardin H, Sarfati J, Traore F, et al: Molecular epidemiology of nosocomial invasive aspergillosis. *J Clin Microbiol* 32:684–690, 1994.

Goodman JL, Winston DJ, Greenfield RA, et al: A controlled trial of fluconazole to prevent fungal infections in patients undergoing bone marrow transplant. *N Engl J Med* 326:845–851, 1992.

Goodwin RA Jr, Owens FT, Snell JD, et al: Chronic pulmonary histoplasmosis. *Medicine* 55:413–452, 1976.

Hardy AM, Wajszczuk CP, Suffredini AF, et al: *Pneumocystis carinii* pneumonia in renal transplant patients treated with cyclosporin and steroids. *J Infect Dis* 149:143–147, 1984.

Hughes WT: Pneumocystis Carinii *Pneumonitis.* New York, CRC, 1987.

Hughes W, et al: Comparison of atovaquone (566C80) and trimethoprim-sulfamethoxazole to treat *Pneumocystis carinii* pneumonia in patients with AIDS. *N Engl J Med* 328:1521–1527, 1993.

Hughes WT, McNabb PC, Makres TD, et al: Efficacy of trimethoprim and sulfamethoxazole in the prevention and treatment of *Pneumocystis carinii* pneumonitis. *Antimicrob Agents Chemother* 5:289–293, 1974.

Kovacs JA, Hiemenz JW, Macher AM, et al: *Pneumocystis carinii* pneumonia: A comparison between patients with the acquired immunodeficiency syndrome and patients with other immunodeficiencies. *Ann Intern Med* 100:663–671, 1984.

Labadie EL, Hamilton RH: Survival improvement in coccidioidal meningitis by high-dose intrathecal amphotericin B. *Arch Intern Med* 146:2013–2018, 1985.

Larsen RA, Bozzette SA, Jones BE, et al: Fluconazole combined with flucytosine for treatment of cryptococcal meningitis in patients with AIDS. *Clin Infect Dis* 19:741–745, 1994.

Loyd JE, Tillman BF, Atkinson JB, Des Prez RM: Mediastinal fibrosis complicating histoplasmosis. *Medicine* 67:295–310, 1988.

Masur H, Gill VJ, Ognibene FP, et al: Diagnosis of *Pneumocystis* pneumonia by induced sputum technique in patients without the acquired immunodeficiency syndrome. *Ann Intern Med* 109:755–756, 1988.

Mendelson EB, Fisher MR, Mintzer RA, et al: Radiographic and clinical staging of allergic bronchopulmonary aspergillosis. *Chest* 87:334–339, 1985.

Murray HW: Pulmonary mucormycosis with massive fatal hemoptysis. *Chest* 68:65–68, 1975.

Nightingale SD, Cal SX, Peterson DM, et al: Primary prophylaxis with fluconazole against systemic fungal infections in HIV-positive patients. *AIDS* 6:191–194, 1992.

Pappas PG, Threlkeld MG, Bedsole GD, et al: Blastomycosis in immunocompromised patients. *Medicine (Baltimore)* 72:311–325, 1993.

Patterson R, Greenberger PA, Radin RC, Roberts M: Allergic bronchopulmonary aspergillosis: Staging as an aid to management. *Ann Intern Med* 96:286–291, 1982.

Pizzo PA, Robichaud KJ, Gill FA, et al: Empiric antibiotic and antifungal therapy for cancer patients with prolonged fever and granulocytopenia. *Am J Med* 72:101, 1982.

Powderly WG: Cryptococcal meningitis and AIDS. *Clin Infect Dis* 17:837–842, 1993.

Powderly WG, Saag MS, Cloud GA, et al: A controlled trial of fluconazole or amphotericin B to prevent relapse of cryptococcal meningitis in patients with the acquired immunodeficiency syndrome. *N Engl J Med* 326:793–798, 1992.

Rex JH, Bennett JE, Sugar AM, et al: A randomized trial comparing fluconazole with amphotericin B for the treatment of candidemia in patients without neutropenia. *N Engl J Med* 331:1325–1330, 1994.

Rosenberg M, Patterson R, Roberts M, Wang J: The assessment of immunologic and clinical changes occurring during corticosteroid therapy for allergic bronchopulmonary aspergillosis. *Am J Med* 64:599–606, 1978.

Saag MS, Powderly WG, Cloud GA, et al: Comparison of amphotericin B with fluconazole in the treatment of acute AIDS-associated cryptococcal meningitis. *N Engl J Med* 326:83–89, 1992.

Sarosi GA, Parker JD, Doto IL, Tosh FE: Chronic pulmonary coccidioidomycosis. *N Engl J Med* 283:325–330, 1970.

Sharkey PK, Graybill JR, Johnson ES, et al: Amphotericin B lipid complex compared with amphotericin B in the treatment of cryptococcal meningitis in patients with AIDS. *Clin Infect Dis* 22:315–321, 1996.

Stevens DA: Coccidioidomycosis. *N Engl J Med* 332:1077–1082, 1995.

Sugar AM: Agents of mucormycosis and related species, in Mandell GL, Bennett JE, Dolin R (eds), *Mandell, Douglas and Bennett's Principles and Practice of Infectious Diseases,* sec. G, *Mycoses,* vol 2. New York: Churchill Livingstone, 1995, pp 2311–2321.

Walzer PD: *Pneumocystis Carinii Pneumonia.* New York: Marcel Dekker, 1994.

Walzer PD, Perl DP, Krogstad DJ, et al: *Pneumocystis carinii* pneumonia in the United States: Epidemiologic, diagnostic, and clinical features. *Ann Intern Med* 80:83–93, 1974.

Watanabe J, Hori H, Tanabe K, Nakamura Y: Phylogenetic association of *Pneumocystis carinii* with the "Rhizopoda/Myxomycota/Zygomycota group" indicated by comparison of 5S ribosomal RNA sequences. *Mol Biochem Parasitol* 32:163–167, 1989.

Wardlaw A, Geddes DM: Allergic bronchopulmonary aspergillosis: A review. *J R Soc Med* 85:747–750, 1992.

Wheat J: Endemic mycoses in AIDS: A clinical review. *Clin Microbiol Rev* 8:146–159, 1995.

Wheat J: Histoplasmosis: Recognition and treatment. *Clin Infect Dis* 19(suppl 1):S19–S27, 1994.

Wheat J, Hafner R, Korzun AH, et al: Itraconazole treatment of disseminated histoplasmosis in patients with the acquired immunodeficiency syndrome. *Am J Med* 98:336–342, 1995.

Winn W: Coccidioidomycosis. *Med Clin North Am* 47:1131–1148, 1963.

Young RC, Bennett JE, Vogel CL, et al: Aspergillosis. The spectrum of disease in 98 patients. *Medicine* 49:147–173, 1970.

64 | Viral Infections of the Lungs and Respiratory Tract*

Jay A. Fishman

OVERVIEW

Respiratory viral infections are the most common illnesses afflicting humans. In the United States, more than 500 million acute respiratory illnesses are estimated to occur yearly, accounting for half of all ill-child visits to physicians. The estimated cost of medical care, unnecessary antibiotics, and time lost from work and school is estimated to be more than $7 billion per year.

Many viruses can infect the respiratory tract and produce symptoms and signs of upper or lower respiratory tract infection. In healthy persons, respiratory viral infections produce acute morbidity but little increased mortality. Persons with underlying illness or immunosuppression exhibit increased mortality as well as morbidity after acute lower respiratory viral infections. The number of viruses accounting for lower respiratory tract infection is considered to be modest. Serious viral infections below the larynx are reported predominantly in infants and children and in immunocompromised or high-risk adults. Upper respiratory tract viral infections are associated with a larger number of viruses, chiefly because of the more than 100 types of rhinovirus that can cause the common cold.

Upper respiratory tract viral infections include the common cold, pharyngitis, sinusitis, acute otitis media, and laryngitis. Lower respiratory viral infections include acute laryngotracheobronchitis (croup), influenza, bronchitis, bronchiolitis, and pneumonia. Complications of respiratory virus disease include secondary bacterial infections, Reye's syndrome, Guillain-Barré syndrome, myositis, encephalopathy, myopericarditis, and febrile seizures. Comon respiratory viruses have been associated with unusual manifestations (e.g., influenza virus and toxic shock syndrome) and newly described viruses (*Hantavirus,* swine influenza) have been associated with fatal disease.

Diagnosis

To identify the virus causing a respiratory illness, a respiratory tract specimen or acute and convalescent sera must be analyzed in a clinical virology laboratory. Even if a virus is not identified, the most likely candidate can often be deduced from clinical and epidemiologic data. Patient age, time of year, clinical presentation (laryngitis, croup, or pneumonia), and knowledge of community surveillance are useful as aids to narrow the viral etiology for a given patient (Table 64-1).

*Edited from Chaps. 151 to 154, "Viral Infections of the Lung and Respiratory Tract," by Greenberg SB; "The Lung in Human Immunodeficiency Virus Infection," by Rich EA; "Emerging Infectious Diseases and Hantavirus Pulmonary Syndrome," by Butler JC, Zaki SR; "Poliovirus and Other Enterovirus Infections," by Melnick JL. In: *Fishman's Pulmonary Diseases and Disorders,* 3d ed., edited by Fishman AP, Elias JA, Fishman JA, Grippi MA, Kaiser LR, Senior RM. New York, McGraw-Hill, 1998, pp 2333–2378. For fuller discussion of topics dealt with in this chapter, the reader is referred to the original text, as noted above.

TABLE 64-1 Modes of Detection for Respiratory Viruses

Virus	Detection by Culture	Direct detection	Serology	Comments
Adenoviruses	+	+/–	+	Culture and IF are preferred methods of diagnosis; significance of isolate must be interpreted in relationship to serotype and clinical findings.
Coronaviruses	–	–	+	Diagnosis not routinely available.
Enteroviruses	+	–	–	Significance of isolate must be interpreted in relationship to type isolated and clinical findings.
EBV	–	–	+	Nonspecific heterophilic antibodies (e.g., Monospot) are most readily available but not reliable in children <4 years old; serology for virus-specific antigens is also available.
CMV	+	+/–	+	Culture is most readily available. Rapid diagnostic methods reported include IF, molecular hybridization, and electron microscopy.
HSV	+/–	+	+	Culture and IF are both preferred to serology; significance of isolate must be interpreted in relationship to clinical findings.
VZV	+/–	+	+	Direct detection by nonspecific (e.g., Tzanck preparation, electron microscopy) and specific (e.g., IF) techniques often superior to culture in speed and sensitivity; FAMA is the most sensitive serologic method; enzyme immunoassay and anticomplement IF also are sufficiently sensitive for most uses.
Orthomyxoviruses (influenza A, B, and C,) Paramyxoviruses (parainfluenza, RSV)	+	+	+	For RSV, direct detection (IF, ELISA) approaches the sensitivity and specificity of viral culture; DFA on nasal swabs in influenza A and B, parainfluenza, RSV.
Rhinovirus	+	–	–	Culture is the only routinely available method for rhinovirus detection.

KEY: +, Available methods using commercially obtainable reagents; –, not routinely available or not consistently reliable; IF, immunofluorescence; FAMA, fluorescent antibody to membrane antigen; RSV, respiratory syncytial virus; ELISA, enzyme-linked immunosorbent assay; DFA, direct fluorescent antibody staining.

Diagnosis of respiratory viral infections relies on tissue culture techniques immunostaining, and serologic tests. Tissue culture cells can sustain viral growth and demonstrate cytopathic effects. A combination of tissue culture cell lines is used, much in the same way the bacteriology laboratory uses selective media for detecting specific bacteria. Serologic tests are performed on acute and convalescent sera obtained 2 to 4 weeks apart. Standard tests include complement fixation (CF), neutralization (Nt), hemagglutination-inhibition (HAI), and enzyme-linked immunosorbent assay (ELISA). Tests that measure specific IgM antibodies are available for a few viruses, but most assays detect IgG antibodies. In most test assays, a fourfold or greater rise in serum antibody between acute and convalescent sera is needed to demonstrate recent infection. For some respiratory viruses, culture is superior to serologic methods; for others, serology is most useful for diagnosis (Table 64-2).

Newer diagnostic techniques—such as direct fluorescent antibody (DFA) staining and quantitative polymerase chain reactions (PCR)—provide rapid identification of specific viral agents and the assessment of responses to antiviral therapies.

Prevention and Treatment

Although a number of antiviral agents have been approved for use in respiratory viral infections, their clinical utility has been best demonstrated when they have been given as prophylaxis rather than as treatment. For example,

---

TABLE 64-2 Target Groups for Influenza Vaccination Programs

Groups at Increased Risk for Influenza-Related Complications
Persons ≥65 years of age
Residents of nursing homes and other chronic-care facilities that house persons of any age with chronic medical conditions
Adults and children with chronic disorders of the pulmonary or cardiovascular systems, including children with asthma
Adults and children who have required regular medical follow-up or hospitalization during the preceding year because of chronic metabolic diseases (including diabetes mellitus), renal dysfunction, hemoglobinopathies, or immunosuppression (including immunosuppression caused by medications)
Children and teenagers (6 months to 18 years of age) who are receiving long-term aspirin therapy and therefore might be at risk for developing Reye's syndrome after influenza

Groups That Can Transmit Influenza to Persons at High Risk
Persons who are clinically or subclinically infected and who care for or live with members of high-risk groups can transmit influenza virus to them. Some persons at high risk (e.g., the elderly, transplant recipients, and persons with AIDS) can have a low antibody response to influenza vaccine. Efforts to protect these members of high-risk groups against influenza might be improved by reducing the likelihood of influenza exposure from their caregivers. Therefore, the following groups should be vaccinated:
  Physicians, nurses, and other personnel in both inpatient and outpatient-care settings; employees of nursing homes and chronic-care facilities who have contact with residents
  Providers of home care to persons at high risk (e.g., visiting nurses and volunteer workers)
  Household members (including children) of persons in high-risk groups

SOURCE: Data from the CDC.

amantadine and rimantadine have far superior anti-illness effects when given prophylactically than when begun once influenza symptoms are present.

Prevention of certain respiratory viral infections has depended on vaccine use, and the development of new respiratory virus vaccines is of increasing importance. Improved influenza virus vaccines are being tested for widespread utilization. Postexposure prophylaxis with immune globulin therapy has not been effective except in childhood respiratory syncytial virus (RSV), measles, and varicella infections. Because of the multitude of immunotypes of rhinoviruses, it is unlikely that vaccines will be easily constructed for this group.

UPPER RESPIRATORY TRACT VIRAL INFECTIONS

The Common Cold

A self-limited, acute coryzal illness has come to be known as the *common cold*. As a leading cause of physician office visits and of absence from work or school, the common cold is caused by one of several families of respiratory viruses. The five most commonly reported virus families retrieved from infected patients are orthomyxovirus (influenza A and B), paramyxovirus (parainfluenza virus and RSV), adenovirus, picornavirus (rhinovirus), and coronavirus. Often, the etiology of colds is undiagnosed.

Epidemics of upper respiratory tract infections occur worldwide, usually in the fall, winter, and spring in temperate climates. Rhinoviruses are recovered predominantly in early fall and late spring but are also isolated throughout the rest of the year. Coronaviruses are documented chiefly in the winter months. Yearly or biannual communitywide outbreaks of influenza virus, parainfluenza virus, or RSV are also common throughout the world. In the United States, children average six to eight colds each year and adults two to four. An increase in the incidence of colds is associated with the beginning of the school year and indoor crowding. Children are often infected in day care centers or school and pass the infection to other family members. Prolonged exposure leads to increased secondary attack rates, so that parents and other children in the home are most likely to acquire these infections.

Shedding of common cold viruses is usually short-lived, lasting a few days to a week. Large quantities of rhinovirus are detected in nasal secretions at the time of maximal illness. Asymptomatic infections do occur but are uncommon. Recent studies have suggested that chemical mediators and neurologic reflexes are important in common cold symptomatology, especially secondary to rhinoviruses. Transmission of these viruses is secondary to contact with infected secretions or droplet nuclei in the air. Experiments have demonstrated that hand-to-hand transmission of rhinoviruses from contaminated skin can take place. Other human volunteer challenge models have shown the ability to transmit other viruses through large- and small-particle aerosols.

Symptoms of the common cold usually begin 1 to 3 days after infection. Sneezing, sore throat, and cough are commonly experienced in addition to nasal discharge and obstruction. Most cold symptoms last 1 week but not uncommonly can persist for up to 2 weeks. Physical examination rarely provides specific clues to the diagnosis. Most cold diagnoses are self-reported. In persons with hay fever and vasomotor rhinitis, it may be difficult to distinguish an allergic pattern from viral infection.

Rhinoviruses and influenza viruses are readily isolated from nasopharyngeal specimens. Serologic studies will often be needed to document recent infection with parainfluenza virus, RSV, coronavirus, and adenovirus.

Symptomatic relief of the common cold is currently the only effective approach to treatment (see "Influenza," below). Antibiotics are not effective in the absence of proven secondary bacterial infection. Nasal symptoms can be diminished with decongestants or vasoconstrictors. Cough may be suppressed with codeine or nonsteroidal anti-inflammatory drugs such as naproxen. Mild fever and sore throat may respond to antipyretics. Most controlled studies have failed to document an anti-illness effect due to vitamin C ingestion.

In experimentally induced and naturally acquired colds, prophylactic administration of recombinant interferon alpha was shown to be effective. However, interferon was not effective when given therapeutically. The adverse local effects of intranasal interferon have limited the widespread use of recombinant interferon. Interruption of transmission by handwashing or disposable nasal tissues may decrease secondary transmission.

Pharyngitis

Most cases of viral pharyngitis occur in conjunction with other clinical signs and symptoms of colds or influenza. Bacteria, especially group A beta-hemolytic streptococci, can also cause pharyngitis that is clinically indistinguishable from viral pharyngitis. Many cases of pharyngitis have no identifiable cause. Peak prevalence of pharyngitis is from fall to spring, when most respiratory viral infections occur. Family spread of infection is common, especially in households with young children.

Among the viral causes of pharyngitis, rhinoviruses are probably the single most commonly isolated pathogen. Adenoviruses often cause pharyngitis in combination with conjunctivitis and fever. Herpes simplex virus has been documented as a cause of pharyngitis—especially in susceptible, nonimmune college students. Coronaviruses, influenza viruses, and parainfluenza viruses have been isolated from cases of acute respiratory disease and pharyngitis. Epstein-Barr virus (EBV) and cytomegalovirus (CMV) can cause a mononucleosis syndrome in which pharyngitis is a prominent clinical feature. During primary infection with HIV, pharyngitis and a mononucleosis-type syndrome have also been reported to occur.

Pharyngeal exudates are not commonly seen with rhinovirus, influenza, parainfluenza, coronavirus, or HIV-related pharyngitis. However, exudates have been documented in cases of adenovirus, herpes simplex virus, and EBV-associated cases. Clinically, these viral types of exudative pharyngitis are indistinguishable from those due to group A streptococci, *Mycoplasma pneumoniae,* or *Chlamydia pneumoniae.* The presence or absence of other respiratory signs and symptoms can be helpful in making a presumptive etiologic diagnosis.

Rapid antigen detection tests for group A streptococci are sensitive and specific enough to warrant widespread use. A positive test is sufficient for initiating specific antibiotic treatment; a negative test is an indication for throat culture. If a test is negative in a patient with exudates and fever, a careful examination for unusual and potentially serious bacterial infections (e.g., diphtheria) must be considered.

Specific viral cultures are available for most of the commonly associated respiratory viruses. However, coronaviruses, EBV, and CMV require serologic tests. At the time of pharyngitis secondary to HIV, a serum p24 antigen test may be positive, but the screening ELISA or Western blot will be negative. Special cultures are needed to recover diphtheria, *Arcanobacterium hemolyticus, M. pneumoniae,* or *C. pneumoniae.*

Patients with streptococcal pharyngitis should receive penicillin treatment. Mycoplasmal or chlamydial pharyngitis will respond to oral macrolides. Most cases of viral pharyngitis will require symptomatic therapy only. Fluids, analgesics, and bed rest constitute the basic treatment. In one study, a nonsteroidal anti-inflammatory drug relieved pain faster than acetaminophen in children with pharyngitis and tonsillitis. Hospitalization is needed only if life-threatening complications or serious systemic illness is documented.

Routine tonsillectomy is not recommended for children with recurrent pharyngitis. If patients are at risk of rheumatic fever, penicillin prophylaxis is recommended. Vaccines for influenza viruses are recommended for annual use in targeted groups.

Laryngitis

Laryngitis or hoarseness secondary to laryngeal inflammation occurs in 20 percent of common respiratory viral illnesses, often associated with cough and pharyngitis. The most commonly documented viruses causing laryngitis are influenza viruses, rhinoviruses, adenoviruses, parainfluenza viruses, and RSV. In adults with acute laryngitis, *Moraxella (Branhamella) catarrhalis* has been recovered in 50 percent of cases. Laryngitis has also been described in a few cases caused by group A streptococci. Rare cases of laryngitis have been reported to be due to *Mycobacterium tuberculosis,* varicella zoster virus, *Histoplasma capsulatum,* and *Candida* species.

Treatment is symptomatic in most cases of laryngitis. Resting the voice is advocated. In one controlled trial, there was a faster return of normal voice in erythromycin-treated patients than in those receiving a placebo. The isolation of *M. catarrhalis* was also significantly reduced in the antibiotic-treated group. Studies employing penicillin have, however, failed to demonstrate a clinical benefit for patients with laryngitis.

Hoarseness lasts 10 days to 2 weeks for most patients. If the symptoms persist, laryngoscopic examination is suggested to look for tumors or other chronic conditions.

Acute Laryngotracheobronchitis (Croup)

Laryngotracheobronchitis (croup) is a viral infection of both the upper and lower respiratory tract in young children; it is associated with dyspnea and inflammation of the subglottic region. Characteristic findings are inspiratory stridor, hoarseness, and cough. Most children have only one episode of croup in a lifetime, but there are sometimes recurrences. Most cases of croup occur in boys during the second year of life.

Parainfluenza virus type 1 is the most commonly documented infectious agent causing croup in the United States and usually occurs in the fall of every other year. Parainfluenza virus type 3, influenza viruses A and B, and RSV are the next most frequently isolated viruses. Cases of croup secondary to RSV usually occur in the first year of life. Outbreaks of croup in the winter and spring are most commonly associated with influenza viruses and less commonly with RSV. Adenoviruses are uncommon causes of croup. Rhinoviruses, enteroviruses, and parainfluenza virus type 4 rarely cause croup. When parainfluenza virus type 1 and influenza viruses occur in epidemics, there are usually concomitant increases in croup cases in the community. With RSV outbreaks, there are no increases in community croup cases.

Clinical Manifestations

Before the clinical onset of croup, most children have symptoms of upper respiratory infection for one or more days. Fever is common, and a nonproductive cough is usual. The child often awakens at night with the distinctive raspy cough, tachypnea, and inspiratory stridor. The respiratory rate is usually greater than 40 per minute. On physical examination, rales, rhonchi, or wheezes can be heard or, if late in the course, decreased breath sounds. Children tend to feel better in the morning and worse in the evening. A typical case lasts 3 to 4 days but occasionally up to 2 weeks. During the acute illness, hypoxemia is documented in 80 percent of hospitalized croup patients and hypercapnia in 50 percent.

The differential diagnosis of croup includes foreign-body aspiration, smoke inhalation, angioneurotic edema, and anaphylaxis—all of which are associated with cough, hoarseness, and stridor. Two other infections must be considered in the differential diagnosis of croup: epiglottitis and bacterial tracheitis. Rhinorrhea and laryngitis are not found with epiglottitis. Marked dysphagia and drooling are common with epiglottitis but not croup. A helpful finding on radiographs of the neck is subglottic swelling. Bacterial tracheitis occurs more commonly in older children and is associated with purulent sputum in addition to fever, stridor, and dyspnea. Organisms most commonly identified in bacterial tracheitis are *Staphylococcus aureus,* group A beta-hemolytic streptococci, and *Haemophilus influenzae* type b. There is often a rapidly progressive clinical course that responds to antibiotics.

Complications of croup include occasional postintubation subglottic stenosis and, rarely, noncardiogenic pulmonary edema. In most published series of hospitalized cases, mortality has ranged up to 2.7 percent. In long-term follow-up studies, an increase in hyperactivity of the airways has been documented.

Diagnosis

The diagnosis of croup is usually made clinically. Routine laboratory tests are not helpful. A specific virus has been identified in only 30 to 60 percent of cases. Virus cultures are available for parainfluenza viruses, influenza viruses, and RSV in most diagnostic virology laboratories. Rapid diagnosis may be achieved via DFA (fluorescent antibody staining of nasal swabs or other respiratory secretions) for RSV, influenza, and parainfluenza viruses. Because parainfluenza viruses may be shed for weeks, obtaining specimens for virus culture several days into a typical illness may be helpful. Cultures usually become positive in 5 to 10 days but may take as long as 3 weeks. Type-specific serologic rises to parainfluenza viruses may not be found because of cross-reactivity with the other parainfluenza viruses.

Prevention and Treatment

Steam or mist vaporizers are of unproven benefit. Animal experiments suggest that cold dry, cold moist, or dry air may be more effective than warm moist air. Nebulized epinephrine led to clinical improvement in some studies. The use of steroids is more controversial. Some investigators have reported fewer intubations and more rapid clinical improvement in hospitalized croup patients who received two to four doses of dexamethasone (0.3 to

0.6 mg/kg). Antibiotics are not warranted unless a bacterial superinfection is proven.

Since hypoxemia is common, hospitalized patients should have oximetry measurements and supplemental oxygen provided. If the Pa_{CO_2} rises and respiratory failure is imminent, nasotracheal intubation should be performed. *Tracheostomy is generally associated with more complications than nasotracheal intubation and is not recommended.*

INFLUENZA

Epidemiology

Influenza viruses are members of the Orthomyxoviridae family. Influenza viruses type A and type B are two genera. Influenza virus type C has not been classified and uncommonly induces illness. Antigenic variations in influenza type A and, to a lesser extent, influenza type B account for the yearly epidemics. Influenza type C has not demonstrated antigenic variation. Minor changes in the two external glycoproteins, the hemagglutinin (HA) and neuraminidase (NA), occur frequently and lead to seasonal strain differences. These minor antigenic variations are termed *antigenic drift* and account for the yearly updating of vaccine strains to be employed. Major changes in the HA or NA antigens are associated with pandemic influenza that causes severe disease in susceptible populations.

Yearly epidemics of influenza begin abruptly and last 5 to 6 weeks. Epidemics occur from December to April in the Northern Hemisphere and from May to September in the Southern Hemisphere. Immunocompromised hosts are the first indicators of an impending epidemic, followed by increased numbers of febrile respiratory illnesses in children. Later indicators of influenza in a community are increased school and industrial absenteeism and deaths due to pneumonia. Two strains of a single subtype or two subtypes have been isolated simultaneously in a single epidemic period. Subtype A may be prevalent in 1 year and subtype B in the next year. There is no easy way to predict which "new" variant will circulate in the next epidemic period, but strains isolated at the end of an epidemic period may "herald" the epidemic virus for the following year and are used in vaccine construction.

Worldwide influenza pandemics occur when a new virus emerges for which there is no immunity. Three of the pandemics of the twentieth century (1957, 1968, and 1977) began in China. One hypothesis for this geographic source of pandemics is that, in China and other parts of Asia, influenza viruses can be isolated throughout the year and the proximity of birds, swine, and humans increases the opportunity for recombination of animal and human influenza viruses, leading to new antigenic shifts in HA or NA.

Pathogenesis

Transmission of influenza virus probably occurs by small-particle aerosol. Virus deposited in the lower respiratory tract attaches to and infects columnar epithelial cells. Replication of virus takes 4 to 6 h, so that infection of new, adjacent susceptible cells takes place in a short time. Thus, the incubation period may be as short as 18 h or last up to 3 to 4 days.

Infected patients begin shedding virus a day before the onset of illness and continue shedding for 5 to 10 days. Although fever and systemic symptoms are quite common, recovery of influenza virus from blood has been rare. A biopsy of nasal or bronchial epithelium in persons with acute influenza will demonstrate desquamation of the ciliated columnar epithelium. In the rare cases of influenza virus pneumonia, alveolar hemorrhage and hyaline membrane formation are common. At the time of clinical improvement, interferon can be measured in nasal secretion samples.

Clinical Manifestations

A typical case of influenza is characterized by an abrupt onset of symptoms that include fever, chills, headache, malaise, and myalgias. Dry cough and nasal discharge become progressively worse over a 3- to 5-day period. The cough is usually nonproductive, is associated with chest pain, and may persist for weeks after other symptoms have disappeared. Fever as high as 104°F typically persists for 1 to 3 days and occasionally 1 week. With the disappearance of fever, the systemic symptoms usually resolve. Some studies have suggested that influenza B illness is less severe than influenza A illness. Influenza C infection produces the influenza syndrome rarely and commonly presents as an afebrile common cold.

Complications from influenza are most common in adults, especially the elderly. Pulmonary complications include primary influenza pneumonia and secondary bacterial pneumonia. Primary influenza pneumonia is uncommon but is associated with a high mortality. The pneumonia is often bilateral and manifest by severe hypoxia, negative Gram's stain of respiratory secretions, and lack of response to antibiotics. Preexisting cardiovascular disease and pregnancy are two settings in which influenza pneumonia may occur with increased frequency.

Secondary bacterial pneumonia has been described in patients who appear to be recovering from influenza but experience recurrence of fever and worsening of respiratory symptoms 1 to 2 weeks later. On physical examination, there is evidence of pulmonary consolidation. Sputum cultures usually grow *Streptococcus pneumoniae, Staph. aureus,* or *H. influenzae.* The elderly and patients with chronic obstructive pulmonary disease (COPD) are at increased risk of pneumonia. Most patients recover after appropriate antibiotic therapy.

Abnormalities in gas exchange and small airway function are common in influenza infection and may persist for weeks to months after clinical illness. Exacerbation of chronic bronchitis, asthma, and cystic fibrosis has been reported with both influenza virus type A and type B infections. In children, influenza A and occasionally influenza B outbreaks have led to increased cases of croup, but at a lower frequency than with parainfluenza virus infections.

Central nervous system complications occur with both influenza virus type A and type B infections. Influenza A infections have been associated with Guillain-Barré syndrome, transverse myelitis, and encephalitis. Reye's syndrome is a complication of influenza B and occasionally influenza A. These complications occur predominantly in children, has a high mortality, and is seen in conjunction with aspirin ingestion. Many other viruses, especially varicella zoster virus, have been reported in Reye's syndrome, but confirmed influenza B cases are most common. In addition to altered mental status leading to coma, hepatic dysfunction is common. Recovered patients will often have serious neurologic sequelae. With the recommendation that *acetaminophen should be used in place of aspirin in children with influenza or varicella virus infections,* cases of Reye's syndrome have declined.

Influenza B is occasionally associated with myositis and myoglobinuria in children. Tender leg muscles and an apparent inability to walk are noted for a few days during the acute illness. Recently, toxic shock syndrome in children and adults has been reported during outbreaks of influenza. Rarely, myopericarditis is related to acute influenza A and B infections.

Diagnosis

Influenza viruses can be isolated from respiratory tract specimens. Nasal wash, throat swab, or sputum specimens will yield virus if transported to the laboratory in viral transport medium. Several tissue culture cells sensitive to influenza virus growth are available. Approximately 70 percent of cultures are positive for virus within 72 h of inoculation. Most are positive within 10 days. In the first few days of infection, rapid diagnosis may be achieved via DFA for influenza, RSV and parainfluenza viruses. During the second week of illness, type-specific serum antibodies are detectable. Specific antibodies can be detected by HAI, CF, or ELISA methods. Specific influenza virus antibodies persist for months to years but decline gradually after the acute illness. The primary benefit of anti-HA antibody may be to inhibit infection. Anti-NA antibody appears to reduce illness but not affect infection. Secretory IgA to influenza virus develops after infection and is apparently an important component of protection from reinfection. Specific influenza virus antibody can be detected 2 to 4 weeks after acute illness. Specific antibodies can be detected using HAI, CF, or ELISA techniques. In epidemiologic surveys, combined use of tissue cell cultures and serologic assays documented more influenza virus illnesses than did either method alone.

Prevention and Treatment

Amantadine and rimantadine are available for prophylaxis and treatment of influenza A (not influenza B) infection. In uncomplicated influenza A, both amantadine and rimantadine reduce the duration of clinical signs and symptoms. The lower frequency of (central nervous system) CNS side effects reported with rimantadine than with amantadine suggests that rimantadine is the preferred antiviral agent, especially in elderly patients. Resistant influenza A isolates have been detected from patients treated with amantadine and rimantadine. The clinical impact of these resistant isolates is yet to be fully defined. Because rimantadine is extensively metabolized, there is significantly less accumulation than with amantadine in the elderly and in patients with renal insufficiency. Therefore the daily dose of amantadine should be reduced in the elderly and in patients with renal failure. The recommended dose of rimantadine for acute illness is 100 mg once daily for 3 to 5 days.

In selected unvaccinated high-risk patients, daily administration of rimantadine or low-dose amantadine should be considered for prophylaxis. If vaccine is given simultaneously with either amantadine or rimantadine, the antiviral agent can be discontinued 2 weeks after the presumed rise of a specific influenza antibody. The level of protection for amantadine and rimantadine given prophylactically is equivalent to vaccine, or 75 to 90 percent. These agents may also be used to control institutional outbreaks. Amantadine may cause anorexia, nausea, peripheral edema, and CNS toxicity, including restlessness, confusion, insomnia and uncommonly seizures, particularly in the elderly. Rimantidine causes adverse effects less commonly than with amantidine, but is associated with anorexia and a lower incidence of CNS toxicity.

Oseltamivir is an oral neuraminidase inhibitor which, when started within 36 h of symptoms, can reduce the severity and duration of symptoms as well as the incidence of respiratory complications due to both influenza A and B. It is about 75 percent effective in preventing symptoms and 87 percent effective in preventing culture-proven influenza. Nausea and vomiting may occur and are reduced by taking the drug with food. Zanamivir is an inhaled neuraminidase inhibitor which, when started within 30 h of symptoms, can reduce both the duration of symptoms and the incidence of respiratory complications due to both influenza A and B. It is about 67 percent effective in preventing symptoms and 84 percent effective in preventing culture-proven influenza. Some patients with asthma develop bronchospasm with this agent.

Supportive treatment for acutely ill patients includes adequate fluid intake and bed rest. Fever should be controlled with acetaminophen, not aspirin. Nasal sprays and cold-mist vaporization may provide local relief. Cough suppressants may be useful. Suspected bacterial superinfection requires hospitalization.

Inactivated influenza virus vaccines have been in use for 50 years. The composition of the vaccine is updated yearly and depends on the circulating virus. For at least 15 years, influenza virus vaccine has contained H1N1, H3N2, and B antigens. Children who are eligible for vaccine should receive two doses and adults one dose yearly. When the circulating virus matches a vaccine strain, influenza vaccine has a 75 percent protection rate against illness in healthy persons less than 65 years of age. Hospitalizations for pneumonia and influenza are also reduced by 30 to 70 percent in the elderly. Side effects are minimal with current influenza vaccines. Local reactions at the injection site occur in 25 to 50 percent of recipients within 24 h. In a few cases, these reactions may be severe. Systemic reactions including fever are more common in children than in adults. The excess rate of Guillain-Barré syndrome reported in 1976 during the swine influenza vaccine program has not recurred in any other year.

The targeted groups for influenza virus vaccine include those at increased risk for influenza-related complications and those who can transmit influenza to persons at high risk (Table 64-2). In addition, physicians should provide vaccine to any persons who want to reduce the risk of becoming ill with influenza. Vaccination of pregnant women is considered safe at any stage of pregnancy. The severity of influenza in HIV-infected patients does not appear to be different from that in uninfected persons. The intensity of infection and the incidence of superinfection appear to be greater in organ transplant recipients. Influenza has been associated with episodes of graft rejection in lung transplant recipients. Recent reports suggest that influenza virus vaccine administration may be associated with transient increases in HIV replication. The clinical significance of this observation has not been determined.

Contraindications to the administration of influenza virus vaccine include anaphylactic hypersensitivity to eggs or to other components, such as the preservative of the vaccine. Acute febrile illnesses in adults should abate before vaccine is given. However, children with minor illnesses can be vaccinated, although it is preferred to wait until the resolution of acute febrile illnesses.

BRONCHIOLITIS

Epidemiology

Bronchiolitis is characterized by wheezing and other lower respiratory tract symptoms in children less than 2 years of age. RSV accounts for more than half the cases, with parainfluenza viruses, adenoviruses, rhinoviruses, and *M. pneumoniae* accounting for an additional one-third. Most cases are reported in winter and early spring, when RSV is often prevalent. The attack rate peaks in the first 6 to 8 months of life and declines thereafter. Hospitalizations in the first year of life are often due to bronchiolitis, more often in boys than girls.

The pathogenesis of bronchiolitis results from direct effects of the virus and exaggerated host responses to the infection. The edema and mucous plugging of small airways cause severe lower respiratory symptoms. Leukotrienes and eosinophil cationic protein are detected in increased quantities in secretions from wheezing children. Studies have shown increases in specific IgE antibody to RSV and augmented histamine release in infants with clinical bronchiolitis.

Clinical Manifestations

For several days before the tachypnea and wheezing that characterize bronchiolitis appear, mild fever and coryza are commonly observed. Nonspecific symptoms such as anorexia and irritability as well as cough usually are also present. Poor oral intake, vomiting, and tachypnea often result in dehydration. Full recovery usually takes 10 to 14 days, with significant improvement in as little as 3 to 4 days.

Hypoxemia is a very common finding in hospitalized infants with bronchiolitis. Hyperinflation and depressed diaphragms are characteristic findings on chest radiographs. It may be impossible to differentiate bronchiolitis from pneumonia, since atelectatic areas may be confused with infiltrates.

Premature infants or infants with serious cardiopulmonary disorders are at increased risk of a complicated course. Apnea is a common complication, especially in RSV-associated bronchiolitis. Recurrent episodes of bronchospasm often occur after bronchiolitis. The full impact of bronchiolitis on pulmonary function in later life has not been defined, but several longitudinal studies reveal small airway abnormalities that persist for years. The importance of RSV infection occurring early in life versus genetic factors in determining the long-term consequences of bronchiolitis is currently under study.

Rarely, acute bronchiolitis due to measles, influenza viruses, or adenoviruses leads to bronchiolitis obliterans, and over weeks to months, patients have repeated bouts of bronchiolitis. The course can be rapidly fatal over several weeks or can develop more slowly. Chronic pulmonary disease develops in most recovering children. No specific therapy appears to be effective.

Diagnosis

Virus isolation from respiratory secretions is helpful in most cases of bronchiolitis. Rapid immunofluorescent diagnostic tests are available for RSV detection within a few hours. Routine tissue cell culture will isolate respiratory viruses. Because maternal antibody is present in young infants, serum antibody tests are not helpful for a specific diagnosis.

Prevention and Treatment

Since hypoxemia is common with bronchiolitis, oxygen administration and mechanical ventilation are often required. Immunoprophylaxis for premature infants and young children (<2 years) has demonstrated utility against RSV. With RSV bronchiolitis, aerosolized ribavirin has proved useful. Administration of this antiviral agent for 2 to 5 days improves clinical scores and alleviates hypoxemia. Studies of intravenous ribavirin are under way. Whether bronchodilators are beneficial for bronchiolitis patients remains questionable. Some studies have shown improvement with either aerosolized or parenteral bronchodilators; others have not shown a benefit. Neither corticosteroids nor antibiotics are of benefit in the treatment of bronchiolitis. The role of antibodies in therapy (monoclonal or polyclonal) is not yet established but merits investigation.

VIRAL PNEUMONIA

Viral pneumonia occurs in children and adults who are immunocompetent or immunocompromised. Most respiratory viruses have been implicated in cases of pneumonia, with influenza viruses and RSV particularly common causes. Most cases occur in the winter months, in closed populations, and in patients with cardiac or pulmonary disease. In children, RSV, parainfluenza viruses, and influenza A and B are the major causes of viral pneumonia. Schoolchildren and infants in day care centers are important epidemiologic units for transmission. Approximately 50 percent of viral pneumonias in children less than 3 years of age are caused by RSV. Like bronchiolitis, RSV pneumonia is most commonly reported between 2 and 6 months of age. In adults, influenza virus types A and B, adenoviruses, parainfluenza viruses, and RSV are the major causes of pneumonia. In hospitalized patients with community-acquired pneumonia, approximately 8 percent of cases are caused by viruses. Mixed infections with bacteria are commonly identified. Of all the cases of community-acquired viral pneumonia in adults, more than 50 percent are due to influenza A. RSV pneumonia is reported less often in adults than in children, but it is being diagnosed more often in the elderly and in transplant recipients. Other common respiratory viruses have been reported to cause pneumonia, but only rarely in adults.

Immunocompromised patients are infected with the entire array of viral pathogens. Influenza, parainfluenza viruses, and RSV are common forms of community-acquired pneumonia in these populations. These infections are of greater severity and more often complicated by superinfection (e.g., nosocomial infections) in the solid organ and hematopoietic transplant recipients. In addition, the immunocompromised host is susceptible to a range of life-threatening herpesvirus pulmonary infections. During the 1 to 6 months after organ transplant and following marrow engraftment in bone marrow transplant recipients, CMV causes significant systemic infection and invasive disease often affecting the graft and the lungs. Patients will often present with a "flu-like" illness and relative leukopenia with a nonproductive cough. This may occur in the setting of recent graft rejection, heightened immune suppression, graft-versus-host disease, or other systemic febrile illness. They may have ongoing varicella zoster virus (VZV) infection (chickenpox or shingles), recent varicella vaccination, oral herpes simplex virus (HSV) infection, or rarely a mononucleosis-like illness caused by Epstein-Barr virus. All may cause devastating pneumonia in the nonimmune host. The potential effects of viral infection are also diverse in this population. These viruses may cause (1) direct infection and tissue injury, including hepatitis and pneumonia (CMV, RSV); (2) cellular effects (upregulation of histocompatibility antigens or adhesion proteins) or systemic inflammation which (via mediators TNF-α and NFκb) contributes to the incidence of immunologic graft rejection and may necessitate increased immune suppression, with the increased risk of opportunistic infection; or (3) enhanced systemic immunosuppression and an increased likelihood of infections, including those due to *Pneumocystis carinii, Aspergillus species,* or *Nocardia asteroides* in the absence of an unusual epidemiologic exposure.

CMV pneumonia reflects uncontrolled CMV replication with tissue invasion in the solid organ transplant recipient—as compared with viral secretion. The risk is greatest in the CMV-seronegative recipient of an organ from a seropositive donor (the "D+/R− patient"). In bone marrow transplant (BMT) patients, the seropositive recipient expresses CMV antigens in the lungs in the face of seronegative transplanted marrow elements. Much of the pneumonitis seen in BMT patients is incited by CMV (50 percent), while the lung injury results from immune attack on infected lung cells in addition to direct effects of the virus. Thus, CMV prevention and the utilization of diagnostic techniques for CMV infection [e.g., antigenemia assays, polymerase chain reaction (PCR) testing, and shell vial cultures with early antigen detection] are critical. Superinfection with bacteria, fungi, and protozoa has been documented in approximately 50 percent of CMV pneumonia patients. Biopsy is essential to differentiate secretion from invasive disease in CMV infection.

The appearance of the airways in HSV and VZV pneumonia is characteristic (vesicular lesions are often present) so as to allow early diagnosis (DFA, PCR, and cultures) by bronchoscope and treatment of infection. Factors for dissemination and pneumonitis in herpes simplex virus (HSV) and varicella zoster infections include bone marrow and organ transplantation, malignancy, chemotherapy, malnutrition, and severe burns. In organ transplant and cancer patients, mortality secondary to HSV and varicella zoster pneumonitis ranges from 10 to 25 percent. Children with acute leukemia and varicella have a 33 percent incidence of pneumonitis. Pneumonia after herpes zoster occurs at a lower incidence than after varicella. Bacterial superinfection following varicella zoster pneumonia with long-term lung dysfunction is commonly described. Tracheobronchitis secondary to HSV has been well described, especially in ventilated burn patients. The possible association of HSV infection of the lung and adult respiratory distress syndrome remains controversial and will require further confirmatory studies. Nevertheless, HSV activation may have a role in acute lung injury in ventilated patients.

Less common causes of viral pneumonia include adenoviruses, measles, and the recently described hantavirus pulmonary syndrome (HPS) (see below). Adenovirus pneumonia in military recruits is uncommon but serious. Solid organ and bone marrow transplant recipients are susceptible to RSV, parainfluenza, adenovirus, and CMV pneumonia.

In children with measles, pneumonia is an uncommon complication. Although rarely seen in adults, measles pneumonia has a high mortality, especially during pregnancy. Whether bacterial superinfection is the primary reason for the high mortality due to measles pneumonia is unknown. Sixty percent of deaths in infants with measles are secondary to pneumonia. Measles in immunocompromised patients is associated with a high percentage of pneumonia and death. Immunocompromised patients exposed to measles have developed giant-cell pneumonia without the typical rash. Measles encephalitis is another serious complication in immunocompromised hosts.

In the summer of 1993, an outbreak of respiratory illness with a case fatality rate of 76 percent was reported in the southwestern United States. An influenza-like illness, followed by unexplained respiratory failure, was reported in most of the cases. The differential diagnosis of the illness included community-acquired pneumonia and pulmonary edema. Chest radiographs were consistent with noncardiogenic pulmonary edema. Autopsied lung tissue revealed intraalveolar edema with few neutrophils and no viral inclusions. A previously unknown hantavirus, Muerto Canyon virus, was isolated from the lungs of these patients and represents the first known cause of human disease by a hemorrhagic fever virus in North America.

Pathogenesis

With the exception of CMV and varicella zoster virus, viruses causing pneumonia spread from the upper to the lower respiratory tract. Necrosis and sloughing of epithelium lead to loss of the normal mucosal surface. Production of mucus increases, leading to bronchiolar plugging. One week after infection, alveoli fill with fluid and leukocytes. Mononuclear cells are noted in peribronchial areas, and intranuclear inclusions may be seen in alveoli. In measles and parainfluenza virus pneumonia, multinucleated giant cells have been reported.

Recovery from respiratory viral infection relies on both specific and non-specific host defenses. High concentrations of interferon are detected in the lungs at the time of maximal virus concentration. Specific antiviral antibody can be found in the lower respiratory tract secretions by the third day of infection. Cytotoxic T lymphocytes appear at the same time and destroy virus-infected epithelial cells. Thus, the humoral and cell-mediated immune responses are necessary for full recovery from viral pneumonia.

Bacterial superinfection in the lung often occurs after respiratory viral infection. The increased adherence and colonization of gram-positive and negative bacteria in virus-infected epithelial cells are thought to be due to alterations of host cell surfaces, induction of receptors on exposed surfaces, and changes in the extracellular environment, allowing for increased bacterial attachment. Virus-induced suppression of the immune response and alterations in phagocytic function probably contribute to increased bacterial growth and decreased bacterial clearance from the respiratory tract. Virus growth in the lower respiratory tract is associated with altered bactericidal mechanisms of alveolar macrophages and neutrophils. Animal models of viral pneumonia demonstrate reduced lung phagocytic function at a time when bacterial superinfection is likely to develop.

Clinical Manifestations

Infants and children with viral pneumonia usually present with 1 or 2 days of cough and low-grade fever. Young infants may present with minimal fever and apneic spells. Wheezing is found when bronchiolitis is present. Myalgia, anorexia, and malaise in addition to upper respiratory tract symptoms are often reported. Air trapping and perihilar infiltrates are found on chest radiographs. Lobar involvement is seen mainly in older children. Small pleural effusions are uncommon. Peripheral leukocytosis is common. Cultures of blood and sputum should be obtained for diagnosis of bacterial lung infections.

RSV pneumonia in infants is associated with hypoxia and apnea. Chest radiographs often demonstrate air trapping and multilobar patchy infiltrates. A high percentage of patients with RSV pneumonia demonstrate right-upper-lobe collapse or consolidation. However, no radiographic pattern is specific for this or any other respiratory virus.

In the immunocompromised host, manifestations of infection are muted and the radiologic picture is often nonspecific. In seronegative recipients of solid organs, the risk of VZV, CMV, and EBV infection is high and must be considered in the differential of acute febrile illness.

Diagnosis

Respiratory viruses are rarely isolated from asymptomatic persons and therefore are considered to be significant if recovered from cultured specimens. The most frequently positive specimens are nasal washes, nasopharyngeal swabs, and throat swabs. Specimens from bronchoscopy secretions or lung biopsy may be useful in diagnosis. Nonrespiratory specimens such as stool, urine, or blood may be sent for virus isolation, but the yield is low and positive results should be interpreted carefully.

There are several rapid tests for viral antigen detection. Immunofluorescent staining or ELISA kits are rapid but not as sensitive as tissue culture systems. PCR techniques are available for HSV, EBV, CMV, and RSV infections. Histology is needed to distinguish viral secretion (CMV) from invasion. Standard serologic tests are often available through local or state laboratories. Acute and convalescent sera are needed to demonstrate a significant antibody rise but are often absent in compromised hosts. IgM antibody assays are not routinely available.

Prevention and Treatment

Most antiviral agents approved for viral infections are not yet well studied in viral pneumonia. Ganciclovir therapy for CMV pneumonia is effective in the absence of other causes of disease—graft rejection or superinfection. Similarly, foscarnet and cidofovir are effective but associated with electrolyte abnormalities, nephrotoxicity, and neutropenia. Combination therapy using reduced doses of ganciclovir and foscarnet are highly effective. Acyclovir, famciclovir, and valacyclovir have been used in presumed HSV and varicella pneumonia, but there have been no controlled studies of its effectiveness. An aerosol formulation of ribavirin is approved for severe RSV disease in young children. More rapid resolution of hypoxia and decreased virus shedding were found in ribavirin-treated infants than in the control group.

Employing antibiotics prophylactically in viral pneumonia has not proved effective in preventing bacterial pneumonia. However, when influenza illness is followed by signs and symptoms of pneumonia, antibiotic treatment of the most common bacterial causes is appropriate. If immunocompromised patients are exposed to measles or varicella, hyperimmune globulin should be given. Infants born to women with clinical measles should receive immune globulin. Nonimmunocompromised persons exposed to measles can be given live measles vaccine instead of immune globulin to prevent measles infection. No approved antivirals are available for treating measles, although ribavirin has been tried.

HANTAVIRUS

In May 1993, several cases of acute febrile illness with respiratory failure, shock, and high mortality were identified by physicians in the southwestern United States. Immunoglobulin (Ig) M and G antibodies against several hantaviruses were detected in the sera of patients by enzyme immunoassay (EIA), suggesting that illness was due to a previously unrecognized but serologically cross-reactive hantavirus. The hantavirus associated with the 1993

outbreak, Sin Nombre virus (SNV; previously called Four Corners virus and
Muerto Canyon virus) was determined to be unique by nucleotide sequence
analysis of amplified viral genetic material. Before the 1993 hantavirus pulmonary syndrome (HPS) outbreak, all hantaviruses known to cause human
disease (Hantaan, Seoul, Puumala, and Dobrava) were associated with hemorrhagic fever with renal syndrome (HFRS), an illness with variable degrees
of fever, hemorrhagic manifestations, and acute renal failure, or nephropathia
epidemica (NE), a usually benign form of HFRS. Although primary pulmonary edema can occur and subtle pulmonary radiographic abnormalities
may be observed, respiratory symptoms are generally not prominent in HFRS
and NE. At least three additional hantaviruses associated with HPS in North
America were recognized after the 1993 outbreak.

Epidemiology and Transmission

In the first 30 months after HPS was recognized, more than 125 cases occurring in at least 24 states were identified. Of cases reported to the Centers
for Disease Control and Prevention more than 50 percent were fatal; persons
with HPS who died and those who survived were similar in age, sex, and
race/ethnicity. Most patients lived in rural areas. The peak incidence occurred
during the late spring and early summer. Like other hantaviruses, those causing HPS appear to be maintained in nature by chronic, asymptomatic infection of a specific rodent species. Transmission to humans generally occurs
after inhalation of aerosolized rodent excreta or contaminated particulates or,
rarely, from the bite of an infected rodent. The deer mouse *(Peromyscus maniculatus)* was identified as the primary reservoir of SNV. The likely primary
rodent reservoirs for other HPS-associated viruses are the rice rat *(Oryzomys
palustris)* for Bayou virus, the cotton rat *(Sigmodon hispidus)* for Black Creek
Canal virus, and the white-footed deer mouse *(Peromyscus leukopus)* for New
York virus. The collective ranges of *P. maniculatus, S. hispidus, O. palustris,*
and *P. leukopus* cover most of North America, indicating that the potential
for HPS transmission exists in any region of the continent. The incubation
period for HPS is not known but is presumed to be similar to that of HFRS—
4 to 42 days (average, 12 to 16 days).

Activities associated with contracting HPS included cleaning areas of the
home used for food storage, cleaning barns and other outbuildings, plowing
with hand tools, and animal herding. Exposure to rodents, generally within the
home, has been found in roughly half of reported cases. There is no evidence
for person-to-person transmission of HPS. Among pregnant women who have
survived HPS, transmission of SNV to their newborns has not been detected.

Microbiology and Pathogenesis

The etiologic agents of HPS are single-stranded, negative-sense RNA viruses
of the family *Bunyaviridae.* Virus particles are 70 to 120 nm in diameter. A
lipid envelope with glycoprotein spikes surrounds a core consisting of the
trisegmented genome and its associated nucleocapsids. Climatic factors leading to a sudden increase of the deer mouse population in the Southwest may
have played a role in facilitating increased transmission of SNV during the
spring and summer of 1993.

Postmortem examination of tissue from HPS victims has routinely revealed
serous pleural effusions and heavy, edematous lungs. Histopathologic changes
characteristic of HPS are mainly seen in the lung and spleen, but the degree

of involvement varies among patients. In most cases, microscopic examination of the lung reveals mild to moderate interstitial pneumonitis with variable amounts of mononuclear infiltrates in alveolar septa, congestion, septal and alveolar edema, and focal hyaline membranes. In typical cases, neutrophilic infiltrates are scanty and the respiratory epithelium is intact, with no evidence of cellular debris, nuclear fragmentation, or type II pneumocyte hyperplasia. As the disease progresses, proliferation of reparative-type pneumocytes, edematous and fibroblastic thickening of the alveolar septa, with airspace disorganization and distortion of the lung architecture suggestive of diffuse alveolar damage, may be seen, particularly among patients who survive for more than a few days in the hospital before death. Large mononuclear cells with the appearance of immunoblasts are found in the lungs, red and periarteriolar white pulp of the spleen, and hepatic portal triads.

The virus is present in the capillary endothelium of numerous organs. The pathophysiologic role of endothelial involvement in the increased vascular permeability, which is the hallmark of this syndrome, remains to be elucidated. Although endothelial cell infection is typical of the hantaviruses, SNV appears to have a unique trophism for the pulmonary vasculature, possibly explaining the pronounced respiratory manifestations of HPS.

Clinical Manifestations

The course of HPS generally progresses through three distinct clinical phases: prodromal, cardiopulmonary, and convalescent (Table 64-3). Fever is an almost universal feature during the prodrome, and myalgias are also common. Early in the course of illness, respiratory symptoms are frequently absent. Distinguishing prodromal-phase HPS from other febrile illnesses, such as influenza or aseptic meningitis, may be difficult; however, sore throat, coryza, and meningismus are unusual in HPS.

Progression to the cardiopulmonary phase is heralded by shock and respiratory distress. Clinical and radiographic deterioration may ensue over a period of hours. Tachypnea may precede the auscultatory finding of rales and abnormalities of the chest radiograph. Leukocytosis may be marked (more than 25,000 cells per cubic millimeter). Fibrinogen levels are generally normal, although disseminated intravascular coagulation has been reported occasionally in HPS. Frank renal failure is not a feature in most cases associated with SNV, and mild creatinine elevations (usually greater than 2.5 mg/dL) occur only in severe cases. Conversely, in the reported cases of HPS associated with Black Creek Canal or Bayou virus, acute renal insufficiency was a prominent characteristic, suggesting that there may be a group of genetically related hantaviruses causing illness somewhat intermediate between HPS and HFRS.

Radiographic abnormalities during the cardiopulmonary phase include prominent interstitial edema, manifest by Kerley's B lines, hilar indistinctness, or peribronchial cuffing, with rapid development of airspace disease. Certain radiographic findings in patients with HPS, including the early prominence of interstitial edema and the lack of a peripheral distribution of initial airspace disease, are uncommon among patients with adult respiratory distress syndrome (ARDS) and may be useful in distinguishing patients with HPS. Lobar infiltrates, commonly seen in patients with pneumococcal sepsis and pneumonia, have not been observed among patients with HPS.

Patients with HPS often require intubation and mechanical ventilation for progressive hypoxemia during the cardiopulmonary phase. In some cases,

TABLE 64-3 Clinical and Laboratory Characteristics of Hantavirus Pulmonary Syndrome Associated with Sin Nombre Virus Infection

Phase	Average duration	Predominant signs and symptoms	Common laboratory findings	Chest radiograph
Prodrome	3–6 days	Fever, myalgia, malaise, headache, dizziness, nausea, vomiting, abdominal pain	WBC normal, slight left shift occasionally seen Platelet count normal, declining count may be seen with repeated testing	Generally normal
Cardiopulmonary	5–10 days	Same as prodrome, plus tachypnea, tachycardia, hypotension	Hypoxemia; leukocytosis, frequently with left shift and slight atypical lymphocytosis Thrombocytopenia Hemoconcentration Metabolic acidosis Prolonged PTT Elevated LDH and AST Mild to moderate proteinuria	May be normal initially; rapidly developing interstitial edema, progressing to alveolar infiltrates Normal cardiac silhouette Pleural effusions common
Convalescent	1–2 weeks	Resolution of shock and respiratory distress, diuresis common	Improving oxygenation, often rapid normalization of laboratory abnormalities Mild anemia occasionally noted	Clearing

KEY: WBC, peripheral white blood cell count; PTT, partial thromboplastin time; LDH, lactate dehydrogenase; AST, aspartate aminotransferase.

large volumes of clear, proteinaceous fluid are obtained by endotracheal tube suctioning. Bronchoalveolar lavage (BAL) specimens from patients with HPS generally contain few cells but have high protein concentrations. In patients who have had Swan-Ganz catheters inserted, normal or elevated systemic vascular resistance and depressed cardiac output were observed, in contrast to the typical findings in bacterial sepsis. Initial pulmonary artery wedge pressures were low. Pronounced left ventricular dysfunction demonstrated by transthoracic echocardiography was noted in some cases. Depressed myocardial function and intractable hypotension terminating with cardiac dysrhythmia are the most common causes of death in patients with HPS. Death generally occurs within 1 week after onset of symptoms. Progressive hypotension in spite of adequate arterial oxygenation is common, suggesting that hypotension was not solely the result of hypoxemia.

Progression to the convalescent phase can be remarkably rapid. Apparently moribund patients requiring maximal ventilatory and inotropic support may progress to extubation and withdrawal of vasoactive agents over a period of a few days. Although no data on the long-term sequelae of HPS are currently available, recovery has been apparently complete in patients surviving the cardiopulmonary phase. Serologic testing of persons with minimal or no symptoms suggestive of HPS indicates that clinically mild or asymptomatic infection rarely occurs.

The diagnosis of HPS should be entertained for any previously healthy person presenting with a febrile prodrome followed by the development of pulmonary compromise and shock.

Diagnosis

Laboratory diagnosis of HPS is made by serologic tests detecting hantavirus IgM antibodies in serum or a fourfold or greater rise in hantavirus IgG antibodies, detection of hantavirus antigen in tissue by immunohistochemistry, and amplification of hantaviral nucleotide sequences by reverse-transcription polymerase chain reaction (RT-PCR). Results of these three diagnostic methods are almost always concordant when adequate material is available for testing. Serologic tests for SNV are generally diagnostic at the time of hospital admission and are available at several sites, including many state public health laboratories. Because SNV RNA is present within circulating mononuclear white blood cells of patients with HPS, RT-PCR testing of blood specimens may be a useful diagnostic tool. Only one of three BAL fluid cell pellets from patients with HPS tested by RT-PCR were positive, probably reflecting the low cellularity of the BAL fluid and the endothelial localization of the virus. Isolation of hantaviruses in cell culture has been very difficult and is not practical for diagnosis.

Treatment

The cornerstone of medical management of HPS is close monitoring of patients in an intensive care unit. Hypoxemia and shock should be treated with oxygen administration, intubation, and mechanical ventilation. Inotropic and vasopressor agents should be used as needed. Capillary leak appears to play a central role in pathogenesis; therefore it seems rational that fluids should be given cautiously if HPS is suspected. The survival rate among HPS patients receiving ribavirin in the open-label trial was similar to that of those not receiving the drug. Untoward effects of intravenous ribavirin therapy include reversible hemolytic anemia and suppression of erythropoiesis, sometimes requiring transfusion.

POLIOMYELITIS

Sporadic cases of paralytic poliomyelitis have occurred for at least as long as human history has been recorded. From ancient times until the late 1800s, polioviruses were widely distributed in most of the world's populations, surviving in an endemic fashion by continuously infecting susceptible infants newly born into the community. Because most poliovirus infections were subclinical, only rare sporadic cases of poliovirus-caused paralysis were noted. A syndrome retrospectively identifiable as paralytic poliomyelitis—almost always in infants or young children—began to be mentioned in the medical literature in the mid-1700s, but it was not fully recognized and described as a clinical entity until the later part of that century and the first half of the next. In the mid-1800s, outbreaks of paralytic polio began to be seen. For the next century, in urban, industrialized parts of Europe and North America, there followed epidemics that grew more severe, more frequent, and more widespread. Cases of what had been called *infantile paralysis* began to be observed also in adolescents and even in young adults. Large epidemics spread across the United States and Europe in the first half of the twentieth century. In the United States in the summer of 1916, more than 27,000 persons were reported to have been paralyzed, with 6000 deaths. In New York City during this one season, more than 9000 cases and more than 2000 deaths were recorded.

Classification and Properties

Poliovirus belongs to the enterovirus group, which includes polioviruses, coxsackieviruses, and echoviruses. These agents—which share a number of clinical, epidemiologic, and ecologic characteristics as well as physical and biochemical properties—are classified as the *Enterovirus* genus of the family Picornaviridae. Poliovirus type 1 is the type species of the genus. Enteroviruses are transient inhabitants of the human alimentary tract and may be isolated from the throat of the infected person (from just before disease onset to 1 week after onset) or from the lower intestine (from just before onset to several weeks after onset). Healthy carriers are common; they usually excrete virus in the feces for several weeks.

The typical enterovirus is approximately 28 nm in diameter and consists of a capsid shell of 60 subunits, each with four proteins (VP1–VP4) arranged in icosahedral symmetry around a genome made up of a single strand of positive-sense RNA. Enteroviruses replicate in the cytoplasm of the infected cell. In the diagnostic laboratory, virus is cultivated in primary or continuous-line cell cultures from various human or monkey tissues. The typical enterovirus infects only primate cells that contain a specific membrane receptor for the virus on the cell surface.

Clinical Presentations

When a person susceptible to infection is exposed to poliovirus, one of the following responses may occur: inapparent infection without symptoms, mild (minor) illness ("abortive poliomyelitis"), aseptic meningitis ("nonparalytic poliomyelitis"), and paralytic poliomyelitis. As the infection progresses, one response may merge with a more severe form: a minor illness may be followed by a few symptom-free days and then by a major, severe illness. This biphasic course is more commonly seen in children than in adults. Only about 1 percent of poliovirus infections result in a paralytic illness.

> *Asymptomatic Infection* By far the most common form of infection is asymptomatic or is marked by no more than minor malaise.
>
> *Minor Illness ("Abortive Poliomyelitis")* The most common form of disease caused by poliovirus is characterized by fever, malaise, drowsiness,

headache, nausea, vomiting, constipation, or sore throat in various combinations.

Aseptic Meningitis or Transient Mild Paresis ("Nonparalytic Poliomyelitis")
In addition to the symptoms and signs described above, the patient has stiffness and pain in the back and neck. Occasionally, there may be mild muscle weakness or transient paralysis. The disease lasts 2 to 10 days, and recovery is almost always complete. About 1 or 2 percent of infections take this course during epidemics. In a small percentage of cases, meningitis advances to paralysis. It should be noted that a number of other viruses—particularly other members of the enterovirus family— also produce this syndrome.

Paralytic Poliomyelitis The major illness comprises the manifestations listed above for aseptic meningitis, along with persisting weakness of one or more muscle groups, either skeletal or cranial. It accounts for about 1 percent of poliovirus infections. The onset of paralysis may follow the minor illness after a symptom-free interlude, or it may occur without an antecedent phase of illness. The predominant sign is flaccid paralysis resulting from damage to the lower motor neurons. Incoordination secondary to brainstem invasion may also occur, and there may be painful spasms of nonparalyzed muscles. The amount of damage varies widely, and the respiratory muscles are not spared. Usually muscle impairment is maximal within a few days after the paralytic phase begins. Maximal recovery usually occurs within 6 months, with residual paralysis lasting much longer, often for life.

The late-onset postpolio syndrome (PPS) consists of muscle weakness, muscle pain, and unaccustomed fatigue. This has occurred with increasing frequency among former poliomyelitis patients. The incidence peaks at an interval of about 30 to 40 years after the acute poliomyelitis. It seems that PPS results from the neuromuscular disease process initiated at the time of the acute illness. The disease is not caused by a reactivation of the original poliovirus or by a reinfection with a current strain; it develops when the patient's remaining motor units in the CNS start to respond poorly to their overuse through many years.

Diagnosis

The diagnostic procedure of choice is isolation of virus from throat swabs, stools, rectal swabs, and, in aseptic meningitis, cerebrospinal fluid. If an agent is isolated in tissue culture, it is tested with specifically designed combination pools of antisera against enteroviruses. Rapid methods, particularly those based on the polymerase chain reaction, have been used for direct detection of poliovirus and other enteroviruses in clinical specimens but few are standardized. For cultivating poliovirus, cultures of human or monkey cells should be used. Cytopathic effects usually appear in 3 to 6 days. Paired serum specimens are required in order to show a rise in antibody titer. Neutralizing antibodies appear early.

Pathogenesis and Pathology

The portal of entry of the virus is the mouth. Primary multiplication takes place in the oropharynx or the intestine, and for a few days virus may appear in the blood. The virus can be isolated regularly from the throat just before and at the first signs of illness. The incubation period is usually between 7 and 14 days but may range from 3 to 35 days. By 1 week after onset, there is little virus in the throat, but large amounts of virus continue to be excreted in the stools for several weeks, even though humoral antibodies usually develop during the same period. By 3 to 5 days after exposure, virus can be recovered from blood, throat, and feces. At this time symptoms of the "minor illness" may appear, or the infection may remain asymptomatic. Viremia is present for a few days before the onset of CNS signs in those who develop either "nonparalytic polio" (aseptic meningitis) or the paralytic disease. After initial multiplication in the tonsils, the lymph nodes of the neck, Peyer's patches, and the small intestine, poliovirus then spreads by way of the bloodstream to other susceptible tissues, namely other lymph nodes, brown fat, and the CNS. Poliovirus can also spread along axons of peripheral nerves to the CNS, whence it continues to progress along the fibers of the lower motor neurons to invade the spinal cord and parts of the brain. Tonsillectomy or other surgery in the oropharynx increases the risk of CNS impairment at times when polioviruses are prevalent.

The anterior horn cells of the spinal cord are most prominently involved, but in severe cases the intermediate gray ganglia and even the posterior horn and dorsal root ganglia are often affected. Lesions are found as far forward as the hypothalamus and thalamus. In the brain, the reticular formation, the vestibular nuclei, the cerebellar vermis, and the deep cerebellar nuclei are most often affected. The cortex is virtually spared with the exception of the motor cortex along the precentral gyrus. Although flaccid paralysis is the hallmark of poliomyelitis, the virus does not multiply in muscle in vivo. The changes that occur in peripheral nerves and voluntary muscles are secondary to destruction of nerve cells within the CNS. Cells that are not killed but lose function temporarily may recover completely within 3 to 4 weeks after onset. Inflammation occurs secondary to the attack on nerve cells.

Respiratory failure resulting from paralysis of the diaphragm and intercostal muscles represents the most serious complication of paralytic poliomyelitis (see Hodes reference). Aspiration pneumonia, pulmonary edema, myocarditis, paralytic ileus, gastric dilatation, and ileus of the bladder may also complicate acute paralytic disease. Poliomyelitis may affect respiration adversely in several ways. Invasion of the motor nerve cells by the virus causes loss of discharge, the basic stimulus that activates striated muscles, including diaphragm, intercostals, and accessory muscles of respiration. The degree of weakness produced is proportional to the number of motor cells that have lost their capacity to function. There results partial or complete loss of the ability to produce the rhythmic changes in the thoracic volume that bring about pulmonary ventilation. Poliomyelitis virus may also injure the regulatory neurons in the medulla.

Epidemiology

Human beings are the only known reservoir of poliovirus infection. At times when a poliovirus is widely prevalent in an area, houseflies become contaminated and may passively distribute virus to food. The usual source of transmission is infectious feces spread by contaminated fingers. The disease occurs in all age groups, but children are usually more susceptible than adults because of the acquired immunity of the adult population.

Vaccination

Both live and killed vaccines are available for polio, but most countries have relied almost entirely on live OPV. Most recently, the cases of polio identified in developed regions have been revertants of OPV strains. Therefore, in the United States, OPV has been replaced by inactivated polio vaccine (IPV). Polio remains active in South Asia and sub-Saharan Africa, which would be the sole areas in which OPV is appropriate for general use, in the eradication of outbreaks and in nonimmune populations. Routine use of polio vaccination is no longer recommended except in those traveling to endemic regions who are either unvaccinated or have been vaccinated more than 10 years earlier.

NOSOCOMIAL RESPIRATORY VIRAL INFECTIONS

Nosocomial respiratory viral diseases are recognized predominantly in children but are also seen in elderly persons and chronically ill adults. Increased morbidity, mortality, and hospital costs have been documented as a result of these hospital-acquired infections. Respiratory viruses account for approximately 70 percent of nosocomial viral illnesses, including that due to RSV, influenza, parainfluenza, adenoviruses, and rhinoviruses.

Outbreaks of nosocomial respiratory viral infections can be detected during seasonal respiratory viral epidemics in the community. Respiratory viruses are introduced to hospitalized patients by infected patients, visitors, or personnel. Transmission occurs through infected hospital staff or patients as well as transfer of virus from hands, aerosols, or fomites. Nosocomial respiratory viral infections can occur in any exposed person, whether at "high risk" or not.

BIBLIOGRAPHY

Barker WH, Mullooly JP: Pneumonia and influenza deaths during epidemics: Implications for prevention. *Arch Intern Med* 142:85–89, 1982.

Chanock RM, Parrott RH, Connors M, et al: Serious respiratory tract disease caused by respiratory syncytial virus: Prospects for improved therapy and effective immunization. *Pediatrics* 90:137–143, 1992.

Dolin R, Reichman RC, Madore HP, et al: A controlled trial of amantadine and rimantadine in the prophylaxis of influenza A infection. *N Engl J Med* 307:580–584, 1982.

Duchin JS, Koster FT, Peters CJ, et al: Hantavirus pulmonary syndrome: A clinical description of 17 patients with a newly recognized disease. *N Engl J Med* 330:949–1005, 1994.

Englund JA, Sullivan CJ, Jordan C, et al: Respiratory syncytial virus infection in immunocompromised adults. *Ann Intern Med* 109:203–208, 1988.

Greenberg SB: Respiratory herpesvirus infections: An overview. *Chest* 106:1S–2S, 1994.

Gwaltney JM Jr, Moskalski PB, Hendley JO: Hand-to-hand transmission of rhinovirus colds. *Ann Intern Med* 88:463–467, 1978.

Hierholzer JC: Adenoviruses in the immunocompromised host. *Clin Microbiol Rev* 5:262–274, 1992.

Hodes HL: Treatment of respiratory difficulty in poliomyelitis, in *Poliomyelitis: Papers and Discussions Presented at the Third International Poliomyelitis Conference.* Philadelphia: Lippincott, 1955, pp 91–96.

Koprowski HL, Jervis GA, Norton TW: Immune responses in human volunteers upon oral administration of a rodent-adapted strain of poliomyelitis. *Am J Hyg* 55:108–126, 1952.

Melnick JL: Live attenuated poliovaccines, in Plotkin SA, Mortimer EA Jr (eds), *Vaccines,* 2d ed. Philadelphia: Saunders, 1994, pp 155–204.

Oda Y, Katsuda S, Okada Y, et al: Detection of human cytomegalovirus, Epstein-Barr virus, and herpes simplex virus in diffuse interstitial pneumonia by polymerase chain reaction and immunohistochemistry. *Am J Clin Pathol* 102:495–502, 1994.

Taber LH, Knight V, Gilbert BE, et al: Ribavirin aerosol treatment of bronchiolitis due to respiratory syncytial virus infection in infants. *Pediatrics* 72:613–618, 1983.

Wallace JM: Pulmonary infections in human immunodeficiency disease: Viral pulmonary infections. *Semin Respir Infect* 8:534–536, 1989.

65 | Parasitic Infections of the Lungs*

Jay A. Fishman

Although debilitating and even fatal protozoal infections are among the most prevalent infections worldwide, they rarely involve the lungs and pleura. Protozoal involvement of thoracic structures generally occurs as a complication of infection at other sites, which leads to signs and symptoms that usually dominate the initial clinical presentation.

AMOEBIASIS

Etiology and Epidemiology

Entamoeba histolytica is the causative agent of amoebiasis. A number of other *Entamoeba* species—such as *E. coli, E. gingivalis, E. hartmani,* and *E. polecki*—are found as commensals in the intestinal tracts of humans and other hosts, but they have rarely if ever been convincingly incriminated in invasive intestinal disease. Liver abscess and the associated complication of thoracic disease can be considered exclusively caused by *E. histolytica.* This amoeba is found worldwide, both in humans and in ground waters such as lakes and streams. It has been found throughout North America, Europe, Asia, Africa, Central and South America, the Caribbean, and South and Southeast Asia. Indeed, the clinician should think of the parasite as ubiquitous.

E. histolytica is the cause of much morbidity and mortality in the developing world, where infection rates of approximately 50 percent are common. Recent epidemics of disease in the developed world have been related to both point-source and multicentric propagative outbreaks in institutions and in specific populations. Risk groups in North America include migrant workers, immigrants, travelers, sexually active male homosexuals, lower socioeconomic groups in the southern United States, and institutionalized groups, such as prisoners, orphans, children in day care centers, and the mentally ill or retarded. Within some of these risk groups, such as practicing male homosexuals and institutionalized persons, carriage rates may exceed 50 percent. In North America, the populationwide infection rate is thought to be about 4 to 5 percent. Globally, about 10 percent of the world's population is infected with *E. histolytica,* and about 100,000 deaths per year occur secondary to amoebiasis. Persistence of infection in a population is a complex interaction between sanitation, personal hygiene, water and food supplies, socioeconomic status, and crowding.

Environmentally robust cysts are ingested by the human host; after surviving passage through the stomach, trophozoite forms of the parasite are released in

---

*Edited from Chaps. 155 and 156, "Protozoan Infections of the Thorax," by Griffiths JK, Wyler DJ; and "Helminthic Diseases of the Lungs," by Malmoud AAF, In: *Fishman's Pulmonary Diseases and Disorders,* 3d ed., edited by Fishman AP, Elias JA, Fishman JA, Grippi MA, Kaiser LR, Senior RM. New York, McGraw-Hill, 1998, pp 2379–2412. For fuller discussion of topics dealt with in this chapter, the reader is referred to the original text, as noted above.

the small intestine. Trophozoites are carried to the ileum and colon, where they reproduce by binary fission. Cysts are formed only in the colon, and it has been theorized that encystation is due to unfavorable colonic conditions that do not support further trophozoite growth. Cysts are able to survive in the environment for weeks to months, whereas trophozoites die rapidly after leaving the body.

Cysts of the parasite are spherical and are 5 to 20 μm in diameter, with a mean of 12 μm, and are found in the fecal stream of infected individuals. Depending on the maturity of the cyst, it contains one to four nuclei, which are identical to the nucleus found in the trophozoite. Trophozoites are the motile replicating forms that breach the intestinal barrier and cause invasive disease. They are 12 to 60 μm in diameter, with a mean of approximately 25 μm. The circular nucleus contains clumped, or beaded, peripheral nuclear chromatinin and a central prominent karyosome (nucleolus). Only one nucleus is seen in the trophozoite form. The trophozoite cytoplasm contains vacuoles and often has a granular characteristic. Movement is accomplished by the extension of cytoplasmic pseudopods, which differentiate *E. histolytica* from the free-living amoebae *Naegleria* and *Acanthamoeba;* these can also cause invasive disease, as discussed below. *E. histolytica* is the only intestinal amoeba that ingests red blood cells, which process, seen in a section or biopsy from tissue, secures the diagnosis. The invasive manifestations of amebiasis include dysentery, liver abscess, and the uncommon extraintestinal infections of the lung, brain, skin, and other rarer sites. Despite the ability of the parasite to do all this, the vast majority of individuals with intestinal *E. histolytica* suffer no adverse consequences.

In recent years, much has been written on the biochemical and genetic evidence separating *E. histolytica* into distinct pathogenic and nonpathogenic strains. The former are uniformly found in invasive disease and the latter in asymptomatic individuals. However, about 1 percent of infected, asymptomatic people carry the invasive type of *E. histolytica,* and about 10 percent of this group (1 in 1000 overall) will eventually develop invasive amebiasis. Those who carry the nonpathogenic strains tend to clear the infestation within 1 year. Differentiation into pathogenic and nonpathogenic strains has been accomplished by zymodene analysis, genomic DNA differences, and restriction fragment [polymerase chain reaction (PCR)] techniques. Some have suggested that the pathogenic organisms be reclassified into a new species, *Entamoeba dispar,* but there is no clinically available method to differentiate *"dispar"* isolates from *"histolytica"* isolates. In the absence of symptoms or signs of illness, it is pointless to eradicate the organism from patients in heavily contaminated environments where reinfestation and reinfection are likely.

Transmission

The organism is classically spread through fecal-oral contamination. Routes of transmission include contaminated food and water, person-to-person contact with cyst passage, and sexual practices that include fecal-oral contact. In the United States, person-to-person spread is now considered more important than contaminated food or water. With very rare exception, the form of the parasite that is responsible for transmission is the cyst. Cases of transmission of amebiasis after colonic irrigation or endoscopy may be the exceptions that prove this rule. Attempts to stop transmission in institutions via mass treatment or by quarantining cyst passers have in general failed. In addition to the high-risk groups mentioned earlier, one must note that malnourished individuals and children tend to suffer more acutely than do their well-nourished or older peers.

Pleuropulmonary complications have been estimated to occur in 1 in 1000 patients; when the liver is involved, the incidence rises substantially to 15 to 20 percent. For unknown reasons, men outnumber women by 10- to 15-fold in many published series, and the peak ages for pulmonary amebiasis are between 20 and 40 years. It is unclear whether these predilections are real or if they represent reporting bias.

Pathophysiology

Entry into the thorax is most commonly the result of extension of liver disease, such as abscess. Other routes exist, such as hematogenous spread that can lead to metastatic brain, lung, and other abscesses, although the frequency of these pathways is far lower. Amoebae that have broached the mucosal barrier are thought to gain entry to the liver via the portal vein. Subsequent liver abscesses can be either purely amoebic or mixed bacterial and amoebic. Because normal defenses against amoebae are far less efficient than defenses against less complex creatures such as bacteria, these abscesses tend to progress and may extend or rupture into the pleural space or the peritoneum in 10 to 20 percent of cases if not treated. There is some evidence to suggest that extension of amoebic infections across the diaphragm via lymphatics may occur.

E. histolytica has a large array of pathogenic properties. It produces a surface lectin that allows it to adhere to mucosal epithelial cells, leukocytes, erythrocytes, submucosal colonic cells, and even bacteria that have galactose-containing lipopolysaccharides. Amoebae kill cells only after direct contact. Once contact has been made, the host cell suffers a marked and sustained elevation of intracellular calcium. In addition, a parasitic saponin-like compound has been identified in parasite granules that may contribute to dissolution of host cell membranes. Proteolytic enzymes are released into the extracellular milieu and may help in dissolving the host. Targeted host cells may also die via apoptosis. The initial host cell response is that of host polymorphonuclear leukocytes; when they are lysed by the amoebae, neutrophil contents contribute to the inflammatory and destructive lesion.

Individuals cured of invasive amoebiasis develop high titers of antibody and appear resistant to *subsequent* infection. However, the serum responses of the host during *primary* invasive disease do not appear to be protective. By the end of the first week of illness, naive hosts will develop an amoebicidal antibody that will inhibit amoebic attachment in vitro, but they will nonetheless have progressive, unremitting disease. Antibody to amoebae appears to act via activation of the classic and alternate complement system—but trophozoites purified from invasive lesions are resistant to complement-mediated lysis. In contrast, trophozoites found in the intestinal lumen are sensitive to complement, perhaps explaining the mechanism by which antibody is able to prevent reinvasion in the experienced host. Thus, the host antibody response is useful in preventing subsequent invasive episodes but is not of much use in the initial event. Similarly, cell-mediated immunity is of some benefit but is not paramount. For example, people with AIDS do not appear to have a higher incidence of invasive amoebiasis than HIV-seronegative individuals, suggesting that the mucosal immune response is not tightly associated with cellular immunity. Nonetheless, amoebic disease can be fulminant in the malnourished, in the very young, in those given steroids, and in pregnant women, in whom cell-mediated responses are blunted. The reader should take away from this discussion a healthy respect for how poor the human immune response to this pathogen is.

CLINICAL PRESENTATIONS OF THORACIC AMOEBIASIS

True thoracic disease complicates 7 to 20 percent of hepatic disease and about 2 percent of intestinal disease. Three major forms of pleuropulmonary disease have been well described. Perhaps most common is a *sympathetic* or *neighbor* reaction to an unruptured abscess within the liver. Another common presentation is empyema, after rupture of the liver abscess into the pleural space. Rupture of a liver abscess can also result in the third major presentation, that of parenchymal involvement with abscess, consolidation, or hepato-bronchial fistula. Because the major route of invasion into the lung and thorax is the liver, elevation of the right hemidiaphragm is one of the earliest signs of thoracic involvement. Indeed, most thoracic disease is within the right hemithorax, since 80 percent of liver abscesses are located within the right lobe of the liver. Dyspnea (5 percent), cough (10 percent), right hemithoracic pain (10 percent), and right shoulder pain (about 30 percent) have been reported in individuals with liver abscess. The pain may be pleuritic or abdominal, and many people with liver abscess will appear to have a predominantly pulmonary disease, with fever, chills, chest pain, cough, and weight loss. Right-lower-lobe consolidative signs and/or effusion may be present in nearly half of all patients with liver abscess.

Clinical signs helpful to the diagnosis of an amoebic liver abscess include pain and tenderness in the right upper quadrant, a palpable liver, and fever; each of these signs is found in about 75 percent of patients. Localized intercostal pain is present between the midaxillary and midclavicular lines on the right in most patients. Hepatobronchial fistula formation may be marked by the presence of foul, "anchovy paste" or "chocolatey" sputum. Approximately half of those with thoracic disease will develop a hepatobronchial fistula, versus about 30 percent who develop an effusion and empyema. Lung abscess occurs in about 14 percent and true consolidation alone in about 10 percent of patients.

Individuals with thoracic disease should *always* be evaluated for possible pericardial infection. The latter can lead to cardiac tamponade and death, congestive heart failure or pericarditis, or simply to a slow, unremitting clinical deterioration. Pericardial disease is thought to occur most frequently after rupture of an adjacent abscess, often from the left lobe of the liver, into the pericardium. Pericardial effusions should be seen as a warning of impending rupture. In Mexico City, Ibarra-Perez noted pericardial disease in about 10 percent of patients referred for thoracic complications. In contrast, in Adams and MacLeod's series of more than 5000 patients, it was a complicating factor in just over 1 percent of the patients.

Diagnosis of Hepatic and Thoracic Amoebiasis

Radiographic and ultrasonic investigations may be very helpful in delineating the architectural confines of the disease, as may computed tomography (CT). Liver abscess may be confirmed with ultrasound or CT evaluations; most disease is in the right lobe of the liver (about 80 percent), and the abscesses are usually spherical. Differentiation between bacterial, amoebic, and mixed bacterial and amoebic infections may be difficult. Happily for the diagnostician, serologic tests are usually positive (about 95 percent) in those with invasive disease and negative in those without invasion. Given the availability of serologic testing, the hoary tradition of making the diagnosis by aspiration of the abscess is now usually needed in only a small percentage of patients. Therapeutic drainage in toxic patients is required in only about 5 percent of individuals.

Early on, elevation of the right hemidiaphragm is found in more than half the patients. As noted above, atelectasis and sympathetic effusion may be seen in association with subdiaphragmatic abscess. When present, effusions must be delineated, as they may represent empyema, and aspiration of fluid for diagnostic studies is required. More convincing evidence of extension into the thorax includes overt consolidative changes, abscess, or fistula formation. As noted above, pericardial disease may occur, usually after rupture of an adjacent abscess into the pericardial space, and ultrasonic or CT evaluation of the pericardium is warranted if there is any question of pericardial disease.

Treatment

Treatment for hepatic or pulmonary disease consists of drainage when indicated (toxemia, empyema, pericarditis) and drug therapy. Metronidazole, given at a dose of 750 mg three times daily orally or by vein for at least 10 days, is both inexpensive and effective. Iodoquinol (650 mg three times daily orally for 20 days), paromomycin (500 mg four times daily orally), chloroquine, or diloxanide are used to eliminate parasites from the gut. Very serious complications of abscess, such as rupture into the abdomen with peritonitis or pericardial disease, can be treated with dehydroemetine.

FREE-LIVING AMOEBAE: *NAEGLERIA* AND *ACANTHAMOEBA*

Free-living amoebae rarely infect humans, but when they do, the results are devastating and the outcome is almost always death. Three conditions have been classically associated with these organisms: primary meningoencephalitis due to *Naegleria fowleri,* subacute meningoencephalitis after hematogenous spread of dermal or pulmonary disease with an *Acanthamoeba* species, and keratitis secondary to *Acanthamoeba.* Infection with one of these agents, unlike *E. histolytica,* does not appear to be related to sanitation and hygiene levels, nor is any vector for these organisms known. It appears that transmission to the human occurs after contact with the amoeba in its natural, free-living state. These amoebae are discussed here because the diagnosis of pulmonary disease with *Acanthamoeba* may allow the institution of lifesaving therapy before meningoencephalitis begins. *Leptomyxid* species of amoebae behave similarly to *Acanthamoeba* species, have rarely been isolated from humans with granulomatous subacute meningoencephalitis, and should be mentioned in passing, as they appear to act identically to *Acanthamoeba.*

N. fowleri is found worldwide in soil, surface, river, and lake waters, and in thermally polluted wastewater sites. Its presence is directly related to temperature, and it thrives at temperatures up to 45°C. Acquisition of the disease often occurs in children and young adults after swimming in fresh water. In the United States, it has been reported most frequently in the southeastern states, probably because of the presence there of warm, fresh waters. *Naegleria* probably invades the central nervous system (CNS) after disruption of the olfactory mucosa, penetration of the submucosal nervous plexus and the cribiform plate, and subsequent entrance into the CNS. This disease is acute in onset and rapidly progressive.

In contrast, *Acanthamoeba* species cause CNS infections after hematogenous spread of amoebae from the skin, lungs, or other sites. *Acanthamoeba* species have also been isolated from soil and water of diverse origins. The hosts for these infections also differ: *N. fowleri* infections occur in normal hosts in excellent health, whereas *Acanthamoeba* infections tend to occur in those with AIDS, diabetes mellitus, pregnancy, liver disease, malignancies with or without steroid or chemotherapy treatment, and transplantation. *Acanthamoeba* infections are probably more common than recognized and have been reported in a variety of animal species as well as in humans.

The onset of *Acanthamoeba* disease is insidious, and focal neurologic deficits are common. Classically the host response is granulomatous, but if the host is immunosuppressed, this may be absent. Usually the primary site in the lungs or skin has been present for weeks to months before the CNS disease becomes apparent. Lesions in the brain spare the leptomeninges except when there are overlying areas of cortical involvement. Cerebral edema is common, as is death from uncal or tonsillar herniations. The necrotizing granulomatous lesions contain perivascular motile trophozoites and cysts. The perivascular nature of the lesions has suggested hematogenous spread. *Acanthamoeba* keratitis is associated with the use of contact lenses and minor corneal trauma; it occurs in normal hosts, as *N. fowleri* infections do.

Two patients with *Acanthamoeba* meningoencephalitis after bone marrow transplantation were recently described. They presented with fever and nodular pulmonary infiltrates 6 and 9 months after transplantation for leukemia. Both patients had a history of sinusitis and had been treated with steroids. One of the two had painful subcutaneous nodules that ulcerated. Mental obtundation, seizures, and coma occurred, and CT scan findings included hydrocephalus. Cerebrospinal fluid (CSF) findings included low glucose and elevated protein levels and little or no pleocytosis. At autopsy, one patient was found to have necrotizing meningoencephalitis, pneumonitis, and adrenalitis; the second had meningoencephalitis and dermatitis. Thus the clinician should include this amoebic disease in the differential diagnosis of nodular pulmonary infiltrates in the immunosuppressed patient.

Diagnosis is made by finding the amoeba in histological samples; unhappily, diagnosis has almost always been at autopsy. Brain—or by extension lung or skin—biopsy is the only way to make the diagnosis during life, as the organism has not been isolated from the CSF of a patient with granulomatous amoebic encephalitis. Lumbar puncture is often contraindicated because of the risk of herniation.

At times, culture is the only way to diagnose the infection. A nonnutrient agar overlaid with killed *E. coli* or *Aerobacter aerogenes* will support the growth of *Acanthamoeba,* often when biopsy material is negative. Cysts and trophozoites can be visualized with Wright, Giemsa, hematoxylin-eosin, and periodic acid–Schiff stains. Calcofluor white, a fluorescent laundry detergent brightener, will also stain the organisms in biopsy specimens.

Treatment of *Acanthamoeba* infections has produced dismally poor results in cases of meningoencephalitis; cases of keratitis have been more successfully treated. This is likely to be the result of earlier recognition of ocular disease, the fact that debridement of the cornea can be undertaken easily, and the ability to achieve high local concentrations of drugs using topical therapy. None of these observations apply to systemic forms of *Acanthamoeba*. Amphotericin B, neomycin, 5-flucytosine, paromomycin, ketoconazole, fluconazole, pentamidine, and miconazole have in vitro activity. In general, each clinical isolate should be tested for sensitivities to these drugs as well as the most effective class, the diamidine group, which includes propamidine and pentamidine.

MALARIA

Infection with *Plasmodium falciparum* (falciparum malaria) should be considered a medical emergency because a delay in diagnosis and in the institution of appropriate therapy can result in death. Examination of appropriately stained blood smears is the only conclusive way to establish the diagnosis. Smears should be negative on 3 consecutive days if malaria is to be ruled out.

Symptoms and signs of respiratory disease frequently accompany even uncomplicated falciparum malaria, whereas respiratory failure is an uncommon, potentially fatal complication of infection. Typically, but not exclusively, respiratory failure accompanies other complications such as renal failure and encephalopathy (cerebral malaria) and is best understood in the context of an overview of falciparum malaria.

Biology of *Plasmodium falciparum*

Like the other *Plasmodium* species that infect humans, *P. falciparum* is transmitted primarily by the bites of mosquitoes. Only rarely does infection result from inoculation of infected blood via blood transfusion, contaminated hypodermic needles, organ transplantation from infected donors, or breaches in barriers of maternal-fetal circulation (congenital malaria). Infected mosquitoes inject sporozoites while taking a blood meal. These extracellular-stage parasites rapidly circulate to the liver, where they invade hepatocytes and differentiate as tissue schizonts (also called *hepatic exoerythrocytic* forms). After an incubation period of approximately 2 weeks, thousands of extracellular malaria parasites called *merozoites* are released from the tissue schizonts into the circulation. These merozoites rapidly invade erythrocytes, wherein they undergo a cycle of asexual reproduction (schizogony) during a 48-h period, growing at a logarithmic rate. The cycle culminates in the rupture of merozoite-laden erythrocytes. The next cycle is initiated when the just-released merozoites invade other erythrocytes. Schizont rupture is associated with the dramatic features of the malarial paroxysm, most notably high fever and rigors.

In addition to the asexual-stage parasites, gametocytes develop from a subpopulation of merozoites; when they are ingested by vector mosquitoes, the sexual cycle is initiated and culminates in the formation of infective sporozoites. The gametocytes are not pathogenic and may persist in the circulation even after successful chemotherapeutic eradication of the asexual-stage parasite.

Pathophysiology of Falciparum Malaria

The intravascular location of the infection makes virtually every organ susceptible to insult, but the typical targets are the brain, kidneys, lungs, and gastrointestinal tract. Tissue hypoxia develops by at least two identified mechanisms: reduced oxygen-carrying capacity that results from severe hemolytic anemia, and obstruction to microcirculation that results from the adherence of infected erythrocytes to the postcapillary endothelium of the microcirculation.

Hemolysis occurs when schizont-infected erythrocytes rupture, releasing the many merozoites that give rise to the next generation of intraerythrocytic parasites. Additional mechanisms play secondary roles in the pathogenesis of anemia in malaria. Because asexual parasite replication is logarithmic, a rapid rise in parasitemia is possible, as is the ensuing extensive hemolysis. *P. falciparum* can grow in erythrocytes of all ages, so theoretically there is no limit to the magnitude of parasitemia that can be attained. In contrast, infection with the *Plasmodium* species that cause nonlethal human malaria is restricted to subpopulations of erythrocytes (e.g., young erythrocytes for *P. vivax* and *P. ovale*), which limits the attainable parasitemia and consequently also morbidity.

P. falciparum parasites produce adhesion molecules as they mature within the erythrocyte. The adhesion molecules are translocated to, and become inserted in, the erythrocyte plasma membrane, where they mediate binding of the infected cell to the surface of endothelial cells in postcapillary venules. The cytoadherence that results takes place primarily in postcapillary venular beds and physically obstructs the microcirculation. Obstruction to blood flow, combined with the reduced oxygen-carrying capacity from anemia, compromises normal tissue metabolism. A third component in the pathogenesis is the substantial elaboration of tumor necrosis factor alpha (TNF-α) during the infection. These pathogenic elements converge to damage endothelial integrity, leading to adult respiratory distress syndrome (ARDS).

Respiratory Failure in Falciparum Malaria

Estimates from the 1940s suggested that some form of pulmonary complication occurs in 3 to 10 percent of patients with falciparum malaria. However, noncardiogenic pulmonary edema occurred in only 3 of 3300 cases of falciparum malaria in military personnel stationed in Vietnam in the mid-1960s. This may represent a more contemporary complication rate, which could be expected in cases diagnosed rapidly and treated with appropriate antimalarial therapy and adjunctive supportive care. The potentially dire consequences of delay in the diagnosis and in institution of appropriate management of respiratory insufficiency in patients with falciparum malaria argues for their early admission to an intensive care unit when respiratory symptoms develop. Noncardiogenic pulmonary edema can develop very suddenly, even after appropriate antimalarial therapy has been instituted and even after parasites are no longer detected on blood smears. An appropriate parasitologic response to antimalarial chemotherapy is no assurance that the patient will not develop late pulmonary complications.

The risk of developing noncardiogenic pulmonary edema in falciparum malaria is greatest in patients who have developed renal failure, cerebral malaria, or hyperparasitemia (greater than 5 percent infected erythrocytes) or who are pregnant or immediately postpartum. Evidence of disseminated intravascular coagulation is a frequent finding. The specific therapeutic approaches in malaria are like those for adult respiratory distress syndrome of other causes. Intravenous quinidine (with continuous electrocardiographic monitoring) should be instituted for antimalarial therapy. Exchange transfusion can achieve the desired rapid reduction in parasitemia and might be lifesaving.

CRYPTOSPORIDIUM PARVUM

Epidemiology and Life Cycle

Cryptosporidium parvum is an ubiquitous organism that appears to be able to infect most if not all mammalian species. Like many other coccidian organisms, *C. parvum* is acquired by ingestion of infectious oocysts in contaminated food and water and has been responsible for major outbreaks of disease in normal and immunosuppressed hosts throughout North America and Europe as well as Africa and other continents. Unlike other coccidians, however, no specific treatment exists for *C. parvum* and it is often lethal in the immunosupressed host. Increasing recognition has been given to its role in infections of the respiratory tract as well as its well-documented role in diarrhea and wasting in AIDS patients, organ transplant recipients, and children. Pneumonia can be the presenting complaint in immunocompromised individuals with cryptosporidiosis, and it is a common though mild complication of intestinal cryptosporidiosis in the immunocompetent host.

The life cycle of the organism is that of most coccidians. Sporozoites are released from the infectious oocysts once they have passed the barrier of the stomach and its acidic milieu. The tissue tropism of the organism appears to be limited to epithelial cells, such as those of the respiratory tree and the intestine; the initial attachment event is probably mediated by a parasite lectin. These sporozoite forms invade intestinal villus cells and undergo several cycles of asexual replication (schizogony) before micro- and macrogametocytes form and fuse to produce the ookinete, or fertilized sexual form. The result of this sexual union is a new oocyst, which may be shed in the fecal stream to infect anew. Thus, the organism is acquired and shed in a classic fecal-oral pattern. The parasite's intracellular location is unique. It is intracellular yet extracytoplasmic. The parasite enters the host cell and becomes covered by the host-cell membranes, making it intracellular, yet it does not enter the cytoplasm. At the site of the initial attachment to the host cell, the parasite fuses its membranes with that of the host cell, so that its cytoplasm is separated from that of the host cell by a membrane of dual origin.

The oocyst stage is extremely robust and is essentially unaffected by chlorination. Indeed, researchers routinely resuspend fecal samples containing oocysts in dilute bleach to rid the sample of bacteria and other infectious agents, leaving viable intact oocysts behind. Water supplies can (realistically) be rendered free of *C. parvum* oocysts only by filtration, as the oocysts are 3 to 5 μm in size. Unhappily, filtration does not appear to lower the risk to zero.

Pathophysiology of Cryptosporidiosis

During infection, the architecture of the intestinal villus is altered. The villus becomes short and blunt, contributing to the decreased absorptive capacity of the intestine, and the intestinal crypts may become hyptertrophied. In animal studies of intestinal function, secretory capacity is relatively spared and absorptive capacity is decreased. Localized prostanoid production contributes to the diarrhea by inhibiting Na+ absorption and inducing net chloride secretion.

Presentations of Intestinal Cryptosporidiosis

Intestinal symptoms tend to present in one of two forms. In the first, the naïve host (usually a child) is infected and has an influenza-like illness with mild systemic complaints and watery diarrhea. The illness is usually dismissed by medical workers as a viral diarrhea, although its resolution over several weeks is at the far end of the temporal spectrum for viral diarrhea. Mild malabsorption is common. In the second major form of the disease, it may present as overwhelming fulminant watery diarrhea that is life-threatening. Parenteral fluids are lifesaving in this circumstance, and eventual use of parenteral hyperalimentation and fluid replacement is a common fate for the immunosuppressed individual. Persistent infection is seen in AIDS and in solid organ transplant recipients. Persistent infection of the biliary and pancreatic ducts can occur, leading to acalculous cholecystitis, obstructive hepatic failure, and pancreatitis.

Respiratory Cryptosporidiosis

The other major manifestation of cryptosporidiosis includes cough and other respiratory symptoms. This is not surprising given the tens or hundreds of billions of oocysts that are excreted by a normal host during infection and the ability of the parasite to invade the respiratory tract epithelium. In studies of childhood cryptosporidiosis, cough is one of the most commonly reported symptoms, reported in about one-fifth to one-third of normal children. In humans with AIDS, respiratory infection is marked by severe persistent cough and dyspnea. One individual with AIDS and immunosuppressive therapy after allogeneic kidney transplantation has been found to have been infected with *Cryptosporidium baileyi*, with involvement of the trachea, larynx, lungs, and intestines at autopsy.

Respiratory cryptosporidiosis is manifest by cough, copious tracheal secretions, and dyspnea. Although respiratory tract infection was followed by diarrhea in most, the cause of death in most was respiratory in nature. Chest radiographs usually reveal diffuse interstitial infiltrates with bronchial accentuation, which may be difficult to distinguish from other processes, such as *Pneumocystis carinii* pneumonia (PCP). Histologic samples show parasites in the ciliated epithelium and a mononuclear cell infiltrate. Death from respiratory cryptosporidiosis can also occur in individuals with other immunosuppressive conditions, such as malignant lymphoma or bone marrow transplantation.

Diagnosis of Respiratory Cryptosporidiosis

The clinician should have a high suspicion of this process in a patient with intestinal cryptosporidiosis. Humans infected with *C. parvum* can have the infection diagnosed by several methods, such as biopsy or stool sampling. Biopsies stained with classic hematoxylin-and-eosin stain should be examined under high oil magnification ($\times 600$ to $\times 1200$), as the parasites are small, seen only on the epithelial surface, and can be mistaken for debris or yeast unless the slide reviewer is attuned to this possibility. Nonetheless, the parasites are easily recognized when looked for. The organism can also be detected by performing a modified acid-fast staining of the expectorated sputum, which is classically nonpurulent, or of bronchial brushings or biopsy material obtained at bronchoscopy. The diagnosis of cyptosporidial pneumonia has been made when acid-fast stains have been performed in a quest for tuberculosis. The parasite oocysts are 4 to 5 μm in diameter and avidly acid-fast; when observed under phase microscopy, the oocyst wall may appear somewhat birefringent. A fluorescent monoclonal antibody to the parasite is also commercially available.

Treatment Options

Treatment of cryptosporidiosis is problematic, as no consistently effective drug therapy exists. Paromomycin is an aminocytol (aminoglycoside) type of antibiotic that is too toxic for systemic use but has found limited use for specific parasitic infections. It is the most commonly effective agent available, although other agents such as azithromycin and atovaquone have had anectodal success. Immunotherapy has been tried with varying degrees of success. One agent has been hyperimmune bovine colostrum administered orally at high doses. Other immunomodulatory measures—such as placing the patient on antiretroviral drugs for HIV infection, thus reducing exogenous immune suppression—have proved beneficial and at times lifesaving. Malnutrition is characterized by a defect in cell-mediated immunity that normalizes with refeeding.

TOXOPLASMOSIS

Etiology and Epidemiology

Toxoplasma gondii is an ubiquitous coccidian parasite that infects all mammals and avians. Its definitive host is the feline (Felidae), be it the house cat or the tiger. Not all *Toxoplasma* infection results in disease, however, and the term *toxoplasmosis* is reserved for those with illness due to the parasite. The parasite persists in the infected host after infection, and thus disease can be either acute or recurrent. The latter is particularly important in the immunosuppressed host, where reactivation can occur as immunity wanes. Pulmonary disease is significant only in the immunosuppressed or congenitally incompetent host.

The life cycle of the parasite is important to understanding its clinical presentations. In its definitive host, the feline, an *intestinal* intraepithelial sexual cycle leads to the passage of oocysts that are 10 to 20 μm in size in the fecal stream. An infected house cat can pass millions of oocysts per day, and the oocysts can persist in the soil for more than a year. They are infectious after sporulation occurs, several days after excretion. In nonfeline hosts such as humans, infection is extraintestinal and asexual. Humans usually acquire the infection by the ingestion of infectious oocysts or by the ingestion of poorly cooked meat that contains cysts filled with the parasite. Vegetables and other crops contaminated with oocysts have also been incriminated in transmission. Unless cannibalism is practiced, human-to-human transmission does not occur except as the result of mother-to-fetus transmission. The ingestion of oocysts or cysts by humans leads to tissue invasion and systemic dissemination of the parasite, as these transmission forms are relatively resistant to stomach acid. Commonly infected mammalian tissues include skeletal and cardiac muscle and brain. Seropositivity rates in France are high, often over 90 percent of the adult population, in contrast to far lower rates in the United States (3 to 70 percent depending on the region). Infection rates are highest in warm and wet climates with a high density of cats; rates are lowest in high, dry, arid climates with few felines. Congenital infection of the fetus, a major public health problem, almost always occurs as a result of infection during gestation, although rare reports of congenital infection after maternal infection just before conception exist. Other rare modes of transmission include transfusion and organ transplantation.

The invasive active asexual form of *T. gondii* is the tachyzoite, which is 3 by 7 μm in size and obligatorily intracellular. The tachyzoite invades host cells, where it multiplies within an intracellular parasitophorous vacuole. Unlike many other intracellular parasites, the tachyzoite can infect nearly any mammalian cell. Eventually the cell lyses, and the motile tachyzoites invade new host cells. In active acute or recurrent disease in immunocompromised humans, this may be the form seen at diagnosis. In the normal host, cysts eventually form, filled with metabolically quiescent bradyzoite parasites. These cysts persist for life, and are 10 to 200 μm in diameter. The bradyzoites can be killed by heating (cooking) above 65°C for 4 min or longer, freezing at −20°C for 24 h or longer with subsequent thawing, or irradiation. Cysts act as a source of infection to the next animal that eats the host or as a source of recrudescent infection should immunity wane.

Immunocompromised people are at great risk of dying from either severe acute or severe recurrent disease. In particular, the receipt of organs from a *Toxoplasma*-seropositive donor by a seronegative recipient has been identified as a major risk. On the basis of experience with cardiac transplantation, it has been theorized that acute infection in the seronegative recipient host is far more dangerous than reactivation of latent disease in the seropositive host. In this latter group, residual antibody may limit disease. Because of the risk of fatal toxoplasmosis in high-risk patients, "baseline" serologic studies for toxoplasmosis are warranted and recommended in those with HIV infection and with lymphomas or leukemias and in patients prior to organ transplantation. In contrast to the organ transplantation recipient, the HIV-seropositive individual who is *Toxoplasma* seropositive (a marker of latent infection) is at much greater risk than the HIV-seropositive, *Toxoplasma*-seronegative person. The estimated risk of an HIV-infected, latently *Toxoplasma*-infected person developing recurrent disease is about 25 to 50 percent. In contrast, the incidence of acute toxoplasmosis in the *Toxoplasma*-seronegative, HIV-seropositive person in the United States is only about 3 percent.

Serologic Testing and Other Diagnostic Methods

Older serologic methods for the detection of *Toxoplasma* antibodies have been replaced in many settings by the availability of enzyme-linked immunosorbent assay (ELISA)–based assays. These include the Sabin-Feldman dye test, the complement fixation test, hemagglutination tests, and the IgM fluorescent antibody test. More modern techniques include ELISA assay methods for both IgG and IgM antibodies, which can assist the clinician in differentiating acute from past exposure. Falling antibody titers in immunocompromised hosts have been associated with active disease, and antibody titers can be unreliable guides in the host with dysregulation of the humoral response. In hosts of this nature, a definitive diagnosis rests upon the histologic demonstration of parasites or the detection of *T. gondii*

DNA using molecular techniques. The molecular assays are fundamentally still research tools. An aggressive attitude toward obtaining biopsy samples is often crucial to the survival of an immunocompromised patient. In rare instances, body fluids or ground tissues from biopsies can be used to inoculate mice or tissue culture cells to make a diagnosis when serologic methods are unreliable.

Clinical Syndromes and Diagnostic Features

Congenital Infection

This is the result of infection in utero. CNS disease is the major sequela, with chorioretinitis, strabismus, blindness, epilepsy, psychomotor or mental retardation, anemia, encephalitis, pneumonitis, microcephaly, intracranial calcification, hydrocephalus, hepatosplenomegaly, and thrombocytopenia reported. Approximately 1 percent of cases are fatal, about 10 percent are severe, 40 percent are mild, and about 50 percent are asymptomatic in the infantile period. Congenital toxoplasmosis in pregnant women with HIV has been reported to be quite virulent. Infection early in gestation appears to result in increased fetal loss and more severe fetal disease. Recent studies suggest that significant disease such as blindness will occur in a majority of the asymptomatic group with the passage of time, and that anti-*Toxoplasma* drug therapy is indicated. This disease is termed *ocular* or *reactivation toxoplasmosis* and is nearly always the result of congenital infection. Scarring of the retina and underlying choroid occurs, and rupture of cysts later in life may result in new disease.

Acute Acquired Toxoplasmosis in the Immunocompetent Host

This is usually of little long-term concern—80 to 90 percent of these cases are asymptomatic, and asymptomatic cervical lymphadenopathy is the hallmark of this disease. It may be confused with mononucleosis caused by Epstein-Barr virus or cytomegalovirus. Fever, malaise, sore throat, and hepatosplenomegaly are also seen, and the peripheral blood may manifest atypical lymphocytosis. Chorioretinitis may be the most significant long-term problem. Very rarely, acute acquired disease may present with severe dissemination, marked by pneumonitis, hepatitis, encephalitis, polymyositis, or myocarditis. This may be the result of an inadequate host immune response.

Histologically, follicular hyperplasia with cortical and paracortical clusters of epithelioid cells that encroach upon the germinal centers is a classic finding in lymph nodes. Sinus histiocytosis is also seen. In cases of dissemination, pulmonary histologic findings include interstitial pneumonitis with focal necrosis and a mononuclear cell infiltrate. Tachyzoites can be found both within and without host cells, and cysts may also be seen. The latter are only rarely found in the normal host when histologic samples are obtained.

Acute Toxoplasmosis in the Immunocompromised Host

This is manifest most often by necrotizing encephalitis as a result of brain cyst reactivation. Myocarditis, hepatosplenomegaly, fever, and interstitial pneumonitis are also common, especially if the disease is the result of acute infection and not reactivation of old latent disease. Toxoplasmic encephalitis usually presents subacutely with focal symptoms in about 90 percent of patients. CT or magnetic resonance imaging (MRI) usually shows discrete focal low-density lesions in the brain with ring enhancement with the administration of an enhancing agent. Indeed, focal neurologic deficits with this set of findings in the *Toxoplasma*-seropositive patient should be initially treated as toxoplasma encephalitis, without performance of a brain biopsy. Diffuse encephalitis can occur with toxoplasmosis in this population, though it is uncommon. Pulmonary disease due to toxoplasmosis is being increasingly recognized.

Pulmonary Disease in the Immunocompromised Host with AIDS

This is usually manifest by prolonged fever, cough, and dyspnea. Rales and a decrease in the percussion note have been observed. Other symptoms and signs of dissemination such as hepatosplenomegaly, headache, myocarditis, and encephalitis may also be present. Blood-borne tachyzoites have been isolated from AIDS patients with this syndrome, supporting the concept of a disseminated disease. Indeed, infection of the bone marrow, adrenals, lymph nodes, kidneys, and nearly every other organ has been documented in this process. *Toxoplasma* pneumonia may be hard to differentiate from PCP, and the two may coexist. The mortality rate in this disease is about one in three. The differential diagnosis in the HIV-seropositive individual includes PCP, disseminated *tuberculosis,* cryptococcosis, leishmaniasis, coccidioidomycosis, and histoplasmosis. Pulmonary cryptosporidiosis or microsporidiosis is usually far milder and is not associated with fevers of the magnitude seen in *Toxoplasma* pneumonitis.

Radiographic patterns include interstitial pneumonia, micronodular infiltrates, nodular densities, cavitation, pleural effusion, and lobar pneumonia. Hilar or mediastinal adenopathy is unusual. Histologically, large numbers of parasites may be seen both free and intracellularly, the latter within epithelial cells or pulmonary macrophages. Hyaline membrane formation, thickened alveolar septa with mononuclear infiltrates, and necrosis due to infarction are found.

Given the large differential diagnosis, bronchoscopy with bronchoalveolar lavage and biopsy are extremely useful in obtaining a secure diagnosis when characteristic CNS disease is lacking or if there is doubt about a single pathogenic process being present. Organisms may be seen within macrophages or other cells, or free in the tissues, and must be differentiated from other intracellular pathogens such as *Leishmania* in the appropriate clinical setting. Bronchoalveolar lavage alone will not detect all cases of *Toxoplasma* pneumonitis, and biopsy should be undertaken expeditiously if lavage alone does not reveal the cause of disease.

Pulmonary Disease in the Immunocompromised Host without AIDS

This is similar to that in AIDS patients with several small differences. In a recent series of 121 patients with organ transplants or underlying malignancies, 23 percent had pulmonary involvement. Most (76 percent) had CNS involvement, and 38 percent had cardiac disease. In the subset that had received transplants, 58 percent had myocarditis. Death or serious morbidity was nearly inevitable if the correct diagnosis was not accomplished (88 of 89 patients).

MICROSPORIDIOSIS

Microsporidia are a diverse group of obligate intracellular pathogens that form spores. They lack mitochondria and have the small subunit ribosomal structures usually found in prokaryotes, suggesting that they diverged from eukaryotes at a very early evolutionary stage. Historically they have been recognized as important pathogens of bees, silkworms, and fish. Over 100 genera and 1000 species are recognized. In the last decade, Microsporidia have emerged as pathogens of humans with AIDS. Though usually thought of as intestinal pathogens, Microsporidia have been found to cause disseminated disease including pneumonia in many immunocompromised hosts.

Transmission and Life Cycle

Details of transmission in humans are quite scanty. Given that a number of the five species that have been described in humans have primarily intestinal manifestations, the suspicion has been that the pathogen is primarily acquired through the ingestion of spores. Pulmonary infections also suggest that aerosol or inhalation transmission is possible. Sexual transmission has also been considered, since spores can be found in the urine in disseminated disease. In laboratory animals such as rabbits, ingestion of urine can efficiently transmit *Encephalitozoon cuniculi.* Vertical transmission to nonhuman species has been documented but not in humans to date.

There is suggestive but not conclusive evidence that fecal-oral transmission is important with Microsporidia. Four microsporidial genera have clearly been involved in human disease: *Nosema* (usually pathogens of bees and other insects), *Encephalitozoon* (*E. cuniculi, E. hellem*), *Enterocytozoon bieneusi* (only found in humans to date), and *Pleistophora* (usually a pathogen of fish). *Septata intestinalis* has now been reclassified as *Encephalitozoon intestinalis* and is found only in humans. Several other infections have not been classifiable, although they resembled the genus *Nosema. E. cuniculi* has been found in mammals and birds, whereas *E. hellem* has only been found in humans. *Nosema* infections have been described in an immunologically privileged site, the corneum, in normal hosts.

Pathology

In the first autopsy conducted on an AIDS patient with disseminated microsporidiosis, the striking finding was the presence of *E. hellem* in the eyes, urinary tract, and respiratory tract. Numerous organisms were found lining the tracheobronchial tree, suggesting respiratory acquisition of the infection. Pulmonary microsporidiosis appears to present with bronchiolitis and with infiltrates. Slight fibrosis of the alveolar walls, and intraepithelial infiltration of bronchioli by lymphocytes, has been found. Clusters of spores found in the supranuclear region of bronchial epithelial cells are characteristically seen with *E. bieneusi* infections.

Presentation and Diagnosis

Intestinal microsporidiosis presents with profuse, watery diarrhea. Patients may also present with sterile pyuria, visual loss, or seizures. Patients with pulmonary microsporidiosis have presented with dyspnea on exertion, cough, wheezing, small interstitial infiltrates on chest radiographs, small infiltrates, and small pleural effusions. An increased alveolar-arterial oxygen gradient has also been seen.

Sputa, bronchoalveolar lavage fluid, stool, urine, biopsy samples, and impression smears have all been useful in making the diagnosis. The diagnosis of microsporidiosis is difficult in the typical clinical laboratory. Methods that have proved useful include a modified trichrome stain and fluorescent dye techniques, which take advantage of the fact that the wall of the microsporidial cyst contains chitin and binds the dye. Electron microscopy is the diagnostic "gold standard," but its expense makes its routine use impractical.

Treatment

No known drug treats all genera of Microsporidia. Albendazole and other benzimidazoles have been used in a variety of settings and appear to be useful in the treatment of *E. bieneusi, E. (Septata) intestinalis,* and other *Encephalitozoon* species. Reduction in immune compromise is key. Newer agents are under study.

LEISHMANIASIS

Leishmaniasis has emerged as a rare pulmonic infection, usually in the HIV-infected individual or in the organ transplant recipient. *Leishmania* species, protozoa of the order Kinetoplastida, cause distinctive syndromes: cutaneous disease with nonhealing ulcerations ("Aleppo sore," "Delhi boil"), diffuse cutaneous disease, mucosal and facial disease with rather severe disfigurement ("espundia"), and visceral or systemic leishmaniasis ("kala-azar"). These diseases are rare and usually imported into North America or northern Europe; however, there are important foci around the Mediterranean, the Balkans, the Middle East, and northern Africa. In Central and South America, leishmaniasis is endemic, as it is in South Asia, China, and the Himalayan countries, such as Pakistan and Iran. Leishmaniasis has been reported from every country on the continental Americas except Canada, Chile, and Uruguay; Brazil and Peru are the countries with the highest incidence in South America. Given the expanding HIV pandemic, pulmonary leishmaniasis will be seen more and more frequently. For example, increasing numbers of reports from France, Italy, and Spain describe visceral leishmaniasis in HIV-seropositive individuals.

Leishmania species have a dimorphic life cycle. In mammalian hosts, such as humans, canines, and rodents, the organisms live within macrophages. Canines are an important reservoir host for *Leishmania,* and canine control programs have proved crucial to the elimination of this chronic and debilitating disease. Parasites are ingested by the bite of the insect vector, usually a sandfly of the genus *Lutzomyia* in the Western Hemisphere and *Phlebotomus* elsewhere. Within the sandfly, the parasite transforms from the intracellular amastigote form through a series of flagellated intermediate stages into infectious promastigotes over the course of an ensuing week. These motile stages migrate to the proboscis of the sandfly and occlude the lumen of the proboscis. They are then injected when the insect probes the next host, hoping for a blood meal. The injected promastigotes invade mononuclear phagocytes, and, once within a parasitophorous vacuole, transform back into the amastigote (nonflagellar) stage. Amastigotes then replicate by asexual fission. Eventually cell death occurs, and released amastigotes infect other mononuclear phagocytic cells recruited to the area of inflammation. In local disease, the lesions are limited, but in visceral or disseminated disease, parasites can be found throughout the reticuloendothelial system. No sexual stage has been identified in *Leishmania* to date.

CLINICAL MANIFESTATIONS AND DIAGNOSIS

Disseminated or Visceral Disease (Kala-Azar)

In this syndrome, fever and abdominal organomegaly are the rule. Kala-azar is the older but still pleasing term for generalized involvement including the spleen, bone marrow, liver, and other organs. The usual incubation period is 3 to 8 months but can be as long as 3 years. Fever, weight loss, pallor, anorexia, anemia, hypergammaglobulinemia, and hepatosplenomegaly are the major consequences. Death is frequently due to concomitant infections, such as tuberculosis, pneumonia, sepsis, or dysentery, or to the effects of the infection itself with malnutrition, cachexia, and progressively severe anemia.

Individuals with HIV typically present with fever, hepatosplenomegaly, and pancytopenia, although atypical presentations occur without all these three findings. Involvement of the lungs and other thoracic structures, oral mucosa and esophagus, intestine, skin, and bone marrow has been reported. In addition to the other manifestations of disseminated disease, cough and dyspnea are hallmarks of pulmonary leishmaniasis. Chest radiographs usually show a diffuse and subtle interstitial process unless a second pneumonic process is present. Respiratory distress syndrome, disseminated intravascular coagulation, and hepatic and renal insufficiency with subsequent death have occurred after antileishmanial therapy was begun for disseminated leishmaniasis. Leishmaniasis has also been seen in organ transplant recipients.

Cutaneous and Mucosal (Localized) Disease

Phrases such as *Delhi boil* and *Aleppo sore* date to colonial times in India and the Middle East and describe cutaneous nonhealing ulcers due to *Leishmania* species. These all refer to localized disease, found at the site of a sandfly bite and inoculation. In general this form of leishmaniasis is not life-threatening, and resolution of the ulcer occurs with the development of immunity to the strain of infecting *Leishmania*. Cutaneous disease is far more common than mucosal disease in the Old World.

In contrast, in the New World, mucosal disease is relatively more common and more worrisome and is a major public health hazard in some countries. *Espundia* is a Brazilian word describing mucosal disease. Mucosal disease may include destructive lesions of the oropharynx that prevent the ingestion of foods, and death from inanition may result. In addition, aspiration pneumonia is a common event in the late stages of oronasal destruction.

BABESIOSIS

Babesiosis is caused by tick-borne parasites of the genus *Babesia*. Clinically this disease most resembles malaria, as the organism is a parasite of erythrocytes. In most people, this is a relatively mild disease. In the splenectomized or otherwise immunosuppressed person, the disease can be fatal. The diagnosis of ARDS due to *Babesia* is just as much an emergency as it is for falciparum malaria, and drug therapy and exchange transfusion are likely to be lifesaving.

In the normal host, babesiosis is self-limited, and probably of little long-term consequence. Nonetheless it is manifested by fever, myalgias, anorexia, hemolysis, and occasionally jaundice and hemoglobinuria. It is said that a dry cough is not uncommon in babesiosis. The fever of babesiosis is usually not cyclical, as it may be in established malaria caused by a single brood of parasites. Thrombocytopenia is common in moderate to severe disease, as is renal dysfunction. The diagnosis is made by examination of blood smears, which show typical intraerythrocytic ring forms or tetrads of parasites. Malaria and babesiosis are often confused by the inexperienced reviewer of the peripheral blood smear. However, the lack of gametocytes in babesiosis, parasites that fill the erythrocyte in malaria, or malarial pigment help to distinguish *Babesia* from *Plasmodium* parasites.

In severe cases, especially in those people with no spleen, the presentation can mimic sepsis and include respiratory failure with ARDS. The mechanism of respiratory embarrassment is unknown, though it acts like ARDS both radiologically and clinically. In endemic areas, evaluation of the cause of the sepsis syndrome should include the review of a blood smear for *Babesia* parasites. The diagnosis is often serendipitously made by hematology laboratory technologists who are performing a manual differential leukocyte count.

Treatment, if warranted, usually consists of clindamycin 600 mg (intravenous or oral, thrice daily) combined with quinine (650 mg thrice daily) for at least 7 days. Therapy may need to be extended in the very ill, immunosuppressed, or splenectomized host.

PARASITIC HELMINTHS

Parasitic helminths are a distinct group of infectious agents that are responsible for worldwide morbidity and mortality in humans. People with helminthic infections of the lungs often seek medical advice because of one or more common chest complaints—cough, pain, or breathlessness. In humans, worms produce a variety of pulmonary parenchymal and vascular diseases (Table 65-1).

Biology and Immunology

A basic biologic generalization about helminthic infections is that the worms, as a rule, cannot multiply within the mammalian host. There are exceptions to this rule. For example, *Strongyloides stercoralis* and *Echinococcus granulosus* can increase their numbers within a host. This ability of *S. stercoralis* to autoinfect the same subject and cause a hyperinfection syndrome is of considerable clinical significance in immunosuppressed patients. A different example is that of *Echinococcosis,* in which dissemination is usually a consequence of leakage or rupture of a hydatid cyst—thereby releasing its contents, which seed sites elsewhere and initiate similar lesions.

Another biologic characteristic of worm infections, particularly those migrating in host tissues such as the lungs, is the association with eosinophilia in the peripheral blood and tissue. When eosinophilia is marked, this association provides a clinically useful sign of a migratory worm infection. The mechanism and specificity of this eosinophilic response depend on the integrity of the *cellular* immune response of the host: sensitized T lymphocytes produce mediators that induce differentiation in the bone marrow or progenitor cells into mature eosinophils; this is done either directly or via other cell products from mononuclear phagocytes. Eosinophilia does not occur in athymic nude mice infected with *Trichinella spiralis* or *Schistosoma mansoni.* Similarly, eosinophilia often does not feature prominently when strongyloidiasis occurs in immunosuppressed persons. In vitro, eosinophils along with antibodies or complement kill the larval forms of several helminths. The killing of parasites is accompanied by a respiratory burst in these cells and evacuation of the contents of their granules onto the surface of the helminth. In vivo, depletion of eosinophils in experimental animals leads to loss of their acquired resistance to infection from several helminths, such as *T. spiralis* and *S. mansoni.* Both oxidative and nonoxidative products of eosinophil granules have been implicated in target killing.

TABLE 65-1 Pulmonary Parenchymal and Vascular Diseases Produced by Worms

Major pulmonary presentation	Infection	Causative organism	Infective stage	Pathogenic stage
Loeffler-like syndrome	Ascariasis	*Ascaris lumbricoides*	Embryonated eggs in soil	Migrating larvae
	Hookworms	*Ancylostoma duodenale, Necator americanus*	Larvae in soil Larvae in soil	Migrating larvae
	Strongyloidiasis	*Strongyloides stercoralis*	Larvae in soil	Migrating rhabditiform larvae
	Hyperinfection with *S. stercoralis*	*S. stercoralis*	Larvae in bowel	Migrating filariform larvae
Pulmonary eosinophilia	Lymphatic filariasis	*Wuchereria bancrofti, Brugia malayi*	Larvae in mosquito	Microfilariae
Space-occupying lesions	Echinococcosis Hydatid cysts	*Echinococcus granulosus*	Eggs in soil	
	Paragonimiasis	*Paragonimus westermani*	Metacercariae	Adult worms
	Schistosomiasis	*Schistosoma mansoni, S. japonicum, S. haematobium*	Cercariae in fresh water	Eggs

DISEASES DUE TO NEMATODES (ROUNDWORMS)

Ascariasis, Hookworms, and Strongyloidiasis

Human infections with *Ascaris lumbricoides,* with the hookworms *Ancylostoma duodenale* and *Necator americanus,* and with *S. stercoralis* are among the most prevalent helminthiases worldwide. Transmission also occurs in the southeastern United States.

Epidemiology and Life Cycle

Human ascariasis results from ingestion of embryonated *A. lumbricoides* eggs that are contained in feces-contaminated soil. Ingestion of contaminated vegetables and fruits that have not been properly washed is the most frequent transmission vehicle. *Ascaris* eggs hatch in the gastrointestinal tract, producing larvae that penetrate the gut wall and migrate via venous blood and the right side of the heart to the lungs. Hookworms (*A. duodenale* and *N. americanus*) and *S. stercoralis* infect humans when infective larvae, found in soil, penetrate intact skin. Larvae of hookworms or of *S. stercoralis* travel via the bloodstream to the lungs (Table 65-1). The parasite larvae migrate via pulmonary capillaries into alveolar spaces. They then ascend toward the trachea to be swallowed en route to their final habitat in the small intestine. Although larvae are sometimes found in the sputum of infected persons, more often the eggs (*A. lumbricoides, A. duodenale,* and *N. americanus*) or the larvae *(S. stercoralis)* are found in stools. Passage to the outside environment, where the stool forms develop into stages infective for humans, completes their life cycle.

Pathogenesis and Pathology

In nematode infections, the most prominent pulmonary pathologic changes occur in persons with ascariasis or with the hyperinfection syndrome of strongyloidiasis. *Ascaris* pneumonia may occur in 1 to 2 weeks after infection. Portions of larvae are seen in the pulmonary parenchyma, surrounded by patchy infiltrate of neutrophils and eosinophils. The alveoli contain a serous exudate; the production of bronchial mucus is increased. Later, migrating larvae are destroyed within aggregates of eosinophils. The nature of the inflammatory process in *Ascaris* pneumonia suggests hypersensitivity. The intensity of the reaction depends on the number of parasite larvae and on previous sensitization. In areas in which transmission of *Ascaris* eggs occurs seasonally, pulmonary reactions are usually more in evidence during these periods.

In *immunocompetent* subjects, pulmonary disease caused by hookworms or *S. stercoralis* is unremarkable. However, infection with *S. stercoralis* can be life-threatening in *immunocompromised* subjects. Filariform larvae seem to develop prematurely in immunocompromised persons and invade the gut wall or the perianal skin. Tissue migration occurs through most body organs, including the lungs. Initially, the pulmonary lesions resemble those of *Ascaris* pneumonia. In some patients, bronchopneumonia and lung abscesses develop. The lungs of fatal cases show intraalveolar hemorrhages and inflammatory changes.

Clinical Features

The major clinical manifestations caused by infection of the lungs with the larval forms of intestinal nematodes resemble those of Loeffler's syndrome;

these manifestations occur typically in patients with seasonal or *Ascaris* pneumonia. The symptoms include persistent, irritating, and nonproductive cough, substernal pain, and, in the severely ill, hemoptysis and dyspnea. Eosinophilia is the most consistent laboratory finding. Radiographic signs—e.g., patchy or miliary infiltrate—are sometimes seen.

The onset of the Loeffler-like syndrome caused by intestinal nematodes usually occurs 2 to 3 weeks after infection, coincident with larval migration from the pulmonary circulation to the alveoli. This coincidence was illustrated by the occurrence of the syndrome in a group of students exposed to eggs of the pig roundworm *(A. suum)*. Typical symptoms occurred 10 to 15 days later; some of the students developed marked respiratory failure. In locations where transmission of ascariasis is cyclic because of environmental factors, pneumonitis occurs seasonally. Mild symptoms are occasionally encountered in persons with hookworm infection or in immunocompetent subjects who have strongyloidiasis.

The most clinically significant pulmonary syndrome induced by intestinal nematodes is caused by hyperinfection with *S. stercoralis*. As a rule, the syndrome occurs in patients with compromised cell-mediated immunity, although it is occasionally encountered in normal persons. Immunosuppression is usually caused by neoplastic diseases, such as Hodgkin's, other lymphomas and leukemias, or nonmalignant conditions that are being treated with corticosteroids—e.g., organ transplantation. The sequence of events in immunosuppressed patients indicates that a change has occurred in the reproductive cycle of the parasite: in nonimmunosuppressed subjects, the rhabditiform larvae have to go to the outside world to transform into the infective filariform organisms; in immunosuppressed patients, the change to infective larvae occurs within the host. The organisms penetrate the intestinal mucosa, resulting in massive invasion of almost every organ including the lungs. The major clinical features include asthma, pulmonary opacities and cavitation, consolidation, and diffuse focal infiltrates. Usually, widespread dissemination of the nematode is accompanied by secondary infection caused by gram-negative organisms carried along with *S. stercoralis*. Eosinophilia is often absent in patients with the *S. stercoralis* hyperinfection syndrome, probably because of defective cell-mediated immunity. The *S. stercoralis* hyperinfection syndrome is often fatal: mortality occurs in up to 77 percent of people with such infections.

Management

Definitive diagnosis of infection due to intestinal nematodes is often delayed for weeks, until the adult worms mature in the small intestine. At this stage, fecal examination will disclose the characteristic eggs of hookworms or *Ascaris* or the larvae of *S. stercoralis*. The management of patients with the pulmonary manifestations of these parasitic worms is nonspecific and symptomatic. Reduction of exposure in areas where transmission of ascariasis is seasonal will decrease the prevalence and severity of clinical presentations. Specific antihelminthic therapy is ineffective during the pulmonary stage but can cure the infection once the parasites reach maturity in the small intestine.

Mebendazole is the drug of choice for treating ascariasis and hookworms. It is given orally, 100 mg per day for 2 to 3 days. Thiabendazole, 25 mg/kg body weight, twice daily for 2 days, is the recommended treatment for intestinal strongyloidiasis. In patients suspected of having the hyperinfection syndrome, early diagnosis, modification of the immunosuppressive therapy, and prompt anti-*Strongyloides* chemotherapy are the important elements in averting a fatal outcome. Therapy should be directed at gastrointestinal bacteria as well as the worms. Some preference for ivermectin (200 μg/kg/day for 1 to 2 days) has developed, particularly in the organ transplant recipient in whom hepatotoxocity associated with thiabendazole may not be acceptable. Most instances of strongyloidiasis in these patients are diagnosed at autopsy or shortly before death. Aggressive efforts at demonstrating *S. stercoralis* larvae entail repeated examination of stools and duodenal aspirates. Sputum and bronchial washings are examined for parasite larvae. Serology may be of help. Alternatively, thiabendazole is started as early as possible and continued for 10 to 15 days.

Pulmonary Filariasis (Tropical Pulmonary Eosinophilia)

Persons living in areas endemic for *Wuchereria bancrofti* and *Brugia malayi* may present with an acute or chronic lung disease usually referred to as *tropical pulmonary eosinophilia*. This is still a poorly defined clinical entity. Its main features are a history of residence in filaria-endemic areas, particularly India, chronic nocturnal paroxysmal cough, marked eosinophilia, positive serologic evidence, and a therapeutic response to the administration of diethylcarbamazine.

Epidemiology and Life Cycle

Human infection with the tissue nematodes *W. bancrofti* or *B. malayi* can cause several amicrofilaremic syndromes, including tropical pulmonary eosinophilia. Infection is transmitted by the bite of several species of mosquitoes, thereby introducing the infective third-stage larvae. These organisms undergo ill-defined maturational stages culminating in the development of adult male and female worms that are usually situated in lymphatic vessels and lymph nodes. Mature worms deposit microfilariae that appear in peripheral circulation, often at maximum numbers at specific times of the day. However, some filariae show no periodicity with respect to the appearance of their microfilariae in peripheral blood. Microfilariae are taken up by mosquitoes during their bites, thereby completing the life cycle of the parasite.

Despite negative blood examinations, microfilariae have been found in lung and lymph node biopsies, confirming the filarial origin of this syndrome. Serologic or histopathologic evidence of infection can be obtained, even though larvae cannot be found in the blood.

Pathogenesis and Pathology

Patients with pulmonary filariasis *(tropical pulmonary eosinophilia)* show evidence of humoral hyperreactivity manifest as increased serum levels of total IgE and antifiliarial IgG and IgE. The possibility has been raised that these antibodies play a causal role in producing the pulmonary symptoms by inducing clearance of microfilariae and acute IgE-mediated responses, which are manifest clinically as asthma and eosinophilic pulmonary infiltrates. Histopathologically, the earliest lesions are histiocytic infiltrates in the interstitium and alveolar spaces. In established cases, the cell infiltrate consists predominantly of eosinophils, lymphocytes, and histiocytes, and it assumes a nodular configuration.

Clinical Features

Young males are predominantly afflicted with tropical pulmonary eosinophilia. The syndrome is characterized by episodes of dry night cough, low-grade fever, and general fatigue. Examination of the chest may reveal coarse rales and rhonchi, along with wheezing. In many patients, pulmonary function tests disclose a restrictive pattern in which vital and total lung capacity and residual volumes are all decreased. Some patients with chronic disease have perfusion impairment. Radiographically, the syndrome may be associated with reticulonodular opacities and increased bronchovascular markings. The sera of these patients usually demonstrate high IgE levels and specific antibodies to the parasite. Eosinophil counts in peripheral blood generally exceed 3000/mm^3.

Management

Diagnosis is based on the typical clinical, radiographic, functional, and immunologic findings in the setting of an appropriate epidemiology history—i.e., previous residence in a filaria-endemic area. A favorable response to diethylcarbamazine therapy confirms the diagnosis. The drug is usually administered as 5 mg/kg/day in divided doses for 2 to 3 weeks. Recurrences of tropical pulmonary eosinophilia are rare. If they do occur, a second course of antihelminthic chemotherapy is indicated.

Dirofilariasis

Another filarial parasite, *Dirofilaria immitis* (dog heartworm), may accidentally be transmitted to humans by the bites of the mosquito intermediate vector. In most, the infection is discovered as a coin lesion on the chest radiograph. In some, cough, chest pain, hemoptysis, and eosinophilia were manifest. Definitive diagnosis is usually obtained from microscopic examination of excised lesions.

Toxocariasis (Visceral Larva Migrans)

Toxocariasis is due to human infection with animal parasites (dog or cat ascarids). It is most commonly encountered in children. The invading parasite larvae migrate in human tissues, but cannot mature to adult worms. *Toxocara canis* and *T. cati* are the two recognized etiologic agents of human visceral larva migrans. They both are widely distributed, in both developing and developed countries.

Etiology

The eggs of *T. canis* and *T. cati* are passed in the stools of dogs and cats, respectively. Transmission to humans occurs by ingestion of embryonated eggs in the soil or by contamination of food. Larvae hatch in the small intestine, penetrate the gut wall, migrate to the liver, and are then carried via systemic veins to the systemic arterial circulation for distribution throughout the body. Larval migration through the host tissues and the associated inflammatory responses are considered responsible for the manifestations of disease. Most of these manifestations relate to liver pathology, eosinophilia, and pulmonary invasion. The concentrations in serum of total and specific immunoglobulins are also increased.

Pathogenesis and Pathology

It is not clear whether tissue injury results from the invasion of different organs by the parasite larvae or from death and encapsulation of some organisms by an eosinophilic response of the host. The most commonly affected organ is the liver, in which granulomas surround parasite larvae. Similar lesions can be induced in experimental animals. In the few fatal cases of toxocariasis, autopsy revealed that the major pathologic lesions were in the CNS.

Clinical Features

Toxocariasis is a disease of children 1 to 4 years of age. It is particularly common in those with a history of pica. The two main presenting features relate to the chest and abdomen. Pulmonary complaints, such as cough and wheezing, and pulmonary infiltrates occur in more than one-third of symptomatic children. Peripheral eosinophilia is usually marked and may persist for years. Hepatomegaly is common.

Management

Toxocariasis is a cosmopolitan infection of children. Diagnosis is suspected because of the clinical presentation and serologic evidence of anti-*Toxocara* antibodies. Since the disease is usually benign and self-limiting and since the efficacy of most antihelminthics against *Toxocara* infection is doubtful, no specific therapy is recommended. Corticosteroids may be necessary to limit the inflammatory response in patients with extensive disease of the lungs or central nervous system.

Rare Nematode Infections

In severe human *T. spiralis* infection, pneumonitis is accompanied by eosinophilia. The pulmonary syndrome follows the intestinal phase of infection and is usually associated with other allergic manifestations of trichinosis, including periorbital edema, muscle swelling, and weakness.

Anisakiasis—due to the roundworm *Anisakis marina*—in humans results from infection with the larval form of a nematode of marine mammals. The disease has been reported in Japan and Western Europe. Although it is usually manifested as an intestinal eosinophilic disorder, it has also been implicated as the probable cause of cough, eosinophilia, and pleural effusion.

DISEASES DUE TO CESTODES (SEGMENTED WORMS)

Echinococcosis

Human infection with the larval stage of the canine tapeworm *Echinococcus granulosus* is one of the most important helminthic pulmonary diseases. *E. granulosus* is worldwide in distribution; it occurs most commonly in sheep- and cattle-raising areas, particularly in Australia, South America, the Mediterranean, and some parts of Africa. The infection has also been reported in the United States.

Epidemiology and Life Cycle

Adult *E. granulosus* worms are found in the intestines of dogs and wolves; they release eggs from their gravid segments that are passed in the feces. Humans acquire the infection by ingesting the eggs; embryos are then released and migrate to the liver, where most cysts in humans are found. Embryos may also migrate to the lungs or other tissues. Once the parasite has lodged in human tissues, it may develop in a space-occupying hydatid cyst. The inner lining of these cysts is a germinal layer capable of producing daughter cysts that may seed other organs upon spontaneous rupture or surgical manipulation of the original cyst.

Pathogenesis and Pathology

Hydatid cysts are more frequently found in the lungs of children than those of adults. In most instances, the slowly enlarging space-occupying lesion is well tolerated. Cysts in the lungs are usually discovered early in the course of the disease because radiographic examinations of the chest are now so common. Pulmonary cysts are usually solitary. The classic unilocular hydatid cyst is usually fertile: cyst contents can seed other sites and start new cysts. The cyst is surrounded early in the course of infection by a granulomatous reaction on the part of the host; later, the inflammatory reaction is succeeded by fibrosis. Rupture of a fertile hydatid cyst may occur through a bronchus, leading to expectoration of scolices in the sputum. Rupture into the mediastinum or pleural cavity can lead to secondary implantations. The fluid content of a hydatid cyst is believed to be immunogenic, and leakage of the cyst may evoke an anaphylactic response. Occasionally eosinophilia has been reported to accompany hydatid disease of the lung.

Clinical Features

Hydatid cysts are usually asymptomatic; approximately half of the clinically diagnosed cysts are in the lungs. Most patients with pulmonary hydatid disease are children. In about three-fourths of patients, the cysts are in one lobe. Approximately half of the patients present with cough; smaller fractions present with dyspnea or chest pain. On chest radiography, the lesions vary in diameter from 1 to 20 cm; sometimes the cyst is surrounded by an area of pneumonitis or atelectasis. Less often, a fluid level, the "water lily sign," or calcification is seen. Other diagnostic procedures—e.g., serology and computed tomography—may be useful in improving characterization of the lesions.

Management

In most instances, diagnosis of the hydatid nature of a pulmonary cyst depends on immunologic procedures. Surgery is the treatment of choice for hydatid disease of the lungs, but spillage must be prevented. There is no satisfactory medical treatment for hydatid disease. This is particularly the case in pulmonary hydatid disease. Albendazole is the current recommended therapeutic agent.

DISEASES DUE TO TREMATODES (FLATWORMS)

Schistosomiasis

Schistosomal infections of humans represent one of the major endemic helminthiases in Southeast Asia, the Middle East, Africa, the Caribbean, and South America. Five species represent the most common and clinically significant infections: *Schistosoma haematobium, S. mansoni, S. japonicum, S. mekongi,* and *S. intercalatum.*

Epidemiology and Life Cycle

The schistosomes are blood flukes; in humans, they inhabit the venous system around the urinary bladder or the small and large intestines. Human infection is initiated by penetration of intact skin by the free-living cercariae that are shed by specific freshwater snails. The cercariae change within a few hours into schistosomula, which migrate from the subcutaneous tissues to the lungs and then the liver, where they mature into adult worms. Fecund adult parasites then migrate to their final habitat: the veins around the ureters and urinary bladder *(S. haematobium)* and the mesenteric veins (all other species). Adult worms deposit eggs that are intended to pass through the lumens of ureters or gut to the outside environment in order to complete the life cycle of the parasite. However, some of these ova may be trapped in the host tissues. Other ova may be carried by the venous circulation to the heart and then lungs. In *S. haematobium* infection, schistosome eggs reach the pulmonary circulation via the inferior vena cava. Eggs of the other species reach the systemic circulation after the development of portal hypertension and portosystemic anastomosis.

Pathogenesis and Pathology

Schistosome eggs reach the pulmonary circulation by routes that depend on the species of the parasite, their final habitat, and the stage of infection. Because *S. haematobium* worms parasitize the vesical plexus, which connects directly with the inferior vena cava, egg seeding to the lungs may occur at any phase of infection. By contrast, the anatomic location of adult worms of the other species in the mesenteric veins does not allow parasite ova to travel through the portal to the hepatic, and subsequently systemic, circulations. Eggs of these species are believed to reach the lungs only in the late stages of infection, after portal hypertension develops and anastomotic channels open between the portal and systemic circulations.

Upon reaching the pulmonary circulation, schistosome eggs usually gather in small arterioles, where they induce the formation of delayed-hypersensitivity granulomas, made up of eosinophils, lymphocytes, and macrophages. In addition, deposition of fibrous tissue causes narrowing, thickening, and occlusion of pulmonary arterioles. In an autopsy study of 32 cases of *S. mansoni* cor pulmonale, two characteristic histopathologic lesions were identified: (1) focal changes, related directly to the presence of schistosome eggs, that were located either within the alveolar tissue or within the pulmonary arteries or arterioles, and (2) plexiform or angiomatoid lesions consisting of several thin-walled and dilated vessels. The most prominent vascular lesions were associated with the focal changes surrounding mature schistosome eggs in the lumens of pulmonary arteries or arterioles. These were accompanied by fibrin deposition and remarkable proliferation of endothelial cells. Fibrosis surrounds most focal lesions. Because of the curtailment of the pulmonary vasculature and the decreased distensibility caused by the perivascular fibrosis, pulmonary hypertension and cor pulmonale ensue. Pulmonary function is predominantly restrictive and is accompanied by a decrease in the diffusing capacity.

Clinical Features

It is not clear whether schistosomal infection during its early phases in humans is associated with appreciable pulmonary disease. Migration of schistosomula through human lungs is not known to cause detectable symptoms or signs. By contrast, after the onset of oviposition, some ova may reach the lungs, particularly in *S. haematobium* infection. Furthermore, chronic infection with the other schistosome species may be associated with sufficient deposition of eggs in the lungs to cause the development of cor pulmonale. The clinical and radiographic findings in schistosomal pulmonary hypertension and cor pulmonale are not distinctive. In Egypt, 7.5 percent of patients hospitalized with schistosomal hepatomegaly had cor pulmonale; in Brazil, 23 percent of similar patients had pulmonary hypertension (i.e., >20 mmHg).

Management

Diagnosis of pulmonary disease due to schistosomiasis may be achieved by finding the parasite eggs in urine or stools of persons with suggestive clinical manifestations. However, pulmonary disease may occur several years after infection, and finding parasite ova may be difficult. Under these circumstances, demonstrating the characteristic pathologic changes and ova in tissues or positive serology may settle the diagnosis. Active schistosome infections are treated with praziquantel, which kills adult worms and stops further destruction of tissue by ova deposition. The drug is administered as a single oral dose of 40 mg/kg body weight for *S. mansoni* and *S. haematobium* infection and in a dose of 20 mg/kg body weight three times a day for *S. japonicum* infection. Reversal of pathologic lesions in the lungs after antischistosomal chemotherapy has not been documented.

Paragonimiasis

Human infection with species of the lung fluke *Paragonimus* is prevalent in the Far East, Africa, and South and Central America. Infection is maintained in endemic areas through contamination of water sources, with feces or sputum of infected individuals resulting in infection of the intermediate snail and crustacean hosts. Symptomatic paragonimiasis is initially characterized by cough and bloody sputum that may lead to bronchiectasis or lung abscesses.

Epidemiology and Life Cycle

Human infection with *Paragonimus* is acquired from eating raw or pickled crustaceans (freshwater crayfish and crabs) that harbor the infective parasite stage (metacercariae). These forms excyst in the duodenum, penetrate the intestinal wall, and migrate via the diaphragm and pleural cavity to the lungs, where they mature into adult worms (12 × 6 × 5 mm). Adult *Paragonimus* worms are hermaphroditic; they produce golden-brown eggs, which are coughed up and voided through either sputum or feces. The life cycle of the parasite outside the human host goes through a specific snail intermediate host; metacercariae then encyst on freshwater crustaceans.

Pathogenesis and Pathology

The primary site of infection in humans is the lung. The worm is also found in the brain in 25 percent of patients and less often in many other tissues. During invasion of the lungs by the maturing adult worms, parasite tunnels in the pulmonary parenchyma can usually be demonstrated, particularly in peripheral areas. The tunnels and parasites are surrounded by a granulocytic reaction made of eosinophils and neutrophils. Charcot-Leyden crystals are often seen. In patients with encysted worms, the parasites are enclosed with cystic lesions that may communicate with each other or with a bronchus. Death of the worms usually leads to collapse of the cyst, disintegration of the parasite, and fibrosis or calcification. The surrounding pulmonary tissue may show evidence of atelectasis, bronchiectasis, or compensatory emphysema.

In some patients, secondary infection and lung abscess develop in the cystic lesions surrounding adult parasites. The radiographic changes correspond roughly to the three stages of parasite development within the lungs: (1) on arrival in the lungs, maturing worms are associated with the development of radiographic opacities; (2) these are succeeded by nodules that correspond to the parasite cysts; (3) fibrosis or calcification ensues.

Clinical Features

The incubation period between infection and the development of maturing adults in the lungs is 2 to 20 days. Few specific symptoms have been described during this stage. In persons with established infection, the worm load seems to determine the extent of clinical features. In moderate to heavy worm loads, complaint of cough and respiratory discomfort (particularly upon rising in the morning) and rusty, blood-tinged sputum containing parasite eggs, necrotic material, and Charcot-Leyden crystals are common. Frank hemoptysis, sometimes severe, also occurs in patients with pulmonary paragonimiasis. The chest radiograph is normal in 10 to 20 percent of infected persons. Radiographic signs in the others include infiltrate, cavitation, fibrosis, and pulmonary thickening. The characteristic ring shadow with a crescent corona occurs in some infected persons.

Management

The diagnosis of paragonimiasis is made from detection of the characteristic eggs in the sputum or stools of infected persons. Serologic testing may be helpful in egg-negative cases. The drug of choice for treating paragonimiasis is praziquantel. It is administered orally, 75 mg/kg per day for 2 days. Chemotherapy usually leads to cessation of egg passage in sputum and stools, some clearing of the chest radiograph in almost two-thirds of treated patients, and a decrease in serum IgG antibodies against the parasite.

BIBLIOGRAPHY

Adams EB, MacLeod IN: Invasive amebiasis: I. Amebic dysentery and its complications. *Medicine* 56:315–323, 1977.

Adams EB, MacLeod IN: Invasive amebiasis: II. Amebic liver abscess and its complications. *Medicine* 56:325–334, 1977.

Adkins RB, Dao AH: Pulmonary dirofilariasis: A diagnostic challenge. *South Med J* 77:372–374, 1984.

Boustani MR, Lepore TJ, Gelfand JA, Lazarus DS: Acute respiratory failure in patients treated for babesiosis (review). *Am J Respir Crit Care Med* 149:1689–1691, 1994.

Current WL, Garcia LS: Cryptosporidiosis. *Clin Microbiol Rev* 4:325–358, 1991.

Force L, Torres JM, Carrillo A, Bass I: Evaluation of eight serological tests in the diagnosis of human echinococcosis and follow-up. *Clin Infect Dis* 15:473–480, 1992.

Gachot B, Wolff M, Nissack G, et al: Acute lung injury complicating imported *Plasmodium falciparum* malaria. *Chest* 108:746–749, 1995.

Garcia LS, Shimizu RY, Bruckner DA: Detection of microsporidial spores in fecal specimens from patients diagnosed with cryptosporidiosis. *J Clin Microbiol* 32:1739–1741, 1994.

Gelpi AP, Mustafa A: Ascaris pneumonia. *Am J Med* 44:377–389, 1968.

Gentile G, Venditti M, Micozzi A, et al: Cryptosporidiosis in patients with hematologic malignancies. *Rev Infect Dis* 13:842–846, 1991.

Gleich G, Adolphson C, Leiferman K: The biology of the eosinophilic leukocyte. *Annu Rev Med* 43:85–101, 1993.

Glickman LT, Magnaual J-F: Zoonotic round worm infection. *Infect Dis Clin North Am* 7:717–732, 1993.

Goldstein ST, Juranek DD, Ravenholt O, et al: Cryptosporidiosis: An outbreak associated with drinking water despite state-of-the-art water treatment. *Ann Intern Med* 124:459–468, 1996.

Gomez Morales MA, Atzori C, Ludovisis A, et al: Opportunistic and non-opportunistic parasites in HIV-positive and negative patients with diarrhoea in Tanzania. *Trop Med Parasitol* 46:109–114, 1995.

Gozal D: The incidence of pulmonary manifestations during *Plasmodium falciparum* malaria in non-immune subjects. *Trop Med Parasitol* 43:6–8, 1992.

Gunnarsson G, Hurlbut D, DeGirolami PC, et al: Multiorgan microsporidiosis: Report of five cases and review. *Clin Infect Dis* 21:37–44, 1995.

Ibarra-Perez C: Thoracic complications of amebic abscess of the liver. Report of 501 cases. *Chest* 79:672–677, 1981.

Jensen BN, Gerstoft J, Hojlyng N, et al: Pulmonary pathogens in HIV-infected patients. *Scand J Infect Dis* 22:413–420, 1990.

Jerray M, Benzarti M, Garrouch A, et al: Hydatid disease of the lungs: Study of 386 cases. *Am Rev Respir Dis* 146:185–189, 1992.

MacKenzie WR, Hoxie NJ, Proctor ME, et al: A massive outbreak in Milwaukee of Cryptosporidium infection transmitted through the public water supply. *N Engl J Med* 331:161–167, 1994.

Mahmoud AAF: Praziquantel for the treatment of helminthic infections. *Adv Intern Med* 32:193–206, 1987.

Mahmoud AAF: Strongyloidiasis. *Clin Infect Dis* 23:949–953, 1996.

Marsden PD, Nonata RR: Mucocutaneous leishmaniasis—A review of clinical aspects. *Rev Soc Bras Med Trop* 9:309–326, 1975.

Moulin B, Ollier J, Bouchouareb D, et al: Leishmaniasis: A rare cause of unexplained fever in a renal graft recipient. *Nephron* 60:360–362, 1992.

Pomeroy C, Filice GA: Pulmonary toxoplasmosis. A review. *Clin Infect Dis* 14:863–870, 1992.

Sadigursky M, Andrade ZA: Pulmonary changes in schistosomal cor pulmonale. *Am J Trop Med Hyg* 31:779–784, 1982.

Weber R, Bryan RT, Schwartz DA, Owen RL: Human microsporidial infections (review). *Clin Microbiol Rev* 7:426–461, 1994.

66

Pulmonary Infection in Immunocompromised Hosts*

Jay A. Fishman

OVERVIEW

Prolonged survival of a variety of patients—individuals with AIDS, those who have undergone solid organ and bone marrow transplantation, patients with "connective tissue diseases" or primary immune deficiencies, and people who have completed intensive chemotherapeutic regimens for cancer—have greatly expanded the population of "immunocompromised hosts." These patients are defined by their susceptibility to infection with organisms that have little native virulence for the normal host. The detection of underlying immune compromise has been facilitated by improvements in microbiologic techniques, particularly molecular assays, and by advances in radiologic imaging. Survival has also been improved by the availability of new antimicrobial agents, including antifungal agents, macrolides, antivirals (ganciclovir, foscarnet, oral agents) and highly active antiretroviral therapies (HAART) for HIV infection. The clinical use of cytokines and growth factors has also strengthened approaches to the compromised host. The newest challenges in these populations include systemic infections for which adequate therapies have not yet been developed (e.g., hepatitis virus C) and the progressive antimicrobial resistance of common pulmonary pathogens including *Staphylococcus aureus,* the enterococci, *Pseudomonas* species, and *Stentotrophomonas* (formerly *Xanthomonas*) species. In addition, strains of the pneumococcus resistant to trimethoprim-sulfamethoxazole or quinolone antibiotics routinely used for posttransplant prophylaxis are seen with greater frequency. With the changing health care scene, the medical care of immunocompromised individuals is increasingly managed outside of academic centers. Therefore information about the clinical management of these patients has become increasingly important to the entire spectrum of medical practitioners.

*Edited from Chaps. 134 to 141, "Introduction: Pulmonary Infection in Special Hosts," by Fishman JA; "HIV Infection and Opportunistic Pulmonary Infections in AIDS," by Fishman JA; "Pulmonary Infections in Neutropenia and Cancer," by Fishman JA; "Respiratory Disease in Bone Marrow and Hematopoietic Stem Cell Transplantation," by Crawford SW; "Pneumonia in the Organ Transplant Patient," by Fishman JA, Rubin RH; "Pulmonary Infections in Patients with Primary Immune Defects," by Hill HR, Pfeffer KD; "Postoperative Pneumonia," by Nichols RL, Hardin WD Jr; and "Respiratory Infections in the Economically Disadvantaged," by Nardell EA, Kent D. In: *Fishman's Pulmonary Diseases and Disorders,* 3d ed., edited by Fishman AP, Elias JA, Fishman JA, Grippi MA, Kaiser LR, Senior RM. New York, McGraw-Hill, 1998, pp 2095–2198. For fuller discussion of topics dealt with in this chapter, the reader is referred to the original text, as noted above.

GENERAL PRINCIPLES

Opportunistic Infection

Opportunistic infection is defined as an infection occurring in an individual as a result of a compromised immune function that would not be expected to occur or would cause disease of lesser intensity in the presence of normal immune function. Thus, immunocompromised individuals are subject to the common infections that are present in the community, but these infections are likely to affect them with greater frequency and severity than would be the case in the immunologically normal host. In addition, infection in these patients may be caused by organisms that are considered to be either *non-pathogens* or are generally causes of insignificant disease in the normal host, including such organisms as *Pneumocystis carinii* and cytomegalovirus.

The risk of infection in any patient is determined by the interaction of two factors: the potential pathogens to which the individual is exposed (epidemiologic exposures) and a measure of the individual's susceptibility to infection, termed the *net state of immunosuppression* (Table 66-1). The occurrence of infection in an individual at a time when his or her immune status is thought to be nearly normal is evidence that either an excessive environmental exposure has occurred or that the person's immune status is depressed. Conversely, even minimal environmental exposures can cause invasive infection in an individual who is maximally immunosuppressed.

Epidemiologic Exposures

Epidemiologic exposures of importance to the immunocompromised patient can be divided into two general categories: those occurring within the community and those occurring within the hospital. Exposures within the community will vary based on such factors as geography and socioeconomic status. Thus, opportunistic pathogens acquired in the community include the geographically restricted systemic mycoses (blastomycosis, coccidioidomycosis, and histoplasmosis), *Mycobacterium tuberculosis*, *Strongyloides stercoralis*, *Leishmania donovani*, *P. carinii*, *Legionella* species, and community-acquired respiratory viral infections (e.g., influenza, respiratory syncytial virus, and

---

TABLE 66-1 Factors in the Net State of Immune Suppression

Immunosuppressive therapy: dose, duration, temporal sequence
Underlying immune deficiency: autoimmune disease, functional
   immune deficits
Mucocutaneous barrier integrity: catheters, epithelial surfaces,
   devitalized tissue, fluid collections
Neutropenia, lymphopenia
Metabolic conditions
  Uremia
  Malnutrition
  Diabetes
  Alcoholism with cirrhosis
Viral infection:
  Cytomegalovirus
  Epstein-Barr virus
  Hepatitis B and C
  Human immunodeficiency virus

---

parainfluenza). Common viral agents may include herpes simplex virus, cytomegalovirus, and hepatitis B and C viruses. Owing to the limited effectiveness of many vaccines in immunocompromised individuals, infections due to *Streptococcus pneumoniae* and *Haemophilus influenzae* are common.

Within the hospital, excessive environmental exposures can be divided into two general categories: domiciliary and nondomiciliary. Domiciliary exposures occur on the hospital unit where the patient is housed. When the air, food, equipment, or potable water supply is contaminated with pathogens such as *Aspergillus* species, *Legionella* species, or vancomycin-resistant enterococci, clustering of cases of infection in time and space will be observed. As a result, an increased incidence of nosocomial pneumonia or catheter and wound infections may be seen. Nondomiciliary exposures occur when the patient is transported to contaminated operating rooms, radiology suites, or catheterization laboratories for procedures. Nondomiciliary outbreaks, although possibly more common, are more difficult to detect because of the lack of clustering on a particular hospital unit. The leading clue to the presence of a nosocomial hazard is the occurrence of opportunistic infection in a patient whose net state of immunosuppression would not normally lead to such an event, or nosocomial infection with organisms not known to be present on the clinical unit on which the patient is housed.

Net State of Immunosuppression

The net state of immunosuppression (Table 66-1) is a complex function determined by the interaction of several factors: the dose, duration, and temporal sequence in which immunosuppressive drugs are deployed; injuries to the primary mucocutaneous barrier to infection (e.g. indwelling catheters, gastrointestinal or bronchial anastamoses in transplant patients); neutropenia or lymphopenia; underlying immne deficiency; pulmonary aspiration injury; metabolic problems including protein-calorie malnutrition, uremia, and, perhaps, hyperglycemia; the presence of devitalized tissues, hematomas, effusions, or ascites; and infection with immunomodulating viruses [cytomegalovirus (CMV), Epstein-Barr virus (EBV), hepatitis B (HBV), and hepatitis C (HCV), and the human immunodeficiency viruses (HIV-1 and 2)], which predispose to other opportunistic infections, graft rejection, and graft-versus-host disease. The sum of the congenital, metabolic, operative, and transplant-related factors is the patient's net state of immune suppression. Generally more than one factor is present in each host; the identification of the relevant factors, and correction when possible is central to the prevention and treatment of infection in these hosts.

For example, in the alcoholic patient with hepatitis C and cirrhosis who has undergone liver transplantation, the so-called net state of immune suppression is the sum total of all the factors that place the patient at increased risk for infection. Among these are the immune suppression needed to maintain graft function, immune deficits caused by cirrhosis and chronic illness; immunologic and inflammatory effects of infection by hepatitis C virus; exposure to, and colonization with, community-acquired and nosocomial organisms; and new infections (e.g., spontaneous peritonitis) that may occur during the prolonged waiting period for a compatible organ. When the organ for transplantation does become available, it may arrive contaminated by organisms acquired by the donor during hospitalization. This gravely ill patient is then subjected to a major surgical procedure. After the operation, the lungs are apt to be compromised; recovery of function in the allograft is apt to be subnormal; immune-suppressive drugs are initiated; biliary (T-tube), intravenous, and urinary catheters are placed; and major incisions have to heal. Drug toxicities at this stage are common, resulting in neutropenia and hepatitis. Biliary function and anastomotic integrity are assessed by injecting contrast dye into ducts and tubes (e.g., for a T-tube cholangiogram) that are colonized by native and nosocomial organisms. The sum of the underlying, operative, and transplant-related factors is the *net state of immune suppression.* Thus, the spectrum of susceptibility to infection is a *continuum* from individual deficits (e.g., viral upper respiratory infection that paves the way for bacterial superinfection) to multiple simultaneous deficits (e.g., the transplant recipient).

Timetable of Infection

In the broad spectrum of immunocompromised hosts, the risks of infection may be *relatively stable* over time, as in the diabetic with vasculopathy and neuropathy who is prone to skin and soft tissue infections caused by trauma to insensate limbs with diminished tissue integrity and neutrophil function. The risks of infection may be *time-limited,* as in the postsurgical patient without complications or in the autologous bone marrow transplantation recipient with engraftment. The risk of infection may be *cumulative and progressive,* as in the AIDS patient, in whom infection is a function of declining immunity (without therapy), falling CD4+ lymphocyte counts, rising viral loads, and the effects of other persistent infections (CMV, *Crytosporidium*). In these individuals the occurrence of new infections suggests the progression of immune compromise. The risks may also be *progressive but not cumulative.* Thus, the risks of infection in the recipient of allogeneic bone marrow or of a solid organ *change predictably with time* as a function of the changing condition of the patient. For example (Fig. 66-1), in the early phase after bone marrow transplantation, infection is a result of nosocomial exposures and neutropenia. Subsequently, with engraftment, viral pneumonitis (CMV) and hepatic venoocclusive disease may occur. Finally, during the development of, and treatment for, acute and chronic graft-versus-host disease, susceptibility to infection is largely a function of immune suppression and mucosal injuries. As immunosuppressive and chemotherapeutic regimens have become more standardized in recent years, it has become apparent that the specific type of infections that occur most often will vary in a predictable pattern as a reflection of the specific risk factors (surgery, immune suppression, acute and chronic rejection, reemergence of underlying diseases, viral infections) (see Fig. 66-1) present at each phase of the posttransplantation course. The main determinant of infection is the exogenous immune suppression or chemotherapy and the extra immune suppression used to treat either graft rejection or graft-versus-host disease (Fig. 66-2). Superimposed viral infections will enhance the risk of infection at any point along the time line.

Because each risk factor renders the patient susceptible to infection by new groups of pathogens, *infections occurring with the wrong pathogen or at the wrong time suggest an undiscovered immune deficit or an unusual epidemiologic exposure.* The occurrence of specific infections can be prevented by the use of antibiotic prophylaxis, vaccines, and behavioral modifications (e.g., no raw vegetables or digging in a garden without a mask). This will result in a shift to the right of the infection time line. Infections generally observed later in the course of disease or therapy will be observed at the appropriate

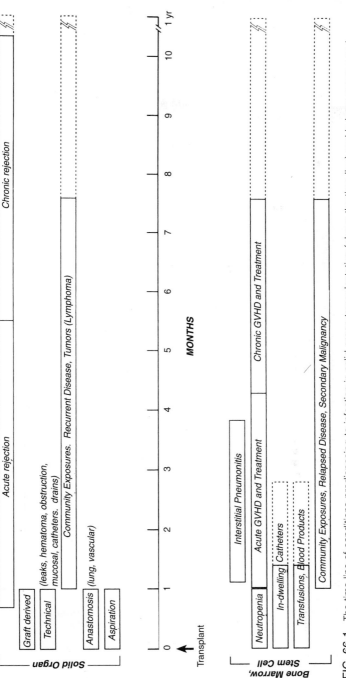

FIG. 66-1 The time line of conditions predisposing to infection in solid organ transplantation (above the time line) and in bone marrow and stem cell transplantation (below the time line). Patients will vary in individual susceptibility patterns.

Bacterial

Oral anaerobes, Enterobacteriaceae, S. aureus, Pseudomonas sp. (aspiration and nosocomial)

Listeria, Nocardia, Legionella, Mycobacteria sp. (atypical pneumonias)

Community acquired: H. influenzae, S. pneumoniae, S. aureus

Viral

HSV

EBV, Adenovirus, Papovavirus. Parvovirus

Respiratory viruses (RSV)

CMV Pneumonitis (BMT, lung)

CMV (systemic, with anti-rejection therapy)

VZV

Viral oncogenesis

Parasitic Pneumocystis, Fungal

Pneumocystis, Strongyloides (hyperinfection)

Candida, Aspergillus, Mucoraceae

Cryptococcus, Histoplasma, Coccidioides

MONTHS

0   1   2   3   4   5   6   7   8   9   1

Transplant

946

FIG. 66-2   The time line of infections commonly observed following solid organ transplantation and in bone marrow and stem cell transplantation. Although the specific factors contributing to the net state of immune deficiency differ between individuals and various forms of immune suppression, the general temporal presentation of infection is similar in the two groups. Individual patients may deviate from the predicted pattern based on specific predisposing conditions. Infections occurring out of sequence should suggest the presence of an excessive epidemiologic exposure or an undetected immunosuppressive condition.

time *in the absence of infections that tend to occur earlier* but have been prevented by a variety of preventative measures. The timetables represented in Figs. 66-1 and 66-2 are useful in a number of regards:

1. Development of a differential diagnosis for infectious syndromes by time posttransplant—what type of infections are most likely at various times after transplantation.
2. Identification of excess epidemiologic hazards.
   a. Nosocomial: *Aspergillus,* methicillin-resistant *Staphyloccus aureus* (MRSA), vancomycin-resistant enterococcus (VRE)—clustered in time and space, by inpatient unit, by procedures or surgical suite.
   b. Community: Influenza, RSV, *Legionella* outbreaks.
   c. Individual: Unique exposures, travel, occupational hazards.
3. Excessive immune suppression: Too many infections, too severe, or at the wrong time on the time line suggest that a problem exists with immunosuppressive regimens used by a program.

VIRULENCE AND INFECTION

The risk of infection in any individual patient depends not only on the sum of the immune deficits and the nature, duration, and intensity of the exposures to potential pathogens but also on the *virulence* of the organism. Recent data suggest that the *specific host-pathogen interactions* are a critical factor in the development of infection. Host cells may *enhance* the virulence of the invading organism by the *induction of genes in that organism* that contribute to bacterial persistence or invasion. Thus, resistance to phagocytosis is induced by target cells in *Yersinia* infections. Also, the survival of uropathogenic *Escherichia coli* in urine and the growth of pili for attachment are induced by contact with the targeted uroepithelial cells. Another example of the host-pathogen interaction is the role of CMV in transplantation. CMV is the cause of common clinical syndromes that frequently occur in immunocompromised patients. Among these are pneumonitis, hepatitis, glomerulonephritis, gastritis, colitis, retinitis, and mononucleosis-like syndromes. CMV also induces an array of host responses (i.e., neutropenia, immune suppression, upregulation of histocompatibility antigens and other cell surface antigens, TNF-α secretion, cardiac allograft atherogenesis, and graft rejection) that contribute to the host's susceptibility to infection (Table 66-2). Thus, the concept of immune status balanced against epidemiologic exposure may be incomplete: the immunoregulatory effects of some pathogens and the interaction of the organisms with the "correct" target cells of the host are best regarded as only part of the response to opportunistic infection.

Physical defects may also contribute to virulence. Foreign materials (vascular grafts, sutures, eye or limb prostheses) may provide a nidus for infection

TABLE 66-2 Effects of Viral Infection in the Immunocompromised Host

Direct causation of invasive viral infection
Immunomodulatory effects
  Systemic immune suppression, opportunistic Infection
  Allograft injury
  Cellular effects, upregulation of surface antigens and graft rejection
Oncogenesis
  Hepatitis B: hepatocellular carcinoma
  Epstein-Barr virus: B-cell lymphoproliferative disease (PTLD)
  Papillomavirus: squamous cell carcinoma, anogenital cancer
  HHV8 (KSHV): Kaposi's sarcoma, effusion lymphoma

by an organism which would not be capable of causing infection under normal conditions. Local immune defects coupled to physical factors may predispose to life-threatening infection. Thus, corticosteroid eye drops used for inflammation due to prosthetic lens implants may lead to eye infections with *Streptomyces, Bartonella, Sporothrix,* and *Fusarium* species. *Salmonella* infection in the organ transplant recipient "homes" to vascular anastomoses and may persist despite appropriate therapy, causing mycotic aneurysms.

Protecting the Patient from Infection

Although the clinical care of the compromised host has improved, flaws in the armamentarium against infection have been highlighted by the emergence of bacteria and fungi that are resistant to common antimicrobial agents. For example, increasingly *Streptococcus pneumoniae* and *Neisseria gonorrhoeae* are detected that are resistant to penicillins; enterococci that are resistant to penicillin, tetracycline, vancomycin, teicoplanin, streptomycin, and gentamycin; *Pseudomonas* and the enteric gram-negative bacteria that are resistant to broad-spectrum beta-lactamases; and the azole-resistant yeasts, all of which are routinely isolated both in the community and in hospitalized patients. Moreover, decreases in the aquisition of infection by compromised hosts can only be accomplished by *complete* reverse precautions that entail the use of laminar-airflow rooms and access to the patient only via glove ports or the use of gowns, gloves, masks, caps, and shoe covers. This practice reduces the incidence of hospital-acquired infection (as distinguished from spread of endogenous infection) by up to 50 percent, to the approximate rate of such infections in granulocytopenic patients.

However, the practice of *complete* reverse precautions is very costly. Consequently, protection against both acquired and endogenous infections has fallen onto the broad use of prophylactic antibiotics. Such oral agents as trimethoprim-sulfamethoxazole, quinolones, acyclovir (and related agents), and azole antifungal drugs now have widespread use in the management of both inpatients and outpatients. Oral decontamination regimens (i.e., nonabsorbable antibiotics), although useful for limited periods of time, are poorly tolerated because of taste, consistency, malabsorption of glucose and xylose bases, and cost. Moreover, the use of such prophylactic agents may contribute to the emergence of antibiotic-resistant organisms.

Recognition of New Syndromes

The identification of *new* infectious disease syndromes has often occurred in individuals with immune deficits. Thus, the cluster of cases of *P. carinii* pneumonia in homosexual males was the first indicator of a new viral pathogen (HIV-1), and the role of *Cryptosporidium* as a common cause of diarrhea in both normal and compromised individuals was elucidated as a result of diarrheal disease in AIDS patients in the 1980s. Similarly, many uncommon bacteria (*Bartonella* species, *Rhodococcus equi*), viruses (Kaposi's-associated human herpesvirus 8, polyomaviruses), fungi (*Penicillium*), and parasites (*Microsporidia*) have been identified in immunocompromised patients. Thus, a continuing lookout for new pathogens or novel presentations of known pathogens is essential for the care of the immunocompromised patient. Often, infection in immunocompromised hosts presents without the expected signs and symptoms of infection. This lack of clinical manifestations may delay identification of the critically ill patient. In the outpatient setting, the practitioner must have a low threshold for performing tests (e.g., blood counts, cultures, radiographs) on patients with minimal complaints.

Multiple Simultaneous Processes

Early and aggressive therapy of infection is required in the immunocompromised patient. Thus, most febrile or possibly infected patients are treated empirically while awaiting data that identify specific pathogens. The occurrence of multiple simultaneous infections or conditions may complicate and delay appropriate therapy. Thus, CMV infection may complicate the treatment of graft rejection or venoocclusive disease and contribute to the pathogenesis of *P. carinii* or *Toxoplasma* pneumonia.

In the lungs, standard radiographic techniques may not detect the presence of multiple patterns of infection. Similarly, radiographic patterns may change during the care of the patient (e.g., cavitation of pulmonary nodules after the resolution of neutropenia). It is commonly necessary to repeat tests, to utilize computed tomography (CT), or to use invasive diagnostic modalities (biopsy) in the evaluation of the patient who is unresponsive to therapy. In the compromised host with fever and pneumonitis, chest radiographs may be difficult to interpret. Noninfectious causes of pulmonary infiltrates may coexist with infection, and atypical patterns predominate. Drug toxicities (bleomycin, cytoxan, sulfa drugs), leukoagglutinin reactions, radiation injury, pulmonary emboli, and lesions of metastatic cancer may coexist with opportunistic infection. The "typical" evolution of pulmonary infection may be altered by the presence of underlying (e.g., interstitial) pulmonary disease as well as by diminished inflammatory responses.

Complications of therapy may contribute to the development of new infections: Trimethoprim-sulfamethoxazole can cause pneumonitis, hepatitis, or Stevens-Johnson syndrome; ganciclovir can cause renal failure and neutropenia; transfusion reactions can cause pulmonary infiltrates and hemolysis; cyclosporine can cause hemolytic-uremic syndrome; antibiotics can cause thrush or *Clostridium difficile* colitis.

Patient Management

Antibiotics alone may not suffice in the treatment of infection in the immunocompromised host. Many major infections require improvement in the immune responses of the host in order to clear ongoing infection. Infections may respond to a decrease in exogenous immune suppression, to correction of neutropenia by growth factors, or to treatment of simultaneous infections that predispose to superinfection (e.g., respiratory syncytial virus, CMV). Drainage of collections of infected fluid such as a hematoma or a lymphocele or removal of drains or catheters enhances the treatment of infection.

Identification of metastatic sites of infection (e.g., infections of the central nervous system due to *Nocardia* or *Cryptococcus* species) may facilitate management. Synergistic antibiotic therapy must be used when available. Compromises often must be made. The loss of renal function due to antibiotics used in the treatment of fungal infections significantly hinders patient management. However, progression of a fungal infection while on inadequate doses of amphotericin must be avoided.

Infection must be prevented in the susceptible host, since antibiotics are often ineffective during acute infection. Whenever possible, vaccines should be given before immune suppression or splenectomy. During immune suppression, only killed or conjugate vaccines should be used. Repletion of immunoglobulin deficiencies [after bone marrow transplant (BMT) or solid organ transplantation] and the use of specific hyperimmune globulins (i.e., for exposure to varicella or for CMV) may help to prevent infection. Similarly, in patients susceptible to infection, the use of antibiotics to prevent common infections is cost-effective. The use of preemptive therapies based on tests that demonstrate the presence of infection (e.g., the administration of ganciclovir in patients with evidence of CMV infection by antigenemia assays or polymerase chain reaction studies) allows the interruption of infection before disease becomes manifest clinically. Similarly, routine surveillance cultures have been useful to detect specific pathogens in subgroups of patients (e.g., neutropenic patients with *Aspergillus* colonization) or in specific geographic regions.

The clinical *evaluation of the patient prior to immune suppression,* if elective, may be very helpful in preventing disease. Patients with cystic fibrosis or chronic bacterial sinusitis may become colonized in the airways or sinuses with *Pseudomonas* or *Aspergillus* species. These colonizing organisms may reactivate during immune suppression. Careful evaluation by radiography and invasive cultures may prevent major infection. Similarly, patients who are not immune to varicella zoster *may* benefit from vaccination. Patients seronegative for *Toxoplasma gondii* or CMV are at high risk of reactivation in the presence of an organ transplant from a seropositive donor. Similarly, seropositive patients with AIDS or before seronegative bone marrow transplantation are at high risk for reactivation disease due to *Leishmania,* CMV, or *Toxoplasma.* In endemic areas, transfusions and transplants may provide entry of *T. gondii, Trypanosoma cruzi* (Chagas' disease), *Leishmania* species, *Acanthamoeba, Naeglaria, Strongyloides stercoralis, Taenia* species, or *Echinococcus* species with exacerbation of infection by immune suppression. A careful clinical history and pretreatment of known infections or specific antibiotic prophylaxis may prevent such complications of immune deficiency.

INFECTIONS IN SPECIAL HOSTS

The spectrum of common infections varies with the specific immune defects present in each host (Table 66-3).

AIDS

Highly Active Retroviral Therapy and the Immune Reconstitution Syndrome

The management of HIV infection has been dramatically altered for those individuals with access to antiretroviral therapies. However, the HIV epidemic

TABLE 66-3 Infections Associated with Specific Immune Defects

Defect	Common causes	Associated infections
Granulocytopenia	**Leukemia, cytotoxic chemotherapy, AIDS, drug toxicity, Felty syndrome**	Enteric gram-negative rods, *Pseudomonas, S. aureus, S. epidermidis,* streptococci, *Aspergillus, Candida* and other fungi,
Neutrophil chemotaxis	Diabetes, alcoholism, uremia, Hodgkin's disease, trauma (burns) lazy leukocyte syndrome, CT disease	*S. aureus, Candida,* streptococci
Neutrophil killing	CGD, myeloperoxidase deficiency	*S. aureus, E. coli, Candida, Aspergillus, Torulopsis*
T-Cell defects	AIDS, congenital, lymphoma, sarcoidosis, viral infection, organ transplants, steroids	Intracellular bacteria (*Legionella Listeria,* mycobacteria), HSV, VZV, CMV, EBV, parasites (*Strongyloides, Toxoplasma*), fungi (*P. carinii, Candida, Cryptococcus*)
B-Cell defects	Congenital/acquired agammaglobulinemia, burns, enteropathies, splenic dysfunction, myeloma, ALL	*S. pneumoniae, H. influenzae, Salmonella* and *Campylobacter* spp., *Giardia lamblia*
Splenectomy	Surgery, sickle cell, cirrhosis	*S. pneumoniae, H. Influenzae, Salmonella* spp., *Capnocytophaga*
Complement	Congenital/acquired defects	*S. aureus, Neisseria* spp., *H. influenzae, S. pneumoniae*
Anatomic	IV/Foley catheters, incisions, anastamotic leaks, mucosal ulceration, vascular insufficiency	Colonizing organisms, resistant nosocomial organisms

KEY: CT, computed tomography; CGD, chronic granulomatous disease; ALL, acute lymphocytic leukemia; HSV, herpes simplex virus; VZV, varicella zoster virus; CMV, cytomegalovirus; EBV, Epstein-Barr virus.

is continuing without interruption. Anti-HIV therapy should be started before the immune system is irrevocably compromised. Most experts advise starting with a highly potent combination of three or four antiretroviral agents initially to minimize the emergence of resistant viral strains. Adherence levels of less than 90 to 95 percent are often associated with failure. Therapy is indicated for all HIV-infected individuals with CD4+ cell counts below 200/mm³. Controversy exists about what level of virus or CD4+ cell counts to use to initiate therapy, but generally includes those with rapidly rising viral loads or falling CD4+ cell counts. Many delay therapy until the CD4+ cell count is below 350/mm^3.

HAART has resulted in the recrudescence of immunity as manifest by rising CD4+ lymphocyte counts and diminished signs of opportunistic infection and cancer associated with severe T-cell deficits. Treatment of HIV infection with highly active antiretroviral therapy (HAART) *with reversal of immune deficiency* appears to eliminate the risk of *P. carinii* pneumonia (studied up to 2 years) in AIDS patients with and without prior *P. carinii* pneumonia. The risk of *Mycobacterium avium* complex (MAC), tuberculosis, and cytomegalovirus (CMV) has also decreased. Thus, prophylactic (both primary and secondary) and therapeutic regimens must be considered in light of the individual's immune status. Not all patients respoind to HAART or maintain viral suppression during therapy. Immune benefits are not generally expected before 12 to 16 weeks of therapy with normalization of CD4+ cell counts. The specifics of antiviral therapy are not considered here.

One of the features of HAART is a syndrome of intensified inflammatory responses referred to as the immune reconstitution syndrome, which generally occurs within the first 3 months of starting effective antiretrovital therapy. This is thought to represent a hyperacute response to pathogens to which the HIV-infected individual has been exposed. It has been observed in *P. carinii* pneumonia, CMV retinitis and vitritis, disseminated MAC as pneumonitis and lymphadenitis, cryptococcosis with meningitis and necrotizing lymphadenitis, and with acceleration of hepatitis C virus infection including cryoglobulinemia and renal failure. Thus, effective antiviral therapy may result in more intense symptoms and unusual manifestations of some opportunistic infections, while the overall incidence of new infections has declined.

HIV Testing

HIV testing should be considered for all persons in high-risk groups [intravenous drug users, sexually active homosexual or bisexual men, hemophiliacs or individuals requiring blood or clotting factors, persons with sexually transmitted diseases (especially syphilis), pregnant women, health care workers with exposure to body fluids or needle-stick injury, and all patients with conditions commonly associated with AIDS (Table 66-4).

Testing for HIV infection is generally divided into viral culture assays, antibody tests, and specific (molecular) viral tests. Issues of confidentiality, informed consent, and counseling need to be addressed regarding HIV testing. Culture systems for HIV are nonstandardized and are not available in most nonacademic centers. Most patients produce antibodies to HIV within 6 to 8 weeks, and almost 100 percent will have detectable antibodies by 6 months after exposure. These tests are well standardized, easy to perform, and less expensive than culture; however, antibody tests may have false positives (cross-reacting antibodies) and false negatives (e.g., in the early period). The enzyme-linked immunosorbent assay (ELISA) and Western blot tests are in this group. The ELISA test has a sensitivity of 99.7 percent and specificity of 98.5 percent; if results are negative, no further testing is performed unless new, acute infection is suspected. If results are positive, confirmation by Western blot is performed. Between 4 and 20 percent of Western blot tests are *indeterminate* because of seroconversion in progress, loss of antibody in advanced HIV disease, cross-reacting antibodies in pregnancy, blood transfusions, autoantibodies from collagen vascular disease, infection with

TABLE 66-4 When to Suspect HIV Infection

History
 High-risk behaviors or exposures
  Unsafe or promiscuous sex
   Sex with prostitutes
   Sex with person at risk for HIV
  Injection drug use
  Blood or blood product transfusion between 1975 and 1985 (especially
   in high-prevalence areas)
  Transfusion of blood clotting concentrate before January 1985
 Sexually transmitted disease
 Tuberculosis, especially extrapulmonary
 Racial and ethnic minority populations in high-prevalence areas of HIV
  disease
 Homeless persons in high-prevalence areas of HIV disease
 Individuals from high-prevalence areas for heterosexual transmission
Symptoms and signs
 Acute retroviral syndrome
 Unexplained constitutional symptoms
  Fatigue, malaise, fever, diarrhea, night sweats, anorexia, weight loss
 Lymphatic
  Persistent generalized lymphadenopathy
Dermatologic manifestations
 Infectious
  Severe herpes simplex (oral, anogenital), oral or genital candidiasis,
   staphylococcal skin infections, herpes zoster (especially recurrent),
   superficial dermatophytoses (tinea nail infection), molluscum contagio-
   sum, warts, condyloma acuminata, oral hairy leukoplakia (Epstein-Barr
   virus), necrotizing gingivitis or periodontitis
  Kaposi's sarcoma, petechiae (ITP), seborrheic dermatitis, psoriasis (new
   or worsening), eosinophilic folliculitis, severe drug eruptions, aphthous
   ulcers, intraepithelial neoplasia
Neurologic conditions
 Cranial neuropathy, Guillain-Barré syndrome, aseptic meningitis, peripheral
  neuropathy, myopathy, cognitive impairment
Laboratory findings
 Unexplained anemia, leukopenia, lymphocytopenia, atypical lymphocytosis,
  thrombocytopenia
 CD4 lymphocytopenia
 Polyclonal hyperglobulinemia
 Elevated blood urea nitrogen or serum creatinine, proteinuria,
  hypoalbuminemia
 Elevated lactate dehydrogenase
 Hypocholesterolemia and hypertriglyceridemia

HIV-2, recent influenza vaccination, or in recipients of trial HIV vaccines. These subjects should be retested at 2 to 3 and 6 months, and inconclusive assays resolved with specific viral (molecular, p24 antigen, or culture) testing. Western blot test results are considered positive if *two bands* are present from the gp41, gp160/120, or p24 group, indeterminate with a single band, and negative with no bands.

Specific viral tests include the p24 antigen detection, molecular amplification by PCR, and culture-based assays. These are positive earlier than the antibody tests and therefore may be useful in primary infection before the development of antibody; they have high sensitivity (95 to 99 percent) and are often useful when the Western blot is indeterminate. Quantitative techniques are very useful in assessing the response to antiviral therapy and disease progression. These tests tend to be expensive, may require working with infected sera and live virus, are operator-dependent, and are not yet fully standardized between laboratories. The limits of viral detection of the available molecular assays are approximately 500 copies per milliliter for the branched-chain assays (second-generation bDNA) and 50 to 200 copies per milliliter for the PCR tests. P24 assays may be negative in infected persons.

Measures of HIV viral RNA in plasma do not correlate exactly with the CD4+ lymphocyte count. The CD4+ count provides a surrogate marker for the response to antiviral therapy and the risk of infection and death. At present, the best predictive value of testing is the combination of viral load with CD4+ lymphocyte enumeration. Viral RNA levels in long-term nonprogressors are consistently under 10,000 copies per milliliter, while progression and immunologic deterioration are often associated with loads over 50,000 to 100,000 copies. Patients with viral loads of 10,000 to 50,000 are considered at intermediate risk. Viral load changes generally precede CD4+ count changes. Immune alterations due to infection (e.g., CMV) or immune modulation therapy (interferons) are not yet interpretable.

AIDS Patient Management

Details of patient management are beyond the scope of this volume. Laboratory tests are notoriously variable within individual patients and between laboratories. Thus, any important test merits being repeated before being acted upon. This is especially valid for blood counts (white blood cells, CD4+ cell counts, differential counts). Baseline knowledge of the patient's HIV viral load, blood counts, chemistries, CD4+ cell count, PPD status with controls, Pap smear, VDRL, serologies for *Toxoplasma gondii,* cytomegalovirus, hepatitis B, varicella zoster virus, hepatitis C, and chest radiograph will be very valuable for future management. Careful attention to the patient's nutritional status and unique epidemiologic exposures is important in AIDS as for all immunocompromised patients. PPD testing must be interpreted according to modified standards for immunocompromised hosts.

Immunization is a part of the routine management of AIDS. In general, HIV-infected persons are susceptible to the same community-acquired respiratory pathogens (with additions) as the normal host, but with a greater severity of disease. Thus, patients should be vaccinated early in the course of disease when they are clinically stable. Live vaccines are generally contraindicated, but measles vaccine is generally well tolerated in children, and measles-mumps-rubella (MMR) vaccine is recommended for unvaccinated adults born after 1957 or vaccinated between 1963 and 1967. The efficacy of vaccination in this population is not clear; HIV viral loads may temporarily increase after vaccination. However, general practice suggests that pneumococcal, influenza (inactivated whole virus and split virus vaccines), *Haemophilus influenzae,* hepatitis B recombinant vaccine, and MMR be given as indicated.

Underlying lung disease is common in HIV-infected patients even before the development of opportunistic infection. While FEV_1 and FVC are nearly normal, 11 to 13 percent of patients with CD4+ lymphocyte counts below 200/mm^3 or with a history of AIDS-associated extrapulmonary diseases (including thrush and varicella zoster infections) and weight loss have decreased $D_{L_{CO}}$ measurements. Intravenous drug users have a higher incidence of abnormal FVC, FEV_1, and $D_{L_{CO}}$ measurements (33.3 percent), consistent with patterns of cigarette smoking and racial distribution. Thus, susceptibility to pulmonary infection is further exacerbated in this population and the importance of vaccination increased.

Opportunistic Infections

The problem of opportunistic infection in the untreated or newly diagnosed AIDS patient is unique because of the *progressive decline* in immune function when compared with the intermittent compromise seen after chemotherapy or the relatively stable immunosuppression utilized after solid organ transplantation. The specific opportunistic infections that occur depend on the nature and duration of immune suppression as well as on the infectious exposures of the patient (Table 66-5). As a result of the progressive and cumulative risks, the incidence of opportunistic infections *increases* over time. A "time line" exists for the common infections and noninfectious manifestations seen in AIDS, relating to the total CD4+ lymphocyte count as a measure

---

TABLE 66-5 Infectious Agents Commonly Associated with AIDS

Viral (with HIV-1, HIV-2)
  Cytomegalovirus
  Herpes simplex
  Herpes zoster
  Epstein-Barr virus
  Parvovirus B19
  HHV-6, HHV-8
  HTLV-1, HTLV-2
Protozoan
  Toxoplasma gondii
  Cryptosporidium
  Isospora belli
  Microsporidium
  Cyclospora
Fungal
  Candida species
  Cryptococcus neoformans
  Histoplasma capsulatum
  Blastomyces dermatitidis
  Aspergillus species
  Petriellidium boydii
  Coccidioides immitis
  Pneumocystis carinii
  Sporothrix schenckii
Bacterial
  Mycobacterium avium–intracellulare complex
  M. tuberculosis
  Legionella species
  Nocardia asteroides
  Encapsulated gram-positive bacteria
  Salmonella species
  Rhodococcus equi
  Bartonella species
  Campylobacter species

of susceptibility (Fig. 66-3). In an individual, the time line is also related to the patient's viral load, but an exact correlation does not exist. The specific pattern of opportunistic syndromes will change for individual patients, but it reflects the overall progressive immunological deterioration of AIDS.

Many opportunistic pulmonary infections in AIDS patients were initially assumed to be reactivation of latent infection. However, some of these processes—including *P. carinii, T. gondii,* tuberculosis, and histoplasmosis— represent a mix of both new exposures and old disease. For example, by genetic analysis, a number of patients treated for primary infection due to *P. carinii* have been shown to develop "recurrent infection," which has been demonstrated to be due to organisms of a different genotype than the organisms isolated from the initial infection. Similar observations have been made in terms of the drug susceptibility of mycobacterial isolates in recurrent disease. This observation may have implications for the development of prophylactic therapies. The clinical manifestations of opportunistic infections in AIDS are altered by prophylactic and therapeutic regimens, adverse drug reactions, and drug interactions.

Toxicities of both prophylactic and therapeutic drug regimens (particularly rash, marrow suppression, and hepatic toxicities) are much more frequent in HIV-infected patients and are exacerbated by the simultaneous need for antiviral therapies. Given the large number of drugs that patients with advanced HIV disease may be asked to ingest, compliance issues must be addressed realistically with each patient.

Specific Agents of Opportunistic Infection in AIDS

A general approach to the prophylaxis of infection in AIDS is presented in Tables 66-6 and 66-7. The need for continued primary prophylaxis in AIDS patients who have CD4+ lymphocyte counts that rise from below 200/mm^3 to above this level in response to antiviral therapies for infections other than *P. carinii* has not been resolved. Up to 15 to 20 percent of AIDS patients have more than one opportunistic infection at one time. The spectrum of clinical diagnoses in pulmonary disease in AIDS includes bacterial infection (45.5 percent), *P. carinii* pneumonia (27 percent), Kaposi's sarcoma (7 percent), bronchitis (5 percent), *M. tuberculosis* (4.3 percent), other mycobacteria (4 percent), lymphoma (2.1 percent), and a variety of other processes. Common community-acquired upper respiratory infections, manageable on an ambulatory basis, constitute more than 50 percent of respiratory illnesses in HIV-infected persons. The incidence of fungal infections varies by geographic region, while the rate of demonstration of viral pulmonary infection is closely related to the diagnostic testing techniques used at each center and to seasonal variation.

Approaches to the Diagnosis of Opportunistic Pulmonary Infections in AIDS

With the wide array of potential pathogens causing disease in HIV-infected patients, the frequency of atypical and multiple infections, and the urgency to diagnosis of infection in the immunocompromised host, a systematic approach to lung disease in these hosts is imperative. A few general rules are useful.

1. *Prophylaxis is generally effective.* When failure of prophylaxis occurs, it is usually due to noncompliance, malabsorption of drugs, emerging antibiotic resistance, or coinfection or tumor that alters the local environment. For

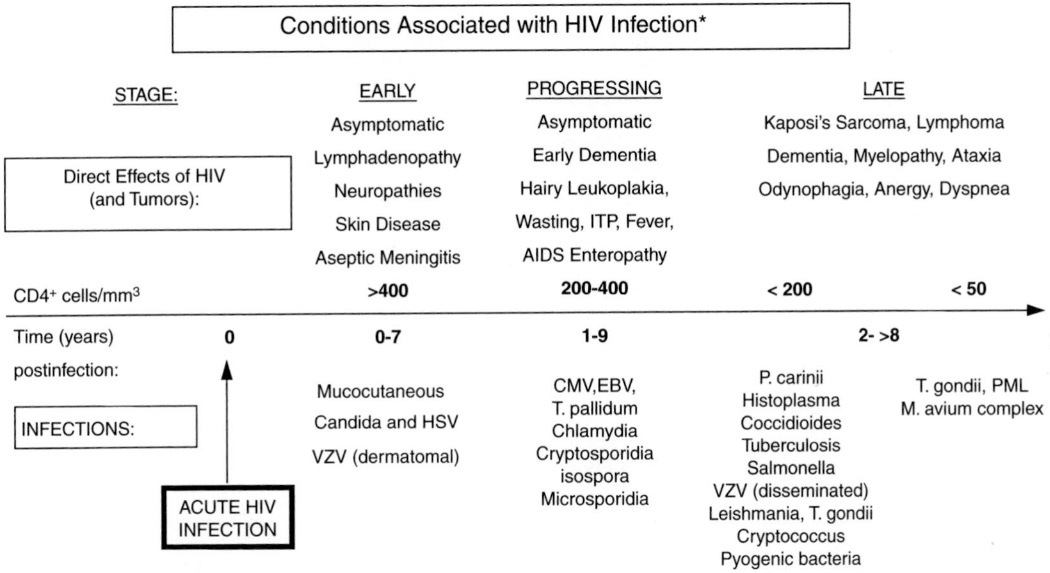

Conditions Associated with HIV Infection*

STAGE:		EARLY	PROGRESSING	LATE	
Direct Effects of HIV (and Tumors):		Asymptomatic	Asymptomatic	Kaposi's Sarcoma, Lymphoma	
		Lymphadenopathy	Early Dementia	Dementia, Myelopathy, Ataxia	
		Neuropathies	Hairy Leukoplakia,	Odynophagia, Anergy, Dyspnea	
		Skin Disease	Wasting, ITP, Fever,		
		Aseptic Meningitis	AIDS Enteropathy		
CD4+ cells/mm³		>400	200-400	< 200	< 50
Time (years) postinfection:	0	0-7	1-9	2- >8	
INFECTIONS:	ACUTE HIV INFECTION	Mucocutaneous Candida and HSV VZV (dermatomal)	CMV,EBV, T. pallidum Chlamydia Cryptosporidia isospora Microsporidia	P. carinii Histoplasma Coccidioides Tuberculosis Salmonella VZV (disseminated) Leishmania, T. gondii Cryptococcus Pyogenic bacteria	T. gondii, PML M. avium complex

*Multiple conditions and infections occur in each host. The risk of infections or conditions from early in the course of disease will persist without specific therapy or prophylaxis. M. tuberculosis may occur at any point in the continuum. HIV-2 may have slower progression than HIV-1.

FIG. 66-3 The progression of AIDS-associated conditions.

TABLE 66-6 Recommended Antibiotic Prophylaxis for First-Episode Opportunistic Infections in HIV-Infected Adults[a]

Pathogen	Indication	Preventive regimens	
		First choice	Alternatives
Pneumocystis carinii	CD4+ cells <200 mm³ or <14%	TMP-SMX 1SS or DS PO qd	Dapsone 50 mg PO qd, *plus* pyrimethamine 50 mg PO qw, *plus* leucovorin 25 mg PO qw
	Unexplained fever for ≥2 weeks	or DS tiw	Dapsone 100 mg PO qd
	Oropharyngeal candidiasis		Aerosolized pentamidine 300 mg q 3–4 weeks
Mycobacterium tuberculosis			
Isoniazid-sensitive	Skin test reaction ≥5 mm or prior positive TST result without treatment or contact with active tuberculosis	Isoniazid 300 mg PO, *plus* pyridoxine 50 mg PO qd ×12 months Isoniazid 900 mg PO, *plus* pyridoxine 50 mg PO biw ×12 months	Rifampin 600 mg PO qd ×12 months
Isoniazid-resistant only	High probability of exposure to isoniazid-resistant tuberculosis	Rifampin 600 mg PO qd × 12 months	Rifabutin 300 mg PO qd × 12 months
Multidrug-resistant (isoniazid and rifampin)	High probability of exposure to multidrug-resistant tuberculosis	Choice of drugs requires consultation with infectious disease experts	None
Toxoplasma gondii	IgG antibody positive to *Toxoplasma* and CD4+ cells <200 mm³	TMP-SMX 1 DS PO qd	TMP-SMX 1 SS PO qd or 1 DS PO tiw Dapsone 50 mg PO qd *plus* pyrimethamine 50 mg PO qw, *plus* leucovorin 25 mg PO qw Atovaquone 1500–3000 suspension PO qd (investigational)
Streptococcus pneumoniae[b]	All patients	Pneumococcal vaccine 0.5 mL IM × 1	None
Mycobacterium avium PO qd (A1)complex[b]	CD4+ cells <75 mm³	Clarithromycin 500 mg PO bid Azithromycin 1200 mg PO weekly	Rifabutin 300 mg

[a]Not all agents are approved for all indications by the U.S. Food and Drug Administration.

[b]Recommended for consideration. Proven survival advantage to prophylaxis of MAC with clarithromycin (not to exceed a total of 1 g per day).

TABLE 66-7 Suggested Prophylaxis of Opportunistic Infections in HIV-Infected Adults

Pathogen	Indication	Preventive regimens	
		First choice	Alternatives
Bacteria	Neutropenia, recurrent infection	Granulocyte colony-stimulating factor (G-CSF) (with oral TMP-SMX or quinolone)	Granulocyte-macrophage colony-stimulating factor (GM-CSF)[a]
Candida species	CD4+ cells <50 mm^3	Fluconazole 100–200 mg PO qd	Ketoconazole 200 mg PO qd
Cryptococcus neoformans	CD4+ cells <50 mm^3	Fluconazole 100–200 mg PO qd	Itraconazole 200 mg PO qd
Histoplasma capsulatum	CD4+ cells <50 mm^3, endemic area	Itraconazole 200 mg PO qd	Fluconazole 200 mg PO qd
Coccidioides immitis	CD4+ cells <50 mm^3, endemic area	Fluconazole 100–200 mg PO qd	Itraconazole 200 mg PO qd
CMV	CD4+ cells <50 mm^3, CMV antibody$^{(+)}$	Ganciclovir 1 g PO tid	(Under study)
Hepatitis B virus	All susceptible patients	Energix-B, 20 μg IM × 3 Recombivax HB, 10 μg IM × 3	None
Influenza virus	All patients (annually)	Whole or split virus, 0.5 mL IM per year	Rimantadine 200 mg PO bid
Herpes simplex virus	Any CD4+ cell count History of recurrences	Acyclovir 400–800 mg PO bid	Valacyclovir, famciclovir

KEY: CMV, cytomegalovirus; TMP-SMX, trimethoprim-sulfamethoxazole.
[a]M-CSF or GM-CSF *may* stimulate HIV replication.

example, it is often impossible to eradicate *Candida* esophagitis unless erosive esophageal herpes simplex virus infection is also treated. *Pneumocystis* is difficult to treat in the presence of CMV infection or bronchial obstruction.

2. Specific therapies for individual infections have a *high incidence of adverse reactions in the HIV-infected patient.* Thus, presumptive or empiric therapy without microbiologic confirmation, though often appropriate, has a greater risk in this population than in the normal host.

3. The *utilization of newer diagnostic tests* has improved the care of AIDS patients. The interpretation of some tests (e.g., PCR for CMV or *P. carinii*) is unclear, and the availability of some tests (urinary *Histoplasma* antigen or immunoperoxidase stains for *T. gondii*) is not universal. The

induced sputum examination has been very useful in the early, noninvasive diagnosis of *P. carinii* infection, and for mycobacterial disease in the absence of spontaneous sputum production. The sensitivity of sputum induction for *P. carinii* infection approaches 90 percent, but the negative predictive value of the test is only 50 percent. The cost and sensitivity of this procedure cannot be justified for the routine diagnosis of bacterial infections, particularly in persons capable of producing sputum samples. The use of *more invasive tests,* such as bronchoscopy, with the obvious limitations of cost and risk to the patient, has the advantage of providing subglottic specimens and the potential for diagnosis of a broader range of pathogens. The interpretation of positive cultures for CMV or for MAC may be uncertain without tissue histopathology for confirmation. In patients with a rapidly deteriorating clinical condition or a failure to respond to initial therapy, bronchoscopy with biopsy or needle aspiration may be preferable to bronchoalveolar lavage or sputum induction as an initial procedure. In general, noninvasive, nuclear isotope–based radiologic tests are rarely useful in the diagnostic evaluation of pulmonary disease in AIDS patients.

4. The *rate of progression of infection* is often a clue to the type of disease. Thus, community-acquired pneumonia develops rapidly (in 2 to 5 days), while the initial episode of *P. carinii* pneumonia generally evolves more slowly (over 7 to 12 days). Fungal infection and mycobacterial infection are generally preceded by systemic complaints. Pyogenic pulmonary infection is generally associated with sputum production, while the atypical infections may have little or no sputum despite cough and dyspnea.

5. The *radiographic pattern* is often suggestive of the diagnosis (Table 66-8). All typical patterns are altered by progressive immune deficits and coexisting or prior lung disease. *Diffuse infiltrates* (alveolar or interstitial) may be seen with a homogeneous distribution, as in *P. carinii, T. gondii,* CMV, mycobacterial species, *Histoplasma,* or *Coccidioides.* Drug toxicity may also cause pulmonary infiltrates. Inhomogeneity with these pathogens reflects altered pulmonary parenchyma from previous disease, obstruction (e.g., with tumor, *Strongyloides stercoralis*), or upper-zone disease or pneumothorax in *P. carinii* pneumonia. Tumors may appear with interstitial radiographic patterns in HIV disease. Lymphoid interstitial pneumonitis is an interstitial process of unknown origin that is seen in AIDS patients. Diffuse interstitial infiltrates are often due to *P. carinii,* but not in patients receiving trimethoprim-sulfamethoxazole (TMP-SMX) prophylaxis and rarely without hypoxemia. Thus, the presence of a sepsislike picture with a diffuse interstitial infiltrate in a patient receiving anti–*P. carinii* prophylaxis might suggest mycobacterial disease, *Legionella* infection, or *C. neoformans. Focal airspace disease* is most often seen with bacterial infections (pyogenic, mycobacteria, *Legionella* species), *Mycoplasma pneumoniae* (viral influenza, adenovirus, CMV), and mixed infections (e.g., CMV and *P. carinii*). Occasionally, primary cryptococcal pneumonia, *Aspergillus* infection, or obstructive disease will present with focal infiltrates. Each of these processes may evolve to frank *cavitation,* particularly infections due to pyogenic bacteria (*Staphylococcus, Klebsiella, S. pneumoniae*) or *M. tuberculosis.* Small cavities are seen with *P. carinii,* the mycobacteria, and metastatic tumors. Large cavities are uncommon; *M. tuberculosis* or aspergilloma

TABLE 66-8 Roentgenographic Findings in Opportunistic Pulmonary Diseases in AIDS

Diffuse infiltrates	Cavitary lesions	Hilar adenopathy	Focal infiltrates	Nodular lesions	Pleural effusions
Pneumocystis carinii	Tuberculosis	Tuberculosis	*Legionella* sp.	*C. neoformans*	Tuberculosis
Tuberculosis	Pyogenic bacteria	Lymphoma	Tuberculosis	*H. capsulatum*	Fungal
Toxoplasma gondii	Aspergillosis	Kaposi's sarcoma	*P. carinii*	Tuberculosis	Pyogenic
Histoplasma capsulatum	*Cryptococcus neoformans*	*Cryptococcus neoformans*	*Streptococcus pneumoniae*	*P. carinii;* Kaposi's sarcoma	Lymphoma; Kaposi's sarcoma
P. carinii and other agents	*P. carinii; Rhodococcus equi*	HIV, acute; Epstein-Barr virus, acute	Kaposi's sarcoma; *Nocardia asteroides;*	Lymphoma; Septic emboli	
Lymphocytic interstitial pneumonitis	Septic emboli (addicts)		*C. neoformans*		

961

is most often present. *Nodular lesions* can be seen with any of the metastatic tumors or hematogenous infections. Endocarditis, Kaposi's sarcoma (KS), toxoplasmosis, tuberculosis, MAC, and *Cryptococcus* may all progress from nodules to small cavities. In particular, unusual bacterial pathogens (*Bartonella, Rhodococcus, Candida, Salmonella*) have been observed as pulmonary nodules associated with right-sided endocarditis in AIDS patients. *Intrathoracic adenopathy* is common in AIDS patients, most often with infections earlier in the course of disease (CD4+ cell count greater than 400/mL) and with tumors late in disease. Fungal infections (*Cryptococcus, Histoplasma, Coccidioides*), CMV, and mycobacterial infections may also cause adenopathy. Adenopathy should prompt invasive diagnosis in the absence of a clear etiology in AIDS. *Pleural effusions* are common with tuberculosis, other pyogenic bacterial infections, and tumors.

6. The *CD4+ lymphocyte count* is a good indicator of susceptibility to specific infections, while the viral load is most closely associated with overall disease prognosis. Often, community-acquired pneumonia due to *S. pneumoniae, H. influenzae, Mycoplasma,* or *Legionella* species may be the sentinel infection of HIV disease. As host immunity declines, other opportunistic infections will occur. *M. tuberculosis,* an organism of high virulence, will cause infections at *any* CD4+ lymphocyte count but will occur increasingly as the CD4+ lymphocyte count falls below 500/mL. In contrast, less virulent organisms will cause disease only with greater degrees of immune ompromise. Thus, MAC is more common below CD4+ counts of 200/mL. *P. carinii* causes pneumonia in less than 1 percent of persons with CD4+ counts over 200/mL but in 18 percent per year with CD4+ counts below 200.

7. *Chronic or recurrent sinus infection* may provide a source of *Pseudomonas* or *Aspergillus* for pulmonary infection. Such pathogens as *Microsporida* and *P. carinii* and metastatic Kaposi's lesions with obstruction have also contributed to chronic sinus infections and, probably, to subsequent pulmonary infections with organisms found in the sinuses.

8. The *spectrum of pulmonary disease varies by geographic region* and by HIV transmission category. This reflects both the heightened risk of certain infections in inner-city areas and in intravenous drug users (tuberculosis, *Bartonella* species, endocarditis), in areas with endemic fungal and parasitic infections (*Histoplasma, Coccidioides, Leishmania*), and in developing countries (tuberculosis is increased with a lower rate of diagnosis of *P. carinii*). Similarly, KS tends to be more common in homosexual and bisexual men than in intravenous drug users.

9. *Physical findings* are often useful in establishing a differential for pulmonary disease. The presence of lymphadenopathy or cutaneous lesions of KS may increase the likelihood of pulmonary malignancy. Diffuse rales or rhonchi are more often found in *P. carinii,* cryptococcal, or MAC-related infections than with pyogenic infections.

INFECTION IN CANCER PATIENTS

Defects Due to Tumors and Chemotherapy

The incidence of infection in cancer patients is determined partly by the nature of the underlying neoplasm. Many studies of infection in cancer have focused on patients with leukemia and lymphoma, owing to the severe and predictable nature of the immune deficiencies developed by these people. In a series conducted by Bodey and colleagues, fatal infections in acute leukemics were caused by bacteria in 66 percent, fungi in 33 percent, viruses in 0.2 percent, and protozoa (including *P. carinii,* now considered a fungus) in 0.1 percent. In contrast, fatal infection in lymphoma patients (86 percent) and solid-tumor patients (94 percent) were more often bacterial. In studies of cryptococcal infection in cancer patients, the rate of cryptococcal infection in chronic lymphocytic leukemia was more than double that in Hodgkin's disease (24.3 versus 10.9 per thousand), and the rate in breast cancer was only 0.159 per thousand. Other tumors are also associated with specific infections. For example, lung cancer is associated with tuberculosis at a rate of 92 per 1000, second only to the rate in patients with Hodgkin's disease (96 per 1000), who have a known cellular immune defect. Without therapy, the degree of depression in cellular immunity (delayed-type hypersensitivity) is more prominent in lymphoma, whereas humoral immunity is impaired to a greater degree in diseases affecting B-lymphocyte function, such as multiple myeloma and chronic lymphocytic lymphoma. Thus, the lymphoma patient is particularly susceptible to intracellular organisms including *Listeria monocytogenes, Mycobacterium tuberculosis,* viruses, and fungi, whereas the myeloma patient is more apt to develop pneumonia or bacteremia due to *Haemophilus influenzae, Streptococcus pneumoniae,* and a variety of other acute bacterial infections. Acute leukemia is associated with a depression in the number and function of circulating granulocytes and is associated with severe pyogenic bacterial infections. Patients with acute and relapsed leukemia have demonstrated impaired phagocytosis and killing of fungi and bacteria by these cells, which may appear morphologically normal. *These defects may persist well into periods of remission and may progress along with progression of the underlying disease.*

The impact of the various forms of chemotherapy on host defenses must be added to those caused by the cancer itself. A variety of immune functions are impaired by chemotherapy, including the phagocytosis and killing of bacteria by neutrophils (corticosteroids, carmustine, radiation); antibody production (methotrexate, cyclophosphamide, L-asparaginase, 6-mercaptopurine); uptake and processing of antigen by macrophages (corticosteroids, cyclophosphamide, dactinomycin); recognition of antigens by T and B lymphocytes (corticosteroids, cyclophosphamide); and antigen-driven lymphocyte proliferation (methotrexate, 5-fluorouracil, fludarabine, cytarabine, L-asparaginase, dactinomycin, 6-mercaptopurine, hydroxyurea). Predisposition to infection induced by chemotherapy may mask more subtle defects due to underlying disease—e.g., the effects of granulocytopenia due to intensive chemotherapy will generally predominate over the effects of underlying lymphoma or myeloma.

Neutropenia

The most common predisposing condition for infection in the cancer patient is granulocytopenia, often due to chemotherapy. However, the *function* of inflammatory cells and of other immune (e.g., mucosal) barriers are of equal importance to the *number* of granulocytes. In neutropenia, the risk of infection increases as granulocyte counts decrease. Thus, the risk of infection in the patient with neutropenia (under 1000/mm^3 total granulocytes) increases when granulocyte numbers fall further, to below 500/mm^3; the risk is greatest when counts are lower than 100/mm^3. The many causes of neutropenia differ

TABLE 66-9 Causes of Neutropenia

Iatrogenic
  Cancer chemotherapy
  Drug toxicities (trimethoprim-sulfamethoxazole, chloramphenicol, ganciclovir, AZT)
Infection
  Viral (cytomegalovirus, HIV, Epstein-Barr virus, hepatitis B)
  Parasitic *(Leishmania)*
  Bacteria *(Clostridium)*
  Acute neutropenia of sepsis/endotoxemia (gram-negative sepsis)
  Bone marrow failure of neonatal sepsis
Immune
  Drug-induced autoimmunity (haptenic: penicillins, sulfa drugs)
  Aplastic anemia (includes idiosyncratic reactions: phenothiazines, chloramphenicol)
  Alloimmune neonatal neutropenia (maternal-fetal incompatibility)
  Congenital autoimmune neutropenia
  Primary autoimmune (systemic lupus erythematosus, Felty's syndrome, rheumatoid arthritis)
  Transfusion-induced
  Antineutrophil antibody–mediated
  Cyclic neutropenia (CD57 lymphocyte expansion)
Hereditary
  Infantile genetic agranulocytosis
  Familial neutropenia
  Cyclic neutropenia (autosomal dominant)
  Old age

qualitatively (Table 66-9). They include iatrogenic neutropenias (chemotherapy, drug toxicities), aplastic anemia and other immune neutropenias, the hereditary and acquired cyclic neutropenias, and malignancy-associated (especially acute leukemias) and infection-induced neutropenias. The rate of decline in white blood cell numbers and the duration of neutropenia influence the risk of infection. Thus, the patient with acute leukemia and rapidly falling neutrophil counts is at greater risk than the person in whom counts are falling slowly or are stable.

The Microbiology of Infection in Neutropenia and Cancer

Pulmonary infections in patients with functional or quantitative defects in neutrophils can reach the lungs via inhalation, microaspiration of colonizing organisms, and bacteremia after nonrespiratory penetration and bacteremia (e.g., from vascular catheters or disrupted mucosal surfaces). Decisions about the management of these patients are often made without microbiologic data because of the urgency of therapy in the immunocompromised host. Distinctions between pulmonary and extrapulmonary infections often become blurred in the attempt to treat most of the likely pathogens in a febrile neutropenic cancer patient. Often a specific, unsuspected pulmonary pathogen is detected on routine blood or urine culture or from a biopsy of an extrapulmonary infected site.

Common Infections in Neutropenic Patients

Common infections in the neutropenic host and the cancer patient are most often the result of colonization with, and infection by, pyogenic bacteria, including *S. pneumoniae, Staphylococcus aureus,* the Enterobacteriaceae, *Pseudomonas aeruginosa, H. influenzae,* and *Stenotrophomonas* (formerly *Xanthomonas) maltophilia.* Common fungal pathogens include *Candida albicans, Aspergillus* species, *C. kreusei, C. glabrata, Mucor, Absidia,* and *Rhizopus* species. The emergence of bacteria and fungi with antimicrobial resistance takes on special importance in the neutropenic host because therapy is generally empiric and is started before microbiologic data become available. The common "resistant" organisms include vancomycin- and ampicillin-resistant *Enterococcus faecium* and *faecalis,* methicillin-resistant *S. aureus,* inducible chromosomal and acquired plasmids encoding beta-lactamases in gram-negative bacteria, and azole (i.e., fluconazole) resistance to *C. kreusei* and *C. glabrata.* In individual patients, the spectrum of colonizing organisms also changes over time, especially with antibiotic use (and abuse). Seeding from blood-borne infection (e.g., due to vascular access catheters or localized infection) occurs most often with the organisms described above; other organisms are *Candida* and *Aspergillus* and, occasionally, mycobacteria. Patients with solid lung tumors may develop obstructive pneumonia or pulmonary hemorrhage, followed by superinfection with the flora of the upper respiratory tract and oropharynx.

Fungi and Less Common Pathogens

Combined cellular and granulocytic deficiencies are often present after chemotherapy. As a result, in addition to the common pathogens described above, pathogens normally controlled by cellular immune mechanisms (especially intracellular pathogens) can be detected; among these are *M. tuberculosis, Brucella* species, the geographic fungi, *Cryptococcus neoformans, Strongyloides stercoralis, Salmonella,* and *P. carinii.* Unusual pathogens have been identified in increasing numbers of cancer patients with neutropenia. The classic presentations of pneumonia, inflammation and perforation of the cecum (often with *Pseudomonas* and anaerobes), and "typhlitis" (often *Clostridium septicum*) may be the first signs of life-threatening infection in a neutropenic patient. Atypical presentations of infection may be from a portal of entry other than the gastrointestinal tract or the lungs. Thus, the first clinical signs of infection may be "spontaneous" or line-associated bacteremia (*S. aureus, S. epidermidis, Clostridium, Bacillus, Clostridium jeikeum, S. maltophilia, Candida* species, *Fusarium*), skin lesions (gram-negative sepsis, *Candida* species, *Nocardia asteroides, C. neoformans,* herpes simplex or varicella zoster), gingivitis (anaerobes), hepatic dysfunction (hepatosplenic candidiasis), or seizures (*N. asteroides* in brain abscess associated with slowly progressive pneumonia).

Because of the widespread use of antibacterial agents, mucosal injury, use of intravenous catheters and bone marrow transplantation, fungal infections have occurred with increasing frequency, most often in acute leukemia patients (see Table 66-10). *Candida glabrata* and *C. krusei* that are resistant to fluconazole develop during antibiotic treatment. Although Mucoraceae *(Rhizopus, Mucor, Absidia),* like the *Aspergillus* species, may present with invasive disease of the sinuses and periorbital and frontal cortex in diabetics, they can also cause rapidly progressive hemorrhagic pneumonia with infarction and fungemia. Invasive disease of the sinuses and periorbital and frontal cortex is especially prevalent in neutropenic diabetics and in patients treated with desferoxamine, with prolonged corticosteroid therapy, or with broad-spectrum

---

TABLE 66-10 Factors in the Development of Fungal Infections in Cancer Patients

---

Age/performance status
Prior chemotherapy or radiotherapy: Dose and duration
  Steroids
  Purine analogues
Prior infections (specific isolates)
Recent antibiotic use (resistance)
  Broad-spectrum antibiotics
  Prophylactic agents
Functional immune status (cell number, activity)
Hematopoietic transplantation–related
  Delayed engraftment or function of marrow
  Graft-vs-host disease and treatment
  Degree of donor-recipient histocompatibility mismatch
  Insufficient dose of stem cells (CD34+)
  Total T-cell number
Integrity of mucosal barriers (catheters, gastrointestinal)
Neutropenia (severity, duration $\geqslant$2 weeks)
Hospital environment
Nonhematopoietic organ failure (e.g., dialysis)
Other simultaneous infections (e.g., cytomegalovirus)

---

antibiotics. The treatment of this invasive disease is *surgical debridement* in addition to antifungal therapy. In patients with neutropenia or acute leukemia, a group of "benign" dermatophytes—including *Trichosporon beigelii, Aureobasidium, Alternaria, Curvularia, Phialophora, Wangiella,* and *Cladosporium*—have been associated both with disease of the skin and with invasive infection of the lungs, the sinuses, and the central nervous system. Occasionally infections are caused by "atypical fungi" (e.g., *Saccharomyces cerevisiae, Pseudallescheria boydii, Cunninghamella bertholletiae, Drechslera, Fusarium* species, *Geotrichum candidum,* and *Penicillium* species). *Fusarium* causes infection of the bloodstream and lungs that is indistinguishable from that due to *Aspergillus,* but with greater tendency to cutaneous involvement. The cardinal sign of *P. carinii* pneumonia is the presence of arterial hypoxemia out of proportion to physical or radiologic signs.

Viral Infections

Viral infection has become increasingly prevalent in cancer patients. Herpes simplex virus (HSV) and varicella zoster virus (VZV) are frequently reactivated during periods of neutropenia. Patients who are undergoing chemotherapy for Hodgkin's disease or who have received bone marrow transplants are at greater risk than other immunocompromised hosts (35 to 50 percent in the first year). Specific antiviral prophylaxis is effective in reducing the incidence and severity of these relapses. Most often, these viruses cause painful but relatively benign skin or mucosal (especially esophageal, gastrointestinal, and perianal) lesions. These lesions may progress in up to 50 percent of neutropenic cancer chemotherapy patients, and the skin rash may become more diffuse, with hemorrhagic or nonhemorrhagic lesions extending beyond the dermatomal limits. Systemic dissemination to visceral organs occurs in 10 percent of patients with disseminated skin disease commonly involving the liver, lungs, brain, or gastrointestinal tract. Nasal, oropharyngeal, or esophageal HSV or VZV infections may spread directly to the lungs with the development of vesicular lesions in the trachea, or may cause viral pneumonitis in the parenchyma as a result of viremia secondary to cutaneous reactivation. Primary varicella pneumonia may accompany chickenpox in adults and in the compromised host. Pulmonary invasion occurs within the first 7 days of illness, with mortality approaching 18 percent. Chest radiographs reveal nodular or interstitial infiltrates in up to 16 percent of adults with chickenpox, whereas only 10 to 25 of these have clinical symptoms. Pulmonary invasion by HSV and VZV in the neutropenic host should be considered a life-threatening emergency.

In bone marrow transplant (BMT) recipients, pulmonary infection due to CMV occurs in the CMV-seropositive recipient of CMV-seronegative marrow. Because much of the lung injury is due to immune responses to CMV antigens, the full pneumonitis develops not during lymphopenia but, rather, with the engraftment of the marrow and with the reemergence of immune function. Viral replication is not needed for CMV pneumonitis to occur. In the granulocytopenic host, pulmonary CMV infection may be fatal.

Parasitic Infection

The predominant parasitic infection enhanced by immune compromise is that due to *S. stercoralis,* a nematode that infects more than 100 million people worldwide, producing lifelong infection. *Strongyloides* is distinguished by its *ability to complete the replicative cycle within the human host.* Malnutrition is a major cofactor; neutropenia and corticosteroids are common coinducers of parasite replication. In the normal pattern of infection, the filariform larvae penetrate the skin, follow the veins to the lungs, and are then swallowed, entering the small intestine. The "hyperinfection syndrome" is the result of activation in the gastrointestinal tract by immune suppression, which causes penetration or transudation of worms across the wall, carrying gastrointestinal organisms with them. Peritonitis, bacteremia, and gram-negative, eosinophilic meningitis may result. Pneumonia may result from bacteremia or from obstruction of small airways and pneumonitis; the pulmonary infection fails to resolve without therapy directed at eliminating the nematode.

Clinical Approaches to Infection in the Cancer Patient

Clinical Signs of Infection

Identification of the presence of infection is often delayed in the neutropenic or cancer patient because the inflammatory response is diminished (decreased numbers or mobilization of granulocytes) and the usual signs of infection are absent. Thus, in neutropenic patients, pneumonia may not be associated with sputum production and radiologic changes. In the febrile neutropenic patient with leukemia, the source of obscure infection is often the perineal and perirectal areas; less common are infections of the urinary tract, skin (including venous lines and wounds), and lungs. In nonhematopoietic cancer patients, however, pulmonary infections predominate. A site of origin for a febrile episode is undetermined in 20 to 50 percent of patients. Many sites of infection are detected only at autopsy, notably in patients with disseminated fungal or combined fungal and bacterial infections. Mortality in the febrile neutropenic population is 30 to 50 percent. Noninfectious causes of fever are common; among them are pulmonary thromboembolism, tumor, radiation pneumonitis, atelectasis with pulmonary edema, drug allergy or toxicity, and pulmonary hemorrhage. Often, the resolution of fever in response to a trial of antibiotics is the only evidence of infection.

Initial Management of the Cancer Patient with Fever: Stratification of Risk

Each patient presenting with signs of infection must be evaluated in terms of the perceived risks of infection and noninfectious causes of fever and for the presence of neutropenia or other immune dysfunctions. Attempts to manage patients with greater efficiency and to shorten hospital stays have led to the development of *critical pathways,* which include standard patterns of evaluation and treatment for many patients, including those with cancer. Such uniform approaches are useful in establishing a *minimal standard* of care, but they do not address concerns about the pitfalls of failing to individualize therapy.

The safe application of critical pathways for the outpatient management of neutropenic patients necessitates careful stratification of these compromised patients by experienced clinicians in terms of their risk for infectious complications. *Any sign of infection* requires at least a brief hospitalization (1 to 3 days), with careful evaluation. However, many experienced oncologists now manage most febrile neutropenic patients *routinely* as outpatients. Any febrile neutropenic patient—or patient in whom absolute neutrophil count (ANC) is expected to fall below 1000/mm^3—with localizing signs (headache, altered mental status, rash, dyspnea, chest pain, pain over an indwelling catheter site, pulmonary infiltrates) should be considered for emergency admission. In particular, patients with leukemia or lymphoma, uncontrolled metastatic cancer, recent need for antibiotics, or ANC under 100 (or expected to fall below 100) are generally considered "higher-risk" patients and are best managed as inpatients until clinically stable. Patients with a history of frank rigors or hypotension merit admission. Any febrile cancer patient needs an assessment of vital signs, oxygen saturation, complete blood count with differential, electrolytes and blood urea nitrogen and creatinine (for obstruction by tumor or acute drug toxicity), blood cultures (at least one peripheral and one from any indwelling catheter), urine sediment examination and culture, sputum Gram-stain examination and culture, and chest radiograph. After a careful physical examination, the threshold for lumbar puncture and the determination of serum or spinal cryptococcal antigen should be low. The patient's history and medical record should be reviewed, with attention to current drugs, recent chemotherapy (especially corticosteroids), recent microbiologic data and antibiotic use, allergies, and exposures.

Empiric Use of Antibiotics in Fever and Neutropenia

After appropriate smears and cultures have been obtained, empiric antimicrobial therapy in the febrile neutropenic patient is essential, preferably within 1 to 2 h of arrival. The specific antibiotics selected for "routine use" in the febrile neutropenic patient remain controversial. Ultimately, this is because many combinations appear to work equally well, and because there are few studies of various combinations in identical patient populations using the same entry and endpoint criteria. The antibiotics selected must "cover" previously documented infections or surveillance culture data, physical findings, known hospital flora, and potential community exposures.

Initial therapy should assume that the organisms causing infection are likely to be resistant to prophylactic antibiotics currently in use by the patient. Many infections are loculated and require drainage (sinusitis, postobstructive pneumonitis). Patients thought to be at *low risk* for infection or other complications (nonleukemic, underlying cancer not progressing, no serious coexisting illness, no recent infections or courses of antibiotics, expected ANC to remain above 100) may be *considered* for home management after 24 h (to await blood culture data), based on the clinical assessment. In these patients, empiric antibiotics might include ticarcillin (or ticarcillin-clavulanate, piperacillin with or without tazobactam, or ceftriaxone) plus gentamicin (or tobramycin or amikacin). In medical centers in which the rate of infections with *P. aeruginosa* is minimal, a common empiric combination is cefazolin and gentamicin. However, this combination offers little coverage for *Pseudomonas* or resistant *Staphylococcus,* especially in pulmonary infection; therefore, it cannot be generally recommended.

Patients at *high risk* for complications or progression of disease (see above) are treated with ticarcillin and gentamicin (with or without cefazolin) *or* ceftazidime and gentamicin (with or without cefazolin). Monotherapy with ceftazidime or imipenem has also been found to be effective in medical centers that do not have nosocomial flora resistant to these agents. Optimal antibiotic therapy should include synergistic therapy for *Pseudomonas* infection in medical centers in which this organism is prevalent or if the patient is profoundly neutropenic. The routine use of quinolones or aztreonam for initial therapy in high-risk patients has not been well studied and is not recommended.

In the critically ill patient, or if infection due to *Staphylococcus epidermidis,* methicillin-resistant *S. aureus,* or enterococcus is suspected, vancomycin should be added or used to replace cefazolin. Such patients might include those with skin wounds, decubitus ulcers, or indwelling vascular access catheters. Gram-positive bacterial infections generally progress more slowly than do the gram-negative infections. Therefore, the *routine use* of vancomycin in these patients does not appear to be justified, because of the increased risk of vancomycin-resistant enterococci.

If an abdominal or anaerobic bacterial source is suspected, clindamycin or metronidazole (or imipenem or meropenem) can be added. Anaerobic infections other than those due to *Bacteroides fragilis* are uncommon as a source of major morbidity in these patients. Restrictions on the use of clindamycin have been instituted at many centers because of outbreaks of *C. difficile* colitis. Topical oral antifungal therapy (clotrimazole, nystatin) is commonly administered with parenteral antibiotics. Antibiotics may be adjusted on the basis of microbiologic data or if the patient is afebrile for 7 to 10 days with the ANC over 500 and increasing.

Fever and Pulmonary Infiltrates

Pulmonary disease in the cancer patient is clinically challenging, owing to the large array of processes that may cause radiologic infiltrates (Table 66-11). Noninfectious causes of pulmonary infiltrates and fever (edema, cancer, radiation injury, drug toxicity, leukoagglutinin transfusion reaction, pulmonary embolus, hemorrhage, alveolar proteinosis) are common (up to 25 percent) and may closely mimic infection. Conversely, the absence of inflammatory cells or mobilization may mask the signs of significant infection. In the patient

TABLE 66-11 Common Causes of Pneumonia in Cancer Patients Based on Radiographic Abnormalities and Disease Progression

Abnormality on chest radiograph	Common Cause by Rate of Disease Progression[a]	
	Acute (<24 h)	Subacute-Chronic
Consolidation	Bacteria (include *Legionella*) pulmonary embolus, hemorrhage, pulmonary edema	Fungi, *Nocardia*, tuberculosis [drug, virus (RSV), *P. carinii*, radiation]
Interstitial infiltrate	Pulmonary edema (include drug) Leukoagglutinin reaction (bacterial)	Viral, *Pneumocystis*, radiation, drug (fungi, *Nocardia*, tuberculosis, tumor)
Nodular infiltrate	Bacteria, edema (CMV, VZV)	Tumor, fungal, *Nocardia*, TB *Pneumocystis* (CMV)

KEY: RSV, respiratory syncytial virus; CMV, cytomegalovirus; VZV, varicella zoster virus; TB, tuberculosis.
[a]Common causes (and less common in parentheses) in the absence of specific epidemiologic exposures or past history.

undergoing chemotherapy or in the neutropenic host, cough, sputum, radiologic infiltrates or cavitation, and fever may all be absent. Infection may spread to the chest from contiguous structures (e.g., perforation of the esophagus due to *Aspergillus*) or may complicate anatomic changes (e.g., bronchial obstruction in lung cancer).

Radiologic Clues to Diagnosis

A number of clues are available to assist in the differential diagnosis of pulmonary infiltrates in cancer patients. For example, the clinical and radiographic appearance and progression of disease may suggest a diagnosis based on the time course and nature of the infiltrate (Table 66-11). In general, acute processes include both bacterial infections and noninfectious injuries, such as pulmonary embolus or edema. Subacute processes include *P. carinii,* viral, *Mycoplasma, Nocardia,* or *Aspergillus* infections. More chronic processes include drug-induced, radiation-induced, mycobacterial, nocardial, or malignant invasion of the lungs.

In particular, bronchial obstruction by tumor or enlarged lymph nodes may cause atelectasis or postobstructive pneumonia. The underlying process may be suggested by a pneumonia that either fails to respond to antibiotic therapy or recurs in the same location after successful treatment. Tumor masses, especially those due to lymphoma, may cavitate, giving the appearance of a lung abscess. Finally, it is important to bear in mind that a chronic process may be superinfected by an acute bacterial, viral, or drug-induced lung injury.

The clinical assessment coupled with the radiologic pattern of lung disease is usually the basis for forming a differential diagnosis for the patient with fever and pneumonitis. CT scans have greatly improved differentiation of some processes. For example, in patients with simultaneous processes affecting the lung (e.g., aspiration and tumor), CT scans may disclose distinctive patterns of parenchymal involvement (consolidation and infiltrative lesions with associated adenopathy) better than do conventional chest radiographs. Subtle interstitial infiltrates *(P. carinii)* or nodules *(Cryptococcus)* are better detected by CT scans than by conventional radiographs.

Noninfectious Pneumonitis

After a dose of radiation greater than 2000 rads, radiation injury is common. The injury may become evident either acutely or more than 6 months after the initial exposure. The acute form of radiation pneumonitis may present as a bronchitis or esophagitis with dry cough, fever, fatigue, hypoxemia, and dyspnea that develop over 6 to 12 weeks. The histologic picture reveals vascular damage, mononuclear infiltrates, and edema. The severity of lung injury due to radiation appears to correlate with the rapidity of the withdrawal of steroid therapy, but it may also reflect the emergence of the underlying inflammatory response. Radiation fibrosis usually occurs in 6 to 9 months, and pulmonary function may take up to 2 years to plateau.

Acute, drug-induced lung disease may reflect hypersensitivity to chemotherapeutic agents or to sulfonamide agents. Methotrexate, bleomycin, and procarbazine can cause a syndrome of nonproductive cough, fever, dyspnea, and pleurisy with skin rash and blood eosinophilia. Chest radiographs demonstrate diffuse reticular infiltrates. Cytoxan may cause a syndrome of subacute pulmonary disease with interstitial inflammation and pulmonary fibrosis. Fever, dyspnea, fatigue, and cough are common in cytoxan lung. Other common drugs causing lung injury are cytarabine and azathioprine. Drug toxicity for agents such as bleomycin, BCNU, and CCNU may be related to the cumulative dose (for bleomycin, over 450 mg) and to the age of the patient. Synergistic toxicity for the lung occurs between radiation and a variety of chemotherapeutic agents (e.g., bleomycin, mitomycin, busulfan) and supplemental oxygen use. A variety of noninfectious processes may mimic infection. Alveolar proteinosis may be associated with hematologic malignancies or accompany infection due to *Nocardia* or, less often, *Cryptococcus, Aspergillus, M. tuberculosis,* and *Histoplasma.* Pulmonary infarction may mimic infections by causing hemoptysis, leukocytosis, pleuritic chest pain, and segmental pleural-based infiltrates on the chest radiograph.

Approach to Patients on Empiric Therapy

The duration of empiric therapy must be individualized. In a patient receiving empiric therapy who becomes afebrile on antibiotics by 72 h and with a neutrophil count above 500/mm^3, the antibiotics may be stopped after 7 days and the patient reevaluated if no localizing source is found or untreated pathogens detected. Patients who are clinically well and who become afebrile with neutrophil counts of 100 to 500/mm^3 should be afebrile for 5 to 7 days before antibiotics are stopped in order to reevaluate sources of infection. If the patient is not clinically well (e.g., has mucositis, fewer neutrophils than 100/mm^3, or unstable vital signs), the antibiotics should be continued until the patient is stable and afebrile for 48 to 72 h.

Unless a specific source of infection is located and the pathogen(s) are identified, patients with persistent fever and neutropenia should have antibiotics broadened 48 to 72 h after the start of therapy. The options include (1) addition of vancomycin (or other gram-positive agent); (2) addition of antianaerobic therapy for oral mucositis or gingivitis, abdominal pain, or perirectal tenderness; (3) expansion of gram-negative bacterial coverage (generally adding a second agent from a different class of antibiotics); (4) consideration of antiviral therapy in patients with esophagitis or a history of HSV or VZV infections; and (5) addition of fluconazole or amphotericin B for symptoms of esophagitis or for documented or suspected fungal infection. In general, the first dose of amphotericin B should be a full dose (0.6 to 0.8 mg/kg for yeasts, 1.0 to 1.5 mg/kg for suspected *Aspergillus* or *Mucor* infections, full-dose lipid associated formulations). The patient must be well hydrated, and attention must be paid to magnesium and potassium maintenance. Slowly advancing doses of this drug (e.g., from a starting dose of 10 to 20 mg) have been advocated without much supporting data and entail the disadvantage of *days of delay* in achieving tissue levels of the drug.

Special attention must be paid to any symptoms of pulmonary disease, the presence of new pulmonary infiltrates on chest radiographs, or the presence of sinus symptoms in patients with persistent fevers. New infiltrates should prompt examinations of sputum and procurement of specimens (open biopsy, thoracoscopic biopsy, or bronchoscopy, preferably with biopsies, or needle aspirates under tomographic guidance) for histologic and microbiologic evaluation.

BONE MARROW AND STEM CELL TRANSPLANTATION

Temporal Sequence of Pulmonary Disease Syndromes

Specific pulmonary complications may be grouped according to the time of presentation relative to the day of transplantation. "Early" events occur within the first 100 days after transplant, and "late" events occur beyond day 100. The timetable has been altered by stem cell transplantation, where engraftment occurs earlier. The early period can be further subdivided into the period of profound neutropenia, which exists for a variable period after transplantation, and the period of acute graft-versus-host disease (GVHD), which begins 2 to 3 weeks after allogeneic transplantation and extends approximately to day 100. Although this division is clinically useful, overlap occurs in the timing of specific complications, and the categorization of pulmonary complications is often arbitrary, since the cause of many respiratory abnormalities is uncertain.

The most important characteristic that separates patients receiving allografts from those receiving syngeneic or autologous marrow or stem cells is the occurrence of GVHD in the former group. Syngeneic and autograft recipients share early risk factors, such as neutropenia, with patients receiving allogeneic transplants and are at risk of early pulmonary complications, such as bacterial or fungal pneumonia and noninfectious treatment-related pulmonary injury. Transplant recipients who have delayed engraftment or subsequent marrow failure are at continued risk of bacterial or fungal infection. Allogeneic marrow recipients with GVHD have continued abnormalities in immune function that increase the risk of opportunistic infections by mechanisms that are incompletely understood but include suppressive agents to treat the condition (cyclosporine, tacrolimus, rapamycin, corticosteroids, and other agents). Among patients with chronic GVHD, infection and pneumonia due to encapsulated organisms (e.g., *Streptococcus pneumoniae, Haemophilus influenzae,* and *Staphylococcus aureus*) appear related to deficiencies in specific antibody production or perhaps to continued defects in macrophage function.

Common Clinical Presentations

Signs and symptoms of pulmonary disorders related to marrow and hematopoietic stem cell transplantation are often nonspecific. Tachypnea is common, as are fever, cough, and rales. However, any or all of these may be absent at the time of presentation of pulmonary complications. Routine chest radiographs are obtained frequently during the first weeks of neutropenia and often provide the first indication of pulmonary impairment.

Diffuse Infiltrates

Diffuse infiltrates are common radiographic abnormalities noted in marrow recipients. However, these infiltrates are most often nonspecific. Infectious causes for diffuse infiltrates have been documented in fewer than 20 percent of marrow recipients undergoing open lung biopsy within 30 days after marrow transplantation. Within this early period, pulmonary edema syndromes predominate. The edema may be associated with cardiac decompensation or intravascular volume excess, or with adult respiratory distress syndrome (ARDS) and pulmonary capillary leak due to treatment-related toxicities or sepsis syndrome. Infections presenting with diffuse infiltrates within the first weeks after transplantation include respiratory viral causes, such as RSV, whereas CMV is uncommon. Alveolar hemorrhage may contribute to the radiographic infiltrates in the presence of thrombocytopenia, regardless of the cause of the lung injury.

Between 30 days and 180 days after marrow transplantation, infections are a major reason for diffuse radiographic abnormalities. CMV was common, but it is now unusual in patients receiving appropriate prophylaxis. Diffuse pneumonia due to bacterial infections also is unusual; however, diffuse involvement with fungus may occur in as many as 20 percent of diffuse infiltrates and may be extremely difficult to detect.

Focal Lesions

Focal parenchymal infiltrates are frequently due to infection regardless of the time of presentation after transplant. Focal consolidations or masses are related to local fungal infection in 80 percent of marrow transplant recipients receiving broad-spectrum antibiotics. Other causes are *Legionella* species, *Nocardia,* relapse of lymphoma in patients transplanted for that disorder, bronchiolitis obliterans with organizing pneumonia (BOOP), and, rarely, infarct due to thromboembolic disease.

Aspiration

Desquamation of the oropharyngeal mucosa is a frequent complication after intensive chemotherapy, and the stomatitis is often referred to as "mucositis." It develops within the first week after radiotherapy and reaches its greatest severity after 10 to 14 days, and impaired mucociliary clearance is common. Recurrent aspiration of oropharyngeal contents is common among transplant recipients with oral mucositis due to sedation, poor cough reflex, and dysphagia. These patients may present with basilar infiltrates or consolidation.

Pleural Effusions

Pleural effusions are common in the first weeks after marrow transplantation and are rarely related to an identifiable infectious source. Pleural effusions may be associated with fluid retention of any cause, especially with ascites secondary to hepatic venoocclusive disease (HVOD). HVOD may occur in as many as 60 percent of patients after total-body irradiation or in association with GVHD. Characteristics include weight gain within the first weeks after transplantation and elevation of the serum bilirubin, which usually precede the development of pleural effusions. The effusions are frequently bilateral. Bilateral pleural effusions in the presence of weight gain can be approached conservatively without diagnostic thoracentesis. Cautious diuresis coupled with treatment of GVHD often produces satisfactory results. Small effusions are common and may be associated with treatment-related pleuropericarditis or thromboembolic events, but a specific cause is seldom determined. A large unilateral or rapidly accumulating effusion in the presence of fever or ipsilateral chest pain may represent hemorrhage or infection and should be evaluated promptly by thoracentesis.

Noninfectious Etiology

Noninfectious causes of lung injury after marrow and hematopoietic stem cell transplantation include a spectrum of syndromes: idiopathic pneumonia, alveolar hemorrhage, pulmonary edema, obliterative bronchiolitis, and BOOP. Idiopathic pneumonia is characterized as a syndrome of hypoxemia and radiographic nonlobar infiltrates in the absence of congestive heart failure and without evidence of an infectious origin. It is included as a form of "interstitial" pneumonia. The term *interstitial pneumonia* in marrow transplant recipients refers to the syndrome of diffuse inflammatory pulmonary disease presenting with fever and tachypnea. This term includes noninfectious causes, as well as infectious pneumonia due to viruses (CMV) or protozoa. To avoid the ambiguity of the term *interstitial* in relation to inflammatory disorders of the lung, it is preferable to classify the clinical conditions as *diffuse* pneumonia on the basis of the radiographic presentation. Most noninfectious causes of lung injury are attributed to treatment-related toxicities. Alkylating chemotherapy agents and ionizing irradiation are likely contributors; however, ARDS secondary to sepsis syndrome also may occur. While pneumonia is associated with the presence of GVHD, whether GVHD causes a direct lung injury is unproved. The role of unrecognized infections remains a concern (Table 66-12).

Idiopathic Pneumonia Syndrome

Incidence and Epidemiology

The largest studies of idiopathic pneumonia after allogeneic marrow transplantation estimate the incidence at 12 to 17 percent. The spectrum of idiopathic lung injury was referred to as a "syndrome" [idiopathic pneumonia syndrome (IPS)] by a National Institutes of Health–sponsored workshop on idiopathic lung injury after marrow transplantation in recognition of the probability of multiple causes and varied clinical presentation (Table 66-13). The diagnosis of IPS is defined by a bronchoalveolar lavage (BAL) that does not reveal an infection in the presence of nonlobar radiographic infiltrates and physiologic changes consistent with pneumonia. A common series of laboratory evaluations is presented in Table 66-14. Many clinicians use IPS only to describe noninfectious lung injury occurring within the first 3 to 4 months after transplantation.

TABLE 66-12 Pulmonary Complications in Bone Marrow Transplantation

Early Complications (<100 days)	Approx. Incidence (%)
Pulmonary edema syndromes	0–50
Infectious pneumonia	20–30
Bacterial	2–30
Fungal	4–13
Viral	4–10
Protozoa	<5
Idiopathic pneumonia	7–12
Oral mucositis	50–70
Pulmonary venoocclusive disease	Rare
Late complications (>100 days)	
Bronchopneumonia	20–30
Idiopathic pneumonia	10–20
Viral pneumonia	0–10
Airflow obstruction (obliterative bronchiolitis)	2–11[a]

[a]Obstructive airflow among marrow recipients with chronic graft-versus-host disease.

Pathogenesis

The causes of diffuse idiopathic pneumonia are probably multiple and include treatment-related toxicities due to radiation or chemotherapeutic agents. However, sepsis-related pulmonary toxicity may account for a proportion of cases of diffuse idiopathic pneumonia with histology consistent with ARDS. While GVHD is associated with an increased incidence of idiopathic lung injury, it is unclear whether this is a cell-mediated immune response to the lung or related to an increased incidence of sepsis in these immunosuppressed patients. Also, administration of large volumes of blood products during the transplantation procedure may lead to pulmonary vascular injury through leukoagglutination reactions. Other unusual causes of noninfectious diffuse pneumonia after marrow transplantation are leukemic infiltration due to relapse of primary malignancy, injection of malignant cells with reinfused autologous marrow, and fat embolization due to marrow infusion. Several cases of fat embolization were associated with pulmonary hemorrhage and steroid administration.

TABLE 66-13 Criteria for Diagnosis of Idiopathic Pneumonia Syndrome

Evidence of widespread alveolar injury
 Multilobar infiltrates on chest radiograph or computed tomography
 Symptoms and signs of pneumonia
 Evidence of abnormal physiology and absence of active lower respiratory tract infection documented by negative bronchoalveolar lavage
Lung biopsy or autopsy with examination of stains and cultures for bacteria, fungi, and viruses, including cytomegalovirus (CMV) centrifugation culture, cytology for viral inclusions and *Pneumocystis carinii,* and immunofluorescence monoclonal antibody staining for CMV, respiratory syncytial virus, influenza virus, parainfluenza virus, and adenovirus

TABLE 66-14 Routine Laboratory Evaluation of Bronchoalveolar Lavage
Specimens in Marrow and Stem Cell Transplant Recipients

Pathology[a]
Wright-Giemsa stain
Papanicolaou stain
Silver stain
Modified Jimenez stain (or other stain suitable for detecting *Legionella*)
Consider: monoclonal fluorescent antibody stain for *Pneumocystis*
Microbiology
Stains:
  Gram's
  Wet mount KOH or calcofluor white
  Modified acid-fast
  Fluorescent antibody stain for *Legionella*
Culture:
  Bacterial (aerobic), semiquantitative method
  Fungal
  Legionella (chocolate yeast extract)
  Acid-fast
Virology
Fluorescent antibody stains[b]:
  CMV
  HSV
  RSV, parainfluenza and influenza viruses pooled antibodies[c,d]
Culture (rapid centrifugation technique preferred)[e]:
  CMV
  HSV
  Adenovirus
  RSV, parainfluenza, and influenzaviruses (in appropriate clinical setting)

KEY: CMV, cytomegalovirus; HSV, herpes simplex virus; RSV, respiratory
syncytial virus.
[a]Studies usually reviewed by a pathologist.
[b]Studies may be performed in virology or pathology laboratory.
[c]Separate studies for each virus should be performed if the study
 with pooled antibodies is positive.
[d]Fluorescent antibody stains may be supplemented or replaced by enzyme immunoassays (EIA) as available.
[e]If available. Culture may be replaced with fluorescent antibody stains or
 EIA alone if culture facilities are unavailable.

Clinical Presentation

The clinical presentation of IPS is nonspecific. Most patients develop a syndrome of fever, nonproductive cough, and tachypnea. Hypoxemia with hyperventilation is common. The onset is most often rapid, occurring over a
few days. Occasionally, insidious onset similar to that of idiopathic pulmonary fibrosis is seen. Median onset is within the first 3 weeks of transplantation, but it may occur up to months later. The chest radiograph shows
diffuse intraalveolar and/or interstitial infiltrates. The presentation is not
sufficiently distinct to be readily differentiated from that of pulmonary
edema syndromes or diffuse infectious pneumonia. Marked tachypnea in
the absence of radiographic infiltrates should raise the suspicion of
obstructive airway disease or pulmonary venoocclusive disease rather than
idiopathic pneumonia.

Pathology

IPS after marrow transplantation represents a histologic spectrum ranging from a primarily interstitial reaction with diffuse or focal widening of the alveolar septa and interstitial spaces with mononuclear inflammatory cells and edema to diffuse alveolar damage (DAD) with alveolar epithelial necrosis, intraalveolar hyaline membranes, edema and hemorrhage, and type 2 cell hyperplasia. The predominantly interstitial presentation has been referred to as *idiopathic interstitial pneumonia,* whereas the pathology of diffuse alveolar damage is identical to that of ARDS. Variable degrees of alveolar hemorrhage may be seen with either of these presentations. Elements of both histologic pictures may be seen in any pathologic specimen. Recent experience from Seattle found that the interstitial pattern predominated in more than 50 percent and DAD in one-third of lung biopsies from marrow recipients with idiopathic pneumonia. By definition, all microbiologic and histologic evaluations for infectious agents (viral, protozoal, fungal, and bacterial) are negative in idiopathic pneumonia. The importance of a thorough microbiologic examination lies in the fact that these histologic presentations are similar to those of infectious pneumonia, especially CMV pneumonia.

Course of Disease and Treatment

The mortality from idiopathic lung injury after marrow transplantation remains over 70 percent. The diagnosis of idiopathic lung injury rests largely on the results of BAL. Lung biopsy (transbronchial or open) appears to add little to the diagnostic sensitivity of BAL for infection in the presence of diffuse parenchymal infiltrates. At present, histopathology does not help to direct therapy in idiopathic lung injury after hematopoietic stem cell transplantation. Lung biopsy should be considered in cases with patchy or multifocal infiltrates because of the higher incidence of infection and concern for false-negative results from BAL. There are no randomized studies of treatment of idiopathic lung injury after marrow transplantation. High-dose corticosteroids (ranging from 1 to 16 mg/kg per day of methylprednisolone) and other forms of intensive immune suppression are commonly used.

Pulmonary Hemorrhage

Incidence and Clinical Syndrome

Diffuse alveolar hemorrhage (DAH) is a syndrome of progressive dyspnea, hypoxemia, cough, and a progressively bloodier return from BAL in autologous marrow recipients, usually within 2 weeks of transplant. The incidence of DAH is up to 20.5 percent and associated with age over 40 years, fever, transplantation for a solid tumor, severe mucositis, white blood cell recovery, and renal insufficiency. Thrombocytopenia is a common finding, and patients with DAH receive more platelet transfusions than patients without this condition. It is unclear whether this hemorrhagic pneumonia represents a unique syndrome or rather severe lung injury in the presence of a bleeding diathesis.

Pulmonary Edema Syndromes

Biventricular failure after transplantation is often iatrogenic and associated with excessive fluid administration. However, an increase in total body weight may also be the first indication of GVHD. Radiographic evidence of pulmonary edema after marrow transplantation has been reported in up to 50 percent of patients, most occurring in the second week. Close attention to the total amount of sodium and fluids administered can lead to dramatic reduction in the incidence of pulmonary edema. Also, pulmonary edema may be associated with left ventricular decompensation related to cardiotoxic cytoreductive regimens, including anthracyclines in excess of 500 mg/m^2 and high-dose cyclophosphamide. Posttransplantation cardiac and pericardial toxicity occur in 4 to 10 percent of cases, usually associated with total-body irradiation and cyclophosphamide, often in the setting of prior anthracycline administration. The utility of cardiac imaging studies before transplantation to predict heart failure is limited.

The most frequent noncardiac association with pulmonary edema states is HVOD. The syndrome is often associated with interstitial pulmonary edema, the formation of pleural effusions, and renal failure. Noncardiac pulmonary edema also develops in association with acute GVHD and may be due, in part, to DAD and capillary leak. The presentation of pulmonary edema is nonspecific and usually occurs within 30 days after marrow infusion. Marrow recipients are often febrile and tachypneic at this time in the transplant course, and recipients of allogeneic marrow may display evidence suggestive of acute GVHD. Thus, the distinction between pulmonary edema and idiopathic pneumonia often cannot be made with certainty without pulmonary artery catheterization. However, recent increase in total body weight appears to correlate well with total-body fluid accumulation and should prompt a trial of diuretic therapy and a search for other signs of GVHD (gastrointestinal tract, liver, skin) before consideration of invasive diagnostic procedures. Noninvasive assessment of cardiac function with ultrasonographic or radionuclide techniques is often warranted to guide treatment.

New-Onset Airflow Obstruction and Obliterative Bronchiolitis

Epidemiology and Incidence

About 10 percent of allogeneic marrow recipients with chronic GVHD are likely to develop airflow obstruction consistent with obliterative bronchiolitis. However, the reported incidence of obliterative bronchiolitis varies, in part, with the method used to identify the presence of the disease, possibly because of decreased airway diameter. The onset of progressive airflow disease more than 100 days after allogeneic marrow transplantation is strongly related to the development of GVHD. Factors associated with the increased risk of GVHD, such as increasing age and HLA-nonidentical marrow grafts, are not independent risk factors for the development of obliterative bronchiolitis. The cause of obliterative bronchiolitis after marrow transplantation is unknown.

Clinical Presentation

The usual clinical manifestation of new-onset airflow obstruction is the insidious onset of tachypnea, dyspnea on exertion, and dry, nonproductive cough. Fever is uncommon. Although the chest radiograph is commonly interpreted as normal, high-resolution chest CT often reveals parenchymal hypoattenuation and segmental bronchial dilatation. Auscultation of the chest may reveal scattered expiratory wheezing and occasionally diffuse inspiratory crackles, but results are sometimes normal. Arterial blood-gas analysis reveals moderate hypoxemia and, in the later stages, hypercarbia. When the presentation is beyond 150 days after marrow grafting, evidence of GVHD is usually present. However, the disorder may occur at any time after transplantation, and some cases are recognized only after several years. The major differential diagnoses of the gradual onset of nonspecific respiratory symptoms in the presence of a normal chest radiograph include pulmonary venoocclusive disease and pulmonary embolism. Obliterative bronchiolitis is characterized by reduction in expiratory airflow on spirometry and increases in residual lung volumes not found in the other two diseases.

Course of Disease and Treatment

Prospective evaluation of pulmonary functions after marrow transplantation identified marrow recipients with variable courses of disease progression. Patients with onset of airflow obstruction within the first 150 days after marrow transplantation tend to have a rapid decline in pulmonary function and a fatal outcome. These patients may not survive long enough to develop manifestations of chronic GVHD but usually display acute GVHD after marrow grafting. It is possible that infection plays a role in the development of the airflow obstruction in some of these patients. Marrow recipients with the onset of airflow obstruction beyond 150 days after transplantation tend to have a more gradual decline in lung function. Airflow may stabilize in 50 percent of these patients.

There are no prospective trials of treatment for new-onset airflow obstruction. At present, the accepted approach to these patients is to aggressively control with immunomodulating agents the chronic GVHD that most often accompanies the airflow obstruction. Treatment usually consists of increased immunosuppression. Reversal of the airflow obstruction is uncommon. The usual goal of management is stabilization of the obstruction. For this reason, prompt recognition and treatment for this progressive process are critical. Supportive measures include prophylaxis against *P. carinii* pneumonia and *S. pneumoniae* infection, inhaled bronchodilators, supplemental immunoglobulin administration to maintain normal serum levels, and prompt treatment of intercurrent infections.

Pulmonary Venoocclusive Disease

Pulmonary venoocclusive disease (PVOD) is a rare complication of treatment with chemotherapeutic regimens, and as a solitary pulmonary complication, PVOD is very uncommon after marrow grafting. The primary histologic lesion of PVOD—obstruction of the pulmonary veins and venules by loose intimal fibrosis proliferation—may be difficult to detect with hematoxylin-and-eosin stains alone, and specific stains for elastic tissues, such as Verhoeff–van Gieson stain, are required to demonstrate the fibrotic reaction in the veins. The typical presentation of PVOD is that of insidious dyspnea on exertion and resting tachypnea within 3 to 4 months after transplantation. Significant hypoxemia may occur along with hyperventilation. The chest radiograph is often unrevealing. On cardiac examination, there is evidence of pulmonary hypertension. Auscultation of the lungs is often normal, although scattered inspiratory crackles may be heard. Noninvasive examinations, echocardiography, perfusion/ventilation nucleotide scans, and electrocardiograms are nondiagnostic. Pulmonary function testing may be consistent with mild restrictive defect, but airflow obstruction, suggesting obliterative bronchiolitis, is absent. BAL has failed to demonstrate pathogens or inflammatory cells. The diagnostic procedure of choice is a pulmonary angiogram. Right heart catheterization reveals elevated pulmonary artery pressure, with normal pulmonary artery wedge pressures. Angiography excludes the presence of thrombi as a cause of the pulmonary hypertension.

In most cases presenting after treatment for malignancy, the disease has followed an insidious course, with progressive hypoxemia and dyspnea on exertion due to pulmonary hypertension. Some patients recover with high-dose corticosteroid therapy or other immunosuppressive therapy.

Pulmonary Infection

Viral Pneumonia: Cytomegalovirus

Incidence and Epidemiology The incidence of cytomegalovirus (CMV) pneumonia has declined significantly in recent years. The rates now appear to be approximately 4 percent for both allogeneic and autologous transplantation. The decline is attributable to effective prophylaxis and preemptive treatment. It is presumed that most if not all CMV infection occurring in seropositive patients is due to reactivation of latent infection. The risk of infection in seronegative patients with seronegative marrow donors is attributable to blood product exposure, and this risk can be virtually eliminated by use of screened seronegative or filtered blood products.

Clinical Presentation The clinical presentation of CMV pneumonia is not distinct from that of other entities that cause diffuse pneumonia. Patients with CMV pneumonia may have nonproductive cough, dyspnea, hypoxemia, or fever, with a median onset of 60 days after marrow transplant. Onset within the first 2 weeks is unusual. The period of risk of CMV pneumonia generally ends by approximately the fourth or fifth month after transplant, although later cases occur among patients with chronic GVHD or after autologous transplant. Chest radiograph generally shows bilateral infiltrates; in later stages, diffuse consolidation occurs. Unilateral, focal, and even nodular infiltrates have been seen in the early stages.

Course of Disease Historically, CMV pneumonia was an inexorable process leading to death within 2 to 4 weeks (usually less) in 85 percent of patients with biopsy-proven disease. Treatment with a variety of antiviral agents, including ganciclovir, did not change the course. At present, survival of 30 to 70 percent can be expected with the combination of ganciclovir and intravenous immunoglobulins. While improved survival rates are encouraging, it remains possible that this change is in part due to treatment earlier in the disease course. Survival of patients with respiratory failure at time of initial treatment remains uncommon.

Treatment and Prevention Recent studies suggest that the combination of ganciclovir and/or foscarnet and intravenous hyperimmune CMV immunoglobulins substantially improves survival from CMV pneumonia compared to experience with a variety of antiviral agents, including vidarabine, acyclovir, and leukocyte or lymphoblastoid interferons, alone or in various combinations. CMV pneumonia can be prevented in most cases with the prophylactic administration of ganciclovir to all seropositive recipients. Most seropositive patients who are at the highest risk of developing CMV pneumonia can be prospectively identified by routine studies of body fluids. Patients with positive blood, throat, urine, or BAL cultures have a significantly increased probability of developing CMV pneumonia. Detection of CMV antigens in blood leukocytes (using peroxidase-labeled monoclonal antibodies) or CMV DNA in plasma or blood leukocytes (using PCR) are sensitive and specific in the identification of patients at highest risk for CMV pneumonia. The negative predictive value of such testing approaches 100 percent. Prospective use of these techniques after allogeneic transplantation permits preemptive treatment with ganciclovir, which appears to eliminate the incidence of CMV pneumonia.

Other Viral Infections: RSV, Parainfluenza, Adenovirus, HSV, HHV-6

Incidence and Epidemiology   Viral pneumonias other than CMV may occur after marrow transplantation at an incidence that is lower and usually poorly defined. The most common of these is due to adenovirus. Adenovirus infection occurs in 5 percent of patients within the first 3 months after transplantation, attributable in almost all cases to reactivation of latent virus. Approximately 20 percent of marrow transplant patients with adenovirus infection develop pneumonia. Pneumonia due to herpes simplex virus (HSV) or varicella zoster virus (VZV) occurs uncommonly. HSV pneumonia is generally due to contiguous spread of virus to the trachea or aspiration from the oropharynx, although it may be due to generalized infection with viremia. Pneumonia due to VZV occurs among patients with disseminated infection and viremia. Both situations have become exceedingly uncommon with the advent of acyclovir treatment and, in the case of HSV, acyclovir prophylaxis.

Pneumonia due to "typical" respiratory viruses—including parainfluenza types 1 and 3, influenza A and B, and respiratory syncytial virus (RSV)—occurs sporadically as in other immunocompromised patients and in normal persons and is (except with parainfluenza type 1) more common during the winter months. Nosocomial transmission from infected health care workers has been documented. The incidence of respiratory virus infection may be higher than previously appreciated. Recently described members of the herpesvirus family have been noted in lung tissues of patients with pneumonia and blood of febrile recipients after transplantation. Human herpesvirus 6, the cause of childhood roseola (exanthema subitum), has been detected in the lungs of some patients with idiopathic pneumonia. It is unclear whether this virus is a cause of pneumonia or merely latently reactivated, since virtually all adults are seropositive for the virus.

Fungal Infections

Incidence and Epidemiology   Major risk factors for invasive fungal infections are the level and duration of neutropenia, age of the patient, the presence of GVHD, total number of other infections, and corticosteroid administration after marrow grafting. The frequency of *Aspergillus* infections is reportedly similar in recipients of allogeneic and autologous transplants. Allogeneic recipients may have more prolonged neutropenia and immune dysfunction, a greater risk of CMV infection, and enhanced risk of invasive fungal disease. Atypical fungal infections are increasing.

Bacterial Infections

Pathologic specimens rarely confirm bacterial bronchopneumonia after marrow transplantation. However, this may represent a selection bias of patients undergoing biopsy, since bacterial pneumonia has been reported in as many as 28 percent of autopsies of marrow recipients in some centers. The distribution of bacteria responsible for pulmonary infections during the neutropenic period is unknown. Aerobic gram-negative organisms are frequently detected during episodes of bacterial pulmonary infection. Half of the cases of bacteremia after marrow transplantation are due to gram-positive organisms, especially coagulase-negative *Staphylococcus,* with the rest due primarily to aerobic gram-negative Enterobacteriaceae.

Uncommon Nonbacterial Infections

P. carinii pneumonia occurs in as many as 10–15 percent of marrow transplant recipients without the use of trimethoprim-sulfamethoxazole prophylaxis, although regional and center-to-center variations exist. Except for patients being treated for chronic GVHD or CMV (who remain at risk and who should continue to receive prophylaxis), the risk period for *P. carinii* pneumonia ends approximately 120 days after transplantation. Because it is highly effective, trimethoprim-sulfamethoxazole is the prophylactic regimen of choice. Other regimens have been discussed elsewhere. Patients with allergies to sulfa may undergo desensitization so that prophylaxis with trimethoprim-sulfamethoxazole can be administered.

Most marrow transplant patients with *Toxoplasma gondii* infection have had only central nervous system disease diagnosed and treated during life or involvement of heart and brain documented at postmortem. However, several have had more generalized disease, diagnosed only at autopsy, in the myocardium, lungs, and brain. Chest radiographs in these patients showed diffuse, patchy involvement. These patients also had concomitant bacterial or viral infection, and the contribution of *Toxoplasma* to either the signs or symptoms of pulmonary disease is uncertain. Most infections have been fatal.

Pulmonary Function Testing in Hematopoietic Stem Cell Transplantation

Pretransplant Testing

Pulmonary function testing (PFT) is a standard part of the pretransplant evaluation at many centers. The results form baseline data for comparison with later testing, and have been used as an indication to exclude a candidate for transplantation. Abnormalities in the measures of airflow, lung volume, and diffusing capacity have been associated with increased risk of pulmonary complications after transplantation. After accounting for other clinical characteristics associated with death after transplantation (age, relapsed malignancy, HLA-mismatched graft), restrictive lung defect (decreased total lung capacity), hypoxemia, and reduced diffusing capacity are associated with statistically increased risk of death, especially within the first few months after transplant. The risks associated with these PFT results are applicable to autologous as well as allogeneic marrow recipients, suggesting that they predict mortality due to treatment-related toxicities. Hypoxemia and reduced diffusing capacity were independently associated with death, each carrying risk.

Posttransplant Testing

PFT performed after marrow transplantation has consistently revealed reductions in lung volumes and diffusing capacities associated with total-body irradiation and intensive chemotherapy. PFT abnormalities have been reported to include declines in lung volume, gas diffusion, and airflow. Losses of lung volume are more pronounced among patients who survive pneumonia after transplant. The declines in lung volume may be at least partly reversible within 2 years after transplantation, while the low diffusing capacity reportedly persists for several years. Development of airflow obstruction has been seen in approximately 10 percent of allogeneic marrow recipients in the presence of chronic GVHD and most often is related to obliterative bronchiolitis. Such PFT results strongly suggest that lung parenchymal and vascular injury are common features of marrow transplant, even in the absence of recognized infection or idiopathic pneumonia.

SOLID ORGAN TRANSPLANTATION

Timetable of Infection

As immunosuppressive regimens have become standardized in recent years, it has become apparent that *different infectious processes occur at different points in the posttransplant course.* That is, although pneumonia can occur at any point in the posttransplant course, the etiology of pneumonia will vary depending on the amount of time that has passed since transplantation (Fig. 66-1).

Infections in the First Month after Transplantation

In the first month after transplant, two major causes of pulmonary infection apply to all forms of organ transplantation. The first is the recurrence of pneumonia that was present prior to transplantation (in the lung allograft donor or in the recipient) but was incompletely treated, and which may be exacerbated after transplant due to superinfection with nosocomially acquired gram-negative bacilli and fungal species. This is most commonly seen in patients with end-stage liver or cardiac disease who require critical care support prior to transplant. Second, infection due to aspiration of nosocomial flora is often the result of postoperative vomiting (because of gastric distention or metabolic dysfunction) or a technical problem with the endotracheal tube in the perioperative period. The risk of antibiotic-resistant pneumonia will increase with the duration of the pretransplant hospitalization as well as with the duration of posttransplant intubation or ventilatory restriction (following the transplant operation).

Extensive pulmonary injury before transplant places the patient at high risk for postoperative pneumonia that is poorly responsive to therapy. In the special case of the lung transplant patient who may require prolonged intubation, bacterial pneumonia and infection that threatens the bronchial anastomosis, particularly with fungi, are special concerns. These patients require exquisite attention to the technical aspects of the transplant procedure, to the management of the endotracheal tube, and the maintenance of pulmonary toilet (including, on occasion, repeated therapeutic bronchoscopy). Notable by their absence in the first posttransplant month are the opportunistic infections, despite the fact that the highest daily doses of immunosuppression are administered during this first month. This emphasizes that it is the *sustained exposure to immunosuppressive therapy,* "the area under the curve," that is the major determinant of the net state of immunosuppression.

Infections 1 to 6 Months after Transplantation

In the period 1 to 6 months after transplant, the nature of pulmonary infection changes markedly. During this time period, the immunomodulating viruses, particularly CMV, exert their maximal effects. Thus, CMV can directly cause pneumonia itself; CMV may contribute to the incidence of graft rejection, necessitating increased exogenous immune suppression and increasing the risk of opportunistic infection; or CMV and the other immunomodulating viruses may be globally immunosuppressive, enhancing the likelihood of pulmonary infections due to *P. carinii, Aspergillus* species, and *Nocardia asteroides* in the *absence* of an unusual epidemiologic exposure. Unlike the bone marrow transplant recipient, the risk of active CMV *disease* (as compared with viral secretion) in the solid organ transplant recipient is greatest in the CMV-seronegative recipient of an organ from a seropositive donor. Thus, CMV prevention and the utilization of diagnostic techniques for CMV viremia (e.g., antigenemia assays, polymerase chain reaction testing, shell vial cultures with early antigen detection) are important parts of the therapeutic program.

During this period, *in the absence of specific prophylaxis,* significant nonviral pulmonary infections—including those due to *P. carinii, Aspergillus* species, and *N. asteroides*—are common at most transplant centers. There is important regional variation in the occurrence of each of these pathogens. At centers with high endemicity of these infections, low-dose trimethoprim-sulfamethoxazole prophylaxis (which effectively eliminates *P. carinii* and nocardial infection) and epidemiologic protection against *Aspergillus* (as with a HEPA-filtered air supply within the hospital) are effective, particularly in the context of effective CMV prevention.

Infections beyond 6 Months after Transplantation

In the period more than 6 months after transplant, patients can be divided into two groups in terms of the forms of pulmonary infection that can develop. Most patients will have had a good result from their transplant and will have good allograft function and receive relatively modest levels of maintenance immunosuppression. These patients are subject to community-acquired respiratory virus infection, particularly influenza, and RSV and pneumococcal pneumonia. The remaining patients have had a less positive outcome from their transplant; these individuals have less satisfactory graft function and require far more intensive acute and chronic immunosuppressive therapies to manage rejection. These patients, often termed "chronic ne'er do wells," are the subgroup of transplant patients at highest risk for pulmonary infection with such organisms as *P. carinii, Cryptococcus neoformans, N. asteroides,* and *Aspergillus* species. For this subgroup of patients, prolonged trimethoprim-sulfamethoxazole prophylaxis, epidemiologic protection, and a consideration of fluconazole prophylaxis are indicated. Notable among the "n'er do well" group is the liver transplant recipient with recurrent hepatitis C infection, the lung transplant patient with cystic fibrosis and resistant *Pseudomonas* or *Stentotrophomonas* infections, and the one with a kidney transplant who has chronic allograft dysfunction.

Radiologic Clues to the Diagnosis of Pneumonia in the Organ Transplant Patient

The presentation and evolution of the chest radiograph provide important clues to both the differential diagnosis of pulmonary infection in the transplant patient and the appropriate diagnostic workup that should be undertaken.

The following radiologic parameters are useful in developing clinical-radiologic-pathologic correlations:

1. Time of appearance, rate of progression, and time to resolution of pulmonary roentgenographic abnormalities in relation to clinical events.
2. Distribution of radiologic abnormalities. An abnormality confined to one anatomic area is considered *focal,* whereas widespread lesions are considered *diffuse.* Abnormalities that are present in more than one area but are countable are termed *multifocal.* As visualized particularly on CT scan, abnormalities may be located *centrally, peripherally,* or both.
3. Which of three types of pulmonary infiltrate is present. The first type is a *consolidation,* in which there is substantial replacement of alveolar air by material of tissue density, typically with air bronchograms and a peripheral location of the abnormality. The second type is *peribronchovascular* (or *interstitial*), in which the infiltrate is predominantly oriented along the peribronchial or perivascular bundles. Finally, *nodular* lesions are space-occupying, nonanatomic lesions with well-defined, more or less rounded edges surrounded by aerated lung.
4. Other characteristics. These include pleural fluid, atelectasis, cavitation, lymphadenopathy, and cardiac enlargement. Pleural fluid is a clue to congestive heart failure and fluid overload when it is bilateral and to necrotizing or granulomatous infection when it is unilateral, especially when associated with lymphadenopathy or cavitation.

By combining this classification with information concerning the rate of progression of the illness (Table 66-15), a useful differential diagnosis is then generated. Thus, focal or multifocal consolidation of acute onset will quite likely be caused by bacterial infection. Similar multifocal lesions with subacute to chronic progression are more likely secondary to fungal, tuberculous, or nocardial infections. Large nodules are usually a sign of fungal or nocardial infection in this patient population, particularly if they are subacute to chronic in onset. Subacute disease with diffuse abnormalities, either of the peribronchovascular type or miliary micronodules, are usually caused by viruses (especially CMV) or *P. carinii* (or, in the lung transplant patient, rejection). Additional clues can be found by examining the pulmonary lesion for the development of cavitation, with cavitation suggesting such necrotizing infections as those caused by fungi, *Nocardia,* and certain gram-negative bacilli (most commonly with *Klebsiella pneumoniae* and *P. aeruginosa*). The depressed inflammatory response of the immunocompromised transplant patient may greatly modify or delay the appearance of a pulmonary lesion on radiograph, particularly if neutropenia is complicating the effects of the antirejection therapy. CT of the chest has revolutionized the evaluation of these immunocompromised patients, and CT is particularly useful when the chest radiograph is negative or when the radiologic findings are subtle or nonspecific. An additional important application of CT in this patient population is defining the extent of the disease process. Particularly with opportunistic fungal and nocardial infection, precise knowledge of the extent of the infection at diagnosis, and the response of all sites to therapy, will lead to the best therapeutic outcome, as therapy should be continued until all evidence of infection is eliminated, not just the primary site. CT findings are also quite useful in defining which invasive diagnostic procedure should be utilized to obtain diagnostic samples and in identifying the anatomic site at which sampling should be directed to optimize the diagnostic yield.

TABLE 66-15 Differential Diagnosis of Fever and Pulmonary Infiltrates in the Organ Transplant Recipient According to Roentgenographic Abnormality and the Rate of Progression of the Symptoms

| Chest radiographic abnormality | Etiology According to the Rate of Progression of the Illness | |
	Acute[a]	Subacute-chronic[a]
Consolidation	Bacterial (including Legionnaire's disease) Thromboembolic	Fungal Nocardial Tuberculous Viral,
	Hemorrhage (pulmonary edema)	(Drug-induced, radiation, *Pneumocystis* tumor)
Peribronchovascular	Pulmonary edema (leukoagglutinin, reaction bacterial)	Viral *Pneumocystis* (Fungal, nocardial, tuberculous, tumor)
Nodular infiltrate[b]	Bacterial, pulmonary edema	Fungal Nocardial Tuberculous *(Pneumocystis)*

[a]An acute illness develops and requires medical attention in a matter of relatively few hours (<24). A subacute-chronic process develops over several days to weeks. Note that unusual causes of a process are in parentheses.
[b]A nodular infiltrate is defined as one or more large (>1 cm^2 on chest radiography) focal defects with well-defined, more or less rounded edges, surrounded by aerated lung. Multiple tiny nodules of smaller size, as sometimes caused by such an agent as CMV or varicella zoster virus, are not included here.

PRIMARY IMMUNE DEFECTS

Primary immunodeficiencies are defined as alterations in the immune system that are congenital, as opposed to those related to chemotherapy, autoimmune disease, organ transplant, or chronic systemic disease. Clinical problems that require evaluation of the immune system include chronic or recurrent bacterial or fungal infections of the skin, sinuses, and respiratory and digestive tracts and repeated infections with unusual viruses. Other suggestive signs and symptoms are persistent atypical rashes, chronic diarrhea, failure to thrive, paucity of lymphoid tissue, lymphadenopathy, chronic conjunctivitis, and unusual reactions to live virus vaccines. The evaluation of recurrent infections should analyze all compartments of the host defense system, including anatomic structures, mucociliary function, B- and T-cell activity, phagocytic cell function, and complement activity. Table 66-16 outlines both initial and confirmatory screening tests available to most clinicians.

Antibody (B-Cell) Deficiency

Antibody deficiency states are among the most common of the primary immunodeficiency diseases. Although the defect in immunoglobulin production can occur at any point in B-cell maturation/activation or secretion of antibody, or even in T- and B-cell interaction, the end result is a decrease in serum

TABLE 66-16 Immunologic Workup of Primary Immune Deficiencies

Suspected abnormality	Screening tests	Confirmatory tests
Antibody deficiency	Serum IgM, IgG, IgA levels IgG antibody response to protein (diphtheria,tetanus, influenza) and polysaccharide (pneumococcus, Haemophilus influenzae) antigens Isohemagglutinin titers for IgM antibody response Serum IgG subclass levels	B-cell enumeration [total B (CD20) surface IgM-, IgG-, IgA-, IgD-bearing B cells)] In vitro immunoglobulin synthesis
Cell-mediated immunodeficiency	Total lymphocyte count Delayed hypersensitivity skin tests (diphtheria, tetanus, Candida, PPD, SK/SD for T-cell function) Tests for HIV antibodies	Enumerate total T cells and T-cell subsets (CD3, CD4, CD8) Measure T-cell function with mitogenic, antigenic, and allogeneic (mixed lymphocyte reaction) responses,- lymphokine production, cytotoxic assay Assays for Th and Ts activity Enzyme assay (ADA, PNP) for ADA or PNP deficiency
Complement deficiency	CH_{50} or CH_{100} for classic pathway activity APH_{50} for alternative pathway activity Serum C2, C3, C4, C5, and factor B levels	Other specific component levels C1 esterase inhibition levels C1 esterase functional component
Phagocyte defects	NBT test for respiratory burst activity (defect in CGD) Serum IgE levels for HIE	Leukocyte adhesive protein analysis: (CD11a/CD18, CD11b/CD18, and CD11c/CD18) Adherence and aggregation Chemotaxis and random motility Phagocytosis Assays for respiratory burst activity (chemiluminescence, oxygen radical production) Bacterial killing test Enzyme assay (MPO, glucose-6-phosphate dehydrogenase) for phagocyte enzyme defects Cytochrome b or cytosolic protein measurement for CGD.

antibody levels or the inability to respond to antigens with specific antibody. Patients typically present with recurrent sinopulmonary infections caused by encapsulated bacteria such as *S. pneumoniae, H. influenzae* (both type b and nontypable), and *S. aureus.* Diseases caused by mycoplasma, enteroviruses, and intestinal parasites are also occasionally seen. The incidence of autoimmune abnormalities and hematologic malignancies is also significant in patients with these defects. Treatment for most of these defects relies on the administration of gamma globulin. Annual chest radiographs and pulmonary function tests are especially helpful, given that the lung disease in patients with hypogammaglobulinemia may be insidious in onset and progression.

X-Linked Agammaglobulinemia

X-linked agammaglobulinemia (XLA, or Bruton's agammaglobulinemia) is a relatively common inborn error of immunity, occurring in 1 per 50,000 live births. A block in the normal maturation of immunoglobulin-producing B cells (block in VHDJH recombination) results in the absence or severe reduction of serum immunoglobulin, absence of circulating mature B cells, and absence of plasma cells in all lymphoid tissue. T-cell number and function are intact. Inheritance is sex-linked recessive, although a clinically indistinguishable syndrome with autosomal recessive inheritance has been observed in some patients. Recent studies have localized the defect to a protein tyrosine kinase gene (Bruton's tyrosine kinase, *btk*) on the proximal region (q21.3–q22) of the X chromosome. After maternal antibody is consumed (usually after the first 4 to 6 months of life), patients develop sinopulmonary infections, bacteremia, and meningitis with encapsulated gram-positive and gram-negative bacteria, such as *H. influenzae, S. pneumoniae, S. aureus, P. aeruginosa,* and *M. pneumoniae.* Respiratory disease due to *P. carinii* or gastrointestinal infection with *Giardia lamblia* is also commonly observed. Although viral infections are not typical, enterovirus (polio and echo) and hepatitis viruses may cause severe or fatal disease. Autoimmune diseases, such as rheumatoid arthritis, occur in up to 20 percent of patients, while lymphomas and other lymphoreticular malignancies occur in approximately 5 percent of cases. IgG levels are very low (less than 100 mg/dL), and IgA and IgM are often undetectable.

Common Variable Immunodeficiency

Common variable immunodeficiency (CVI) is a not uncommon defect due, in general, to various B-cell activation or differentiation defects, resulting in low serum levels of IgG and depressed levels of IgA or IgM. B cells may be normal, high, or low, and T-cell number and function, although usually normal at diagnosis, deteriorate with time. Although the disease is familial, it is not strictly X-linked or autosomally inherited. In some patients, the genomic defects of both CVI and isolated IgA deficiency appear to be localized to the major histocompatibility complex region of chromosome 6. The disease is characterized by the development of recurrent sinopulmonary infections or chronic bronchiectasis in childhood or adulthood. Chest radiograph findings consistent with atelectasis, bronchiectasis, and/or interstitial markings, along with pulmonary function tests revealing mild to severe obstruction and restrictive disease, are seen in 60 to 80 percent of CVI patients. A few patients with CVI present with infections with unusual organisms, such as *P. carinii,* mycobacteria, or fungi. Recurrent attacks of both herpes simplex and zoster are not uncommon.

Selective IgG Subclass Deficiencies

Patients with selective IgG subclass deficiencies have recurrent sinopulmonary infections associated with normal or decreased total concentrations of serum IgG, but with selective deficiencies of IgG subclass 1, 2, 3, or 4. Patients with IgG2 subclass deficiency can make antibody, but the spectrum of the response is decreased, resulting in recurrent infection. Recent studies suggest a critical role for interleukin-6 (IL-6) and interferon gamma (IFN-γ) in enhancing IgG subclass production. Titers to bacterial polysaccharide antigens are low even after immunization, since antibody responses to polysaccharides reside predominantly in the IgG2 subclass. Titers to protein antigens such as tetanus or diphtheria toxoids may be normal. IgG2 subclass deficiency may be associated with IgG4 subclass deficiency, IgA deficiency, Wiskott-Aldrich syndrome, and ataxia-telangiectasia. Persons with low or absent IgG2 or IgG4 appear to be particularly predisposed to recurrent or severe pneumonias and middle ear infections. Selective IgG3 deficiency is also associated with recurrent sinopulmonary infections, but the mechanism is not clear. These IgG3-deficient patients have normal responses to both common protein (Dt) and polysaccharide antigens; however, responses to influenza or rubella vaccine may be abnormal. Treatment is based on clinical findings of recurrent infections rather than isolated laboratory abnormalities. It is important to document not only a low concentration of a subclass but also failure to make specific antibody when the individual is immunized, before immunoglobulin therapy is contemplated.

Selective IgA Deficiency

This most common of all the inborn defects of humoral immunity, occurring in 1 per 700 persons, accounts for more than 1 percent of recurrent infections in children. The defect is assumed to be a differentiation block affecting IgA-committed B cells. Typically, peripheral counts of patients with IgA deficiency show normal numbers of mature B lymphocytes as well as normal numbers and proportions of CD4 and CD8 cells. Selective IgA deficiency has been defined as serum IgA less than 5 mg/dL in severe deficiency and greater than 5 mg/dL but less than 2 SD below the age normal mean in partial IgA deficiency. The diagnosis and treatment of IgA deficiency depend not only on the serum level of IgA but also on the history and results of related diagnostic studies, particularly the immune workup. In general, treatment relies on the administration of appropriate antibiotics for acute infection or chronic suppressive therapy for chronic infection. When IgA deficiency is associated with IgG2 deficiency, intravenous immune globulin (IVIG) depleted of IgA may be indicated.

Hyper-IgM Immunodeficiency

These patients have absent or markedly reduced IgA, IgE, and IgG levels, elevated levels of IgM, circulating mature B lymphocytes bearing IgM or IgD and plasma cells, as well as hyperplastic lymphoid tissue. Recurrent neutropenia, probably secondary to autoimmune phenomena, may coexist with the humoral defect. Because antibody protection for the gastrointestinal and respiratory tracts is normally provided by IgA and IgG isotypes, patients with this syndrome are especially prone to respiratory and gastrointestinal infections with pyogenic organisms. They are also predisposed to *P. carinii* pneumonia. As with other immunoglobulin deficiencies, patients with the hyper-IgM syndrome have very high rates of autoimmune (involving the formed elements of the blood) and lymphoproliferative disorders.

Complement Disorders

Disorders due to primary deficiencies of complement components are rare causes of pulmonary infections. Complement function can be assessed by determining the total hemolytic activity in serum (CH50), which measures the ability of serum to lyse antibody-coated sheep cells. A low to absent CH50 suggests a deficiency in a classic pathway complement component. Levels of specific complement components can then be determined.

Congenital absence of C3 or consumption of C3 due to deficiency of factor I (C3b inactivator) results in a clinical picture like that seen in deficiency of the critical antibody opsonins, including infections due to pyogenic bacteria including severe and recurrent pneumonias due to *S. pneumoniae, H. influenzae,* and Enterobacteriaceae.

The terminal complement components, C5–9, form the cytolytic membrane attack complex (MAC), and deficiency of any one of these will block its formation. C5–9 deficiencies predispose to disseminated infection with *Neisseria meningococcus* and *N. gonococcus.*

C1 esterase inhibitor deficiency results in persistent consumption of C2 and C4 by the C1 esterases, resulting in release of vasoactive kinins and the development of nonpruritic angioedema. Although angioedema can occur in any tissue, including the gastrointestinal tract, edema of the upper airway can be life-threatening. Diagnosis is suggested by family history (autosomal dominant state), edema without pruritus, and chronically decreased C4 and C2 levels, especially during the 24 to 72 h of the episode. Patients with the familial form of the disease will have low to absent C1 esterase inhibitor concentrations. Angioedema with later onset, without a familial pattern, may be due to the absence of the functional component of the inhibitor, which may be associated with malignancy. Treatment is with danazol or purified C1 inhibitor for acute attacks.

Cell-Mediated Immunity

Although the most characteristic infections in patients with cellular immune deficiency are those caused by opportunistic intracellular pathogens, including protozoa (*P. carini* and *Toxoplasma gondii*), fungi (*Candida* and *Aspergillus* species), viruses (particularly those of the herpesvirus family), and some intracellular bacteria (including *Listeria* and *Mycobacteria* species), defects in humoral or phagocyte defense mechanisms can also be seen.

DiGeorge's Syndrome

DiGeorge's syndrome (DGS) is a constellation of abnormalities resulting from dysmorphogenesis of the third and fourth pharyngeal pouches. Patients have hypoplasia or aplasia of the thymus and the parathyroid glands, complex cardiac malformations, esophageal atresia, bifid uvulas, cleft palate, short philtrums, mandibular hypoplasia, hypertelorism, and low-set notched ears. The severity of immunologic manifestations varies from severe forms with complete thymic aplasia, resembling severe combined immunodeficiency disease (SCID), to only latent hypoparathyroidism, which may also be seen in relatives of patients with DGS. Most patients have partial T-cell function, which may improve with age, presumably due to the adaptation of functional extrathymic sites for T-lymphocyte maturation. T-cell numbers are typically reduced, with reduced percentages of CD3+ and CD4+ cells, but CD8 cells may be normal or even elevated. Patients with more significant CD4+ T-cell deficiency seem to have more frequent and severe infections requiring hospitalization. B-lymphocyte counts are usually normal; antibody production is also usually normal, but of poor biologic quality. Some patients may have low IgA or elevated serum IgE levels. Surviving infants often have the tendency to acquire parathyroid function, cell-mediated immunity, and functional T cells. Patients are prone to severe viral pneumonias, particularly those of the herpes and measles family. Pneumonias due to fungal and gram-negative bacilli and *P. carinii* also occur.

Severe Combined Immunodeficiency Disease

SCID is a syndrome of heterogeneous lymphocyte stem cell defects that affect both T- and B-cell function, resulting in profound hypogammaglobulinemia and absence of T-cell function. Laboratory analysis may reveal lymphopenia (10 to 20 percent) and normal or increased numbers of circulating B cells, but severely reduced IgG levels. In general, SCID syndrome patients present with a triad of mucocutaneous candidiasis, intractable diarrhea, and *P. carinii* pneumonia, evident shortly after birth or within 6 to 9 months of life and progressing to severe failure to thrive. Within a few days after birth, patients may also develop a morbilliform rash that is probably a manifestation of graft-versus-host disease (GVHD) from passively transferred maternal lymphocytes. Infections with a wide range of microbes occur in all forms of SCID, including viral pathogens, particularly herpesviruses (herpes simplex, cytomegalovirus, varicella), adenovirus, measles, influenza, and *Legionella*. Fatal giant cell pneumonia has resulted from measles infection and live measles vaccination, and progressive vaccinia has occurred after smallpox vaccination.

Purine Nucleoside Phosphorylase

Absence of the enzyme purine nucleoside phosphorylase (PNP) is associated with marked cell-mediated immunodeficiency but intact humoral immunity. The gene encoding the enzyme is localized to chromosome 14q13.1. Patients are prone to disseminated viral infections, *P. carinii* infection, mucocutaneous candidiasis, and chronic diarrhea. Neurologic disorders afflict more than 50 percent of patients, and more than one-third of PNP patients develop autoimmune diseases.

Wiskott-Aldrich Syndrome

Wiskott-Aldrich syndrome (WAS) is caused by a defect localized to the short arm of the X chromosome (Xp11.22–11.3), resulting in severely impaired production of antibodies to polysaccharide antigens, as well as variable reductions of T-cell numbers and impaired mitogen responses that tend to worsen with age. Both T-cell numbers and function progressively decrease, and profound lymphopenia becomes apparent at approximately 6 years of age. Most patients have abnormalities of serum immunoglobulin levels, with low IgM and isohemagglutinin concentrations, a tendency toward elevated IgA and IgE levels, and normal or slightly depressed IgG levels. Males afflicted with this syndrome suffer from a triad of recurrent infections, thrombocytopenia, and a skin disease indistinguishable from atopic dermatitis. Typical infections include pyoderma or cellulitis associated with eczematoid eruptions, chronic otitis media with persistent otorrhea and/or mastoiditis, and chronic pneumonitis. Encapsulated pyogenic bacteria, such as *S. pneumoniae, H. influenzae,* herpesvirus, and *P. carinii,* are the most frequently identified pathogens.

Ataxia-Telangiectasia

This syndrome (AT) is characterized by profound deficiencies of cellular immunity [including lymphopenia, defects in cutaneous anergy, decreases in Th:Ts (T-cell helper:T-cell suppressor) ratios, decreases in cytotoxic T cells, and an increase in immature T cells with increased gamma/delta TCR expression], impaired humoral responses (thymic hypoplasia associated with IgA deficiency, IgE deficiency, and IgG2 and IgG4 subclass deficiency), and a constellation of progressive cerebellar ataxia with degeneration of Purkinje cells. The defective genes of the two most common AT variants map to chromosome 11q22.3, which may result in a recombination defect that interferes with the rearrangement of T-cell and B-cell genes, an inability to repair damaged DNA, and a failure of normal organ maturation. Telangiectasias, particularly ocular and cutaneous, and a high incidence of malignancies, particularly non-Hodgkin's lymphoma, and breast cancer (in heterozygous female carries of the AT allele) are seen. AT is also associated with insulin-resistant diabetes mellitus, gonadal agenesis, premature aging, elevated levels of serum $alpha_1$-fetoprotein and carcinoembryonic antigen, and hypersensitivity of fibroblasts and lymphocytes to ionizing radiation, reflecting an inability to repair damaged DNA. Patients suffer from an increased incidence of bacterial and viral sinopulmonary infections, and many eventually develop chronic bronchiectasis. The most frequent pulmonary pathogens are *S. aureus* and other encapsulated bacteria. Concurrent IgG2 (50 percent), IgG4, and IgA deficiencies (70 percent) may be associated with the tendency toward recurrent infections of the respiratory tract. Approximately 80 percent of patients have depressed IgE levels.

Phagocytic Defects

Disorders of Phagocyte Numbers

These disorders include cyclic neutropenia, Felty's syndrome, Kostmann's syndrome, Shwachman-Diamond syndrome, and autoimmune neutropenia. They are characterized by absolute counts of polymormonuclear neutrophils (PMNs) as low as 50 to $200/mm^3$ but typically lower than $1000/mm.^3$ Owing to the presence of a compensatory monocytosis, these disorders are associated with a low incidence of severe respiratory infections, although pneumonia is seen—as are furunculosis, subcutaneous abscess, and otitis media. Typical pathogens include *S. aureus, P. aeruginosa,* and enteric bacteria.

Defects of Phagocyte Function

Chronic Granulomatous Disease   CGD is caused by a defect in a membrane-associated nicotinamide adenine dinucleotide phosphate (NADPH) oxidase in phagocytic cells, resulting in the failure of phagocytic cells to produce superoxide, hydrogen peroxide, and other reduction products of oxygen that are necessary for killing certain microbial species. Diagnosis is made by the inability of neutrophils to reduce nitroblue tetrazolium (NBT) from yellow to blue-black formazan and by the inability of neutrophils to kill staphylococci or other catalase-positive microorganisms. Additional laboratory findings suggestive of CGD include leukocytosis, elevation of erythrocyte sedimentation rate, abnormal chest radiographs, and hypergammaglobulinemia. Onset is typically in infancy, childhood or, less commonly, early adolescence, with a male-to-female ratio of 6:1. All forms of CGD are characterized by abscess formation at sites of bacterial tissue invasion and in lymph nodes, liver, and lung. Patients present with severe recurrent lymphadenitis and infections of the skin as well as the sinopulmonary gastrointestinal tracts. Severe and recurrent pulmonary infections occur in almost all patients with CGD, including bronchopneumonia, empyema, lung abscess, and hilar adenopathy syndromes. Most young adult patients demonstrate chronic bilateral infiltrates, pulmonary fibrosis, or pulmonary calcifications associated with restrictive/obstructive disease. Aggregates of granulomas, leading to mechanical obstruction, may form as a response of activated macrophages to microbial persistence and chronic antigenic stimulation. *S. aureus* represents by far the most common cause of infections in CGD. Other catalase-positive and non–H_2O_2-producing organisms include *Escherichia coli, Klebsiella,* and *Enterobacter* species, *Serratia marcescens,* and *Salmonella* and *Pseudomonas* species. Pneumonias in CGD patients may be caused by *Mycobacterium tuberculosis,* atypical mycobacteria, and *P. carinii.* In specific geographic locations, such as the southeastern United States, *Chromobacterium violaceum* has been recognized as the cause of infection in several CGD patients. *Nocardia* infection, particularly of the respiratory system, is also relatively common, as are fungal infections. Antibiotics and interferon gamma have been useful in therapy.

Glucose-6-Phosphate Dehydrogenase Deficiency This is a variant of CGD, in which G6PD levels are less than 1 percent, and results in an inability to generate oxygen by-products and a slightly milder form of disease than that in patients with CGD.

Chediak-Higashi Syndrome CHS is a rare autosomal recessive defect characterized by abnormal fusion of azurophilic lysosomes of neutrophils and cytoplasmic granules of monocytes and lymphocytes. This defect results in impaired microbicidal activity of phagocytes due to the presence of giant lysosomal granules, which have abnormal postphagocytic phagolysosomal fusion and degranulation. In addition, neutrophil counts tend to be low, secondary to their rapid turnover. Chemotactic defects and impaired natural killer cell activity have also been noted. Patients present with recurrent skin and upper and lower respiratory tract infections, including recurrent or chronic otitis media, sinusitis, and pharyngitis, in addition to lower respiratory tract infections, including bronchopneumonia. Segmental or lobar lung involvement can account for up to 30 percent of documented infections. Most infections are due to *S. aureus, H. influenzae,* group A streptococcus, and gram-negative enteric organisms (*Klebsiella, Proteus, Shigella, Pseudomonas*). *Aspergillus* and *Candida* represent less common etiologic agents. Respiratory failure can occur with extensive histiocytic infiltration of the lungs during an accelerated lymphoma-like proliferative phase marked by widespread tissue infiltrates of lymphoid and histiocytic cells, usually without malignant histologic characteristics. Anemia, hypersplenism, and platelet dysfunction, associated with the accelerated phase, and albinism or hypopigmentation, due to abnormal fusion of melanocyte pigment organelles, are also seen.

Leukocyte Adhesion Deficiency

Patients with this autosomal recessive disease lack or have markedly reduced beta$_2$ integrins, essential glycoprotein constituents of the CD11/CD18 receptor complex that mediates leukocyte adhesion. Recurrent necrotic and indolent infections of soft tissues, primarily in skin, mucous membranes, and the intestinal tract, are the clinical hallmarks of this disease. The recurrent infections reflect a profound impairment of leukocyte mobilization into extravascular inflammatory sites, despite peripheral blood granulocyte counts of 15,000 to 161,000/mm^3. A wide spectrum of gram-positive or negative bacteria (*S. aureus* and gram-negative enteric bacteria) and fungal microorganisms (*Candida* and *Aspergillus*) infect LAD patients, as in the case of those with neutropenia syndromes.

Hyperimmunoglobulin E Syndrome

Also known as the hyper-IgE (HIE) recurrent infection, or Job's syndrome, this unusual disorder, which appears to be autosomal dominant with incomplete penetrance, is lacking an exact immunologic defect. Serum levels of polyclonal IgE are markedly elevated (above 2000 IU/mL), but immunoglobulins other than IgE are normal. Complete blood counts and differentials are mildly abnormal, with occasional borderline neutropenia. Most patients have mild to moderate eosinophilia, despite lacking a significant history of classic allergic diseases. All patients have chronically elevated erythrocyte sedimentation rates. Diagnosis of HIE can be established in patients (usually during infancy) with a history of staphylococcal infections of the skin and sinopulmonary tract, and IgE levels at least 10 times normal. Coarse facies, chronic eczematoid eruptions, cold cutaneous or subcutaneous abscesses, eosinophilia, and mucocutaneous candidiasis are also seen, as are recurrent bone fractures and osteopenia. "Cold abscesses" are not seen in all HIE patients, but they are rare in other immunodeficiency states. They can present in any part of the body as fluctuant masses, with little evidence of inflammation and often without fever. Drainage of these abscesses usually reveals large volumes of purulent material, which almost always grow *S. aureus*. Otitis externa and chronic otitis media, occasionally complicated by mastoiditis, are common in HIE patients. Recurrent bronchitis represents the most common pulmonary manifestation of HIE. Patients often suffer several days a month of productive cough, rarely associated with fever. Less commonly, pneumonia, with or without associated complications—including bronchiectasis, lung abscess, empyema, pneumatocele formation, and bronchopleural fistula formation—may represent serious and potentially devastating features in HIE patients. *S. aureus* and *H. influenzae* are the most frequent causes of pneumonias in HIE. Management relies on the use of narrow-spectrum antistaphylococcal prophylaxis, such as cloxacillin or dicloxacillin. Trimethoprim-sulfamethoxazole may also be employed as a prophylactic agent.

BIBLIOGRAPHY

American Society of Clinical Oncology: Recommendations for the use of hematopoietic colony-stimulating factors: Evidence-based, clinical practice guidelines. *J Clin Oncol* 12:2471–2508, 1994.

American Society of Clinical Oncology: Update of recommendations for the use of hematopoietic colony-stimulating factors: Evidence-based, clinical practice guidelines. *J Clin Oncol* 14(6):1957–1960, 1996.

Badier M, Guillot C, Delpierre S, et al: Pulmonary function changes 100 days and one year after bone marrow transplantation. *Bone Marrow Transplant* 12:457–461, 1993.

Bodey G, Buckley M, Sathe Y, et al: Quantitative relationships between circulating leukocytes and infection in patients with acute leukemia. *Ann Intern Med* 64:328–340, 1966.

Bodey G, Rodriguez V, Chang H, et al: Fever and infection in leukemic patients: A study of 494 consecutive patients. *Cancer* 41:1610–1622, 1978.

Bowden RA, Sayers M, Flournoy N, et al: Cytomegalovirus immune globulin and seronegative blood products to prevent primary cytomegalovirus infection after marrow transplantation. *N Engl J Med* 314:1006–1010, 1986.

Carlson K, Backlund L, Smedmyr B, et al: Pulmonary function and complications subsequent to autologous bone marrow transplantation. *Bone Marrow Transplant* 14:805–811, 1994.

Carpenter CC: Antiretroviral therapy in adults: Updated recommendations of the International AIDS Society USA Panel. *JAMA* 283:381–390, 2000.

Chan CK, Hyland RH, Hutcheon MA, et al: Small-airways disease in recipients of allogeneic bone marrow transplants. *Medicine* 66:327–340, 1987.

Chao NJ, Duncan SR, Long GD, et al: Corticosteroid therapy for diffuse alveolar hemorrhage in autologous bone marrow transplant recipients. *Ann Intern Med* 114:145–146, 1991.

Chou S: Newer methods for diagnosis of cytomegalovirus infection. *Rev Infect Dis* 12(suppl 7):S727–S736, 1990.

Clark JG, Crawford SW, Madtes DK, Sullivan KM: Obstructive lung disease after allogeneic marrow transplantation: Clinical presentation and course. *Ann Intern Med* 111:368–376, 1989.

Cohen IM, Galgiani JN, Potter D, et al: Coccidioidomycosis in renal replacement therapy. *Arch Intern Med* 142:489–494, 1982.

Collins LA, Samore MH, Roberts MS, et al: Risk factors for invasive fungal infections complicating orthotopic liver transplantation. *J Infect Dis* 170:644–652, 1994.

Crawford SW, Fisher L: Predictive value of pulmonary function tests before marrow transplantation. *Chest* 101:1257–1264, 1992.

Crawford SW, Hackman RC: Clinical course of idiopathic pneumonia after marrow transplantation. *Am Rev Respir Dis* 147:1393–1400, 1993.

Dykewitz CA: Summary of the guidelines for preventing opportunistic infections among hematopoietic stem cell transplant recipients. *Clin Infect Dis.* 33:139–144, 2001.

Ettinger NA, Trulock EP: Pulmonary considerations in organ transplantation. *Am Rev Respir Dis* 143:1386–1405, 144:213–223, 144:433–451, 1991.

Ezekowitz RAB, Dinauer MC, Jaffe HS, et al: Partial correction of the phagocyte defect in patients with X-linked chronic granulomatous disease by subcutaneous interferon gamma. *N Engl J Med* 319:146–151, 1988.

Feld R: Vancomycin as part of the initial empirical antibiotic therapy for febrile neutropenia in patients with cancer: Pros and cons. *Clin Infect Dis* 29:503–507, 1999.

Fishman JA: Pneumocystis carinii and parasitic infections in transplantation. *Infect Dis Clin North Am* 1005–1044, 1995,

Fishman JA, Rubin RH: Infection in the Transplant Patient, *N Engl J Med* June 1998.

Fishman JA, Rubin RH, Koziel MJ, Pereira BJG: Hepatitis C virus and organ transplantation. *Transplantation* 62(2):147–154, 1996.

Hackman RC, Madtes DK, Petersen FB, Clark JG: Pulmonary veno-occlusive disease following bone marrow transplantation. *Transplantation* 47:989–992, 1989.

Hadley S, Karchmer AW: Fungal infections in solid organ transplant recipients. *Infect Dis Clin North Am* 1045–1074, 1995.

Hadley S, Samore MH, Lewis WD, et al: Major infectious complications after orthotopic liver transplantation and comparison of outcomes in patients receiving cyclosporine or FK506 as primary immunosuppression. *Transplantation* 59:851–859, 1995.

Hannah GJ, Hirsch MS: Antiretroviral therapy of HIV infection. In Mandell GL, Bennett JE, Dolin R. eds: *Principles and Practice of Infectious Diseases*, 5th ed. New York: Churchill Livingstone 2000, pp 1479–1500.

Hooper DC, Pruitt AA, Rubin RH: Central nervous system infections in the chronically immunosuppressed. *Medicine* 61:166–188, 1982.

Hughes W: Guidelines for the use of antimicrobial agent in neutropenic patients with unexplained fever. *J Infect Dis* 161:381–396, 1995.

Ljungman P, Gleaves CA, Meyers JD: Respiratory virus infections in immunocompromised patients. *Bone Marrow Transplant* 4:35–40, 1989.

Luft BJ, Noat Y, Arauja FG, et al: Primary and reactivated toxoplasma infection in patients with cardiac transplants. Clinical spectrum and problems in diagnosis in a defined population. *Ann Intern Med* 99(1):27–31, 1983.

Meyers JD, Flournoy N, Thomas ED: Nonbacterial pneumonia after allogeneic marrow transplantation: A review of ten years experience. *Rev Infect Dis* 4:1119–1132, 1982.

Paya CV: Fungal infections in solid organ transplantation. *Clin Infect Dis* 16:677, 1993.

Pizzo P: Fever in immunocompromised patients. *N Engl J Med* 341:893–900, 1999.

Quadri TL, Brown AE: Infectious complications in the critically ill patient with cancer. *Semin Oncol* 27:335–346, 2000.

Rubin RH, Wolfson JS, Cosimi AB, Tolkoff-Rubin N: Infection in the renal transplant patient. *Am J Med* 70:405–411, 1981.

Singer C, Kaplan M, Armstrong D: Bacteremia and fungemia complicating neoplastic disease: A study of 364 cases. *Am J Med* 62:731–742, 1977.

Troussard X, Bernaudin JF, Cordonnier C, et al: Pulmonary veno-occlusive disease after bone marrow transplantation. *Thorax* 39:956–957, 1984.

Vose J, Armitage J: Clinical application of hematopoietic growth factors. *J Clin Oncol* 13:1023–1033, 1995.

Wade J, Schimpff S, Newman K, et al: *Staphylococcus epidermidis:* An increasing cause of infection in patients with granulocytopenia. *Ann Intern Med* 97:503–508, 1987.

Wingard JR, Mellits ED, Sostrin MB, et al: Interstitial pneumonia after allogeneic marrow transplantation. *Medicine (Baltimore)* 67:175–186, 1988.

Wingard JR, Merz WG, Rinaldi MG, et al: Increase in *Candida krusei* infection among patients with bone marrow transplantation and neutropenia treated prophylactically with fluconazole. *N Engl J Med* 325:1274–1277, 1991.

Winston DJ, Chandrasekar PH, Lazarus HM, et al: Fluconazole prophylaxis of fungal infections in patients with acute leukemia: Results of a randomized placebo-controlled, double-blind, multicenter trial. *Ann Intern Med* 118:495–503, 1993.

Winston DJ, Emmanouilides C, Busuttil RW: Infection in liver transplant recipients. *Clin Infect Dis* 21:1077–1089, 1995.

Young LS, Martin WJ, Meyer RD, et al: Gram-negative rod bacteremia: Microbiologic, immunologic, and therapeutic considerations. *Ann Intern Med* 86:456–471, 1977.

67 | Zoonotic and Unusual Pneumonias*

Jay A. Fishman

ZOONOTIC BACTERIAL PNEUMONIAS

A wide variety of domestic and wild vertebrates are colonized by bacteria capable of producing pneumonia in humans (Table 67-1). There are few unique distinguishing clinical features that reveal the etiologies of these infections. Clues derived from a careful history of immunologic competence, travel, occupation, hobbies, and animal and arthropod contact are invaluable aids to the correct diagnosis, and therapy and can be lifesaving. Some of these organisms are among the potential agents of bioterrorism (see Appendix).

Pasteurella multocida Respiratory Infections

Pasteurella multocida is a common commensal of the oral cavity of most felines and many dogs and a frequent respiratory pathogen in animals and birds. In the United States, domestic associations are responsible for many cases of cellulitis following cat or dog bites. Respiratory infections are probably underreported, with fewer than 50 cases on record. Sputum isolates, however, are not infrequent in patients with chronic pulmonary disease. Immunocompromised patients may be prone to infection without traumatic dog or cat exposures.

Bacteriology

P. multocida is a small gram-negative bipolar-staining coccobacillary organism that resembles *Haemophilus* species and may form pairs and chains. Rapid growth on blood agar and inhibition by MacConkey medium help to separate this microorganism from other common components of the respiratory flora, including *Haemophilus* species. The organism produces a capsule that interferes with phagocytosis. Besides cell-envelope endotoxin, no other pathogenic properties have been identified.

Ecology and Epidemiology

In cats and other felines, the organism resides periodontally in the anterior regions of the mouth. Isolates from dogs are characteristically from the posterior pharynx. Many birds and domestic and wild animals worldwide harbor this organism as a commensal in oral or gastrointestinal areas. *P. multocida* is occasionally found in the secretions of persons with chronic lung disease, especially those with bronchiectasis and a history of domestic animal contacts. Human-to-human transmission has been documented from mother to newborn infant, resulting in neonatal aspiration pneumonia. The organism can survive in soil and water for more than 3 weeks and in animal carcasses for

---

*Edited from Chap. 157, "Zoonotic and Other Unusual Bacterial Pneumonias," by Weinberg AN, Heller HM. In: *Fishman's Pulmonary Diseases and Disorders,* 3d ed., edited by Fishman AP, Elias JA, Fishman JA, Grippi MA, Kaiser LR, Senior RM. New York, McGraw-Hill, 1998, pp 2413–2430. For fuller discussion of topics dealt with in this chapter, the reader is referred to the original text, as noted above.

TABLE 67-1 An Overview of Zoonotic and Other Unusual Pneumonias

Environmental niche	Microorganism	Disease	Epidemiologic associations	Distribution
Live animal contact or via arthropod	*Francisella tularensis*	Tularemia	Contact with animals, birds, or arthropods, bioterrorism	North America, Europe, Asia
	Pasteurella multocida	Pasteurellosis	Feline and dog contact; chronic lung disease	Worldwide
	Rhodococcus equi	*Rhodococcus* pneumonia	Airborne; contact with soil contaminated with horse, cow, or swine excrement	Worldwide
	Yersinia pestis	Plague	Contact with rodents, fleas; contact with plague pneumonia case; bioterrorism	Worldwide, including Asia, southwestern U.S.
Soil, stagnant water, and inert animal products	*Bacillus anthracis*	Inhalation anthrax or wool-sorter's disease	Industrial; use of animal products in hobbies; bioterrorism	Worldwide in warmer regions
	Brucella species	Brucellosis	Ingestion or contact with infected animal products	Worldwide
	Burkholderia pseudomallei	Melioidosis	Direct penetrating contact with soil, water	Latitude 20°N to 20°S, especially rural Asia
	Yersinia enterocolitica	Yersiniosis	Ingestion of contaminated foods, water; cirrhosis	Worldwide
Obligate human commensal	*Neisseria meningitidis*	Meningococcal pneumonia	Airborne, human to human; postviral, nosocomial	Humans worldwide
	Moraxella catarrhalis	*Moraxella* pneumonia	Aspiration, especially individuals with underlying lung disease	Humans worldwide

approximately 2 months. In about half the cases of respiratory disease, no clue to airborne spread exists, but there are usually cats in the local environment.

Pathogenesis and Pathophysiology

Pathogenic strains have a polysaccharide capsule that inhibits phagocytosis, and they contain endotoxin in the cell envelope. Exotoxins and other pathogenicity-promoting factors have not been identified. Almost all patients who develop respiratory infections have underlying chronic pulmonary disease and/or immune compromise. Aspiration probably initiates active infection. Necrosis and lung abscess, empyema, septicemia, and transbronchial spread to other lung segments have been described.

Clinical and Radiologic Features

The clinical features of *P. multocida* respiratory disease include worsening of the patient's baseline respiratory function—especially when high fever, tenacious secretions, and pleural effusions develop. Radiologic changes include lobar, multilobar, or diffuse patchy infiltrates, usually sparing the upper lobes, superimposed on underlying chronic lung disease. Effusions have been noted in approximately 20 percent of cases.

Diagnostic Features

The diagnosis depends on isolation of the organism from sputum, pleural fluid, or blood. The pathogen can usually be identified with the routine methods of the diagnostic laboratory. The bipolar gram-negative staining bacilli resemble *Brucella* species, *Yersinia pestis, Francisella tularensis, Burkholderia* (formerly *Pseudomonas*) *pseudomallei,* and *Haemophilus* species, but the clinical history and bacteriologic characteristics can rapidly clarify the identification.

Treatment

Most strains are exquisitely susceptible to penicillin or ampicillin. The third-generation cephalosporins, cefotaxime and ceftriaxone, are as active as penicillin and more potent than earlier-generation relatives. Tetracycline and chloramphenicol are useful when a history of immediate-type allergic reactions precludes use of a beta-lactam agent. Oral preparations of cephalosporins and penicillins are not recommended for treating pneumonias due to *P. multocida.* (See Table 67-2 for specific dosages of useful agents.) Fluoroquinolones are very active in vitro, and although they have been used successfully in animals with *Pasteurella* pneumonia, there have been no reports of their use in treating the disease in humans.

Pneumonia Due to *Yersinia pestis*

This organism was the cause of three major pandemics from the sixth through the nineteenth centuries. Pulmonary disease in a few victims led to aerosol spread to countless others, resulting in acute primary pneumonia and the "black death" of epidemic plague. In the United States, approximately 20 cases of plague are reported yearly, of which 1 in 5 have lung involvement.

Bacteriology

Y. pestis is a bipolar-staining, gram-negative bacillus closely related to *Escherichia coli* and other Enterobacteriaceae. It grows well on blood or

TABLE 67-2 Diagnostic Studies and Treatment Recommendations in Zoonotic Pneumonias[a]

Disease	Gram's stain morphology	Culture methods	Identifying tests	Therapy total dose/number of doses[b]
Anthrax	Large gram-positive bacillus (rarely seen)	BAP, blood cultures	FA	PCN (12–18 mu/6), CL (4–6 g/6) CIP (iv or po) or FQ D (200 mg/2)[a]
Brucellosis	Small gram-negative coccobacillus (rarely seen)	Media enriched with serum, $CO_2 + O_2$	Rise in AA, Prozone	TMP-SMX (480 mg + 2.4 g/3) + SM (1 g/2) D (200 mg/2) + RI (600 mg/L)
Melioidosis	Bipolar staining gram-negative bacillus	BAP, MAC	Morphology, FA, AA	TMP-SMX (640 mg + 3.2 g/4) and ceftazidime (6–9 g/3) or CL (4–6 g/4) + D (200 mg/2)
Pasteurellosis	Small bipolar staining gram-negative bacillus	BAP, CO_2	Inhibited by MAC, biochem. tests	PCN or A (6 mu or 8 g/4) or cefotaxime (6–8 g/4) or CL (3 g/4)
Plague	Enteric bipolar staining gram-negative bacillus	BAP, MAC, enteric media, blood cultures	Biochem. tests, FA, AA	SM (2 g/2) and D (200 mg/2) or CL (4–6 g/4)
Rhodococcus	Gram-positive coccobacilli (slightly acid-fast positive)	BAP	Biochem. tests	E (2 g/4) or CLA (1 g/2) or AZ (500 mg) and CIP (1.5 g/2) and RI (600 mg)
Tularemia	Small gram-negative coccobacillus	Enriched media with cysteine, serum	FA, AA, rarely cultured	SM or gentamicin (2 g/2 or 4.5 mg/kg/3) or CL (3–4 g/4) or D (200 mg/2)
Yersiniosis	Enteric gram-negative bacillus	BAP, MAC, enteric media, blood cultures	Biochem. tests, motility 25°C	A (8 g/4) or 2d or 3d gen. cephalosp. (4–6 g/4) or CL (3 g/4)

[a]See Appendix for treatment of bioterrorism-based exposures of "weaponized" agents.
[b]Expressed as million units (mu), grams (g), or milligrams (mg) divided by number of doses in 24 h.
KEY: BAP, blood agar; MAC, MacConkey agar; FA, fluorescent antibody; AA, agglutinin antibody. Antibiotics include A, ampicillin; AZ, azithromycin; CIP, ciprofloxacin; CL, chloramphenicol; CLA, clarithromycin; D, doxycycline; E, erythromycin; FQ, fluoroquinolone; PCN, penicillin; RI, rifampin; SM, streptomycin; TMP-SMX, trimethoprim-sulfamethoxazole.

MacConkey agar and is identified definitively with differential biochemical tests, agglutination reactions, and direct fluorescent antibody staining.

Ecology and Epidemiology

In the United States, *Y. pestis* is endemic in rock squirrels, prairie dogs, and other ground animals. Spread among animals occurs via several species of rodent fleas. Domestic animals that wander outdoors, like cats, can become infected by direct contact with sick rodents or via rodent flea bites. In addition, cats and dogs can inadvertently carry fleas into the home. Occasionally rodent die-offs, called epizootics, occur, and many dead animals can be found with viable organisms in carcasses and in the soil surrounding ground dwellings. In the United States, spread to humans occurs in the endemic areas west of the Rockies—especially in California, northern Arizona, and New Mexico—when a hungry flea feeds on a susceptible person. Living or working in proximity to local enzootic "hot spots" places certain groups (such as Native Americans, geologists, hikers, veterinarians, and pet owners) at risk. Bubonic and cutaneous plague is usually acquired by contact with infected fleas, but aerosols from ill animals or from carcasses can lead to primary pneumonia, pharyngitis, or conjunctivitis. Several cases of cat-to-human aerosol spread have been associated with respiratory infection or submandibular abscess in pets. Plague is considered a potential agent of bioterrorism (see Appendix).

Pathogenesis and Pathophysiology

Once the organism gains access to human tissues at 37°C, rapid multiplication occurs, with formation of a polysaccharide capsule. The capsule imparts virulence properties that include resisting phagocytosis and persistence of bacteria within nonsensitized monocytes. Virulence factors impacting on the host also include a potent endotoxin and V and W antigens of the cell envelope, which also influence intracellular survival. Bacteremic spread usually follows initial multiplication in regional nodes or at the local flea bite site. Secondary pneumonia involving the well-perfused basal segments can follow. When a person with plague pneumonia coughs, there may be aerosol spread to persons nearby, resulting in primary pneumonia and rapidly developing adult respiratory distress syndrome (ARDS).

Clinical and Radiologic Features

The clinical presentation of pneumonia depends on the mechanism of spread. In contemporary experience in the United States, cases have all been secondary to bubonic plague, to primary septicemia without an overt skin lesion, or to inhalation of droplets from an infected pet cat. The onset of respiratory disease follows after days to a week of a febrile illness, and is ushered in by the gradual onset of cough, dyspnea, and increasing toxicity. A hemorrhagic productive cough, pleurisy, and increasing respiratory distress are additional symptoms. The unique feature in most cases of pneumonia is the epidemiologic association with classic bubonic plague in a person recently in an endemic area or who has had contact with a pet cat ill with respiratory symptoms or a facial abscess. From cases of primary inhalation pneumonia described previously, exposure to an index case may be followed by the rapid development of a fulminating respiratory illness, with dyspnea, cyanosis, and thin, watery sputum that rapidly becomes hemorrhagic. The clinical picture is not unlike that of overwhelming pneumococcal pneumonia, with marked toxicity and mental torpor associated with progressive cyanosis.

The radiologic features of secondary pneumonia include basal segment nodular to hazy airspace infiltrates, hilar and mediastinal node hypertrophy, and occasionally pleural effusions. In primary pneumonia, infiltrates may be minimal during the first 24 h, followed by progressive airspace disease resembling ARDS or pulmonary edema.

Diagnosis and Differential Diagnosis

The presence of characteristic bipolar-staining gram-negative bacilli in sputum supports the diagnosis when epidemiologic factors are suggestive. Cultures of blood, sputum, and lymph node aspirates often yield positive results. Direct fluorescent antibody staining, if available, can provide immediate etiologic confirmation. A passive hemagglutination test can be performed as a confirmatory study on acute and convalescent sera at selected reference laboratories of the Centers for Disease Control and Prevention. Other acute respiratory infections caused by microorganisms that appear as gram-negative bacilli with bipolar staining must be considered, including *F. tularensis* and *P. multocida*.

Treatment and Prevention

The combination of streptomycin and tetracycline has been the treatment of choice for serious plague infections. Gentamicin can be substituted for streptomycin if intravenous therapy is necessary or streptomycin is not available. In patients with impaired renal function, chloramphenicol should be used in place of tetracycline. (See Table 67-2 for dosage schedules.)

Persons suspected of having plague pneumonia should be rapidly isolated, and strict contact, respiratory, and conjunctival precautions instituted. Anyone exposed face to face with a coughing patient, including health care workers, should be given preventive tetracycline, 2 g daily, divided into four doses, for 5 to 10 days. Isolation procedures are continued until productive cough is no longer present or sputum cultures are negative for *Y. pestis.*

A vaccine is available for laboratory workers and others with frequent exposure to the microorganisms or to hyperendemic areas. Careful surveillance of ground rodent populations, posting warnings in endemic regions, watching for die-offs that indicate epizootic spread, and spraying for local flea control may also be effective preventive measures.

Pneumonia Due to *Francisella tularensis*

Tularemia is a common animal disease in the United States. The causative agent, *F. tularensis,* is ubiquitous, distributed among many species of wild and domestic animals and birds. Bloodsucking arthropods, especially ticks and deer flies, serve an important role in transmission to humans. As with plague, the major clinical manifestations include skin lesions and swollen or draining regional lymph nodes. Pulmonary impairment occurs secondary to bacteremia or as a primary inhalation or aspiration pneumonia. Approximately 150 human cases are reported in the United States yearly, but this is probably an underestimate. Pulmonary invasion is seen in 10 to 15 percent of ulceroglandular cases and in more than 50 percent of patients with the typhoidal syndrome in addition to primary inhalation pneumonia.

Bacteriology

F. tularensis is a fragile-appearing gram-negative coccobacillary organism that grows poorly on artificial media unless fortified with serum and cysteine (or sulfhydryl compounds). The potential for laboratory-acquired inhalation or ingestion-associated disease is great. Most routine laboratories will not attempt to culture the organism, leaving this to special reference centers. Identification is on the basis of morphologic and biochemical determinants, but direct fluorescent staining or agglutination reactions with specific antisera are also useful.

Ecology and Epidemiology

The organism is associated with more than 100 species of wild and domestic animals and birds, but most clinical cases arise from contact with rabbits, squirrels, or arthropods. Aquatic mammals and their immediate water and mud living environments can also be contaminated with *F. tularensis*. Bloodsucking arthropods, especially ticks and deerflies, act as reservoirs capable of harboring the pathogen for long periods and are responsible for dissemination among wildlife species. Domestic cats represent a potentially increasing problem. Most human cases are acquired from contact with infected animals during hunting, trapping, and other outdoor pursuits, especially during colder months. In southern areas, or in the summer season in northern latitudes, bloodsucking arthropods, especially ticks and deerflies, constitute a significant mode of spread. Ingestion of contaminated food, animal bites, conjunctival contact, and aerosol dissemination are also important mechanisms for acquiring the pathogen. In recent years, cases secondary to arthropods have been more frequent than those associated with direct animal contact, although domestic cat bites and airborne spread appear to be increasing. Human-to-human transmission is not recognized, in contrast to the significant theoretical potential for spread of pneumonic plague. Tularemia is considered a possible agent of bioterrorism (see Appendix).

Pathogenesis and Pathophysiology

F. tularensis contains a number of protein and polysaccharide antigens in the cell envelope and an endotoxin component that is similar to endotoxins of other gram-negative microorganisms. Very little is known about other mechanisms of pathogenesis. The organism is capable of remaining viable in reticuloendothelial cells of nonimmune subjects and in macrophages that have not been stimulated by recent exposure to intracellular pathogens. As few as 10 to 50 organisms can initiate disease following cutaneous penetration or by inhalation, but a significant number are required when the challenge is through ingestion of contaminated foods. Local growth usually is followed by regional node suppuration and occasionally bacteremic dissemination to many organs, including the lungs. Rhabdomyolysis of uncertain cause may accompany bacteremia and pneumonia. Ingestion may result in pharyngeal infection, involvement of the gastrointestinal tract, or subclinical disease followed by the typhoidal syndrome. Primary pneumonia follows inhalation of organisms, resulting in numerous areas of inflammation, necrosis, a tendency to granuloma formation, and pleural inflammation.

Clinical and Radiologic Features

Respiratory disease is heralded by the onset of a nonproductive cough, usually in a febrile patient ill with the ulceroglandular form of tularemia. In the absence of a local chancriform lesion or tender swollen lymph node (bubo), the disease may be dominated by constitutional symptoms, with high fever and shaking chills (typhoidal tularemia). Pneumonia following an inhalation exposure results in cough, dyspnea, and occasionally pleurisy. Respiratory disease can be subtle, and the diagnosis may be apparent only if a chest radiograph is done.

Radiologic changes include evidence of parenchymal and pleural disease, which is often out of proportion to the physical findings. Diffuse areas of bronchopneumonia occur, with hilar node enlargement. Unilateral or bilateral pleural effusions are often noted. Central oval infiltrates, described as characteristic in early reports, are seldom observed today. Lobar airspace disease and lung abscess are unusual additional patterns that have been described.

Diagnosis and Differential Diagnosis

Any febrile patient with animal or arthropod exposure in an endemic region, especially presenting with a skin lesion or tender lymph nodes, should be evaluated for tularemia. Respiratory involvement is confirmed by radiologic study. Cough, when present, is usually nonproductive, and blood cultures are seldom positive. Characteristic organisms are rarely seen in pleural fluid or aspirates of suppurating nodes. Direct fluorescent antibody staining of exudates can confirm the diagnosis, but this method is not widely available. Other rapid diagnostic tests—including urine antigen detection, polymerase chain reaction, and a ribosomal probe—are in development. Serologic testing remains the method of choice for confirming a diagnosis. Currently the enzyme-linked immunosorbent assay (ELISA) and microagglutination methods are preferred to tube agglutination testing. A single convalescent titer of 1:160 or greater is considered highly suspect for active disease, but a fourfold rise in titer between acute and convalescent (1 to 5 weeks) sera is more reliable, since antibodies of the IgM and IgG class can persist for many years after infection. An elevated blood level of creatine phosphokinase is a sign that tularemia-induced rhabdomyolysis is the cause of the acute infection, especially in highly endemic areas. Skin testing can be helpful in diagnosis, but the antigen is not commercially available.

Among the respiratory infections that are confused with tularemia, perplexing diseases, which are also associated with outdoor and animal exposures such as psittacosis and Q fever, are especially important. Legionnaires' disease and mycoplasmal pneumonia can present with similar clinical courses, without diagnostic sputum. Plague, tuberculosis, and systemic fungal infections produce a spectrum of acute to chronic respiratory manifestations that can be confused with pulmonary tularemia.

Treatment and Prevention

Streptomycin was the first effective antibiotic for treating all forms of tularemia, and it remains the agent of choice. Gentamicin appears to be equally potent and has the advantage of a broader spectrum of activity if one is initiating treatment when the etiologic diagnosis is less secure. *Tobramycin, however, appears to be unreliable and therefore should not be substituted.* Recent experience confirms that results of therapy are optimal when an aminoglycoside is chosen early in the clinical illness. Tetracycline and chloramphenicol are useful alternatives when an aminoglycoside is contraindicated, but relapse rates are higher, especially when tetracycline is given for less than 2 weeks. The use of fluoroquinolones, imipenem, and erythromycin have not been evaluated. β-Lactam antibiotics are not effective. The prognosis is excellent with appropriate antimicrobial therapy. (See Table 67-2 for specific dosages.)

TABLE 67-3 Diagnosing *Rhodococcus equi* Respiratory Infection

History of exposure to horses, cattle, or their environment
Immunocompromised host: malignancy, steroids, HIV
Cavitary or nodular infiltrates on radiograph
Gram-positive pleomorphic bacilli
Modified acid-fast
Pale-pink or salmon-pink mucoid colonies
Grows rapidly, aerobically on most media
Differential diagnosis includes *Nocardia* species, mycobacteria

Pneumonia due to *Rhodococcus equi*

Rhodococcus equi, formerly known as *Corynbacterium equi,* has been most commonly reported as causing pneumonia in immunocompromised hosts, especially those receiving corticosteroid therapy. In recent years, the majority of recognized cases of *R. equi* disease have been in patients infected with the human immunodeficiency virus (Table 67-3).

Bacteriology and Immunology

Rhodococcus is a pleomorphic gram-positive bacillus in the order Actinomycetales. It grows well on most media aerobically, at 37°C, as mucoid pale-pink or salmon-pink colonies that are usually observed by 48 h after incubation. *R. equi* has a high cell wall mycolic acid content and, as a result, like *Nocardia* species and Mycobacteriaceae, is weakly acid fast. Some strains will ferment glucose, but most will not ferment carbohydrates. Most produce catalase and hydrogen sulfide. Beta-lactamase is present in some strains.

R. equi is a facultative intracellular pathogen that survives within macrophages. Prevention of phagosome-lysosome fusion is a major pathogenic mechanism. Humoral response as well as cell-mediated immunity has been demonstrated in animals, but it is unclear how much of a protective role each plays. In equine models, administration of antibody decreases the severity of pneumonia in foals challenged with aerosol inoculation of organisms. Protection was not seen in a murine model when the animals were infected with intravenous inoculation of organisms. In murine models, depletion of both CD4 T cells and CD8 T cells impairs the ability to clear the infection.

Epidemiology

Most of the reported cases occurring in humans without HIV infection have been in patients who had significant contact either with livestock (often horses) or with soil and environment that were heavily contaminated with livestock waste. In contrast, in AIDS and in other immunocompromised hosts, *Rhodococcus* disease occurs in patients who do not have any particular environmental exposure history—implying a wide distribution of the organism. There is no geographic endemicity.

Pathogenesis and Pathophysiology

R. equi usually enters the body by direct inhalation, although soft tissue infections after cutaneous inoculation can occur. It is an intracellular pathogen and causes disease in patients with impaired cell-mediated immunity and defects in phagocytic processing of organisms. Affected tissue usually shows a necrotizing granulomatous reaction, with histiocytes and macrophages frequently containing bacteria. Unlike lesions infected with *Mycobacterium tuberculosis* and systemic fungi, there is also a prominent infiltration of neutrophils in the affected areas, a characteristic shared with *Actinomyces* species.

Clinical and Radiologic Features

Patients most frequently complain of indolent symptoms, such as fever, nonproductive cough, and mild dyspnea. Typically there is a paucity of findings on physical examination of the chest, but signs of consolidation and pleural friction rubs may be present. Often it is found concurrent with other pulmonary infections. Extrapulmonary dissemination occurs in both HIV-infected and non–HIV-infected patients, but there appears to be a significantly greater rate of recovery of the organism from blood cultures in HIV patients. The central nervous system is a recognized site of metastatic infection, as it is for *Nocardia* species.

The most common radiographic abnormalities are lobar infiltrates, which usually evolve into nodular or cavitating lesions within weeks or months, similar to those seen with *Nocardia* infection. There is no predilection for involvement of any particular lobe. Pleural effusions are common.

Diagnosis and Differential Diagnosis

R. equi can readily be cultured from sputum, bronchial lavage, pleural fluid, or other infected tissue and often from blood. Since the organisms stain as pleomorphic gram-positive bacilli, grow readily on most media, and are usually catalase producers, they can be mistaken for "diphtheroid" or "coryneform" contaminants unless further testing is done. It is therefore important for the clinician to alert the microbiology laboratory staff if the possibility of *R. equi* is entertained. They are slightly acid fast when stained with Ziehl-Neelsen stain.

Rhodococci share many microbiologic features with *Mycobacteria* and *Nocardia*. The high mycolic acid content of their cell walls results in their acid-fast staining properties and may also play a role in their similar clinical and pathologic manifestations. *Nocardia* species, *M. tuberculosis,* and nontuberculous mycobacteria should also be considered when acid-fast organisms are found in clinical specimens, especially in immunocompromised patients with nodular or cavitary pneumonia.

Treatment

Antibiotic therapy alone is usually adequate to achieve cure. As with mycobacterial infections, multidrug regimens and therapy of 2 to 6 months' duration may be needed. Erythromycin, rifampin, ciprofloxacin and other quinolones, chloramphenicol, sulfonamides, and aminoglycosides are active against most isolates. *R. equi* is an intracellular pathogen that is capable of multiplying in phagocytes. Therefore, antibiotics that are capable of achieving high intracellular levels, such as rifampin or quinolones, but especially erythromycin and the expanded-spectrum macrolides, clarithromycin or azithromycin, are preferred. (See Table 67-2 for specific dosage recommendations.) In some patients, surgical resection of a nodular or cavitating lesion may be necessary to achieve cure.

ENVIRONMENTAL AND ANIMAL PRODUCT PNEUMONIAS

Anthrax Respiratory Disease

Inhalation anthrax was once referred to as Bradford's disease and wool sorter's disease. Inhalation anthrax has become rare. An epidemic of anthrax occurred in the area of Sverdlovsk, in the former Soviet Union, in 1979, as a result of studies of anthrax as a biologic weapon. "Weaponized" anthrax was implicated in bioterrorist-associated outbreaks in the United States in 2001 (see Appendix).

Bacteriology

B. anthracis is a large (red-blood-cell diameter), square-ended bacillus that stains gram-positive and has a tendency to form chains. Growth on sheep blood agar results in dull, sticky, irregularly shaped colonies within 24 h. The organism possesses a polyglutamic acid capsule, produces a complex potent exotoxin, and, under adverse conditions, forms highly refractile, centrally located spores that are very resistant to extremes of temperature and moisture. More than a century ago, Louis Pasteur used serial passage at 43°C to develop an effective, safe vaccine for animals, and it is now known that toxin production is mediated by a temperature-sensitive plasmid that is killed at 43°C.

Ecology and Epidemiology

Anthrax is primarily a disease of herbivores. The resistant spores are present after animals dying of the disease contaminate the soil. The optimal conditions for germination of spores and multiplication of bacilli include alkaline soils containing adequate calcium and low areas that are wet for prolonged periods, termed *incubator areas,* with thick vegetation that produces heat with decay. Periods of extreme drought after a rainy season favor spore formation. Animals grazing in these areas can inhale or ingest spores or pick them up on their fur. The cycle is completed when an animal develops the disease and dies, returning organisms to the soil, where they eventually sporulate under adverse conditions. Inhalation anthrax rarely occurs from contact with live infected animals, and there is no human-to-human transmission. Working in the animal hide industry, being exposed to bone meal fertilizer, and using imported raw wool in home crafts can lead to inhalation of spores and clinical disease in susceptible persons. The unvaccinated person who occasionally enters a goat-wool or hide-processing plant to do needed repairs is at greatest risk for an inhalation exposure. Anthrax spores may be "weaponized" to facilitate aerosolization as an agent of biologic warfare (see Appendix).

Pathogenesis and Pathophysiology

Inhalation results in activation of bronchial clearing mechanisms and entrapment of spores in hilar and mediastinal nodes, where reversion to vegetative bacilli can occur. The number of spores needed to cause pneumonia depends on the nature of the aerosol (10^2–10^4 for weaponized spores) and the host immune states. The polyglutamic acid capsule is antiphagocytic, and the extracellular microorganisms produce a tripartite protein exotoxin that leads to profound local edema acutely, accompanied by hemorrhage in the mediastinal and hilar areas. Compromise of airflow results. Recent studies have elucidated the mechanism of edema formation. The protective antigen fragment of the toxin is the binding domain, essential for cell penetration by the edema factor portion of the molecule. Edema factor is a potent adenylate cyclase. Activation within mammalian cells stimulates production of cyclic AMP, and the resultant flux of sodium, potassium, and water leads to profound local edema. When this process takes place in hilar and mediastinal nodes and surrounding tissues, profound airway obstruction ensues, with pooling of secretions and, if the patient survives, secondary bacterial pneumonia. The pathogen rarely invades lung tissue, as death from asphyxia occurs rapidly, usually associated with pleural effusions (secondary to lymphatic obstruction) and hemorrhagic septicemic lesions in many organs, including the central nervous system. Typical thoracic pathologic findings include hemorrhagic mediastinitis with hemorrhagic mediastinal lymphadenopathy.

Clinical and Radiologic Features

The onset of inhalation anthrax is insidious, usually resembling a nonspecific febrile influenza-like illness. Malaise and muscle aches, mild headache, coryza, pharyngitis, and chest pains have been described as early symptoms. Cough, if present, is usually mild and nonproductive, and fever is low grade. At this stage, it is hardly possible for the physician to entertain a presumptive or possible diagnosis of anthrax unless a history of industrial or craft-related exposure to imported animal hair or hides or to animal products such as bone meal is obtained. A number of the nonspecific features described above may be relevant. Watery nasal discharge can be indicative of nasal or paranasal sinus edema. Cough may represent hilar and mediastinal node swelling, and careful auscultation may reveal prolonged expiration or wheezes. Chest pain may be the first clue that hilar and mediastinal inflammation is present.

Within hours to a few days, the mild complaints abruptly worsen and acute airway obstructive features dominate the clinical picture. Any activity precipitates severe dyspnea, stridor, and wheezing. Impairment of the nervous system (hemorrhagic meningitis) and hypoxemia result in decreasing levels of consciousness. Edema of the pharynx, neck, and anterior chest may develop. Chest pain, fever, and cyanosis are progressive changes. Worsening airway obstruction can lead to intercostal space retraction, and pleural effusions are noted on examination. Death usually occurs within hours to a day once acute respiratory symptoms are present.

Inhalation anthrax is primarily a mediastinitis, and the radiologic features mostly reflect the pathologic findings. Widening of the mediastinum or prominence of hilar nodes is the earliest radiologic finding, sometimes accompanied by pleural effusions. In advanced cases, the mediastinal shadow is greater than 9 cm in width and sharply demarcated from surrounding lung tissue because of absence of airspace consolidation. There may be perihilar and peribronchial streaking associated with edema and hemorrhage.

Diagnostic Features

A physician alerted to the possibility of inhalation anthrax has few laboratory studies to rely on. Nasal secretions and sputum rarely reveal the characteristic bulky gram-positive bacilli. Half of the reported cases of inhalation disease are complicated by meningitis, and hemorrhagic cerebrospinal fluid with observable organisms will confirm the diagnosis. There are no available data on examination of buffy-coat smears, and therapy must be instituted before blood culture results become available. Unfortunately, the most commonly recognized form of anthrax, the cutaneous chancriform necrotic lesion, does not usually accompany inhalation cases.

Treatment and Prevention

Intravenously administered penicillin is the treatment of choice for non-military exposures. Fluoroquinolone, chloramphenicol, tetracycline, or doxy-cycline is an effective substitute (see Appendix and Table 67-2 for specific dosage recommendations). Unfortunately, the lower-airway obstructive man-ifestations are often not reversible once acute respiratory manifestations have developed. Assisted ventilation, drainage of pleural effusions, and use of diuretics are all useful support efforts.

Mortality in inhalation anthrax is high without early diagnosis, compared to the rarity of death from cutaneous disease. In the animal hide industry, prevention is the cornerstone of dealing with anthrax. Plant workers and others in contact with potentially infected animal products should be immunized with the currently available vaccine. A genetically engineered vaccine based on toxin specificity is in the development stage. Animal products imported from endemic regions of the world (such as the Near East and the Indian subcontinent) are steam-sterilized, and modern ventilation is in the workplace. At-risk subjects, then, are people who service these plants, such as ventilation workers and other transients. Bone meal is another vehicle for carrying inert spores. It should be treated by heat sterilization before packaging for use by commercial and home gardeners. Those who import craft yarn from endemic areas are at special risk unless the rules for commercial hide sterilization are also imposed on casual imports.

Pneumonia due to *Brucella* Species

In the approximately 200 cases of brucellosis that are reported yearly in the United States, acute respiratory manifestations are usually insignificant. Bru-cellosis is often an indolent illness and in chronic cases, pleurisy, hilar adenopathy, and nodular lung lesions are encountered. Exposure to animals or to animal foods or residence in an endemic region is usually present when sought for in the history.

Bacteriology

Brucellae are small coccobacillary, gram-negative, nonmotile, aerobic, nonen-capsulated organisms that are now classified with the alpha-proteobacteria, closely related to *Rochalimaea* and *Bartonella* species. Carbon dioxide is es-sential for growth of *Brucella abortus,* and all four pathogenic species require growth medium enriched with vitamins and serum. With the aid of a battery of biochemical, metabolic, and immunologic criteria, brucellae pathogenic for humans can be classified as *B. abortus, B. suis, B. melitensis,* and *B. canis.*

Ecology and Epidemiology

Brucella species are distributed worldwide, wherever their natural hosts reside. Infection and disease occur primarily in domestic animals in geo-graphic regions such as the Mediterranean littoral (*B. melitensis*), worldwide except in areas of Europe and Japan (*B. abortus*), in the midwestern United States (*B. suis*), and in North and Latin America (*B. canis*). Spread from one region to another occurs with live animal movements and when infected an-imal products are commercially or privately shipped. Rigorous control meas-ures such as herd inspections and vaccination procedures have dramatically reduced enzootic and epizootic disease in many regions.

The epidemiology of brucellosis is intimately related to the association of susceptible persons with infected animals and animal products. Abattoir workers (especially slaughterers) and others in the meat-processing industry, farmers, dairy workers, veterinarians, and bacteriology laboratory technicians account for most cases in the United States and a preponderance of male victims. Also at risk are travelers to endemic regions who eat local foods and people who consume imported goat cheese, sausage, and other unpasteurized edibles from endemic areas. The organisms are usually acquired by ingestion, through skin abrasions and lacerations, or via conjunctival inoculation. Evidence indicates that aerosol spread can be a route in abattoir workers. No human-to-human transmission has been reported.

Pathogenesis and Pathophysiology

Organisms invade the local reticuloendothelial system and lymph nodes, followed by bacteremic spread to many organs during the following weeks. There is increasing evidence that the aerosol route may be especially efficient as a portal of entry. The distribution of nodular lesions in lung tissue is primarily in basal segments, however, which argues for bacteremia rather than primarily an inhalation mechanism for most cases of pulmonary disease. Species and strain differences account for the wide variety of tissue reactions encountered, including granulomas, necrosis, and abscess formation of lymph nodes, liver, and spleen. Lipopolysaccharide endotoxin is present in the cell envelope and may be responsible for profound metabolic and cardiovascular effects initially and as organisms are killed during therapy. *Brucella* species are able to survive within nonstimulated macrophages and can destroy these cells while escaping host antibodies and antibiotic therapy. The development of host immunity appears to be primarily cell-mediated, just as in *M. tuberculosis* disease. Impairment of cell-mediated immunity can lead to activation of latent *Brucella* or to greater susceptibility and severity of a primary infection. Brucella is a potential agent of biologic warfare (see Appendix).

Clinical and Radiologic Features

The clinical expression of brucellosis is dominated by nonspecific flu-like constitutional manifestations, including fever and headache. Nonproductive cough has been described in 10 to 33 percent of cases, but other indicators of respiratory involvement are rarely or poorly described. In one review of 59 cases, dyspnea and pleuritic chest pain were present in 10 percent of the patients. Hoarseness, bronchitis, and, rarely, mucopurulent, purulent, or hemorrhagic sputum have been noted. The most frequent radiologic findings have been perihilar and peribronchial infiltrates or solitary granulomas. Unilateral hilar adenopathy, nodular basilar infiltrates, and pleural effusions occur occasionally.

Diagnostic Features

During the acute illness or in relapse, blood cultures may be positive—especially if kept for a minimum of 14 days. In the presence of an infiltrate or pleural effusion, material for Gram's stain and culture should be obtained, even though the yield from these studies is small. A positive culture may be obtained from a lymph node or pulmonary granuloma biopsy. In most cases the diagnosis is made from a fourfold rise or a single value of at least 1:160 in the agglutination titer. Occasionally "inhibitory" or blocking antibodies are present in the serum, and a positive titer will be discovered only if the serum is further diluted (so-called prozone phenomenon). The standard tube agglutination test utilizes *B. abortus* as the antigen and will detect antibodies to *B. suis* and *B. melitensis,* but not to *B. canis.* Diagnostic confusion and numerous alternative diagnoses are the rule in cases of brucellosis. Acute disease can be confused with miliary tuberculosis, endocarditis, tularemia, disseminated histoplasmosis, and lymphoproliferative diseases. Subacute and chronic cases must be differentiated from subacute bacterial endocarditis, tuberculosis, histoplasmosis, and other systemic fungal infections and sarcoidosis.

Treatment and Prevention

The combination of doxycycline with rifampin for 4 to 6 weeks is the most effective oral antibiotic regimen. Doxycycline combined with streptomycin 1 g daily or with trimethoprim-sulfamethoxazole is also an effective alternative regimen. Fluoroquinolones are active in vitro, but they are associated with an unacceptably high relapse rate. (See Table 67-2 for specific dosage schedules.)

Preventive measures for cattle have been successful utilizing vaccination programs and destruction of diseased animals. Quarantine and inspection activities have diminished the risk of importing infected animals into the United States, and this reduction of disease in cattle has resulted in a decline in human cases. The program for *B. suis* eradication has been ineffective, and human cases of *B. suis* now outnumber those due to *B. abortus*. The efficacy of human vaccines is marginal.

Pneumonia due to *Burkholderia (Pseudomonas) pseudomallei*

Melioidosis is primarily an acute necrotizing or, in the later stage, a chronic fibronodular cavitating process indistinguishable from tuberculosis. It is a disease of tropical latitudes, and most cases have been seen in Southeast Asia, associated with rural settings. Infection with *Burkholderia pseudomallei* has been seen almost exclusively in individuals with exposures in Southeast Asia and northeastern Australia.

Bacteriology

The organism is an aerobic, bipolar-staining gram-negative bacillus that is motile and lacks a well-defined capsule. Similar to the pseudomonads, *B. pseudomallei* grows well on minimal as well as enriched media, including blood and MacConkey agar, used in most routine laboratories. Typical colonies are distinctive in appearance, rough or wrinkled, and cream to orange in color; they may resemble a flower with folds radiating from a central core. Colonies have the typical musty, fruity odor of the pseudomonads but lack pyocyanin and other pigments that characteristically color the surrounding medium. Identification rests on a battery of biochemical reactions, and confirmation is based on agglutination or fluorescent antibody studies.

Ecology and Epidemiology

B. pseudomallei occupies an environmental niche that includes moist soils, rice paddies, and other stagnant water in tropical and subtropical regions, approximately subtended by latitude 20 degrees north to 20 degrees south. Evidence of subclinical and clinical disease occurs in wild and domestic animal populations, as well as in humans living permanently or transiently in rural endemic areas, especially in Southeast Asia and northeastern Australia. As many as 10 to 30 percent of native populations have evidence of prior infection from serologic data.

Transmission is mainly by direct contact with contaminated soil or water through minor abrasions or major wounds. Ingestion and inhalation are probably less frequent modes of spread, but common source outbreaks occur in animals and humans. Animal-to-human disease has not been seen, and the only reported human-to-human spread has been associated with Foley catheter contamination and venereal transmission. In endemic regions, lack of previous exposure and debilitating circumstances, including malnutrition and uncontrolled diabetes, may increase susceptibility to infection and disease.

Pathogenesis and Pathophysiology

There is no information available on the mechanisms of pathogenicity of *B. pseudomallei*. Acute infections are associated with necrotic lesions containing polymorphonuclear neutrophils (PMN) in lung and in other tissues. Chronic infections, especially in the respiratory tract, resemble tuberculosis with granuloma formation, Langhans' or foreign-body giant cells, central caseation necrosis, and occasionally a PMN response in the necrotic area. Activation of latent infection after a period of months to even decades occurs. This "awakening" can be in the wake of influenza and other acute infections, acute stress (trauma, thermal burn, surgery, etc.), and immunosuppressing illnesses or therapies, but spontaneous activation also occurs. The location of dormant microorganisms and the specific molecular events that stimulate recurrent disease are unknown.

An antecedent local infection in an area of broken skin can be followed by acute septicemia in nonimmune subjects. Initial pulmonary lesions occur predominantly in the better-vascularized basal segments, but eventually other areas of the lungs and other tissues are affected. Subacute and chronic disease may result from a subclinical primary focus, often localized in an apical segment, resembling tuberculosis in location and propensity for granuloma formation and cavitation. Subpleural invasion can result in empyema or sympathetic sterile effusions.

Clinical and Radiologic Features

Primary melioidosis occurs within a few days to 2 weeks of exposure, usually in persons present in or recently from an endemic area. Military personnel with outdoor injuries constitute a potential group for delayed active disease. In the United States, the acute phase of melioidosis is rarely seen. The portal of entry may be present as a small necrotic skin lesion in an area of known trauma, with accompanying cellulitis or lymphangitis. In addition to marked toxicity and high fevers, the respiratory complaints include cough, dyspnea, pleuritic pain, and purulent sputum. Bibasilar rales may be heard, but objective findings are often minimal in the face of severe toxicity. Mortality approaches 75 percent, even when the diagnosis is suspected and appropriate therapy immediately instituted.

Milder types of subacute and chronic pneumonia are usually seen in patients developing clinical illness after leaving an endemic area. In addition to fever, productive cough, and pleuritic pain, many patients experience marked weight loss and a clinical picture resembling tuberculosis or fungal disease. Secondary skin manifestations are rarely seen unless bacteremia ensues. Physical changes are often subtle but can include localized rales, a pleural friction rub, signs of an effusion, and manifestations of disease localized to soft tissues, lymph nodes, bones, or joints.

Radiologic findings reflect the stage of disease present. In acute fulminant infections, airspace disease can be absent or miliary to larger nodular densities seen in basal segments. In subacute and chronic cases, fibronodular or cavitary apical lesions are found.

Diagnostic Features

Melioidosis should be seriously entertained in any febrile patient with a history of residence in a major endemic region such as Southeast Asia or northeastern Australia. If sputum is available, the gram-negative bipolar staining bacilli may be seen, and the organisms can be readily cultured and identified by the routine laboratory. Blood and urine cultures are frequently positive in acute cases. In more indolent infections, biopsy may be necessary. Serologic studies can be helpful in active and recrudescent disease. A specific IgM immunofluorescence test is often positive in recent infections and recrudescent disease. Complement fixation and indirect hemagglutination tests are available and require testing of paired sera over several weeks to confirm active disease.

Differential Diagnosis

In patients from Southeast Asia, acute fulminating infections with pneumonia may be due to traditional bacteria and viruses, but it may also be caused by infection with *Y. pestis* (plague) and *F. tularensis* (tularemia) (see above).

Chronic forms of melioidosis resemble tuberculosis and fungal infections such as histoplasmosis and blastomycosis. Occupation, travel, and history of respiratory illness should help to clarify the cause. Confirmation usually requires biopsy with special stains and culture, or serologic data.

Treatment and Prevention

During the Vietnam War, mortality greater than 50 percent occurred, even with use of three-drug regimens in massive doses. In subacute and chronic pneumonias and recrudescent disease, cure rates approach 100 percent. Treatment must be prolonged, and surgical intervention for drainage or removal of cavitary lesions is sometimes necessary to prevent relapse. Since the mid-1970s, a number of reports have confirmed the efficacy of trimethoprim-sulfamethoxazole for acute and other forms of respiratory disease. Strains from some geographic areas, however, may be resistant to trimethoprim-sulfamethoxazole. A recent study of clinical isolates from Thailand demonstrated an 81 percent resistance rate among 200 isolates tested.

Ceftazidime in high doses is effective therapy, but first- and second-generation cephalosporins are not. Imipenem, amoxicillin-clavulanate, ampicillin-sulbactam, and ticarcillin-clavulanate have good activity in vitro, but clinical experience with these drugs is limited. *B. pseudomallei* is an intracellular pathogen. When beta-lactam antibiotics are used, an antimicrobial that achieves good intracellular levels, such as trimethoprim-sulfamethoxazole, should be administered concurrently. The tetracyclines and chloramphenicol are effective therapy and also are generally used in combination. Kanamycin, but not other aminoglycosides, is active. Fluoroquinolones are not active at levels achievable in serum.

Although contemporary experience is limited and in vitro data must serve as a guide, specific recommendations for acute and chronic infections are outlined in Table 67-2. It should be emphasized that this is a controversial area, dosages are enormous, and drug toxicity can limit the usefulness of many recommended agents. Modifications in these programs must be guided by clinical circumstances and await more definitive studies.

There are no prophylactic antimicrobial studies available, nor has a vaccine been developed. People traveling, living, or working in endemic regions should be advised of this soil- and water-dwelling organism.

Pulmonary Infections due to *Yersinia enterocolitica*

Most infections caused by *Y. enterocolitica* are in the gastrointestinal tract, resulting in a self-limited gastroenteritis- or appendicitis-mimicking mesenteric and terminal ileum adenitis. Septicemias and involvement of the lungs and other viscera are extremely rare, usually occurring in persons suffering from cirrhosis or who are immunocompromised.

Yersinia belong to the family Enterobacteriaceae. *Y. enterocolitica* is a gram-negative, facultative bacillus that resembles many other enteric microbes. Identification procedures include the ability to grow and exhibit motility at room temperature plus a battery of biochemical and serologic tests. Although occasionally overlooked in stool because it is confused with many other members of the fecal flora, the organism is readily identified in blood and respiratory specimens. Most strains are nonlactose or slow lactose fermenters, causing confusion with *Y. pestis, Salmonella, Shigella,* and several other members of the Enterobacteriaceae family. Cold enrichment techniques and highly selective media, extensively used to identify this organism in fecal specimens, are not necessary in nonfecal material. Various serotypes and biotypes, with distribution in geographically distinct regions, have been described.

Y. enterocolitica has been isolated from a variety of rodents and other wild animals, and from cats and dogs. There is little evidence for direct transmission or for spread among people other than by the fecal-oral route. Most cases occur singly, but epidemics involving families and hundreds of people have been described. Disease is initiated by ingestion of contaminated milk or other food. Most cases of respiratory disease have been reported in immunocompromised hosts, alcoholics, and cirrhotics.

Direct aspiration may be the mechanism for initiation of pulmonary disease, following an initial pharyngeal focus. Bacteremia can complicate pharyngeal disease, although the most likely mechanism entails ulceration of Peyer's patches in the terminal ileum, mesenteric adenitis, and portal bacteremia. Systemic shunting to the lungs can follow, especially in cirrhotics, the group that most frequently develops septicemia. Mechanisms of pathogenesis are not clarified, but strains virulent for animals and causing human disease have plasmid-mediated V and W envelope antigens, temperature-sensitive calcium dependency (as with *Y. pestis*), a factor that enhances cell penetration, and endotoxin. An enterotoxin, similar to stable toxin of *E. coli,* is also produced, but an extragastrointestinal role has not been established for this material. The development of immune-complex manifestations such as erythema nodosum and nonsuppurative polyarthritis may contribute to pathogenicity.

During the past decade, concomitant with greater recognition of this pathogen as a cause of gastroenteritis, cases of pneumonia and lung abscess have been reported. Respiratory infections occur in association with an acute febrile septicemic illness or as a primary respiratory process, with cough, dyspnea, and signs of consolidation. The history is usually vague for gastrointestinal symptoms, animal exposure, or unusual food intake. There may be signs of increasing hepatic failure with ascites or peritonitis in patients with underlying cirrhosis. Radiologic findings include nodular basilar densities consistent with septicemic spread, dependent segment infiltrates suggesting an aspiration mechanism, occasionally with cavitation, and fluffy widespread densities consistent with septic emboli. Immunocompromised patients may be especially prone to severe necrotizing pulmonary infections.

The diagnosis often depends on information obtained from blood or sputum cultures. Enteric-like gram-negative bacilli can be seen in sputum. Pharyngeal cultures should be done if signs of local inflammation are present. Suppurating nodes and peritoneal or joint fluids are other sources of material that may contribute to the diagnosis when sputum is not available.

Cases of respiratory infection have responded well to a variety of antibiotics, including ampicillin or second-generation cephalosporins. Third-generation cephalosporins, chloramphenicol, and aminoglycosides are also effective. Underlying diseases influence the outcome, but when pneumonia is the major problem, prognosis is excellent. Treatment is usually continued for a total of 3 to 6 weeks. (See Table 67-2 for dosage details.)

Preventive measures include avoiding rodent or domestic animal contamination of food and water supplies. Opportunities for susceptible persons to come in contact with this zoonotic microorganism may be increasing as well, as immunocompromised people look to natural foods and mineral waters for improved health.

PNEUMONIAS CAUSED BY OBLIGATE HUMAN COMMENSALS

Neisseria meningitidis

Bacteriology

More than 100 cases of *N. meningitidis* pneumonia have been reported during the past 15 years. *Neisseria* are oxygen-requiring, gram-negative–staining cocci recognized from their characteristic pairing as kidney-shaped diplococci. They are fastidious, succumbing rapidly to the external environment and to dry or cold conditions. Although *Neisseria* can grow on blood agar, optimal conditions include enriched media, such as chocolate agar, and incubation in an atmosphere of 6 percent CO_2 at 35 to 37°C with 50 percent humidity. *N. meningitidis* is distinguishable from other *Neisseria* species that are residents of the oral-respiratory region by sugar-fermentation reactions and by serologic identification, which depends on specific capsular polysaccharides. Isolation and identification of *N. meningitidis* in sputum are facilitated by the use of a selective medium, such as modified Thayer-Martin agar (MTM), which contains antibiotics that suppress more rapidly growing microorganisms. The presence of *Neisseria*-like diplococci in a Gram-stained smear of sputum should provide the impetus to culture the specimen on MTM media as well as on less selective media, such as blood and chocolate agar.

N. meningitidis is a typical gram-negative organism containing a potent lipopolysaccharide endotoxin in the outer membrane layer of the cell envelope. Exterior to this layer is a polysaccharide capsule, by which *N. meningitidis* can be separated into at least 13 chemically defined serogroups. Groups A, B, C, X, Y, Z, and W-135 are currently the most important clinically. Persons lacking bactericidal or capsular antibody to a specific serogroup are susceptible to colonization and to disease caused by that serogroup. With increasing age, acquisition of protective antibodies is associated with less likelihood of developing clinical disease.

Epidemiology

Nasopharyngeal carriage of various serogroups of meningococci occurs in approximately 5 to 15 percent of subjects. Convening and crowding large numbers of young persons from widely separated geographic areas, as occurs in the military or in boarding schools, can result in significant and rapid spread of an individual serogroup from a few asymptomatic carriers to many susceptibles. Spread is probably by aerosol droplets during close contact, since drying rapidly kills meningococci. People ill with influenza or adenoviral respiratory infections appear to be more susceptible—as occurs with other respiratory pathogens, such as *S. pneumoniae* and *Staphylococcus aureus*.

Pathogenesis and Pathophysiology

Initiation of infection begins when an encapsulated strain colonizes the nasopharynx of a person lacking immunity to that serogroup. Attachment to mucosal cells is facilitated by filamentous pili and perhaps by the action of bacterial IgA1 protease. The lower respiratory tract is invaded by aspiration or inhalation of droplet particles. A preceding viral infection can stimulate excessive airway secretions, damage surface epithelial structures, and interfere with clearance of microorganisms. Septicemia, petechial eruptions, meningitis, diffuse intravascular coagulation, and ARDS rarely accompany pneumonia, supporting a postulated aspiration mechanism. Bronchopneumonia, lobar extension, and necrosis and abscess formation are seen. Modern pathologic correlations are lacking, since there are no animal models of meningococcal pneumonia and histopathologic material is essentially nonexistent.

Clinical and Radiologic Features

The clinical presentation of meningococcal pneumonia resembles that of pneumococcal infection. Productive cough, pleuritic pain, chills, and fever are associated with physical changes of rales with consolidation. In contrast to the picture of pneumococcal disease, pleural rubs and hemoptysis are unusual. Suspicion of meningococcal disease is enhanced if many cases of bacterial pneumonia erupt in closed populations such as military or school groups or among hospital patients. Pharyngitis is often an early complaint.

Radiologic features are nonspecific and include patchy bronchopneumonia and lobar airspace infiltrates, usually located in a lower or right middle lobe, accompanied by an effusion in about 20 percent of cases. Occasionally the radiologic appearance resembles diffuse pulmonary edema or an antecedent viral infection.

Diagnostic Features

Diagnosis depends on isolation of predominantly *N. meningitidis* from a carefully collected sputum specimen that has characteristic gram-negative diplococci and PMNs on the stained smear. Attention to these criteria is essential, since pathogenic and nonpathogenic *Neisseria* and *Moraxella* species are part of the normal respiratory flora. Invasive procedures, such as transtracheal aspiration, are not necessary if a valid sputum is available, and the Gram's stain appearance prompts culturing the specimen on MTM media. Alternative methods of identification include the capsular swelling technique (Quellung), latex bead coagglutination, and fluorescent antibody staining. Recent purification of all of the major group-specific capsular polysaccharides should lead to expansion of these rapid diagnostic methods. Blood and cerebrospinal fluid cultures are rarely positive in meningococcal respiratory disease (Table 67-4).

TABLE 67-4 Diagnosing Meningococcal Pneumonia

Antecedent viral respiratory infection
Multiple community or hospital respiratory cases
Purulent or frothy sputum
Kidney-shaped gram-negative diplococci on smear
Culture sputum on modified Thayer-Martin medium
Incubation with CO_2 enrichment

Treatment and Prevention

Low-dose penicillin is effective for most cases, although those complicated by cavitation or empyema should be treated with a minimum of 6 million units daily. Patients allergic to penicillin can be given chloramphenicol. The third-generation cephalosporins also are effective. In contrast to meningitis or meningococcemia, respiratory infections appear to respond uniformly well to treatment.

Meningococci spread via aerosols, so isolation of suspected cases is essential, especially during the first 24 h of treatment. Chemoprophylaxis and immunoprophylaxis have been found effective in epidemics of meningitis, but no data are available for respiratory disease protection. Penicillin, the drug of choice for treating active disease, does not reliably eradicate the carrier state or protect intimately exposed contacts. Probably because of its transport into oral and respiratory tract secretions in high concentrations, rifampin is an effective prophylactic agent. The usual protective dose is 600 mg orally, twice daily for 2 days. Fluoroquinolones such as ciprofloxacin, at a dose of 500 mg twice daily for 5 days, is also effective. Minocycline diffuses into upper respiratory secretions in high concentrations and is a useful alternative to rifampin. Labyrinthitis, a frequent toxic side effect, prevents wider use of this agent, however.

Immunoprophylaxis has been safe and effective when given systematically to large at-risk groups in military installations, schools, day care centers, or defined communities. A quadrivalent vaccine, containing serogroups A, C, Y, and W-135, is commercially available, and an octavalent preparation is in development. Although group Y and W-135 isolates have commonly been causal, there are no data for efficacy of the vaccine for respiratory infections. Children below the age of 2 years respond poorly to the group C vaccine and unpredictably to the other polysaccharide products. This younger age group remains vulnerable, and protection must be provided, when necessary, with chemoprophylaxis. Immunizing persons with influenza viral vaccines should eliminate some cases of secondary bacterial infections, including those caused by *N. meningitidis.*

Moraxella (Branhamella) catarrhalis

Formerly considered a nonpathogenic respiratory commensal, *M. catarrhalis* has aroused renewed interest as an opportunist and primary pathogen. Resemblance to *Neisseria* on Gram's stain and penicillin resistance of many clinically significant isolates are features that encourage inclusion in this section.

Bacteriology

Moraxella are gram-negative cocci that pair as kidney-shaped diplococci; hence they cannot be distinguished morphologically from *Neisseria.* The organisms grow well on nonselective media such as sheep blood agar and enriched chocolate agar, especially when supplemented with added CO_2. Growth of *Moraxella* is variable on selective media such as MTM—in contrast to pathogenic *Neisseria,* which thrive on that medium. They fail to utilize a variety of sugars. These and other biochemical tests help to distinguish them from *Neisseria.* Many clinical isolates produce β-lactamase and, therefore, are resistant to penicillin.

Epidemiology

A member of the resident microflora of the nasopharynx and pharynx, *M. catarrhalis* can also colonize the mucosa of the genital tract. Among persons with chronic lung disease it can be found, along with other bacteria, in respiratory secretions.

Pathogenesis and Pathophysiology

Aspiration of nasopharyngeal secretions, stimulated by an acute viral upper respiratory infection, is the most common proposed pathophysiological factor. Contributing conditions that are immunocompromising—such as steroid therapy, malignancy, hypogammaglobulinemia, and neutropenia—are present in a large number of patients. Paranasal sinus and ear infections occur predominantly in children, probably because of compromised drainage ducts in anatomically crowded areas. Rarely, *Moraxella* produce primary invasive diseases outside the respiratory tract, including meningitis, endocarditis, septic arthritis, and, in immunocompromised patients, septicemia.

Clinical and Radiologic Features

Most people who develop respiratory infections are adults with chronic lung disease associated with smoking, industrial exposures, or bronchitis and bronchiectasis. Purulent bronchitis or bronchopneumonia can follow an intercurrent viral infection. Respiratory distress, if present, may be related to the acute process, with bronchospasm and fever superimposed on the chronic underlying disease. Signs of consolidation or pleural fluid may be present, along with persistent obstructive changes. Evidence has been accumulating that normal adults may develop primary laryngitis and children a nonproductive cough as other manifestations of clinical respiratory tract disease, but primary pneumonia is very uncommon at any age in subjects with healthy lungs.

The radiologic appearance is influenced by the underlying chronic lung disease. No acute changes may be observed, but usually increased markings are seen superimposed on the findings of obstructive lung disease and fibrosis. Patchy consolidation is often noted. Lobar infiltrates, cavitation, and pleural effusions are distinctly unusual findings and suggest mixed infections or other complications of the underlying disease.

Diagnostic Features

The unique feature in cases of *M. catarrhalis* respiratory infections is the finding of gram-negative kidney-shaped diplococci associated with PMN exudate cells. Diagnosis depends on careful examination of an adequate expectorated sputum sample and culturing the specimen on nonselective blood and enriched chocolate agar as well as on selective MTM. The use of several media assures that these fastidious organisms will be identified in a crowd of other commensals. Blood cultures should be obtained in cases associated

TABLE 67-5 Diagnosing *Moraxella* Pneumonia

Underlying chronic lung disease
History of aspiration
Kidney-shaped gram-negative diplococci on smear
Culture sputum on sheep blood and enriched chocolate media
Culture sputum on selective modified Thayer-Martin medium

with immunosuppression or malignancy, and pleural effusions aspirated and examined bacteriologically. Transtracheal aspiration rarely adds to the examination of an adequate expectorated sputum. Serologic methods are not available to help verify a pathogenic role for *Moraxella* in mixed infections (Table 67-5).

Treatment

As the pathogenic role for *M. catarrhalis* was recognized, it became apparent that many isolates produced beta-lactamase and were resistant to penicillin and ampicillin due to beta-lactamase production. Therapy should be initiated with either a second generation or the macrolides clarithromycin or azithromycin, the combination of amoxicillin-clavulanic acid, a fluoroquinolone, or trimethoprim-sulfamethoxazole until beta-lactamase activity is determined.

BIBLIOGRAPHY

Abramova FA, Grinberg LM, Yampolskaya OV, Walker DH: Pathology of inhalational anthrax in 42 cases from the Sverdlovsk outbreak of 1979. *Proc Natl Acad Sci USA* 90:2291–2294, 1993.

Barnes PF, Appleman MD, Cosgrove MM: A case of melioidosis originating in North America. *Am Rev Respir Dis* 134:170–171, 1986.

Cohen MS, Steere AC, Baltimore R, et al: Possible nosocomial transmission of group Y *Neisseria meningitidis* among oncology patients. *Ann Intern Med* 91:7–12, 1979.

Drabick JJ, Gasser RA Jr, Saunders NB, et al: *Pasteurella multocida* pneumonia in a man with AIDS and nontraumatic feline exposure. *Chest* 103:7–11, 1993.

Emmons W, Reichwein B, Winslow DL: *Rhodococcus equi* infection in the patient with AIDS: Literature review and report on an unusual case. *Rev Infect Dis* 13:91–96, 1991.

Greer AE: Pulmonary brucellosis. *Dis Chest* 29:508–519, 1956.

Harvey RL, Sunstrum JC: *Rhodococcus equi* infection in patients with and without human immunodeficiency virus infection. *Rev Infect Dis* 13:139–145, 1991.

Putsch RW, Hamilton JD, Wolinsky E: *Neisseria meningitidis:* A respiratory pathogen? *J Infect Dis* 121:48–54, 1970.

Sookpranee M, Boonma P, Susaengrat W, et al: Multicenter prospective randomized trial comparing ceftazidime plus co-trimoxazole with chloramphenicol plus doxycycline and co-trimoxazole for treatment of severe melioidosis. *Antimicrob Agents Chemother* 36:158–162, 1992.

Weinberg AN, Heller HM: Unusual bacterial pneumonias, in Pennington JE (ed): *Respiratory Infections: Diagnosis and Management,* 3d ed. New York, Raven, 1994, pp 485–513.

Part Fifteen | Acute Respiratory Failure

evolves over 12 to 48 h, but it may take several days. Dyspnea, hypoxemia, and rapid, shallow breathing are seen. The majority of patients require intubation and mechanical ventilation within hours.

No laboratory findings are pathognomonic for ARDS. Usually, the chest radiograph reveals diffuse bilateral infiltrates consistent with pulmonary edema; the infiltrates may be mild or dense, interstitial or alveolar, patchy or confluent. The infiltrates may develop quickly and symmetrically, even before arterial hypoxemia, or more gradually and asymmetrically. Early in the course, the chest radiograph may show focal infiltrates which progress over hours or days to a complete "whiteout." Radiographic distinction between cardiogenic pulmonary edema and ARDS may be difficult.

Arterial blood gas measurements are abnormal. The ratio of arterial P_{O_2} to the fraction of O_2 in inspired air ($Pa_{O_2}/F_{I_{O_2}}$) is reduced to below 200. Initially, respiratory alkalosis is generally seen due to an increase in the number of lung dead-space units. However, as dead-space ventilation and the work of breathing increase, CO_2 elimination declines and respiratory acidosis develops. In the later phases of ARDS, oxygenation may improve, while increased minute ventilation and respiratory acidosis persist.

Leukocytosis or leukopenia, anemia and thrombocytopenia (a reflection of systemic inflammation and endothelial injury) may be observed. Disseminated intravascular coagulation occurs less frequently; usually, it is due to sepsis, severe trauma, or head injury. Renal function may be abnormal due to decreased renal perfusion or acute tubular necrosis. Liver function tests can be abnormal, showing a hepatocellular or cholestatic pattern of injury. These abnormalities reflect multiorgan dysfunction and may be entirely related to the underlying systemic inflammation that accompanies ARDS.

The differential diagnosis of ARDS includes congestive heart failure, diffuse pulmonary infections, and many other specific causes of acute respiratory failure associated with parenchymal infiltrates on chest radiograph.

MANAGEMENT

Management goals include treatment of the underlying cause, cardiopulmonary support, and therapy specific for lung injury.

Mechanical Ventilation

The traditional ventilatory strategy for ARDS included volume-cycled ventilation using tidal volumes of 10 to 15 mL/kg body weight and a respiratory rate sufficient to maintain a normal pH. Positive end-expiratory pressure (PEEP) was applied and adjusted to achieve the "target" Pa_{O_2} and $F_{I_{O_2}}$. An attempt was made to keep the Sa_{O_2} >90 percent and the $F_{I_{O_2}}$ in a nontoxic range (e.g., <0.7). However, none of these elements of the strategy were studied prospectively, and a "safe" level of $F_{I_{O_2}}$ in acute lung injury has not been defined.

More recently, animal studies have shown that high stretch due to high tidal volumes, accompanied by relatively high peak and plateau pressures, is associated with injury. Because the lung injury in ARDS is heterogeneous, some (normal) lung regions with preserved compliance may be exposed to high regional inflation volumes. In addition, cyclic reopening of atelectatic alveoli has been postulated as an additional mechanism of injury in ARDS. Partial protection appears to be afforded if PEEP is added at levels that circumvent the cyclic opening and closing (i.e., levels greater than that corresponding with the "lower inflection point" of the volume-pressure curve).

The current ventilator strategy in patients with acute lung injury is predicated on the belief that further lung injury can be minimized by avoiding tidal volumes resulting in plateau pressures that exceed the "upper inflection point" of the volume-pressure cure (the point above which a significant percentage of alveoli are probably overdistended), and using a level of PEEP slightly above the lower inflection point. Pressure-*targeted* ventilation (either pressure- or volume-controlled ventilation) employs limited tidal volumes (4 to 8 mL/kg) and plateau pressures (less than 35 cmH$_2$O). P$_{CO_2}$ is allowed to increase, if necessary, to meet the above objectives (*permissive hypercapnia*). PEEP is adjusted for Pa$_{O_2}$/F$_{I_{O_2}}$ and maintained above the lower inflection point of the volume-pressure curve. The combination of low stretch and PEEP above the lower inflection point, the *open lung approach,* has been demonstrated to improve mortality and increase the number of ventilator-free days during the first month of mechanical ventilation in ARDS.

Drug Therapy

At present, there is no specific drug treatment for ARDS. A variety of pharmacologic approaches have been tried.

Corticosteroids are not of benefit in early treatment or prevention of ARDS. Furthermore, corticosteroid use early in ARDS and sepsis is associated with a poorer outcome. In contradistinction, corticosteroids may have a beneficial effect on the fibroproliferative stage of ARDS. A large, multicenter, randomized, controlled trial is under way to assess the effect of corticosteroids in late-phase ARDS.

Inhaled nitric oxide (NO) selectively vasodilates lung regions in which the NO is distributed. Intrapulmonary shunting and pulmonary artery pressures are reduced, and ventilation/perfusion matching and arterial oxygenation are improved. NO has been administered for extended periods in ARDS, enabling reduction in F$_{I_{O_2}}$. The anticipated reduction in the risk of pulmonary oxygen toxicity may have a beneficial effect on clinical outcome. To date, however, there are no data to indicate that NO improves survival in ARDS.

Perfluorocarbons are biologically and chemically inert liquids that have low surface tension, high density, and high solubility for oxygen and carbon dioxide. Clinical trials using perfluorocarbons have demonstrated their safety and efficacy in a technique called "partial liquid ventilation" (PLV). The liquid is introduced to fill the functional residual capacity, and ventilation is conducted using tidal volumes of gas. PLV has been reported to improve oxygenation and survival in infants with severe RDS after surfactant replacement and conventional management have failed. PLV has also been reported to be safe, to improve pulmonary compliance, and to decrease physiological shunting in patients with ARDS receiving extracorporeal life support. Complications of therapy include pneumothorax and mucus plugs. A randomized clinical trial is currently under way in acute lung injury and ARDS to determine whether outcomes are also improved by PLV.

Surfactant replacement by aerosol has been studied in sepsis-induced ARDS and has been demonstrated to be ineffective. Almitrine (a respiratory stimulant that also improves ventilation-perfusion matching by enhancing hypoxic pulmonary vasoconstriction) has not been shown to produce persistent improvement in gas exchange in ARDS. Prostaglandin E$_1$ (PGE$_1$), a vasodilator with weak anti-inflammatory properties, has not been demonstrated to reduce ARDS severity, duration, or mortality. Finally, ketoconazole, a commonly used antifungal agent, which inhibits several proinflammatory pathways in macrophages in vitro and blocks production of prostaglandins and leukotrienes, has been demonstrated to be ineffective in early acute lung injury and ARDS.

Fluid Management

In both noncardiogenic and hemodynamic pulmonary edema, hydrostatic forces may contribute to increases in extravascular lung water (EVLW). A commonly employed practice in management of ARDS is reduction of intravascular volume (and pressures) through diuresis. The inherent danger in this approach is that the reduction in plasma volume may lead to reduced cardiac output and compromised blood flow to peripheral organs. Multiple organ failure is a much more common cause of death in ARDS than is respiratory failure, and care must be taken not to compromise organ perfusion. Whether fluid loss improves outcome or is simply a marker of resolving pulmonary vascular injury is unclear.

Another previously employed approach included administration of albumin intravenously in an attempt to increase intravascular oncotic pressure and reduce EVLW. Unfortunately, albumin traverses the leaky alveolar-capillary barrier, increasing tissue oncotic forces and, as a result, EVLW. Routine use of albumin in ARDS is not recommended.

Prone Positioning

Turning patients with ARDS from the supine to prone position has been shown to improve oxygenation in most. The improvement usually occurs within minutes, and it may persist after the patient is returned to the supine position. Studies suggest that the improvement occurs in response to prone positioning-related recruitment of lung regions that are perfused but not well ventilated when the patient is supine. With turning to the prone position, lung expansion becomes more uniform, and there is a reduction in the forces that cause collapse of dorsal airspaces in the supine position; minimal changes occur in the regional distribution of perfusion.

CLINICAL COURSE AND PROGNOSIS

The course of ARDS is variable, with a range of a few days to several months. The mean duration of mechanical ventilation is generally 10 to 14 days; approximately 10 to 20 percent of patients remain ventilator-dependent for longer than 3 weeks. Most deaths occur within the first 2 weeks. The duration of mechanical ventilation is inversely correlated with survival rate.

Multiple complications may punctuate the clinical course. Barotrauma, including pneumothorax, is related to the level of peak airway pressure and use of large tidal volumes; it does not appear to be independently associated with a poor outcome. Nosocomial pneumonia, sinusitis, and local airway damage are also common complications. Laryngeal injury may develop early in the course and is probably not related to the duration of intubation. For patients requiring prolonged mechanical ventilation, tracheostomy may improve patient comfort. Early tracheostomy probably does not decrease the risk of laryngeal trauma. With the use of low-pressure, high-volume endotracheal tube cuffs, tracheomalacia, tracheoesophageal fistulas, and innominate artery erosion are seen less frequently than previously.

Previously reported fatality rates in ARDS exceeded 50 percent, particularly in sepsis and in patients more than 60 years of age. Contributing factors included severe underlying illness (as reflected in the injury severity score in trauma patients), advanced malignancy, and presence or development of multiple organ failure. Although severity of initial lung injury (measured as an index of gas exchange, such as the Pa_{O_2}/Fi_{O_2} ratio or composite lung injury score) is not predictive of outcome, improvement in Pa_{O_2}/Fi_{O_2} over the first 3 to 7 days is associated with improved survival. More recent data suggest a decrease in ARDS-related fatality over the last decade, particularly in sepsis-induced ARDS and in those less than 60 years of age.

Nearly all survivors of ARDS reach maximal recovery by 6 months after extubation; only a few undergo further improvement. Although pulmonary function markedly improves in most patients during their recovery, approximately half continue to have some abnormality at the 6-month point. The abnormality generally consists of either a mild restrictive impairment or, more often, a mild impairment in diffusing capacity; however, more marked abnormalities may be observed. Patients who have continuing pulmonary dysfunction are more likely to have had a severe course, as reflected in failure of physiologic variables to improve over the first several days of the illness or in the need for prolonged mechanical ventilation. Rarely, patients continue to have severe pulmonary dysfunction and require long-term oxygen therapy. Although survivors of ARDS may continue to have impairments in overall physical and psychosocial function, these sequelae are usually mild and are not perceived by the patients to be related to their pulmonary condition.

BIBLIOGRAPHY

Acute Respiratory Distress Syndrome Network, The: Ventilation with lower tidal volumes as compared with traditional tidal volumes for actue lung injury and the acute respiratory distress syndrome. *N Engl J Med* 342:1301–1308, 2000.

Amato MBP, Barbas CSV, Medeiros DM, et al: Beneficial effects of the "open lung approach" with low distending pressures in acute respiratory distress syndrome. *Am J Respir Crit Care Med* 152:1835–1846, 1995.

Ashbaugh DG, Bigelow DB, Petty TL, Levine BE: Acute respiratory distress in adults. *Lancet* 2:319–323, 1967.

Bernard GR, Artigas A, Brigham KL, et al, and the Consensus Committee: The American-European Consensus Conference on ARDS: Definitions, mechanisms, relevant outcomes, and clinical trial coordination. *Am J Respir Crit Care Med* 149:818–824, 1994.

Doyle RL, Szaflarski N, Modin GW, et al; Identification of patients with acute lung injury—Predictors of mortality. *Am J Respir Crit Care Med* 152:1818–1824, 1995.

Garber BG, Hébert PC, Yelle J-D, et al: Adult respiratory distress syndrome: A systematic overview of incidence and risk factors. *Crit Care Med* 24:687–695, 1996.

Gattinoni L, Mascheroni D, Tomesin A, et al: Morphological response to positive and expiratory pressure in acute respiratory failure: Computerized tomography study. *Intensive Care Med* 12:137–142, 1986.

Ghio AJ, Elliott CG, Crapo RO, et al: Impairment after adult respiratory distress syndrome: An evaluation based on American Thoracic Society recommendations. *Am Rev Respir Dis* 139:1158–1162, 1989.

Hudson LD, Milberg JA, Anardi D, Maunder RJ: Clinical risks for development of the acute respiratory distress syndrome. *Am J Respir Crit Care Med* 151:239–301, 1995.

Hudson LD, Steinberg KP: Epidemiology of acute lung injury and ARDS, *Chest* 116 (1 suppl):74S–82S, 1999.

Marini JJ: Evolving concepts in the ventilatory management of acute respiratory distress syndrome. *Clin Chest Med* 17:555–575, 1996.

Milberg JA, Davis DA, Steinberg KP, Hudson LD: Improved survival of patients with acute respiratory distress syndrome (ARDS): 1983–1993. *JAMA* 273:306–309, 1995.

69 | Systemic Inflammatory Response and Multiple Organ Dysfunction Syndromes*

Michael A. Grippi

INTRODUCTION AND DEFINITIONS

The *systemic inflammatory response syndrome* (SIRS) and *multiple organ dysfunction syndrome* (MODS, previously called *multiple system organ failure*) occur in patients who have experienced a catastrophic event, including severe trauma, or who have progressive infection or other major, acute medical problems. With the acute stress response, neurohumoral and other physiologic adaptations direct metabolic substrate to the heart and brain. Vasoconstriction and fluid retention occur. An inadequate response leads to death from shock unless the patient is supported. With successful resuscitation, hypermetabolism is associated with mobilization of fuel sources, including glucose reserves. Muscle breakdown generates precursors for hepatic gluconeogenesis. Ineffective glucose utilization (by tissues other than blood cells and neurons) necessitates metabolism of amino acids and fat to support the liver, heart, and other organs. A generalized capillary leak, further fluid retention, vasodilatation, and an increase in cardiac output are observed. Several days later, neovascularization of damaged tissue occurs, capillary leak decreases, and the excess extracellular fluid is excreted.

While most patients recover, in some, the inflammatory process persists (beyond 4 or 5 days) and progresses to SIRS (Table 69-1). SIRS is characterized by a persistent inflammatory source (e.g., localized infection); when a source of infection is evident, the disorder is defined as sepsis (Table 69-2). Hypotension, metabolic acidosis (lactic acidosis), or acute respiratory distress syndrome (ARDS) may complicate SIRS/sepsis; when organ dysfunction arises in SIRS/sepsis, the syndrome is termed MODS.

MECHANISMS AND PATHOPHYSIOLOGY

As in simple stress (e.g., the postoperative state), SIRS and MODS are characterized by hypermetabolism; however, the hypermetabolic state of SIRS or MODS persists for 3 to 4 weeks rather than a few days, as in simple stress. Furthermore, in both simple stress and early in SIRS, the increase in metabolic demand can be met by an increase in oxygen supply or in oxygen extraction. As the disease progresses toward MODS, however, the ability to extract, and perhaps, utilize, oxygen is lost in some tissue beds.

---

*Edited from Chap. 168, "The Systemic Inflammatory Response Syndrome and the Multiple Organ Dysfunction Syndrome," by Deutschman CS. In: *Fishman's Pulmonary Diseases and Disorders*, 3rd ed., edited by Fishman AP, Elias JA, Fishman JA, Grippi MA, Kaiser LR, Senior RM. New York, McGraw-Hill, 1998, pp 2567–2574. For fuller discussion of topics dealt with in this chapter, the reader is referred to the original text, as noted above.

TABLE 69-1 Criteria for the Diagnosis of the Systemic Inflammatory Response Syndrome[a]

Temperature >38°C or <36°C
Heart rate >90 beats/min
Respiratory rate >20 breaths/min or P_{CO_2} <32 mmHg
White count >12 × 10^9/L or <4 × 10^9/L or >10% immature forms

[a]Presence of two or more criteria defines SIRS.
SOURCE: Bone RC, Balk RA, Cerra FB, et al: Definitions for sepsis and organ failure and guidelines for the use of innovative therapies in sepsis. *Chest* 101:1644–1655, 1992.

A block in cellular glucose utilization is also seen in both stress and SIRS and MODS, although this glucose intolerance is more marked in the latter, possibly because of a defect in the enzyme pyruvate dehydrogenase. An increase in Krebs cycle activity and aerobic glycolysis results in an increase in pyruvate and proportionate increase in lactate. If a microcirculatory perfusion deficit develops, increases in lactate exceed increases in pyruvate. These changes in glucose metabolism become progressively less responsive to modulation by insulin. Ultimately, futile cycling of alanine and lactate between the liver and the periphery occurs. Fat metabolism is markedly altered as well. In stress, a level of ketosis occurs that is disproportionately low for the degree of starvation; increased hepatic gluconeogenesis and hyper-insulinemia develop, along with increased lipolysis, decreased lipogenesis, and increased oxidation of long- and medium-chain triglycerides. In early SIRS or MODS, lipogenesis is decreased further; however, oxidation of long-chain triglycerides by the liver decreases in association with a decrease in expression of key beta-oxidative enzymes. Ultimately, this process results in fat intolerance as the liver continues to fail. Amino acids become an important fuel source. As oxidation of amino acids increases, urea production does too. Exogenous protein can be an important energy source, but ultimately, hepatic failure compromises ureagenesis and limits this energy source as well.

In SIRS or MODS, vasodilatation and peripheral edema become more pronounced. Cardiac output increases as afterload decreases, but ultimately the heart also fails as energy sources are depleted. Renal mechanisms are then

TABLE 69-2 Subclassifications of Sepsis

Sepsis: Systemic inflammatory response to infection
Severe sepsis: Sepsis associated with organ dysfunction, hypoperfusion, or hypotension (including lactic acidosis, oliguria, altered mental status)
Septic shock: Sepsis-induced hypotension despite adequate fluid resuscitation and presence of perfusion abnormalities. If pressors or inotropes are required to maintain normotension or normal perfusion, the patient is in septic shock.
Sepsis-induced hypotension: Systolic blood pressure <90 mmHg or a reduction of ≥40 mmHg from baseline in the absence of other causes of hypotension

SOURCE: Bone RC, Balk RA, Cerra FB, et al: Definitions for sepsis and organ failure and guidelines for the use of innovative therapies in sepsis. *Chest* 101:1644–1655, 1992.

called upon to conserve fluid, but also to excrete urea. The generalized edema limits the ability to concentrate the urine maximally. As insulin-mediated glucose uptake decreases, the ability of catecholamines to modulate vascular tone decreases and blood pressure becomes vasopressor-refractory.

Several hypotheses have been advanced to account for the aforementioned pathophysiology.

A variety of cytokines have been implicated in SIRS and MODS, including tumor necrosis factor alpha (TNF-α), interleukin-1 (IL-1), interleukin-6 (IL-6), and interferon gamma (INF-γ). TNF or IL-1, produced either by inflammatory cells that have migrated to the site of injury or by local endothelial cells, are released into the circulation and affect distant organs. In the liver, TNF stimulates Kupffer cells to produce more TNF and other cytokines (IL-1 and IL-6) which induce hepatocytes to express the genes for a number of acute-phase reactants. The low levels of TNF (and IL-1) released from the initial site of inflammation result in a self-limited process. According to the *cytokine hypothesis* of MODS, overproduction of TNF, IL-1, or IL-6 results in uncontrolled inflammation, characterized by prolonged, excessive vasodilatation and organ damage by activated macrophages and other inflammatory cells. Since many pathways are activated in SIRS, cytokines appear to be important, but not exclusive, mediators of certain aspects of SIRS and MODS.

Another hypothesis, the *microcirculatory hypothesis,* is based on the concept that failure of cells or organs to receive adequate levels of oxygen or some important nutrient or substrate triggers SIRS or MODS. Low flow contributes to cellular dysfunction, and release of vasoactive mediators and vascular congestion secondary to microthrombi and leukocytes are considered important. Reperfusion of ischemic tissue may be as important as decreased flow itself, and generation of oxygen free radicals and peroxidation of membrane lipids following reperfusion may contribute to tissue injury.

The release of endotoxin by gram-negative bacteria or other organisms has long been implicated in the genesis of SIRS. However, in many patients, the putative source of bacteria is never identified, raising the possibility that the inflammation arises from an endogenous source—bacteria in the gastrointestinal tract (or their associated endotoxins) that translocate to the mesenteric lymph nodes, the liver, and the circulation. The *gut hypothesis* holds that bacteria or endotoxins activate white cells and induce cytokine production and release of cytokines by hepatic macrophages (Kupffer cells).

Other hypotheses include the *two-hit hypothesis* (an initial period of hypotension "primes" the trauma patient for SIRS or MODS; i.e., the initial insult activates other processes that amplify the effects of the initial event, however mild), the *connectionist hypothesis* (the transition from SIRS to MODS arises when different organs lose the ability to communicate with one other), and the *transcription hypothesis* (the abnormalities in SIRS and MODS may be related to deficits in hepatic metabolism, with alterations due, in part, to decreases in the transcription of genes coding for key enzymes).

CLINICAL FEATURES AND EPIDEMIOLOGY

In one of the two general forms of SIRS and MODS, development of acute lung injury or ARDS (see Chap. 68) is the earliest manifestation, and the lungs are the predominant or only organ system affected until late in the course. Patients most often present with a primary pulmonary disorder (e.g., pneumonia, aspiration, lung contusion, pulmonary embolism, etc.) or with an illness associated with development of ARDS (e.g., burns, trauma, or surgery). Pulmonary dysfunction may persist for 2 to 3 weeks or longer, and the patient then shows evidence of recovery, chronicity of lung involvement, or progression to other organ dysfunction, most often hepatic, renal, or cardiovascular.

In the second form of SIRS and MODS, although the earliest manifestations remain pulmonary, patients most often have an extrapulmonary source for the syndrome. Examples include patients with major trauma (including isolated head injury), intraabdominal sepsis, extensive blood loss, pancreatitis, and vascular catastrophes such as ruptured or dissecting aneurysms. Acute lung injury and ARDS develop early, but dysfunction in other organs soon becomes evident. The liver is the second most commonly affected organ; gastrointestinal, cardiovascular, and renal systems are equally cited as the next most involved organ systems. Patients typically remain in a pattern of compensated dysfunction for several weeks and then either recover or succumb to their illness. The diversity of the population at risk makes early diagnosis of this form of SIRS or MODS difficult. Many of these patients have undergone a surgical procedure during which development of mild hypoxemia and an increase in lung water are not uncommon. Under the circumstances, incipient ARDS may go unrecognized.

Due to the diverse etiologies of SIRS and MODS, the incidence is difficult to determine. The incidence of the primary pulmonary form (i.e., ARDS) is estimated in excess of 150,000 cases per year. In the multiorgan form of SIRS or MODS, the incidence following trauma severe enough to warrant admission to an ICU appears to be about 14 percent.

Estimated mortality from ARDS alone is approximately 50 percent. Involvement of additional organ systems worsens the prognosis; organ dysfunction involving more than three systems is associated with virtually 100 percent mortality, although some studies have reported lower death rates, perhaps reflecting the lack of consensus on definitions of organ dysfunction. Mortality appears to be a function of the length of time that patients are in organ failure.

MANAGEMENT

Pulmonary dysfunction in SIRS or MODS most often takes the form of ARDS, the management of which is discussed in Chap. 68.

Inadequate tissue perfusion potentiates SIRS and may catalyze progression to MODS, particularly as reflected in renal insufficiency, as the kidneys are quite sensitive to hypoperfusion. While liberal fluid administration may be required in SIRS or MODS, assessment of effects of fluid administration is problematic, since end-organ dysfunction is already present. Blood pressure support may also be challenging, since catecholamine resistance characterizes SIRS and MODS. Hypotension requiring vasopressors can be treated with norepinephrine or phenylephrine. Norepinephrine has the theoretic advantage of preferential constriction of the somatic (muscle) beds over the splanchnic, thereby transferring fluid from the periphery into the central, visceral compartment. Dopamine, long a preferred agent, is no longer routinely advocated.

As SIRS progresses to MODS, the intrinsic metabolic defect associated with the disorder worsens. Glucose and fat intolerance develop, as does progressive azotemia. Most clinicians rely on a nutritional formula that is relatively hypocaloric and protein-rich. Although the blood urea level may rise with this formula, the increase in blood urea nitrogen is generally well tolerated in adequately hydrated patients. If the increase in blood urea nitrogen is a manifestation of uremia rather than an isolated consequence of protein overfeeding, dialysis may be necessary.

BIBLIOGRAPHY

Barie PS, Hydo LJ, Fischer E: A prospective comparison of two multiple organ dysfunction/failure scoring systems for prediction of mortality on critical surgical illness. *J Trauma* 37:660–666, 1994.

Beal AL, Cerra FB: Multiple organ failure syndrome in the 1990s: Systemic inflammatory response and organ dysfunction. *JAMA* 271:226–233, 1994.

Bone RC, Balk RA, Cerra FB, et al: Definitions for sepsis and organ failure and guidelines for the use of innovative therapies in sepsis. *Chest* 101:1644–1655, 1992.

Deitch EA: Multiple organ failure: Pathophysiology and potential future therapy. *Ann Surg* 216:117–134, 1992.

Marshall JC, Cook DJ, Christou NV, et al: The multiple organ dysfunction score: A reliable descriptor of complex clinical outcome. *Crit Care Med* 23:1638–1652, 1995.

70 | Acute Respiratory Failure in the Surgical Patient*

Michael A. Grippi

INTRODUCTION

Advances in surgery, anesthesia, and perioperative care have enhanced the opportunity for surgical intervention in patients with significant comorbid conditions. These higher-risk patients may experience a variety of pulmonary complications, which account for approximately one-quarter of postoperative deaths and contribute substantially to health care costs.

ANESTHESIA-RELATED RESPIRATORY EFFECTS

Although anesthesia-related pulmonary effects in the operating room are generally minor, persistent postoperative effects may delay extubation or precipitate respiratory failure.

Inhaled or intravenously administered anesthetics decrease respiratory muscle tone and produce a decrease in lung volume (20 percent decline in FRC). The resulting atelectasis occurs during both spontaneous breathing and mechanical ventilation; it disappears with application of positive end-expiratory pressure (PEEP). Atelectasis alters ventilation/perfusion relationships, increases shunt fraction, and widens the alveolar-arterial oxygen gradient. Shunt may be further accentuated by impairment of hypoxic pulmonary vasoconstriction induced by certain inhalational anesthetics. Increased age, obesity, and chronic obstructive pulmonary disease (COPD) predispose to general anesthesia–related hypoxemia. Inhalational anesthetics also blunt the response to hypoxemia and hypercapnia. The hypoxemic drive is markedly attenuated, even at very low, subanesthetic concentrations. Fat and muscle drug depots depress hypoxic drive for several hours after termination of anesthesia.

Spinal anesthesia preserves diaphragmatic function and does not affect hypoxic pulmonary vasoconstriction or impair the ventilatory response to CO_2. However, a clinically significant benefit over general anesthesia has not been demonstrated consistently. Regional anesthesia should not be viewed as clearly superior to general anesthesia in the high-risk patient.

Postoperative pain can cause splinting, retention of secretions, atelectasis, and hypoxemia. Hence, use of parenteral or epidural opiates has become standard practice. However, severe respiratory depression may occur with epidural narcotics; risk factors include advanced age, concomitant administration of systemic opiates or other central nervous system depressants, and extensive surgery. Hydrophilic narcotics (e.g., morphine) have a greater tendency than lipophilic compounds (e.g., fentanyl) to remain in the cerebrospinal fluid and

*Edited from Chap. 170, "Acute Respiratory Failure in the Surgical Patient," by Kotloff RM. In: *Fishman's Pulmonary Diseases and Disorders,* 3d ed., edited by Fishman AP, Elias JA, Fishman JA, Grippi MA, Kaiser LR, Senior RM. New York, McGraw-Hill, 1998, pp 2589–2604. For fuller discussion of topics dealt with in this chapter, the reader is referred to the original text, as noted above.

to spread cephalad to the respiratory center located in the floor of the fourth ventricle. Respiratory depression complicating epidural narcotic administration almost invariably occurs within the first 24 h. Treatment consists of administration of naloxone and ventilatory support using a face mask and ambu bag. Intubation is necessary if the situation cannot be reversed pharmacologically.

EFFECTS OF SURGERY ON PULMONARY FUNCTION

Following lower abdominal procedures, vital capacity (VC) falls by 25 percent and returns to normal by the third postoperative day. In contradistinction, VC declines by 50 percent within 24 h of upper abdominal surgery; a marked reduction persists for as long as 7 days. Upper abdominal and thoracic procedures are associated with a fall in lung volumes and development of atelectasis and hypoxemia. Transdiaphragmatic pressures are reduced, possibly due to a reduction in diaphragmatic contractility caused by inflammation, surgical trauma, or pain or perhaps due to diminished phrenic nerve output.

With coronary artery bypass grafting (CABG), lung volumes decrease by approximately 30 percent; return to baseline may take several months. Lung function may decline to a greater degree when internal mammary harvesting and grafting are employed. Hypoxemia and significant widening of the alveolar-arterial oxygen gradient are usually seen following cardiac surgery. Shunt fraction may increase severalfold on the basis of atelectasis, which is seen consistently postoperatively, especially on the left. The atelectasis may be due to alterations in chest wall compliance resulting from division of the sternum and surgical trauma to the ribs and costovertebral joints. Intraoperative lung retraction may directly injure the left lower lobe; alternatively, left-lower-lobe atelectasis may arise from intraoperative injury to the left phrenic nerve, which courses along the lateral surface of the pericardium. The basis of the phrenic nerve dysfunction may be thermal injury induced by cardioplegic techniques or stretch and ischemic injury to the nerve as a result of sternal retraction, dissection of the internal mammary artery, or prolonged distention of the pericardium. Electrophysiologic studies of phrenic nerve function following cardiac surgery suggest that nerve injury is an uncommon cause of postoperative pulmonary dysfunction.

An additional potential cause of pulmonary dysfunction with cardiac surgery is use of cardiopulmonary bypass, which may lead to abnormal surfactant production, as well as induce a capillary leak syndrome. Presumably, exposure of blood to nonendothelial surfaces results in complement activation, triggering of inflammatory cascades, and neutrophil sequestration in the microvasculature ("postperfusion lung" or "pump lung").

Atelectasis and impaired oxygenation are common after lung surgery. The magnitude of pulmonary function loss due to resectional lung surgery can be estimated from preoperative spirometry and quantitative lung scanning. Chest wall trauma contributes to the decline in function. Respiratory system compliance may fall by as much as 75 percent; work of breathing increases, and lung volumes decline dramatically, out of proportion to the surgical loss of functional lung. Following standard thoracotomy and lung resection, FEV_1 and FVC fall to 30 percent of preoperative values by 24 h. Limited, muscle-sparing incisions have less of a negative impact on pulmonary function.

RISK OF POSTOPERATIVE PULMONARY COMPLICATIONS

The overall incidence of postoperative pulmonary complications is approximately 5 percent. Several well-defined risk factors have been identified (Table 70-1) and relate to the type of operative procedure and the presence of underlying lung disease.

Upper abdominal and thoracic procedures carry the highest risk of postoperative pulmonary complications (Table 70-2), probably because of alterations in pulmonary mechanics accompanying these procedures (see above). Thoracoabdominal aneurysm repair is associated with the highest risk; other high-risk procedures include abdominal aortic aneurysm repair, upper gastrointestinal surgery, thoracotomy, and open heart surgery. The risk with lower abdominal procedures is smaller, and the risk with procedures involving the extremities is negligible. Use of a transverse abdominal incision appears to carry less risk than a vertical midline incision. Laparoscopic cholecystectomy may have a lower rate of pulmonary complications than the conventional open approach. Median sternotomy or muscle-sparing lateral thoracotomy are better tolerated than the standard posterolateral thoracotomy. Whether video-assisted thoracoscopic surgery (VATS) carries a diminished risk of postoperative pulmonary complications remains unanswered.

Postoperative respiratory failure occurs in 5 percent of patients with COPD and develops principally after upper abdominal and thoracic procedures. A

TABLE 70-1 Risk Factors for Postoperative Pulmonary Complications

Factors related to the patient
  Chronic obstructive pulmonary disease
  Advanced age
  Extensive (and recent) smoking history
  Obesity
  High physical status category per American Society of Anesthesiologists (ASA)
Factors related to the surgery
  Thoracic and upper abdominal procedures
  Emergency surgery
  Prolonged anesthesia time (>3 h)
  Large intraoperative blood transfusion requirements

TABLE 70-2 Incidence of Respiratory Failure following Surgery

Procedure	Incidence of postoperative respiratory failure
TAAA repair	8–33%
AAA repair	5–24%
Lung resection	4–15%
CABG	5–8%
All types[a]	0.8%

KEY: TAAA, thoracoabdominal aortic aneurysm; AAA, abdominal aortic aneurysm; CABG, coronary artery bypass grafting.
[a]Refers to general survey of gastrointestinal, urologic, gynecologic, and orthopedic procedures.

preoperative $FEF_{25-75\%}$ <50 percent predicted, in conjunction with an FVC <75 percent predicted, defines a high-risk group. For patients with severe COPD undergoing lung resection, the risk of postoperative respiratory failure or death is 50 percent when the predicted postresection FEV_1 is <40 percent predicted (versus 4 percent when the predicted postresection FEV_1 is >40 percent predicted). Patients with good performance status appear to do better. Patients with a predicted postresection FEV_1 <30 percent predicted who have a peak oxygen consumption equal to or greater than 15 mL/kg/min during exercise testing are more likely to have an uncomplicated course.

Patients with moderate to severe lung disease undergoing coronary artery bypass grafting (CABG) appear to have a greater incidence of pulmonary complications and longer length of stay in the intensive care unit. Following major abdominal vascular surgery, including abdominal aortic aneurysm repair and aortobifemoral bypass grafting, approximately one-quarter of patients require ventilatory support for more than 24 h. An extensive smoking history and low preoperative Pa_{O_2} appear to be predictive, but the severity of COPD is not; no prospective evaluation of patients undergoing abdominal surgery has shown that pulmonary function studies can reliably identify high-risk patients.

Severe COPD is not an absolute contraindication to abdominal or nonresectional thoracic surgery. The patient's lung disease should be carefully assessed and the surgery carefully planned when it is deemed likely to extend the patient's survival or to markedly improve quality of life. Prior to surgery, patients with COPD should be advised regarding smoking cessation. Smoking is an independent risk factor for general postoperative pulmonary complications and prolonged ventilatory support. A minimum of 8 weeks of abstinence is required to achieve risk reduction in postoperative pulmonary complications. The institution or intensification of inhaled bronchodilators and use of oral antibiotics for purulent secretions or productive cough should be considered. Incentive spirometry or cough and deep breathing techniques should be taught prior to surgery. A short course of oral corticosteroids may be useful for significant bronchospasm.

ETIOLOGIES OF POSTOPERATIVE RESPIRATORY FAILURE

The many causes of acute respiratory failure in the surgical patient are not mutually exclusive. A systematic search for the precipitating factor(s) is always warranted. The most common etiologies are discussed below.

Atelectasis

Atelectasis, usually segmental and seen at the bases radiographically as obscuration of the diaphragms, is the most common postoperative pulmonary complication. Less common is atelectasis due to plugging of central airways by retained secretions. Postoperative atelectasis can lead to severe hypoxemia, which may be potentiated by impaired hypoxic pulmonary vasoconstriction induced by vasodilatory drugs used commonly in surgical patients. The clinicoradiographic picture resembles pneumonia; fever and elevated white blood cell count suggest pneumonia but are not specific. Proximal airway plugging with atelectasis may induce rapid development of hypoxemia and respiratory distress.

Treatment includes supplemental oxygen delivered via nasal prongs or face mask; however, severe respiratory distress, hypoxemia, hypercapnia, or inability of the patient to clear airway secretions necessitates intubation and mechanical ventilation. When the patient's clinical status permits, delivery of continuous positive airway pressure (CPAP) via a nasal or face mask may be effective. Fiberoptic bronchoscopy is equivalent to standard chest physiotherapy in treatment of acute lobar atelectasis; each is very effective in the absence of an air bronchogram (which indicates proximal airway obstruction as the cause of the atelectasis). Fiberoptic bronchoscopy should be reserved for those situations where chest physiotherapy is contraindicated (e.g., chest trauma, immobilized patient), poorly tolerated, or unsuccessful. Other potentially beneficial measures include mucolytics, nasotracheal suctioning, cautious use of analgesia and sedation, and, when possible, discontinuation of vasoactive drugs. Prophylactic maneuvers (e.g., cough, deep breathing exercises, and incentive spirometry) should be initiated in high-risk patients prior to surgery and used frequently in the postoperative period. Early ambulation of the postoperative patient is an important measure.

Pneumonia

Nosocomial pneumonia is associated with a mortality rate of 20 to 50 percent. The incidence is about 15 to 20 percent following thoracic and upper abdominal surgery, 5 percent following lower abdominal surgery, and less than 5 percent following nonthoracoabdominal procedures. Risk factors include low serum albumin, COPD, heavy smoking history, advanced age, protracted preoperative hospital stay, high status according to the American Society of Anesthesiologists (ASA) preanesthesia classification, prolonged surgery, presence of a nasogastric tube, use of antacids or H_2 blockers, immunosuppression, impaired consciousness, witnessed aspiration, and the need for prolonged mechanical ventilation.

Microaspiration of oropharyngeal secretions, frequently colonized with gram-negative aerobic bacilli in critically ill or postoperative patients, appears to be the predominant mechanism for nosocomial pneumonia. An endotracheal tube impairs swallowing, allows pooling of secretions above the inflated cuff and passage of secretions beyond the cuff into the lower airways. Postextubation swallowing dysfunction, gastroesophageal reflux, and anesthesia-induced depressed consciousness potentiate the risk. Use of H_2 blockers and antacids promotes gastric colonization with gram-negative enteric organisms.

Diagnosis is based on the nonspecific findings of fever, leukocytosis, purulent sputum, and radiographic infiltrates. Because cultures of sputum and tracheal aspirates do not accurately reflect distal airway flora, bronchoscopy using a sterile brush technique or bronchoalveolar lavage has sometimes been employed as an adjunctive diagnostic measure. Treatment is broad and empirically directed at *Staphylococcus aureus* and gram-negative organisms, including *Pseudomonas* (aerobic bacilli of the Enterobacteriaceae family account for approximately one-third of all nosocomial pneumonias). Often the pneumonia is polymicrobial. Prophylactic strategies include abstinence from cigarette smoking for a minimum of 8 weeks prior to elective surgery, expeditious removal of nasogastric and endotracheal tubes postoperatively, careful titration of postoperative analgesia, and, in the intubated patient, maintenance of a semierect position. Selective digestive decontamination (SDD) using topical antibiotics applied to the oropharynx and stomach has not been clearly demonstrated to be of benefit.

Aspiration of Gastric Contents

Mendelson's syndrome, the aspiration of gastric contents first described in pregnant women undergoing anesthesia, occurs when upper airway protective mechanisms and cough are compromised. In the perioperative period, risk is significant from the time of general anesthesia induction to full return of consciousness postoperatively. Impaired consciousness, gastric distention during induction, and vomiting induced by noxious stimulation of the posterior oropharynx during intubation or extubation add to the risk, as do drug-induced relaxation of the lower esophageal sphincter, placement of the patient in a supine position, and surgical manipulation of the bowel. While the risk of aspiration diminishes beyond the immediate perioperative period, it remains a concern in the patient receiving narcotic analgesia. The incidence of general anesthesia–associated aspiration during the immediate perioperative period is about 0.03 percent; the incidence is nearly fourfold higher in the setting of emergency surgery. Predisposing factors include gastrointestinal obstruction, swallowing dysfunction, altered sensorium, previous esophageal surgery, and a recent meal. The majority of events occur during laryngoscopy (prior to insertion of the endotracheal tube) and tracheal extubation.

Aspirated acidic fluid produces a chemical pneumonitis within minutes. The magnitude of injury is directly related to the pH and volume of aspirated material. In experimental animals, a pH of less than 2.5 and a volume in excess of 0.4 mL/kg have been defined as critical threshold values. The presence of food particles contributes to lung injury by inducing an inflammatory reaction within the airways. Large food particles may also cause airway obstruction and atelectasis. The chemical pneumonitis enhances the risk of subsequent bacterial superinfection.

Diagnosis is based on witnessed vomiting and recovery of gastric contents from the airways or a compatible clinicoradiographic picture. Findings include fever, tachypnea, and diffuse crackles developing within several hours of the event. Wheezing may be due either to obstruction of airways by particulate matter or reflex bronchospasm. Hypoxemia is usually severe. Initial radiographic patterns include extensive bilateral consolidation resembling diffuse pulmonary edema, widespread but discrete patchy infiltrates, and focal consolidation usually localized to one or both lung bases. Uncommonly, a fulminant course with shock and death within several days is seen. Most patients recover fully, although some develop ARDS or nosocomial pneumonia. The overall mortality rate in massive aspiration is approximately 30 percent; it exceeds 50 percent in those patients with initial shock or apnea, secondary pneumonia, or ARDS.

Treatment is supportive and includes mechanical ventilation and use of PEEP if necessary. Bronchoscopy is indicated only when large airway obstruction by particulate matter is suspected. Bronchoalveolar lavage is not helpful, and administration of systemic corticosteroids has proved ineffective. Prophylactic antibiotics are not advised. However, up to 40 percent of patients will develop a superimposed bacterial pneumonia within several days, as reflected in a recurrent fever, new or progressive radiographic infiltrates, or purulent sputum. Antibiotic treatment directed toward gram-positive and gram-negative aerobes and anaerobic mouth flora is warranted at that time.

Prevention of aspiration is important. Standard practice includes overnight fasting prior to elective surgery. However, despite prolonged fasting, up to one-third of patients maintain a gastric volume in excess of 0.4 mL/kg (approximately 25 to 30 mL in the average adult), and up to three-quarters have a gastric pH below 2.5—meeting critical thresholds for the potential of inducing severe lung injury. Since administration of H_2 blockers can effectively raise the pH and reduce the volume of gastric contents, some clinicians now advocate their use during the 12 h preceding surgery, often in combination with a prokinetic agent; the cost-effectiveness of this approach is questionable. In the high-risk patient undergoing emergency surgery, rapid sequence induction of anesthesia should be employed to shorten the time between loss of consciousness and tracheal intubation. During induction, manual pressure can be applied to the cricoid cartilage (Sellick maneuver) and maintained until the endotracheal tube is in proper position and the cuff inflated. Postoperatively, extubation should be performed when consciousness and the gag reflex have returned to a level sufficient to permit airway protection.

Acute Lung Injury and Acute Respiratory Distress Syndrome

The hallmark of acute lung injury is the presence of noncardiogenic pulmonary edema or acute respiratory distress syndrome (ARDS) (see Chap. 68). Management is supportive. Several risks for acute lung injury are particularly notable in surgical patients.

Fulminant noncardiogenic pulmonary edema may rarely complicate use of cardiopulmonary bypass. Risk is greatest when bypass duration exceeds 150 min. Proposed mechanisms include neutrophil accumulation within the damaged pulmonary capillary bed and release of proteolytic enzymes and other toxic mediators. Exposure of blood to nonendothelialized surfaces may also cause complement activation, contributing to neutrophil sequestration and activation within the lung. In some instances, acute lung injury may actually represent an idiosyncratic reaction to protamine, used to reverse the effects of heparin at the end of the pump "run." The syndrome evolves gradually over 3 to 4 days. Pulmonary involvement may occur in isolation or may be accompanied by fever, leukocytosis, renal insufficiency, bleeding diathesis, or transient neurologic impairment. This form of acute lung injury appears to carry a more favorable prognosis than that typically associated with ARDS.

Pulmonary edema, probably on a noncardiogenic (i.e., permeability) basis, may develop rapidly in the remaining lung following pneumonectomy. The incidence is approximately 2.6 percent.

ARDS also has been described following cardiac and noncardiac surgery in patients treated with the antiarrhythmic agent amiodarone. Amiodarone-induced pulmonary toxicity usually presents as a subacute illness characterized by cough, dyspnea, fever, and patchy pulmonary infiltrates. In most reported cases, amiodarone was administered preoperatively for varying periods of time. Most patients had no evidence prior to surgery of the more indolent form of amiodarone pulmonary toxicity. However, ARDS has been described in patients whose only exposure to amiodarone occurred postoperatively.

Mild, self-limited pulmonary edema is common in fresh lung allografts. However, in approximately 15 percent of cases, the allograft is severely injured, with widespread, persistent alveolar edema and profound hypoxemia.

This *primary graft failure* is nonimmunologic in nature and thought to represent an extreme form of ischemia-reperfusion injury. Primary graft failure occurs despite acceptable ischemic times below 6 h. Injury is confined to the allograft. Ventilator management is complicated, particularly in the presence of underlying COPD. Positive-pressure breaths and PEEP are preferentially applied to the highly compliant emphysematous lung, leading to progressive hyperinflation, mediastinal shift, and impaired gas exchange and hemodynamics. Use of a double-lumen endotracheal tube and independent lung ventilation, with selective application of PEEP to the edematous allograft, are employed.

Pulmonary thromboendarterectomy for treatment of chronic thromboembolic pulmonary hypertension may be complicated by reperfusion pulmonary edema in one-third of cases. Reperfusion edema may occur intraoperatively or evolve over the first several postoperative days. The chest radiograph shows edema limited to lung zones supplied by formerly obstructed vessels. Blood is redistributed from previously perfused segments to newly endarterectomized vessels supplying edematous areas of lung, exacerbating shunt physiology (*pulmonary artery steal*).

Finally, massive blood transfusion (>15 U/24 h) has been associated with ARDS, but a causal relationship has not been proved. Induction of acute lung injury by the passive transfer in transfused blood products of donor antibodies directed against recipient leukocytes has been described—so-called *transfusion-related acute lung injury* (TRALI) or the *leukoagglutinins reaction*. The incidence is 0.02 percent per unit and 0.16 percent per patient transfused. Respiratory distress, hypoxemia, and diffuse pulmonary infiltrates occur within 2 to 4 h of transfusion. Fever, chills, and hypotension may be present; urticaria is observed in a minority. The reaction tends to be self-limited and is typically characterized by rapid clearing of infiltrates and improved oxygenation within several days. However, a more protracted course of more than 1 week has been reported. When TRALI is suspected, the blood bank should be notified and all units transfused should be assayed for the presence of leukoagglutinating antibodies.

Phrenic Nerve Injury and Diaphragmatic Paralysis

Phrenic nerve injury complicating cardiac surgery arises chiefly from use of cold cardioplegic solution. Unilateral injury, usually on the left, occurs in approximately 10 percent of patients having CABG. The injury is usually inconsequential, except in the marginal patient with significant underlying pulmonary disease. Bilateral injury, which is rare (estimated incidence of 1 to 3 percent), results in marked impairment in pulmonary function and may cause respiratory failure.

Phrenic nerve injury is also seen in cardiac valve replacement, pulmonary thromboendarterectomy, and lung transplantation. In lung transplantation, the hemithorax is typically packed with ice to preserve the allograft during reimplantation, possibly accounting for reversible phrenic nerve dysfunction. Diaphragmatic paralysis is permanent when secondary to actual transection of the nerve.

Bilateral phrenic nerve injury should be suspected when weaning attempts result in progressive hypercapnia or atelectasis. Orthopnea (in the spontaneously breathing patient) arises due to further impairment in diaphragmatic function secondary to loss of gravitational assistance in diaphragm descent. Inspiratory thoracoabdominal paradox (inward movement of the abdominal wall with concurrent expansion of the thorax) is frequently observed and is best evoked in the supine position. The chest radiograph shows nonspecific findings of small lung volumes and bibasilar atelectasis. The vital capacity falls by greater than 25 percent with assumption of the supine position. Transdiaphragmatic pressure (not routinely available as a bedside diagnostic test) approximates zero.

With unilateral diaphragm paralysis, fluoroscopy reveals paradoxical upward movement of the affected hemidiaphragm with a maximal inspiratory effort ("sniff"). With bilateral dysfunction, patients often assume an altered breathing pattern marked by active contraction of the abdominal muscles during expiration, forcing the flaccid hemidiaphragms upward. With subsequent inspiration, the abdominal muscles relax and the hemidiaphragms descend briefly, potentially creating the false impression that they are functional. Because of this, fluoroscopy is confirmatory in only a minority of these patients.

The "gold standard" for confirmation of phrenic nerve injury is electrophysiologic testing using transcutaneous phrenic nerve stimulation in the neck and surface recording of the diaphragmatic electromyogram (EMG). A prolonged latency between nerve stimulation and diaphragmatic action potential, consistent with a demyelinating injury, confirms the diagnosis. Diminished amplitude of the diaphragmatic EMG in the face of normal latency may represent either an axonal degenerative neuropathy or failure to precisely localize the diaphragm for electrode placement.

Management of patients with respiratory failure due to phrenic nerve dysfunction is supportive. Recovery occasionally requires 6 to 12 months.

Pulmonary Embolism

Risk of pulmonary embolism (PE) is increased in a variety of surgical procedures. Obesity, immobility, and underlying malignancy potentiate the risk. The clinical findings of dyspnea, tachypnea, and tachycardia are nonspecific, particularly in postoperative patients. Evidence of acute cor pulmonale or electrocardiographic findings of an "S1Q3T3" pattern or new right bundle-branch block may provide helpful diagnostic information. The chest radiograph is most suggestive of pulmonary embolism when it is normal in the face of severe hypoxemia. When it is abnormal, its greatest utility is in identifying other causes of hypoxemia such as pneumonia, pneumothorax, or ARDS. Diagnostic and management considerations in pulmonary embolism are discussed in Chap. 40.

Obstructive Sleep Apnea

Obstructive sleep apnea (OSA) is present in 2 to 4 percent of the adult population. The use of volatile anesthetics, opioids, and sedatives diminishes the activity of the upper airway musculature and increases the frequency and duration of obstructive apneas, making the perioperative period a dangerous time for patients with OSA. Use of nasal CPAP immediately after extubation facilitates safe administration of anesthetic, analgesic, and sedative agents, without undue risk of precipitating life-threatening airway obstruction. A high index of suspicion for OSA in the perioperative period is necessary to prompt appropriate intervention when upper airway obstruction is observed.

BIBLIOGRAPHY

Bolliger CT, Jordan P, Soler M, et al: Exercise capacity as a predictor of postoperative complications in lung resection candidates. *Am J Respir Crit Care Med* 151:1472–1480, 1995.

Cohen A, Katz M, Katz R, et al: Chronic obstructive pulmonary disease in patients undergoing coronary artery bypass grafting. *J Thorac Cardiovasc Surg* 109:574–581, 1995.

Cunnion KM, Weber DJ, Broadhead WE, et al: Risk factors for nosocomial pneumonia: Comparing adult critical care populations. *Am J Respir Crit Care Med* 153:158–162, 1996.

Dureuil B, Cantineau JP, Desmonts JM: Effects of upper or lower abdominal surgery on diaphragmatic function. *Br J Anaesth* 59:1230–1235, 1987.

Hudson LD, Milberg JA, Anardi D, Maunder RJ: Clinical risks for development of the acute respiratory distress syndrome. *Am J Respir Crit Care Med* 151:293–301, 1995.

Jayr C, Matthay MA, Goldstone J, et al: Preoperative and intraoperative factors associated with prolonged mechanical ventilation: A study in patients following major abdominal vascular surgery. *Chest* 103:1231–1236, 1993.

Kroenke K, Lawrence VA, Theroux JF, Tuley MR: Operative risk in patients with severe obstructive pulmonary disease. *Arch Intern Med* 152:967–971, 1992.

Morice RC, Peters EJ, Ryan MB, et al: Exercise testing in the evaluation of patients at high risk for complications from lung resection. *Chest* 101:356–361, 1992.

Polk HC, Mizuguchi NN: Multifactorial analysis in the diagnosis of pneumonia arising in the surgical intensive care unit. *Am J Surg* 179(2A suppl):31S–35S, 2000.

Sykes LA, Bowe EA: Cardiorespiratory effects of anesthesia. *Clin Chest Med* 14:211–226, 1993.

71 | Respiratory Distress Syndrome of the Newborn*

Michael A. Grippi

INTRODUCTION

Respiratory distress syndrome (RDS) is caused primarily by insufficiency of pulmonary surfactant in the immature lung at birth and is the most common pulmonary disease of newborns. RDS is the most common cause of morbidity and death in the first month of life. The worldwide incidence is about 1 percent. RDS is related to prematurity, rarely occuring after 38 weeks gestation; the incidence is 60 percent at gestational age less than 29 weeks. The disorder is more common in males and in Caucasians. A familial pattern exists. At any given gestation, the incidence of RDS is higher for abdominal delivery without labor than for vaginal delivery with labor. Risk is increased if elective cesarean section is performed prior to 39 weeks of gestation. The incidence is significantly higher in infants of diabetic mothers, especially if the infant is large for gestational age.

PATHOLOGY AND PATHOPHYSIOLOGY

At birth, normal newborns have five to seven times more surfactant than adults. In RDS, an inability to package and transport surfactant to the alveolar surface results in insufficient quantities of the material in the terminal airspaces. Each of the surfactant proteins (SP-A, SP-B, SP-C, SP-D) plays an important role in the functioning of surfactant. SP-B deficiency is lethal. SP-A deficiency leads to susceptibility to infection. Diffuse atelectasis, decreased lung compliance, respiratory bronchiole injury, and surfactant inactivation by plasma proteins are seen. Lamellar bodies are decreased, as is tubular myelin in the air spaces. Autopsy findings include diffuse atelectasis and pulmonary edema. The respiratory bronchioles are dilated and lined with hyaline membranes consisting of plasma proteins and epithelial debris.

Physiologic assessment reveals reduced functional residual capacity and static lung compliance and increased airway resistance. The alveolar-arterial oxygen gradient is increased, as is right-to-left shunt. Right-to-left shunts occur at the ductus arteriosus and the foramen ovale and within the lung's interstitial compartment. Alveolar ventilation is decreased (despite an increased minute ventilation) and significant hypercarbia is seen.

DIAGNOSIS AND CLINICAL MANIFESTATIONS

Within a few minutes of birth, infants with RDS demonstrate labored breathing, with tachypnea, nasal flaring, expiratory grunting, intercostal and subcostal retractions, and cyanosis. In the preterm infant, the differential diagnosis

*Edited from Chap. 169, "Respiratory Distress Syndrome in Premature Newborn Infants," by Long WA, Corbet A. In: *Fishman's Pulmonary Diseases and Disorders,* 3d ed., edited by Fishman AP, Elias JA, Fishman JA, Grippi MA, Kaiser LR, Senior RM. New York, McGraw-Hill, 1998, pp 2575–2587. For fuller discussion of topics dealt with in this chapter, the reader is referred to the original text, as noted above.

includes transient tachypnea of the newborn (delayed clearance of lung water), pneumonia, and sepsis. Additional diagnostic considerations in the near-term infant include meconium aspiration pneumonia, persistent pulmonary hypertension of the newborn, postasphyxial pulmonary edema, and, rarely, congenital alveolar proteinosis (SP-B deficiency).

The chest radiograph shows diffuse reticular-granular densities and decreased lung volume, consistent with widespread microatelectasis. Arterial blood gases reveal hypoxemia, hypercarbia, and mild lactic acidosis. Generalized edema, reduced urine output, poor peripheral perfusion, and systemic hypotension are often seen.

Typically, an inspired fraction of oxygen (F_{IO_2}) of 0.4 or greater is required during the first 24 h. Many infants require mechanical ventilation. Usually, the disease peaks by age 72 h, after which spontaneous diuresis and improved oxygenation occur. In favorable cases, the need for supplemental oxygen may resolve within a week. In complicated cases, prolonged mechanical ventilation and oxygen therapy are necessary. Episodes of recurrent apnea, systemic bacterial infection, patent ductus arteriosus (PDA), cerebral intraventricular hemorrhage, or bronchopulmonary dysplasia may further complicate the course.

Bronchopulmonary dysplasia (BPD), an inflammatory response to the barotrauma or volutrauma of mechanical ventilation and high concentrations of oxygen used in treating RDS, may occur in very immature infants requiring prolonged mechanical ventilation. Significant BPD occurs when supplemental oxygen is required when the infants are at 36 weeks postmenstrual age (term is 40 weeks). The incidence of BPD increases with decreasing gestational age. BPD is a major clinical problem, contributing substantially to infant morbidity and mortality and to health care costs.

PREVENTION

Prevention of RDS is based on prevention of premature labor and delivery. Prenatal use of corticosteroids in women presenting in preterm labor and prophylactic administration of exogenous surfactant have decreased mortality and morbidity from RDS significantly in the past decade.

Since fetal lung liquid enters the amniotic cavity through the fetus's nasopharynx, prenatal assessment of surfactant is possible using several techniques based on amniocentesis. Gestational age is most important in evaluating risk.

In premature labor, corticosteroid treatment reduces the incidence of RDS and neonatal death by 50 percent and greatly reduces the incidence of cerebral intraventricular hemorrhage. The effects of prenatal corticosteroids and postnatal exogenous surfactant (see below) are additive; use of both agents improves survival of premature infants.

TREATMENT

Death due to RDS is now uncommon in infants weighing more than 750 g. Selected aspects of management are discussed briefly below.

General Measures

Prompt resuscitation of asphyxiated newborns is important. Lung expansion at birth stimulates surfactant secretion. Early intubation, mechanical ventilation, administration of exogenous surfactant, and use of positive end-expiratory pressure (PEEP) are employed in infants under 1000 g birth weight and in larger premature infants who make poor respiratory efforts at birth. Lung expansion also may be achieved by early application of nasal continuous positive airway pressure (CPAP).

Since pulmonary edema characterizes RDS, it is usual to restrict fluid intake to 50 to 70 mL/kg per day.

Group B streptococcal infection can mimic or coexist with RDS. As a result, it is prudent to obtain blood cultures and begin appropriate antibiotics in all infants with apparent RDS.

A patent ductus arteriosus (PDA) is common in RDS. Initial right-to-left shunting through the PDA is replaced by left-to-right shunting by the end of the first day of life. With reduction in pulmonary vascular resistance by 3 or 4 days of age, the PDA may predispose the infant to the development of BPD. Treatment with indomethacin is warranted; indomethacin failure should prompt surgical ligation.

Mechanical Ventilation

Infants with RDS needing an F_{IO_2} of at least 0.4 are intubated and treated with mechanical ventilation and exogenous surfactant. PEEP levels between 4 and 8 cmH$_2$O are typically employed. Ventilator respiratory rates of 60 per minute appear to produce less lung injury than rates of 30 per minute. The faster respiratory rate permits use of smaller tidal volumes, reducing the risk of overdistention in the distal airways. The tidal volume should be maintained at 4 to 6 mL/kg birth weight, requiring a peak inflation pressure (PIP) of 15 to 30 cmH$_2$O. The arterial P_{O_2} should be maintained between 50 and 70 mmHg by adjusting F_{IO_2} or by adjusting mean airway pressure through increases in PEEP or PIP. Permissive hypercapnia (arterial P_{CO_2} of 45 to 55 mmHg) is frequently employed. If an infant with RDS develops pulmonary interstitial emphysema during conventional mechanical ventilation, institution of high-frequency ventilation (HFV)—including high-frequency flow-interrupter ventilation (HFIV) or high-frequency oscillator ventilation (HFOV)—may be employed. HFOV also may be tried if conventional ventilation for RDS fails and the infant deteriorates with severe hypoxemia.

Surfactant Replacement Therapy

Prophylactic exogenous surfactant is administered within 15 to 30 min of birth in infants under 750 g birth weight. In larger infants, treatment is initiated in those with evidence of RDS. Use of a mammalian surfactant is currently preferred. The agent is instilled directly into the endotracheal tube using bag-tube ventilation; in general, two to three doses are instilled at 8- to 12-h intervals until the F_{IO_2} requirement is less than 0.3.

Surfactant instillation may transiently reduce blood pressure and cerebral blood flow; transient hypercarbia and an increase in cerebral blood flow may follow. The incidence of hemorrhagic pulmonary edema appears to be increased after exogenous surfactant, while that of symptomatic PDA is not.

The beneficial effect of exogenous surfactant in premature infants in reducing the severity of RDS and neonatal mortality (by approximately 50 percent) is maintained through 1 year of age. In the smallest infants (500 to 699 g birth weight), evidence that surfactant is effective in reducing mortality is not convincing. In infants with birth weights over 1500 g, surfactant therapy is associated with significant reductions in the incidence of BPD and hospital costs. A poor response to surfactant is associated with high risk for development of BPD.

ACKNOWLEDGMENT

The author gratefully acknowledges the expert review of Dr. Roberta Ballard in preparation of the manuscript.

BIBLIOGRAPHY

Dekowski SA, Holtzman RB: Surfactant replacement therapy: An update on applications. *Pediatr Clin North Am* 45:549–572, 1998.

Fujiwara T, Maeta H, Chida S, et al: Artificial surfactant therapy in hyaline membrane disease. *Lancet* 1:55–59, 1980.

McGettigan MC, Adolph VR, Ginsberg HG, Goldsmith JP: New ways to ventilate newborns in acute respiratory failure. *Pediatr Clin North Am* 45:475–509, 1998.

NIH Consensus Development Conference Statement: Effect of corticosteroids for fetal maturation on perinatal outcomes. *Am J Obstet Gynecol* 173:246–252, 1995.

Rodriguez RJ, Martin RJ: Exogenous surfactant therapy in newborns. *Respir Care Clin North Am* 5:595–616, 1999.

MANAGEMENT AND THERAPEUTIC INTERVENTIONS

72 | Oxygen Therapy and Pulmonary Oxygen Toxicity*

Lisa M. Bellini

INTRODUCTION

Supplemental oxygen is frequently prescribed. Established guidelines and clinical criteria delineate its proper use.

OXYGEN DELIVERY AND TISSUE UTILIZATION

At rest, the average adult male consumes about 225 to 250 mL of oxygen per minute, a rate which may increase as much as tenfold during exercise. P_{O_2} in tissues is markedly lower than that in ambient atmosphere. Furthermore, the measured basal tissue P_{O_2} (i.e., mixed venous P_{O_2} or $\bar{v}_{O_2}$) is only marginally greater than the threshold value for mitochondrial anaerobic metabolism. Consequently, tissue hypoxia develops whenever oxygen delivery is inadequate to meet tissue metabolic demands, as occurs within approximately 4 to 6 min of cessation of spontaneous ventilation.

Oxygen delivery to the periphery (D_{O_2}) is determined as the product of the oxygen content of arterial blood (Ca_{O_2}) and cardiac output (CO). The oxygen content of arterial blood is a function of hemoglobin concentration, its degree of saturation, and the fractional amount of oxygen dissolved in solution. The amounts of both bound and dissolved oxygen are directly related to the oxygen tension in arterial blood (Pa_{O_2}): $Ca_{O_2} = ([Hg] \times 1.34Sa_{O_2}) + (Pa_{O_2} \times 0.0031)$ where [Hg] = hemoglobin concentration, g/dL; 1.34 = O_2 carrying capacity of hemoglobin at 37°C, mL/g hemoglobin; Sa_{O_2} = measured % O_2 saturation of hemoglobin; and 0.0031 = solubility coefficient for oxygen.

Aerobic metabolism requires a balance between oxygen delivery (D_{O_2}) and O_2 utilization ($\dot{V}_{O_2}$). With normal aerobic metabolism, oxygen transport and oxygen utilization are independent variables. While the amount of O_2 delivered to tissues per unit time defines the upper limit of oxygen available for the body's total metabolic needs, normally, oxygen delivery always exceeds

*Edited from Chap. 172, "Oxygen Therapy and Pulmonary Oxygen Toxicity," by Beers MF. In: *Fishman's Pulmonary Diseases and Disorders,* 3rd ed., edited by Fishman AP, Elias JA, Fishman JA, Grippi MA, Kaiser LR, Senior RM. New York, McGraw-Hill, 1998, pp 2627–2642. For fuller discussion of topics dealt with in this chapter, the reader is referred to the original text, as noted above.

peripheral oxygen utilization. Oxygen consumption is "supply-independent," commensurate with the rate of adenosine 5'-triphosphate (ATP) production, and reflective of cellular energy requirements. However, if oxygen delivery falls below a critical threshold (D_{O_2} critical), or if utilization exceeds delivery (e.g., with strenuous exercise), tissues shift from aerobic to anaerobic metabolism for metabolic needs. Excessive lactic acid production ensues, cellular metabolism is disrupted, and oxygen consumption is no longer supply-independent.

MECHANISMS OF HYPOXEMIA

Tissue hypoxia results from arterial hypoxemia, reduced oxygen delivery, or excessive or enhanced tissue utilization.

Hypoxemia is a deficiency of oxygen tension in the arterial blood. It results from either reduction of the inspired oxygen tension or from respiratory dysfunction. The most common pulmonary causes of hypoxemia include ventilation/perfusion mismatch, true shunt, diffusion barrier, and, occasionally, low mixed venous oxygen tension. Alveolar hypoventilation increases alveolar P_{CO_2} and secondarily decreases alveolar P_{O_2}. Most causes of arterial hypoxemia can be improved by administration of supplemental oxygen.

In the setting of a normal Pa_{O_2}, tissue hypoxia may result from abnormalities in any of the determinants of oxygen delivery. *Circulatory hypoxia* results when fully oxygenated blood is delivered to tissues in insufficient quantity or at an inadequate level to support tissue metabolic needs. Usual etiologies include low cardiac output states, systemic hypovolemia, and arterial insufficiency of peripheral tissues. Compensation is partially effected at the tissue level initially by increased oxygen extraction from blood, resulting in lowering of mixed venous oxygen tension ($\bar{v}_{O_2}$). Thus, a low $\bar{v}_{O_2}$ is the hallmark of circulatory hypoxia. Because Pa_{O_2} may be normal and the hemoglobin normally saturated, oxygen administration is unlikely to be of great benefit.

Tissue hypoxia may also result from *reduced blood-oxygen transport* (e.g., anemia) or abnormal hemoglobin-O_2 affinity (e.g., hemoglobinopathies, low levels of 2,3-diphosphoglycerate, carbon monoxide poisoning, or methhemoglobinemia). Under these circumstances, cardiac output is increased as an adaptive response, and $\bar{v}_{O_2}$ is normal or decreased. Although not a primary therapy, oxygen administration (including hyperbaric oxygen therapy) may play an adjunctive role.

Tissue hypoxia may result from *maldistribution* of a normal or supranormal cardiac output. Examples include microvascular perfusion defects observed in septic shock or the systemic inflammatory response syndrome (SIRS). The hallmark of maldistribution hypoxia is development of precapillary shunting in peripheral tissues. Cardiac output is normal or increased, and $\bar{v}_{O_2}$ is usually low. Because of the presence of peripheral shunting, supplemental oxygen is usually not effective.

Hypoxia may also arise from misutilization of oxygen at the tissue level due to inhibition of either intracellular enzymes or oxygen-carrying molecules involved in intermediary metabolism and energy generation. An example is hydrogen cyanide poisoning, in which Pa_{O_2}, hemoglobin concentration, percentage of hemoglobin saturation, and tissue perfusion are normal, but peripheral O_2 utilization is impaired. The cyanide binds to cytochrome oxidase and inhibits intramitochondrial transport of electrons to molecular oxygen, resulting in a lactic acidosis. In addition, oxygen extraction is often impaired, leading to a normal or increased $\bar{v}_{O_2}$. Oxygen therapy is usually not effective.

Finally, "demand hypoxia" results when tissue oxygen utilization is supernormal, exceeding the rate of oxygen delivery. Common causes include maximal exercise and hypermetabolic states, such as thyrotoxicosis. As in circulatory hypoxia, $\bar{v}_{O_2}$ is decreased; however, cardiac output is normal or, more likely, increased. Because oxygen-carrying capacity is normal, oxygen administration is often ineffective; definitive treatment requires control of the underlying disorder.

CLINICAL MANIFESTATIONS OF HYPOXIA

Clinical manifestations of hypoxia depend on whether the hypoxia is acute or chronic and on the individual's clinical status. Manifestations include changes in mental status, dyspnea, tachypnea, respiratory distress, and cardiac arrhythmias. Cyanosis, often considered a hallmark of hypoxia, occurs only when the concentration of reduced hemoglobin in the blood is 1.5 g/dL or greater. However, this is not a reliable sign, given its absence in anemia and during periods of poor peripheral perfusion.

The $\bar{v}_{O_2}$ represents an approximation of mean tissue P_{O_2}, and a level of less than 30 mmHg indicates overall tissue hypoxia. Measurements of $\bar{v}_{O_2}$ require pulmonary artery catheterization and therefore are limited to intensive care settings. In most clinical situations, direct determinations of Pa_{O_2} or arterial oxygen saturation are the major parameters available to the clinician. These determinations are made either invasively with arterial blood samples or noninvasively by infrared pulse oximetry. Both are useful in excluding arterial hypoxemia; neither directly measures tissue P_{O_2}. Inadequate tissue oxygen delivery is inferred from acute decreases in Pa_{O_2} to less than 50 mmHg. Patients with chronic hypoxemia have developed compensatory mechanisms. In addition, assumptions about the adequacy of tissue oxygenation may not be warranted in clinical settings in which factors other than arterial hypoxemia are responsible for the development of hypoxia.

INDICATIONS FOR OXYGEN THERAPY

Recommendations for administration of supplemental oxygen, based upon published guidelines, are outlined in Tables 72-1 and 72-2. Indications can be categorized as acute or chronic.

TABLE 72-1 Guidelines for the Institution of Acute Oxygen Therapy

Accepted indications
  Acute hypoxemia (Pa_{O_2} <60 mmHg; Sa_{O_2} <90%)
  Cardiac and respiratory arrest
  Hypotension (systolic blood pressure <100 mmHg)
  Low cardiac output and metabolic acidosis (bicarbonate <18 mmol/L)
  Respiratory distress (respiratory rate >24/min)

Questionable indications
  Uncomplicated myocardial infarction
  Dyspnea without hypoxemia
  Sickle cell crisis
  Angina

KEY: Pa_{O_2}, partial pressure of arterial oxygen; Sa_{O_2}, arterial oxygen saturation.
SOURCE: Fulmer JD, Snider GL: ACCP-NHLBI National Conference on Oxygen Therapy. *Chest* 86: 234–247, 1984.

TABLE 72-2 Indications for Long-Term Oxygen Therapy

Continuous oxygen
Resting Pa_{O_2} of 55 mmHg or oxygen saturation 88%
Resting Pa_{O_2} of 56–59 mmHg or oxygen saturation of 89% in the presence
  of any of the following indicative of cor pulmonale:
    Dependent edema suggesting congestive heart failure
    P pulmonale on the electrocardiogram (P wave greater than 3 min in
      standard leads II, III, or aVF)
Polycythemia (hematocrit >56%)
Resting Pa_{O_2} >59 mmHg or oxygen saturation >89% reimbursable only
  with additional documentation justifying the oxygen prescription and a
  summary of more conservative therapy that has failed
Noncontinuous oxygen[a]
During exercise: Pa_{O_2} of 55 mmHg or oxygen saturation 88% with a low
  level of exertion
During sleep Pa_{O_2} of 55 mmHg or oxygen saturation 88% with associated
  complications, such as pulmonary hypertension, daytime somnolence,
  and cardiac arrhythmias

[a]Oxygen flow rate and number of hours per day must be specified.

Acute Indications

In the acute setting, the most common indication for supplemental oxygen is
arterial hypoxemia, which for a middle-aged adult is defined as a Pa_{O_2} less
than 60 mmHg (corresponding to a hemoglobin saturation of about 90%).
Because of the sigmoidal shape of the oxyhemoglobin dissociation curve, a
further decrease in oxygen tension results in a considerable drop in oxygen
saturation. In certain clinical situations, the target Pa_{O_2} may be adjusted upward or downward. For example, in patients with low O_2-carrying capacity
(e.g., severe anemia), or in flow-limited states (e.g., angina pectoris), increases
in Pa_{O_2} above 60 mmHg may result in marginal but potentially important
increases in tissue O_2 delivery. Conversely, the target Pa_{O_2} may be set lower
in patients in whom hypoxemia constitutes a more important chemical drive
to breathe [e.g., those with chronic hypercapnia due to chronic obstructive pulmonary disease (COPD)].

Hypoxemia is extremely common in acute myocardial infarction. In such
patients, oxygen administration is of unquestioned benefit. Data supporting use of oxygen therapy in nonhypoxemic patients with acute myocardial infarction are controversial. Double-blinded studies of the value of
oxygen in uncomplicated myocardial infarction demonstrate no significant
effects on morbidity or mortality. Similarly, while supplemental oxygen
has been recommended for temporary treatment of inadequate systemic
perfusion resulting from cardiac failure, supporting clinical studies are
lacking.

In carbon monoxide poisoning, the Pa_{O_2} is a poor guide to the need for
oxygen therapy. Despite a normal or "supranormal" Pa_{O_2}, a state of significant tissue hypoxia exists, as often indicated by a severe metabolic acidosis.
Because of the high concentration of carbon monoxide–bound hemoglobin
(carboxyhemoglobin), administration of supplemental oxygen does not increase tissue oxygen delivery, but it does markedly shorten the half-life of
circulating carbon monoxide (80 min versus 320 min on room air). Hyperbaric oxygen administration (see Chap. 23) represents the current standard

of care for those patients with high carboxyhemoglobin levels and evidence of end-organ ischemia-reperfusion damage.

Oxygen has been advocated as adjunctive therapy in the setting of acute trauma. Increasing the supply of circulating hemoglobin best treats the low-flow state induced by acute hemorrhage. However, supplemental oxygen as supportive therapy seems warranted until red blood cells become available for transfusion.

Use of supplemental oxygen as adjuvant therapy in sickle cell crisis to accelerate resorption of air in pneumothorax and for relief of dyspnea without hypoxemia remains controversial.

Chronic Indications

Many patients currently receive long-term oxygen therapy for arterial hypoxemia. Patients with COPD represent the largest group. Early studies of oxygen therapy in COPD showed that continuous supplemental oxygen administered for 4 to 8 weeks decreased the hematocrit, improved exercise tolerance, and lowered pulmonary vascular pressures. Studies from the 1980s documented significant reduction in mortality in patients receiving supplemental oxygen compared with controls. The greatest efficacy is seen with polycythemia, pulmonary hypertension, or hypercapnia. Although data are not available in other groups of patients with chronic hypoxemia, use of long-term supplemental oxygen in these circumstances is widely accepted.

Table 72-2 lists the currently accepted indications for long-term oxygen therapy. In addition to chronic arterial hypoxemia at rest, continuous-flow oxygen therapy is indicated for patients with exercise-induced hypoxemia and those exhibiting nocturnal desaturation. In all patients, the need for additional supplemental oxygen should be based on measurements of arterial saturation. Strategies for delivery of long-term oxygen should include early follow-up for assessing efficacy, followed by routine reevaluation at 6-month intervals.

TECHNIQUES OF OXYGEN ADMINISTRATION

The major types of oxygen delivery systems can be divided into low-flow and high-flow varieties. Both can deliver humidified gases; each offers advantages and disadvanatages.

Low-Flow Systems

Low-flow oxygen delivery systems provide a fraction of the patient's minute ventilation as pure oxygen; the remainder is usually supplied as entrained room air. Flow through these devices is less than 6 L/min, and inspired oxygen concentration varies, since small fluctuations in tidal volume produce variations in the amount of entrained room air. Consequently, when the ventilatory pattern is abnormal or variable, marked variation in the fraction of inspired oxygen may be seen. When the delivery of a constant $F_{I_{O_2}}$ is required—e.g., in patients with chronic carbon dioxide retention—low-flow systems should not be used.

Nasal catheters and cannulae are the most widely used low-flow devices. Low-flow nasal cannulae deliver oxygen to the nasopharynx at flows between 1 and 6 L/min, with the corresponding $F_{I_{O_2}}$ ranging from 0.24 to 0.44. Higher flows do not significantly increase $F_{I_{O_2}}$ above 44 percent and may result in drying of mucous membranes.

Simple oxygen masks that cover the nose and mouth can deliver oxygen concentrations up to 60%. These devices provide a self-contained reservoir of 100 to 200 mL of additional gas, thereby facilitating increases in the achievable fraction of inspired oxygen above 0.44. Simple face masks require an oxygen flow of 5 to 6 L/min to avoid accumulation of carbon dioxide within the mask. Conventional masks interfere with drinking, eating, and expectorating; in addition, they can become displaced, particularly during sleep, and they increase the risk of aspiration by concealment of vomitus. Drying of respiratory mucous membranes is alleviated by humidification of the inspired gas.

When an $F_{I_{O_2}}$ of greater than 0.6 is required in a nonintubated patient, a reservoir bag (600 to 1000 mL) is attached to a simple face mask and flushed continuously with oxygen at flow rates of 5 to 8 L/min. If there are no one-way valves on the reservoir bag, the apparatus is referred to as a *partial nonrebreathing mask*—a device that can deliver oxygen in concentrations of 80 to 85%. A true nonrebreathing mask makes use of a one-way valve between the mask and the bag so that the patient inhales exclusively from the reservoir bag and exhales through separate valves on either side of the mask. A very high $F_{I_{O_2}}$ can be achieved when the mask fits tightly against the patient's face. However, tight-fitting molded masks, including those used to deliver continuous positive airway pressure (CPAP), are often uncomfortable and are not suitable for use for more than a few hours.

Low-flow delivery devices are frequently used for long-term oxygen therapy, along with oxygen concentrators and compressed gas or liquid oxygen sources. Most patients requiring a stationary source of supplemental oxygen use oxygen concentrators. Unless patients are immobile or confined to bed, both stationary and mobile oxygen delivery systems should be employed. Both compressed gas and portable liquid oxygen systems are available, but the liquid system containers are easier to refill than high-pressure cylinders. The major disadvantages of liquid oxygen are higher cost and the requirement for pressure-relief venting.

Oxygen "conserving" devices include reservoir nasal cannulae, electronic demand devices, and transtracheal catheters. The reservoir nasal cannula has a pouch that stores 20 mL of extra oxygen during expiration and delivers the oxygen as a bolus at the onset of the next inspiration. Electronic demand devices, triggered by the onset of inspiration, deliver a pulse of oxygen early in the breath. Both types of devices are prone to failure. Transtracheal catheters improve oxygen delivery by bypassing the anatomic dead space of the upper airway, using the upper airway as an oxygen reservoir during inspiration and expiration. Transtracheal oxygen is delivered directly into the trachea via a hollow catheter implanted surgically under local anesthesia or inserted percutaneously using the Seldinger technique. Transtracheal catheters effect reductions in total oxygen usage of 50 to 75 percent, are inconspicuous, do not produce nasal or facial irritation due to oxygen flow, and are infrequently displaced during sleep. However, there is an increased incidence of infection, and potentially fatal "mucus balls" occluding the airway and catheter have been described.

High-Flow Systems

High-flow oxygen delivery systems maintain the selected $F_{I_{O_2}}$ by incorporating a reservoir whose volume exceeds the patient's anatomic dead space or by delivering oxygen at a very high flow. The flow of all high-flow systems exceeds fourfold the patient's actual minute volume; otherwise, entrainment of room air at peak inspiration occurs. High-flow systems are used to treat hypoxic patients who depend on their hypoxic drive to breathe or hypoxemic patients who have an abnormal ventilatory pattern and whose ventilatory requirements exceed the delivery capabilities of low-flow systems.

The *Venturi mask* is a high-flow oxygen delivery device in which a jet of 100% oxygen flows into the mask through a fixed constrictive orifice, past open side ports, thereby entraining room air. The amount of air entrained, and therefore the resultant F_{IO_2}, depend on the size of the side ports and flow of oxygen. Since both of these variables are fixed, the resultant O_2–room air mixing ratio is held steady, resulting in a well-controlled, constant F_{IO_2}. Exhalation occurs through valved exhalation ports. Venturi masks deliver an F_{IO_2} between 0.24 and 0.50. Water drops may clog the oxygen injector device, resulting in changes in gas flow. In addition, development of back pressure by occluded exhalation ports may lead to decreases in the volume of entrained room air and a resultant increase in F_{IO_2}.

Other high-flow systems include reservoir nebulizers, humidifiers, T tubes, tracheostomy collars, aerosol masks, face tents, CPAP masks, and air-oxygen blenders. Air-oxygen blenders consist of precision metering devices that convert high-pressure wall sources of compressed air and oxygen (at 50 to 70 psi) to usable, predictable flows of up to 100 L/min at an F_{IO_2} ranging from 0.21 to 1.0.

OXYGEN TOXICITY

Changes in both pulmonary and extrapulmonary homeostasis occur in response to exposure to high concentrations of oxygen. Extrapulmonary physiologic effects of hyperoxia are usually clinically insignificant: suppression of erythropoiesis, systemic vasoconstriction, and depression of cardiac output. In contrast, the pulmonary effects of hyperoxia are clinically relevant and include depression of hypoxic ventilatory drive, pulmonary vasodilation, and absorption atelectasis. In addition to adverse physiologic effects, oxygen in high concentrations is cytotoxic. Whereas all respiring cells are potentially susceptible to the toxicity derived of hyperoxia, the major clinical adverse effects are related to lung damage.

Pathophysiology

The mechanism of tissue oxygen toxicity is believed to be formation of reactive free radicals. The most significant mechanism of pulmonary cellular toxity is lipid peroxidation and protein oxidation secondary to the direct effects of O_2 radical toxicity. The toxic effects of oxygen on the lung occur when free radical production during hyperoxic exposure overwhelms intrinsic antioxidant defenses. Excess free radicals interact with cellular components, resulting in cytotoxic events that produce a characteristic cascade of biochemical, cellular, morphologic, and physiologic changes. The biochemical reactions, in turn, result in a sequence of characteristic cellular and morphologic changes. Since oxygen concentration is directly proportional to partial pressure, breathing 100% O_2 at an altitude of 5000 ft (0.8 atm), 80% O_2 at sea level (1 atm), or 40% O_2 in a hyperbaric chamber (2 atm) for the same duration results in a similar toxicity profile.

Four phases in the development of pulmonary oxygen toxicity have been recognized: initiation, inflammation, destruction, and proliferation and fibrosis. The first three occur during exposure to both lethal and sublethal doses of hyperoxia; the fourth phase occurs if there is reexposure to sublethal oxygen levels. If lethal exposure persists, ongoing tissue destruction and death are observed. In the aggregate, the pathophysiologic and morphologic changes associated with hyperoxic stress are similar to other forms of diffuse alveolar damage. An initial inflammatory response (exudative phase) is followed by fibrosis and repair (proliferative phase), a sequence not dissimilar to that in other forms of acute lung injury, including acute respiratory distress syndrome (see Chap. 68).

Clinical Manifestations

Normal volunteers exposed to 100% O_2 experience symptoms within 12 to 24 h. The earliest manifestations include substernal chest pain, tachypnea, and nonproductive cough. Measurements of tracheobronchial function show decreased particle clearance as early as 6 h after the start of exposure to 100% O_2. Systemic symptoms—including malaise, nausea, anorexia, and headache—may be seen. The presence of crackles, suggestive of interstitial or alveolar edema, may be noted as a nonspecific finding. The onset of acute pulmonary oxygen toxicity usually follows an asymptomatic period during which no physiologic changes are seen.

The best-known clinical syndrome of chronic pulmonary oxygen toxicity occurs in newborns receiving oxygen for treatment of neonatal respiratory distress syndrome (see Chap. 71). Persistent morphologic changes with healing may produce bronchopulmonary dysplasia, a chronic disorder.

Although reversible physiologic, anatomic, and biochemical changes can be detected following short exposure to hyperoxia, humans can tolerate 100% oxygen at sea level for 24 h without serious pulmonary injury. Currently, the diagnosis of oxygen poisoning depends on the nonspecific symptom complex described previously or abnormal pulmonary function tests in the proper clinical setting.

Susceptibility of cells or organisms to oxygen toxicity can be modified by factors other than intrinsic cellular antioxidant mechanisms. Many drugs act synergistically with hyperoxia, accelerating free radical production and worsening oxygen toxicity. The metabolism of nitrofurantoin and paraquat, as well as bleomycin, have been shown to increase lung injury and fibrosis through enhanced production of O_2 radicals. Potentiation of oxygen toxicity by disulfiram occurs through inhibition of cytosolic superoxide dismutase by diethyldithiocarbamate. Variability of dietary intake can also modify oxygen tolerance. Protein malnutrition, as well as dietary deficiency of any of the antioxidant quenchers, may alter the response to hyperoxia. The adverse effects of deficiencies of vitamins A and E are also well described.

Prevention

Because early detection of O_2 toxicity is difficult and specific therapy lacking, avoidance of pulmonary toxicity during oxygen therapy remains the cornerstone of management. Based upon general consensus, the following guidelines can be offered regarding oxygen administration at 1 atmosphere. Oxygen in concentrations up to 100% can be administered during cardiopulmonary resuscitation and in the transport and initial management of critically ill patients. If needed, an $F_{I_{O_2}}$ of 1.0 can be used for up to 24 h without significant lung injury. During this period, management should be directed toward improving pulmonary gas exchange, optimizing oxygen delivery, and limiting tissue metabolic demands, so that inspired O_2 concentration can be decreased to the lowest possible levels. Oxygen at an $F_{I_{O_2}}$ of 0.5 or less can be administered safely to most patients for weeks, although factors specific to individual patients (e.g., prior bleomycin use) may dictate a lower tolerance. The maximal safe duration for oxygen exposures between an $F_{I_{O_2}}$ of 0.5 and 1.0 is less certain, although these concentrations can probably be tolerated longer than 24 h. The upper safe limit of $F_{I_{O_2}}$ for chronic O_2 therapy in the ambulatory setting is largely undefined.

BIBLIOGRAPHY

Christopher K, Spofford BT, Brannin P, Petty T: Transtracheal oxygen delivery. *JAMA* 256:494–497, 1986.

Dunne PJ: The demographics and economics of long-term oxygen therapy. *Respir Care* 45:223–230, 2000.

Kacmarek RM: Delivery systems for long-term oxygen therapy. *Respir Care* 45:84–94, 2000.

Medical Research Council Working Party: Long-term domiciliary oxygen therapy in chronic hypoxic cor pulmonale complicating chronic bronchitis and emphysema. *Lancet* 1:681–686, 1981.

Nocturnal Oxygen Therapy Trial Group: Continuous or nocturnal oxygen therapy in hypoxemic chronic obstructive lung disease: A clinical trial. *Ann Intern Med* 93:391–398, 1980.

Oba Y, Salzman GA, Willsie SK: Reevaluation of continuous oxygen therapy after initial prescription in patients with chronic obstructive pulmonary disease. *Respir Care* 45:401–406, 2000.

Petty TL, Bliss PL: Ambulatory oxygen therapy, exercise, and survival with advance chronic obstructive lung disease (the Nocturnal Oxygen Therapy Trial revisited). *Respir Care* 45:204–213, 2000.

Tarpey SP, Celli BR: Long-term oxygen therapy. *N Engl J Med* 333:710–714, 1995.

73 | Intubation and Upper Airway Management*

Lisa M. Bellini

INTRODUCTION

The oropharynx and nasopharynx join at the level of the base of the skull to form the hypopharynx. The nasopharynx is separated from the oropharynx by the soft palate, which is a freely mobile structure, and the adenoids or nasopharyngeal tonsils. The hypopharynx includes the vallecula, which is the space posterior to the tongue and anterior to the epiglottis, and the openings to the esophagus and the trachea. In adults, the epiglottis is typically crescentic, reasonably stiff, and thin. The U-shaped infant epiglottis is longer and floppier. In addition, the infant larynx is also more cephalad and the cords angled relative to the airway (rather than perpendicular, as in the adult).

Before any procedure on the airway, a directed history and thorough physical examination should be performed. A history of nasal polyps, nasal septal deviation, or change in voice—or the presence of hoarseness, stridor, tachypnea, or coughing—should be noted. The patient's ability to breathe through a single nostril (when the mouth is closed and the other nostril occluded) indicates the relative patency of that passage. Mouth opening may be limited with temporomandibular joint disease, fibrosis of the temporalis muscle (e.g., from radiation), or mandibular fractures; an inability to open the mouth more than 40 mm is considered significant. Protruding maxillary incisors interfere with direct laryngoscopy. Caps and other dental prostheses may be damaged during laryngoscopy, while severe dental caries or periodontal disease make it easier to dislodge teeth during instrumentation of the airway. The edentulous patient often has an atrophic mandible and a large tongue and is difficult to ventilate by mask because of poor mask fit. Intubation of the trachea becomes difficult because the tongue is no longer constrained by the teeth and interferes with visualization of the larynx; enlargement of the tongue may also be problematic. Burns, scars, or radiation of the submandibular soft tissue prevent displacement of the tongue into this space during laryngoscopy. Similarly, retrognathia makes it difficult to displace or flatten the tongue during laryngoscopy. A hyomental distance (i.e., the distance from the hyoid bone to tip of the mandible) of less than 6 cm is indicative of potential difficulties with intubation. Enlarged tonsils, intraoral and hypopharyngeal tumors and cysts, or an infiltrated, inflamed, or floppy epiglottis also interfere both with laryngoscopy and mask ventilation. The retropharyngeal and lateral pharyngeal spaces are continuous with the mediastinum and, therefore, are subject to expansion by processes affecting this

---

*Edited from Chap. 174, "Intubation and Upper Airway Management," by Hanson CW III. In: *Fishman's Pulmonary Diseases and Disorders,* 3d ed., edited by Fishman AP, Elias JA, Fishman JA, Grippi MA, Kaiser LR, Senior RM. New York, McGraw-Hill, 1998, pp 2661–2672. For fuller discussion of topics dealt with in this chapter, the reader is referred to the original text, as noted above.

structure (e.g., formation of edema, blood, pus, emphysema). The oral and pharyngeal mucosae are swollen and bleed easily during pregnancy; when compounded by a diminished functional residual capacity and increased volume of acidic gastric contents, this makes intubation of the gravid patient quite hazardous.

Other considerations include cervical spine abnormalities such as cervical osteophytes, ankylosing spondylitis, rheumatoid arthritis (that affects the cervical spine of 25 to 90 percent of patients), injuries to the cervical spine, and the presence of a cervical collar or halo fixation. Patients with short, muscular necks have limited neck mobility, as well as redundant soft tissue in the mouth and submandibular space. The normal range for flexion and extension of the neck ranges from 90 to 165 degrees. Normal aging results in as much as a 20 percent reduction in mobility of the C-spine mobility by the age of 75 years.

GENERAL MANAGEMENT PRINCIPLES

The most important principle of airway management is that a source of oxygen and a means of ventilation should be available whenever possible. In addition, a backup plan for airway management should be considered at the outset in the event the primary plan goes awry. Usually, the first clinical consideration is whether endotracheal intubation is necessary.

The decision regarding intubation is influenced by the patients' level of consciousness, clinical context (e.g., perioperative, emergency), anticipated duration of the respiratory problem, risk of gastric aspiration, patency of the airway, concurrent medical problems, and appropriateness of noninvasive airway management. For example, if neurologic depression is due to central nervous system injury, noninvasive management is often inappropriate, owing to potential hypercarbia, hypoxia, or exacerbation of the primary injury. Conversely, sedation or obtundation secondary to drugs or seizure is often brief, and temporizing, noninvasive measures may be appropriate.

The volume and acidity of the patient's gastric contents must be considered in any decision about airway management. Aspiration of solid food can be catastrophic, as can large volumes of acidic, enzymatically active gastric fluid. Most studies have indicated that aspirated contents with pH lower than 2.5 or volume greater than 0.5 to 1.0 mL/kg are likely to cause lung damage. Pain and narcotics can alter gastric emptying or change gastric pH—as can a number of disease states, such as intestinal obstruction, diabetic gastroparesis, and obesity. Unless the patient has fasted for more than 8 h and is not subject to the aforementioned confounding factors, a full stomach should be presumed, and airway management handled accordingly.

Some degree of airway obstruction can be managed without intubation by head positioning and use of oral and nasal airways or positive airway pressure by mask. A rolled towel or small pillow placed behind the neck or occiput reproduces the sniffing position (head extended on the neck with the neck flexed on the thorax). Anterior displacement of the jaw can be accomplished by pulling it forward or by placing pressure on the angle of the mandible (the jaw thrust maneuver). This serves to further open up the retrolingual space. Grasping the tongue with gauze or an instrument and pulling it forward accomplishes the same end. This position is appropriate for spontaneous respiration because it limits soft tissue obstruction to airflow.

Oral and nasal airways alleviate airway obstruction due to redundant airway soft tissue or muscle relaxation. The application of positive pressure to the mouth and nose (mask continuous positive airway pressure, or "mask CPAP") stents open the airway. These measures can be used as short-term, temporizing alternatives to intubation in the spontaneously breathing patient. True ventilation by mask is readily accomplished in the anatomically normal patient, whereas features such as a beard, a flat or sharp nose, and sunken cheeks (in the edentulous patient) can make mask-assisted ventilation difficult or impossible. Saliva and blood interfere with mask ventilation, direct airway visualization, and fiberoptic procedures. Pretreatment with an antisialogogue, such as atropine, glycopyrrolate, or scopolamine, when time permits, significantly diminishes saliva production. Suction must be available before initiation of any elective procedure, and suction equipment should be available on any emergency cart for clearing secretions and use in the event of regurgitation.

Nasotracheal intubation is easiest in the sniffing position, because the tip of the endotracheal tube is best aligned with the larynx and least likely to be deflected by the walls of the pharynx. Nasal and oral fiberoptic procedures are easier in this position as well, with the oral, pharyngeal, and tracheal axes well aligned. The sniffing position is modified by additional head extension and flattening of the back of the tongue with the laryngoscope blade during oral intubation. Small, titrated doses of sedatives, topical anesthesia, and vasoconstrictor agents markedly alter the ease with which awake procedures—such as fiberoptic, nasotracheal, and oral intubation—are performed. Narcotics are more likely than other agents to obtund the cough reflex. Topical cocaine has anesthetic and vasoconstrictor properties, but because of its classification as a controlled agent, the combination of lidocaine and phenylephrine is often used as an alternative.

NONINVASIVE TECHNIQUES OF AIRWAY MANAGEMENT

Commonly used noninvasive airway management techniques are based on use of nasal and oral airways, resuscitation bags, and face and laryngeal masks.

A variety of nasal and oral airways are available. Nasal airways are generally made of flexible rubber and have a beveled tip. Oral airways are curved to lie over and behind the tongue. Some are fashioned with slots for ready passage of a suction catheter; others have a central channel designed to accommodate a fiberoptic scope. Binasal airways are designed to fit in a ventilation circuit, permitting ventilation without endotracheal intubation in anesthetized patients.

Resuscitation bags are self-inflating and, therefore, can be used without a pressurized gas source. An internal flap valve system directs inflowing gas to the patient or reservoir, permitting application of positive pressure by mask or endotracheal tube and venting exhaled gas to the atmosphere. Many bags are equipped with oxygen reservoirs. Inspired oxygen concentration is ordinarily limited to 40 to 60% when oxygen inflow is 10 L/min and bag reinflation is rapid, since room air is entrained with each breath. The addition of an oxygen reservoir permits administration of oxygen concentrations between 75 and 90% at flows of 10 to 15 L/min. Some bags are equipped with adjustable valves for application of positive end-expiratory pressure (PEEP).

The wide variety of face masks have three common features: a body, a seal, and a connector. The body is usually made of malleable material which adjusts to differing facial anatomy. The body of some masks is made of clear plastic in order to allow diagnosis of regurgitation. The seal is usually a cushioned rim that can be inflated or deflated and is attached to the body, although some are detachable. Some seals are flanged and not cushioned. The connector is designed with a universal fitting (22-mm internal diameter) for attachment to any ventilating circuit; many are equipped with retaining straps for attachment to mask straps, which pass behind the patient's head, freeing the hand of the operator.

The laryngeal mask airway has a compliant cuff that is applied to the dorsal surface of the larynx, isolating the airway from the mouth and esophagus. Although its most extensive use has been in surgical patients, the device has also been used for bronchoscopy in the awake patient, in the intensive care unit, and in emergency resuscitation. The airway is inserted via the mouth into the hypopharynx; its correct position is verified by chest auscultation.

ENDOTRACHEAL INTUBATION

In the intensive care unit, endotracheal intubation is effected through either the nasal or oral route. Nasal intubation is associated with a higher incidence of bleeding; the increase in equipment dead space is minimal (less than 10 mL). The conflicting literature on the incidence of sinusitis and pneumonia with nasotracheal and orotracheal intubations includes data showing no difference between the two.

Nasal intubation can be done blindly or with use of a laryngoscope and forceps. The blind technique allows for rapid airway control in an awake patient with minimal depression of protective airway reflexes. Initially, the nasal passages are examined for patency, septal deviation, or presence of polyps. In a cooperative patient, the larger nasal passage is selected by alternately occluding each nostril and choosing the one with better airflow. Topical anesthetic and vasoconstrictor agents are sprayed in the nostril or applied with cotton pledgets. The anesthetic is also sprayed into the back of the mouth to anesthetize the hypopharynx. An appropriate-size tube (6 to 7 mm for women, 7 to 8 mm for men) is selected and lubricated. With the patient in the sniffing position, the tube is advanced through the nostril with slow, firm pressure. The natural curve of the tube is oriented so that the tip initially points toward the occiput and curves in a caudad direction as it advances. If the procedure is done blindly in an awake patient, the operator listens for breath sounds as the tip approaches the cords. A whistle attachment is available to enhance the operator's ability to hear breath sounds. The tube is passed into the airway on inspiration. Slight rotation of the tube at the nose can be used to correct for lateral misalignment. When the procedure is performed in an anesthetized patient, the endotracheal tube is passed into the hypopharynx above the cords; laryngoscopy is performed and the tube is advanced into the trachea under direct visualization. A Magill forceps is often used to grasp the tube and to direct the tip between the cords. Care must be taken to avoid grasping the tube with the cuff, which is easily perforated.

With orotracheal intubation, the patient's head is placed in the sniffing position and a Macintosh or Miller blade inserted into the right side of the mouth using the left hand (regardless of the handedness of the operator). The Miller blade is better with an anatomically anterior larynx; however, most operators become familiar with one blade or the other and use it preferentially. The blades of both instruments are flanged to keep the tongue to the left side of the oropharynx, out of the visual field. Larger adult blades (Macintosh #4 or Miller #3) are used for patients with long mandibles; shorter blades (Macintosh #3 or Miller #2) are used in patients whose anatomy is of average size. The right hand is used to pull upper and lower lips out of the way, so that these structures are not caught and injured between the blade and the teeth. The tip of the laryngoscope blade is advanced along the tongue until the epiglottis is visible. If the Macintosh blade is used, it is advanced between the tongue and the epiglottis; if the Miller blade is used, the epiglottis is elevated directly. The vocal cords should be visible immediately below the epiglottis.

Correct endotracheal tube position can be verified by a number of methods. Audible or palpable air passage (in the spontaneously breathing patient), a visible vapor trail within the tube, or auscultatory evidence of breath sounds over the lung fields are standard approaches. End-tidal capnometry showing phasic variation in the level of carbon dioxide is the "gold standard." This method has become more feasible in nonsurgical settings since the development of portable and disposable devices.

Alternative approaches in patients who are difficult to intubate because of anatomic considerations include fiberoptic laryngoscopy (the trachea is entered with the bronchoscope and an endotracheal tube advanced over the bronchoscope), use of a flexible light wand (the airway is transilluminated and an endotracheal tube advanced into the airway using the wand as a stylet), and retrograde techniques (percutaneous cannulation of the trachea in the neck and retrograde passage of a wire or catheter into the oropharynx, followed by securing of the wire to an endotracheal tube and positioning in the trachea). Percutaneous cricothyrotomy and tracheostomy kits are also available for emergency access to the airway.

Contemporary endotracheal tubes are disposable and have high-volume, compliant cuffs. Pediatric tubes are generally uncuffed because children are more vulnerable than adults to the development of subglottic stenosis due to tube contact with the trachea. Uncuffed tubes also maximize the cross-sectional area of the tube. All single-lumen tubes have a 15-mm outer diameter connector that fits any standard ventilation device. Most tubes also have a radiopaque stripe, permitting tube localization on chest radiographs. The tip of the tube is beveled; the bevel faces the left because endotracheal tubes are generally inserted from the right by right-handed operators. The extra hole opposite the bevel on many tubes is the "Murphy eye," a design that permits suctioning or antegrade gas flow if the bevel is occluded. Special tubes are used for facial or oral surgery, laser surgery, and jet ventilation. In addition, a variety of double lumen tubes are available for thoracic surgical procedures.

BIBLIOGRAPHY

Charters P, O'Sullivan E: The "dedicated airway": a review of the concept and an update of current practice. *Anaesthesia* 54:778–786, 1999.

Depoix JP, Malbezin S, Videcoq M, et al: Oral intubation v nasal intubation in adult cardiac surgery. *Br J Anaesth* 59:167–169, 1987.

Hochman II, Zeitels, Heaton JT: Analysis of the forces and position required for direct laryngoscopic exposure of the anterior vocal folds. *Ann Otol Rhinol Laryngol* 108:715–724, 1999.

Kil HK, Bishop MJ: Head position and oral vs. nasal route as factors determining endotracheal tube resistance. *Chest* 105:1794–1797, 1994.

Mallampati SR, Gatt SP, Gugino LD, et al: A clinical sign to predict difficult tracheal intubation: A prospective study. *Can Anaesth Soc J* 32:429–434, 1985.

O'Conner RE, Swor RA: Verification of endotracheal tube placement following intubation. National Association of EMS Physicians Standards and Clinical Practice Committee. *Prehosp Emerg Care* 3:248–250, 1999.

74 | Hemodynamic and Respiratory Monitoring in Acute Respiratory Failure*

Lisa M. Bellini and Michael A. Grippi

INTRODUCTION

Monitoring of clinical parameters is a core activity in all critical care units. However, with the exception of cardiac monitoring in the setting of acute myocardial infarction, few data are available to support the cost-effectiveness of this practice. Along with routine vital signs, a variety of cardiovascular and respiratory variables are commonly monitored.

CARDIOVASCULAR MONITORING

Assessment of cardiovascular status centers on routine measurements of heart rate, heart rhythm, systemic blood pressure, central venous pressure, and hemodynamic determinations derived from more invasive techniques, including right-heart catheterization.

Cardiac Rate and Rhythm and Systemic Blood Pressure

Heart rate is continually measured in all patients in critical care units. As a nonspecific sign of neurohumoral stress, tachycardia may signal a variety of disorders, from pain or anxiety to shock. Accurate determinations of heart rate are important because this parameter is used to calculate many derived indices of cardiovascular function.

Electrocardiographic (ECG) monitoring decreases morbidity and mortality from acute myocardial infarction, likely reflecting the high prevalence of clinically significant and treatable rate or rhythm disturbances that would otherwise go undetected. The value of arrhythmia monitoring in noncardiac intensive care units is uncertain. Atrial and ventricular tachycardia may occur in about 25 percent of patients in general critical care units; however, the prognostic significance and need for treatment of such arrhythmias are unclear.

Systemic blood pressure may be monitored invasively or noninvasively. Invasive measurement using an indwelling arterial line can result in magnification and diminution of the aortic pressure as it travels down the arterial tree into a fluid-filled catheter connected to a transducer. Typically, as the pressure wave moves from the aortic arch to a peripheral artery, high-frequency components of the waveform (e.g., the dicrotic notch) are attenuated and peak systolic pressures are exaggerated. Hence, radial or dorsalis pedis peak systolic pressures commonly exceed brachial or aortic pressures, while peripheral

*Edited from Chap. 175, "Hemodynamic and Respiratory Monitoring in Acute Respiratory Failure," by Gottlieb J. In: *Fishman's Pulmonary Diseases and Disorders,* 3d ed., edited by Fishman AP, Elias JA, Fishman JA, Grippi MA, Kaiser LR, Senior RM. New York, McGraw-Hill, 1998, pp 2673–2690. For fuller discussion of topics dealt with in this chapter, the reader is referred to the original text, as noted above.

diastolic pressures frequently fall below central diastolic pressures. Mean arterial pressure is a more constant value among various sites of measurement.

Noninvasive measurement of systemic blood pressure uses automated devices that measure and record the pressure at regular intervals. Although different devices have in common an inflatable cuff placed around the patient's arm, methods of signal detection vary considerably from one device to another. The absence of technologic standardization makes recordings partially method-dependent.

Disparate pressures may be obtained in the same patient when measured invasively and noninvasively because the two methods measure different phenomena. Arterial cannulation provides information about pressure within the vessel, regardless of flow. In contrast, indirect manometry detects flow within a vessel as an approximation of pressure. A moderately underdamped catheter system will overestimate peak systolic pressure and therefore may read higher systolic pressures than noninvasive measurements in the same patient. An overdamped catheter system may show the opposite relationship. In addition, shock states may be associated with reduced peripheral flow, leading to an underestimation of the central pressure by noninvasive methods.

Central Venous Pressure

Central venous pressure (CVP) is measured using a transducer-catheter system from which a continuous waveform may be displayed. The major indication for placement of a central venous catheter is securing vascular access for frequent blood sampling, parenteral hyperalimentation, long-term vascular access, administration of certain medications (e.g., potassium, chemotherapy), or placement of other devices, (e.g., a pacemaker, pulmonary artery flotation catheter, or dialysis catheter). The internal jugular approach is preferred for its relative safety, high initial success rate, and ease of access for pulmonary artery catheter placement.

Although CVP is an unreliable surrogate for left ventricular filling pressure, it may provide important clinical information. A low CVP (normal, 0 to 7 mmHg) usually indicates reduced central blood volume. Rapid administration of 500 mL of saline normally causes a 2- to 4-mmHg rise in CVP, which returns to baseline over 15 min; failure of the CVP to increase or to rapidly return to baseline suggests significant reduction in circulating volume or increased vascular compliance. CVP also reflects right ventricular preload. An elevated CVP must be interpreted carefully, as it may suggest a variety of conditions, including right ventricular volume overload or failure, pulmonary embolism, right ventricular infarction, or left ventricular failure, each of which requires a different therapeutic approach. An elevated CVP may occur in the presence of systemic hypertension or hypotension, hypervolemia, or relative hypovolemia.

Measurement of CVP is helpful in calculating systemic vascular resistance (SVR):

$$\text{SVR} = \frac{\text{mean arterial pressure} - \text{CVP}}{\text{cardiac output}}$$

The effect of positive end-expiratory pressure (PEEP) on CVP interpretation is complex. When chest wall and lung compliances are equal, approximately half the level of applied PEEP may be transmitted to the surrounding intrathoracic structures. Thus, a PEEP of 10 cmH_2O may result in an increase of up to 5 cmH$_2$O (about 3 mmHg) in CVP. However, the concurrent effect of PEEP in reducing venous return may result in no change or an actual reduction in transmural CVP. In addition, in disease states characterized by decreased lung compliance (e.g., ARDS, pulmonary edema), the effect of PEEP on CVP may be even smaller. Hence, calculation of "true" CVP in the setting of PEEP is not reliable.

Right-Heart Catheterization

The basic *pulmonary artery flotation catheter* (Swan-Ganz catheter) includes a proximal port, located approximately 30 cm from the tip, through which right atrial pressure can be monitored, and a distal port at the tip, used to measure pulmonary artery and pulmonary artery occlusion pressures. The same caveats that apply to measurement of systemic arterial pressure apply to measurement of pulmonary artery pressures. In addition, lack of catheter fixation distally in the artery, coupled with beat-to-beat movement of the heart and great vessels, may produce exaggerated ringing of the pulmonary artery signal (catheter "whip" or "fling").

Pulmonary artery diastolic pressure (PAD) may be assumed to reflect left ventricular end-diastolic pressure (LVEDP) as a function of left ventricular volume and compliance. Underlying assumptions include a short time constant for emptying of the pulmonary artery; a continuous column of blood between the distal catheter port and the left ventricle; an intraluminal pressure that reflects volume and transmural pressure rather than altered compliance or altered surrounding pressure; and no flow between the measurement site and the left ventricle.

The gradient between PAD and *pulmonary artery occlusion pressure* (PAOP) is less than 4 mmHg in the absence of significant pulmonary disease. However, when pulmonary vascular resistance is elevated (e.g., in emphysema, interstitial lung disease, pulmonary embolism or other pulmonary vascular disease), the gradient between PAD and PAOP may be as much as 20 to 30 mmHg, and PAD does not reflect LVEDP.

An additional problem with interpretation of hemodynamic measurements arises when the pulmonary artery catheter lies in a lung region where alveolar pressure exceeds both pulmonary artery and venous pressures (zone 1) or pulmonary venous pressure, alone (zone 2). Under these circumstances, measurements are affected by alveolar pressure, as reflected in respiratory variations in alveolar pressure and PAOP of similar magnitudes. Fortunately, increased pulmonary blood flow to lung regions where pulmonary artery and venous pressures exceed alveolar pressure (zone 3) usually carries the catheter into those regions. In addition, in critically ill supine patients, the variation in vertical height of the lung is reduced. Nevertheless, high-PEEP or low-flow states may enlarge zones 1 and 2, creating the potential for hemodynamic misinterpretation. A cross-table lateral chest radiograph can be used to verify that the catheter is in a dependent portion of the lung (zone 3).

PAOP may also overestimate LVEDV in myocardial ischemia, left ventricular hypertrophy, or mitral stenosis, when the ventricular septum impinges on the left ventricular cavity due to right ventricular distention, when vasopressors are used (vasopressors may decrease left ventricular compliance, resulting in a higher left ventricular transmural pressure and PAOP for any given LVEDV), or when the distal opening of the catheter is directed against an arterial wall. PAOP underestimates true LVEDP when the tracing is underdamped or when LVEDP continues to rise after mitral closure, as in aortic insufficiency (Table 74-1).

TABLE 74-1 Sources of Error in the Interpretation of Wedge Pressure and Pulmonary Diastolic Pressure

Artifact	Mechanism	Comment
Wedge pressure overestimates left ventricular end-diastolic volume	Flow through a resistance downstream from site of measurement	Mitral stenosis, pulmonary venous anastomosis, pulmonary venous hypertension
	Decreased compliance of left ventricle	Ischemia, left ventricular hypertrophy, catecholamines, pericardial disease, right ventricular interdependence due to distended right ventricle
	Increased pressure surrounding left ventricle	Positive end-expiratory pressure; subtract no more than 50% of PEEP
	Interrupted column of blood between catheter and left ventricle	Zone 1 or 2 conditions exist, so that alveolar pressure is the effective back pressure to pulmonary artery; observe for equal airway and pulmonary artery (PA) catheter pressure swings with inspiration
	Catheter is "overwedged" from balloon overdistention	Use smallest volume of air to inflate balloon
PA diastolic overestimates left ventricular end-diastolic volume	All of the above	
	Increased time constant for emptying of pulmonary circulation	Insufficient time for equilibration of PA diastolic and wedge pressure, particularly with tachycardia and pulmonary hypertension
Wedge pressure underestimates left ventricular end-diastolic volume	Closure of mitral valve before end diastole	Aortic insufficiency
PA diastolic underestimates left ventricular end-diastolic volume	Underdamped system	Overestimation of PA systolic and underestimation of PA diastolic

1067

Calculation of *cardiac output* and systemic vascular resistance using a pulmonary artery flotation catheter may be valuable in differentiating cardiogenic shock from other hypotensive states. A variety of methods are available for measuring cardiac output, including thermodilution, dye dilution, Fick, continuous, and bioimpedance techniques. Bioimpedance techniques have not been used widely and are not considered further here.

The *thermodilution method* is based on temperature of the trace indicator. Following injection of a bolus of saline, a thermistor located several millimeters from the catheter tip records the passage of the bolus as a time-temperature curve. In general, the smaller the area under the curve, the larger is the cardiac output. Calculation of the cardiac output is performed using a microprocessor.

The thermodilution technique has limitations. Tricuspid or pulmonic regurgitation may cause recirculation of the cooled solution, producing a large area under the curve and an erroneously low calculated cardiac output; severe tricuspid regurgitation may overestimate cardiac output. An atrial septal defect or other right-to-left shunt can result in loss of saline sensed at the thermistor and an erroneously elevated calculated output. Three determinations have about a 90 percent likelihood of obtaining a result that lies within 10 percent of the true cardiac output; six determinations may provide a 90 percent chance of a result that lies within 5 percent of the true value. During mechanical ventilation, 40 percent variability (20 percent greater or lower than the mean) in measurement may be seen in any given patient, depending on the point in the respiratory cycle when the bolus is injected. To reduce variability, injection should be performed at end-expiration.

In the *dye dilution method,* a dye (e.g., indocyanine green) is injected into the right atrium, and blood is slowly and steadily withdrawn from a distal systemic artery. The concentration of dye is plotted over time, yielding a curve that looks similar to a thermodilution curve. A computer is used to adjust for recirculation of the dye. From a knowledge of quantity of dye injected and the area under the curve, cardiac output can be calculated. This method is seldom employed clinically because of the need for special equipment and the inconvenience of arterial sampling.

The *Fick method* is based on measurement of oxygen consumption and arterial and mixed venous oxygen contents. A value for oxygen consumption can be assumed (e.g., 200 mL/min), but, ideally, oxygen consumption is measured directly using a metabolic cart. Arterial and venous oxygen contents are derived from blood samples from systemic and pulmonary arteries, respectively. The general Fick equation is used to calculate cardiac output ($\dot{Q}$, in liters per minute):

$$\dot{Q} = \frac{V_{O_2}}{Ca_{O_2} - Cv_{O_2}}$$

In acute respiratory failure, Fick determination of cardiac output is limited primarily by technical inaccuracies in measuring oxygen consumption when the inspired oxygen fraction exceeds 0.6.

Some pulmonary artery catheters permit measurement of cardiac output continuously, using constant detection of temperature changes. One method employs a heated coil (44°C) placed upstream from the thermistor. In most experimental situations, correlation between values from bolus injection and continuous thermodilution methods is good. Advantages of the continuous method include near-continuous availability of cardiac output and derived parameters (e.g., systemic vascular resistance) and reduced errors from manual bolus injection. Disadvantages include interference by intravenous infusions of cool solutions and a response time that renders the method too slow to serve as an instantaneous monitor.

RESPIRATORY MONITORING

In addition to respiratory rate, routine respiratory measurements in the critical setting include assessments of respiratory mechanics, gas exchange, and overall integrated function of the cardiovascular and respiratory systems.

Respiratory Mechanics

Airway pressure measurements are made regularly during mechanical ventilation. *Peak inspiratory pressure* reflects both respiratory system compliance and resistance and therefore depends on tidal volume and flow. Barotrauma has been correlated with peak inspiratory, plateau, and mean airway pressures. In mechanically ventilated patients with obstructive airway disease, especially asthma, deleterious effects of hyperinflation may correlate better with lung volume at end-inspiration above functional residual capacity (FRC) than with any particular pressure. In acute respiratory failure, monitoring of peak inspiratory pressure, intrinsic PEEP, plateau pressure, and mean airway pressure is routinely employed. In the absence of elevated plateau or mean airway pressures, high peak inspiratory pressure, particularly in the presence of high inspiratory flow, is probably of no great concern. However, a source of increased resistance should be sought, such as a kinked or obstructed endotracheal tube or airway narrowing.

Reduced *static respiratory system compliance* characterizes many diffuse parenchymal lung disorders, including pulmonary fibrosis and pulmonary edema (cardiogenic and noncardiogenic). Static respiratory system compliance, normally about 100 mL/cmH$_2$O, may fall below 25 mL/cmH$_2$O in patients with acute lung injury. Accurate measurement depends on accurate determination of tidal volume and static or "plateau" pressure (see Chap. 2). Determination of tidal volume is accomplished by integrating the area under the flow–time curve; flow is measured using a pneumotachograph or ultrasonic flowmeter incorporated into the ventilator circuit.

When intrinsic PEEP is present, end-expiratory pressure measured at the trachea may underestimate alveolar pressure, as resistance between the alveolus and trachea results in slowly emptying areas of lung at low flows (see Chap. 2). Underestimation of end-expiratory pressure results in underestimation of compliance. Measurement of intrinsic PEEP is accomplished by manual occlusion of the expiratory port at end-expiration, or, with modern ventilators, electronically.

Dynamic respiratory system compliance reflects the total impedance to volume change of the respiratory system; it includes static compliance and resistive components. Dynamic compliance is calculated as tidal volume divided by peak inflation pressure. Changes in compliance of the lungs or chest wall or changes in airway resistance (including resistance of the artificial airway) can affect dynamic compliance.

Airway resistance is calculated as the difference between peak inspiratory and plateau pressures divided by flow.

Gas Exchange

Although measurement of arterial blood gas values continues to be critically important in monitoring patients in critical care settings, advances in *pulse oximetry* have revolutionized clinical practice. Reliable interpretation of pulse oximetry data requires careful consideration of the clinical circumstances. Falsely low recordings may be seen with carboxyhemoglobinemia or methemoglobinia, following injection of methylene blue, or in the presence of fingernail polish, onychomycosis, or severe anemia. In acute respiratory failure, pulse oximetry may be inaccurate because of peripheral vasoconstriction from shock or the use of vasopressors.

In critically ill infants, *transcutaneous oxygen (Tc_{O_2}) measurements* are commonplace. Electrodes are placed against skin warmed to 41°C; the heat increases blood flow to cutaneous capillaries, "arterializing" the capillaries. Tc_{O_2} generally provides a reliable estimate of P_{O_2} in neonates. In adults, correlation of Tc_{O_2} with Pa_{O_2} depends on several factors, including age, cardiac output, local perfusion, skin thickness, and various disease states; marked variation in the relationship between Tc_{O_2} and Pa_{O_2} may be observed. Regional differences in peripheral perfusion accompanying acute respiratory failure and adult respiratory distress syndrome (ARDS) make use of trancutaneous oxygen monitoring unreliable in this setting.

Capnography refers to detection of CO_2 in expired gas. Methods employ either mainstream or sidestream sampling of the expirate. Mainstream sampling utilizes a detector in line with the main expiratory circuit. Advantages include rapid response time and large detector diameter, thereby minimizing increases in airway resistance. Drawbacks include the need to manipulate the expiratory circuit directly for cleaning. Sidestream sampling does not interfere with the main breathing circuit and may be used with a nasal cannula in spontaneously breathing patients. Disadvantages include slow response time and a tendency for the small sampling port to become obstructed with secretions. The primary utility of capnography is detection and confirmation of lung ventilation during intubation. In addition, the technique can be used to monitor changes in pulmonary blood flow accompanying thromboembolism or cardiac arrest, in which decreased pulmonary perfusion results in a decrease in CO_2 clearance and increase in the gradient between end-tidal P_{CO_2} and Pa_{CO_2}. End-tidal P_{CO_2} may be used as a surrogate for Pa_{CO_2} in the spontaneously breathing, or mechanically ventilated, healthy patient. However, with cardiovascular instability or lung injury, alterations in the distribution of pulmonary blood flow and dead-space ventilation negate its usefulness.

Measurements of Integrated Cardiovascular and Respiratory Function

Several "oxygen indices" constitute useful measures of the integrated gas exchange and oxygen delivery functions of the lungs and cardiovascular system. Commonly employed measurements or calculations include physiologic shunt fraction, alveolar-arterial oxygen gradient, oxygen transport, mixed venous oxygen saturation, serum lactate level, and gastric tonometry.

Physiologic shunt fraction (Q_S/Q_t), a conceptual representation of the fraction of cardiac output flowing by nonventilated alveoli, is calculated as:

$$\frac{Qs}{Qt} = \frac{Cc_{O_2} - Ca_{O_2}}{Cc_{O_2} - Cv_{O_2}}$$

where Cc_{O_2} is pulmonary capillary oxygen content, Ca_{O_2} is arterial oxygen content, and Cv_{O_2} is mixed venous oxygen content. Pa_{O_2} is used to calculate arterial oxygen content, Pv_{O_2} to calculate venous oxygen content, and alveolar P_{O_2} (from the alveolar air equation) to calculate pulmonary capillary oxygen content. Shunt fraction may be helpful in monitoring a patient with respiratory failure over time, but only if the $F_{I_{O_2}}$ and mixed venous P_{O_2} remain constant and the $F_{I_{O_2}}$ is high.

Unlike shunt fraction, the *alveolar-arterial oxygen gradient* (PA_{O_2}-Pa_{O_2}) may fluctuate in a biphasic manner with $F_{I_{O_2}}$, depending on the degree of actual shunt and $F_{I_{O_2}}$. Increasing $F_{I_{O_2}}$ may decrease PA_{O_2}-Pa_{O_2} in lung regions with variable ventilation/perfusion ratios; PA_{O_2}-Pa_{O_2} increases significantly with increasing $F_{I_{O_2}}$ in the presence of true shunt. In the setting of changing $F_{I_{O_2}}$ requirements, the *alveolar-arterial P_{O_2} ratio and the Pa_{O_2}-$F_{I_{O_2}}$ ratio* have been used as measures of the lung's oxygenating ability. Each shows less fluctuation with $F_{I_{O_2}}$ than does PA_{O_2}-Pa_{O_2}.

Oxygen delivery (D_{O_2}) is the product of cardiac output and arterial oxygen content; the range of normal is 500 to 600 mL/min/m². Therapy aimed at increasing oxygen delivery beyond normal levels has had mixed results, perhaps reflecting different patient populations studied or different strategies in attempting to prevent (vs. reverse) low oxygen consumption.

Some pulmonary artery catheters have *reflectance oximetry* capabilities. The principle underlying their use is based on the assumption that the contribution of dissolved oxygen to oxygen content is negligible and that arterial and venous hemoglobin levels are equal. Any reduction in mixed venous oxygen saturation must result from a reduction in arterial oxygen saturation, an increase in oxygen consumption, or a decrease in cardiac output. Unfortunately, several of these variables may change simultaneously, often with unpredictable results. For example, in some cases of sepsis, a decrease in oxygen consumption may balance reduced oxygen delivery, leading to no change in mixed venous oxygen saturation. The lack of specificity and low sensitivity of the technique limit its usefulness.

Originally believed to be a sensitive and specific marker of tissue hypoxia, *serum lactate* may not be elevated despite severe local ischemia. Conversely, serum lactate may be greatly elevated due to decreased hepatic clearance, even in the absence of anaerobic metabolism. Nonetheless, some authors have noted the poor prognosis associated with a lactate level greater than 10 times the upper limit of normal. In the absence of liver disease, an elevated serum lactate suggests inadequate tissue perfusion. If cardiac output appears adequate, a search for ischemic tissue (e.g., the gut or an extremity) is indicated.

Another method proposed to assess the local balance between tissue oxygen delivery and consumption is *gastric tonometry*. The technique detects intramucosal pH—which, in turn, is directly proportional to splanchnic perfusion. The method says little about states of perfusion of other tissues. Gastric tonometry requires insertion into the stomach of a fluid-filled balloon attached to a nasogastric tube. Equilibration of tissue P_{CO_2} with gas in the gastric lumen occurs; CO_2 passes through the semipermeable balloon wall. Fluid within the balloon is withdrawn and analyzed using a carbon dioxide electrode. Tissue pH is calculated from measured P_{CO_2} and arterial bicarbonate using the Henderson-Hasselbalch equation. Gastric tonometry correlates with other measures of splanchnic perfusion. Limitations include falsely low mucosal pH when arterial bicarbonate is low (e.g., in non–anion gap metabolic acidosis) and decreased clearance of carbon dioxide from low blood flow.

BIBLIOGRAPHY

Bernard GR, Sopko G, Cerra F, et al: Pulmonary artery catheterization and clinical outcomes: National Heart, Lung, and Blood Institute and Food and Drug Administration Workshop Report. Consensus Statement. Consensus Development Conference. *JAMA* 283:2568–2572, 2000.

Fegler G: Measurement of cardiac output in anaesthetized animals by a thermo-dilution method. *Q J Exp Physiol* 39:153–164, 1954.

Haller M, Zollner C, Briegel J, Forst H: Evaluation of a new continuous thermodilution cardiac output monitor in critically ill patients: A prospective criterion standard study. *Crit Care Med* 23:860–866, 1995.

Ivanov R, Allen J, Calvin JE: The incidence of major morbidity in critically ill patients managed with pulmonary artery catheters: A meta-analysis. *Crit Care Med* 28: 615–619, 2000.

Marini JJ: Lung mechanics in the adult respiratory distress syndrome—Recent conceptual advances and implications for management. *Clin Chest Med* 11:673–690, 1990.

Saarela E, Kari A, Nikki P, et al: Current practice regarding invasive monitoring in intensive care units in Finland: A nationwide study of the uses of arterial, pulmonary artery and central venous catheters and their effect on outcome. *Intens Care Med* 17:264–271, 1991.

75 | Mechanical Ventilation*

Michael A. Grippi

INTRODUCTION

The modern era of mechanical ventilation began in the 1950s, during the poliomyelitis epidemic. Although ventilators have become much more sophisticated over the last several decades, the objectives of mechanical ventilation remain the same: relief of dyspnea, improvement in respiratory mechanics and pulmonary gas exchange, and facilitation of lung and airway healing.

While mild or moderate hypoxemia can be managed by administration of oxygen through a face mask, treatment of severe hypoxemia usually necessitates intubation. Positive-pressure ventilation recruits collapsed lung units and improves matching of ventilation, perfusion, and oxygenation. Furthermore, many patients who benefit from mechanical ventilation have relatively normal arterial blood gases but also have clinical signs of increased work of breathing. These patients are at risk of developing respiratory muscle fatigue. Increased respiratory work increases the O_2 cost of breathing to account for as much as 50 percent of total O_2 consumption. In such circumstances, mechanical ventilation decreases the work of breathing.

TRADITIONAL MODES OF MECHANICAL VENTILATION

The following represent "traditional" modes of mechanical ventilation.

Controlled Mechanical Ventilation

In controlled mechanical ventilation (CMV), the ventilatory rate is preset; the patient cannot trigger the machine. In the volume-targeted mode, the breaths have a preset volume (*volume-controlled* ventilation); in the *pressure-controlled* mode, the breaths are pressure-limited and time-cycled. Volume-controlled ventilation is now uncommonly used and largely restricted to apneic patients.

Assist-Control Ventilation

In the *assist-control* (AC) mode, the ventilator delivers a breath when triggered by the patient's inspiratory effort, or does so independently when the effort does not occur within a preselected time period; the patient's triggering rate may exceed the preset rate. If the spontaneous rate drops below the preset backup rate, controlled ventilation is provided. The ventilator cycles off when the preset tidal volume is reached. The amount of active work performed by a patient ventilated in the AC mode depends on the trigger sensitivity and inspiratory flow settings.

*Edited from Chaps. 176 and 177, "Mechanical Ventilation: Conventional Modes and Settings," by Tobin MJ, and "Mechanical Ventilation: Physiological Considerations and New Ventilatory Techniques," by Marini JJ. In: *Pulmonary Diseases and Disorders,* 3rd ed., edited by Fishman AP, Elias JA, Fishman JA, Grippi MA, Kaiser LR, Senior RM. New York, McGraw-Hill, 1998, pp 2691–2708, 2709–2726. For further discussion of topics dealt with in this chapter, the reader is referred to the original text, as noted above.

Intermittent Mandatory Ventilation

With *intermittent mandatory ventilation* (IMV), the patient receives periodic positive-pressure breaths from the ventilator at a preset volume and rate, but the patient can also breathe spontaneously between mandatory breaths. Synchronization of patient inspiratory effort and machine-delivered breaths is achieved by incorporation of a patient-triggered demand valve. The valve allows delivery of a machine breath if the patient makes an inspiratory effort while a timing window is open (Fig. 75-1). If no effort occurs by the time the window closes, the ventilator delivers a controlled positive-pressure breath.

Compared with controlled mechanical ventilation, IMV is associated with a lower incidence of barotrauma and, when left ventricular function is normal, a higher cardiac output (because of increased venous return during spontaneous breaths). With poor left ventricular function, cardiac output is lower with IMV because of the negative intrathoracic pressure–associated increase in left ventricular afterload (the predominant effect with poor cardiac reserve). Inspiratory effort appears equivalent for spontaneous and assisted breaths during IMV. Respiratory center output may be preset, fixed, and insensitive to breath-to-breath changes in mechanical load, as occur during IMV. As a result, IMV may potentiate respiratory muscle fatigue or prevent its recovery.

Pressure Support Ventilation

Pressure support (PS) ventilation is patient-triggered but pressure-targeted and flow-cycled. The clinician sets the level of pressure that augments every spontaneous breath, but the patient can alter respiratory frequency, inspiratory time, and tidal volume. The pressure setting, patient effort, and pulmonary mechanics determine tidal volume. The absence of patient effort can result in apnea.

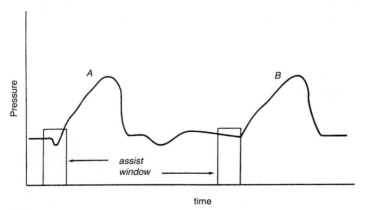

FIG. 75-1   Synchronization of intermittent mandatory ventilation (IMV) through use of an assist window. If the patient makes an effort during a window of time, the ventilator senses this effort and delivers a breath in synchrony with the patient's effort (A). If no effort is made while the window is open, a controlled breath is delivered (B). (From Kacmarek RM, Hess D: Basic principles of ventilator machinery, in Tobin MJ (ed), *Principles and Practice of Mechanical Ventilation.* New York, McGraw-Hill, 1994, pp 65–110, with permission.)

Exhalation is triggered by a decrease in inspiratory flow to a preset level, designated in terms of an absolute flow or percent of peak inspiratory flow.

Noninvasive Positive-Pressure Ventilation

Noninvasive positive-pressure ventilation (NIPPV) can sometimes be used in patients who are able to cooperate and follow instructions; it should not be used following respiratory arrest, with hypotension or uncontrolled arrhythmias, or with excessive secretions or high risk of aspiration. Success appears more likely if NIPPV is used early in the progression of acute respiratory failure. Patients who do well with NIPPV typically show considerable improvement within the first hour of therapy. Facial discomfort and trauma, including skin ulceration (especially over the bridge of the nose), and lack of direct access to the patient's airway generally limit continuous use of NIPPV to 1 to 2 days. An excessive leak at the bridge of the nose causes intolerance as a result of air blowing into the patient's eyes. If patients complain of excessive nasal dryness, humidification can be added; rhinorrhea can be reduced by use of ipratropium bromide nasal drops; nasal blockage may respond to ephedrine nasal drops. A chin strap can be used when there is a large leak through the mouth. Aerophagia and gastric distension can occur, especially in those who breathe out of synchrony with the ventilator. If these problems are suspected, a nasogastric tube should be inserted.

STANDARD VENTILATOR SETTINGS

Ventilator settings are based on the patient's size and underlying clinical status.

Trigger Sensitivity

With most mechanical ventilators, a decrease in circuit pressure triggers a machine-delivered breath. A trigger setting more sensitive than 1 to 2 cmH_2O frequently causes ventilator autocycling; a less sensitive setting increases the work of breathing significantly. With increased end-expiratory lung volume, the patient must first generate sufficient pressure to offset the elastic recoil associated with hyperinflation and then overcome the sensitivity threshold of the ventilator.

Tidal Volume

While use of tidal volumes in the range of 10 to 15 mL/kg had been used routinely in the past, recent studies in acute lung injury indicate that alveolar overdistention may produce endothelial, epithelial, and basement-membrane injuries associated with increased microvascular permeability. The new ventilator strategy in acute lung injury calls for use of smaller tidal volumes (4 to 8 mL/kg) to achieve plateau pressures no higher than 35 cmH_2O. Although Pa_{CO_2} is likely to rise under such circumstances, the increase is permitted (*permissive hypercapnia*), and the clinical focus is the pH, rather than the Pa_{CO_2}. If the pH falls below 7.20, some recommend use of intravenous bicarbonate (an unproved and controversial approach).

Respiratory Rate

The optimal ventilator rate depends on the mode of ventilation. With AC ventilation, the ventilator supplies a breath in response to each patient effort.

If the patient has a sudden decrease in respiratory center output, a low machine rate results in hypoventilation. In addition, if a large discrepancy exists between the patient's spontaneous rate and the machine's back-up rate, a respiratory cycle with an inverse inspiratory-to-expiratory time (I:E) ratio arises. Inverse-ratio ventilation is uncomfortable and usually necessitates increased sedation or neuromuscular blockade. With AC ventilation, the backup rate should be set approximately 4 breaths less than the patient's spontaneous rate.

With IMV, the ventilator or mandatory rate is initially set high and then gradually reduced according to patient tolerance. Unfortunately, titration is often based on data from arterial blood gases. Even a small number of ventilator breaths will result in acceptable values for Pa_{O_2} and Pa_{CO_2} but will achieve little or no respiratory muscle rest in patients with increased work of breathing. In ventilator-dependent patients, work of breathing at IMV rates of 14 breaths per minute or less may be sufficient to induce respiratory muscle fatigue.

Inspiratory Flow Rate

In most patients receiving AC ventilation or IMV, the initial inspiratory flow is set at 60 L/min. In chronic obstructive pulmonary disease (COPD), increasing the flow to 100 L/min produces better gas exchange, as reflected by decreases in venous admixture and V_D/V_T, probably as a result of more complete emptying of "slow spaces" due to increased expiratory time. A high inspiratory flow setting is also needed for patients with increased respiratory drive. Otherwise, the delivered flow may be insufficient to meet a patient's ventilatory requirements and result in increased work of breathing.

Fractional Inspired Oxygen Concentration ($F_{I_{O_2}}$)

Initially, $F_{I_{O_2}}$ is set at a high value, often 1.0, to ensure adequate oxygenation. Thereafter, the lowest $F_{I_{O_2}}$ that achieves satisfactory arterial oxygenation should be selected. The usual target is a Pa_{O_2} of 60 mmHg or an arterial saturation (Sa_{O_2}) of 90%; higher values do not substantially enhance tissue oxygenation. Due to the potential of O_2 toxicity, the clinical strategy is to reduce the $F_{I_{O_2}}$ to the lowest level compatible with adequate systemic oxygenation. Although excessive O_2 administration should be avoided, there is more to fear from severe hypoxemia than from the potential damage that might result from hyperoxia.

Positive End-Expiratory Pressure (PEEP)

PEEP is typically used in the setting of diffuse lung injury in an attempt to reduce the required $F_{I_{O_2}}$. Beneficial effects include improved arterial oxygenation, enhanced lung compliance, reduced work of breathing due to auto-PEEP (see below) in patients with airflow limitation, and, possibly, decreased lung injury from repeated alveolar collapse and reopening. The major mechanism for the increase in Pa_{O_2} with PEEP is an increase in end-expiratory lung volume. If cardiac output decreases disproportionally more than Pa_{O_2} increases, PEEP results in an overall decrease in delivery of O_2 to tissues.

Auto-PEEP, the difference between alveolar pressure and the set airway pressure at end-exhalation, is most commonly observed with dynamic hyperinflation due to severe airflow obstruction. It can be measured during passive ventilation as the difference between end-expiratory airway occlusion pressure (total PEEP) and the set level of PEEP. The lung distention caused by auto-PEEP increases the risk for barotrauma and may cause cardiovascular instability and increased work of breathing. By reducing right ventricular preload and increasing right ventricular afterload, alveolar overdistention can reduce left ventricular filling and impair cardiac output. In addition, dynamic hyperinflation increases respiratory muscle oxygen demands during spontaneous ventilation and increases the ventilating pressures required during machine-assisted breathing.

NEWER MODES OF VENTILATORY SUPPORT

A number of new ventilatory techniques may find clinical use in treatment of respiratory failure.

High-Frequency Ventilation

With *high-frequency ventilation* (HFV), CO_2 elimination is effected using tidal volumes smaller than the anatomic dead space. The lower peak airway pressures and tidal volume excursions may reduce the risks of barotrauma. The two types of HFV devices in clinical use are jet ventilators and oscillators. With jet ventilation, a high-velocity stream of humidified gas is directed phasically and at rapid frequencies into the endotracheal tube, entraining additional fresh gas during each insufflation. Current indications for its use include bronchoscopy, upper airway surgery, and some cases of bronchopleural fistulas. High-frequency oscillation has been used primarily in infants. The airway gas column is caused to vibrate in a semiclosed system at frequencies exceeding those used in jet ventilation. Fresh gas is directed across the external breathing circuit. Oscillatory vibrations facilitate gas exchange largely by nonconvective mechanisms (e.g., through facilitated diffusion).

Airway Pressure Release Ventilation

In *airway pressure release ventilation* (APRV), mean airway pressure is elevated by maintaining a moderately high level of CPAP. Periodic, rapid depressurization of the airway allows exhalation, which is followed by replacement with fresh gas as the baseline level of CPAP is reestablished.

Proportional-Assist Ventilation

With *proportional-assist ventilation* (PAV), the power output of the ventilator is adjusted by the clinician to offset flow-resistive or elastic pressure breathing requirements. Pressure assistance by the machine is proportional to a variable combination of inspired volume (the elastic assist) and inspiratory flow (the resistive or frictional assist). Proportionality is accomplished by monitoring flow and volume, the two key components of the simplified equation of motion of the respiratory system that describes the inspiratory pressure (P) across the respiratory system. PAV couples the ventilator's output with the patient's neuromuscular control mechanisms and continuously changing ventilatory needs. Tidal volume and flow are fully controlled by the patient, and the "gain factors" determining the elastic and flow-resistive assist proportions are the independent variables. When the patient inspires harder, the machine boosts its output; as the patient relaxes, the machine cuts back in parallel.

Extracorporeal Techniques: Membrane Oxygenation and CO_2 Elimination

The first extracorporeal circuits for gas exchange used venoarterial bypass intended primarily to accomplish oxygen transfer in support of acute lung injury. To significantly enhance arterial oxygenation, a large fraction of the total cardiac output must be diverted to the membrane oxygenator. *Extracorporeal membrane oxygenation* (ECMO) allows major reductions of supplemental oxygen and ventilator inflation pressure, but it is a resource-intensive procedure.

The primary objective of venovenous *extracorporeal CO_2 removal* (ECCO$_2$R) is to rest the lungs. A highly efficient membrane clears almost all CO_2 from a much smaller blood flow than ECMO requires (approximately 25 percent of the total cardiac output). Unlike ECMO, ECCO$_2$R directs all venous return, diverted and undiverted, through the lung, where most oxygen exchange continues to occur. With ECCO$_2$R, circulating volume can easily and quickly be adjusted by ultrafiltration. ECCO$_2$R is extremely effective in reducing the lung's exposure to injurious airway pressures.

Intravenous Gas Exchange

With *intravenous gas exchange* (IVOX), a large-diameter venacaval catheter composed of numerous hollow fibers effects substantial O_2 and CO_2 exchange intravenously, external to the native lungs. As oxygen is drawn through the fibers and past venous blood en route to the right heart, gas exchange takes place across the gas-permeable walls of fibers. Unfortunately, the results of the first large-scale clinical studies of IVOX have been disappointing.

Tracheal Gas Insufflation

Tracheal gas insufflation (TGI) is a technique in which the anatomic dead space of the upper airway is reduced or bypassed by continuous or phasic injection of fresh gas near the carina. Most benefit is derived from use of modest flows of fresh gas and appears to be greatest when the anatomic component exceeds the alveolar component of the physiological dead space. For the present, the technique remains experimental.

Independent (Differential) Lung Ventilation

Differential or *independent lung ventilation* (ILV) is based on separate ventilation to each lung using a cuffed, double-lumen endotracheal tube. Levels of ventilation, inspired oxygen, and end-expiratory pressure appropriate to each lung can be individually adjusted, improving O_2 and CO_2 exchange. However, double-lumen tubes usually require bronchoscopy for correct placement, and tube movement can result in occlusion of a major bronchus or failure of lung isolation. Nasal intubation is not feasible, and deep sedation is invariably required.

Inverse-Ratio Ventilation

With *inverse-ratio ventilation* (IRV), the inspiratory period is set to more than half the respiratory cycle time. Improved oxygenation may be due to increases in alveolar pressure and lung volume, development of auto-PEEP, or recruitment of collapsed alveolar units or units with long time constants. Clinically utilized inverse ratios range from 1:1 to 4:1. At more extreme ratios, hemodynamic instability and the potential for barotrauma increase significantly.

Partial Liquid Ventilation

An exciting approach to recruitment of collapsed lung units is to fill the units with a gas-exchanging liquid perfluorocarbon (PFC). Full liquid breathing would be exceedingly difficult to implement clinically. *Partial liquid ventilation,* however, is feasible. With partial liquid ventilation, routine tidal gas ventilation is performed using a conventional ventilator and a PFC which partially or completely fills the functional residual capacity. PFCs dissolve considerable volumes of O_2 and CO_2; they distribute easily throughout the lung and gravitate to the lung regions most at risk for airway closure and alveolar collapse. The risks, indications, doses, and appropriate methods for implementing partial liquid ventilation have yet to be fully elucidated.

VENTILATOR-INDUCED LUNG DAMAGE

Ventilator-induced lung damage includes pneumothorax, interstitial emphysema, and tension cysts. A more recently recognized entity is endothelial and epithelial damage and resultant edema formation, which occurs as a result of alveolar overdistention in the setting of underlying acute lung injury.

The exact safe upper limit for tidal transalveolar ("transpulmonary") pressure is unknown. Based on experimental data, limiting it to approximately 30 cmH_2O (or limiting the inspiratory plateau pressure to 35 cmH_2O) seems reasonable. Peak tidal alveolar pressures as low as 30 cmH_2O applied for several days can produce diffuse alveolar damage in experimental animals. Transpulmonary (transalveolar) pressures higher than those corresponding to total lung capacity (approximately 30 to 35 cmH_2O) create excessive alveolar stress; fragile alveoli may undergo endothelial separation, increased permeability, capillary stress fractures, or overt rupture, at even lower pressures.

WEANING

About one-quarter of patients fail initial attempts at discontinuing mechanical ventilation. Weaning failure most commonly results from respiratory muscle dysfunction, problems with oxygenation, or psychological difficulties. Respiratory muscle dysfunction results from an imbalance between respiratory neuromuscular capacity and the mechanical load on the respiratory system. Hypoxemia is less commonly a primary cause of weaning failure, perhaps because weaning is usually not attempted in patients who are significantly hypoxemic or at risk for hypoxemia.

Initiation of Weaning

A basic tenet of weaning is that the underlying condition necessitating mechanical ventilation has been reversed. A variety of bedside tests may helpful in predicting the chance of a successful wean.

In general, cardiopulmonary instability or persistent hypoxemia (e.g., Pa_{O_2} less than 55 mmHg with $F_{I_{O_2}}$ of 0.40 or higher) mitigate against initiation of weaning. Many patients fail attempts at weaning despite satisfactory oxygenation. A minute ventilation of less than 10 L/min has been used as a standard weaning parameter, as has a maximal inspiratory pressure of at least -20 cmH_2O (preferably, -30 cmH_2O). More recently, assessment for rapid shallow breathing has proved useful in deciding when to attempt weaning. Rapid shallow breathing can be quantitated as the *respiratory frequency–tidal volume ratio* (f/V_T). A value less than 100 breaths per minute per liter indicates that rapid shallow breathing is absent and that weaning is likely to be successful (Fig. 75-2).

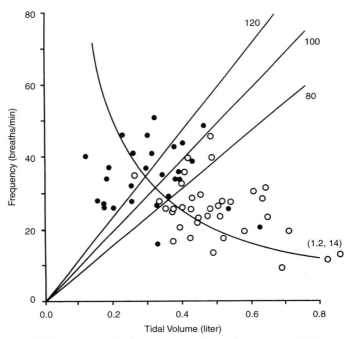

FIG. 75-2 Isopleths for the ratio of respiratory frequency to tidal volume (f/VT), each representing different degrees of rapid shallow breathing. Patients who fell to the left of the 100 breaths per minute per liter isopleth had a 95 percent likelihood of failing a weaning trial, whereas patients who fell to the right of this isopleth had an 80 percent likelihood of a successful weaning outcome. The hyperbola represents a minute ventilation of 10 L/min, a criterion commonly used to predict weaning outcome; clearly this criterion was of little value in discriminating between patients who were successfully weaned (open circles) and those who failed weaning (solid circles). Values for one patient (VT = 1.2 L, f = 14 breaths per minute) lay outside the graph. (From Yang KL and Tobin MJ: A prospective study of indexes predicting the outcome of trials of weaning from mechanical ventilation. *N Engl J Med* 324:1445–1450, 1991, with permission.)

Weaning Techniques

IMV and PS ventilation are the most popular methods of weaning. With IMV-based weaning, the ventilator rate is reduced in steps of one to three breaths per minute, and an arterial blood gas is obtained approximately 30 min following each change. Unfortunately, adjusting the IMV rate based on results of arterial blood gases may result in a false sense of security. Several positive-pressure breaths per minute can effect acceptable blood gases and may obscure the patient's true work of breathing, which may be excessive.

When PS ventilation is used for weaning, the level of pressure is reduced gradually, in decrements of 3 to 6 cmH$_2$O, and is titrated on the basis of respiratory frequency. PS ventilation can be used to counteract the work of breathing imposed by the endotracheal tube and ventilator circuit. Consequently, the notion has arisen that if a patient can sustain spontaneous ventilation at this "compensatory level" of pressure support, successful extubation is likely. Unfortunately, there is no reliable method for accurately determining the required level of compensatory pressure support in an individual patient.

The oldest method of weaning involves the use of spontaneous breathing trials of increasing duration several times daily. Brief trials (e.g., 5 min) are gradually increased in accordance with the patient's performance, as assessed clinically. The patient is rested for several hours between trials. When the patient is able to sustain spontaneous ventilation for 1 to 2 h, extubation is performed.

Finally, another method of weaning is to employ a single daily trial of spontaneous breathing through a T-tube circuit. The trial is conducted while the physician is in the intensive care unit. If the patient can sustain spontaneous ventilation for 30 to 60 min without undue distress, he or she is extubated. If the patient develops signs of distress on physical examination, the trial is stopped and mechanical ventilation is reinstituted. A weaning strategy based on a once-daily trial of spontaneous breathing simplifies patient management.

Extubation

Patients who can sustain spontaneous ventilation without distress may have difficulty following extubation owing to upper airway obstruction, inability to protect the upper airway, or inability to clear secretions. In contrast to the many parameters that have been introduced to predict the outcome of a weaning trial, indices that reliably predict the likelihood of complications following extubation have not been developed. Instead, evaluation consists of clinical assessment of factors such as the patient's level of consciousness, volume of secretions, and ability to cough.

BIBLIOGRAPHY

Acute Respiratory Distress Syndrome Network: Ventilation with lower tidal volumes as compared with traditional tidal volumes for acute lung injury and the acute respiratory distress syndrome. *N Engl J Med* 342:1301–1308, 2000.

Brochard L: Pressure support ventilation, in Tobin MJ (ed): *Principles and Practice of Mechanical Ventilation.* New York, McGraw-Hill, 1994, pp 239–257.

Brochard L, Mancebo J, Wysocki M, et al: Noninvasive ventilation for acute exacerbations of chronic obstructive pulmonary disease. *N Engl J Med* 333:817–822, 1995.

Esteban A, Frutos F, Tobin MJ, et al: A comparison of four methods of weaning patients from mechanical ventilation. *N Engl J Med* 332:345–350, 1995.

Gammon RB, Shin MS, Groves RH Jr, et al: Clinical risk factors for pulmonary barotrauma: A multivariate analysis. *Am J Respir Crit Care Med* 152:1235–1240, 1995.

Gattinoni L, Pelosi P, Crotti S, Valenza F: Effects of positive end-expiratory pressure on regional distribution of tidal volume and recruitment in adult respiratory distress syndrome. *Am J Respir Crit Care Med* 152:1807–1814, 1995.

Marini JJ: Evolving concepts in the ventilatory management of ARDS. *Clin Chest Med* 17:555–575, 1996.

Sandur S, Stoller JK: Pulmonary complications of mechanical ventilation. *Clin Chest Med* 20:223–247, 1999.

Tobin MJ: Mechanical ventilation. *N Engl J Med* 330:1056–1061, 1994.

Villar J, Winston B, Slutsky AS: Non-conventional techniques of ventilatory support. *Crit Care Clin* 6:579–603, 1990.

Yang KL, Tobin MJ: A prospective study of indexes predicting the outcome of trials of weaning from mechanical ventilation. *N Engl J Med* 324:1445–1450, 1991.

76 | Nutrition in Acute Respiratory Failure*

Lisa M. Bellini

INTRODUCTION

Nutrition is an important aspect of the care of all critically ill patients, particularly those with acute respiratory failure. *Nutritional status* is assessed by whether or not malnutrition is present; *hypermetabolism* is the degree of excess metabolic activity in a disease state. Clinical prototypes based on these nutritional considerations in acute respiratory failure include the patient with severe chronic obstructive pulmonary disease (COPD) who is malnourished but not hypermetabolic and the septic patient with acute respiratory distress syndrome (ARDS) who is well nourished but extremely hypermetabolic.

CONSEQUENCES OF MALNUTRITION

In fasting humans, glycogen, protein, and fat stores represent potential energy sources. Glycogen stores are limited and are expended within 1 to 3 days of fasting. While body proteins represent a large potential energy source, their nonfuel functions necessitate their conservation. Hence, starvation involves adaptive mechanisms by which fat and fat-derived fuels become the major energy sources, glucose utilization is reduced, and protein is conserved.

In critical illness, protein, particularly that derived from muscle, is catabolized for energy production. Respiratory muscles, including the diaphragm and intercostals, are susceptible to this catabolic requirement. Malnutrition reduces diaphragm strength, maximal voluntary ventilation, and vital capacity. Starvation causes a parallel fall in metabolic rate and hypoxic ventilatory response. The ventilatory response returns to normal with refeeding. Consequences of decreased respiratory strength and ventilatory drive in respiratory disease may include impaired cough, increased risk of atelectasis and pneumonia, and prolonged mechanical ventilation in the setting of acute respiratory failure.

Protein-calorie malnutrition is one of the most frequent causes of acquired immunodeficiency. Chemotaxis, opsonization, and phagocytosis usually remain normal or are mildly depressed; intracellular killing is decreased. The thymus, spleen, and lymph nodes become markedly atrophic, and lymphocyte numbers may decrease. Although immunoglobulin levels remain normal or are slightly increased, antibody responses may be depressed. Consequences of altered immune function include increased respiratory infections, such as pneumonia.

*Edited from Chap. 178, "Nutrition in Acute Respiratory Failure," by Pingleton SK. In: *Fishman's Pulmonary Diseases and Disorders,* 3d ed., edited by Fishman AP, Elias JA, Fishman JA, Grippi MA, Kaiser LR, Senior RM. New York, McGraw-Hill, 1998, pp 2727–2738. For fuller discussion of topics dealt with in this chapter, the reader is referred to the original text, as noted above.

MALNUTRITION IN COPD

The effect of nutritional status on respiratory muscle function in COPD is controversial. In COPD, inspiratory muscle weakness results from the mechanical disadvantage at which inspiratory muscles are placed due to hyperinflation and, perhaps, generalized muscle weakness. The potential additive role of undernutrition in causing inspiratory muscle weakness is debated. In addition to diminished muscle mass and hyperinflation, other nutritional factors may reduce diaphragm strength, including hypophosphatemia, hypocalcemia, and hypomagnesemia.

As many as 25 percent of patients with COPD are malnourished. Almost 50 percent of hospitalized patients with COPD have evidence of malnutrition; in critically ill patients with COPD and acute respiratory failure, the incidence is 60 percent. Fifty percent of patients with COPD with either chronic hypoxemia or normoxemia with severe airflow obstruction (FEV_1 <35%) demonstrate malnutrition; the incidence is 25 percent with moderate airflow obstruction.

Hypercapnia is found in the majority of patients with COPD when inspiratory pressures are less than one-half of normal. Hypercapnia occurs with much less respiratory muscle weakness in the presence of other mechanical abnormalities. Dyspnea may worsen with malnutrition in the spontaneously breathing patient with COPD. Hypercapnic respiratory failure may be precipitated by malnutrition, and weaning from mechanical ventilation is made more difficult compared with the nonmalnourished patient with COPD.

Nutritional repletion can improve diminished respiratory muscle strength. Intensive, nocturnal, enterally administered nutrition can result in weight gain and improved respiratory muscle and pulmonary function. The mechanisms underlying improved muscle performance with supplemental nutrition are not clear.

MALNUTRITION IN ARDS

Although patients with ARDS may be hypermetabolic during any phase of their illness, hypermetabolism in ARDS is most commonly associated with infection, especially sepsis. When ARDS is a component of multiple system organ failure (MSOF) syndrome, clinical symptoms and signs of hypermetabolism are common.

The characteristic metabolic responses to injury or severe infection include changes in carbohydrate, fat, and protein metabolism not normally seen in simple starvation. Increased glucocorticoid and glucagon levels stimulate gluconeogenesis at the expense of lean body tissues, predominantly skeletal muscle. Protein synthesis is increased, although the rate of catabolism is also accelerated. Net protein loss, manifest as high urinary nitrogen excretion and low serum visceral protein concentrations, is observed. The starved patient loses approximately 75 g of muscle protein per day, or about 200 to 300 g of muscle tissue daily. The stressed patient can lose as much as 250 g of muscle protein, or 750 to 1000 g of muscle mass each day. With an increase in protein catabolism, energy needs are met by deamination of amino acids, which provide carbon skeletons for glucose production at sites of gluconeogenesis. Ineffective peripheral utilization of glucose occurs, evident as elevated plasma glucose despite normal or elevated levels of insulin. Fatty acids are utilized increasingly for fuel. The magnitude of these abnormalities is directly proportional to the extent of injury.

The metabolic state following injury includes "ebb" and "flow" phases. The ebb phase is a period of initial metabolic dormancy, characterized by decreased oxygen consumption, inadequate circulation, and fluid imbalance. Lasting 24 to 36 h, the ebb phase gives way to a metabolic peak or flow phase, which is a hyperdynamic period in which substrates are mobilized for energy production. Increased cellular activity and hormonal stimulation characterize the flow phase. Metabolic rate increases, body temperature rises, and nitrogen loss accelerates. Clinical signs include increased cardiac output, tachycardia, bounding peripheral pulses, and widened pulse pressure. In hypermetabolic patients, both cardiac index and oxygen consumption are proportional to severity of illness. Hypermetabolic patients are generally febrile; an increase in body temperature is associated with an increase in metabolic rate of approximately 10 percent per degree above 37°C. Hypermetabolic patients have increased metabolic expenditure and, therefore, increased energy (caloric) needs.

Upregulation of metabolism in the stressed patient is at least partly regulated by hormonal and inflammatory mediators. Inadequate insulin levels and elevated levels of glucagon, glucocorticoids, and catecholamines generate glucose at the expense of nitrogen stores (i.e., protein catabolism occurs). Hyperglycemia and insulin resistance follow. The hypothalamic-pituitary axis is stimulated. Growth hormone augments the insulin response to glucose mobilization and use of fat stores and improves nitrogen balance. In addition to the alterations in hormonally mediated processes, multiple inflammatory mediators promote hypermetabolism.

NUTRITIONAL ASSESSMENT

The clinical utility of nutritional assessment in intensive care settings is limited to identification of patients in whom malnutrition is suspected upon admission. Nutritional assessment techniques are much less helpful during the course of a critical illness but include evaluation of clinical, anthropometric, chemical, and immunologic parameters that reflect altered body composition.

Loss of body weight universally accompanies protein-calorie malnutrition and provides an indication of altered nutritional status. Weight loss in excess of 10 percent of ideal body weight suggests malnutrition. Unfortunately, many critically ill patients are edematous, and measured weight does not reflect the real body cell mass.

Hepatic secretory proteins, such as albumin, transferrin, retinol-binding protein, and prealbumin, are markers of visceral protein stores and are used in nutritional assessment. Hepatic protein production is influenced by numerous factors in addition to nutritional status, including hepatic dysfunction, protein-losing states, acute infection, and inflammation. Frequent coexistence of these conditions in critically ill patients limits their use as markers of nutritional deficiency or the effectiveness of nutritional support.

Anthropometry involves measurement of skinfold thickness, body circumferences, and skeletal breadths to determine the body's proportions of fat, muscle tissue, and skeletal mass. Primary advantages of anthropometry over more complex body composition measurements include simplicity, safety, cost, and widespread applicability. Although techniques of measurement are standardized, interpretation of results remains controversial and of limited value in the critical care setting.

The *creatinine-height index* is a theoretic estimate of lean body mass derived from measurement of the 24-h urinary creatinine excretion, compared to standard values based on height. Limitations include the effects of age, diet, exercise, stress, and renal disease on interpretation of the index.

Cellular immunity and *delayed cutaneous hypersensitivity* are commonly tested by assessing recall to skin-test antigens, such as *Candida,* mumps, *Trichophyton,* and streptokinase-streptodornase. Depression of cellular immunity is seen consistently in malnutrition; nutritional repletion is associated with improved immunocompetence. In critically ill patients, utility of skin testing is limited by multiple factors, e.g., sepsis, malignancy, radiotherapy, chemotherapy, burns, and other immunocompromising conditions.

Multiparameter nutritional indexes have been proposed in an attempt to overcome the difficulties with sensitivity and specificity of single tests of nutritional assessment. The *prognostic nutritional index* (PNI) is a mathematical formula that combines measurements of serum albumin, triceps skinfold thickness, transferrin levels, and measurement of delayed hypersensitivity skin testing. The PNI may predict major morbidity in surgical patients, but its utility in critically ill medical patients has been less well studied.

Muscle function tests have also been used as markers of nutritional status. Clinical investigations have focused on assessment of the abductor pollicis, handgrip dynamometry, and respiratory muscle strength. Limitations of these techniques in the critical care setting include the need for an awake, alert patient, metabolic factors, such as hypercapnia and hypoxia, use of medications, and intrinsic muscle disease.

ASSESSMENT OF NUTRITIONAL REQUIREMENTS

General indications for nutritional support in any critically ill patient include inadequate or absent oral intake, malnutrition, or anticipated prolonged clinical course. In acute respiratory failure, the need for mechanical ventilation is often the first consideration in assessment of nutritional support.

General nutritional goals include attaining and maintaining energy (calorie) requirements and nitrogen balance. Energy balance is achieved when sufficient calories are provided to equal energy expenditure. Positive nitrogen balance occurs when protein is supplied at a rate to balance protein catabolic rate. To avoid nutritional depletion, total calories in an amount that approximates total energy expenditure should be provided. *Total energy expenditure* (TEE) is the amount of energy in calories consumed in a 24-h period. Several methods exist for estimating TEE. Some are based on calculations using formulas or nomograms; others are derived from measurements of energy expenditure.

An estimate of basal metabolic rate based on *resting energy expenditure* (REE) can be obtained using the *Harris-Benedict equation,* which relates energy expenditure to sex, weight (W, in kilograms), height (H, in centimeters), and age (A, in years).

$$REE \text{ (males)} = 66.47 + 13.75 \text{ (W)} + 5.0 \text{ (H)} - 6.76 \text{ (A)}$$
$$REE \text{ (females)} = 655.1 + 9.56 \text{ (W)} + 1.7 \text{ (H)} - 4.68 \text{ (A)}$$

A "stress factor" or percent increase in energy requirement based on severity of the patient's illness is then added to this determination; TEE is calculated as REE plus the stress factor. Stress factors are based on estimated metabolic needs beyond resting need; they vary with body temperature, degree of physical activity, and extent of injury. Most critically ill patients with respiratory disease have an average stress factor of 1.2. Severely nutritionally depleted or starved patients with COPD may have a smaller stress factor, or no stress factor at all if they are receiving totally controlled ventilation. Severely hypermetabolic patients with acute respiratory failure may have a stress factor of 1.2 to 1.4 during periods of hypermetabolism. The utility of the Harris-Benedict equation in clinical practice is controversial. Caloric needs may be inaccurate, and overestimation of caloric requirements has been noted. However, application of the equation remains a relatively simple method of estimating caloric requirements.

The most accurate method of determining energy requirements is indirect measurement of actual energy expenditure using a metabolic cart. Caloric requirements are assessed by measuring the rate of oxygen consumption; each liter of oxygen consumed represents approximately 4 to 5 kcal. Metabolic carts can be used to measure oxygen consumption in both mechanically ventilated and spontaneously breathing patients, but they are expensive and require technical expertise and stringent conditions not typically present in critical care settings.

Energy expenditure can also be measured using a pulmonary artery catheter by assessing the rate of oxygen consumption from the measured cardiac output (using thermodilution technique) and the oxygen content difference between arterial and mixed venous blood (see Chap. 74).

SUPPLEMENTAL NUTRITION IN COPD

Malnourished, spontaneously breathing patients with COPD have increased resting energy requirements; values are approximately 15 percent above those predicted by the Harris-Benedict equation, representing a far greater energy requirement than that of malnourished patients without COPD. This is due to the increased energy needs of the ventilatory muscles, which can be approximated from assessment of the severity of lung hyperinflation. Energy requirements in COPD depend on whether the patient is breathing spontaneously or is mechanically ventilated. Calculation of nutritional requirements in the spontaneously breathing patient with COPD should also consider the limitations that such patients have in augmenting caloric intake due to early satiety, anorexia, bloating, and fatigue.

Once total energy requirements are determined, the nutritional substrate mix must be considered (i.e., the percentage of total calories supplied as carbohydrate, fat, and protein). Protein (nitrogen) requirements in pulmonary disease are not significantly different than in the absence of lung disease. Optimal support establishes neutral or positive nitrogen balance, depending on the need for protein repletion. In the critically ill patient with acute respiratory failure, protein balance can be accomplished by giving 1 to 3 (generally, 1.5 to 2.0) g of protein per kilogram of body weight per day, or approximately 20 percent of total calories administered as protein. In acute respiratory failure, higher levels of protein may increase the work of breathing, resulting in further patient fatigue. Protein administration has been shown to increase minute ventilation, oxygen consumption, and the ventilatory response to hypoxia and hypercapnia. However, a prolonged lack of dietary protein contributes to nutritional deficiency.

The most appropriate carbohydrate-fat substrate mix for patients with COPD is controversial. Although the critically ill patient with respiratory failure uses lipids preferentially as a fuel source, glucose oxidation is not impaired, and lipid infusion probably does not change the pattern of fuel oxidation. Glucose and lipids provide no benefit over one another in the protein "sparing" effect. Fat calories may be supplied during nutritional support to provide essential fatty acids. Intravenously administered lipids, even when given slowly, may cause hemodynamic changes in injured lungs, although the clinical significance of these changes may be small. Lipids, especially long-chain triglycerides, can impair reticuloendothelial clearance functions, even when hypertriglyceridemia is absent. The proportion of fat calories, as well as glucose calories, in excess of caloric needs significantly influences hepatic steatosis. Despite the many disadvantages of intravenous lipids, fats in enteral feeding formulations are well tolerated and are associated with few adverse effects.

Disadvantages of carbohydrate administration include hyperglycemia, especially in diabetics or patients receiving glucocorticoid therapy. Excess administered glucose is not oxidized but rather is stored as body fat. This can result in increased fat deposition in the liver as well as in nutrition-associated hypercapnia. While recommendations for an appropriate substrate mix of carbohydrates and fats vary, generally, a mixture of carbohydrates to provide 60 to 70 percent of caloric needs, along with fats to provide 20 to 30 percent of caloric needs, is recommended.

MONITORING ENERGY BALANCE

The goal of assuring positive energy balance during acute respiratory failure can be assessed in several ways. Serial monitoring of body weight (over days to weeks) is an important and useful method. Unfortunately, fluid shifts in acutely ill patients complicate assessment of tissue accretion or depletion. However, in the critically ill patient, weight loss, in the absence of diuresis, strongly suggests inadequate caloric support.

Nitrogen balance, which should be assessed in any patient receiving nutritional support, is the difference between nitrogen intake and output:

$$\text{Nitrogen}_{\text{balance}} = \frac{\text{protein(g)}_{\text{intake}}}{6.25} - \text{nitrogen(g)}_{\text{output}}$$

Urinary nitrogen is measured as 24-h urine urea nitrogen excretion (UUN). Urine urea nitrogen generally makes up about 80 percent of total urinary nitrogen losses. Therefore, multiplication of the measured UUN by 1.25 approximates urinary nitrogen losses. Unfortunately, UUN is not accurate when the creatinine clearance is less than 20 ml/min. Measurement of total urinary nitrogen is available in many hospital laboratories.

ROUTE OF NUTRIENT DELIVERY

Nutritional support can be administered systemically as *total parenteral nutrition* (TPN) or *total enteral nutrition* (TEN). Although TPN remains an important route of nutrient delivery in critically ill patients who are unable to tolerate enteral nutrition, recent data suggest the importance of using TEN in patients with functioning gastrointestinal tracts.

TEN restores intestinal integrity and preserves the barrier function of the gut. Direct contact of the gut with nutrients preserves enteral mucosal integrity and corrects the pH balance of the gut, helping to reduce bacterial overgrowth. TEN also reduces gastrointestinal bleeding. Early enteral feeding may enhance motility by minimizing the delay in gastric emptying. Randomized trials have indicated that in the intensive care unit, early enteral feeding following onset of illness (within 3 days) is safe, efficient, cost-effective, and associated with improved outcome. In patients with acute respiratory failure who do not have functioning gastrointestinal tracts, TPN should be administered.

COMPLICATIONS OF SUPPLEMENTAL NUTRITION

Complications of TPN primarily include infection and traumatic complications of central venous line placement.

Mechanical complications of TEN relate to the size and position of the feeding tube and include inadvertent nasotracheal passage, interference with sinus drainage, and obstruction of the tube. Adverse pleuropulmonary sequelae that can potentially worsen respiratory disease include pneumothorax, pneumomediastinum, and subcutaneous emphysema. Neurologically impaired or sedated patients are at high risk for errant feeding tube placement. Radiographic confirmation of tube position after placement is essential.

Aspiration of enteral feedings can be disastrous in patients with respiratory disease. Large-volume aspiration of enteral feedings may precipitate or worsen respiratory failure; small-volume aspiration may cause nosocomial pneumonia. The reported frequency of aspiration is extremely variable. Risk factors include presence of an endotracheal tube or other artificial airway, reduced level of consciousness, ileus, and gastroparesis. Feeding tube size is probably much less important than patient position. Maintaining the patient in a semierect position minimizes aspiration risk. Gastric residual volumes should be checked frequently, especially in those at risk for delayed gastric emptying.

Gastrointestinal complications of TEN are related to altered motility and include vomiting, abdominal distention, and diarrhea. Early correction of electrolyte abnormalities, reduction in narcotic dosages, and use of gastrointestinal suction decrease morbidity from progressive bowel dilation. Withholding TEN in the presence of abdominal pain or distention, or in the absence of bowel sounds, is controversial. Jejunal tube feeding may result in less abdominal distention than feeding through the gastric route.

The incidence of diarrhea in acute respiratory failure may approach 50 percent. Causes include infection, especially due to *Clostridium* species. Diarrhea is frequent in mechanically ventilated patients receiving TEN, although the precise cause is unknown. Severe diarrhea with TEN may also be a symptom of deranged metabolism. Lumen absorptive capacity may be affected by hypotension and reduced mesenteric circulation, toxemia, or cellular derangements associated with multiple system organ failure. Hypoalbuminemia associated with volume expansion and severe catabolism has also been noted in conjunction with diarrhea in critically ill patients. Adverse effects of diarrhea include patient discomfort, compromised skin integrity, and loss of nutrients, water, and electrolytes.

Metabolic complications of nutritional support include hyperglycemia and hypophosphatemia. Hypophosphatemia can worsen or precipitate acute respiratory failure. Nutrition-associated hypercapnia may be an important metabolic complication in acute respiratory failure. The cause is generally thought to be related to *total* calories administered, rather than the percentage of calories from carbohydrate when total calories are not excessive. The problem of excessive CO_2 production caused by feeding can be avoided by identifying patients at risk, especially those with respiratory disease. Enteral formulations with altered carbohydrate-fat ratios have been developed and promoted for patients with COPD. However, they appear to be of little additional value when total calories administered are appropriate.

BIBLIOGRAPHY

Askanazi J, Rosenbaum SH, Hyman AI, et al: Respiratory changes induced by the large glucose loads of total parenteral nutrition. *JAMA* 243:1444–1447, 1980.

Cataldi-Betcher EL, Seltzer MH, Slocum BA, Jones KW: Complications occurring during enteral nutrition support: A prospective study. *J Parenter Enteral Nutr* 7:546–552, 1983.

Cerra FB: Hypermetabolism, organ failure, and metabolic support. *Surgery* 101:1–14, 1987.

Covelli HD, Black JW, Olsen MS, Bechman JF: Respiratory failure precipitated by high carbohydrate loads. *Ann Intern Med* 95:579–581, 1981.

Donahoe M: Nutritional support in advanced lung disease. The pulmonary cachexia syndrome. *Clin Chest Med* 18: 547–561, 1997.

Gadek JE, DeMichele SJ, Karlstad MD, et al: Effect of enteral feeding with eicosapentaenoic acid, gamma-linolenic acid, and antioxidants in patients with acute respiratory distress syndrome. Enteral Nutrition in ARDS Study Group. *Crit Care Med* 27:1409–1420, 1999.

Saudny-Unterberger H, Martin JG, Gray-Donald K: Impact of nutritional support on functional status during an acute exacerbation of chronic obstructive pulmonary disease. *Am J Respir Crit Care Med* 156 (pt 1): 794–799, 1997.

77 | Sedation and Analgesia in the Intensive Care Unit*

Michael A. Grippi

INTRODUCTION

Critically ill patients frequently have impaired communication, loss of normal diurnal sleep-wake cycles, sleep deprivation, or pain. Increased recognition by clinicians of these uncomfortable circumstances has resulted in widespread use of sedatives, anxiolytics, and analgesics in the intensive care unit. Use of neuromuscular blocking agents has also become common practice in management of mechanically ventilated patients.

INDICATIONS FOR SEDATIVES IN THE CRITICAL CARE SETTING

Commonly used sedatives in the intensive care unit include benzodiazepines, opioids, neuroleptics, and intravenous anesthetics. Each class of agents, either alone or in combination, can produce obtundation, and, except for the neuroleptics, each can suppress respiration. Indications for use of sedating drugs during mechanical ventilation (Table 77-1) include relief of agitation and distress and provision of anesthesia and analgesia.

Agitation is excessive, nonproductive, potentially harmful motor activity. Occasionally, the motor activity is purposeful—e.g., attempts at self-extubation. New onset of agitation warrants a search for its cause. Although mild agitation does not necessarily warrant treatment, severe agitation may be hazardous in the mechanically ventilated patient who has indwelling intravascular or other catheters or an endotracheal tube. In addition, severe agitation may produce metabolic acidosis, hypoxemia, or marked hemodynamic fluctuations. Severe agitation is treated pharmacologically (see below) as a search for the underlying cause, and its correction, are undertaken. *Distress* refers to physical or mental suffering and is usually associated with agitation in the intensive care unit. Distress may arise because of pain, dyspnea, anxiety, or delirium.

Pain is a subjective, unpleasant physical and emotional sensation. Because the patient's speech and behavior may be modified greatly in the critical care setting, the clinician's recognition of pain may hindered. New pain may herald a new problem, e.g., pneumothorax, ischemic bowel, peripheral arterial occlusion, or intracranial bleeding. Additional common sources of pain include endotracheal tubes, chest tubes, and urinary bladder catheters.

Dyspnea, the subjective sensation of shortness of breath, is a common symptom in mechanically ventilated patients. Patients may be quite dyspneic despite perfectly normal arterial blood gases. In some, a likely source of the

---

*Edited from Chap. 179, "Treatment of Agitation and Distress in Mechanically Ventilated Patients," by Hansen-Flaschen J. In: *Fishman's Pulmonary Diseases and Disorders,* 3d ed., edited by Fishman AP, Elias JA, Fishman JA, Grippi MA, Kaiser LR, Senior RM. New York, McGraw-Hill, 1998, pp 2739–2752. For fuller discussion of topics dealt with in this chapter, the reader is referred to the original text, as noted above.

TABLE 77-1 Indications for Sedating Drugs in the Treatment
of Mechanically Ventilated Patients

Control patient *agitation*
Alleviate patient *distress,* particularly:
  Pain
  Anxiety
  Delirium
  Dyspnea
Provide *anesthesia* for neuromuscular blockade
Provide *sedation* or *analgesia* for procedures and special
situations, including:
  Endotracheal intubation
  Bedside procedures, such as cardioversion and percutaneous
  tracheostomy
  Diagnostic imaging studies, such as CT and MRI
  Alcohol or sedative drug withdrawal
  Acute brain injury associated with increased intracranial
  pressure
  Terminal withdrawal of mechanical ventilation

dyspnea is discoordination between the ventilator and the patient's spontaneous respiratory efforts. In addition, delay in onset of flow at the initiation
of a spontaneous inspiratory effort or insufficient flow during the breath may
be contributing factors. Dyspnea is commonly experienced during prolonged
weaning.

Anxiety is a generalized sense of apprehension unassociated with a specific
threat, while *fear* is the emotional response to a defined external threat or
danger. Anxiety is fostered by the patient's loss of control, pain, dyspnea,
and delirium. Palpitations, diaphoresis, tachycardia, tachypnea, systolic
hypertension, nausea, insomnia, or confusion may be elicited by anxiety.

Delirium, the most common organic brain syndrome seen in the intensive
care unit, is an acute, fluctuating, reversible disturbance of consciousness and
cognitive function. Perception and short-term memory are altered; confusion,
disorientation, hallucinations (predominantly visual) and impaired reasoning
are seen. Delirium is often most severe in the evening and early morning
hours. Periods of clouded sensorium may alternate with periods of lucidity.
Marked fluctuations in autonomic function may be observed. Causes include
neurologic injuries, neoplastic syndromes, severe cardiovascular, hematologic, and respiratory disorders, endocrine and metabolic disturbances, and a
variety of toxins. Acid-base or metabolic disturbances and drugs, especially
narcotics, benzodiazepines, and anticholinergics, can cause or exacerbate
delirium. Sleeplessness is a common contributing factor to the development
of delirium in the intensive care unit. Other causes include intermittent partial
seizures and drug withdrawal. The possibility of drug or alcohol withdrawal
should be considered whenever delirium appears abruptly during the first 2 or
3 days of hospitalization.

PATIENT ASSESSMENT

The patient's spontaneous behavior should be observed, ideally by clinicians
who have an opportunity to repeatedly assess him or her over time. The ability
to see, hear, understand, and respond appropriately to simple questions should
be determined. An awake patient who does not respond appropriately to

commands, despite adequate hearing, vision, and muscle strength, is likely to be delirious or otherwise neurologically impaired. Responsive patients should be asked about their comfort with direct questions that intubated patients can answer by shaking their head or by some other unambiguous movement. Quantification of distress is often useful in planning and monitoring a therapeutic response. Visual analog scales are useful for measuring the intensity of subjective experiences, such as pain, anxiety, and dyspnea.

DRUGS USED TO TREAT AGITATION AND DISTRESS

Drugs used to treat agitation and distress during mechanical ventilation include opioids, benzodiazepines, neuroleptics, and intravenous anesthetics. All depress the central nervous system in a dose-dependent fashion.

Opioids

Opioids produce dose-related sedation and analgesia. They are less effective anxiolytics and amnestic agents than are benzodiazepines. Important respiratory effects of opioids include depression of respiration (a dose-related effect), cough suppression, and rarely, at high doses, induction of noncardiogenic pulmonary edema. Through histamine release, morphine can increase bronchospasm in asthmatics. Respiratory muscle rigidity and impaired ventilation sometimes are seen when anesthetic doses of fentanyl are given rapidly.

Multiple systemic effects of opioids are well known. Cardiovascular effects include venodilation, reduction in systemic vascular resistance, reduced venous return to the heart, and hypotension (especially in volume-depleted patients). Profound hypotension should be anticipated in patients with significant right-heart failure. Gastrointestinal effects include decreased gastrointestinal motility and resulting constipation, ileus, and gastroesophageal reflux. Morphine constricts the sphincter of Oddi and may exacerbate biliary colic. Opioids can also cause nausea and vomiting. Opioids inhibit the urinary voiding reflex and increase the tone of the external sphincter. They can cause pruritus, skin flushing, miosis, and, occasionally, delirium.

Two commonly used opioids are morphine and fentanyl. Morphine is available in both oral (long- and short-acting) and parenteral forms. Morphine is metabolized in the liver; the metabolites are excreted in the urine. The effects of morphine can be prolonged considerably with hepatic or renal insufficiency or poor perfusion of either organ. Fentanyl, a synthetic opioid, demonstrates a more rapid peak effect (5 to 15 min) and shorter duration of action (30 to 60 min) than morphine. However, with prolonged administration, fentanyl, as a highly lipid-soluble drug, gradually moves out of fat stores after administration is discontinued. Fentanyl causes considerably less histamine release than morphine, and therefore, may be preferable for patients with hypotension or right heart failure. Since fentanyl does not produce active metabolites which can accumulate in renal insufficiency, the drug may be preferable to morphine when the serum creatinine is greater than 2 mg/dL or in acute oliguria.

Benzodiazepines

Benzodiazepines produce sedation, anxiolysis, amnesia, hypnosis, and muscle relaxation; they also possess anticonvulsant activity. They are not analgesics. Intravenous administration can cause transient respiratory depression, hypotension, or tachycardia, especially when combined with an opioid or neuromuscular blocking agent. Benzodiazepines sometimes produce a paradoxical increase in anxiety, irritability, or agitation. This effect may be observed transiently as the dose is increased. In some critically ill patients, benzodiazepine administration is closely associated with the onset of delirium. Physical dependence can occur with prolonged administration.

Benzodiazepines commonly used in the intensive care unit include diazepam, lorezepam, and midazolam. Diazepam is the least expensive benzodiazepine available for intravenous administration. After a single bolus injection, diazepam's duration of action is 40 to 95 min. The drug is highly lipid-soluble, so that full recovery may require 5 to 7 days or longer after prolonged infusion, particularly in critically ill patients who have impaired hepatic or renal function. Lorazepam has a slower onset of action (15 to 30 min) than diazepam. The duration of action is approximately 6 to 8 h after single intravenous bolus injection. The drug is less lipid-soluble than the others and has no active metabolites. The elimination half-life is not measurably prolonged after single injection in elderly patients or those with renal insufficiency. Although lorazepam can be given safely by continuous intravenous infusion, the drug sometimes precipitates in the bag or tubing when administered by continuous infusion. In addition, large volumes of fluid are required for continuous infusion. Considerably lower total doses may be required to maintain adequate sedation when lorazepam is given intermittently, rather than continuously. Midazolam, the most lipid-soluble benzodiazepine, has a more rapid onset (1 to 5 min) and shorter duration of sedative effect (30 to 120 min) than lorazepam after single intravenous bolus. Midazolam and its active metabolites can accumulate in critically ill patients. Like lorazepam, midazolam requires large volumes of fluid for continuous infusion.

Neuroleptics

Neuroleptic drugs are useful in the critical care setting for treatment of agitation associated with delirium. Although they lack analgesic properties and have minimal amnestic effects, they decrease motor activity and aggression. The drowsiness associated with initial use is mild and abates with time. The neuroleptics, to some extent, protect against catecholamine-induced cardiac arrhythymias, decrease intracranial pressure, and effectively reduce nausea and vomiting.

The butyrophenone, haloperidol, is the most commonly used neuroleptic in the intensive care unit. The drug produces no significant respiratory depression and has little adverse effect on cardiovascular function of patients in the supine position. Following intravenous administration, drug effect appears in 10 to 15 min, with a peak effect in 40 to 60 min. The half-life for elimination is 10 to 19 h in healthy subjects. Haloperidol is metabolized in the liver and excreted in the urine. The drug can be used safely in multiple organ failure, although metabolism may be delayed with severe liver disease.

Important neurologic and cardiovascular side effects can occur with use of haloperidol. Extrapyramidal reactions (less common when the drug is given intravenously than orally) include acute dystonia, akathisia, or akinesia. The *neuroleptic malignant syndrome,* an uncommon, life-threatening reaction that resembles a severe form of Parkinsonism, has also been described. Younger men appear to be at higher risk. Patients develop diffuse muscle spasms that can cause metabolic acidosis or myoglobinuria. Catatonia, stupor, autonomic instability, and persistent fever are also frequently observed. This reaction can occur at any time during use of a neuroleptic drug and may persist for days after the drug is stopped. Intravenous haloperidol can also cause dysmorphic ventricular tachycardia (torsade de pointes). This potentially life-threatening dysrhythmia is usually, but not always, preceded by progressive widening of the Q-Tc interval on the electrocardiogram. Women and patients with preexisting prolonged Q-Tc intervals may be at higher risk.

Intravenous Anesthetics

Only one general anesthetic agent, propofol, is currently widely used in intensive care units. Propofol is a central nervous system depressant with an extremely high lipid-aqueous partition ratio. Delivered intravenously as an oil-in-water emulsion in 10% Intralipid, its anesthetic effects are very rapid in onset and offset. Titration of the drug can rapidly change the patient's status along the continuum of mild sedation to surgical anesthesia. At lower doses, propofol does not have analgesic or amnestic properties, but it may have anxiolytic effects. Recovery of consciousness is quick (within minutes) after stopping the drug, even after prolonged infusion or in the setting of hepatic or renal dysfunction.

Rapid injection of propofol sometimes causes precipitous hypotension in critically ill patients. The Intralipid vehicle can cause enhanced intrapulmonary shunting when a large dose is infused rapidly into patients with acute respiratory distress syndrome (ARDS). Hypercholesterolemia may be seen, and blood cholesterol should be monitored at 2- to 3-day intervals during prolonged infusions. The lipid calorie content of the formulation is often sufficient to warrant adjustment of the prescription for total parenteral nutrition during a continuous infusion of the drug. Special precautions are required to protect against sepsis associated with rapid bacterial growth in the lipid base. Isolated case reports suggest that propofol may increase the risk of seizures or opisthotonus. Because propofol is expensive compared with other available intravenous sedating drugs, many intensivists reserve this drug for short-term use in special situations.

NEUROMUSCULAR BLOCKING DRUGS

Neuromuscular blocking drugs are used in the intensive care unit to treat life-threatening agitation and facilitate mechanical ventilation. They must be used in conjunction with anesthetic doses of one or more sedating drugs. Both depolarizing and nondepolarizing (competitive) blocking agents are available, but only the latter are used to sustain muscle relaxation during mechanical ventilation. In the critical care setting, pancuronium, vecuronium, atracurium, and cisatracurium are the most commonly prescribed agents.

Pancuronium and vecuronium are structurally related to curare. Pancuronium can sometimes cause tachycardia and hypertension after bolus injection. Pancuronium can also cause histamine release, resulting in hypotension. Vecuronium does not cause histamine release and is not associated with important adverse cardiovascular effects. Both agents are cleared primarily by hepatic metabolism. In contrast, atracurium is degraded spontaneously to inactive metabolites in the blood at a rate that is unaffected by kidney, liver, or cardiovascular dysfunction. Like pancuronium, atracurium can cause histamine release. The *cis* isomer of atracurium, cisatracurium, does not cause this problem. Of the four muscle relaxants noted, pancuronium is the least expensive.

Serious complications can arise when these drugs are given by repeated injection or prolonged, continuous infusion in the intensive care unit. Patient disconnection from the ventilator can lead to cardiopulmonary arrest. An inability of the patient to alter respiratory rate in response to changing metabolic needs may result in severe respiratory acidosis or alkalosis. Inability to swallow or cough jeopardizes the airway. Inability to blink makes patients prone to corneal abrasions, and inability to shiver predisposes to hypothermia. Immobilization gives rise to pressure sores or contractures unless the patient is repositioned frequently and joints are appropriately splinted. Improper handling can cause hyperextension injuries and nerve compression damage.

Another important complication of neuromuscular blocking drugs is failure to regain muscle strength for hours to many days after the agents are discontinued. One mechanism is related to accumulation of active metabolites of pancuronium, vecuronium, and other aminosteroid blocking agents in the presence of renal failure. Neuromuscular blockade may continue for a week after drug administration is stopped. Prolonged paralysis can be prevented by using benzylisoquinoline agents, such as atracurium or cisatracurium, in favor of aminosteroid blocking drugs in renal failure.

Another mechanism underlying prolonged paralysis, described in asthmatics treated with mechanical ventilation for several days or longer, is skeletal muscle atrophy and necrosis. Usually, these patients have been treated with repeated or continuous administration of a nondepolarizing neuromuscular blocking agent in combination with moderate to high doses of corticosteroids. Originally thought to occur exclusively with the aminosteroid muscle relaxants, pancuronium and vecuronium, the benzylisoquinoline agents, such as atracurium, can produce the syndrome. The duration of neuromuscular blockade appears to be the most important predictor of persistent muscle weakness. The mechanism is uncertain, although data suggest that denervation of skeletal muscle unmasks or amplifies a form of corticosteroid-induced myopathy. Muscle biopsies show selective loss of myosin filaments not observed in other forms of acute muscle injury. Muscle function recovers over weeks after denervation is reversed.

TREATMENT OF AGITATION AND DISTRESS

While mild agitation does not necessitate pharmacologic intervention in every case, severe agitation requires immediate attention to prevent patient harm. Treatment occurs shortly after clinical evaluation of the cause of the agitation or concurrent with it.

An opioid, a benzodiazepine, or a neuroleptic agent should be given intravenously to treat moderate, sustained agitation. The dose is titrated to effect using repeated bolus injections at intervals appropriate to the onset of action of the drug. A maintenance dose is established only after adequate control of agitation is achieved. Very large doses (10 to 50 times usual) are sometimes needed to suppress agitation, particularly in patients who have developed tolerance to sedating drugs or alcohol. However, the likelihood of adverse effects increases with increasing dose. Addition of a second or third sedating drug may be appropriate in refractory cases in an attempt to limit side effects from high doses of any one drug.

If an immediately correctable cause for life-threatening agitation is not apparent, fentanyl may be administered at a dose of 0.05 to 0.1 mg by intravenous bolus every 2 to 5 min, up to 0.4 mg or more. If alcohol, benzodiazepine, or barbiturate withdrawal is suspected, lorazepam should be considered (1- to 2-mg boluses, repeated at 10- to 15-min intervals, to a total of 10 mg or more as needed). If either of these drugs fails, the patient should be paralyzed with an intravenous injection of pancuronium, 0.1 mg/kg. If the patient was conscious beforehand, the paralyzing agent should be followed as soon as possible by bolus loading doses of an opioid and a benzodiazepine at doses sufficient to induce analgesia, deep sedation, and amnesia (e.g., fentanyl, 0.3 to 0.4 mg, and lorazepam, 3 to 6 mg). The patient should then be thoroughly reassessed to identify the problem that precipitated the agitation.

Neuromuscular blockade should be continued beyond the initial phase of acute management only if necessary. Some patients in severe respiratory failure, particularly those with acute asthma or severe ARDS, require continued paralysis to maintain adequate ventilation and oxygenation. If renal function is normal, a continuous infusion of pancuronium can be used. To avoid prolonged neuromuscular blockade (see above), cisatracurium can be substituted if the patient is acutely oliguric or if the serum creatinine exceeds 2.0 mg/dL. The muscle relaxant should be administered at the lowest dose that achieves the therapeutic goal; in many instances, complete paralysis is not necessary. Overdose can be avoided by use of a peripheral nerve stimulator to monitor the degree of junctional blockade. In all cases, and particularly when a corticosteroid is administered concomitantly, neuromuscular blockade should be discontinued as soon as possible—ideally within 24 h—to minimize the likelihood of prolonged muscle weakness. Many intensivists recommend withdrawal of pharmacologic paralysis once every 24 h whenever possible to allow a complete physical examination, including assessment of the level of sedation and to determine whether paralysis is still necessary.

Intravenous infusion of propofol is another alternative for control of acute, moderate to severe agitation, particularly in patients who are expected to require mechanical ventilation for only a few days or when rapid recovery from sedation is required. Because of hypotension occurring with rapid infusion, propofol must be loaded in a controlled fashion, and the time required for initial control of agitation is similar to that of benzodiazepines and opioids. The depth of hypnosis can be increased temporarily to produce a brief period of anesthesia for an uncomfortable procedure, or decreased temporarily to allow for a complete neurologic examination. Even after 1 to 2 weeks, a patient receiving propofol can be awakened within 30 to 60 min before extubation.

TREATMENT OF DELIRIUM

Neuroleptic drugs appear effective in calming agitated delirium in the intensive care unit. Because of its favorable hemodynamic and respiratory profile, haloperidol is commonly used. Benzodiazepines can have a similar calming effect on patients who are agitated and delirious, particularly when delirium results from withdrawal of alcohol or some other sedating substance.

Haloperidol may be administered by intravenous bolus injection (5 mg, or 2 mg for patients more than 65 years old). Additional intravenous doses of 2 to 10 mg may be administered every 20 min, at an injection rate not exceeding 5 mg per minute, until agitation is controlled. During loading, the Q-Tc interval should be monitored continuously, and the loading regimen should be discontinued if the interval exceeds 480 ms in order to reduce the risk of torsades de pointes. The patient should also be monitored for development of extrapyramidal side effects and the neuroleptic malignant syndrome. If trismus or other forms of acute dystonia occur, benzotropine may be administered intravenously. Other extrapyramidal reactions can be treated with diphenhydramine. Akathisia responds poorly to either of these drugs, but may abate after administration of a benzodiazepine.

No upper limit has been defined for a loading dose of haloperidol. Quantities in excess of 400 mg/24 h have been given without apparent adverse effect, although the efficacy of such high doses is uncertain. Addition of lorazepam should be considered if more than 20 mg of haloperidol is needed in 24 h. Control of agitated delirium is maintained by giving one-fourth the total loading dose of haloperidol every 6 h by intermittent intravenous injection for the first 24 to 48 h. The dose is then decreased by 25 to 50 percent per day, as tolerated.

Benzodiazepines are preferred for the treatment of delirium associated with alcohol or sedative withdrawal because they are effective for the prevention and treatment of withdrawal seizures, whereas haloperidol and most other neuroleptic drugs appear to lower the seizure threshold. For moderate or severe agitation associated with alcohol or drug withdrawal, unusually large doses of benzodiazepines are often required initially (e.g., lorazepam, 6 to 12 mg). Once control of agitation is achieved, the dose can often be reduced by 25 percent or more each day, thereafter.

TREATMENT OF PAIN

Local approaches to pain control are sometimes appropriate in the intensive care unit. Intravenously administered opioids should be used for most diffuse or persistent types of pain and for patients who are too agitated or delirious to cooperate with local forms of pain control. Opioid analgesics, in general, should not be given subcutaneously or intramuscularly to critically ill patients because the injections are painful, drug absorption is erratic, and relief of discomfort is delayed. Bolus intravenous administration is appropriate for painful procedures; continuous infusion prevents lapses in pain control common with intermittent dosing regimens. Fentanyl is preferable to morphine for patients with renal insufficiency, systemic hypotension, or right ventricular failure. Lower maintenance doses are used for patients in hepatic failure.

A continuous infusion of morphine or fentanyl should be initiated by administration of an adequate loading dose. Boluses are repeated at 5- to 10-min intervals, guided by a visual analog or numeric pain scale, until pain is relieved. Transient hypotension can be treated with an infusion of fluid or a vasopressor (e.g., phenylephrine).

The goal of continuous intravenous analgesia is to achieve and sustain a blood level of opioid that equals or exceeds the minimum effective analgesic concentration (MEAC) for the drug. A patient-controlled infusion pump can be employed to maintain appropriate opioid dosing for mechanically ventilated patients who are sufficiently awake and alert.

BIBLIOGRAPHY

Bone R, Hayden W, Levine R, et al: Recognition, assessment, and treatment of anxiety in the critical care patient. *Dis Mon* 41:293–360, 1995.

Hansen-Flaschen J: Improving patient tolerance of mechanical ventilation: Challenges ahead. *Crit Care Clin* 10:659–672, 1994.

Hanson C: Pharmacology of neuromuscular blocking agents in the intensive care unit. *Crit Care Clin* 10:779–797, 1994.

Kress JP, Pohlman AS, O'Connor MF, Hall JB: Daily interruption of sedative infusions in critically ill patients undergoing mechanical ventilation. *N Engl J Med* 342:1471–1477, 2000.

Leatherman J, Fluegel W, David W, et al: Muscle weakness in mechanically ventilated patients with severe asthma. *Am J Respir Crit Care Med* 153:1686–1690, 1996.

Lowson SM, Sawh S: Adjuncts to analgesia. Sedation and neuromuscular blockade. *Crit Care Clin* 15:119–141, 1999.

Osterman ME, Keenan SP, Seiferling RA, Sibbald WJ: Sedation in the intensive care unit: A systematic review. *JAMA* 283:1451–1459, 2000.

Schwab R: Disturbances of sleep in the intensive care unit. *Crit Care Clin* 10:681–695, 1994.

Young C, Knudson N, Hilton A, Reves JG: Sedation in the intensive care unit. *Crit Care Med* 28:854–866, 2000.

78

Pulmonary Pharmacotherapy*

Lisa M. Bellini and Michael A. Grippi

INTRODUCTION

A wide spectrum of therapeutic agents is currently employed in the treatment of respiratory disorders. Included are bronchodilators, anti-inflammatory agents, leukotriene modifiers, mast cell stabilizers, mucokinetic agents, physiologic replacements, and respiratory stimulants.

BRONCHODILATORS

The bronchodilators include beta-adrenergic agonists, anticholinergics, methylxanthines, and several less commonly used classes of drugs.

Beta-Adrenergic Agonists

The beta-adrenergic agonists or *sympathomimetics* mimic the actions of norepinephrine at neuroeffector and synaptic junctions. Beta-adrenergic agonists are indicated in the treatment of bronchospasm associated with acute and chronic asthma, bronchitis, emphysema, and other obstructive pulmonary diseases. Selection of a specific agent and route of administration depend on underlying patient risk factors and the receptor specificity of the drug.

The short-acting catecholamines epinephrine and ephedrine were the first adrenergic agonists to be marketed; each has alpha-, beta$_1$-, and beta$_2$-adrenergic receptor activity. Subsequently added to the therapeutic armamentarium were metaproterenol and terbutaline; the latter is selective for beta$_2$-adrenergic receptors. The newest agents, albuterol and salmeterol, have a longer duration of action and beta$_2$-adrenergic receptor specificity (particularly salmeterol).

None of the currently marketed agonists is completely specific for beta$_2$-adrenergic receptors; many of the agents have significant alpha- and/or beta$_1$-adrenergic agonist activity. The alpha-adrenergic receptor responses include constriction of arteries and veins, and contraction of the uterus, radial and sphincter muscles of the iris, urinary bladder, and stomach. Beta$_1$-adrenergic effects include increased heart rate, atrial and ventricular contractility, and cardiac conduction velocity. Beta$_2$-adrenergic effects include relaxation of bronchial and uterine smooth muscle, dilatation of arteries and veins, glycogenolysis, gluconeogenesis, and induction of hepatic pancreatic beta cell secretion.

The beta-adrenergic agonists may be administered orally, subcutaneously, intravenously, or by inhalation. Systemic administration decreases

*Edited from Chap. 173, "Pulmonary Pharmacotherapy," by Manaker S, Tietze KJ, Wittbrodt ET. In: *Fishman's Pulmonary Diseases and Disorders,* 3d ed., edited by Fishman AP, Elias JA, Fishman JA, Grippi MA, Kaiser LR, Senior RM. New York, McGraw-Hill, 1998, pp 2643–2660. For fuller discussion of topics dealt with in this chapter, the reader is referred to the original text, as noted above.

the beta$_2$-adrenergic receptor selectivity. The preferred route of administration is by inhalation. Local application of small amounts of drug directly to the airways decreases the amount available for systemic absorption minimizing systemic side effects. Inhaled beta-adrenergic agonists are available in several dosage forms, including wet aerosols, aerosols from metered-dose inhalers, and dry powders. Nebulized drug delivery is labor-intensive; significant cost savings can be realized without sacrificing efficacy by using metered-dose inhalers coupled with spacer devices. Patients too dyspneic or tachypneic to control their inspiratory flow and coordinate use of the devices respond best to nebulized drug delivery.

Drug delivery by metered-dose inhaler is highly dependent on administration technique. Less than 10 percent of the dose is delivered to the lung using optimal inhalation technique; the rest is deposited in the mouth. Spacer devices eliminate the split-second timing necessary with proper metered dose inhaler technique and decrease the amount of drug deposited in the oropharynx; however, they do not provide a therapeutic advantage over correct use of a metered dose inhaler alone.

The beta$_2$-adrenergic agonists are considered first-line drugs in the treatment of both asthma and chronic obstructive pulmonary disease. In asthma, the short acting inhaled beta$_2$-adrenergic agonists are preferred for treating acute symptoms and for preventing exercise-induced bronchospasm. Although the indications for beta$_2$-adrenergic agonists in chronic obstructive pulmonary disease are less well defined, they provide modest symptomatic relief and improvement in pulmonary function. Standard doses of inhaled beta$_2$-adrenergic agonists appear as effective as inhaled anticholinergic drugs for relief of acute exacerbations of chronic obstructive pulmonary disease (COPD).

The intensity and duration of response to beta$_2$-adrenergic agonists is dose- and frequency-dependent. For patients with asthma, higher doses result in incrementally greater bronchodilation. This led to the development of intensive inhaled beta$_2$-adrenergic agonist drug regimens for the treatment of severe, acute exacerbations. Typically, the nebulized drug is administered every 20 min for three to six doses. The dose-response relationships are less well defined for COPD.

The long-acting beta$_2$-adrenergic agonists are add-on agents for patients with moderate or severe asthma when usual doses of inhaled corticosteroids are inadequate or to control nocturnal symptoms. These drugs have no role in the treatment of acute symptoms; all patients should have a short-acting inhaler and should be instructed on how and when to use each type of beta$_2$-adrenergic agonist. The value of long-acting beta$_2$-adrenergic agonists in the treatment of COPD remains undefined. Tolerance to the long-acting drugs may make patients less responsive to short-acting beta$_2$-adrenergic agonists during an acute attack or may mask inadequate control of inflammation.

Beta-adrenergic agonist use has increased coincident with the increase in asthma morbidity and mortality. This observation has promoted interest in the possible relationship between asthma mortality and use of these agents. Although currently available data do not support an association between the use of short-acting beta-adrenergic agonist and an increased risk of death, deaths have been reported in patients who unsuccessfully used a long-acting beta-agonist to treat acute symptoms of asthma.

Anticholinergics

Anticholinergic alkaloids from plant extracts have been used for thousands of years to relieve respiratory symptoms in humans with airway diseases. Atropine, a prototypic anticholinergic antagonist, is nonselective for the five different molecular forms of muscarinic receptors. Ipratropium bromide, a quaternary ammonium congener of atropine, is poorly absorbed, rapidly excreted, and does not cross the blood-brain barrier, markedly reducing the potential for systemic side effects. It is available by both metered-dose inhaler and nebulizer solution.

Inhalation of ipratropium bromide produces bronchodilation in seconds to minutes, with a peak effect after 1 to 2 h. The drug completely reverses bronchoconstriction induced by methacholine or other cholinergic agonists, and it partially relieves bronchospasm induced by a broad spectrum of common bronchoconstrictor stimuli, including beta-adrenergic antagonists, histamine, serotonin, exercise, and cold air.

Ipratropium bromide is most efficacious in COPD, where it is equally or more effective than beta-adrenergic agonists in increasing forced expiratory volume in 1 second (FEV_1) and in reducing airway resistance. Many patients demonstrate bronchodilation in response to the anticholinergics but not to beta-adrenergic agonists. This observation demonstrates that many patients with COPD who fail to respond to beta-adrenergic agonists have bronchospasm attributable to heightened cholinergic tone rather than fixed airway disease. Chronic ipratropium bromide inhalation does not lead to development of tolerance or tachyphylaxis.

The combination of ipratropium bromide (or other anticholinergics) with beta-adrenergic agonists produces greater improvement in FEV_1 and specific conductance than does administration of either agent alone. Because of its greater efficacy and longer duration of action than beta-adrenergic agonists, ipratropium bromide is considered appropriate initial bronchodilator therapy for patients with COPD. Ipratropium bromide is less effective than beta-adrenergic agonists in the treatment of asthma.

After optimal bronchodilation is achieved with maximal doses of beta-adrenergic agonists, the addition of submaximal doses of ipratropium bromide produces additional bronchodilation. The combination of submaximal doses of ipratropium bromide and beta-adrenergic agonists may provide superior bronchodilation, fewer side effects, and greater compliance. Also, the rapid bronchodilation achieved with beta-adrenergic agonists and the prolonged action of ipratropium bromide may lead to substantial symptomatic relief from bronchospasm. These observations have resulted in the development of metered-dose inhalers combining fixed doses of ipratropium bromide and various beta-adrenergic agonists.

Methylxanthines

Theophylline and aminophylline, the ethylenediamine salt of theophylline, have been used for many years in the treatment of asthma and COPD. Potentially beneficial therapeutic effects include bronchial smooth-muscle relaxation, enhanced mucociliary transport, inhibition of mediator release, suppression of permeability edema, decreased pulmonary hypertension, increased right ventricular ejection fraction, improved diaphragmatic contractility, and central stimulation of ventilation.

The mechanism of theophylline-induced bronchodilation is unknown. The drug is a nonselective and weak phosphodiesterase inhibitor. Phosphodiesterase inhibition does not occur at usual therapeutic ranges but may account for some of the anti-inflammatory effect—an effect that appears to be qualitatively different from that of corticosteroids. Adenosine antagonism is unlikely to mediate the bronchodilatation but is likely responsible for the extrapulmonary effects. Theophylline may act by stimulating adrenomedullary secretion of catecholamines, which may contribute to the early bronchodilatory effects of the drug as well as increases in diaphragmatic strength and contractility.

Theophylline may be potentially most beneficial in hypoxic and hypercapnic COPD when dosed to midtherapeutic plasma concentrations (10 to 15 mg/dL). Approximately 50 percent of maximal bronchodilation is achieved at a serum level of 10 mg/dL, with only an additional 17 percent increase at 20 mg/dL. The clinical role for theophylline remains to be determined, but some indications include severe bronchodilator-dependent chronic obstructive pulmonary disease; severe, systemic, corticosteroid-dependent asthma; nocturnal asthma uncontrolled with adrenergic agonists; and acute, severe asthma progressing to respiratory failure.

Adverse effects associated with theophylline include nausea, vomiting, diarrhea, irritability, insomnia, supraventricular tachycardia, ventricular arrhythmias, and seizures. Although the risk of adverse effects increases at serum concentrations greater than 20 mg/dL, patients also may experience serious adverse effects within the usual therapeutic range.

Magnesium Sulfate

Magnesium, a physiological antagonist to calcium, blocks calcium entry into smooth-muscle cells, relaxing muscle fibers. Magnesium may also block calcium-dependent mast cell degranulation and mediator release, as well as acetylcholine release at the neuromuscular junction. Case reports describe the benefit of intravenous magnesium sulfate in acute, life-threatening asthma refractory to nebulized beta-agonists, parenteral corticosteroids, and parenteral terbutaline. More information is needed to better define the subgroup of asthmatics who might benefit from magnesium sulfate therapy.

Inhaled Diuretics

Furosemide inhibits release of chloride into the bronchial lumen; in addition, it may attenuate the sensory nerve response to irritant substances. It significantly blunts the bronchoconstrictive response to cold air in atopic asthmatics, but it also significantly slows airway rewarming. In children with exercise-induced asthma, inhaled furosemide is effective at preventing bronchoconstriction. Inhaled furosemide has no role in the treatment of exacerbations of acute asthma. Furosemide may be useful in the prevention of asthma provoked by exercise and some irritating substances, but additional information is needed before the use of inhaled diuretics can be recommended.

Inhaled diuretics improve sputum rheology and clearance in cystic fibrosis by antagonizing sodium absorption from airway epithelial cells, thus decreasing sputum viscosity. Patients appear not to experience adverse effects from inhaled diuretic therapy, but the efficacy of therapy remains to be proven.

ANTI-INFLAMMATORY AGENTS

The anti-inflammatory agents used in the treatment of lung disease include corticosteroids and "corticosteroid-sparing" agents. The latter category is much less commonly used, and in the broadest definition, includes the immunosuppressive agents, methotrexate, cyclosporine, and gold.

Corticosteroids

Corticosteroids are clearly useful in the management of asthma and may be efficacious in COPD. The role of airway inflammation in asthma is well established, and high-dose systemic (parenteral or oral) corticosteroids have become standard therapy for patients experiencing acute exacerbations. Parenteral administration is often used due to the inability of some patients to swallow medications while in respiratory distress or because of lack of oral access after intubation. Oral corticosteroids are as effective as parental corticosteroids in the treatment of acute asthma.

The minimum effective dose of intravenous corticosteroids in acute asthma has not been established. As little as 120 mg/day of methylprednisolone (in divided doses administered every 6 h) is effective in adults. The time to initial response (increase in FEV_1) begins as early as 1 h after administration; maximal response occurs in 8 to 12 h. Parenteral corticosteroid therapy is usually maintained for 24 to 72 h; oral prednisone at 60 mg daily is begun when the FEV_1 reaches a threshold of 50 percent of predicted normal. This dose may be maintained for 2 to 7 days, followed by gradual tapering of the dose over 1 to 3 weeks. Parenteral methylprednisolone is the corticosteroid of choice, due to its relatively low mineralocorticoid and high glucocorticoid effects.

Patients with asthma who are unresponsive to usually sufficient doses of corticosteroids are described as *steroid-resistant.* Steroid resistance has been formally defined as a less than 15 percent increase in FEV_1 after 7 days of oral prednisolone administered at a dose of 20 mg daily in bronchodilator-responsive asthmatics. Steroid resistance must be distinguished from steroid dependency, defined as the need for systemic corticosteroids for maintaining control of asthma. Steroid-resistant asthmatics may be appropriate candidates for empiric therapy with corticosteroid-sparing agents (see below).

Short-term use (less than 14 days) of systemic corticosteroids is associated with mild glucose intolerance, fluid retention that may progress to edema and hypertension, proximal muscle weakness (especially with large parenteral doses), and mood alteration. Long-term systemic corticosteroids prolong the short-term effects; in addition, peptic ulcer disease, cataracts, increased risk of infection, and impaired wound healing occur. Truncal obesity, hirsutism, acne, moon-shaped facies, striae, and ecchymoses contribute to a cushingoid appearance. Disruption of bone metabolism predisposes patients to osteoporosis and resultant vertebral and long-bone fractures; inhibition of long-bone growth is the major complication in children who receive systemic corticosteroids. Suppression of the hypothalamic-pituitary-adrenal axis diminishes body cortisol stores, which, in turn, reduces the capacity of the body to confront stress, such as trauma, surgery, or infection.

Inhaled corticosteroids offer direct delivery to the lung with reduced risk of systemic effects. Inhaled fluticasone and beclomethasone at high doses allow discontinuation of oral prednisone in the vast majority of previously steroid-dependent patients. To achieve the same effect as higher potency agents, the lower potency inhaled agents are given in higher doses. Escalating doses of fluticasone provide excellent control of asthma, with negligible adrenal suppression. The lack of systemic effects from fluticasone allow much higher doses to be used, providing greater therapeutic benefit. A linear dose-response curve for fluticasone has been demonstrated. Fluticasone propionate is the most lipophilic of the currently available inhaled corticosteroids, having the greatest receptor binding affinity and steroid-receptor complex half-life; beclomethasone, budesonide, triamcinolone acetonide, and flunisolide follow in descending order.

The most common adverse effects of inhaled corticosteroids are irritation of the oropharynx, cough, and bronchospasm. Dysphonia may arise from vocal cord myopathy. Thrush is easily avoided by rinsing the mouth after each use of a corticosteroid inhaler, using a spacer device to decrease deposition of drug particles in the mouth, and keeping the inhaler mouthpiece clean. Newer inhaled corticosteroids, such as fluticasone, undergo extensive first-pass metabolism to inactive substances, thereby decreasing concentrations of active drug and the potential for systemic adverse effects. Long-term studies of inhaled corticosteroids have not documented significant adrenal suppression.

The mechanism underlying the beneficial effects of corticosteroids in chronic obstructive pulmonary disease (COPD) is not fully known. It may be based upon effects on phosphodiesterase activity leading to augmentation of inhaled beta-adrenergic agonist activity, such as increased mucus mobilization and bronchodilation. Patients experiencing an acute exacerbation of COPD show a more rapid improvement in FEV_1 when methylprednisolone is added to their regimen.

Oral corticosteroids for chronic management of COPD may significantly improve mean FEV_1 or FVC. Patients with steroid-responsive COPD have significant symptom resolution after bronchodilator administration, suggesting co-existing asthma. In such patients, alternate-day oral corticosteroid regimens are as effective as daily regimens. Oral corticosteroids do not improve exercise tolerance in stable patients, as measured by minute ventilation, oxygen consumption, and heart rate achieved during maximal exercise. Thus, a minority of patients with stable COPD may benefit from systemic corticosteroids.

The role of inhaled corticosteroids in COPD is unclear. Young (age under 40 years), atopic nonsmokers are most likely to have steroid-responsive disease. Inhaled corticosteroids significantly increase FEV_1 in some patients; a positive bronchodilator response may be a useful screening technique for identifying those patients with COPD that are steroid-responsive. A trial of inhaled corticosteroids appears to be the safest method for assessing benefit in COPD.

Corticosteroid-Sparing Agents

The macrolide antibiotic troleandomycin has long been reported to reduce the need for corticosteroids in severe steroid-dependent asthma. Although the steroid-sparing mechanism of troleandomycin is unknown, the drug is known to reduce theophylline metabolism as well as methylprednisolone clearance by approximately 60 percent, with little effect on prednisolone clearance. Because of these effects on corticosteroid metabolism, patients treated with troleandomycin experience increased complications of systemic corticosteroids. The weight of evidence suggests that troleandomycin has little or no clinical effect at relieving airway obstruction or inflammation independent of its effects on corticosteroid metabolism. Since significant complications may occur, troleandomycin has little role in the current therapy of severe, steroid-dependent asthma.

Initial observations in patients with coexisting rheumatoid arthritis and asthma suggested the potential usefulness of methotrexate as a steroid-sparing agent. However, most studies report no significant difference in corticosteroid dosage during methotrexate therapy or placebo administration. Numerous and serious side effects of methotrexate have been well described.

Cyclosporine inhibits lymphokine synthesis, thereby blocking the activation of T cells; the drug is used widely in organ transplantation. Cyclosporine has no significant drug interactions with beta-adrenergic agonists, corticosteroids, or theophylline, making it potentially attractive for use in asthma. Cyclosporine has been shown to increase peak expiratory flow and FEV_1, reduce exacerbations of airway obstruction, and reduce oral prednisolone dosage by over 60 percent. Side effects include hypertrichosis, hypertension, and reversible nephrotoxicity, as well as a large number of nonspecific side effects. Additional studies are required to confirm the efficacy of cyclosporine in the treatment of asthma, as well as to define its role as a steroid-sparing adjunct or an independent immunosuppressant.

Gold has been shown to decrease bronchial hyperreactivity in mild asthmatics not receiving corticosteroids. Parenteral gold salt administration, usually through intramuscular injection, has a broad spectrum of toxicities. Oral auranofin is associated with less severe and less frequent side effects that include diarrhea, rash, and stomatitis. At this time, there is no clear demonstration that gold administration improves pulmonary function, reduces flares of obstructive airway disease, or reduces the need for systemic corticosteroid therapy. Therefore, use of gold salts in obstructive airway disease should be restricted to well-designed, controlled clinical trials.

Leukotriene Modifiers

The leukotriene antagonists and inhibitors are the first new class of asthma drugs to be developed in several decades. Leukotrienes are synthesized from arachidonic acid, a fatty acid stored in phospholipids of cell walls. Numerous stimuli, including IgE receptor activation, antigen-antibody interactions, and activation of phospholipase A_2, induce the release of arachidonic acid from phospholipids. Arachidonic acid is converted to a variety of products via several unrelated pathways; the 5-lipoxygenase pathway is the pathway of importance in asthma. Either selective receptor blockade or interference with synthesis may inhibit leukotriene action. Most clinical experience has been with the LTD_4 receptor antagonists. The first-generation LTD_4 receptor antagonists had little clinical efficacy, but the second-generation LTD_4 receptor antagonists are highly potent and selective. Zafirlukast, a short-acting oral agent, and montelukast, a long-acting oral agent, have been extensively studied. Other oral, parenteral, and inhaled receptor antagonists are under investigation. In addition, inhibition of 5-lipoxygenase (5-LO) reduces the generation of all leukotrienes, and numerous 5-LO inhibitors are under investigation. Long-term efficacy and safety data are not available. Initial data suggest that LTD_4 receptor antagonists and 5-LO inhibitors are well tolerated. Some concern has arisen over appearance of pulmonary vasculitis (Churg-Strauss syndrome) in patients treated with leukotriene antagonists in whom systemic corticosteroids were tapered or withdrawn. However, the leukotriene antagonists and inhibitors show promise in the management of chronic moderate asthma and, possibly, in exercise-induced asthma.

MAST CELL STABILIZERS

Cromolyn sodium was the first mast cell stabilizer to be approved for clinical use. Nedocromil also stabilizes mast cells in the bronchial mucosa, but it has a broader anti-inflammatory spectrum than cromolyn sodium.

Cromolyn sodium is a potent inhibitor of inflammatory responses, diminishing early phase reactions in asthma by blocking the release of intracellular calcium and inhibiting the enzymes responsible for mast cell degranulation. Cromolyn also reduces late phase reactions in asthma by inhibiting production of the enzymes necessary for superoxide generation. Cromolyn sodium may also exhibit tachykinin antagonism, accounting for some of its anti-inflammatory properties. The pharmacology of cromolyn sodium and nedocromil is similar.

Cromolyn sodium is indicated for the management of asthma in children and in atopic young adults. Cromolyn sodium, alone or in combination with beta$_2$-adrenergic agonists, improves exercise tolerance, enhances sleep quality, reduces asthma exacerbations, and facilitates patient acceptance of therapy. Patients diagnosed with asthma prior to the age of 4 years, patients less than 17 years of age, and patients with long-term asthma (>5 years) may experience maximal benefit from cromolyn sodium therapy.

Cromolyn sodium significantly improves seasonal allergic asthma symptoms and reduces bronchial hyperresponsiveness after direct challenge with histamine or acetylcholine. Long-term use of cromolyn sodium (at least 12 weeks) four times daily is recommended for effective control of chronic bronchial hyperresponsiveness, while a shorter treatment duration (up to 6 weeks) usually suffices for control of seasonal allergic attacks. Cromolyn sodium prophylaxes against exercise-induced asthma in children as efficaciously as beta$_2$-agonists. Premedication with cromolyn sodium, inhaled beta$_2$-adrenergic agonist, or both, 15 to 30 min prior to vigorous exercise is recommended for children and adults. Additionally, it is a useful adjunct to bronchodilators in adults with atopic asthma, and it may provide added benefit when administered in conjunction with inhaled corticosteroids.

Nedocromil is useful prophylactically against asthma exacerbations, but not therapeutically for acute bronchospasm. Nedocromil delays the late-phase response to methacholine and allergen challenges in stable asthmatics and has no effect on the magnitude of bronchoconstriction. Nedocromil appears to be more effective as a bronchodilator-sparing agent than cromolyn sodium in adults, but it provides a similar level of protection against exercise-induced asthma in children. Lack of long-term experience with nedocromil relegates it to second-line status as an adjunct to bronchodilators in the management of asthma.

MUCOKINETIC AGENTS

Purulent, viscous airway secretions are problematic in patients with cystic fibrosis, chronic bronchitis, and bronchiectasis. High concentrations of mucus contribute to the increased viscosity of bronchial secretions in these conditions. Recruited polymorphonuclear leukocytes degenerate in the airway, releasing DNA into the extracellular environment. Although human deoxyribonuclease I metabolizes DNA liberated from airway leukocytes, the high concentration of DNA released in these chronic conditions overwhelms the endogenous ability of the lungs to clear the DNA. Exogenous administration of DNAse assists in the clearance of airway DNA, reducing mucus viscosity, increasing mucus clearance, and diminishing airway obstruction.

The use of nebulized DNAse as short-term adjunctive therapy in cystic fibrosis offers modest dose-dependent improvement in pulmonary function and reduction in symptoms. The use of DNAse in adults with bronchiectasis not attributable to cystic fibrosis, or in those with chronic bronchitis, results in prolonged antibiotic therapy requirements, no enhancement of pulmonary function, and no improvement in quality of life.

N-acetylcysteine (NAC) lyses disulfide bonds in mucus proteins, reducing airway mucus viscosity. NAC is metabolized to the potent antioxidants, glutathione and cysteine. Studies in COPD and acute lung injury have demonstrated no objective benefit of treatment with NAC.

Some iodinated compounds have mucolytic-expectorant properties. Ingested iodide is liberated and stored in secretory glands of the tracheobronchial tree. Upon stimulation by coughing or inhalation of irritant substances, iodide promotes secretion of respiratory tract fluid and mucoproteins and augments ciliary activity. Increased mucus mobilization and decreased mucus viscosity result. Adverse events appear to be infrequent, although thyroid dysfunction may be induced by the iodine load and has been reported after long-term use in elderly patients with chronic obstructive pulmonary disease. Clinicians should use iodinated compounds with caution in elderly patients or those with preexisting thyroid dysfunction.

Sodium bicarbonate solutions (2 to 7.5%) are frequently used as vehicles for bronchodilators and N-acetylcysteine. By raising the pH of the respiratory tract fluids, aerosolized sodium bicarbonate weakens the saccharide structure of airway mucus, increasing its susceptibility to proteases and promoting its removal through enhanced ciliary activity. These effects are additive when used with N-acetylcysteine and cause reduction in mucous viscosity. Local irritation from hypertonic sodium bicarbonate solutions may occur, cough and bronchospasm have been observed in some patients. Therefore, bronchodilators should be given prior to sodium bicarbonate aerosols.

Guaifenesin remains the only agent approved by the U.S. Food and Drug Administration (FDA) as an expectorant. Guaifenesin appears to reduce sputum volume and improve sputum quality, resulting in subjective relief of respiratory congestion. No adverse effects have been reported.

PHYSIOLOGIC REPLACEMENTS

Physiologic replacement therapy is used in treatment of patients with alpha$_1$-antityrpsin deficiency or deficiency of pulmonary surfactant.

Alpha$_1$-Antitrypsin

Alpha$_1$-antitrypsin is a glycoprotein synthesized and secreted by hepatocytes. As a protease inhibitor, alpha$_1$-antitrypsin blocks the actions of neutrophil-derived elastase in the lung. Inherited deficiency of alpha$_1$-antitrypsin promotes development of emphysema in adulthood; tobacco smoking rapidly accelerates the clinical presentation and severity of emphysema (see Chap. 7).

Since 1988, alpha$_1$-antitrypsin replacement therapy has been available for intravenous administration as a purified product prepared from pooled human plasma. Recombinant alpha₁-antitrypsin has also been produced but suffers from rapid renal excretion. Nonetheless, recombinant alpha$_1$-antitrypsin may be efficacious when directly administered by aerosol. Weekly or monthly intravenous infusion of alpha$_1$-antitrypsin to deficient patients increases alpha$_1$-antitrypsin levels in serum and bronchoalveolar lavage specimens. Such infusions concomitantly restore antielastase activity in serum and alveolar lining fluid. Whether alpha$_1$-antitrypsin replacement reduces the accelerated rate of decline in pulmonary function associated with alpha$_1$-antitrypsin-deficiency is unclear.

Alpha$_1$-antitrypsin replacement therapy is remarkably nontoxic, and current preparations have few side effects other than mild fever. Despite the lack of efficacy data, alpha$_1$-antitrypsin replacement therapy is recommended for patients with alpha$_1$-antitrypsin deficiency who are older than 18 years of age, who have abnormal pulmonary function tests, and whose serum alpha$_1$-antitrypsin level is less than 11 mmol. Replacement therapy for alpha$_1$-antitrypsin-deficient patients is not recommended after lung transplantation. There has been no demonstrated efficacy in cystic fibrosis.

Pulmonary Surfactant

Endogenous pulmonary surfactant is an emulsion of phospholipids, cholesterol, and apoproteins that reduces surface tension within alveoli. Natural surfactant is commercially available and is prepared from lung tissue or lavages from a variety of species. Synthetic surfactant is available from a number of commercial sources, although the optimal composition of the material remains to be determined.

The administration of pulmonary surfactant to premature infants with, or at risk for, respiratory distress syndrome has become the standard of care in recent years (see Chap. 71). The agent decreases mortality from respiratory distress syndrome by 30 to 40 percent and reduces morbidity due to pneumothoraces, interstitial emphysema, bronchopulmonary dysplasia, and intraventricular hemorrhage. At present, a role for surfactant therapy in adult lung diseases, including acute respiratory distress syndrome, has not been established.

RESPIRATORY STIMULANTS

A number of drugs may have roles as respiratory stimulants in carefully considered clinical circumstances.

Acetazolamide

Acetazolamide is a noncompetitive inhibitor of carbonic anhydrase that induces a weak diuresis and mild metabolic acidosis. Currently, acetazolamide is approved for the prophylaxis of acute mountain sickness (see Chap. 22). It is sometimes used to treat patients with chronic hypercapnia and drug-induced or compensatory metabolic alkalosis. Prophylactic acetazolamide decreases the frequency of acute mountain sickness by about 30 to 50 percent. Side effects, such as somnolence, paresthesias, and gastrointestinal distress, are common. Acetazolamide may improve symptoms in mild obstructive sleep apnea. Unfortunately, acetazolamide may convert central sleep apnea to obstructive sleep apnea or worsen hypoxemia in patients with central or mixed sleep apnea. Long-term safety and efficacy data are unavailable.

Almitrine

Almitrine stimulates peripheral chemoreceptors in the carotid body and improves ventilation-perfusion matching by redistributing perfusion away from poorly ventilated areas. It has no central respiratory stimulant effect. Long-term controlled trials suggest that almitrine bismesylate increases Pa_{O_2} in the range of 5 to 13 mmHg. However, toxicities include right ventricular strain from increased pulmonary artery pressures, peripheral neuropathy, weight loss during long-term therapy, and diuretic activity. The drug is not available in the United States.

Methylxanthines

Aminophylline and theophylline augment the central ventilatory response to hypoxia. The methylxanthines have been used to treat apnea of prematurity and infants with periodic breathing, but they are less useful in the treatment of obstructive sleep apnea. Although aminophylline reduces central apnea and the central component of mixed apneas, it has no effect on obstructive apnea, and it may increase upper airway occlusion during sleep.

Doxapram

Doxapram is a short-acting, parenterally administered peripheral chemoreceptor agonist and central respiratory stimulant. Doxapram has been approved for postanesthesia respiratory depression or apnea, drug-induced central nervous system respiratory depression, and short-term use as a respiratory stimulant in acute respiratory insufficiency superimposed on chronic pulmonary disease. Case reports describe the use of doxapram as a respiratory stimulant in COPD complicated by acute respiratory failure.

Medroxyprogesterone

Medroxyprogesterone is a gestational respiratory stimulant. Although its mechanism of action is unclear, medroxyprogesterone increases minute ventilation and produces hypocapnia in normal subjects. It does not improve breathing disturbances during sleep in normocapnic patients with obstructive sleep apnea.

Protriptyline

Protriptyline is a tricyclic antidepressant that is cited frequently as an effective respiratory stimulant in patients with obstructive sleep apnea, despite lack of supporting data. The mechanism of action may include suppression of rapid-eye-movement (REM) sleep and increased tone in the upper airway muscles. Protriptyline is contraindicated in glaucoma or prostatic hypertrophy; anticholinergic side effects limit its usefulness.

BIBLIOGRAPHY

Bisgaard H: Role of leukotrienes in asthma pathophysiology. *Pediatr Pulmonol* 30:166–176, 2000.

Bowton DL, Goldsmith WM, Haponik EF: Substitution of metered-dose inhalers for hand-held nebulizers. Success and cost savings in a large, acute-care hospital. *Chest* 101:305–308, 1993.

Christian Virchow J, Prasse A, et al: Zafirlukast improves asthma control in patients receiving high-dose inhaled corticosteroids. *Am J Respir Crit Care Med* 162:578–585, 2000.

Fuchs HJ, Borowitz DS, Christiansen DH, et al: Effect of aerosolized recombinant human DNase on exacerbations of respiratory symptoms and on pulmonary function in patients with cystic fibrosis. *N Engl J Med* 331:637–642, 1994.

Kelly HW: Comparative potency and clinical efficacy of inhaled corticosteriods. *Respir Care Clin North Am* 5:537–553, 1999.

Kerstjens HAM, Brand PLP, Hughes MD, et al: A comparison of bronchodilator therapy with or without inhaled corticosteroid therapy for obstructive airways disease. *N Engl J Med* 327:1413–1419, 1992.

McFadden ER Jr: Dosages of corticosteroids in asthma. *Am Rev Respir Dis* 147:1306–1310, 1993.

Mullen M, Mullen B, Carey M: The association between β-agonist use and death from asthma. *JAMA* 270:1842–1845, 1993.

79 | Ethics in Critical Care*

Michael A. Grippi

INTRODUCTION

In the intensive care unit (ICU), advanced technology can keep patients alive for long periods of time. However, this life-sustaining capability is sometimes at odds with the goals of restoration of sufficient functional status to permit discharge from the ICU and achievement of a reasonable quality of life. Hence, a commonly posed, critically important question is whether the advanced technology of the ICU *should* be used to prolong a given patient's life.

UNDERLYING PRINCIPLES

Ethical dilemmas may arise in the ICU when there is conflict among any of the three core biothethical principles of beneficence, respect for patient autonomy, or justice.

Beneficence refers to the goal of health care providers to perform beneficial services for patients. It encompasses the principle of *nonmaleficence*—doing no harm to the patient. Beneficence and nonmaleficence may conflict when beneficial interventions are associated with discomfort—e.g., tracheal suctioning of an intubated patient. From an ethical standpoint, the suctioning is justified because its beneficial effects outweigh the discomfort it causes. The traditional Hippocratic notions of beneficence and nonmaleficence, according to which physicians determine what is best for their patients, have evolved into the more contemporary view that the *patient,* with physician guidance, should determine what interventions are made on his or her behalf. This approach is consistent with the principle of respect for patient autonomy.

Respect for patient autonomy highlights the principle that patients or their surrogate decision makers, including family members, can decide for themselves (*self-determination*) what medical interventions are acceptable and which measures (including life-sustaining ones) they wish to forgo. Patient autonomy constitutes the basis for *informed consent.* Except in life- or limb-threatening circumstances, a competent adult must give informed consent prior to receiving medical care; under true emergency conditions, consent for the intervention is presumed.

Justice refers to an equitable distribution of health care resources (*distributive justice*), at national, regional, or institutional levels.

*Edited from Chap. 181, "Ethics in the Intensive Care Unit," by Lanken PM. In: *Fishman's Pulmonary Diseases and Disorders,* 3d ed., edited by Fishman AP, Elias JA, Fishman JA, Grippi MA, Kaiser LR, Senior RM. New York, McGraw-Hill, 1998, pp 2761–2772. For fuller discussion of topics dealt with in this chapter, the reader is referred to the original text, as noted above.

END-OF-LIFE ISSUES IN THE INTENSIVE CARE UNIT

Based on a number of judicial decisions, societal consensus has evolved over the last 25 years regarding the ethics of withholding or withdrawing life-sustaining therapies. This consensus is reflected in the practical principles summarized below.

- *Informed adults with decision-making capacity can forgo any life-sustaining medical therapy, even if the action results in their death.*
- *Forgoing life-sustaining therapy includes not only the* withholding *of such therapy as cardiopulmonary resuscitation but also its* withdrawal. *Life-sustaining therapies include mechanical ventilation, nutrition, and hydration. There is no significant ethical or legal difference between withholding and withdrawing life-sustaining therapy.*
- *Surrogate decision makers should make decisions to forgo life-sustaining therapy on behalf of patients who have lost decision-making capacity as long as the decisions are based on knowledge of what the patient would have wanted under similar circumstances. In the absence of such knowledge, decisions should be based on the patient's best interests.*

A *durable power of attorney* for health care designates someone (family member or not) as the patient's surrogate decision maker. In the absence of a valid durable power of attorney, the patient may designate, in writing or verbally, a health care decision maker, and this choice should be respected. In the absence of such a designation, and where state statutes do not specify the hierarchy determining selection of a surrogate, a close family member who knows the patient well should ideally assume the role. A surrogate decision maker's decisions are guided by the standards of *substituted judgment* (the surrogate decision maker expresses what the patient would have preferred under the circumstances) and *best interests* (when knowledge of the patient's preference is lacking, the surrogate decision maker must weigh the benefits of life-sustaining therapy against its burdens).

- *When in doubt about a patient's preferences, health care providers should err on the side of sustaining life.*

A therapeutic trial of life support may be started, despite uncertainty about its effectiveness, in order to determine whether the therapy will be beneficial.

- *As long as the patient or surrogate decision maker has given informed consent, it is appropriate to provide medication to relieve pain and other suffering, such as dyspnea, even if the medication has the potential to hasten the patient's death.*

Administering medication to relieve pain and suffering should not be confused with active euthanasia or assisted suicide.

- *It is inappropriate to force physicians or other health care providers to comply with a patient's request to forgo life-sustaining therapy if compliance violates the health care provider's personal moral values. Under these circumstances, responsibility for care of the patient should be transferred to another provider who can respect the patient's request.*
- *Health care professionals are not obligated to provide medical care that they judge as futile, even if requested by the patient or family. Futile life support can be limited without consent of the patient or surrogate decision maker.*

The consensus around these principles is not as strong as that around the preceding ones. An intervention that is judged to be *physiologically futile* is one that is not expected to, or does not, achieve the relevant physiological function as an end point (e.g., cessation of cardiopulmonary resuscitation (CPR) when there is no prospect of success). A *medically futile* intervention is more difficult to define. One definition is based on the conclusion, supported by experience and reasoning, that the intervention would have a high likelihood of failing to result in "meaningful survival." How one defines "high likelihood" and "meaningful survival" is, however, problematic.

• *Each individual's life is equally valuable.*

According to this principle, access to ICU resources should not be prioritized according to perceptions of relative social worth.

• *Vulnerable members of the community should be protected.*

This principle highlights the importance of additional safeguards to ensure that society's vulnerable members are treated equitably.

• *Access to intensive care should be based on the patient's medical need and the potential benefit of such care; judgments about whether a benefit is worthwhile should reflect not only the values of the patient and health care providers but also the values of the community.*

The admission of patients to the ICU and their care there should be based principally on medical appropriateness. However, this principle acknowledges the fact there is a broad range of potential benefits to patients with similar medical needs, and that critical care should be provided only when there is sufficient medical need and a reasonable likelihood of potential benefit.

• *Although health care providers have a primary obligation to benefit their patients, this duty has limits when it unfairly compromises the availability of resources for others.*

DO-NOT-RESUSCITATE (DNR) ORDERS IN THE INTENSIVE CARE UNIT

For critically ill patients, DNR orders are common. Ideally, a patient's preferences for withholding or withdrawing life support have been articulated well before admission to the ICU, with a written advance directive and designated surrogate decision maker or durable power of attorney. If the advance directive indicates that life support should be withdrawn when there is no reasonable hope for meaningful recovery, the patient's interpretation of "reasonable" and "meaningful" needs to be understood. In the absence of an advance directive, family or close friends may be able to provide the patient's previously communicated verbal wishes or their sense of what he or she would have wanted under the circumstances, based on knowledge of the patient's goals and values.

Within the context of critical illness, the definitions of competency and capacity assume importance. While *competency* is defined legally, a patient's decision-making *capacity* is his or her functional ability, as determined by an attending physician. Many critically ill, legally competent patients lack adequate decision-making capacity. Conversely, a patient who is legally incompetent may retain some decision-making capacity (e.g., a teenager who has opinions about his or her medical care). A patient has adequate decision-making capacity in relation to a specific decision when the patient demonstrates comprehension of the issue, can exercise comparative judgment, and can communicate his or her decision.

When a patient in the ICU lacks decision-making capacity, the physician must turn to a surrogate decision maker. In some states, the choice of proxy is legally mandated. Alternatively, a valid durable power of attorney for health care decisions may specify the decision maker. In the absence of a legal directive, if the patient has informally designated someone as surrogate decision maker, that choice should be recognized. In most cases, the surrogate decision maker is a close family member. The appropriate individual should make decisions on the patient's behalf, based on his or her knowledge of the patient's preferences, values, and life goals (substituted judgment). Under circumstances in which no individual knows the patient or is willing to serve as a surrogate decision maker, a neutral party (generally not a hospital employee) should act as surrogate (e.g., the chairperson of a hospital's ethics committee).

As a first step in the decision-making process regarding DNR orders, health care providers should meet with the patient's family or surrogate decision maker to inform them of the patient's current medical status, therapeutic goals, and progress toward those goals. The discussion should include the patient, unless he or she lacks decision-making capacity. After deciding on the limits of therapy, the attending physician should document in the medical record the deliberations and the basis for the decision. Patient comfort should be assessed and appropriate pharmacologic agents administered, as needed. If communication during the decision-making process is good, conflicts occur infrequently. Resolution of conflicts begins with open communication among all parties.

BIBLIOGRAPHY

American Thoracic Society: Withholding and withdrawing life-sustaining therapy. *Am Rev Respir Dis* 144:726–731, 1991.

Asch DA, Hansen-Flaschen JH, Lanken PN: Decisions to limit or continue life-sustaining treatment in the United States: Conflicts between physicians' practices and patients' wishes. *Am J Respir Crit Care Med* 151:288–292, 1995.

Lanken PN: Critical care medicine at a new crossroads: The intersection of economics and ethics in the intensive care unit. *Am J Respir Crit Care Med* 149:3–5, 1994.

President's Commission for the Study of Ethical Problems in Medicine and Biomedical and Behavioral Research: Deciding to forego life-sustaining treatment: Ethical, medical and legal issues in treatment decisions. Washington, DC: U.S. Government Printing Office, 1983.

Waisel DB, Truog RD: The cardiopulmonary resuscitation-not-indicated order: Futility revisited. *Ann Intern Med* 122:304–308, 1995.

Appendix | Agents Potentially Associated with Bioterrorism

Jay A. Fishman

The occurrence of inhalational anthrax in the United States has prompted concern over the preparedness of the medical community to recognize and treat this uncommon infection and other potential bioterrorism-related infections (Table A-1). Specific agents of bioterrorism are considered below. In the fall and winter seasons, many individuals not known to be at increased risk for anthrax but who have symptoms of influenza-like illness merit evaluation. These patients present with fever, fatigue, cough, malaise, and other symptoms (Table A-2). Common viruses—including rhinoviruses, respiratory syncytial virus (RSV), adenoviruses, and parainfluenza viruses—cause the majority of such infections. Less common causes include influenza A and B, agents of "atypical" pneumonitis (*Legionella* spp., *Chlamydia pneumoniae*, *Mycoplasma pneumoniae*), and *Streptococcus pneumoniae*. Annually, the average individual may have between one and three (adults) or more frequent (children) infections.

ANTHRAX

Anthrax is caused by infection with *Bacillus anthracis*, a spore-forming, gram-positive rod. There are three clinical syndromes of anthrax that follow, respectively, cutaneous, gastrointestinal, or inhalational exposure. The clinician should suspect anthrax if an individual has any of the following:

- An established or probable exposure or flu-like illness with gastrointestinal symptoms, chest pain, and sweats. Note: most recent cases have followed exposure to contaminated mail.

TABLE A-1 Biological Agents with Potential for Use in Bioterrorism

Bacterial Agents

Anthrax
Plague
Tularemia
Brucellosis
Glanders/meliodosis
Q fever

Viral Agents

Smallpox
Venezuelan equine encephalitis
Viral hemorrhagic fevers

Biological Toxins

Botulinum toxin
Ricin
Staphylococcal enterotoxin B

TABLE A-2 Possible Agents of Bioterrorism

Agent/Disease	Symptoms	Diagnostic Tests	Treatment
Anthrax	Flu-like symptoms—fever, headache, and cough (not nasal congestion)	Blood samples; serology; cultures of sputum, blood, or skin lesions	Antibiotics. Vaccine for military personnel.
Botulinum toxin	Blurred vision, difficulty swallowing and speaking	Blood, stool, and gastric samples	Anti-toxin available through public health authorities.
Plague	Fever, cough, and shortness of breath	Sputum and blood samples	Antibiotics. Since plague can be spread from person to person, antibiotics also prescribed for close contacts.
Smallpox	Fever, rash, headache, backache, and muscle pain	Blood samples and tissue samples	Supportive care. Vaccine may become available.
Tularemia	Fever, chills, headache, muscle weakness	Sputum and blood samples	Antibiotics.

- A typical skin lesion with black eschar, often with dense edema.
- Unexplained sepsis with respiratory failure, bloody pleural effusions, or chest radiograph showing widened mediastinum or chest computed tomography (CT) scan showing hyperdense mediastinal and hilar nodes and mediastinal edema.
- Detection of unidentified gram-positive bacilli in an uncontaminated specimen (blood, pleural fluid, cerebrospinal fluid).

Inhalational anthrax begins with a flu-like illness of fever, sweats or chills, severe fatigue, cough, nausea, vomiting, and abdominal pain; coryza and purulent sputum are often absent. Chest x-ray or chest CT may show a widened mediastinum because of mediastinal lymphadenopathy and/or mediastinitis. Bacteremia and shock rapidly ensue, as well as hemorrhagic meningitis in some patients. The incubation period of inhalational anthrax is usually 1 to 7 days after exposure, but illness may occur as many as 60 days later. The estimated human LD_{50} is between 2500 and 55,000 inhaled anthrax spores. Cutaneous anthrax presents with skin lesions that ulcerate, have substantial surrounding edema, and go on to form a black eschar; cutaneous anthrax is much less serious than inhalational anthrax. Anthrax, including inhalational disease, is *not* spread from person to person.

Evaluation

Serum samples should be obtained for serologic testing. Patients with suspected inhalational anthrax should have blood cultures drawn as well as a Gram's stain of a blood buffy coat examined. If meningeal signs are present, lumbar puncture may also suggest the diagnosis. Gram's stain and culture of respiratory secretions are of lower yield, since pulmonary parenchymal involvement is less common than infection of the mediastinal lymph nodes. For patients with suspected cutaneous anthrax, a swab of the ulcer for Gram's stain and culture and, in some situations, a biopsy of the lesion for stains and culture are appropriate. A punch biopsy at the margin of the lesion may be useful if antibiotics have been given previously or for suspicious lesions. Biopsy may be submitted in saline for culture and in formalin for polymerase chain reaction and immunohistochemistry.

In asymptomatic patients, a culture of a nasal swab or of uninvolved skin to assess possible colonization by *B. anthracis* is not known to accurately predict subsequent risk of clinical illness. Public health authorities may decide that such cultures are warranted for epidemiologic purposes.

Treatment

Inhalational Anthrax

Initial antimicrobial therapy of suspected inhalational anthrax should be begun as rapidly as possible.

Antibiotics   Initial treatment with ciprofloxacin 400 mg IV q12h (other fluoroquinolones likely effective) *or* doxycycline 100 mg IV q12h; combine either with one or two of the following: rifampin, clindamycin, imipenem/meropenem, vancomycin, or chloramphenicol. When the patient is stable and IV therapy ≥14 to 21 days, switch to oral ciprofloxacin (500 mg PO bid) or doxycycline (100 mg PO bid), either one with or without rifampin 300 mg PO bid to complete 60 days of therapy.

- There are few data regarding the duration of therapy; careful follow-up is recommended.
- Steroids have been used to treat pulmonary and mediastinal edema; pleural effusions are common.
- Isolates of *B. anthracis* tested in recent patients have had an inducible beta-lactamase that may reduce the efficacy of penicillin when organism density is high. Prolonged use of doxycycline is associated with dental staining in children less than 8 years of age. Fluoroquinolones are not licensed for use in children but appear to be safe; their use in these exceptional circumstances is appropriate and can be modified as susceptibility results allow.

Cutaneous Anthrax

For systemic involvement with extensive edema or facial involvement, the patient merits parenteral antibiotics as recommended for inhalational anthrax (above) with corticosteroids (for edema) for 7 to 10 days, then oral treatment. For limited or localized disease, oral treatment with doxycycline 100 mg PO bid or ciprofloxacin 500 mg PO bid should be effective. A 60-day course is recommended for confirmed disease.

Anthrax Prophylaxis

Individuals (adults) defined on the basis of suspected exposures to *B. anthracis* should receive doxycycline 100 mg PO bid or ciprofloxacin 500 mg PO bid × 60 days. If the risk of exposure is not substantial, prophylaxis is discontinued. For pregnancy or breast-feeding, amoxicillin 500 mg PO bid may be used after 10 to 14 days. The total duration is 60 days based on the assumption of inhaled *B. anthracis* as well. Vaccine availability for anthrax is limited at present and is not recommended for the public or for health care workers, but it is used for U.S. military personnel. If vaccine were available, vaccination might be used after exposure to inhalation of anthrax spores in selected patients, giving doses at 0, 2, and 4 weeks and shortening the duration of antibiotic prophylaxis from 60 to 30 days.

BOTULISM

Botulinum toxin is a potent neurotoxin produced by strains of *Clostridium botulinum*, an anaerobic gram-positive rod. There are seven serologically distinct types of botulinum toxin, groups A to G; serotypes A, B, E, and F produce human disease. Botulinum toxin may be ingested in food or may be inhaled or ingested in water as part of a bioterrorist event. Botulism is characterized by symmetrical cranial neuropathies (manifesting as ptosis, extraocular muscle palsies, blurred vision, and—in approximately half the patients—dilated pupils), followed by a symmetrical descending flaccid paralysis. There is no fever or sensory abnormality. The deep tendon reflexes are reduced or absent. The incubation period of botulism is generally 1 to 5 days after ingestion or inhalation of the toxin. Botulism is *not* transmitted from person to person. The differential diagnosis of botulism includes Guillain-Barré syndrome, myasthenia gravis, tick paralysis, and Lambert-Eaton syndrome.

As in all suspected bioterrorism-associated illnesses, an acute sample of serum should be drawn and the physician should indicate the agent(s) suspected so as to facilitate work-up. In association with public health authorities, botulinum toxin may be detected in serum, stool, gastric contents, or vomitus.

Treatment

Therapy for botulism includes supportive care and *prompt* administration of trivalent equine botulinum antitoxin (types A, B, and E). Mechanical ventilation may be needed for several months. There is no established value of antimicrobial therapy. There is an investigational pentavalent vaccine, but this takes 12 weeks to elicit immunity and is not useful in post-exposure prophylaxis. Similarly, antitoxin is not known to have an effect if it is given prophylactically after exposure. Instead, patients who have been exposed should be observed carefully and given antitoxin if clinical symptoms appear.

PLAGUE

Plague is caused by the gram-negative bacillus *Yersinia pestis*, which appears as a gram-negative rod with bipolar staining. Although naturally occurring plague most commonly presents as a localized lymphadenitis (a bubo), bioterrorism-related plague would present as pneumonia, producing pneumonic plague. This form of plague presents as a flu-like illness with fever, cough, and dyspnea followed by chest pain and hemoptysis. Bacteremia, shock, and disseminated intravascular coagulation ensue shortly. The incubation period following inhalation is 1 to 6 days. The pneumonic form of plague can be spread from person to person by large droplets that require close exposure for transmission to occur.

As in all suspected bioterrorism-associated illnesses, an acute sample of serum should be stored. In suspected pneumonic plague, respiratory secretions can be sent for Gram's stain and culture; blood should also be cultured.

Treatment

The preferred therapy for plague is an aminoglycoside, either streptomycin 1 g IM q12h (for children, 15 mg/kg IM q12h, not to exceed 1 g q12h) or gentamicin 1.5 mg/kg IV q8h (2.5 mg/kg IV q8h for neonates), both for 10 days and both adjusted if needed for renal function. Alternatives include doxycycline 100 mg IV q12h (in children, 2.2 mg/kg IV q12h, not to exceed 100 mg per dose), ciprofloxacin 400 mg IV q12h (in children, 15 mg/kg IV q12h, not to exceed 400 mg per dose) (other flouroquinolones such as levofloxacin, gatifloxacin, or moxifloxacin are likely suitable alternatives), or chloramphenicol 1 g IV q6h (for plague meningitis) (in children, 25 mg/kg IV q6h, not to exceed 1 g per dose). Prolonged use of doxycycline is associated with dental staining in children less than 8 years of age. Fluoroquinolones are not licensed for use in children but appear to be safe; their use in these exceptional circumstances is appropriate and can be modified according to susceptibility results.

Individuals exposed to plague via bioterrorism or close contact with patients having untreated but documented pneumonic plague merit prophylaxis. If identified within 6 days of exposure, such individuals should receive post-exposure antibiotic prophylaxis for 7 days. Choices for post-exposure prophylaxis include doxycycline 100 mg PO bid (in children, 2.2 mg/kg PO bid, not to exceed 100 mg per dose) or ciprofloxacin 500 mg PO bid (in children, 10–15 mg/kg PO bid, not to exceed 500 mg per dose) (other fluoroquinolones, as above, are likely suitable alternatives). Vaccination against plague is not easily available, is not known to be effective against pneumonic plague, and is not useful following exposure.

SMALLPOX

Smallpox is caused by infection with the variola major virus. The clinical syndrome of smallpox begins with a brief prodomal illness of fever, headache, backache, and myalgias, followed quickly by the appearance of a maculopapular rash. The rash appears first on the face and forearms, including the tongue and roof of the mouth, extending afterwards to the legs, palms, soles, and trunk. The maculopapular lesions evolve quickly to vesicles and then to pustules in a synchronous fashion. In smallpox there is greater involvement of the face and extremities as well as the palms and soles than in chickenpox; also, the lesions are more uniform in appearance and synchronous in nature. The incubation period for smallpox is 7 to 17 days. Patients are infectious at the time of onset of the rash. Smallpox is spread from person to person by droplets, droplet nuclei, and direct contact with infected skin lesions. Patients with suspected smallpox should be placed in a negative-pressure room on airborne and contact precautions. Patients are infectious for approximately 3 weeks or until all lesions have scabbed over. Laboratory confirmation of smallpox requires special care. Fluid from a vesicle and/or scab can be examined directly for virus by electron microscopy or by culture *in a high-containment BL-4 laboratory*. There is no known effective antiviral therapy for patients infected with smallpox. While intravenous cidofovir has some activity against cowpox virus infection (a related virus) in mice, this might be considered only for the most severely infected smallpox patients. Cidofovir is contraindicated in patients with a creatinine above 1.5 mg/dL. Because of lack of any data on efficacy, the need for IV dosing, and renal toxicity, cidofovir is *not* used for prophylaxis.

Prophylaxis

Individuals who received smallpox vaccination prior to 1972 (the last year of general vaccination in the United States) should be considered nonimmune. At present, there is an insufficient supply of vaccine to recommend routine vaccination of the public and/or health care workers. If patients with smallpox are identified, household members and others with face-to-face contact with the patient after the onset of fever and rash might be offered smallpox vaccination within 4 days of exposure. Special consideration is made during a larger outbreak of vaccination for hospital and other emergency personnel. Individuals with immunodeficiencies or eczema or who are pregnant are at higher risk of complications from the vaccine; these individuals might either not be vaccinated or might receive vaccinia immunoglobulin (VIG) in a dosage of 0.3 mL/kg IM (divided at different sites) at the same time as the vaccine. If an individual were to develop a complication of smallpox vaccination, VIG in a dose of 0.6 mL/kg IM may be used to treat this complication.

TULAREMIA

Tularemia is caused by infection with *Francisella tularensis*, a small, pleomorphic, gram-negative coccobacillus. Humans acquire tularemia by direct contact with or ingestion of infected animals, by tick bites, and by inhalation. Inhalational tularemia presents as a flu-like illness, with headaches, myalgias, and cough, often followed by development of respiratory symptoms such as chest pain and shortness of breath. The pulse may be slower than expected for the level of fever. Chest x-ray may show bronchopneumonia and hilar adenopathy. The incubation period of tularemia is generally between 1 and 14 days after exposure. There is no person-to-person transmission of tularemia. Patients suspected of having inhalational tularemia should have a Gram's stain and culture of sputum sent as well as a culture of blood; sputum Gram's stain may show small pleomorphic rods. A serologic test is available for tularemia; antibody responses take 7 to 14 days to develop.

Treatment

Antimicrobial therapies for inhalational tularemia include (1) streptomycin 1 g IM q12h (in children, 15 mg/kg IM q12h, not to exceed 1 g q12h); (2) gentamicin 1.5 mg/kg IV q8h (2.5 mg/kg IV q8h for neonates); (3) doxycycline 100 mg IV q12h (in children, 2.2 mg/kg IV q12h, not to exceed 100 mg per dose); or (4) ciprofloxacin 400 mg IV q12h (in children, 15 mg/kg IV q12h, not to exceed 400 mg per dose) (other fluoroquinolones such as levofloxacin, gatifloxacin, and moxifloxacin are likely suitable alternatives). Doses are adjusted for renal dysfunction. Therapy with streptomycin, gentamicin, or a fluoroquinolone should be continued for 10 days and with doxycycline for 14 to 21 days. In the unlikely event that there is confirmation of a bioterrorism-related exposure of individuals to tularemia prior to the onset of symptoms, prophylactic therapy might be given with doxycycline 100 mg PO bid (in children, 2.2 mg/kg PO bid, not to exceed 100 mg per dose) or ciprofloxacin 500 mg PO bid (in children, 10 to 15 mg/kg PO bid, not to exceed 500 mg per dose) for 14 days (another fluoroquinolone, as above, would be a suitable alternative).

REFERENCES

Centers for Disease Control and Prevention website: http://www.bt.cdc.gov

Expert Panel Consensus Reviews
Anthrax: *JAMA* 1999; 281:1735–1745.
Smallpox: *JAMA* 1999; 281:2127–2137.
Plague: *JAMA* 2000; 283:2281–2290.
Botulism: *JAMA* 2001; 285:1059–1070.
Tularemia: *JAMA* 2001; 285:2763–2773.

Index

Note: Page numbers followed by *f* indicate figures; those followed by *t* indicate tables.